Dedicated to our families.

Contents

PART II   Specific Disease Categories

PART III   Medical-Psychiatric Units

Foreword

There is a growing consensus among psychiatrists concerning future trends in psychiatry. Although all of these developments might not occur precisely as predicted, it appears likely that the following trends will characterize *fin de siècle* psychiatry as well as that of the early 21st century.

1. There will be a sharp diminution in solo practice. Psychiatry has a larger percentage of solo practitioners than any other medical speciality. Practice in groups, institutions and managed care settings will increase.
2. Because basic mental health care will be provided both by nonmedical practitioners, such as psychologists and social workers, and by primary care physicians, particularly general internists and family practitioners, psychiatrists will more and more focus on the care of difficult and complicated cases—the seriously mentally ill, and those with dual diagnosis, that is, with medical illness compounded by mental illness.
3. Consultation-liaison psychiatry, which is presently under widespread criticism, finds its fiscal support is problematic, particularly with current pressures to cut costs. It will undergo major changes or else face an eventual demise. With the present pressure to halt while it is most regrettable, reimbursement increasingly determines how medicine is practiced.
4. An increasing number of the elderly will generate medical encounters disproportionate to their numbers. Elderly patients often suffer from a combination of physical and mental disabilities.
5. Psychiatrists perforce will have to possess skills to care for individuals with co-morbidity, that is, patients who are both physically and mentally ill. Increasingly, the locus of this care will be in general hospitals and tertiary care centers. The training of psychiatrists, which provides them with a broad knowledge of general medicine as well as psychiatry, makes them uniquely prepared to perform this task. Clearly, if psychiatry does not assume this responsibility, primary care physicians will, albeit with less sophistication in their diagnosis and treatment of patients' mental complaints. However, pressures to cut costs may favor the psychiatrist who can simultaneously provide medical and psychiatric care; a

single physician in charge is less costly than a series of consultants, and may be clinically superior. Psychiatrists will provide direct patient care, since whichever specialty can care for the complicated co-morbidity cases will have a competitive advantage. It is a matter not only of economy but also of the appropriateness, utility, and efficacy of the psychiatrist as the primary caretaker of patients with combined illness.

Given these prospects, the very important volume, *Principles of Medical Psychiatry*, by Alan Stoudemire and Barry Fogel is not only timely for the immediate practice of psychiatry but is also particularly prescient. Psychiatrists who are currently involved with dual diagnosis patients or those who wish to undertake such responsibilities will find the book invaluable. The well-written, comprehensive chapters cover virtually all areas of concern to the psychiatrist who treats patients with combined psychiatric and medical problems.

The book abounds with practical guidelines and applications, while not neglecting the theoretical underpinnings of the approaches and procedures it recommends. General principles of diagnosis and treatment are covered in depth. Part II offers delineation of useful and tested procedures for management of specific diseases generally encountered, including an up-to-date chapter on psychiatric and neuropsychiatric aspects of AIDS. A final section on the organization and development of combined medical-psychiatric units rounds out this superb volume. Each chapter is well-documented, and a generous bibliography is supplied for those wishing to further explore the various topics.

The thrust of this book is far beyond the present day practice of consultation-liaison psychiatry. The book advocates that the psychiatrist directly assume both medical and psychiatric responsibility. Thus, the editors and many of the contributors rec-

ommend the development of a new field of psychiatry—*medical psychiatry* or, as it has been termed by some others who think along the same lines, *psychiatric* medicine. This designation is groundbreaking in its direct appeal for new areas of concern by psychiatrists and has widespread implications not only for the practice of psychiatry but also for the future training of psychiatrists. It offers a new way of thinking about the roles of psychiatrists, particularly as medicine in the United States moves into hitherto uncharted waters. The practice of medical psychiatry challenges traditional notions, but the editors and authors make a convincing case for this new direction.

In its sections on treatment, the book is specific in its discussion and suggestions. Facts are presented that will be useful in clinical decision making. Many of us have been concerned by the reluctance of some psychiatrists to treat psychiatric syndromes in the presence of medical illness as vigorously as they would the same syndromes in medically uncomplicated patients. There has been a reluctance, although it appears to be diminishing, to use psychopharmacologic agents in such patients. This issue is taken up in detail by this volume, particularly in the chapter by the two editors on psychopharmacology in the medically ill. Another chapter thoroughly discusses the use of electroconvulsive therapy in the medically ill.

Principles of Medical Psychiatry does not advocate somatic therapy alone. The book is permeated with the idea that the techniques of brief dynamic psychotherapy can be uniquely valuable in working with medically ill patients. The theory is laid out in the chapters on medical psychotherapy and on personality disorders, and specific dynamic issues relevant to specific organ systems are pointed out in the chapters of Part II that address various medical diagnoses.

The emphasis that emerges is that brief psychotherapy skills, combined with specific technical knowledge of diagnosis and drug therapy, yield impressive therapeutic power. The integration of technical details of diagnostic evaluation and drug selection and a profound understanding of the psychosocial dynamics of adaptation to illness give strength to these presentations. One must welcome this reinforcement of the further development of the biopsychosocial model.

The prescience of this book has been stated previously. Even if one takes a cautious view of the future, the substance of this volume will be of vital importance to the practice of psychiatry in the future and may well prove to be indispensable. Some might even characterize this as a "survival manual," since an important part of future psychiatric practice will lie in the area covered by *Principles of Medical Psychiatry*.

In a period in which there is a relative paucity of new clinical ideas and of methods to implement them, Drs. Stoudemire and Fogel have produced a volume that is original and creative and that can serve as a catalyst not only for new ways of thinking but also for new ways of practice.

Alfred M. Freedman, M.D.
Professor and Chairman
Department of Psychiatry
New York Medical College
Valhalla, New York

Acknowledgments

The editors would like to especially acknowledge the dedicated and valiant efforts of their secretaries, Ms. Lynda Mathews and Ms. Rita St. Pierre. Without their help this book could never have been completed. We would also like to thank our editors, Barbara Murphy and Kay Ferguson, at Grune & Stratton for providing us with the opportunity to initiate this project and for shepherding it to completion. Dr. Fogel received support during the editing of this book from NIMH Geriatric Mental Health Academic Award MH00604-02. We would like to acknowledge our mentors whose vision, guidance and leadership have inspired our own intellectual growth and professional development. They include Drs. Troy Thompson, Jeffrey Houpt, Richard Simons, Howard Fields, Stuart Agras, Barry Gurland, and Andrew Slaby. Finally, we are indebted to our families for their forbearance and emotional support.

Introduction

Medical psychiatry may be defined as the diagnosis and treatment of psychiatric disorders in the medically ill. As such it represents the practical clinical application of psychiatric knowledge and therapy to the problems of a medically ill population. The definition of medical psychiatry, however, involves not only the specific population of patients to be treated but also the *process* of treatment. First, the medical psychiatrist assumes a substantial degree of *medical responsibility* for the patient either as primary caretaker or as the coordinator of the care of the patient. While medical psychiatrists do offer consultation, they tend to be more directly involved in the patient's care. Second, medical psychiatrists find it within the scope of their clinical duties to perform physical and neurologic examinations, to interpret laboratory tests and, if qualified, to interpret neuroradiologic, neurophysiologic, and neuroendocrine studies. Third, medical psychiatrists personally integrate a wide range of therapeutic modalities including psychopharmacology, psychodynamic psychotherapy, behavior therapy, family interventions, and electroconvulsive therapy. Medical psychiatrists cannot restrict themselves to particular theoretical biases or treatment approaches, because their patients usually require multimodal interventions.

Medical psychiatry, thus defined, is currently practiced by many clinicians who identify themselves primarily as consultation-liaison psychiatrists. Medical psychiatry, however, is not synonymous with consultation-liaison psychiatry. Medical psychiatrists are in general less concerned about educating other physicians than they are about personally treating patients with combined medical-psychiatric illnesses; in contrast to consultation-liaison psychiatrists, medical psychiatrists are more likely to use medical specialists as *their* consultants rather than vice versa. In addition, because of their involvement with patients with combined medical-psychiatric illnesses, medical psychiatrists are more likely to have an inpatient setting, often a combined medical-psychiatric unit, as a primary site of their clinical activities.

Medical psychiatry is distinguished from behavioral medicine by its broader scope and its emphasis on traditional psychiatric diagnostic assessment and multimodal treatment. While behavioral medicine clinicians apply the techniques of behavioral therapies and biofeedback to influence health-related behavior and psychophysiologic reactions, medical psychiatry is engaged primarily in the diagnosis and treatment of psychiatric and medical *illnesses* by applying integrated pharmacologic therapy, psychodynamic therapy, and other appropriate modalities, as well as behavioral techniques as indicated.

A primary motivation in defining the field of medical psychiatry derives from lessons learned from the consultation-liaison movement. The consultation-liaison concept has foundered not because there is any real question about the value of integrating psychiatric care and medical care but because, in the final analysis, neither the public nor the private sector is willing to reimburse the psychiatrist sufficiently to be *primarily* a consultant or liaison educator. In many settings, the psychiatrist's identity is blurred with that of other nonmedical and nonpsychiatric clinicians who make legitimate claims to be able to manage many aspects of the care of the same medical patient population.

This tendency toward role diffusion between consultation-liaison psychiatrists and other clinicians has led to a perpetual identity crisis within the movement. Moreover, internal controversy within the field has led to arguments as to whether or not the "consultant" or the "liaison" role has the most value. This identity crisis and role diffusion, coupled with serious problems in grant funding and reimbursement, demands a new approach to defining the identity and mission of the psychiatrist who chooses to specialize in the care of the medically ill patient.

Medical psychiatry, therefore, defines the psychiatrist as a medical specialist who assumes primary clinical responsibility for the diagnosis and treatment of psychiatric disorders within the medically ill population. Patients need not necessarily be acutely medically ill for this definition to apply, since the field also embraces chronic illness in which maladaptive behavior may cause or perpetuate illness or its disability.

Likewise, the spectrum of psychiatric disorders treated includes both major primary psychiatric disorders and maladaptive or excessive reactions to illness.

In our opinion, medical psychiatry will grow in importance as a discipline. Factors favoring the further development of this area of clinical psychiatric practice include (1) the increasing prevalence of chronic disease and the aging of the population, (2) advances in neurodiagnostic techniques and psychopharmacology, permitting more rational biological therapy of psychiatric disorders in the medically ill, (3) the development and implementation of brief, focused dynamic psychotherapy techniques appropriate for the medical setting, (4) the development of specialized medical-psychiatric inpatient units, (5) increasing time pressures on other medical specialists, leaving the psychiatrist as the only medical specialist with the time, knowledge, and skills to develop a comprehensive understanding of the emotional dimensions of medical patients' illnesses, and (6) increased competitive pressures from nonmedical psychotherapists, causing psychiatrists to emphasize their medical training and skills.

In this book we offer a first approximation to a knowledge base for the practice of medical psychiatry. The intended audience of this book includes practicing psychiatrists who have an interest in treating the medically ill, resident psychiatrists in training, and other physicians, including those in primary care with an interest in the psychiatric aspects of medicine. Advanced medical students who have completed their basic introduction to psychiatry and internal medicine will also find the book useful. We assume that most of our readers will have some familarity with the basic descriptive diagnostic scheme of DSM-III-R, psychopharmacology, and fundamental concepts of psychodynamic theory and therapy. Nonmedical and nonpsychiatric clinicians will find the book accessible as a reference, even without a specific medical or psychiatric background.

Readers will note that rather than dealing with geriatrics, drug-drug interactions, and psychiatric manifestations of medical illness as separate topics, the book incorporates these aspects of medical psychiatry into the organ system chapters of Part II. In addition, the contributors have considered both biomedical and psychodynamic issues in their approach to case assessment. The editors' purpose will have been accomplished if our readers do the same in fostering more integrated treatment approaches in the care of the medically ill.

Alan Stoudemire, M.D.
Atlanta, Georgia
Barry S. Fogel, M.D.
Providence, Rhode Island
September 1987

Contributors

Gene G. Abel, M.D., Professor, Department of Psychiatry, Emory University School of Medicine, Atlanta, Georgia

David B. Abrams, Ph.D., Assistant Professor, Department of Psychiatry and Human Behavior, Brown University, Providence, Rhode Island

Steven A. Cohen-Cole, M.D., Associate Professor, Department of Psychiatry, Emory University School of Medicine, Atlanta, Georgia

C. Edward Coffey, M.D., Assistant Professor, Department of Psychiatry, Duke University School of Medicine, Durham, North Carolina

Barry J. Coyne, Ph.D., Assistant Professor, Department of Psychiatry/Psychology, Emory University School of Medicine, Atlanta, Georgia

Leah Oseas Cullen, M.D., Assistant Professor, Department of Psychiatry and Human Behavior, Brown University, Providence, Rhode Island

Marcia L. Daniels, M.D., Assistant Professor, Department of Psychiatry and Biobehavioral Sciences, University of California at Los Angeles, Los Angeles, California

Lucy Davidson, M.D., Ed.S., Clinical Assistant Professor, Department of Psychiatry, Emory University School of Medicine, Atlanta, Georgia

Peter J. Fagan, Ph.D., Assistant Professor, Department of Medical Psychology, The Johns Hopkins School of Medicine, Baltimore, Maryland

David Faust, Ph.D., Assistant Professor, Department of Psychiatry and Human Behavior, Brown University, Providence, Rhode Island

Giovanni A. Fava, M.D., Assistant Research Professor, Department of Psychiatry, State University of New York, Buffalo, New York

Barry S. Fogel, M.D., Associate Professor, Department of Psychiatry and Human Behavior, Brown University, Providence, Rhode Island

Michael J. Follick, Ph.D., Associate Professor, Department of Psychiatry and Human Behavior, Brown University, Providence, Rhode Island

Charles V. Ford, M.D., Professor, Department of Psychiatry, University of Arkansas Medical Center, Little Rock, Arkansas

David F. Gardner, M.D., Associate Professor, Department of Medicine, Medical College of Virginia, Richmond, Virginia

Richard J. Goldberg, M.D., Associate Professor, Department of Psychiatry and Human Behavior, Brown University, Providence, Rhode Island

Michael G. Goldstein, M.D., Assistant Professor, Department of Psychiatry and Human Behavior, Brown University, Providence, Rhode Island

Stephen A. Green, M.D., Clinical Associate Professor, Department of Psychiatry, Georgetown University School of Medicine, Washington, DC

Barrie J. Guise, Ph.D., Department of Psychiatry and Human Behavior, Brown University, Providence, Rhode Island

Carol Harpe, M.D., Clinical Assistant Professor, Department of Psychiatry, Emory University School of Medicine, Atlanta, Georgia

Jimmie C. Holland, M.D., Professor, Department of Psychiatry, Cornell University Medical College, New York, New York

Jeffrey L. Houpt, M.D., Professor and Chairman, Department of Psychiatry, Emory University School of Medicine, Atlanta, Georgia

Susan G. Kornstein, M.D., Department of Psychiatry, Medical College of Virginia, Richmond, Virginia

Lynna M. Lesko, M.D., Ph.D., Assistant Professor, Department of Psychiatry, Cornell University Medical College, New York, New York

James L. Levenson, M.D., Assistant Professor, Departments of Psychiatry and Medicine, Medical College of Virginia, Richmond, Virginia

Norman B. Levy, M.D., Professor, Departments of Psychiatry, Medicine and Surgery, New York Medical College, Valhalla, New York

Carol Martin, M.D., private practice, Providence, Rhode Island

Mary Jane Massie, M.D., Associate Professor of Clinical Psychiatry, Department of Psychiatry, Cornell University Medical College, New York, New York

M. Eileen McNamara, M.D., Assistant Professor, Department of Psychiatry and Human Behavior, Brown University, Providence, Rhode Island

Mark J. Mills, J.D., M.D., Professor, Department of Psychiatry and Biobehavioral Sciences, University of California at Los Angeles, Los Angeles, California

George Molnar, M.D., Associate Professor, Department of Psychiatry, State University of New York, Buffalo, New York

Michael G. Moran, M.D., Assistant Professor, Department of Psychiatry and Medicine, University of Colorado School of Medicine, Denver, Colorado

Gregory J. O'Shanick, M.D., Assistant Professor, Departments of Psychiatry and Rehabilitation Medicine, Medical College of Virginia, Richmond, Virginia

Janice L. Petersen, M.D., Assistant Professor, Department of Psychiatry, University of Colorado School of Medicine, Denver, Colorado

Michael A. Raciti, Ph.D., Clinical Assistant Professor, Department of Psychiatry and Human Behavior, Brown University, Providence, Rhode Island

Quentin R. Regestein, M.D., Associate Professor, Department of Psychiatry, Harvard University, Boston, Massachusetts

Anne Marie Riether, M.D., Assistant Professor, Department of Psychiatry, Emory University School of Medicine, Atlanta, Georgia

Joanne-L. Rouleau, Ph.D., Assistant Professor, Department of Psychiatry, Emory University School of Medicine, Atlanta, Georgia

Laurie Ruggiero, M.A., Department of Psychiatry and Human Behavior, Brown University, Providence, Rhode Island

Chester W. Schmidt, Jr., M.D., Associate Professor, Department of Psychiatry, The Johns Hopkins School of Medicine, Baltimore, Maryland

Andrew Edmund Slaby, M.D., Ph.D., M.P.H., Adjunct Professor of Psychiatry and Human Behavior, Brown University, Providence, Rhode Island; Clinical Professor, Department of Psychiatry, New York University, New York, New York

G. Richard Smith, Jr., M.D., Associate Professor, Departments of Psychiatry and Medicine, University of Arkansas Medical Center, Little Rock, Arkansas

Michael S. Sokol, M.D., Department of Psychiatry and Human Behavior, Department of Internal Medicine, Brown University, Providence, Rhode Island

Alan Stoudemire, M.D., Associate Professor, Department of Psychiatry, Emory University School of Medicine, Atlanta, Georgia

Robert M. Swift, M.D., Ph.D., Assistant Professor, Department of Psychiatry and Human Behavior, Brown University, Providence, Rhode Island

Troy L. Thompson II, M.D., Associate Professor, Departments of Psychiatry and Medicine, University of Colorado School of Medicine, Denver, Colorado

Wendy L. Thompson, M.D., Clinical Assistant Professor, Department of Psychiatry, University of Colorado School of Medicine, Denver, Colorado

Richard D. Weiner, M.D., Ph.D., Associate Professor, Department of Psychiatry, Duke University School of Medicine, Durham, North Carolina

Thomas N. Wise, M.D., Professor of Psychiatry, Georgetown University Medical Center, Washington, DC; Associate Professor, Department of Psychiatry, and Assistant Professor, Department of Medicine, The John Hopkins School of Medicine, Baltimore, Maryland

PART I

General Principles of Diagnosis and Treatment

Stephen A. Green

1

Principles of Medical Psychotherapy

Optimal medical treatment requires a comprehensive appreciation of the interplay among the patient's organic pathology, the patient's intrapsychic life, and the positive and negative impact of his or her social environment. This biopsychosocial treatment approach, as discussed by Engel (1977, 1980), is conceptualized by interposing the patient between two hierarchies that combine to form an overall hierarchy of natural systems. The person is at the same time at the highest level of an organismic hierarchy, which ranges from subatomic particles through the nervous system, and at the lowest stratum of a social hierarchy, which ranges from a two-person system to the biosphere (Fig. 1-1). These two hierarchies are in a dynamic equilibrium, since every system (e.g., cell or two-person) within each hierarchy is a distinctive whole that is simultaneously interrelated with every other system. Consequently, disturbances at any system level can alter any other system level.

The biopsychosocial model highlights the inextricable link between mind–body interaction and consequently enhances un-

derstanding of such diverse physiologic processes as endocrinologic function (Haskett & Rose, 1981; Kiely, 1974; Mason, 1975; Whybrow & Silberfarb, 1974), immunologic response (Amkraut & Solomon, 1974; Dorian Garfinkel, Keystone, et al., 1986; Locke, Kraus, Leserman, et al., 1984; M. Stein, 1981; M. Stein, Keller, & Schleifer, 1985), stress response (Cannon, 1920, 1932; Selye, 1950), pathogenesis of disease (Rogers, Dubey, & Reich, 1979; Schindler, 1985; Wolff, Wolf, & Hare, 1950), the course of illness (Engel, 1980; Reiser, 1975), and mechanisms of death (Engel, 1968, 1971; Greene, Goldstein, & Moss, 1972; Lown, Verrier, & Rabinowitz, 1977; Reich, DeSilva, Lown, & Murawski, 1981). It demonstrates that disturbances in physiologic functioning influence, and are in turn affected by, one's psychologic functioning, and it consequently emphasizes the clinical reality that optimal medical treatment requires constant assessment of an individual's affective reaction to illness. A pathologic illness response requires comprehensive study of the patient's "illness dynamics" (Green,

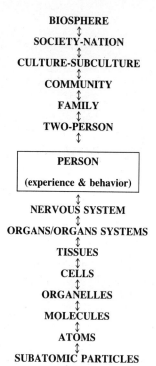

SYSTEMS HIERARCHY
(LEVELS OF ORGANIZATION)

BIOSPHERE
↕
SOCIETY-NATION
↕
CULTURE-SUBCULTURE
↕
COMMUNITY
↕
FAMILY
↕
TWO-PERSON
↕

| PERSON |
| (experience & behavior) |

↕
NERVOUS SYSTEM
↕
ORGANS/ORGANS SYSTEMS
↕
TISSUES
↕
CELLS
↕
ORGANELLES
↕
MOLECULES
↕
ATOMS
↕
SUBATOMIC PARTICLES

Fig. 1-1. Hierarchy of natural systems. (Reprinted from Engel G (1980). The clinical application of the biopsychosocial model. American Journal of Psychiatry, 137, 535–544. With permission.)

1985)—the varied psychosocial factors affecting, and affected by, this organic pathology—information which is then incorporated into a psychotherapeutic approach appropriate to the individual. The following pages discuss diagnosis and treatment of the abnormal emotional states that can afflict patients who enter the health care system for treatment of a medical or surgical illness.

RESPONSES TO ILLNESS

Impaired health, whether it takes the form of a mild upper respiratory infection or a life-threatening cerebrovascular acci-

dent, is a universal condition that precipitates predictable emotional responses. Illness is experienced as a loss—specifically, the loss of health—because it diminishes one's level of functioning. The loss is most obvious when a serious ailment permanently and profoundly changes a person's physical status—for example, when a patient becomes blind or paraplegic. However, even a limited illness may precipitate considerable feelings of loss because of its symbolic significance to the patient. In addition to challenging omnipotent wishes—highlighting the patient's vulnerability to physical ailments whose onset, course, and response to treatment are often unexplainable and unpredictable—an episode of ill health conveys a specific symbolic meaning that derives from a highly personalized interplay among the patient's physical pathology, intrapsychic life, and social environment. That interplay determines how, and to what extent, a patient reacts affectively to a particular loss of health.

Whether illness is experienced in the form of concrete physical restrictions or, more symbolically, is due to implied or anticipated limitations, it promotes the same psychological response—a grief reaction, during which patients mourn the loss of their previous state of health. The process is identical to bereavement. Illness obliges a patient to acknowledge and confront a diminished level of functioning, causing the patient to progress through a series of feeling states—denial, anxiety, anger, depression, helplessness—before resolving the various emotions precipitated by the loss.

This process is most obvious during a medical emergency, such as an acute appendicitis. The initial pain caused by an inflamed appendix, which may be quite severe, is often dismissed as indigestion or the effect of an enterovirus. However, other feelings supplant the early denial as the significance of the symptoms becomes clearer. Anxiety emerges as a patient ruminates on the pain and discomfort (and possible mortality) of surgery, as well as the need to abdicate considerable responsibility for well-being and comfort to anonymous caretakers. This anxiety can persist during the recuperative period, focused on such issues as the restrictions and length of convalescence; however, emerging resentments usually predominate at this stage, during which the patient discharges anger at family members, friends, and even medical personnel who provide succor and support. These feelings eventually give way to a period of helplessness and overt depression, characterized by affective, behavioral, and cognitive changes, when the patient is most aware of the losses brought on by a surgical emergency that has relegated all other activities (e.g., professional and social responsibilities) to positions of secondary importance. Most patients emerge from this phase progressively, reestablishing an emotional equilibrium by working through all of the feelings precipitated by illness. Achieving this equilibrium requires the patient to realistically grasp the specific limitations imposed by the disease, as well as to acknowledge vulnerabilities and ultimate mortality.

An abnormal emotional response to illness occurs when a patient is unable to effectively grieve the losses caused by ill health. For a variety of reasons idiosyncratic to a particular person during a particular period of life, a patient may be unable to recognize, experience, and put into proper perspective some or all of the feelings precipitated by illness. The patient may completely deny all emotions or, more commonly, may experience a specific affect to the relative exclusion of all others. The patient becomes mired in some phase of the grief process, preoccupied with the feelings characteristic of that stage. This preoccupation forestalls attainment of an emotional resolution regarding the loss of health. The situation can evolve into an emotional state similar to pathologic grief, whose symptomatic expression may take the form of an affective disturbance (e.g., excessive anxi-

ety or depression), a behavioral disturbance (e.g., compulsive eating or substance abuse), or impaired object relationships (Brown & Stoudemire, 1983). Subsequent effects on somatic functioning—which may aggravate the initial organic pathology—derive from mind–body interactions. Because of this interdependence, a patient's affective resolution of the loss of health facilitates the restoration of physical, as well as psychological, well-being. Without this grief work, a pathologic illness response emerges, characterized by a psychobiologic disequilibrium generally more disabling than that caused by the initial illness. Descriptions of frequent abnormal psychologic reactions to illness follow.

The Denial Response

Denial, the refusal to perceive or accept external reality, is a common ego mechanism that enables a person to completely ablate distressing cognitions or affects or both. Because of its absoluteness, it is considered a primitive behavior, classified by Vaillant (1977) as a psychotic ego mechanism. It may have an adaptive purpose, for example, to enable an individual to temporarily ignore the overwhelming impact of a stressor that might otherwise threaten psychologic integrity; consequently, denial is often invoked by emotionally healthy persons when extremely stressful circumstances limit the effectiveness of higher-level ego functioning. This type of response is exemplified by the belief that one will survive in battle and is reflected in enhanced short-term psychologic adjustment following a myocardial infarction (Hackett & Cassem, 1974).

Denial becomes maladaptive when it is so excessive that it prevents accurate assessment and acceptance of the realities of life. At that point it is exclusively defensive, providing illusory comfort by prompting actions (or ensuring inactivity) that promote a false sense of well-being—a frequent reaction of medical and surgical patients whose response to illness is actually a nonresponse. Denial may be present throughout the course of illness, beginning at the moment of onset, continuing through the period of initial treatment and convalescence, and extending into the rehabilitative phase. The longstanding cardiac patient who attributes cramping in the left arm to "overwork" and the woman who decides to have her breast mass evaluated "in a few months" exemplify the acute denial of illness. Noncompliance with a therapeutic regimen often reflects continued denial. This can occur in the period of intial hospitalization, as when a patient refuses to maintain bed rest (Reichard, 1964), and in chronic illness, as when patients with diabetes mellitus repeatedly break their diet. It also occurs in terminal patients who adamantly refuse to acknowledge impending death. The unconscious rejection of illness, invoked to maintain emotional stability, may impede accurate diagnosis, interfere with definitive treatment, and, consequently, aggravate the patient's organic pathology.

The Anxiety Response

Signal anxiety, the adaptive expression of this affect, alerts one to danger and thereby prompts purposeful, self-protective behavior. The onset of illness is always accompanied by heightened anxiety as the patient questions the extent and degree of a particular ailment. Common concerns, such as whether or not symptoms signal the beginning of a fatal illness, usually give way to speculation about the diagnostic workup, the course of treatment, and the ultimate prognosis. Patients may wonder how they will be perceived by others if the illness is disfiguring or chronically debilitating. They may ruminate on the toll the illness will take on family relationships, professional responsibilities, friendships, and day-to-day functioning. In short, they may attempt to assess the impact of illness on the overall

quality of life in the near and distant future. Though a difficult and disconcerting exercise, this is usually an adaptive response to illness, spurring a patient to seek timely medical attention and adhere to prescribed treatments.

Illness can also precipitate a pathologic anxiety that causes the patient undue concern about his physical status. As a consequence, the patient becomes hypersensitive to all aspects of care, from diagnostic procedures to therapeutic interventions, developing a preoccupation that has diverse detrimental effects. A new sign or symptom make take on considerable significance, interfering with the patient's ability to provide an accurate medical history, greatly augmenting the apprehension that often accompanies routine examination and treatment, and generally distracting the patient from the pleasures and responsibilities of daily life. If this concern evolves into a chronic anxiety, the patient becomes burdened with an unpleasant affective state in addition to the discomfort of the physical pathology. Moreover, continued demands for reassurance from family, friends, and health professionals may progressively alienate those persons, ultimately isolating the patient from sources of emotional support. In this fashion pathologic anxiety can compromise every phase of medical treatment and decrease the patient's potential for returning to optimal functioning.

The Anger Response

Patients who demonstrate anger as the predominant response to loss of health express the affect in the same way as a person grieving the death of a loved one, focusing feelings of frustration, resentment, and overt hostility in several directions. They may rail at the gods with a diffuse, globally expressed anger, cursing their bad luck and wondering, "Why me?" Alternatively, they may direct that anger toward themselves; a man who herniates a lumbar disk while moving furniture holds himself most responsible for the painful disruption of daily life. Anger is also focused on family members and friends, whose various behaviors often are implicated as contributors to the development or exacerbation of an illness; a patient may view the demands of her spouse as the primary cause of her peptic ulcer disease, hypertension, or migraine headaches. Patients may judge members of their social network as insensitive to their plight or may resent family members because of greater dependency on them. Patients may even blame ancestors for a defective gene pool that predisposes to a particular illness. Finally, health personnel frequently bear the brunt of a patient's hostility. In addition to providing succor and support, caretakers exert considerable control, which often takes the form of deprivation and discomfort. They subject patients to unpleasant diagnostic tests, restrict their diets, limit their activity levels, and prescribe medications that cause unpleasant, sometimes dangerous, side effects. Moreover, practitioners frequently fail to cure disease and often bear grim news about a patient's welfare and mortality. For these reasons, medical personnel are prime targets for patients' angry feelings.

The hallmark of the anger response is interpersonal conflict. Instead of working through feelings connected with illness, patients engage in a variety of struggles with the people in their lives. These may be obvious, such as the debate surrounding the refusal to submit to a diagnostic procedure or to consent to rehabilitative therapy. The impotent pleas of family members urging reconsideration, as well as the frustration of health providers, reflect the patient's considerable hostility. Struggles may also be covert. They can take the form of passive aggression—for example, ignoring dietary restrictions or adhering errati-

cally to a medication regimen—behaviors that afford the patient the pleasure of secret control over caretakers. Displacement is an additional means of disguising anger about the loss of health; for example, the recurrence of old marital disputes permits discharge of the affect without directly identifying illness as its root cause. In sum, the anger response promotes a generalized noncompliance with treatment, progressively transforming the patient's supportive alliances—including those with caretakers—into adversarial relationships. In addition to lowering the level of medical care, this reaction isolates the patient from a support system that usually helps one negotiate the stressful life situation of ill health.

The Depressive Response

Persons who react to physical illness with a depressive response manifest affective, cognitive, and behavioral changes characteristic of a clinical depression (Klerman, 1981; Rodin & Voshart, 1986). These vary in degree, depending on factors idiosyncratic to the patient and the particular disease process; consequently, the intensity of the depressive response may range from a relatively mild adjustment disorder to a major depression.

The clinical presentation encompasses four general areas of objective and subjective signs and symptoms. First, alterations of affect occur. These usually present as a sustained lowering of mood accompanied by pronounced sadness, tearfulness, and anhedonia, though affective changes also may include irritability, agitation, and hypomania. Next, the physiologic sequelae of depression are manifest in wide-ranging somatic symptoms that can affect any organ system (Lindemann, 1944). Third, the depression response causes changes in the patient's usual patterns of behavior, beyond the changes resulting from restrictions of the illness state. Such behavioral changes often take the form of a generalized withdrawal—physical and psychologic—from the social environment. Mounting preoccupation with the loss of health causes patients to retreat from family matters, social relationships, and professional responsibilities. As this isolation grows, the world becomes increasingly joyless. Finally, as with all depression, a prominent aspect of this illness response is diminished self-esteem. The effects of a patient's physical impairment, aggravated by his subsequent mood disturbance, induce fear and doubt about the prospect of regaining the premorbid state of health. This negativism fosters self-criticism characterized by feelings of weakness, self-reproach, and worthlessness.

This illness response affects medical treatment in several ways. Psychophysiologic symptoms of depression complicate the diagnosis of an organic illness, making medical evaluation and treatment more difficult. Depression impedes the immunologic response (Schindler, 1985; Schleifer, Keller, Meyerson, et al., 1984), with possible adverse effects on the patient's ability to battle an illness. Depression can become so severe that it poses a greater threat to patients than their physical pathology. Neurovegetative symptoms, such as extreme anorexia, may progress to the point of passive self-destructive behavior; purposeful suicidal actions also occur (Slaby & Glicksman, 1985). Finally, the characteristic withdrawal of the depressive response progressively isolates an individual from the usual supports of the social environment. It may impair the therapeutic alliance with various health care personnel and may alienate patients from family and friends. It may become so extreme that the patient essentially abandons the will to live (Engel, 1968).

The Dependency Response

Illness limits autonomy because of factors internal to the patient (e.g., restrictions caused by specific symptoms, the individual's general preoccupation with his disease) as well external issues (e.g., limitations imposed by the structured hospital routine, the requirements of a therapeutic regimen). The adaptive aspect of this regression permits the patient to revert to more passive behaviors characteristic of early developmental phases. This allows caretakers to take a necessary degree of control of the treatment and simultaneously provides the patient with the comfort and familiarity of diminished responsibility. (In his discussion of regression, Freud [1924] makes the analogy to the actions of a migrating population under siege; it falls back to previously strengthened positions, revitalizes its forces, and then proceeds with renewed vigor.) The defensive aspect of regression helps patients contend with the distressing emotions precipitated by illness, by assigning to others concern and accountability for their welfare.

Though regression helps one maintain emotional equilibrium during periods of illness, it can interfere with medical treatment if the patient's dependency becomes too extensive, intense, or "fixed." This problem of intractable regression is addressed in Parsons's (1951) description of the dynamics of the sick role, which emphasizes the collaborative aspect of medical treatment. During the early phase of illness, an individual's impairment is legitimized by health care personnel, who identify him as a patient and consequently exempt him from various societal responsibilities. The patient's dependency on caretakers is acknowledged and accepted as they labor towards wellness; however, with improvement the individual is expected to assume increasing levels of independent functioning. This phase of illness, a collaborative endeavor that Parsons terms the "common task" between patient and provider, highlights the fact that individuals bear definite responsibility for important aspects of their health care, which range from adherence to a prescribed diet to active participation in a long-term rehabilitation program. The last phase of the sick role, as outlined by Parsons, has particular relevance to the dependency response. Patients may find the ministrations of others so gratifying that they are disinclined to strive toward the autonomy of his premorbid life. Patients may abdicate increasing responsibility to family, friends, and health care personnel and savor the nurturing pleasures of dependency. Unfortunately, this decline to greater levels of helplessness compromises patients' physical and emotional well-being.

Excessive dependency is often manifest as noncompliance with medical treatment. This may cause an individual to continue harmful habits (e.g., smoking), to be irresponsible with medications, or to allow known symptoms to get worse before seeking medical attention. Whether these motivations are purposeful or unconscious, they yield the same result—prolonged dependency on health personnel, who are obliged to provide the care necessitated by the patient's self-neglect. In addition to possibly aggravating the patient's physical condition, pathologic dependency often subverts supportive relationships. Usual family interactions may be disrupted by the patient's continued regression, which alters established roles in a way that is unpleasant for all concerned. Relationships with professional caretakers may suffer, as medical personnel come to view the regressed individual as a "hateful patient" (Groves, 1978), a countertransference response often triggered by increasingly annoying dependent demands. All these behaviors—which reflect an evolution into a professional patient more concerned with being cared for than with discharging the responsibilities of

adult life—may be overt or covert. It is particularly important for health providers to appreciate a dependency response that might be disguised by a patient's seeming compliance. The longer the patient's wish to remain ill goes unrecognized, the more likely it is that the collaborative doctor–patient relationship will steadily degenerate into an adversarial association harmful to both.

ILLNESS DYNAMICS

Everyone lives within a distinctive context of supports and stressors that influence day-to-day functioning and interpersonal relationships. *Illness dynamics* refers to the diverse factors that affect patients' responses to specific diseases at particular times in their lives (Green, 1985). They derive from conscious and unconscious determinants that converge in the mind, causing the patient to perceive, assess, and defend against the loss of health in a highly subjective manner. The major components of illness dynamics are as follows:

1. Biologic
   a. Nature, severity, and time course of disease
   b. Affected organ system, body part, or body function
   c. Baseline physiologic functioning and physical resilience
   d. Genetic endowment
2. Psychologic
   a. Maturity of ego functioning and object relationships
   b. Personality type
   c. Stage in the life cycle
   d. Interpersonal aspects of the therapeutic relationship (e.g., countertransference of health providers)
   e. Previous psychiatric history
   f. Effect of past history on attitudes toward treatment (e.g., postoperative complications)

3. Social
    a. Dynamics of family relationships
    b. Family attitudes towards illness
    c. Level of interpersonal functioning
        (e.g., educational and occupational
        achievements, ability to form and
        maintain friendships)
    d. Cultural attitudes

Patients' illness dynamics cause them to evaluate all illness-related information in light of their particular values, needs, wishes and fears, thereby shaping a distinctive perception of ill health. Their individual biopsychosocial profiles may help them accommodate to the emotions precipitated by loss of health or, alternatively, may impede that effort.

Illness fosters regression when it "cuts off [one's] major source of gratification, or enhances intrapsychic conflicts by facilitating emergence of repudiated wishes, weakening ego mechanisms of defense or signifying punishment for realistic or neurotic guilt" (Lipowski, 1975). Regression in the face of illness can have widespread impact on the total organism as a result of diffuse mind-body interactions. Reiser (1975) explores the role of the brain as a clearinghouse for the diverse emotional and physiologic reactions, discussing how it "orchestrates, integrates, and at points transduces across the biologic, psychologic, and the social realms," thereby translating idiosyncratic symbolic meanings into physiologic changes throughout the body that may promote the onset of illness, aggravate its clinical course, or help maintain a healthy homeostasis. Reiser describes a "transactional continuity extending from subcellular metabolic processes throughout the body via the brain to the social environment" that suggests how "major life experiences, such as bereavement, can influence even the capacity to sustain the life process itself." This thesis is supported by considerable laboratory and clinical data that include investigation of total body processes, such as immunologic response, and more discrete physiologic activities, such a cardiovascular functioning (Henry, 1975).

Illness dynamics also affect the doctor–patient relationship, as well as sources of support in an individual's social network. According to Lipowski (1975) the process of evaluating the state of ill health "influences the patient's perceptions and mood as well as the content and form of what he communicates concerning his illness, how, to whom, and when. It affects his decision to seek or delay medical consultation, his degree of compliance with medical advice and management, as well as his relationship with his family, employers, health professionals and other concerned people."* These interactions significantly influence an individual's ability to contend with illness.

In sum, illness dynamics derive from the interplay among the singular components of one's biologic, psychologic, and social existence, transforming an episode of ill health into a highly subjective experience. By shaping its meaning in this fashion, they can convert the same disease process into seemingly different illnesses in two individuals requiring the identical diagnostic workup, acute treatment, and ongoing care. Illness dynamics span an enormous and complex range, given the breadth of psychosocial factors influencing and influenced by a specific organic pathology. They may be beneficial or harmful; their ultimate effect depends on whether the idiosyncratic meaning an individual ascribes to his or her disease facilitates the grief work that accompanies a particular loss of health or interferes with that necessary process. When illness dynamics impede grief work, they set the stage for maladapt-

---

*From Lipowski Z (1975). Psychiatry of somatic diseases: Epidemiology, pathogenesis, classification. Comprehensive Psychiatry 16, p. 111. With permission.

ive illness responses, whose psychotherapeutic treatment is addressed in the following pages.

MEDICAL PSYCHOTHERAPY

Reasoned attention by medical personnel to the affects precipitated by an individual's ill health can prevent the onset of an abnormal illness response. However, all therapeutic measures must be carefully tailored to each patient, based on a comprehensive understanding of that patient's illness and illness dynamics. Interventions designed to initiate the grief work accompanying the loss of health are required for some patients, but are contraindicated in patients obviously overwhelmed by their current affective state. The latter group benefits from measures that support adaptive ego functioning, such as supplying an obsessional patient with considerable information about his day-to-day condition.

Unfortunately, many patients do not respond to this aspect of primary medical care, and they become increasingly encumbered by the distressing feelings that characterize a particular pathologic reaction to illness. Continued negative impact on their physical and emotional well-being signals the need for medical psychotherapy, a specialized form of psychotherapeutic intervention. As discussed by Goldberg and Green (1985), medical psychotherapy is based on "the communicated understanding between physician and patient concerning the biologic, psychologic and social aspects" of an individual's illness. The treatment, which can be utilized for crisis situations (e.g., acute onset of illness) or chronic conditions (e.g., persisting or fluctuating illness), can take a supportive or introspective approach.

Despite the correlation between grief work and the usual emotional reaction to illness, helping the patient work through feelings about his loss of health is some-times contraindicated. Such insight-oriented therapy rests on the patient's ability to tolerate the heightened anxiety attending exploratory work, and certain patients have characteristic personality features that render such anxiety-provoking psychotherapy ineffective or harmful. Many persons afflicted with one of the traditional psychosomatic ailments fall into this category (Sifneos, 1973). Attempts to help them resolve the powerful emotions accompanying illness are often frustrated by their diminished ability or motivation for self-examination, a predisposition to hypochondriasis, and limitations on verbal expression (alexithymia)—factors that significantly undermine meaningful attempts to explore and understand affective states. Clinicians' expert knowledge concerning the ideal course of grief work is counterproductive if it prompts them to doggedly confront the defensive structure and maladaptive behaviors of these psychologically immature individuals. Attempts to pressure such patients through the various stages of grief are more likely to foster a clinical regression (Sifneos, 1972–73).

When treating medical and surgical patients unable to contend with the emotions precipitated by illness, the clinician's most important decision concerns a clear delineation of therapeutic goals. The physician must decide whether to (1) commend and encourage the patient's usual style of emotional functioning and thereby foster an atmosphere of support and reassurance, which can be exploited to enhance the physician's positive influence, or (2) pursue a more analytic path, in an attempt to help the patient work through the conflictual feelings precipitated by the illness. Correct treatment of an abnormal illness response therefore requires the clinician to choose between a supportive, anxiety-suppressing approach and an introspective, anxiety-provoking stance as the appropriate form of medical psychotherapy for a particular patient. The clinical data used to make this determination are discussed next, followed by a review of the general characretistics of these distinct therapeutic strategies. Clinical material explicating the two types of medical psychotherapy is presented elsewhere (Green, 1985).

The decision whether a patient suffering from an abnormal illness response requires introspective (anxiety-provoking) investigation of his or her emotions or is more in need of reassurance and support (anxiety-suppressing treatment) is founded on the systematic evaluation of objective clinical findings, particularly a patient's defensive preferences and the maturity of the patient's object relationships. Other useful parameters parallel the more rigid selection criteria for brief psychotherapy proposed by Sifneos (1972). All these factors help establish what Karasu and Skodol (1980) call a "psychotherapy diagnosis," a judgment concerning "the psychotherapeutic approach by which the patient is likely to derive maximal benefit."

General measures of a patient's ego strength include level of sexual development and adjustment, intellectual skills, educational and occupational achievements, and degree of autonomy and ability to assume responsibility. These criteria, which broadly assess psychological strength and weakness, measure the patient's ability to pursue self-selected goals while simultaneously contending with exceptional stresses of life, such as ill health.

A more detailed evaluation of ego functioning, discussed by Vaillant (1977) in his excellent study of basic adaptational styles, derives from a determination of prevailing ego mechanisms. Anxiety-provoking work is definitely contraindicated in an individual who relies heavily on psychotic mechanisms (e.g., denial, delusional projection, and distortion). A middle-aged diabetic patient who responds to the recent amputation of the lower leg by acting as if the limb were still intact is ill suited for introspective work. That patient requires considerable ego support, which can be provided in the form of psychopharmacologic treatment and consistent reality testing. Though immature mechanisms (e.g., schizoid withdrawal, projection, passive-dependent and passive-aggressive behavior, acting out, and hypochondriasis) may not cause such severe regression, they typify a personality structure that is generally unresponsive to an anxiety-provoking approach because of limitations on the capacity to modulate affect and control impulses. Conversely, the presence of neurotic mechanisms (e.g., intellectualization, repression, displacement, reaction formation, and dissociation) and the more sophisticated mechanisms (e.g., suppression, humor, anticipation, altruism, and sublimation) reflect flexibility and resilience of ego functioning sufficient to tolerate the heightened anxiety of emotional self-scrutiny.

The quality of an individual's object relationships provides a general measure of interpersonal functioning, another important indicator of the ability to tolerate anxiety. This information helps define the patient's motivation and ability to become involved in a productive and gratifying manner with others, important data when assessing the capacity for the emotional intensity and mutuality of a therapeutic relationship. The pattern of interaction with family, friends, and professional colleagues may yield a picture of marked passivity, characterized by dependency on most of the people in the patient's life. Other maladaptive modes of relating, such as fight–flight behavior or a series of short-lived superficial encounters involving fluctuating idealization and unreasonable denigration of a partner, may reflect the extreme anxiety emanating from unresolved issues of separation and individuation (e.g., borderline personalities). In the extreme, distorted object relationships are manifested as an inability to differentiate self from nonself. All these patterns suggest the necessity of a supportive approach. Conversely, a patient's interpersonal relationships may reflect the importance that person ascribes to independent functioning, as well as an ability to abdicate autonomy when a need to rely on the support of others is recognized. And the history of at least one meaningful mutual and stable relationship suggests basic trust and a capacity for genuine emotional involvement with others, important criteria for introspective therapy.

Other factors signaling the appropriateness of an anxiety-provoking approach include the patient's willingness for self-scrutiny and desire for emotional change as opposed to symptomatic relief. These are predicated on a requisite degree of intelligence and psychological-mindedness, often evidenced by a patient's insights concerning the illness. They ensure a workable transference relationship, one with sufficient observing ego for the patient to appreciate, and then modulate, the intense affects stirred by distorted perceptions. Attention to the therapeutic relationship can supply other indicators for introspective work, including the patient's realistic expectations concerning the expertise of the therapist and the anticipated goals of treatment, the patient's ability to be affectively and cognitively involved in psychotherapy, and the patient's facility in relating to the therapist throughout encouraging and disheartening phases of the medical illness and psychiatric treatment. A patient's responsiveness to trial interpretations provides data concerning each of these indicators for introspective work. Malan (1976), Sifneos (1972), and Davanloo (1980) detail the diagnostic value of these interventions. Viederman (1984) discusses their therapeutic worth; communicating an empathic and accurate understanding of the patient's plight enhances a sense of trust and, consequently, commitment to the psychotherapy.

Anxiety-Suppressing Psychotherapy

Ever since Freud (1919/1955) praised the "gold" of psychoanalytic interpretations, supportive psychotherapy has been considered an inferior form of treatment to insight-oriented work. This negative, and unfair, reputation derives from a variety of factors, ranging from, the longstanding belief that characterologic change is the primary goal of psychotherapy to, the frustration of practitioners who struggle to successfully implement this taxing treatment modality (Wallace, 1983). The relative inattention afforded anxiety-suppressing psychotherapy over the years reflects this bias, and may explain why it still remains a somewhat nebulous form of treatment. Divergent conceptualizations confuse basic therapeutic issues, such as the distinction between supportive therapy and supportive relationships; consequently, anxiety-suppressing therapy has frequently been explicated by means of "negative definitions," which basically declare what it is not (Buckley, 1986). Winston, Pinsker, and McCullough's (1986) excellent review of the literature significantly clarifies the fundamental goals and techniques of this treatment modality, thus highlighting its relevance to medical psychotherapy.

Anxiety-suppressing psychotherapy requires the clinician to be active and supportive in ways that contain the patient's anxiety within limits that were acceptable premorbidly. The overall treatment is focused on symptomatic relief, as opposed to structural intrapsychic change, an approach based on concrete, sometimes controlling, therapeutic directives. The major goal of treatment is to dissipate the powerful emotions that negatively affect the patient's psychologic well-being. The patient is not guided towards discovery of unconscious motivations and conflicts that have crystallized into the abnormal illness response. Rather, the patient is offered consistent encouragement and support by therapists who wish to maximize their influence by exploiting a working alliance solidified by trust and cooperation. When treating medical patients, the clinician attempts to curtail emotional dysfunction precipitated by illness by altering factors external to the individual, such as prescribing psychoactive medication or effecting changes in their living situations.

Because anxiety-suppressing psychotherapy rests on the clinician's ability to influence and guide the patient, eliciting and maintaining a positive transference is a primary goal of treatment. Careful attention to unconscious issues embodied in an individual's psychodynamics and illness dynamics identifies doctor–patient interactions that may be used by the therapist, whose inherent power (Frank, 1961) can be enhanced in a manner that parallels Alexander and French's (1946) studied manipulation of the transference. Techniques used to foster the positive transference, summarized by Winston, Pinsker, & McCullough (1986), emanate from the clinician's basic posture of being real, giving, and empathically concerned, as opposed to neutral, objective, and analytic. The medical psychotherapist offers advice and reassurance (e.g., opinions concerning the patient's response to a given therapeutic regimen), as well as praise when warranted (e.g., when the patient engages in meaningful discussion about the illness with family members or progresses in a rehabilitative program). The therapist provides an auxiliary ego to the patient. This function may take the form of education in the facts of his illness, identification and justification of the affective and behavioral responses to the sick role, explanation of changes in interactions with friends and family members, and prob-

lem solving of life issues caused by ill health. The therapist communicates all this in a personable style, more conversational than clinical. The negative transference is addressed only when it directly interferes with treatment, and it is interpreted in a circumscribed manner so as to overcome the patient's resistance without mobilizing intense affects that could potentially promote disorganizing levels of anxiety.

Supporting and enhancing a patient's defensive structure is another major goal of anxiety-suppressing psychotherapy. The therapist must identify and maintain those mechanisms that provide the basis for the patient's ego functioning. This knowledge is useful in helping to reinforce the patient's reality testing, particularly if the patient is observed to utilize considerable projection and distortion. It also highlights important defenses that should not be challenged by the clinician. Primitive mechanisms can be adaptive, such as the denial following a myocardial infarction (Hackett & Cassem, 1974); lacking them, a patient may become overwhelmed by emotional distress or may act out in a self-destructive fashion.

In addition to preserving a patient's fundamental defenses, the therapist should also attempt to discover and mobilize healthier ego functioning. For example, the reality testing of a person with diabetes mellitus who is preoccupied with "slipping into coma," despite excellent control of the illness, might be enhanced by working with that individual's obsessional defenses. Repeated review of the patient's insulin needs and blood sugars could afford a greater sense of control over the illness and, consequently, over the emotions it precipitates.

Attending to a patient's diminished self-esteem is the third goal of supportive psychotherapy. When stressed by life events that produce intensely painful affects, individuals may become demoralized and begin to doubt their self-worth. The medical patient needs protection from the isolation attending the sick role and, consequently, benefits significantly from interventions that bolster self-esteem. The therapist's active interest and attention, which communicate concern and respect, can offset feelings of helplessness and hopelessness. Specifically, the clinician is reassuring (c.g., validating the normality of a patient's emotional state) and offers advice (e.g., recommending actions that have helped others plagued by the same illness). These active interventions provide support and educate the patient in a way that legitimizes affective distress. They additionally convey an empathic view of the patient's situation, which serves to bolster self-esteem through the more passive process of identification with the therapist's values.

Two related aspects of supportive psychotherapy, particularly relevant to treatment of an abnormal illness response, are its attention to a specific focus and the structure of the therapeutic environment. The benign neglect afforded unconscious material (e.g., fantasies, dreams, and transference distortions) helps to contain the patient's level of anxiety, permitting the patient to concentrate psychic energies on the here and now. Treatment of a patient in the throes of an anxiety response, for example, would address the worries concerning the potentially debilitating effects of the illness, and not explore the dynamic roots of the patient's considerable separation anxiety. This focus is mirrored in the structure of the therapeutic interaction, which is predominantly characterized by an active give-and-take between the two participants, as opposed to the open-ended communication of introspective work and its characteristic intervals of silence. This structure helps the patient concentrate fully on concrete treatment goals.

The therapeutic maneuvers most often utilized in anxiety-suppressing psychotherapy are suggestion, manipulation, and abreaction. Along with clarification and interpretation, they constitute the fundamental technical interventions described by Bibring (1954) in his study of the therapeutic principles and procedures "considered to be applicable to all methods of psychotherapy independent of their respective ideologies." Bibring defines *suggestion* as "the induction of ideas, impulses, emotions, actions, etc., in brief, various mental processes by the therapist (an individual in authoritative postion) in the patient (an individual in dependent position) independent of, or to the exclusion of, the latter's rational or critical (realistic) thinking." Suggestion promotes change founded on the direct inculcation of beliefs, attitudes, or behavior, as opposed to self-understanding on the part of the patient. The same is true of *manipulation*, which Bibring separates into two forms. *Curative manipulation* involves redirecting "emotional systems" within an individual (e.g., undercutting passive-dependent behavior in an attempt to foster more autonomous functioning); *technical manipulation* helps to "produce favorable attitudes towards the treatment situation or to remove obstructive trends" (e.g., fostering a positive transference). *Abreaction* enables a patient to diffuse intensely disturbing affects within the safety of a therapeutic environment. Patients may also derive support from recognizing that therapists are able to tolerate their exquisitely painful feeling states. Some variations on the themes of suggestion and manipulation are discussed in Chapter 11 of this book.

Anxiety-Provoking Psychotherapy

Insight-oriented psychotherapy seeks to promote psychologic maturation by exploiting the turmoil of an emotional upheaval. The fundamental therapeutic task is to help patients acknowledge, bear, and put into perspective painful feelings that adversely affect their lives (Semrad, 1969), a conceptualization of the treatment that highlights its relationship to the grief process. Patients are first made aware of previously unrecognized emotions that have been kept out of consciousness by their various defensive maneuvers, they then experience those affects within the therapeutic environment, as well as in the context of important relationships. Finally, by recognizing the intensity, diversity, and ambivalence of their feelings, patients achieve some resolution of their conflicts.

Several disciples of the analytic school have tailored the anxiety-provoking model into a variety of brief psychotherapies well suited to the treatment of an abnormal illness response (Alexander & French, 1946; Davanloo, 1980; Malan, 1976; Mann, 1973; Sifneos, 1972). Despite conceptual and technical differences, all these approaches share several characteristics: (1) persistent pursuit of unconscious material (instinctual drives, as well as ego defenses), (2) active, confronting interventions by the therapist, and (3) attention to a central focus, which helps limit the degree of clinical regression. The goal of such treatment is working through, a therapeutic process that guides the patient toward insight and self-understanding to effect significant and lasting behavioral change (Greenson, 1967). Except for time limitations and the circumscribed focus of treatment—such as patients' emotional reaction to physical illness—the process of these therapies is identical to long-term insight-oriented psychodynamic work.

The fundamental task of anxiety-provoking therapy is studied attention to the interrelationship between two general areas of an individual's life: first, libidinal impulses, the anxiety they provoke, and the defenses utilized to contain them and, second, a lifelong pattern of object relationships that characterize one's past, current existence, and the transference relationship. Elucidating the dynamic interaction between these two triads provides the patient with meaningful insight that helps liberate him from longstanding maladaptive patterns.

Though introspective therapy continually challenges defenses that contain unacknowledged affects, it periodically employs supportive techniques when the level of therapeutic tension threatens the treatment. Consequently, all the technical maneuvers discussed by Bibring (1954) come into play, though clarification and interpretation are most often used. *Clarification* "refers to those techniques and therapeutic processes which assist the patient to reach a higher degree of self-awareness, clarity and differentiation of self-observation which makes adequate verbalization possible" (Bibring, 1954). It addresses the patient's emotions, patterns of conduct, attitudes, values, and cognitions, making each issue an object of collaborative study with the therapist. In conjunction with the other technical maneuvers, clarification heightens a patient's psychological-mindedness and prepares the patient for subsequent *interpretations*, which "make conscious the unconscious meaning, source, history, mode or course of a given psychic event" (Greenson, 1967). This insight, an understanding of previously unrecognized forces underlying particular maladaptive behaviors, then undergoes the process of working through. At this point, therapy focuses on the varied resistances that interfere with an individual's ability to utilize insight in a lasting and meaningful way. Though working through has traditionally been regarded as a lengthy process characteristic of long-term treatment, it can occur more rapidly when the focus of therapy is confined to a specific issue, such as the patient's illness dynamics.

CHOICE OF PSYCHOTHERAPEUTIC APPROACH

The type of medical psychotherapy utilized when treating an individual's abnormal illness response generally conforms to either the anxiety-suppressing or the anxiety-provoking approach. By focusing on the theoretical underpinnings and the practice of these two treatment modalities, however, the preceding description neglects some realities of the clinical environment. The actual implementation of supportive and introspective interventions, within the context of a comprehensive treatment plan, requires flexibility and pragmatism on the part of the clinician. The task, which is guided fundamentally by constant attention to the patient's illness dynamics, may be facilitated by the following observations.

First, though a specific type of medical psychotherapy *predominates* in the treatment of an abnormal illness response, it rarely occurs in pure form because of the overlap of anxiety-suppressing and anxiety-provoking techniques. Psychoanalysis, for example, places a premium on therapeutic neutrality. It has always acknowledged the importance of supportive maneuvers, however, most notably as they pertain to the working alliance (Freud, 1913/1955; Greenson, 1967). Alternatively, Winston, Pinsker, and McCullough (1986) discuss "a continuum of supportive therapies" that incorporate expressive (anxiety-provoking) work to a degree determined by the patient's level of ego strength. Pine (1986) emphasizes this point, describing techniques for achieving "interpretive content" in the context of supportive therapy. He outlines specific maneuvers that enable dividuals "generally characterized by a fragility of defense" to tolerate this anxiety-provoking intervention. These observations do not blur the distinction between the supportive and introspective approaches as much as they indicate a positive interaction between aspects of the two approaches, for example, the need to interpret negative transference feelings that arise during anxiety-suppressing therapy. In Pine's words, "supportive and insight therapies are not *counterposed*, in some *opposition* to one another, but are *counterpoised*, in some *balance* with one another." The degree to which this occurs in the treatment of an individual's abnormal illness response is guided by the particulars of the patient's illness dynamics.

Second, though anxiety-suppressing and anxiety-provoking therapy are founded on a psychodynamic understanding of the patient, each of these treatment modalities has distinctive cognitive and behavioral attributes. For example, clarification and interpretation of defenses and unconscious material remain the foundation of insight-oriented work; however, behavioral interventions (e.g., limit-setting maneuvers) may complement the exploratory process. Supportive work can occur within a clinical framework completely apart from psychodynamic psychotherapy. Moos and Schaefer (1984), for example, utilize a cognitive approach based on crisis theory when treating patients unable to cope with the impact of physical illness. They outline two sets of treatment goals for such patients—illness-related tasks (e.g., dealing with pain and incapacitation, dealing with the hospital environment, and developing adequate realtionships with health care staff) and general tasks (e.g., preserving a reasonable emotional balance, preserving a satisfactory self-image and maintaining a sense of competence and mastery, sustaining relationships with family and friends, and preparing for an uncertain future)—and describe the major types of coping skills employed to deal with these various tasks. The treatment includes fundamental interventions of supportive therapy, such as education, reassurance, and abreaction, which are effected by means of cognitive, problem-solving techniques. Anxiety-suppressing therapy can also take the form of behavioral interventions, such as relaxation protocols and desensitization (e.g., to treat excessive anxiety) or positive and negative reinforcement (e.g., to deal with excessive regression).

Third, though supportive and insight-oriented therapy have been discussed in terms of individual treatment, medical psychotherapy is effected in a variety of clinical formats. An individual's abnormal illness response can be treated in the context of family therapy, couples therapy, or group psychotherapy, each of which may be anxiety-suppressing or anxiety-provoking depending on the prevailing illness dynamics. When the psychological well-being of a family is adversely affected by the illness of one of its members (Binger, Alblin, Feuerstein, et al., 1969; Borden, 1962) supportive work can facilitate the family's accommodation to the illness and may be directly therapeutic to the identified patient (Rosman, Minuchin, & Liebman, 1975). Couples therapy is indicated when an individual's abnormal illness response causes increasing distance in the primary relationship and threatens its viability. The psychologic health of each member, their dynamic interaction, and the particular losses imposed by the patient's ill health (e.g., decreased sexual function) determine whether a supportive or an introspective intervention is indicated. The same decision applies to group therapy. Insight-oriented work has traditionally been used in the treatment of classic psychosomatic illnesses (A Stein, 1971) and has been effective in helping patients adjust to terminal illness (Spiegel, 1979; Yalom & Greaves, 1977). However, several attributes of the group process (e.g., diffusion of the transference and greater interpersonal contact) bolster impaired ego functioning and, consequently, favor the use of group therapy as

a supportive form of medical psychotherapy. Group patients benefit from information sharing (Bilodeau & Hackett, 1971), a generalized acceptance of emotional expression (Adsett & Bruhn, 1968; A Stein, 1971), and the mutual support derived from discussing common medical experiences, such as amputation, myocardial infarction, and the impact of a mastectomy or colostomy (Slaby & Glicksman, 1985). As Moos and Schaefer (1984) point out, "a patient may deny or minimize the seriousness of a crisis while talking to a family member, seek relevant information about prognosis from a physician, [and] request reassurance and emotional support from a friend." Because an illness response can take on such complexity, these varied therapeutic modalities are often used in combination to effect a medical psychotherapy that suits the patient's distinctive needs.

Finally, supportive and introspective treatments have been discussed within the context of a single episode of ill health. Most illness is chronic, however, and its elongated time course has implications for the practice of medical psychotherapy. The onset of a long-term illness may so overwhelm an individual that initially the patient can only tolerate an anxiety-suppressing approach; however, this does not suggest that the patient will require support throughout the entire clinical course. Slaby and Glicksman (1985) observe that coping mechanisms appropriate to one stage of life-threatening illness are not necessarily appropriate to later stages. Similarly, while some patients repeatedly require anxiety-suppressing work during exacerbations of a medical disease, others profit from anxiety-provoking therapy during remissions of the medical illness. This may protect the patient against the recurrence of an abnormal illness response during acute clinical exacerbations or subsequent episodes of ill health, as well as generally enhance adaptive ego functioning. It parallels the work of crisis intervention, as described by Caplan (1964), which promotes the acquisition of new coping mechanisms, increased self-esteem, and diminished fear about the recurrence of a particular stressor. The same accommodation may derive from a patient's assessment of his illness over time, which can replace feared fantasies with the reality of symptomatic relief, loving support from family and friends, and a level of functioning that affords some sense of control over the illness.

REFERENCES

Adsett C & Bruhn J (1968). Short-term group psychotherapy for myocardial infarction patients and their wives. *Canadian Medical Association Journal, 99*, 577–581.

Alexander F & French T (1946). *Psychoanalytic Therapy*. New York: Ronald Press.

Amkraut A & Solomon G (1974). From the symbolic stimulus to the pathophysiologic response: Immune mechanisms. *International Journal of Psychiatry, 5*, 541–563.

Bibring E (1954). Psychoanalysis and the dynamic psychotherapies. *Journal of the American Psychoanalytic Association, 2*, 745–770.

Bilodeau C & Hackett T (1971). Issues raised in a group setting by patients recovering from myocarFFdial infarction. *American Journal of Psychiatry, 128*, 73–78.

Binger C, Ablin A, Fruerstein R, Kushner J, ZogerF S, & Mikkelson (1969). Childhood leukemia: Emotional impact on patient and family. *New England Journal of Medicine, 280*, 414–418.

Borden W (1962). Psychological aspects of a stroke: Patient and famliy. *Annals of Internal Medicine, 57*, 689–692.

Brown J & Stoudemire G (1983). Normal and pathological grief. *Journal of the American Medical Association, 250*(3), 378–382.

Buckley P (1986). Supportive psychotherapy: A neglected treatment. *Psychiatric Annals, 16*(9), 515–521.

Cannon W (1920). *Bodily Changes in Pain, Hunger, Fear and Rage*. New York: Appleton-Century-Crofts.

Cannon W (1932). *The Wisdom of the Body*. New York: W. W. Norton.

Caplan G (1964). *Principles of Preventive Psychiatry*. New York: Basic Books.

Davanloo H (Ed) (1980). *Short Term Dynamic Psychotherapy*. New York: Aronson.

Dorian B, Garfinkel P, Keystone E, Gorcynski R, Garner D, & Darby P (1986, March). *Stress, immunity, and illness*. Paper presented at the meeting of the American Psychosomatic Society, Baltimore.

Engel G (1968). A life setting conducive to illness: The giving-up–given-up complex. *Annals of Internal Medicine, 69*, 293–298.

Engel G (1971). Sudden and rapid death during psychological stress. *Annals of Internal Medicine, 74*, 771–782.

Engel G (1977). The need for a new medical model: A challenge for biomedicine. *Science, 196*, 129–136.

Engel G (1980). The clinical application of the biopsychosocial model. *American Journal of Psychiatry, 137*, 535–544.

Frank J (1961). *Persuasion and Healing*. Baltimore: Johns Hopkins University Press.

Freud S (1955). On beginning the treatment. In J Strachey (Ed and Trans), *The Standard Edition of the Complete Psychological Works of Sigmund Freud* (Vol 12, p 121). London: Hogarth Press. (Original work published 1913)

Freud S (1955). Line of advance in psychoanalytic therapy. In J Strachey (Ed and Trans), *The Standard Edition of the Complete Psychological Works of Sigmund Freud* (Vol 17, p 157). London: Hogarth Press. (Original work published 1919)

Freud S (1924). Aspects of development and regression: Etiology. In J Riviere (Ed), *A General Introduction to Psychoanalysis*. New York: Boni and Liveright, pp 348–366

Goldberg R & Green S (1985). Medical psychotherapy. *American Family Physician, 31* 173–178.

Green S (1985). *Mind and Body: The Psychology of Physical Illness*. Washington: American Psychiatric Press.

Greene W, Goldstein S, & Moss, A (1972). Psychosocial aspects of sudden death. *Archives of Internal Medicine, 129*, 725–731.

Greenson RR (1967). *The Technique and Practice of Psychoanalysis* (Vol I). New York: International Universities Press, Inc.

Groves J (1978). Taking care of the hateful patient. *New England Journal of Medicine, 298*, 883–887.

Hackett T & Cassem N (1974). Development of a quantitative rating scale to assess denial. *Journal of Psychosomatic Research, 18*, 93–100.

Haskett R & Rose R (1981). Neuroendocrine disorders

and psychopathology. *Psychiatric Clinics of North America, 4*(2), 239–252.

Henry J (1975). The induction of acute and chronic cardiovascular disease in animals by psychosocial stimulation. *International Journal of Psychiatric Medicine, 6,* 147–158.

Karasu T & Skodol A (1980). VIth axis for DSM-III: Psychodynamic evaluation. *American Journal of Psychiatry, 137,* 607–610.

Kiely W (1974). From the symbolic stimulus to the pathophysiological response: Neurophysiological mechanisms. *International Journal of Psychiatric Medicine, 5,* 517–529.

Klerman G (1981). Depression in the medically ill. *Psychiatric Clinics of North America, 4*(2), 301–318.

Lindemann E (1944). Symptomatology and management of acute grief. *American Journal of Psychiatry, 101,* 141–146.

Lipowski Z (1975). Psychiatry of somatic diseases: Epidemiology, pathogenesis, classification. *Comprehensive psychiatry, 16,* 105–124.

Locke S, Kraus L, Leserman J, et al., (1984). Life change stress, psychiatric symptoms, and natural killer cell activity. *Psychosomatic Medicine, 46,* 441–453.

Lown B, Verrier R, & Rabinowitz S (1977). Neural and psychologic mechanisms and the problem of sudden cardiac death. *American Journal of Cardiology, 39,* 890–902.

Malan D (1976). *The Frontier of Brief Psychiatry.* New York: Plenum.

Mann J (1973). *Time-Limited Psychotherapy.* Cambridge: Harvard University Press.

Mason J (1975). Clinical psychophysiology: Psychoendocrine mechanism. In M Reiser (Ed), *American Handbook of Psychiatry* (Vol 4). New York: Basic Books.

Moos R & Schaefer J (1984). The crisis of physical illness: An overview and conceptual approach. In R. Moos (Ed), *Coping with Physical Illness: Vol 2. New perspectives* (pp. 3–26). New York: Plenum.

Parsons T (1951). *The social system.* Glencoe, IL: The Free Press.

Pine F (1986). Supportive psychotherapy: A psychoanalytic perspective. *Psychiatric Annals, 16*(9), 526–529.

Reich P, DeSilva R, Lown B, & Murawski J (1981). Acute psychological disturbances preceding life-threatening ventricular arrhythmias. *Journal of the American Medical Association, 246,* 233–235.

Reichard J (1964). Teaching principles of medical psychology to medical house officers: Methods and problems. In N Zinberg (Ed), *Psychiatry and Medical Practice in a General Hospital.* New York: International Universities Press.

Reiser M (1975). Changing theoretical concepts in psychosomatic medicine. In M Reiser (Ed), *American Handbook of Psychiatry* (Vol. 4). New York: Basic Books.

Rodin G & Voshart K (1986). Depression in the medically ill: Overview. *American Journal of Psychiatry, 143,* 696–705.

Rogers M, Dubey D, & Reich P (1979). The influence of the psyche and the brain on immunity and disease susceptibility: A critical review. *Psychosomatic Medicine, 41,* 147–164.

Rosman B, Minuchin S, & Liebman R (1975). Family lunch session: An introduction to family therapy in anorexia nervosa. *American Journal of Orthopsychiatry, 45,* 846–853

Schindler B (1985). Stress, affective disorders, and immune function. *Medical Clinics of North America, 69,* 585–597.

Schleifer S, Keller S, Meyerson A, et al, (1984). Lymphocyte function in major depressive disorder. *Archives of General Psychiatry, 41,* 484–486.

Selye H (1950). *Physiology and Pathology of Exposure to Stress.* Montreal: Acta Press.

Semrad E (1969). A clinical formulation of the psychoses. In E Semrad & D van Buskirk (Eds), *Teaching Psychotherapy of Psychotic Patients.* New York: Grune and Stratton.

Sifneos P (1972). *Short-term Psychotherapy and Emotional Crisis.* Cambridge: Harvard University Press.

Sifneos P (1972–73). Is dynamic psychotherapy contraindicated for a large number of patients with psychosomatic diseases? *Psychotherapy and Psychosomatics, 21,* 133–136.

Sifneos P (1973). The prevalence of "alexithymic" characteristics in psychosomatic patients. *Psychotherapy and Psychosomatics, 22,* 255–262.

Slaby A & Glicksman A (1985). *Adapting to Life-Threatening Illness.* New York: Praeger.

Spiegel D (1979). Psychological support for women with metastatic carcinoma. *Psychosomatics, 20,* 780–787.

Stein A (1971). Group therapy with psychosomatically ill patients. In H Kaplan & B Sadock (Eds.), *Comprehensive Group Psychotherapy.* Baltimore: Williams and Wilkins.

Stein M (1981). A biopsychosocial approach to immune function and medical disorders. *Psychiatric Clinics of North America, 4*(2), 203–222.

Stein M, Keller S, & Schleifer S (1985). Stress and immunomodulation: The role of depression and neuroendocrine function. *Journal of Immunology, 135*(Suppl. 2), 827–833.

Vaillant G (1977). *Adaptation to Life.* Boston: Little, Brown.

Viederman M (1984). The active dynamic interview

and the supportive relationship. *Comprehensive Psychiatry, 25,* 147–157.

Wallace E (1983). *Dynamic Psychiatry in Theory and Practice.* Philadelphia: Lea and Febiger.

Whybrow P & Silberfarb P (1974). Neuroendocrine mediating mechanisms: From the symbolic stimulus to the physiological response. *International Journal of Psychiatric Medicine, 5,* 531–539.

Winston A, Pinsker H & McCullough L (1986). A review of supportive psychotherapy. *Hospital and Community Psychiatry, 37*(11), 1105–1114.

Wolff H, Wolf S, & Hare S (Eds) (1950). *Life stress and bodily disease.* Baltimore: Williams and Wilkins.

Yalom I & Greaves C (1977). Group therapy with the terminally ill. *American Journal of Psychiatry, 134,* 396–400.

Steven A. Cohen-Cole
Carol Harpe

2
Diagnostic Assessment of Depression in the Medically Ill

This chapter reviews the wide range of depressive syndromes that physicians may encounter in medical and surgical patients, suggests an approach to the diagnosis of major depression in medical contexts, and offers treatment guidelines for each of the different syndromes.

There are five different depressive diagnoses described in DSM-III-R (American Psychiatric Association, 1987): major depression, organic mood syndrome, adjustment disorder with depressed mood, dementia with depression, and dysthymic disorder. Each of these conditions will be described in detail. A non-DSM-III concept, covert (or masked) depression is an important consideration for medical patients and will be discussed separately.

TERMINOLOGY: ARE THERE "GOOD REASONS" FOR DEPRESSION?

Before each of these different syndromes is described, the use of the word *depression* must be clarified. The word is commonly used in one of three different ways. It is used as a synonym for the affect *sadness*, as a symptom of an illness, and as one of several disease syndromes. For example, medical practitioners often say, "Mrs. Jones is depressed, but she has good reasons to be depressed." This statement is packed with layers of meaning not immediately clear. Does the statement indicate that the patient suffers from a major depression or simply from a normal and expected sadness associated with severe physical illness? Either interpretation could be acceptable. In practice, the phrase usually reflects diagnostic uncertainty between the two poles of meaning. Because the word *depression* has so many overlapping meanings, the statement "Mrs. Jones has good reasons to be depressed" can never be disproved. It has the form of a medical, quasi-scientific statement, but since it cannot be disproved, it is confusing, impressionistic, and nonscientific.

When the phrase is used to indicate that a patient has understandable reasons to be sad, it is tautological because the severe illness and sadness are seen as inextricably linked by the speaker. When the statement is used, however, to indicate that a patient has "good reasons" to have a major depression, the phrase is empirically incorrect. Used in this way, it implies that everyone with such a physical condition will suffer from major depression. This is not supported by research, which demonstrates that less than half of any medically ill population, including terminal cancer patients, meet clinical criteria for major depressive illness (Bukberg, Penman, & Holland, 1984; Maguire, 1984; Rodin & Voshart, 1986; Stoudemire, 1985).

In addition, such statements about the understandability of major depression are dangerous in that they tend to explain away a serious psychiatric disorder that is eminently treatable. When clinicians say that patients have "good reasons" to be depressed, such patients often do not receive independent or aggressive psychiatric treatment for their major depression. This omission is a serious error, since patients with physical illness and major depression usually respond to the standard psychiatric treatments for depression and often remain depressed if not treated adequately (Maguire, Hopwood, Tarrier, & Howell, 1985; Rifkin, Reardon, Siris et al., 1985).

To help with this conceptual and diagnostic muddle, clinicians should avoid the use of the word *depressed* as a synonym for sadness. The terms *depressed* and *depression* should be reserved for distinct clinical entities. Different terms, such as *sad* or *demoralized*, should be used to describe the affect associated with physical illness. (These common feelings of loss and grief are described in detail in Chapter 1 under the heading Responses to Illness.) Distinct psychiatric syndromes can then be appropriately distinguished from more nonspecific affects, and appropriate treatment plans can be developed for each particular depressive syndrome.

MAJOR DEPRESSION

Major depression is the most important depressive syndrome for the psychiatrist to recognize and treat in the medical setting. Depending on the illnesses examined and the methodology employed, prevalence studies indicate that between 5 and 32 percent of medical patients suffer from major depression (Rodin & Voshart, 1986; Schulberg, Saul, McClelland et al., 1985; Stoudemire, 1985). Major depression is also important because of its treatability. Many patients with major depression will improve significantly with appropriate biological or psychological therapy or both. Unfortunately, the diagnosis of major depression in the medical setting is frequently overlooked, and many treatable patients probably never receive appropriate psychiatric treatment. Several studies indicate that about 30–50 percent of major depression is missed in the medical setting (Cavenaugh & Kennedy, 1986; Cohen-Cole et al., 1982; Knights & Folstein, 1977; Schulberg, Saul, McClelland, et al., 1985; Thompson, Stoudemire, & Mitchell, 1983).

The assessment of major depression in the medical setting, however, is problematic. First, since some sad feelings are an acknowledged part of the experience of physical illness, what are the boundaries between these normal sad feelings and the syndrome of major depression? Second, many of the symptoms of physical illness (like decreased energy and anorexia) are identical to symptoms of depression, and the clinician may find it difficult to determine the etiology of the symptoms encountered. These two issues will be considered in detail, with reference to the research literature, in order to provide some guidelines to clinicians taking care of depressed patients in the medical-surgical context.

Major depression, according to DSM-III-R, requires a patient to demonstrate 5 of the 9 symptoms in the following list during the same two-week period of time. These must represent a change from previous functioning. Symptoms clearly due to a physical condition should not be included. One of the 5 must be either a persistent depressed mood (feeling sad, blue, down in the dumps) *or* pervasive anhedonia (the loss of interest or pleasure in all or almost all activities).

1. General symptoms (At least one of these is required for the diagnosis of a major depressive episode.)
   a. Depressed mood most of the day nearly every day for two weeks
   b. Anhedonia (markedly diminished interest or pleasure in all, or almost all, activities most of the day, nearly every day)
2. Physical symptoms (must be present nearly every day)
   a. Insomnia or hypersomnia
   b. Significant weight or appetite change (increase or decrease)
   c. Psychomotor agitation or retardation
   d. Fatigue or loss of energy
3. Psychologic symptoms (must be present nearly every day)
   a. Feelings of worthlessness or excessive or inappropriate guilt
   b. Diminished ability to think or concentrate, or indecisiveness
   c. Recurrent thoughts of death or suicidal ideation

Dysphoric Mood: Neither Necessary nor Sufficient for Diagnosis

Note that dysphoric mood (i.e., sadness), no matter how severe, is not *sufficient* for the diagnosis of major depression by these criteria. The patient must also demonstrate some of the other symptoms. Many, perhaps most, patients with severe physical illness will experience varying degrees of sadness, but the full syndrome of major depression does not necessarily follow. The presence of a dysphoric mood, therefore, may properly be used as a clue for a possible major depression, but the two are not synonymous.

Besides being insufficient for the diagnosis of major depression, dysphoria is not even *necessary* for the diagnosis. Paradoxically, a patient need not be sad to have a major depression. According to DSM-III-R, a patient may present with anhedonia and 4 more symptoms to meet the criteria for major depression. This fact is important clinically because many patients with physical illness will not report feelings of sadness, yet they may meet these other criteria and respond well to treatment. Thus, the question whether or not a patient's dysphoria is a "normal" reaction to the stress of the physical illness is not the key issue in diagnosing major depression. It is far more important to determine whether or not the other symptoms are present.

Four Approaches to the Evaluation of Depressive Symptoms in the Medically Ill

The determination of whether or not the symptoms of depression are present in a medically ill patient is exceedingly complex because some of the apparent symptoms of major depression could be accounted for by the medical illness itself. Should the fatigue, sleep impairment, psychomotor retardation, and anorexia associated with many physical illnesses be interpreted as symptoms of major depression as well? Unfortunately, the literature supplies no clear answer. The research that supported the DSM-III concept of major depression was conducted on patients without significant physical illnesses (J Williams, personal communication, 1986), and there are not yet sufficient studies of medically ill patients to indicate the reliability or validity of different approaches to diagnosis. To date, there have been four major approaches to diagnosing major depression in the physically ill. These approaches are here termed *inclusive*, *etiologic*, *substitutive*, and *exclusive*.

Inclusive Approach

The inclusive approach, used by Rifkin and colleagues, is the simplest. Using the Schedule for Affective Disorders and Schizophrenia (SADS) and Research Diagnostic Criteria (RDC), this group studied physically ill patients and counted symptoms of depression, whether or not they might be attributable to a primary physical problem (Rifkin, Reardon, Siris, et al., 1985). Low energy, if present, was thus considered a symptom of depression whether or not the patient or the physician believed that it was a "normal" response to the physical illness. The approach is conceptually clear and "clean." It is phenomenological, in keeping with the spirit of DSM-III; that is, diagnostic decisions are made on the evaluation of observable phenomena and do not require etiologic inferences. This approach tends to maximize inter-rater reliability in diagnosis; but because so many symptoms of physical illness are also those of depression, it could lead to overdiagnosis by including false positives (i.e., considering people depressed who are only physically ill). Its sensitivity should thus be high, but its specificity lower.

Etiologic Approach

An etiologic approach, advocated by Spitzer, Williams, and Gibbon (1984) and the developers of DSM-III, suggests that diagnosticians count a symptom toward the diagnosis of depression only if it is *not* "clearly due to a physical illness." This is the decision rule for the Structured Clinical Interview for DSM-III (SCID) (Spitzer, Endicott, & Robins, 1978) as well as for the Diagnostic Interview Schedule (DIS) (Robbins, Helzer, Croughan, & Ratcliff, 1981). A recent study of depression in Parkinson's disease patients utilized this approach (Mayeux, Stern, Williams et al., 1986). Unfortunately, the report does not specify how these distinctions were actually made clinically. Since this approach requires inferences of causality from unclear criteria, it seems its reliability would be low.

An important group of studies in stroke patients utilized a similar approach (Lipsey, Robinson, Pearlson et al., 1984; Robinson, Lipsey, & Price, 1985; Robinson, Starr, & Price, 1984). Researchers in those studies used the Present State Examination but made dysphoria a necessary requirement for a diagnosis of major depression. (Anhedonia was not an acceptable alternative.) Their decision rules, moreover, allowed them to count a physical symptom such as fatigue toward the diagnosis of depression *only* if the patient or the physician felt the symptom was in excess of what might be caused by the stroke (RG Robinson, personal communication, 1986). Though the authors report high inter-rater reliability using this approach, it is uncertain whether other psychiatrists could make these same distinctions reliably. The authors were probably able to achieve this reliability because of their close partnership in their research endeavors and the ability to specify decision rules to guide their diagnostic thinking.

It is possible that some psychiatrists working in very specific medical settings (like Robinson and Lipsey's group with stroke patients) might become familiar enough with one specific disease process to be able to reliably differentiate between "normal" symptoms of a physical illness (e.g., fatigue) and "excessive" symptoms, which might be more properly attributed to a depressive syndrome. This determination, however, would be nearly impossible for the general psychiatrist to make in a reliable manner. In addition, the validity of the approach also needs to be established through outcome studies, to determine if major depression diagnosed in this manner has a clinical course different from the outcome for patients who have some symptoms of depression—for example, sadness—but do not meet criteria for major depression.

Substitutive Approach

The substitutive approach suggests changing the criteria for the diagnosis of depression in the medically ill. From a factor analytic study (latent trait analysis) using the Beck Depression Inventory in large numbers of medical patients, Cavenaugh, Clark, and Gibbons found that decreased energy was a poor discriminator of depression and that "indecisiveness" was a relatively good one (Cavenaugh, Clark, & Gibbons, 1983; Clark, Cavenaugh, & Gibbons, 1983). They suggest that psychiatrists incorporate this finding into their clinical work. Though weakened by the lack of clinical interviews and by reliance on an instrument that emphasizes cognitive symptoms, this research is promising in its attempt to reconsider the diagnostic criteria for major depression in the medically ill.

Similarly, Endicott (1984) suggests substituting other symptoms of depression when DSM-III criteria are problematic. For example, if it cannot be determined whether a patient's low energy is due to physical disease or depression, she suggests that we substitute consideration of other depressive symptoms, such as "brooding, self-pity, or pessimism." Endicott does not indicate the source of these other criteria, and it is unclear whether her suggested list would lead to over- or underdiagnosis of depression.

Exclusive Approach

Research on depression in cancer patients by Holland's group at Sloan-Kettering Cancer Institute represents the exclusive approach (Bukberg Penman & Holland, 1984; Plumb & Holland, 1981).

This group simply eliminates anorexia and fatigue from the list of 9 depressive criteria, and requires 4 out of the remaining 7 symptoms for a diagnosis of major depression. This, like the first approach, is relatively "clean" because it specifies how to apply the criteria. It leads to the reverse problem, however, in that it is harder for patients to meet the restricted criteria. Thus, some depressed patients presenting primarily with vegetative symptoms might be missed, leading to false negatives. Specificity is probably high at the cost of a loss of sensitivity.

Clinical Evaluation

All four approaches have specific advantages and disadvantages depending on the particular research or clinical objectives. These advantages and disadvantages are summarized in Table 2-1. For research purposes, the best model to follow is that of the Sloan-Kettering group, which maximizes specificity (i.e., confidence that the true disorder is really present when diagnosed). This approach ensures the most homogenous depressed group possible, with the fewest extraneous or confounding variables, thereby increasing the clinical and statistical significance of the research data.

For the clinician, however, maximizing sensitivity (i.e., detecting all possible disorders within a population) is the most important first step in the proper evaluation of the patient. Although the clinical goal will always be to maximize sensitivity and specificity at the same time, this is not always possible. Depression is generally underdiagnosed in the medically ill (Schulberg, Saul, McClelland, et al., 1985), and the syndrome can be long lasting and debilitating (Maguire, 1984). Furthermore, even when depression is recognized by primary care physicians, the patients are more often than not treated inadequately,

Table 2-1
Approaches to the Diagnosis of Depression in the Medically Ill

Approach	Key Features	Strengths	Weaknesses	Comments
Inclusive	Count all possible symptoms, regardless of whether or not they could be caused by an underlying physical disorder.	Simple, phenomenological, high reliability, high sensitivity	Possible overinclusiveness, possible high number of false positives (low specificity); validity uncertain	Recommended for clinical use, modified case by case with clinical judgment
Etiologic (DSM-III-R)	Do not count a symptom toward the diagnosis of depression if it is "clearly due to a physical condition."	Theoretically sound	In practice, difficulty in attributing etiology of symptoms in a reliable way; validity uncertain	Theoretically sound, but practically difficult to implement
Exclusive	Exclude fatigue and anorexia from list of depressive symptoms.	Lowers the possibility of confounding variables contributing to diagnoses; higher specificity and low false positives	Harder to reach diagnosis; possibly excessive false negatives (low sensitivity); may deny treatment to those who could otherwise benefit	Good for research; too exclusive for clinical use
Substitutive	Substitute cognitive symptoms such as brooding or indecision for fatigue and anorexia.	Reasonable conceptually	Unclear	Conceptually reasonable, but little experience to date

with either anxiolytic medications or subtherapeutic doses of antidepressants (Keller, Klerman, Lavor, et al., 1982). Because of these findings, psychiatrists should lean in the direction of ensuring that depressions are recognized and treated adequately.

For clinical practice, therefore, the best approach seems to be the inclusive approach, which preserves the phenomenological spirit of DSM-III-R. Using this, clinicians diagnose disorders based on the presence or absence of signs and symptoms, without reliance on inferences of intrapsychic dynamics or complex etiological sequences. For an initial working diagnosis as a guide for initiating therapy, relevant symptoms should be counted toward the diagnosis if there is *any* reason to believe that they may be part of a depressive syndrome. Thus, even if the etiology of a particular symptom is questionable (i.e., the symptom may result from both a physical and a psychiatric process), we suggest that it be counted toward those required for the diagnosis. Fatigue, anorexia, and psychomotor changes should be evaluated in the same way. It is worth noting that even if all 4 physical symptoms are present, the patient will still need to demonstrate significant and persistent depressed mood or anhedonia to meet the criteria. This approach may lead to some false positive diagnoses, but such errors are preferable to the alternative: lack of treatment for patients who need it. The risk of treating someone (with psychotherapy or medication) who may not have major depressive illness is small, in general, compared with the risk of neglecting treatment in patients suffering from depression, particularly because most of the false positives will have some other form of depression requiring treatment.

The skilled clinician, however, should not rely solely on the simpleminded application of mechanical formulas. Spitzer, Endicott, and Robins (1978) point out that

"it is important to realize that the use of specified criteria does not eliminate clinical judgment. . . . The criteria involve clinical concepts rather than a mere enumeration of complaints or observations of atomistic behaviors."

In the medically ill, therefore, clinicians should pay particular attention to the psychologic symptoms of depression and anhedonia. Most patients will retain variable affective responses to their environment, some of them pleasurable. Unless they are in extreme, continuous pain or have impaired consciousness, physically ill patients usually can respond to humor, to intimacy from family or friends, or to gestures of support from the staff. That is, they will usually be able to report that they get some degree of pleasure or have some interest in activities around them. They may also smile or laugh at jokes. The patient with major depression, however, may be unable to respond with significant interest, pleasure, or humor to any event.

Questions that can be helpful in this regard are "What are you able to enjoy these days? What interests you now? When did you last have a good time? Have you been able to laugh at anything lately?" Patients who report *pervasive* loss of interest or pleasure for at least two weeks should be considered likely candidates for the diagnosis of major depression. Questions regarding the presence of other psychologic symptoms of depression can also be helpful in problematic circumstances. Patients can be asked about their ability to concentrate, their sense of self-esteem or guilt, and their thoughts about death. As part of the mental status evaluation, tests of concentration and short-term memory need to be utilized as well. Since major depressive illness has been associated with deficits in these areas, the clinician may find that the presence of these cognitive problems may aid in the diagnosis of major depression (Stoudemire, Hill, Kaplan et al., in press).

The Multidimensional Approach to Diagnostic Assessment

The clinician applying DSM-III-R criteria to medically ill patients should remember that the criteria for major depression (as for many other psychiatric illnesses) were established in large part by consensus of expert panel members and have not yet been validated by external standards, such as natural history, family history, response to treatment, and biologic markers (Carroll, 1984). The criteria are cross-sectional in nature and, even under the best of circumstances, are subject to problems of reliability. Therefore, the thorough evaluation of the depressed patient requires a multidimensional approach that includes the following elements:

1. Clinical signs and symptoms (descriptive, cross-sectional)
2. Personal history of depression
3. Previous response to treatment
4. Family history of depression (genetic vulnerability)
5. Response to treatment—current episode
6. Biologic markers
   a. Dexamethasone suppression test (DST)
   b. Thyrotropin-releasing hormone stimulation test (TRHST)
   c. Sleep electroencephalogram (sleep EEG)

The personal and family histories of the patient are of key importance. A prior personal or family history of major depression increases the likelihood of a current episode (Carroll, 1984). Previous response to treatment (of the patient or a family member) is useful information to obtain because successful past treatments can predict similar responses with the same treatments.

The use of the dexamethasone suppression test (DST) as a diagnostic aid has been advocated by Carroll, Feinberg, Greden and others (1981). Used with psychiatric patients, Carroll argues, the DST has a moderately high sensitivity (.6) and an extremely high specificity (.9) for severe depressive disorders. Others have pointed out, however, that medical illnesses (e.g., fever, congestive heart failure, dementia), age, weight loss, stress, and nonpsychiatric medications (e.g., anticonvulsants, benzodiazepines, steroids) all limit its usefulness in physically ill patients by creating many false positives and thereby lowering the specificity (Hirschfeld, Koslow, & Kupfer, 1983). Research in this area continues, however, and changing the cutoff values for different patient populations may turn out to yield promising results (Fogel, Satel, & Levy, 1985). Similarly, the TRH stimulation test and sleep architecture studies (Akiskal, Djenderedjian, Bolinger, et al., 1978) are important biologic markers of depression that are under investigation but cannot yet be advocated for general use in medical populations.

Treatment of Major Depression

The diagnostic distinctions in DSM-III-R and the multidimensional factors described above are important because they have implications for treatment. A patient receiving a diagnosis of major depression usually should be treated aggressively with a balanced combination of biologic and psychologic therapies. In treatment planning, it may be helpful to point to current research suggesting that psychotherapy alone (either cognitive or interpersonal) may be as effective as antidepressant medication alone for the treatment of some ambulatory patients with major depression (Rush & Jarrett, 1986). Combination treatment, however, is the most efficacious. These findings are of importance because some physical illnesses or their treatments present relative contraindications to the use of biologic psychiatric treatments, that is, antidepressants or electroconvulsive therapy (ECT). Although safe and effective somatic therapies can almost always be selected (see chapters 4 and 5), psychotherapy of the depressed medically ill patient should be an important adjunct to the somatic treatments, and it can be the primary treatment in patients without profound vegetative symptoms.

ORGANIC MOOD SYNDROME

The essential feature of an organic mood syndrome is a disturbance in mood, resembling a major depressive episode, that is due to a specific organic factor. The diagnosis is not made if the disturbance occurs in a clouded state of consciousness (as in delirium), if it is accompanied by a significant loss of intellectual abilities (as in dementia), or if there are persistent delusions or hallucinations (as in organic hallucinosis or organic delusional syndromes). A number of medical illnesses and medications have been linked to depressive syndromes, ranging from endocrine conditions (e.g., hypothyroidism and hypoparathyroidism) and cancer of the brain or pancreas to medications such as beta blockers, alphamethyldopa, reserpine, and steroids (Stoudemire, 1987)

Some authors have provided a virtual medical textbook of drugs and medical conditions "associated" with depression. Stoudemire (1985) cites literature revealing more than 200 such causes, but he quite correctly urges caution in interpreting these catalog-style lists, in that one must understand what is meant by *depression* in each situation. For example, vague reports of low energy with a particular drug may be interpreted as a symptom of depression. Furthermore, even a group of such symptoms may not meet clinical criteria for major depression. There are no prospective controlled studies showing an association of any medication with a clinical diagnosis

of major depression. One such study with propranolol failed to reveal the expected association (Stoudemire, Brown, Harris, et al., 1984). One case-control finding recently reported, however, indicated a higher prevalence of antidepressant use among hypertensive patients treated with beta blockers than among patients treated with other hypertension medications (Avorn, Everitt, & Weiss, 1986). Because of these problems, the medications and illnesses reported in the following list are those that have been most commonly reported to be associated with depressive problems. The list represents a selective, but not comprehensive, review.

1. Medical illnesses
   a. Carcinoid syndrome
   b. Carcinomas (pancreatic)
   c. Cerebrovascular disease (stroke)
   d. Collagen-vascular disease (systemic lupus erythematosus)
   e. Endocrinopathies (Cushing's syndrome, Addison's disease, hypoglycemia, hyper- and hypocalcemia, hyper- and hypothyroidism)
   f. Lymphomas
   g. Parkinson's disease
   h. Pernicious anemia (B-12 deficiency)
   i. Viral illnesses (hepatitis, mononucleosis, influenza, Ebstein-Barr virus)
2. Medications
   a. Antihypertensives (reserpine, methyldopa, propranolol)
   b. Barbiturates
   c. Cimetidine
   d. Corticosteroids
   e. Guanethidine
   f. Indomethacin
   g. Levodopa
   h. Psychostimulants (amphetamine and cocaine in the post-withdrawal phase)

Diagnosis of Organic Mood Disorder

DSM-III-R criteria for this diagnosis are loose, in that no length of time is required and only 2 of the 9 associated symptoms of depression (see list, page 25) are required. There are many problems with the DSM-III-R concept of organic mood disorder, the primary one centering on the question of causality. For example, most clinicians would agree that a depression following a leg fracture is not an organic mood disorder but that one associated with hypothyroidism is. But what about depression in the context of Parkinson's disease or Huntington's disease? Many such illnesses are on the boundary between the physical and the psychiatric, and the etiologic issues involved are of sufficient complexity to make us seriously question the overall usefulness of the concept of organic mood disorder. In addition, the loose criteria contribute even further to the lack of usefulness of the category. Despite these problems, it is important for the clinician to always consider occult physical illnesses or medication effects that might be contributing to a patient's depressive symptoms.

Treatment

The treatment of the putative organic mood syndrome should focus first on the medical treatment of the underlying physical condition or on the removal of the offending drug. At times, however, the physical illness cannot be treated, or the drug cannot be removed. In such situations, if the condition meets the clinical criteria for a diagnosis of major depression, clinicians should cautiously initiate the same biologic and psychologic treatments they might use for major depression without an organic etiologic factor. In other cases, even after the illness has been successfully treated or the drug removed, the depressive syndrome remains (as if a depressive process had begun and now is maintained by its own momentum). Such cases should also be treated as major depressions in their own right.

ADJUSTMENT DISORDER WITH DEPRESSED MOOD

The essential feature of an adjustment disorder is the occurrence of a maladaptive reaction to an identifiable stressor. The only criteria for the diagnosis are the presence of the maladaptive or "excessive" reaction and a dysphoric mood. An adjustment disorder, for example, might occur after a patient learned he or she was paralyzed from an automobile accident or a stroke. Grief and demoralization would be expected as normal, but withdrawal associated with hopeless feelings and refusal to participate in potentially effective rehabilitation efforts would be considered maladaptive.

Treatment of adjustment disorders, reviewed in Chapter 1 of this book, is primarily psychologic and social. The focus should be on nonspecific support, education, and psychotherapeutic clarification of the individual's particular conflicts in the context of the physical illness. If patients develop the symptoms of major depression, they should receive biological treatment as well.

In clinical practice, it is worth noting that many patients who do not meet all the criteria for major depression may also respond to antidepressant medication. This seems to be particularly true for patients experiencing continuing sleep disruption or pain associated with their physical problems. A trial of a sedating antidepressant medication (such as doxepin, amitriptyline, or trazodone) is often very helpful, not only in achieving better sleep, but also in improving general mood. Benefit often occurs at relatively low doses, such as 25–100 mg of a tricyclic every night at bedtime. For most patients, these antidepressants are more effective and safer than hypnotic medications.

DYSTHYMIC DISORDER AND DEPRESSIVE PERSONALITY

Patients with dysthymic disorders have experienced depressive symptoms most of the time during the preceding two years. Many such patients become even more dysphoric when they experience physical illnesses. If the symptoms meet the criteria for major depression, these patients should be treated just as any other patient with major depression, with a combination of biologic and psychologic therapies. When they do not meet the criteria for a major depressive diagnosis, the treatment focus rests, as in the adjustment disorders, on psychosocial interventions.

Akiskal, Rosenthal, et al. (1980) have studied dysthymic patients and postulated that two distinct subgroups make up this population: a subaffective dysthymic group and a group with "character spectrum" disorder. The subaffective dysthymic patients were distinguished by their sleep EEGs, their personal and family histories, and their good response to medication. This distinction is difficult to make cross-sectionally on clinical criteria, but it points to the possibility of antidepressant efficacy in groups other than those with major depression. When psychotherapeutic approaches are making little headway in dysthymic patients, we suggest an empirical trial of antidepressants. Rather than the sedating antidepressants (e.g., amitriptyline, doxepin, trazodone), Akiskal, Rosenthal, et al. (1980) claim that secondary amines, such as nortriptyline and desipramine, are better tolerated by patients with dysthymia. Others do best with monoamine oxidase inhibitors (MAOIs). This may be because the secondary amines and MAOIs have fewer troublesome anticholinergic or sedative side effects. Many patients with dysthymic disorders will eventually develop a major depressive disorder (Keller et al., 1982). This condition has been termed *double depression*, that is, major depression superimposed on a dysthymic disorder. Such a condition should be treated like any other major depression.

DEMENTIA WITH DEPRESSION

Many patients with Alzheimer's and other dementias will present with coexisting dysphoric symptoms and may even meet criteria for major depression. DSM-III-R does not provide clear guidelines for the diagnosis of such patients. One of the criteria for major depression is that the depressive symptoms must be "not clearly due to physical illness." If the clinician believes that the dementia plays an etiologic role (i.e., is causing the depressive symptoms), the patient cannot really be diagnosed as having a major depression. This is unfortunate because the only other possible DSM-III-R diagnosis is "dementia with depression." As with adjustment disorders, the criteria are very loose and nonstringent: there are no criteria at all! So the demented patient with mild dysphoria is put into the same category in DSM-III-R as the demented patient with a very severe depressive syndrome that might otherwise meet the criteria for the diagnosis of major depression.

This unfortunate problem is further complicated by the fact that many depressed patients have significant secondary cognitive problems that may be reversed with antidepressant therapy (Stoudemire, Hill, Kaplan, et al., in press). When such depressed patients present with memory problems as a major complaint, clinicians often refer to this syndrome as "pseudodementia." This term is confusing and unfortunate, however, for three reasons: (1) many other psychiatric conditions have secondary cognitive problems, (2) the "pseudo" dementia is a real cognitive problem, and (3) the term pseudodementia suggests a false dichotomy between depression and dementia.

The suggestion has been made to abandon the concept of pseudodementia in favor of two different patterns of mixed cognitive-affective disturbances. Type I refers to a primary affective disorder accompanied by some cognitive disturbance that is reversible, and Type II refers to a primary dementing illness (either Alzheimer's disease or multi-infarct dementia) that is accompanied by a secondary major depression. The treatment of choice, in both situations, is antidepressant medication or ECT with appropriate psychotherapies and psychosocial intervention (Reifler, 1986).

The distinction between these two syndromes can sometimes be very difficult. This is particularly true in the early stages of a dementing illness (e.g., Alzheimer's disease) or with a mild, stable dementia. When the dementia reaches a moderate level of severity, the cognitive problems associated with the dementia usually become qualitatively different from the cognitive problems associated with major depression. The depressed patient with secondary cognitive problems generally has a globally diminished cognitive capacity related to effortful cognitive tasks: the patient cannot perform mental operations requiring a sustained degree of concentration and attention. Automatic cognitive tasks (e.g., naming tasks, word associations, language performance) are generally unimpaired. In contrast, patients with moderately severe dementias begin showing deficits in language skills, naming, word association, and so on. Diagnosis of dementia in the presence of depression has been reviewed in detail recently by Stoudemire, et al. (in press).

In view of these considerations, clinicians should also utilize the DSM-III-R diagnosis of major depression in both Type I and Type II disorders. Since the distinction between the two is often difficult to make before treatment, there is little risk in diagnosing both disorders as major depression. Similarly, since the diagnosis "dementia with depression" is so nonspecific and non-criterion-oriented, it has little usefulness for treatment.

COVERT, MASKED, OR SOMATIZED DEPRESSION

Many depressed patients present to their physicians with primary complaints related to bodily symptoms, for example, pain, fatigue, or "spells." It is likely in fact, that the presentations of depression in primary care settings are routinely masked by other more prominent complaints. Chronic abdominal pain and headaches are extremely common manifestations of depression, as is diarrhea, insomnia, or general nervousness. Primary care physicians unaware of these common depressive equivalents will fail to recognize and properly treat a serious psychiatric disturbance.

Such patients often vigorously deny being depressed and adamantly refuse to see psychiatrists. If they do make it to a psychiatrist's office after strong encouragement from a primary physician, they are often angry because they feel their primary physician does not believe they are suffering physically, and they feel humiliated because their physician believes there is something wrong with their minds.

Such patients can present diagnostic and psychotherapeutic challenges. Successful management usually begins with the communication of an empathic understanding of the reasons for the patient's anger, frustration, and disillusionment with the medical profession. Examples of useful intervention are statements like "I can understand why you are so upset about the referral to a psychiatrist. You're frustrated that your doctor can't find any explanation for your pain and you think the doctor doesn't believe you really hurt. And to make matters worse, you're insulted that your doctor has referred you to a psychiatrist."

Once the anger and frustration have been acknowledged, an explanation can be given of how the psychiatrist might be able to help. An open-minded biopsychosocial approach, emphasizing some of the uncertainties of medical practice, is usually effective. The psychiatrist can point out that many physical problems are never fully resolved, but that the patient has been thoroughly evaluated medically and that no ominous illnesses have been found. The discomfort, distress, and disability may be profound, however. The psychiatrist can point out that many patients with physical illnesses, such as diabetes and cardiac disease, get depressed or have difficulty coping. Psychiatric intervention is often helpful to them. Similarly, psychiatric evaluation may be of assistance with this patient's particular problem.

The most important differential diagnosis in such cases is between masked depression and somatoform disorders. There is a great deal of overlapping symptomatology in the two disorders. Many depressed patients have a wide variety of unexplained physical complaints, and many patients with chronic somatoform disorders (e.g., somatization disorder) have episodes of major depression.

Masked depression is not described in DSM-III-R, but awareness of the problem can often lead to accurate diagnosis and successful treatment. Even if patients deny depressed mood, they may admit to anhedonia. They may say they are unable to experience pleasure because of the physical problem. Four other symptoms of depression often are present. In such cases, the diagnosis can be made relatively easily, and the response to treatment usually is gratifying.

Such patients often respond best initially to a rather biologic medical model of depression. They prefer to think of the illness as a biologic one, with chemical "imbalances" that are corrected with psychotropic drugs, the way insulin helps a diabetic. This rather oversimplified model can be supported temporarily to develop a therapeutic alliance with psychologically resistant or unsophisticated patients, but eventual expansion to a biopsychosocial approach usually is possible and is therapeutically useful. Diabetes is a good example because the psychiatrist can discuss the relevance of psychosocial issues to diabetes management, making the point that psychosocial issues can also contribute to depressive problems and psychosocial intervention is an important adjunct to the treatment of depression.

REFERENCES

Akiskal HS, Djenderedjian AH, Bolinger JM, et al. (1978). The joint use of clinical and biological criteria for psychiatric diagnosis. In HS Akiskal & WL Webb (Eds), *Psychiatric diagnosis: Exploration of biological predictors* (pp. 133–145). New York: Spectrum Publications.

Akiskal H, Rosenthal T, Haykal R, et al. (1980). Characterological depressions: Clinical and sleep EEG findings separating subaffective dysthymias from character spectrum disorders. *Archives of General Psychiatry, 37,* 777–783.

American Psychiatric Association (1987). *Diagnostic and statistical manual of mental disorders* (3rd ed, rev). Washington, DC.

Avorn J, Everitt DE, Weiss S (1986). Increased antidepressant use in patients prescribed beta-blockers. *Journal of the American Medical Association, 255,* 357–360.

Bukberg J, Penman D, & Holland JC (1984). Depression in hospitalized cancer patients. *Psychosomatic Medicine, 46,* 199–212.

Carroll BJ (1984). Problems with diagnostic criteria for depression. *Journal of Clinical Psychiatry, 45,* 14–18.

Carroll BJ, Feinberg M, Greden JF, et al. (1981). A specific laboratory test for the diagnosis of melancholia: Standardization, validation, and clinical utility. *Archives of General Psychiatry, 38,* 15–22.

Cavenaugh S, Clark D, & Gibbons R (1983). Diagnosing depression in the hospitalized medically ill. *Psychosomatics*, *24*, 809–815.

Cavenaugh S & Kennedy S (1986). A successful training program for medical residents. *General Hospital Psychiatry*, *8*, 73–80.

Clark D, Cavenaugh S, Gibbons R (1983). Core symptoms of depression in medical and psychiatric patients. *Journal of Nervous Mental Disorders*, *171*, 705–713.

Cohen-Cole SA, Bird J, Freeman A, Boker J, Palmer R, & Shugerman A (1982). Psychiatry for internists: A study of needs. *Journal of Operational Psychiatry*, *13*, 100–105.

Endicott J (1984). Measurement of depression in patients with cancer. *Cancer*, *53*. 2243–2248.

Fogel B, Satel S, Levy S (1985). Occurrence of high concentrations of postdexamethasone cortisol in elderly psychiatric inpatients. *Psychiatry Research*, *15*, 85–90.

Hirschfeld RMA, Koslow SH, & Kupfer DJ (1983). The clinical utility of the dexamethasone suppression test in psychiatry. *Journal of the American Medical Association*, *250*, 2172

Keller M, Klerman G, Lavori P, (1982). Treatment received by depressed patients. *Journal of the American Medical Association*, *248*, 1848–1855.

Knights E & Folstein M (1977). Unsuspected emotional and cognitive disturbance in medical patients. *Annals of Internal Medicine*, *87*, 723–724.

Lipsey IR, Robinson RG, Pearlson GD, et al. (1984). Nortriptyline treatment of post-stroke depression: A double-blind study. *Lancet*, *1*(8372), 297–300.

Maguire P (1984). The recognition and treatment of affective disorder in cancer patients. *International Review of Applied Psychology*, *33*, 479–491.

Maguire P, Hopwood P, Tarrier N, & Howell T (1985). Treatment of depression in cancer patients. *Acta Psychiatrica Scandinavica*, *72*, 81–84.

Mayeux R, Stern Y, Williams J, et al. (1986). Clinical and biochemical features of depression in Parkinson's disease. *American Journal of Psychiatry*, *143*, 756–759.

Plumb M & Holland J (1981). Comparative studies of psychological function in patients with advanced cancer: 2. Interviewer rated current and past psychological symptoms. *Psychosomatic Medicine*, *43*, 243–254.

Reifler BV (1986). Mixed cognitive-affective disturbances in the elderly: A new classification. *Journal of Clinical Psychiatry*, *47*, 354–356.

Rifkin A, Reardon G, Siris S, et al. (1985). Trimipramine in physical illness with depression. *Journal of Clinical Psychiatry*, *46*, 4–8.

Robbins LN, Helzer JE, Croughan J, & Ratcliff KS (1981). National Institute of Mental Health Diagnostic Interview Schedule. *Archives of General Psychiatry*, *38*, 381–389.

Robinson RG, Lipsey JR, & Price TR (1985). Diagnosis and clinical management of post-stroke depression. *Psychosomatics*, *26*, 769–778.

Robinson RG, Starr LB, & Price TR (1984). A two-year longitudinal study of mood disorders following stroke: Prevalence and duration at six months follow-up. *British Journal of Psychiatry*, *144*, 256–262.

Rodin G & Voshart K (1986). Depression in the medically ill: An overview. *American Journal of Psychiatry*, *143*, 696–705.

Rush AJ & Jarrett RB (1986). Psychotherapeutic approaches to depression. In R. Michels, J Cavenar, J (ed), *Psychiatry* (sec 2, p 65). Philadelphia: J. B. Lippincott.

Schulberg HC, Saul M, McClelland M, et al. (1985). Assessing depression in primary medical and psychiatric practices. *Archives of General Psychiatry*, *42*, 1164–1170.

Spitzer RL, Endicott J, & Robins E (1978). Research diagnostic criteria. *Archives of General Psychiatry*, *35*, 773–782.

Spitzer R, Williams J, & Gibbon M (1984). Instructional manual for the Structured Clinical Interview for DSM-III (SCID). Unpublished manuscript.

Stoudemire A (1985). Depression in the medically ill. Cavenar, J (Ed), *Psychiatry* (Vol 2, sec 99, pp 1–8) Philadelphia: J. B. Lippincott.

Stoudemire A (1987). Selected organic brain syndromes. In R Hales & S Yudofsky (Ed), *Textbook of Neuropsychiatry*. Washington, DC: APA Press, pp. 125–139.

Stoudemire A (in press). Somatoform disorders, factitious disorders and malingering. In J Talbott, R Hales, & S Yudofsky, (Ed), *Textbook of Psychiatry*. Washington, DC: APA Press.

Stoudemire A, Brown JT, Harris R, et al: (1984). Propranolol and depression: A reevaluation based on a pilot clinical trial. *Psychiatric Medicine*, *2*, 211–218.

Stoudemire A, Hill C, Kaplan W, et al. (in press). Neuropsychological assessment of combined depression and dementia in the elderly. *Psychiatric Medicine*.

Thompson TL, Stoudemire A, & Mitchell WE (1983). Underrecognition of patients' psychosocial distress in a university hospital medical clinic. *American Journal of Psychiatry*, *140*, 158–161.

Barry S. Fogel
David Faust

3
Neurologic Assessment, Neurodiagnostic Tests, and Neuropsychology in Medical Psychiatry

**NEUROPSYCHIATRIC
ASSESSMENT IN MEDICAL
PSYCHIATRY**

Because there are a number of different reasons for undertaking neurologic assessment, no "cookbook" approach to neurologic diagnosis is appropriate. Instead, when embarking on neurologic assessment of the psychiatric patient, the psychiatrist should begin with a set of diagnostic hypotheses generated by the psychiatric history and the mental status examination and should form a fairly precise set of questions to be answered by the neurologic assessment. For example, if a patient with suspected senile dementia is referred for a computed tomography (CT) scan with no specific question posed, the radiologist often reports "cortical atrophy, consistent with age." If the psychiatrist poses the question "This patient has severe dementia; is the degree of cortical atrophy compatible with severe Alzheimer's dis-

ease?" it focuses the radiologist on a more quantitative and statistical assessment of the CT scan findings. If multiple sclerosis is suspected in an apparently hysterical patient, specialized history-taking and examination may be needed to detect mild problems with eye movements or visual function that would probably not be tested on a "routine" neurologic examination. Thus neurologic assessment for diagnostic purposes should begin with a differential diagnosis in mind and a specific set of questions upon which to focus with the neurologic consultant.

Specific neurologic tests and examination procedures are best selected with reference to a particular population and a particular set of diagnoses that frequently occur. For example, neurologic examination of elderly patients with psychiatric problems should always include several tests for diffuse cerebral dysfunction, a careful cognitive mental status examination

PRINCIPLES OF MEDICAL PSYCHIATRY
ISBN 0-8089-1883-4

to exclude dementia or delirium, and careful testing of gait, because of the high prevalence of gait disorders in the elderly. By contrast, meticulous sensory examination would rarely be warranted or reliable.

As another example of tailoring evaluation to a specific population, evaluation of alcoholics with acute mental status changes should always include tests of vitamin status and a therapeutic trial of thiamine. Recorded "routine" neurologic examinations of patients with autopsy-proved Wernicke–Korsakoff syndrome were normal in 27 percent of 64 patients undiagnosed in life, and an additional 34 percent of those patients showed mental status changes only, without ataxia or eye signs (Harper, Giles, & Finlay-Jones, 1986). A thiamine trial, though certainly not "routine," is therefore indicated for alcoholics because of their high base rate of thiamine deficiency.

As a final example of population-specific evaluation, patients who have been treated with neuroleptics always require a special examination for abnormal involuntary movements. Published standard neurologic examinations give minimal treatment to the problem of involuntary movements, but it has been demonstrated that a formal movement disorder assessment, such as the Abnormal Involuntary Movement Scale (AIMS), can greatly enhance the detection of tardive dyskinesia and related disorders (Munetz & Schulz, 1986). Because of the extraordinary medical-legal issues raised by prescribing neuroleptics in the face of tardive dyskinesia, the examination for tardive dyskinesia cannot be omitted or abbreviated. The tardive dyskinesia issue illustrates the point of focusing the neurologic examination, particularly if it is to be done by someone else, such as a neurologist or internist. Comments about tardive dyskinesia or its absence often fail to appear in internists' or neurologists' consultation notes unless the psychiatrist has specifically raised the question as one to be addressed in the consultation.

The Role of Formal Consultation with Neurologists and Neuropsychologists

It is becoming more usual for psychiatrists to perform an initial neurologic assessment themselves, and to order the more common ancillary tests, such as the CT scan and the electroencephalogram (EEG). The neurologist usually is called when a definite or potential neurologic problem has been identified by the psychiatrist's initial assessment and further diagnostic confirmation or management is desired. A potential pitfall exists when psychiatrists "sign off" the organic parts of a case after the neurologist has been consulted. First, the psychiatrist, who meets most regularly with the patient, is in the best position to observe changes in status and to collect additional history of neurologic relevance from the patient and significant others. Second, the psychiatrist is also in the most advantageous position to determine whether the neurologic consultation and therapy have adequately addressed the patient's concerns. Third, many neurologic diseases are progressive or episodic, so the disease actually changes after the neurologic consultation. Patients in psychiatric treatment often are comfortable relating new physical problems and symptoms to their psychiatrist, rather than returning to a neurologic consultant they have seen only once or twice. Finally, the psychiatrist is best positioned to assess the overall impact of neurologic therapies on a patient's function, mental status, and quality of life. Appropriate feedback to the neurologist then can lead to an adjustment of management to patients' individual requirements.

When using consultants, the psychiatrist should be aware that neurologists vary greatly in their level of interest in behavior. Some neurologists perform a minimal mental status examination and have a very high threshold for diagnosing any neurologic dysfunction in a patient with known psychiatric problems. Other are trained behavioral neurologists with a deep interest in brain–behavior relationships; they conduct meticulous cognitive mental status assessments and occasionally may even overemphasize the organic components in a patient's neuropsychiatric illness. When a choice of consultants is available, the psychiatrist should bear these distinctions in mind. An individual with gross neurologic disease in need of management does not require a behavioral neurologist, particularly if the behavioral aspects of the problem will be managed by the psychiatrist. On the other hand, the patient with obscure symptoms on the borderline between the neurologic and the psychiatric can profit greatly from a consultation with a behavioral neurologist, particularly if this consultation leads to critical dialogue between the behavioral neurologist and the psychiatrist.

Neuropsychologists also vary in their interests and special skills, and the variation may be even greater than for neurologists, because there are no professional regulations in psychology determining who may call himself or herself a neuropsychologist. Some neuropsychologists restrict their activities to forming an opinion about whether brain damage is present or absent; others go considerably further and address lateralization, localization, and detailed description of the mechanism of cognitive dysfunction. Some neuropsychologists use fixed batteries for all patients; others adapt testing procedures to patient characteristics and referral questions, and may in some cases use clinically based rather than standardized, normed testing procedures. Test batteries themselves differ in their coverage of particular areas of cognitive disorder and are more or less

sensitive or specific depending on the population to whom they are applied.

Neuropsychologists also vary in their involvement in cognitive rehabilitation and in the provision of educational, therapeutic, and rehabilitative services to patients with cognitive disorders and their families. If cognitive rehabilitation or other therapeutic intervention is contemplated, it is generally best to have the neuropsychologic evaluation done by a neuropsychologist with a significant interest in cognitive rehabilitation. The assessment could then be tailored to answer specific questions particularly relevant to rehabilitation or therapy.

The next several sections of this chapter will discuss specific tips for improving the neurologic examination and will review the advantages and limitations of different common neurodiagnostic tests. Neuropsychologic assessment will be treated separately and in greater detail later in this chapter.

Enhancing the Neurologic Examination: A String of Pearls

We assume that the medical psychiatrist will personally perform a neurologic examination. In doing so, the psychiatrist is likely to gain little from the rote application of a textbook neurological examination, but may learn much of value from a hypothesis-testing examination, which tailors tests and observations to the patient's presenting problem and epidemiologic setting. The following subsections provide several "pearls" to assist in more precise and effective neurologic examination of the psychiatric patient.

The sensitivity and specificity of neurologic signs and the detection of occult organic brain disease depend on the clinical population and the diseases suspected. For instance, when multiple sclerosis is suspected, as it ought to be in "hysterics," bedside examination of eye movements may be insensitive to diagnostically relevant abnormalities. Measurement of eye movements in 84 patients with multiple sclerosis and 21 patients with optic neuritis using a simple portable electrophysiologic apparatus revealed a subclinical eye movement disorder in 80 percent of the definite, 74 percent of the probable, and 60 percent of the possible MS patients (Ruelen, Sanders, & Hogeshnis et al., 1983). When subdural hematoma is suspected, as it ought to be when subacute mental status change occurs together with alcoholism, advanced age, or chronic headache, the little-known and seldom-practiced technique of auscultatory percussion may be remarkably sensitive and specific (Guarino, 1982).

Tests infrequently performed may detect confirmatory evidence of an organically based disorder, whereas commonly used screening tests are often insensitive to psychiatrically relevant diffuse cerebral pathology. Jenkyn, Walsh, Culver, et al. (1977) correlated evidence of diffuse cerebral disorder as measured by the Halstead-Reitan Neuropsychological Battery with findings on neurologic examination and found 13 physical signs with a false-negative rate of less than 60 percent. These were the glabellar blink, the nuchocephalic reflex, the suck reflex, impairment of upward gaze, impairment of downward gaze, a tendency to keep the raised arm up after the signal to drop it, impaired visual tracking, impersistence of lateral gaze, trouble accurately recalling three items after a time delay with intervening distraction, paratonia of both arms, difficulty spelling *world* backward, paratonia of both legs, and difficulty in giving past presidents in reverse order. By contrast, they found an extremely high false-negative rate—over 85 percent—for such popularly used tests as the Babinski sign, double simultaneous

stimulation, orientation to place and date, and recall of current presidents.

Enlarged pupils may be the only neurologic sign besides the abnormal mental state in cases of anticholinergic delirium (Brizer & Manning, 1982). In such cases, vital signs are abnormal but somatic motor and reflex signs are absent. In many other acute confusional states that include cognitive, sensory, memory, and attentional aberrations, there are no focal or lateralizing sensory or motor signs because the neurologic disorder is diffuse or multifocal.

Amnesia after an accident with head injury is sufficient for diagnosis of concussion even if there is no history of loss of consciousness (Rimel & Tyson, 1979). Experience in consulting to a busy regional trauma center suggests that evidence of concussion is not always sought by the trauma team when the patient arrives at the emergency room awake and other physical injuries need immediate care. The psychiatrist, if called afterward for assessment of posttraumatic behavior changes, must make the diagnosis retrospectively from evidence of posttraumatic amnesia. If the patient is examined soon enough after the injury, *anterograde* amnesia may still be present. If it is, neurologic dysfunction is unequivocally demonstrated.

The ability to communicate with gestures in the presence of muteness has no value in distinguishing functional from organic etiologies. A study of the 9 mute patients that occurred in 350 consecutive general hospital admissions for head injury revealed that all of the patients with mutism could communicate somewhat with gestures. However, all who were tested showed impaired writing (HS Levin, Madison, Bailey et al., 1983). All 9 recovered some speech, although the 4 with basal ganglion lesions made a less complete recovery. Unlike the ability to gesture, the ability to write a coherent sentence to dictation is, in general, a good high-sensitivity screening test for organically based language disorder.

Specific visual examinations are superior to screening eye examinations. In a review (Ruelen et al., 1983) of 18 patients with probable or definite multiple sclerosis and 20/20 vision, 16 had one or more abnormalities on other measures of ocular function, such as visual evoked potentials and psychophysical tests of contrast sensitivity. Fifty-nine percent of these had pallor of the optic nerve head or changes in the nerve fiber layer on funduscopy. Normal visual acuity does not exclude visual system disorder. Careful funduscopic examination is mandatory to properly screen the visual system. It should certainly be done in all patients suspected of multiple sclerosis—a group that includes all patients suspected of a conversion disorder with neurologic symptoms.

The determination of pallor of the optic nerve head is easy and is frequently valuable in differential diagnosis. A reasonable set of skills for the psychiatrist would thus include examination of the optic disk, assessment of visual fields by confrontation, and assessment of visual acuity. Theoretical knowledge of other parts of the visual examination is helpful in assessing the completeness or incompleteness of examinations done by other physicians. Even eye examinations by ophthalmologists may not include all of the relevant points for assessment of multiple sclerosis, unless the ophthalmologist is specifically asked by the psychiatrist to look for such evidence.

Gait disorder may be the only hard sign of a treatable neurological illness. Dubin, Weiss & Zeccardi (1983) studied 1140 patients evaluated by an emergency psychiatric service after having been cleared medically by an emergency room physician. Thirty-nine of these showed signs of disorientation, abnormal vital signs, or clouding of consciousness, and, of these, 38 were found to have an organic disorder (1 was diagnosed as having paranoid schizophrenia). On review of initial history and physical examination, 14 of the 38 were found to have had gait disturbance, weight loss, hypertension, abnormal vital signs, or a significant medical history.

In a neurological evaluation of 50 patients over the age of 70 with gait disturbance of previously undetermined etiology, 24 percent had an illness that could either be treated or palliated (Sudarsky & Ronthal, 1983). Specific observation of gait is helpful in the diagnosis of Parkinson's disease and cerebellar atrophy. Robins (1983) contends that 10–33 percent of patients presenting for evaluation of dementia have a potentially reversible cause. A summary of six studies involving 503 patients revealed the leading causes of reversible dementia to be normal pressure hydrocephalus, depression, subdural hematoma or intracranial mass, other psychiatric disorders, drugs, and thyroid disease. The neurological conditions on this list may not produce focal motor or sensory signs, but may show only disturbances of mental status and gait. Normal pressure hydrocephalus virtually always affects gait.

For these reasons, examination of gait is essential in any complete psychiatric evaluation. Observation of the patient walking into a room and taking a seat is an easy, unobtrusive part of any psychiatric interview. If subtle abnormalities are noticed, they can be brought out by asking the patient to perform special tasks. Mild weakness of one side can be brought out by having the patient walk on tiptoes and on heels. The foot may droop on the weak side. Patients who appear slightly off balance can be asked to walk on an imaginary line, touching heel to toe, as in the familiar test for intoxication. Patients suspected of Parkinsonism should be observed making turns, stopping and starting on command, and speeding up and slowing down on command. Elderly patients with diffuse cerebral dysfunction and a slow, shuffling gait may not have the same difficulties as Parkinsonian patients do with turning and changing pace.

Finally, it is worth noting that involuntary movements and posturing of the arms are sometimes most evident when the patient is walking. This evidence can sometimes help in the diagnosis of dystonic disorders, Huntington's disease, and tardive dyskinesia with limb involvement.

Neurologic examination of the very elderly patient is best interpreted with knowledge of the norms for neurologic function in advanced age. Cranial nerve examination in normal elderly persons may reveal small pupils, a slowing of pupillary reflexes, diminished upward gaze, sensorineural hearing loss, and diminished sense of smell. Elderly patients may also show a variety of visual problems, related to cataracts, macular degeneration, or glaucoma (Wright & Henkind, 1983). Other abnormalities, such as nystagmus, facial weakness, diminished downward gaze, or hemianopic field defects, cannot be explained by advanced age and are presumptive signs of neurologic disease. Sensory deficits, though they may be due to age-associated changes in sensory organs, are important in the overall management of the patient, as they may significantly affect the patient's ability to communicate and to correctly perceive the environment.

Motor examination of elderly persons shows that as a group they are not as strong as young adults. There is great individual variability, however. The detection of moderate to severe weakness does not pose any problem for the examiner; the problems lie in distinguishing mild but significant weakness from normal age-associated muscular change. In this area, the most useful tests are tests of function, such as having the patient arise from bed, get up from a chair, or climb stairs. Some loss of muscle bulk is normal for age, particularly in the intrinsic muscles of the hand. Mild impairment in coordination is occasionally encountered in normal elderly, although it should not be accepted as age related without a search for other evidence of motor system disease. Bradykinesia is common in patients over 75 but, in the absence of other Parkinsonian signs, does not imply the presence of Parkinson's disease. Action tremors in the elderly usually imply benign essential tremor rather than cerebellar dysfunction. The latter should not be diagnosed without clear-cut ataxia or dysmetria. (Dysmetria is the inability of a patient to target limb movement precisely from one point to another.).

Decreased joint position sense and vibratory sensitivity are common in the elderly and do not necessarily imply posterior column disease, unless the abnormalities are profound. Age-related losses are usually prominent only in the lower extremities, however, and a clear-cut loss of position and vibration sense in upper extremities should warrant careful investigation.

Normal elderly persons may have palmomental or snout reflexes and often do not have ankle jerks. Babinski signs, on the other hand, are rare in normal elderly. It is not uncommon, however, to encounter Babinski signs due to cervical spondylosis with mild cord compression, particularly in elderly individuals with severe degenerative disease of the cervical spine. In the absense of pain, weakness, bladder dysfunction, or gait disorder, the spinal disease would not require a specific treatment. The Babinski sign in this special case does not imply cerebral disease.

Normal elderly persons, even active ones, may be unable to stand on one foot with their eyes closed; this may be due to changes in the proprioceptive system with aging. The bradykinesia that accompanies advanced age may result in a slow, cautious gait, with diminished arm swing. Significant instability of gait, asymmetry of gait, and failure of postural reflexes, however, always imply central nervous system disease. Unfortunately, many elderly people with gait disturbance and a tendency to fall have multifactorial gait disturbance, with sensory, motor, and cognitive factors all contributing. It is nonetheless worthwhile to investigate all elderly persons with gait disturbance for specific etiologies, particularly such treatable ones as B_{12} deficiency, hypothyroidism, normal pressure hydrocephalus, Parkinson's disease, and mild toxic-metabolic delirium.

The material just presented is elaborated and abundantly referenced in a review by Wolfson and Katzman (1983).

Many neurologic disorders are diagnosable more on the basis of history than on the basis of the examination. In this area, psychiatrists may have an edge over neurologists because of their fine history-taking skills and their habit of using collateral information. When a group of neurologists independently performed neurologic histories and examinations on a group of acute stroke patients, there was substantial disagreement between examiners on basic historical points, such as the history of past stroke or transient ischemic attack (TIA), and even on whether the patient had a headache at the time of onset. Interobserver variability was less on the physical examination, particularly regarding weakness and global aphasia; sensory examination was more variable. Disagreement between independent examiners increased when patients were more difficult to examine (Shinar, Gross, Mohr, et al., 1985). When a patient is difficult to examine on initial evaluation, the treating psychiatrist usually has the opportunity to repeat the neurological examination later in the patient's course when there is better cooperation.

Orthostatic hypotension is a feature of many medical and neurologic disorders with behavioral manifestations; it should be carefully sought in all medical-psychiatric patients. Patients should have blood pressures measured while lying down, after lying for at least 3 minutes, and while standing; a drop of more than 10 mmHg diastolic or 20 mm Hg systolic is abnormal. While prescribed medications are probably the most frequent cause of orthostatic hypotension in medical-psychiatric patients, unexpected orthostatic hypotension may be a clue to autonomic neuropathy (diabetes, alcoholism, porphyria, etc.), occult carcinoma, extrapyramidal disorders, or Wernicke's encephalopathy. In patients with dizzy spells or falls, the possibility of delayed orthostatic hypotension should be investigated. This involves having the patient remain standing and rechecking the blood pressure at 5 and 10 minutes.

A systematic examination for tardive dyskinesia should be performed by the psychiatrist on every patient with a history of neuroleptic exposure, and on every elderly patient prior to initiating neuroleptic therapy. A structured examination, such as the AIMS (Baldessarini, Cole, Davis, et al, 1979), is best. In a study at the Western Psychiatric Institute, it was demonstrated that the detection rate of tardive dyskinesia rose substantially when formal screening for tardive dyskinesia was instituted (Munetz & Schulz, 1986). The study is particularly compelling because a consultation service for movement disorders had been actively promoting its services in the baseline year prior to institution of formal screening; evidently many cases had not been identified or referred to the consultation service. Elderly patients are at increased risk for tardive dyskinesia, and occasional elderly patients have dyskinetic or choreatic movements without a history of neuroleptic exposure (D'Allesandro, Benassi, Cristina, et al., 1986). Therefore, a baseline examination for involuntary movements should be done before beginning an elderly patient for the first time on neuroleptic drug therapy.

Specific Neurodiagnostic Procedures

Neurodiagnostic procedures can be subdivided into brain imaging procedures, tests of brain function, cerebrospinal fluid (CSF) examination, and special procedures, such as the isotope cisternogram. In most institutions, brain imaging has meant CT scanning; CT is rapidly being superseded by magnetic resonance imaging (MRI). The most widely available test of brain function is the electroencephalogram (EEG); topographic EEG, brain evoked activity mapping (BEAM), and evoked potential tests represent further developments on the EEG. Positron emission tomography (PET) and single photon emission computed tomography (SPECT) are relatively new nuclear medicine procedures that permit assessment of regional brain function by using radiolabeled, metabolically or pharmacologically active tracers. The sections that follow offer suggestions for the effective use of these ancillary procedures in the medical-psychiatric setting.

Brain Imaging Procedures: The CT Scan

The CT scan is currently the standard radiologic test for anatomic brain abnormalities. The procedure is widely available, and with the rapid action of newer-generation CT scanners, the test can be accomplished in all but the most uncooperative patients. Although eventually CT will probably be supplanted by MRI in many situations, it will retain an important role in the assessment of neurologic emergencies, because it can be done rapidly in an acutely ill patient. At least with current MRI technology, the MRI is unsuitable for an extremely unstable patient, because the patient is inaccessible to medical intervention while inside the MRI scanner.

The CT scan is essential in the workup of dementia, in the evaluation of subacute mental status changes in patients with possible metastatic cancer, in patients with suspected stroke, and in head trauma patients with coma or deteriorating mental status. Although it is extraordinarily valuable in such situations, it is of little use in screening the patient with an uncomplicated delirium, or with a psychiatric disturbance and normal neurologic examination. In the latter circumstances, functional tests, particularly the EEG, are of greatest value. If the EEG or other functional tests suggest a significant focal abnormality, follow-up with a brain imaging study is recommended.

Nonspecific CT abnormalities such as cerebral atrophy or ventricular enlargement may occur in manic-depressive illness, schizophrenia, and eating disorders, as well as in alcoholism and in normal aging. The question remains open whether nonspecific CT abnormalities may be helpful in clinical management or the assessment of prognosis in patients with schizophrenia or bipolar illness (Pandurangi, Dewan, Baucher, et al., 1986). Given the evidence at the time of this writing, however, we would not recommend the routine use of CT scans for this purpose.

In the medical-psychiatric setting, there may be some specific reasons to order a CT scan in the patient with mental status changes and an apparently normal neurologic examination. The most common situation is when the patient suffers from a medical disease that so frequently leads to anatomic involvement of the brain that the yield is high even with a nonspecific clinical picture. For example, mental status changes in patients with acquired immune deficiency syndrome (AIDS), systemic lupus erythematosus, and lung cancer would all require a brain imaging technique such as CT at the first sign of altered mental status, even if there were no focal neurologic or EEG signs at the time.

Psychiatrists often order CT scans in the evaluation of suspected dementia. Because cortical atrophy is a normal finding in nondemented elderly, efforts have been made to develop quantitative criteria that distinguish the atrophy of normal aging from the atrophy of dementia. Ventricular size and shape and quantitative measurements of white-matter density have been investigated; no particular quantitative method has yet been accepted as a standard. Part of the problem in standardizing quantitative CT interpretation is that there are many different generations of CT scanners, each of which leads to a slightly different image on the same patient (Naeser, 1985). If reliable normed quantitative CT interpretation is available at one's institution, results can be used to increase the probability of a correct diagnosis. Thus, if a patient with suspected Alzheimer's disease and moderate dementia shows no atrophy at all by quantitative criteria (e.g., white-matter density), the diagnosis is doubtful. A recent article by Gado and Press (1986) summarizes the appropriate use of CT in the diagnosis of dementia and illustrates the more common quantitative measures of atrophy that are readily measurable on CT films. In evaluating CT evidence of cerebral atrophy, the influence of alcohol and medications should be considered. Even moderate drinkers may show mild cortical atrophy that reverses upon total cessation of drinking (Cala, Jones, Burnes, et al., 1983). Corticosteroid therapy may lead to cerebral atrophy on CT, reversible with discontinuation of steroids (Bentsen, Reza, Winter, et al., 1978; Heinz, Martinex, & Hawnggeli, 1977; Okuno, Nasatoshi, Konishi, et al., 1980).

The CT has two major limitations as a brain imaging method. First, there are many important pathologic processes, particularly demyelination, that do not greatly alter the radiodensity of brain and may be invisible on CT. Second, CT has difficulty distinguishing lesions in brain regions adjacent to bone, because of overshoot artifacts and partial volume effects. Structures such as the anterior and inferior temporal lobe lie adjacent to bone, and often cannot be imaged satisfactorily on CT (Lee, Kieffer, & Montoya, 1983).

Brain Imaging Procedures: Magnetic Resonance Imaging

Nuclear magnetic resonance imaging (NMR or MRI) is a relatively new brain imaging technique with remarkable resolution and sensitivity. To obtain a magnetic resonance image, the patient's head is placed inside a giant superconducting magnet, and a rapidly fluctuating magnetic field is superimposed by coils driven by a radio frequency oscillator. According to the principle of nuclear magnetic resonance, this applied magnetic field alters the spin of protons in tissue water, which relax each time the magnetic field strength is reduced. Electromagnetic radiation is released by the protons and is detected by detector coils placed around the patient's head. Mathematical reconstruction techniques, similar to those used in CT, permit the construction by computer of a brain image based not on radiodensity, but primarily on the water content of the tissue being imaged. Because brain water content differs from normal in a number of pathologic processes that do not alter radiodensity, the MRI is intrinsically more sensitive to these processes than CT.

MRI scanning requires a relatively medically stable patient, because rapid access to the patient is not possible while the patient is in the scanner. A full set of scan slices may take more than half an hour, and considerable cooperation is needed from the patient, or else the patient must be heavily sedated. Metal aneurysm clips are an absolute contraindication to MRI, because the magnetic field may twist or dislodge a clip, leading to cerebral hemorrhage. Cardiac pacemakers are a contraindication to MRI for similar reasons.

Initial studies of MRI show that it is superior to CT scan in the detection of a number of pathologic conditions and only rarely fails to detect lesions found on CT. In a review of 1000 cases of MRI, only one showed an abnormality on CT that was not visualized on MRI—a small, calcified arteriovenous malformation. By contrast, MRI revealed lesions not seen on CT in patients with multiple sclerosis, other white-matter diseases, encephalitis, meningitis, encephalopathy of unknown origin, hydrocephalus, brain contusion, seizure disorders, and psychiatric disorders, (Baker, Berqvist, Kispert, et al., 1985). Strikingly, many of the disorders for which MRI is the superior imaging technique may present psychiatrically, or with prominent psychiatric complications. The unique value of MRI in multiple sclerosis is confirmed by several other studies (Gabarski, Gabrielsen, & Gilman, 1985; Jacobs, Kinkel, Polachini, & Kinkel, 1986; Sheldon, Siddharthan, Tobias, et al., 1985). The diagnostic superiority is not only in detecting abnormality, but also in disclosing the extent of involvement. Multiple cerebral lesions not seen on CT may be visualized with MRI. Patients with multiple sclerosis with personality change, affective disorder, or dementia may thus show the etiologic brain changes on MRI, but not other tests.

Because bone is transparent on MRI, temporal, occipital frontal, and posterior fossa lesions can be clearly seen without the bone artifacts typical of CT.

MRI can detect small subdural hematomas and small brain contusions not visualized on CT (Margulis & Amparo, 1985). This may be helpful to the psychiatrist trying to determine whether a post-head-injury psychosis is "reactive" or due to a frontal or temporal lesion. In complex partial seizures, MRI may reveal anatomic abnormalities in cases where CT is normal (Laster, Penry, Moody, et al., 1985; Lesser Modic, Weinstein, et al., 1986; Sperling, Wilson, Engel, et al., 1986).

Because MRI is extremely sensitive, criteria for normality will need further development, particularly in elderly patients, whose brains may show periventricular changes on MRI not seen in normal young adults (Brant-Zawadski, Fein, Van Dyke, et al., 1985). Other limitations of MRI include the inability to visualize calcifications, difficulty distinguishing tumor from edema, and difficulty differentiating old from new hematomas (DiChiro, 1985). These drawbacks, while important in neurologic differential diagnosis, are irrelevant to the majority of psychiatric cases, in which the main purpose of brain imaging is to establish the presence of cerebral abnormality, rather than to make a specific pathologic diagnosis.

Physiologic Tests: The EEG

The EEG, one of the earliest ancillary physiologic tests in psychiatry, remains one of the most useful in the clinical assessment of the psychiatric patient. Although it lacks the visual impact of brain imaging, it is actually more useful in distinguishing functional from organic etiology in many circumstances. In addition, it is an inexpensive test that is readily available in small hospitals without CT scanners, and in psychiatric hospitals with limited medical laboratory facilities.

In cases of reversible diffuse brain dysfunction on a toxic-metabolic basis, the CT is normal, while the EEG may be diagnostic. The detection of mild deliria presenting psychiatrically, and the differentiation of cognitive dysfunction secondary due to depression from degenerative cerebral disease have been cited as two established indications for the use of the EEG in psychiatry (Kiloh, McComas, Osselton, et al., 1981). Mild diffuse brain damage due to hypoxia and hypotension may contribute to psychiatric disorders following open heart surgery; the EEG may be the only laboratory evidence of such diffuse damage. For example, in a study of 100 patients evaluated following open heart surgery for cardiac valvular disease, 38 thought to be neurologically asymptomatic received EEGs postoperatively; 14 showed abnormalities. In the same study, 15 of the 49 who received careful postoperative neuropsychologic evaluation showed cognitive deficits. Yet, only 4 of the 100 were diagnosed as cognitively disordered by their primary physicians (Sotaniemi, 1983). The "hard" abnormality of an abnormal EEG can be useful diagnostically in linking cognitive disorder to probable hypotensive injury.

Abnormal EEGs are found in two-thirds of untreated patients with pernicious anemia, and in virtually all with significant organic metal findings (Evans, Edelsohn & Golden, 1983). In a patient with a psychiatric disorder and a low B_{12} level, the EEG might thus provide confirmatory evidence that the low B_{12} level was psychiatrically relevant. Hypothyroidism, when it produces an organic mental disorder, is associated with EEG slowing. The EEG may be particularly valuable in linking thyroid disorder and mental symptoms in cases where the serum thyroxine (T4) is normal but the thyroid stimulating hormone (TSH) is elevated (Haggerty, Evans, & Prang, 1986). Herpes simplex encephalitis, which may present with nonspecific symptoms of psychiatric illness, may produce an abnormal EEG in an early stage while the CT is negative and the CSF is not diagnostic. In suspected cases, therefore, all three tests should be done, and the EEG should not be omitted even if the CT and CSF exam are normal (Griffith & Ch'ien, 1983). A recent report (Drury, Klass, Westmoreland, et al., 1985) describes 4 patients with acute psychosis who showed striking periodic EEG abnormalities and who recovered clinically and electroencephalographically within a week. Patients with apparent "brief reac-

tive psychosis" deserve an EEG to exclude unsuspected organic events.

Although routine EEG is an excellent test for metabolic encephalopathy, it is sometimes normal in mild metabolic disorders. For example, 3 out of 12 delirious liver transplant candidates had normal EEGs (Trzepacz, Maue, Coffman, et al., 1986). In many such cases of mild metabolic encephalopathy with normal EEG, a prior baseline EEG tracing may permit a diagnosis. If it is known that a patient's baseline alpha rhythm is at 11–12 Hz, a current alpha rhythm of 9 Hz indicates a significant change compatible with a metabolic encephalopathy (Markand, 1984). For this reason, patients with chronic medical diseases known to cause intermittent metabolic encephalopathies (e.g., liver disease, renal disease) should be considered for a baseline EEG, particularly if they appear vulnerable to psychiatric complications.

An increased rate of EEG abnormalities has been encountered in a number of "functional" mental disorders, including obsessive-compulsive disorder (Marks & Kettl, 1986) and borderline personality (Cowdry, Pickar, & Davies, 1985–86). These EEG abnormalities do not imply a neurologic diagnosis, however, nor do they necessarily have prognostic or therapeutic implications. The relevance of EEG findings must be established empirically for each disorder; mere presence of sharp abnormalities on EEG does not imply a diagnosis of epilepsy or that the psychiatric disorder will improve with anticonvulsants.

The literature on EEG for some psychiatric disorders shows wide variations in the prevalence of abnormality. While some investigators find a high prevalence of EEG abnormalities in borderline personality (Cowdry et al., 1985), others find no significant difference from controls (Cornelius, Brenner, Soloff, et al., 1986). These discrepancies probably reflect differences in the specific populations being studied. Treatment-refractory patients with any psychiatric diagnosis might be expected to have a higher incidence of EEG abnormality than unselected first admissions with that diagnosis.

Proper interpretation of EEGs in elderly patients requires a knowledge of EEG norms for age. The dominant posterior background rhythm in the EEG may slow with age, but does not go below 8 Hz in the absence of disease. Slowing with age is gradual when it occurs, and a decrease of more than 1 Hz in background rhythm over a period of less than one year should arouse suspicion of central nervous system (CNS) disease or metabolic disturbance. The general organization of the EEG is preserved with normal aging. By contrast, patients with Alzheimer's disease may show slowing of the dominant posterior rhythm below 8 Hz, as well as increased theta and delta activity and poorer organization of the record (Nolfe & Giaquinto, 1986; Coben, Danziger, & Storandt, 1985). Some patients with Alzheimer's disease have normal EEGs at a time when clinical and psychiatric evidence suggest a diagnosis of moderate dementia. In these patients, a follow-up EEG in 6–12 months may show additional slow activity, or frank abnormality. In patients with suspected Alzheimer's disease and a normal EEG, an especially careful search for other causes of dementia is essential, and if follow-up EEGs and examinations fail to show progression, the diagnosis is doubtful (Meary, Snowden, Bowen, et al., 1986).

Despite its being a recording of potentials generated by the cerebral cortex, the EEG may not be helpful in distinguishing "subcortical" dementing illnesses such as progressive supernuclear palsy from "cortical" dementias like Alzheimer's disease (Fowler & Harrison, 1986).

Making the Most of the EEG

Brain electrical activity is a dynamic phenomenon that changes with time, circumstances, and the patient's state of arousal. The diagnostic efficacy of the EEG is greatest when the test is timed with this in mind. To take an obvious example, the patient who is said to awaken from sleep with brief episodes of bizarre behavior requires a sleep EEG to be properly investigated for nocturnal epilepsy, and ideally an all-night sleep study would be done, which could in addition assess the patient for abnormalities of sleep architecture. The following subsections elaborate on this theme.

Electroencephalograms are most valuable in the identification of organic brain disease when obtained when patients are symptomatic. A psychiatrist wishing to evaluate a neurologic etiology for suspected paroxysmal hysterical or anxiety symptoms should not only obtain a routine EEG, but also try to get one under the circumstances a patient feels will elicit an attack. Fariello, Booker, Chun, et al. (1983) reported on 32 cases of patients with paroxysmal symptoms who were studied as they reenacted the situations that provoked their paroxysmal attacks while having simultaneous polygraphic recording of EEG, EKG, and respiration. The investigators found it necessary to change the diagnoses in 19 cases, many of which had been previously diagnosed as hysterical. Provocative circumstances included having patients take a bath, stand up quickly, read, and undergo venipuncture. While a careful history and awareness of the existence of unusual seizure types is helpful in diagnosing epilepsy, ictal EEG abnormality during the time of the suspected seizure facilitates an unequivocal diagnosis.

An emergency EEG is a definitive procedure when partial complex status is suspected. Nonconvulsive status epilepticus should be suspected in instances of acute mental status change with diminished responsiveness or automatic behavior, particularly in patients with a past history of seizures. Partial complex status may present as a confusional state, as aphasia, as decreased responsiveness with staring, or as catatonia. Although a history of seizures is often present, there are well-documented cases with no past history of epilepsy. The interictal EEG was abnormal in 8 cases reported by Ballenger, King, & Gallagher (1983) and in 9 of the 12 cases reviewed from literature. The neurologic examination was normal in 4 of the 8 cases reported. The *ictal* EEG, however, was abnormal in every case in which it was performed.

Sleep EEGs, sleep-deprivation EEGs, and EEGs with special leads may help with the diagnosis of temporal lobe epilepsy, but even with these procedures, the EEG may always be normal or nondiagnostic. Temporal lobe epilepsy (TLE) thus remains a clinical diagnosis, to be established by a careful history, clinical observation, and, if necessary, therapeutic trials of anticonvulsants.

Because the clinical manifestations of TLE may overlap with the manifestations of functional psychiatric disorders, psychiatric clinicians tend to attach great importance to the presence or absence of diagnostic EEG abnormalities. Unfortunately, there are patients with definite TLE with no focal spike activity detectable, even with special leads. A typical case is included in a report on electrophysiological correlates of pathology and surgical results in TLE (Engle, Driver, & Falconer, 1975). A patient with no definite spike focus on scalp EEG or spenoidal leads had a definite lateral temporal spike focus on electrocorticography. This patient had total relief of seizures following anterior temporal lobectomy; the pathology was mesial temporal sclerosis.

Different authors disagree on the incidence of negative EEGs in TLE. Much of the disagreement may be explainable by differences in the clinical populations reported upon. For example, the likelihood of a diagnostic EEG is lower for older patients

(Ajmone-Marsa & Zivin, 1970). More optimistic authors believe that, with repeated EEGs, over 90 percent of patients with TLE may eventually admit of an electroencephalographic diagnosis, but three or more recordings, with sleep and other special procedures, may be needed (Driver & McGillivray, 1982).

Of the EEG activation procedures routinely available to the psychiatrist, all-night sleep deprivation probably is the most productive. This procedure involves keeping the patient awake all night without stimulants, and then obtaining at least 90 minutes of EEG on the next day. In a recent French study, 22 patients with clinical diagnoses of partial epilepsy received EEGs before and after sleep deprivation. Twenty-seven percent had normal EEGs before sleep deprivation, but all showed abnormalities afterward. The occurrence of spike activity was 27 percent before and 59 percent after the activation procedure (Arne-bes Calvet, Thiberge, et al., 1982). Another European study showed that all-night sleep deprivation increased the yield of paroxysmal findings by 37.4 percent in a group of 88 patients with clinically diagnosed partial epilepsy (Declerck Sijben-Kiggen, Wauquier, et al., 1982). The technique of the second study required 3–5 hours of EEG recording on the day following sleep deprivation.

Patients with disabling paroxysmal symptoms of questionable etiology and patients with known epilepsy refractory to standard treatment should be referred for intensive neurodiagnostic monitoring (Gumnit, 1986). Intensive neurodiagnostic monitoring, which comprises EEG telemetry—with or without simultaneous video recording—and ambulatory cassette EEG recording, may resolve a diagnostic or therapeutic impasse when routine EEG procedures fail. Simultaneous video EEG describes a procedure in which at least 10 channels of EEG are simultaneously recorded with a video picture of the patient, with the information from the two sources synchronized. Telemetered EEG refers to EEG recording from a wireless transmitter worn by the patient while the patient is normally active in a supervised medical setting. Ambulatory cassette EEG may be recorded on either an inpatient or an outpatient basis, using a Holter monitor–like device.

These procedures can be used to identify the nature of a paroxysmal event, to identify the type of seizure in patients with epilepsy, to locate the part of the brain in which a seizure begins, and to quantify the number of seizures. Intensive neurodiagnostic monitoring is best performed at a comprehensive epilepsy center, or at least under the direction of an experienced electroencephalographer with a major commitment to the procedure. While intensive neurodiagnostic monitoring is extraordinarily sensitive, the presence of numerous artifacts and technical difficulties make it unsatisfactory for occasional use by a neurologist without special involvement in epilepsy.

Selection between inpatient video–EEG telemetry and ambulatory cassette monitoring is best made by an experienced neurologist, considering the specifics of the case. Most patients with a mixture of genuine and psychogenic seizures will best be sorted out by several days of video–EEG monitoring in an inpatient setting with anticonvulsants withdrawn. Relatively mild but frequent paroxysmal events in reliable patients often can be satisfactorily investigated with outpatient ambulatory cassette monitoring.

Ambulatory cassette monitoring and inpatient telemetry are the most sensitive detectors of interictal electrical abnormalities and brief subclinical seizure activity in patients with epilepsy (Ebersole & Bridgers, 1985; Ebersole & Leroy, 1983). They would not ordinarily be employed, however, in a patient with typical epileptic symptoms who responded well to standard anticonvulsant treatment. The expense and inconvenience of long-term monitoring becomes justified when seizure control is difficult to attain, putting either the diagnosis or the therapy in doubt. One particular example is when a patient with automatisms fails to respond to the usual drugs for TLE. Some of these patients turn out, on long-term monitoring, to have generalized spike-and-wave discharges that indicate a form of epilepsy better managed with valproic acid than with carbamazepine or phenytoin.

Nasopharyngeal leads may be helpful in localization, but add little to the EEG diagnosis of psychiatric patients. While nasopharyngeal leads may occasionally disclose medial-basal temporal foci of epileptic activity, these are almost always accompanied by epileptic discharges from other brain regions, occurring either simultaneously or independently (Levin, Leaton, & Lee, 1986). While nasopharyngeal leads may add localizing information if the patient can tolerate them, it is not worth fighting with a patient to place nasopharyngeal leads. Longer recording times and provocative procedures are far more likely to increase the yield of EEG abnormalities in equivocal cases. Even when surface EEG detects seizure discharges, their anatomic location cannot be reliably ascertained. In patients destined for surgery, depth recording or positron emission tomography (PET) scanning (discussed later) is needed to accurately locate the focus. When ictal EEGs are read by experienced electroencephalographers, they correctly locate the lobe of onset less than half the time (Spencer, Williamson, Bridger, et al., 1985). Therefore, if psychiatric understanding of a case is to depend on precise location of the focus of seizure activity, surface EEG cannot be trusted to accurately determine that focus.

Evoked Potentials

Evoked potentials are derived by repeatedly presenting a stimulus to the patient, recording the EEG for a fixed period following each stimulus, and then averaging a large number of responses. The averaging is usually carried out by a microcomputer, which digitizes the EEG signal and calculates the average at a number of points, simulating a smooth curve. The averaging procedure cancels out EEG background activity, leaving a pattern specifically related to the presented stimulus. Stimuli may be simple, such as flashing lights, or complex, such as stimuli for a discrimination task. The auditory, visual, and somatosensory modalities can all be used for the stimulus.

Evoked potentials may be divided into early and late potentials. Early potentials depend on neuronal activity in the primary sensory pathways and are relatively independent of attentional state and even level of consciousness, although pattern-shift visual evoked responses require ocular fixation. By contrast, late evoked potentials depend on level of consciousness, attentional state, and, in certain circumstances, mental set. Evoked responses usually are reported in terms of specific positive or negative waves, described in terms of latency of onset and peak amplitude. Early evoked potentials usually are recorded over the appropriate sensory area for the modality of presentation, although late evoked potentials may be recorded anywhere over the scalp, depending on the purpose of the recording (see the section to come on brain evoked activity mapping [BEAM]).

Early evoked potentials will show delayed latency if there is delayed conduction in the primary sensory pathways; they are particularly sensitive to demyelinating lesions. Visual evoked potentials thus show delayed latency in optic neuritis, which will persist after symptoms have remitted. Auditory evoked potentials may show delayed latency if there is demyelination of auditory pathways. In the case of auditory pathways, it may even be possible to locate the approximate site of the lesion, depending on which waves are delayed.

The early evoked potentials—pattern-shift visual evoked potentials, brain stem auditory evoked potentials, and short-latency somatosensory evoked potentials—can demonstrate abnormal sensory system function when the history and neurological examination are equivocal. They may thus serve to document a second, discrete lesion in suspected cases of multiple sclerosis, assisting the diagnosis and at times averting more invasive tests such as myelography. Evoked potentials may also define the anatomic distribution of the disease process, or monitor objective changes in patients' status (Chiappa & Young, 1985).

Evoked potentials have anatomic specificity but not etiologic specificity. Abnormal latencies for brain stem auditory evoked potentials imply impaired function of brain stem pathways but do not distinguish among vascular, demyelinating, metabolic, and neoplastic etiologies. Symmetrical delays in visual evoked potentials can be produced by B_{12} deficiency, the effects of toxins, inflammatory diseases, and even normal aging (Celesia, 1986). Thus, despite the wide use of evoked potentials in the diagnosis of multiple sclerosis, abnormal evoked potentials should not be equated with the presence of demyelinating disease (Stockard & Iragui, 1984).

Early evoked potentials can be applied to investigate sensory losses suspected to be due to hysteria or malingering. The principle is that sensory losses, if they are sufficiently severe, reliably produce delays in latency of evoked potentials, or occasionally an absence of the evoked potential. Normal pattern-shift visual evoked potentials imply visual acuity of at least 20/120. A patient who claimed only the ability to see light and movement but had normal visual evoked potentials would thus have no organic basis for the symptom. Auditory evoked potentials have latencies dependent on the degree of hearing loss; the audiometric threshold is within 5 or 10 decibels of the threshold for the appearance of the PIV-V complex of the evoked potential. (The PIV-V complex is a particular portion of the brainstem auditory evoked response that appears consistently in the absence of auditory system disease, provided that the auditory stimulus is sufficiently strong.) Hysterical, pretended, or functionally elaborated deafness would thus be detectable as a discrepancy between the audiometric threshold and the threshold for appearance of the PIV-V complex. An exception would exist for patients with cortical deafness or auditory agnosia; however, these patients always show abnormalities on EEG or brain imaging. The somatosensory evoked potential tests the posterior columns and can be expected to be abnormal if there is total anesthesia or significant loss of joint position sense. Sensory deficits not affecting joint position sense are compatible with normal somatosensory evoked potentials. Nonorganic sensory loss would be suspected if normal somatosensory evoked potentials were obtained in a patient who complained of total anesthesia or loss of joint position sense.

Malingering patients may alter their visual evoked potentials by failing to fix their vision on the stimulus; they may alter somatosensory evoked potentials by dislodging the stimulus electrodes. If malingering is suspected, the patient should be continuously observed by a skilled observer throughout the recording process in order to exclude patient-produced artifacts.

For further details, consult the superb review by Howard and Dorfman (1986).

In addition to aiding in the diagnosis of multiple sclerosis and the differential diagnosis of hysteria, early evoked potentials may be useful in demonstrating the physiologic effect of toxins of psychiatric interest. For example, some patients with tardive dyskinesia will have abnormal brain stem auditory evoked responses (Zeitlhofer, Brainin & Reisher, 1984). Chronic alcoholics may show abnormal brain stem auditory evoked responses, and patients with abnormal responses are much more likely to show brain stem or cerebellar atrophy on CT scan (Chu, 1985).

Early evoked responses are reliable when interpreted by an experienced clinical neurophysiologist. The tests are relatively inexpensive and noninvasive and can be administered by a technician. The psychiatrist should consider them when the hypothesis to be tested concerns the intactness of primary sensory pathways.

Late evoked potentials, a subject of endless fascination for researchers in clinical neurophysiology, have yet to establish a secure role in medical psychiatry. The main reason is that no incremental diagnostic or predictive value has been established for any late evoked potential measure. One of the best studied late evoked potentials is the P300, a positive wave recorded at the vertex from 265 to 500 milliseconds following a target auditory stimulus. Decreased amplitude, increased latency, or both have been reported for P300 in dementia (Kraiuhin, Gordon, Meares, et al., 1986), focal brain lesions (Ebner, Haas, Lucking, et al., 1986), borderline personality (Blackwood, St Clair, & Kutcher, 1986), and schizophrenia (Blackwood et al., 1986). Parameters for patient and control groups may overlap, however. In the discrimination of demented patients from normal controls, evoked potentials were less effective than psychometrics (Kraiuhin et al., 1986) or even routine EEG (Visser, Van Tilburg, Hooijer, et al., 1985). The P300 evoked potential, therefore, is of physiologic interest but of limited value as a diagnostic test.

Topographic EEG Spectral Analysis

The EEG contains far more information than can be readily analyzed visually. This is particularly true of EEG background rhythms, which comprise activity in several different frequency bands, combining to produce rather complex wave forms. A mathematical procedure called the fast Fourier transform can readily be done by a computer using digitized EEG signal and can produce an analysis of the EEG in terms of relative power in several different frequency bands. The principle of breaking a complex waveform into frequency bands is familiar to stereo buffs, who use graphic equalizers to vary the volume of music in several different frequency bands to adjust to the acoustics of any given space.

Topographic EEG spectral analysis displays the breakdown of the EEG into several frequency bands at a number of different points on the scalp, corresponding to the different EEG electrodes. Computerized graphic displays interpolate values between actual data points, generating a picture that can be displayed either in black and white or in colors representing different frequencies or levels of intensity. The end result is a graphic display that permits a facile visual analysis of asymmetries and changes in the frequency spectrum of a patient's EEG and also provides a set of quantitative data that can be used for statistical analyses of various kinds.

Topographic EEG methods have been helpful in discriminating groups of patients with Alzheimer's-type dementia from elderly healthy controls (Coben et al., 1985); they can also distinguish dyslexic boys from age-matched controls without reading problems (Duffy, 1985). In both of these situations, visual inspection of the EEG would not have reliably distinguished the two groups.

In the latter case mentioned, topographic EEG revealed differences from controls in the medial frontal region, an unsuspected finding given the previous belief that dyslexia reflected a temporal lobe problem only. Subsequent study of dyslexics by the same group showed that clinically different subtypes of dyslexia had distinguishable topographical EEG patterns.

Topographic EEG spectral analysis is a more powerful physiologic measure than visually interpreted EEG. Since the data come from EEG electrodes on the scalp, however, this study is no more able than a routine EEG to detect deep cerebral events far from the recording electrodes. It also shows considerable test–retest variability due to the physiologic state, vigilance of the patient at the time of recording, various artifacts, and circadian fluctuations. The dominant posterior rhythm, however, shows considerable stability, even with a one-year retest interval (Gasser, Bacher, & Steinberg, 1985).

Because of its ease of interpretation and automatic production of quantitative data, topographic EEG is a popular research tool for investigating drug effects on the EEG and for providing neurophysiologic measures that discriminate different groups of patients. In the medical psychiatric setting, it may find its greatest utility in work with specific, well-defined clinical populations in which a neurophysiologic abnormality may or may not be present. For example, topographic EEG might be useful in a group of patients with chronic lung disease, helping to assess which patients with psychiatric complications had a subtle metabolic encephalopathy, and which were suffering mainly from reactive emotional symptoms. While these applications seem rational and promising, topographic EEG has not been often applied with medically ill psychiatric patients and cannot be advised as a routine clinical test at this time. Clinicians working in hospitals or clinics with experienced clinical neurophysiologists available may wish to adapt topographic EEG to specific clinical problems they encounter in their practice.

Brain Evoked Activity Mapping

Brain evoked activity mapping (BEAM) is a specific modification of topograhic EEG that includes not only EEG spectral analysis, but also a topographic display of evoked potentials. Evoked potentials are calculated every 4 milliseconds for a total of 512 milliseconds after the presentation of a stimulus, and the amplitude of the evoked potential is determined at each point in the EEG electrode montage. Amplitudes are then interpolated between the actual data points, and a colored computer graphic is generated based on those interpolations. BEAM may thus test any form of visual, auditory, or somatosensory evoked potential. The result is presented as an endless-loop animated picture representing the spread of the evoked potential through the brain over the 512-millisecond period of the overall recording. The pictures are fascinating to watch and lend themselves to instant qualitative interpretation, even by the inexperienced observer. A full BEAM study includes both topographic EEG spectral analysis and BEAM evoked potentials in several sensory modalities.

In patients with brain tumor, the BEAM shows delayed arrival of the evoked potential at the tumor site, with late persistence of a potential at that site. BEAM could predict the recurrence of a malignant glioma several weeks before it appeared on CT scan (Duffy, 1985). BEAM studies also can distinguish patients with Alzheimer's disease, dyslexia, and epilepsy from appropriate controls.

Because the BEAM evaluates late potentials, it is vulnerable to all of the confounding variables that affect the conventional late evoked potentials, including attentional state, level of consciousness, cooperation, and mental set.

In general, guidelines for BEAM are similar to those for late evoked potentials and topographic EEG. Specifically, BEAM can be used to test physiologic hypotheses and distinguish among patients suspected to have a specific neurophysiologic dysfunction. It is nonspecific and cannot be regarded as a clinical diagnostic test for any disease entity at this time. Because of the extremely high number of variables measured by the BEAM apparatus, "statistically significant" differences between groups may represent nothing more than the chance effects expected when one has a large number of variables. The ultimate development of the BEAM as a true diagnostic test will hinge on the development of large banks of normative data for different patient populations. Even then, artifacts may arise from failure to adequately standardize the conditions of recording.

At the present time, a psychiatrist should not simply order a BEAM study. Rather, specific hypotheses should be discussed with a competent clinical neurophysiologist, who might then help devise an adaptation of BEAM methodology suitable for investigating the patient or group of patients.

Positron Emission Tomography

Positron emission tomography (PET) is a nuclear medicine procedure. It makes use of a special radionuclide produced in an on-site cyclotron dedicated to the purpose. The radionuclide produces positrons, which collide with nearby electrons and produce a diametrically opposed pair of photons. The photons are detected by an array of detectors, and the fact that they occur in pairs permits location of their source. Technology similar to that used in CT and MRI permits the computer reconstruction of an image. In contrast with CT and MRI, however, the PET scan image does not represent anatomic structures. It is a representation of the distribution of a radionuclide.

By incorporating suitable radionuclides in physiologically or pharmacologically active substances, the PET scan technique permits the collection of data corresponding to physiologic and pharmacologic phenomena, such as glucose metabolism or receptor binding. Most reported studies have been done with ^{18}F fluorodeoxyglucose. This compound is incorporated in metabolically active cells in the brain and remains within those cells. Thus, the distribution of fluorodeoxyglucose permits mapping of the areas of maximum cerebral metabolic activity. Because of the efficiency of the detection process and the high activity of the radionuclides used, PET scanning can be carried out with a very small dose of tracer compound.

The PET scan procedure takes about 30 minutes. At present, it requires an onsite cyclotron to produce the radionuclide, and the overall cost of the procedure is substantially greater than the cost of a CT or an MRI. Experts in the field have predicted that this cost will come down if and when the test becomes more widespread (TerPogossian, 1985).

The fluorodeoxyglucose PET scan, because it measures cerebral metabolic activity, is sensitive to the level of consciousness and the mental and physical activity of the patient being scanned. For example, continual movement of the right hand throughout a PET scan would be expected to produce increased glucose utilization over the left motor strip. Because so many patient variables may affect the PET scan, comparisons between patients and control groups require substantial control over the circumstances of testing. This and the 30-minute scan period limit the utility of the fluorodeoxyglucose PET scan in uncooperative patients.

While the PET scan is inferior to CT and MRI in resolution (TerPogossian, 1985), its unique ability is that it can measure metabolic changes that antedate anatomic changes or occur in their absence.

Patients with Alzheimer's disease may show PET scan changes in the posterior temporal and parietal regions at a time when the CT scan is normal for age or shows only nonspecific diffuse atrophy (Duara, Grady, Haxby, et al., 1984; Haxby, Grady, Duara, et al., 1986; Friedland, Budinger, Brant-Zawadzki, et al., 1984). PET shows diffuse hypometabolism in normal pressure hydrocephalus; this contrasts with temporoparietal hypometabolism in Alzheimer's disease (Jagust, Friedland, & Budinger, 1985). It remains to be seen, however, whether PET scans will be predictive of surgical outcome, or add anything to a careful history and examination in selecting patients for shunts.

The PET scan may show decreased metabolism in a temporal lobe seizure focus that is not visualized on MRI or CT. Subsequent removal of foci shown on PET scan may improve the epilepsy, and pathologic examination may show the underlying cause of the epileptic condition (Sperling et al., 1986).

PET scans may show abnormal caudate metabolism in patients at risk for Huntington's disease, prior to the onset of clinical symptoms. If patients with these findings all subsequently turn out to develop Huntington's disease, the PET scan may prove to be the most sensitive diagnostic test for this disorder (WRW Martin, 1985; Kuhl, Phelps, Markham, et al., 1982). In other movement disorders, such as dystonia, Parkinsonism, and hereditary chorea, PET studies in research context may illuminate the pathophysiology but would not be considered diagnostic tests (WRW Martin, 1985). In rare cases in which it was unclear whether a movement disorder were of organic origin, a positive PET study would document abnormal physiology, but a negative would not be conclusive, because a PET may be normal in some movement disorders of unquestionable organic etiology.

Applied to stroke or trauma patients,

the PET scan may show hypometabolism in larger areas than appear clinically involved by brain imaging techniques (Langfitt, Obrist, Alavi, et al., 1986). Ultimately, PET may aid in the differential diagnosis of the neurobehavioral sequelae of head injury, as it may show persistent functional abnormality in the limbic and the cortical structures at a time when a normal MRI or CT would favor a "functional" diagnosis.

Because PET is a highly sensitive test that permits accurate quantitative measurement of regional radioactivity, it makes possible in vivo pharmacokinetic studies, particularly of receptor binding using radio labeled agonists or antagonists (Maziere, Comar, & Maziere, 1986). In vivo receptor binding has been demonstrated for dopaminergic, serotonergic, opiate, benzodiazepine, and beta-adrenergic receptors. While pharmacokinetic studies at present are currently restricted to research settings, it is likely that such studies may eventually aid in the diagnosis of metabolic encephalopathies and in the understanding of atypical responses to drugs.

In conclusion, the PET scan will probably find a place in the early diagnosis of brain diseases, in the evaluation of refractory focal epilepsy, and, in academic settings, for the documentation of regional cerebral dysfunction associated with specific neurobehavioral syndromes. At present, it has little routine clinical utility. The development of routine clinical uses for the PET scan will require a decrease in the cost, wider availability of the scanners, and the accumulation of data on the relevance of PET scan results in predicting prognosis and treatment response in specific neuropsychiatric disorders.

Single Photon Emission Computed Tomography

Single proton emission computed tomography (SPECT) is a nuclear medicine procedure based on a photon-emitting radionuclide rather than a positron-emitting radionuclide. This difference has several implications. Since photon-emitting radionuclides are readily available and may be fairly stable, an on-site cyclotron is not necessary to conduct SPECT studies. On the other hand, precise quantitation of regional radioactivity is done much more easily with PET than with SPECT. The reason is that with SPECT the intensity of radiation from the single photon-emitting source falls off as the square of the distance and in proportion to the density of the material through which the photon travels. In a structure like the brain, which in not homogenous, precise mathematical reconstruction of regional radioactivity is virtually impossible. PET is based on the detection of photon pairs that are diametrically opposed. Each pair of photons must traverse the entire diameter of the brain, regardless of where in the brain the pair originates. This permits a more straightforward correction for attenuation of photons by tissue and leads to more accurate quantification.

When precise, quantitative counts of receptors or metabolic rates are needed for research purposes, or to establish the pathophysiology of particular conditions, PET would thus be the preferable study. If studies with PET lead to diagnostic tests for particular conditions, it is possible that SPECT may be adapted as a lower-cost substitute. Such efforts are under way, particularly in the study of Alzheimer's disease, for which PET may have value in early diagnosis (Frackowiak, 1986; TerPogossian, 1985).

Lumbar Puncture and Cerebrospinal Fluid Examination

Cerebrospinal fluid (CSF) examination, though less frequently done now than in the past, remains the essential test for the diagnosis of acute and chronic meningitis, for encephalitis, and for neoplastic involvement of the meninges. It is regularly performed by neurologists and internists when infection is suspected; the psychiatrist's role in initiating the CSF examination is that of raising a suspicion of infectious or inflammatory CNS disease based on mental status changes. Mild deliria with mainly psychiatric manifestations may be viewed as functional by nonpsychiatrists, leading to delays in performing needed CSF examinations. In our experience, this is most likely to happen with young adults with acute onset psychoses or personality changes. These patients may have encephalitis or meningoencephalitis, with a raised CSF cell count supporting the diagnosis. Such elevated cell counts were found in almost one-fifth of a recent sample of patients admitted to a Finnish hospital with acute psychosis of less than two weeks' duration (Ahokas, Koskiniemi, Vaheri, et al., 1985). The Finnish investigators also found that 41 percent of their sample had IgG oligoclonal bands in the CSF, suggesting an inflammatory or immunologic process. Although patients with mild lymphocytic pleocytosis in the CSF, or elevated oligoclonal bands, usually do not have specifically treatable CNS infections, their positive CSF findings identify them as a group requiring comprehensive neuropsychiatric assessment and follow-up. It is likely that such patients may have a different course, prognosis, and response to treatment than those without CNS inflammation underlying their psychopathology.

CSF findings in viral meningoencephalitis are nonspecific and do not permit ascertainment of the causal agent (Griffith & Ch'ien, 1984). For this reason, CSF examination is sometimes omitted when a typical systemic viral infection is complicated by headache and mild changes in cognitive mental status. This is appropriate, but psychiatric considerations may indicate CSF examination even when a viral infection such as infectious mononucleosis has already been diagnosed. Specifically, when psychotic-level behavior changes take place, CSF evidence of inflammation helps make the attribution of the mental disorder to organic CNS involvement, rather than to a functional psychosis triggered by the stress of physical illness. Prognostic and management implications follow.

Patients with disorders, such as malignancies, lupus, and AIDS, that are known to frequently involve the CNS may require diagnostic CSF examination if brain imaging, serologic studies, and physical examination cannot establish the presence of CNS involvement in a patient with manifest mental changes. For example, cell count may be elevated or C_4 levels decreased from baseline in patients with CNS lupus (Rodnan & Schumacher, 1983). Psychiatrists involved in the care of such patients should initiate CSF examination when the information would be necessary to determine whether mental symptoms were due to direct CNS involvement. Because psychiatrists must choose treatment strategies based on this determination, their need to know the CSF findings may be greater than that of the primary physician at particular points in the patient's course. When gross, nonmental signs of brain involvement supervene, the neurologist or internist would naturally make decisions regarding the need for CSF examination.

In multiple sclerosis, the CSF IgG may be a particularly useful measure of disease activity (Caroscio, Kochwa, Sacks, et al., 1986). When a patient with psychiatrically complicated multiple sclerosis experiences a decline in functional status, such a measure of disease activity may help the clinician decide on the relative roles of affective disturbance and acute demyelination in producing the decline in function.

Chemical analysis of CSF has a limited role in the diagnosis of toxic-metabolic encephalopathy. CSF glutamine or ammonia levels are elevated in hepatic encephalopathy and Reye's syndrome, and determination of CSF glutamine may make sense in diagnosing a patient with known liver disease and mental status changes, for whom the EEG, physical examination, and blood ammonia level were not decisive (Tarter, Hegedus, Van Thiel, & Schade, 1985).

Measurement of CSF concentrations of neurotransmitters and their metabolites has increasingly been pursued in research laboratories, but as yet no clinical tests have emerged for this research (Stahl, 1985). One might anticipate, however, that appropriately selected CSF neurotransmitter measures would help in distinguishing psychological reactions from altered CNS chemistry in patients with psychiatric complications of systemic disease. Development of such tests would require systematic study of subgroups of patients at risk, much as should be done for BEAM and other sensitive but nonspecific tests.

The diagnosis of fungal infection of the CSF is often considered when subacute mental changes develop in an immunocompromised patient. The psychiatrist may become involved in such cases because the initial CSF examination was normal or nonspecifically abnormal, raising concerns about psychiatric contributions to the change in mental status. In assessing such patients, it is useful for the psychiatrist to know that the diagnosis of fungal meningitis may require multiple lumbar punctures and CSF cultures, with a relatively high volume (5 cc or more) of CSF taken for each culture. The cryptococcal antigen, the most popular CSF test for the most common treatable fungal meningitis, is falsely negative in 42 percent of patients with culture-positive disease. Fungal meningitis thus, *cannot* be ruled out by a single CSF examination, and follow-up examinations should be performed if clinical suspicion is high (McGinnis, 1985). Recent work suggests that CSF ferritin levels are consistently elevated in patients with bacterial and fungal meningitis, but not in patients with viral meningitis (Campbell, Skikne, & Cook, 1986). This work suggests that analysis of CSF proteins might aid in the early diagnosis of CSF infections in immunocompro-

mised patients. Ferritin is also increased in herpes simplex encephalitis (Sindic, Kevers, Chalon, et al., 1985). If CSF ferritin levels are available at one's hospital, they might be considered in patients with acute psychosis and temporal lobe abnormality suggestive of herpes encephalitis, particularly in cases where routine CSF findings are equivocal.

CSF examination is not useful in diagnosing typical cases of Alzheimer's disease (Becker, Feussner, Mulrow, et al., 1985; Hammerstrom & Zimmer, 1985). A lumbar puncture should be performed if there are atypical features, such as rapid progression, fever, meningeal signs, or a positive blood serology for syphilis.

The technique and precautions for lumbar puncture (LP) are described in standard neurology textbooks and will not be repeated here. We will mention, however, that recent work has shown that the amount of fluid removed for CSF studies bears no relation to the subsequent development of headache, so that there is no reason not to obtain sufficient fluid for cultures or biochemical studies in patients for whom an LP is indicated. The subsequent occurrence of headache does depend on the size of LP needle used. Prolonged recumbency does not affect the likelihood of developing a post-lumbar-puncture headache, so outpatient lumbar puncture is reasonable, particularly if a small-gauge needle is used (Gibb, 1984).

Improving the Formulation of the Neurologic Differential Diagnosis

The formulation of a psychosocial diagnosis requires integration of information from the developmental history, the family history, and the clinical interview. The development of a useful and plausible neurologic differential diagnosis similarly requires an integration of diverse information from the history of present illness, the family history, the mental status examination, the neurologic examination, and laboratory tests. Schizophrenia is not diagnosed from mental status findings alone, nor should mental status findings or laboratory tests be used in a simplistic way to categorize a case as either organic or functional. It is more useful to generate for each case a plausible list of organic conditions that might be causal or contributory to the patient's mental disorder. Contributory problems are more common than causal problems and may be more often neglected, because the nonorganic factors in the case may be of impressive magnitude.

A useful discipline is to think in every psychiatric case of three plausible organic conditions the patient might have, given the epidemiologic setting, the history, the examination, and laboratory findings. The points that follow have been useful in formulating neurologic differential diagnoses for psychiatric patients.

Hard neurologic signs should never be dismissed as irrelevant. Borson (1982) described a man recurrently treated for various functional psychiatric diagnoses while receiving a medical diagnosis of inactive Behcet's disease. Despite a deteriorating course, with psychiatric symptoms accompanied at times by abnormal gait and rigid posture, the psychiatric disorder was not related by his physicians to Behcet's disease. This seems puzzling in view of the known involvement of the CNS by that disorder. (Behcet's disease is a form of vasculitis that usually presents with oral and genital ulcers and recurrent ocular inflammation. CNS involvement, which may include meningoencephalitis, occurs in approximately 25 percent of patients [Petersdorf, Adams, Braunwald, et al., 1983].) In another instance (Shraberg & D'Souza, 1982), a woman with coma induced by opiate overdose was misdiagnosed as hysterical because of apparent intermittent alertness and forcible eye closure when the

examiner tried to open her eyes. Hard neurologic signs included hyperreflexia, difficulty swallowing, and coma vigil. The EEG was diffusely abnormal and the CT scan showed cerebral edema. Other cases have been reported of psychotic patients with cerebellar disease on CT scan, dysarthria, ataxia, and unilateral difficulty on tests of coordination who were diagnosed as functional (Hamilton, Frick, Takahashi, et al., 1983) and of a subdural hematoma ultimately diagnosed by EEG and CT scan that presented with depression, ataxia, and fluctuating mental status with periods of relative alertness erroneously taken as evidence for a functional etiology (Alarcon & Thweatt, 1983).

Soft neurologic signs and nonspecific psychiatric symptoms are most meaningful when occurring in combinations suggestive of specific diagnoses. Neurologic signs and symptoms must be interpreted in a proper context. Repeated examinations and a search for independent confirmatory signs may be needed. Organic illnesses that are most frequently misdiagnosed include myasthenia gravis, hyperthyroidism, multiple sclerosis, normal pressure hydrocephalus, brain tumor, chronic subdural hematoma, and pancreatic carcinoma (Martin, 1983). Clues often exist but may be subtle, such as tremor with hyperthyroidism, gait disturbance with normal pressure hydrocephalus, and gait disturbance and headache with subdural hematoma.

There are a number of methods of seeking supporting evidence for suspected neurologic disease (Massey & Scherokman, 1981). These include (1) identifying mild facial asymmetry with the help of old photographs; (2) finding that rapid alternating movements are done more slowly in the dominant hand (the opposite is usually the case); (3) eliciting pathologic posturing of the hand, arm, or shoulder during gait tasks or mental status questions; and (4) finding *unilateral* occurrence of finger flexor reflexes such as the Hoffman sign, together with other motor abnormalities suggestive of neurologic disease. (The Hoffman sign is elicited by holding the patient's hand palm downward and resting the tip of his middle finger on the examiner's index finger. Flicking the middle fingernail with the examiner's thumb evokes flexion of all the fingers on the abnormal side. The sign shows finger flexor reflexes are hyperactive and is suggestive of pyramidal tract disease.)

Although unilateral signs usually are diagnostically meaningful, bilateral signs do not necessarily imply the presence of neurologic disease. Frontal release signs such as the snout reflex are found in a significant proportion of the normal population (Jacobs & Glassman, 1980). Babinski signs are present after strenuous exercise in 7 percent of normal subjects (Elliot & Walsh, 1925; Farrell, 1941).

In patients with considerable abnormality of behavior, it may be impossible to perform the subtle sensory and visual-field examinations that may be needed to identify parietal lobe lesions. In one reported case of parietal infarctions presenting psychiatrically, the onset of psychiatric illness in midlife coupled with a history of hypertension suggested the neurologic etiology (Tippin & Dunner, 1981).

The clinical diagnosis of multiple sclerosis is often based on a diagnostic history plus signs that, in themselves, would be nonspecific. Kellner, Davenport, Post, et al. (1983) reported two cases of patients hospitalized with rapid cycling bipolar illness who eventually were found to have multiple sclerosis. In the first instance, the patient had right-sided muscle spasms at age 22 following an episode in her teens of visual disturbance. She was originally diagnosed as suffering a conversion reaction. The second patient developed a mood disorder at age 46 and at age 49 developed paresthesia and stiffness in her legs and poor coordination. At age 52, in light of a progressive gait disturbance, she received a lumbar puncture, at which time oligoclonal bands were found in the cerebrospinal fluid. Multiple sclerosis may be associated with unipolar or bipolar affective illness. A typical scenario is presentation with "hysteria" and neurologic symptoms out of proportion to neurologic signs, followed after a variable period by harder neurologic findings. The combination of a vague intermittent neurologic history with affective disorder should lead a psychiatrist to consider multiple sclerosis. MS should be pursued with particular vigor if bedside examination shows soft signs such as hyperactive reflexes and mild incoordination. In this situation, ancillary tests such as evoked potentials and special eye examinations are worthwhile.

Patients whose behavioral symptoms get worse on neuroleptics may have an undiagnosed organic disorder. Walker (1982) cites 3 patients with organic disease (1 with a left basal ganglion infarct and 2 with cortical atrophy) who experienced a deterioration of mental status on phenothiazines that was not reversed with anti-Parkinson drugs. Once a neuroleptic is given, significant neurological abnormalities may be attributed to the drug rather than to the possibility of underlying brain disease. The neurologic assessment of the unmanageable catatonic patient, particularly in the emergency setting is facilitated by administering a benzodiazepine rather than a neuroleptic. Neuroleptics may further confuse the clinical picture and cause a clinician to miss a treatable neurologic disease. The neuroleptic malignant syndrome may mimic catatonia. In this instance, a benzodiazepine would help, whereas neuroleptics could worsen the condition (McEvoy & Lohr, 1984).

Diagnostic exclusion of an organic basis for patient's symptoms is impossible early in the course of many illnesses. Psychiatric symptoms may be harbingers of organic illness such as lupus, demyelinating disease (e.g., multiple sclerosis), degenerative brain disease (e.g., Huntington's chorea), and other illnesses—months to years before the emergence of hard neurological signs. Oommen, Johnson & Ray (1982) reported on a case of herpes type II virus encephalitis that presented as a confusional psychosis without other neurologic signs with a normal CT scan and EEG. The CSF was positive and the diagnosis was confirmed at autopsy. Four other such cases were found in the literature. Clinicians cannot assume that viral encephalitis is not present because of the absence of hard neurologic signs and abnormal laboratory tests. Yik et al. (1982) reported a recurrent psychiatric disorder (including exhibitionism) commencing in a woman at age 42 that was ultimately attributable to hepatic encephalopathy. The covert diagnosis of hepatic portal vein occlusion was made 5 years after the onset of psychiatric symptoms. Neurologic signs were present that waxed and waned, but there were no peripheral stigmata of liver disease early in the course of the illness.

Depression with profound weight loss without a past personal or family history of depression raises a suspicion of brain tumor, pancreatic carcinoma, a hormone-producing tumor, or endocrine cancer. Frontal and temporal cerebral metastases are particularly likely to present with psychiatric symptoms (Peterson & Perl, 1982). In one study, 22 percent of patients with frontal tumors presented with psychiatric symptoms (Strauss & Keshner, 1935). Spinal cord tumors may be misdiagnosed as conversion disorders (Epstein, Epstein, & Postel, 1971).

Peroutka (1982) reported a case of a 72-year-old woman with the onset of auditory hallucinations and paranoid delusions due to a right temporoparietaloccipital lesion found on CT scan. Only an isolated neuropsychologic test finding and a history of a focal seizure and reversible focal motor dysfunction pointed toward a neurologic disorder.

Among lupus patients, 20–40 percent develop a psychiatric disorder such as delirium, dementia, or depression (Bresnahan, 1982). EEG and CSF usually show abnormalities but occasionally are normal in definite cases. Neurologic signs pointing to an organic etiology for psychosis may appear some time after the presentation of schizophreniform psychoses in patients with numerous diseases of the basal ganglia and adjacent regions, such as idiopathic calcification, Wilson's disease, Huntington's chorea, postencephalitic Parkinsonism, bilateral subthalamic infarctions, and brain stem encephalitis (Cummings, Gosenfield, Honlihan, et al., 1983). The absence of definite neurologic abnormality on initial screening does not permit the clinician to relax vigilance regarding the subsequent development of neurologic signs. Particularly in cases of Huntington's disease and Wilson's disease, diagnoses have been missed because the subsequent development of Parkinsonism or involuntary movement was attributed to neuroleptics rather than considered as possibly indicating further evolution of an organic disease with psychiatric manifestations.

NEUROPSYCHOLOGIC ASSESSMENT IN MEDICAL PSYCHIATRY

An Overview of the Field and the Purposes of Assessment

The field of neuropsychology is dedicated to the study of brain–behavior relationships in illness and health. Of particular interest are higher-level cortical or intellectual functions, such as memory and reasoning, as opposed to lower-level functions, such as sensation.

Why should a psychiatrist order neuropsychologic services? What is the purpose of neuropsychologic assessment? Perhaps the most important purpose is to provide a detailed and precise description of intellectual or cognitive functions. The practitioner should be aware that what is often referred to as intellectual assessment, comprising one of the standardized intelligence tests (i.e., the Wechsler Adult Intelligence Scale—Revised [WAIS]) and perhaps a very broad screening test for "organicity" (i.e., the Bender Gestalt), provides general information only and, by itself, may be of limited practical value. The Wechsler scales provide scores on a series of subtests that sample a range of functions, as well as overall verbal, performance, and full-scale IQ scores. One certainly can draw some general conclusions, and perhaps more specific hypotheses, based on the results of intelligence testing. For example, in some cases, one might be able to conclude that overall level of intellectual functioning is high or very high and that the patient has generally stronger verbal than nonverbal skills. The problem, however, is what one cannot say.

Suppose one refers a patient with a past history of moderate or severe head injury, primarily involving frontal areas. The patient is presenting with considerable variability in mood, impulsiveness, forgetfulness, and an apparent lack of insight into his condition. The psychiatrist asks for intellectual assessment, or perhaps even for neuropsychologic screening. What comes back is an intelligence test that is completely normal and perhaps a Bender judged to be equivocal for brain damage. The difficulty this creates is that one can only conclude that the individual appears normal, or near normal, in the areas assessed on the intelligence test and the Bender. Moderate or even severe deficits

may exist, however, probably attributable to frontal dysfunction, that were missed by intelligence testing. Because of the lack of comprehensive coverage and the highly structured nature of most of the tasks on intelligence tests, they can be insensitive to deficits associated with frontal dysfunction. Their lack of sensitivity is not limited to frontal disorders. For example, fairly gross, but select, language disorders can also be missed.

The foregoing is not to criticize the intelligence test, which is an exemplary psychometric instrument, but merely to point out that it cannot substitute for neuropsychologic assessment. First, as mentioned already, it may miss significant areas of deficit. Second, it does not provide specific enough information. It may be useful to know that a patient performed poorly on measures emphasizing verbal production, but one needs to know just what the problem is. Is it a difficulty with articulation, fluency, or naming? Does the patient have a general disorder in the retrieval of previously stored information, language material included, that interferes with performance on a wide variety of tasks? Third—a point related to the preceding one—coverage is inadequate. Many areas of cognitive functioning simply are not assessed at all or are assessed in only the most superficial manner. For example, intelligence tests do not sample writing at all; reading or comprehension and production of grammatical structure are not assessed directly, and no scores are derived in these areas. Many authors have described or reported on the limits of intelligence testing as the sole means of assessing cognitive functions (e.g., Lezak, 1983; Reitan, 1985; Warrington, James, & Maciejewski, 1986). For example, Reitan states, "It is . . . clear that general intelligence measures are not as sensitive to the psychological effects of cerebral damage as measures that were developed specifically for this purpose" (p. 245).

Neurophyschological Assessment of Memory

To give the reader some feel for what is meant by comprehensive and detailed coverage of cognitive functions, memory and learning will be used as an example. These are very complex and involved areas of functioning, and disruption can occur in very limited or specific areas. One or a few memory tasks thus cannot provide the sampling that is needed. A comprehensive examination certainly would assess *immediate*, *recent*, and *remote memory*. By *immediate memory*, we mean the simple repetition of material in temporary "storage," or the repetition or reproduction of material that is kept actively in mind. Repeating a phone number given by the information operator is an immediate memory task. Recent memory tasks call for the reproduction of material that has not been kept actively in mind, but rather has been stored and must be retrieved. If one is asked to count backward from 10 to 1 and then repeat the phone number, this becomes a recent memory task. A precise delineation between recent and remote memory is not possible, but remote memory usually refers either to information that has been stored in memory in the past (e.g., the words one knows) or to the recall of newly presented information after some period of delay, usually at least 30 minutes.

There is good reason to assess these three aspects of memory. It is not at all uncommon for a patient to show intact immediate memory but gross problems in recent and remote memory. Further, a patient who performs very poorly on recent memory tasks may do so because immediate memory is highly problematic, perhaps due to gross deficiencies in attention. In fact, the patient's recent memory may be perfectly intact, but because the information never "got in" in the first place, there is nothing available for the recent memory "machine." There can thus be very marked disassociations among immediate, recent, and remote memory deficits, although their superficial features may be similar (e.g., poor retention on a long-term basis), and unless one examines all three, the likelihood of an erroneous classification is high.

A comprehensive memory assessment must also distinguish the storage of information from the retrieval of information. When asked to reproduce presented material, a patient may perform poorly. When cues are provided, however, such as multiple-choice questions about the presented material, a patient may answer most, or even all of these questions correctly. These correct answers would certainly suggest that the presented material was stored in some manner and that the patient's essential problem involves retrieval. A patient who has not stored information cannot retrieve it, but a patient who cannot retrieve information spontaneously has not necessarily failed to store it. Problems in storage are different from problems in retrieval and have different implications for differential diagnosis, treatment, management, and perhaps prognosis as regards activities of daily living.

Comprehensive memory testing must include not only verbal materials, but also visual materials. The patient with intact functioning in one of these two areas has more compensatory options open than the patient with both visual and verbal memory deficits. He or she may be able to learn to rely on the stronger modality or supplement the weaker modality with the stronger one. Further, failure to assess visual memory may result in the misreading or misinterpretation of clinically relevant cognitive and perceptual deficits. For example, a patient's disorientation may be partially due to severe impairments in visual memory, which make adjustment to new surroundings (e.g., the hospital setting) highly problematic.

Another section of a comprehensive memory test would compare memory for rote materials, such as a list of unrelated words, to memory for meaningful materials, such as sentences or narratives. Patients with left temporal abnormalities may have inordinate difficulties memorizing rote verbal materials but may perform at an average or near average level with conceptually based materials (Luria, 1980). With the latter types of materials, context, redundancy, or the potential for storing material as conceptual units may greatly facilitate recall. In contrast, many patients with mild frontal disorders perform normally with rote materials but have marked difficulties with conceptually based materials. The latter may provide a richer field for competing associations or may require a more organized approach, thereby bringing to the fore problems in self-regulation, difficulties resisting the pull of irrelevant associations, or difficulties maintaining or shifting psychologic sets.

Comprehensive assessments of memory functions will also cover incremental learning, or gains in retention following repeated presentations of materials. For example, the examiner may present a list of 15 unrelated words, assess the number of words retained after the first presentation, present the list again, and then again assess retention. The procedure can be repeated until the patient retains all of the words, or it can be terminated after a set number of presentations. Some patients will evidence very poor first-trial learning; that is, they will remember very little information after the first presentation of material. Following subsequent presentations, however, they may show substantial gains in retention, and perhaps by the third or fourth presentation they may retain as much, or nearly as much, as normal individuals. Such patients thus often benefit greatly from an additional repetition or two of information (the physician may wish to keep this fact in mind when explaining a medication schedule), and memory difficulties can often be bypassed in this manner. Other patients will

show normal or near normal retention following the first presentation of information but minimal gains over repeated trials. For example, a patient with frontal disorder and an associated deficit in planning may not utilize even the simplest naturally applied memory strategies for increasing retention following repeated exposure to material. On a second presentation of material, such a patient may fail to attend more closely to the material not initially retained or may fail to rehearse it. In such a case, the problem is not with memory per se; instead, it represents a failure to approach memory tasks with adequate plans. If intervention is implemented to improve memory, it thus must focus on these strategic shortcomings. Obviously, such an approach would be very different from that used with the patient who simply needs an additional presentation of material.

The above discussion shows the level of detail that might be required to achieve a thorough assessment of memory. It also suggests the contrast between this depth and the relatively superficial coverage provided by mental status examination. General intelligence tests, such as the WAIS, offer only indirect coverage of memory, on such items as the digit-symbol task or vocabulary. (For an excellent overall discussion of the assessment of memory and learning, although a critical one, see Mayes [1986].) The same can be said for other areas of functioning, which will be described in a more abbreviated form.

Motor and Sensorimotor Functions

In a comprehensive neuropsychologic examination, motor and sensorimotor functions may be covered in some detail. In the motor area, one wishes to examine speed and dexterity and, in particular, to compare right- and left-sided functioning. Many neuropsychologists will also examine what Luria (1973, 1980) has referred to as *kinetic melody*, or the ability to execute a series of shifting and sequential motor movements. For example, one might have the patient extend an arm and, at the same time, extend one finger, then two fingers, and then the whole hand. Such sequential and shifting movements are obviously pertinent to everyday tasks, such as writing. Sensorimotor functions may be examined by assessing for stereognosis, graphesthesia, or simultaneous discrimination of stimuli presented to both sides of the body simultaneously. It is in the examination of motor and sensorimotor functions that neuropsychologic examinations may most closely resemble neurologic examinations, although many of the techniques or procedures the neuropsychologist employs are standardized and yield quantitative scores.

Visual-Motor Functions

Visual-motor functions are typically examined through copying tasks and spontaneous drawing tasks. The advantage of using both is that the patient may perform well on one but not on the other. For example, on a spontaneous drawing task, patients may produce well-practiced or sparse objects that show no pathognomonic signs, but the same patients may show significant deficits on copying tasks. Abnormal results on visual-motor tasks are almost always nonspecific (Lezak, 1983) because functioning in this general area can be disrupted by a wide range of problems. In order to begin sorting out the factors underlying problem performance, the neuropsychologist might administer parallel tasks that place little or no demand on motor functions and instead stress visual analysis (e.g., the reproduction of designs using easily handled sticks) and parallel tasks that place little or no demand on visual analysis and instead stress motor requirements (e.g., tracing the presented figures).

Language Assessment

In the language area, at minimum, one wishes to asses naming, fluency, repetition, spontaneous speech, oral comprehension, grasp and production of grammatical structure, reading, writing to dictation, and writing spontaneously. Any one of these areas may be assessed in considerable detail. For example, seemingly simple problems in naming may be quite select and involve only certain categories or classes of words. There have been, for example, reports in the literature of very specific naming problems, such as in inability to name inanimate objects only, with intact naming of animate objects. A wide variety of problems can disrupt reading, including impaired visual scanning, impaired spatial analysis, problems forming visual-auditory associations, and various aphasic conditions.

Attention, Concentration, and Vigilance

Attention, concentration, and vigilance also demand detailed assessment. Attention, for example, is not a unitary function, and problems in this area may occur only for selective types of material. Problems include focusing on material, focusing on the most pertinent material, avoiding distraction, sustaining attention over time, and so on. A recent book titled *Varieties of Attention* (Parasuraman & Davies, 1984) discusses various types of attention and their neuropsychologic assessment.

Assessment of Higher Reasoning

The assessment of higher-level reasoning is a major importance. One wishes to determine whether the patient is able to think abstractly, to form concepts, and to generate and test plausible hypotheses. One wishes to assess these functions in both the verbal and nonverbal areas. For example, in the verbal area, one might examine the patient's capacity to form analogies, to define proverbs, and to draw inferences from written material. In the verbal and nonverbal areas, one might examine the capacity to execute a series of consecutive reasoning operations, to think inductively and deductively, and to form and maintain a complex set. As regards the last of these functions, for example, one might wish to determine whether the patient can perform alternating addition by threes and sixes, that is, 1–4–10–13–19, and so on. Not only is higher-level reasoning critical to many areas of everyday functioning, but because it is one of the most advanced and complex of the cognitive functions, it is often one of the first areas to be affected by disease processes.

Executive Functions

Finally, one wishes to examine self-regulation and planning, functions that are often disrupted by frontal disorders but also by a variety of other conditions (e.g., attention deficit disorder). Can the patient inhibit impulsive responses to prominent stimuli and instead deliberate before responding? Does the patient jump to impulsive conclusions in thinking? Does the patient act according to a plan, or does the patient's behavior quickly deteriorate into an essentially random sequence when all but the simplest requirements for action are presented? Assessment of self-regulation and planning shades into some of the areas already mentioned, such as higher-level reasoning, in part because it is a prerequisite for a wide range of intellectual functions.

Practical Use of the Neuropsychologic Test Results

The information obtained through neuropsychological assessment can be put to a number of uses, although not all of these uses are equally well served. Frequently results are used to make a determination, or to form a probability statement, regarding the presence of organically based brain impairment. Along these same lines, one can attempt to distinguish organic from functional disturbances in cognitive functioning. One can also attempt to localize brain damage.

How well does neuropsychologic assessment achieve these aims? More importantly, how well does neuropsychologic assessment compare with other means for detecting and localizing brain damage, such as the CT scan or other neuroinvestigative techniques? The answer depends on the presenting features of the patient, the type of neuropsychologic assessment that is performed, perhaps the skills of the examiner, and of course the accuracy of the competing methods that are available. Different variations of neuropsychologic batteries will be discussed later in this chapter. For now, we will briefly review some findings on the accuracy of one of the more popular batteries, the Halstead-Reitan.

The Halstead-Reitan is a standardized battery that has been researched widely. With certain types of patient populations, the Halstead-Reitan usually detects brain damage and infrequently misidentifies normal individuals as brain damaged. Most typically, studies involve patients who are shown to have brain damage through some independent technique (e.g., CT scan) and patients who are normal according to those techniques. Patients with equivocal findings are often dropped or eliminated from study. For example, a study might involve patients with left-hemisphere tumors and right-hemisphere tumors, who are compared with normal individuals. With such patient populations, "hit rates" at or exceeding 80 percent or even 90 percent are not uncommon. Attempts to determine localization are generally less successful. In these studies, the brain is usually divided into four quadrants: left anterior, left posterior, right anterior, right posterior. This is clearly a rather gross and somewhat arbitrary division, and it is thus rather disappointing that accuracy rates in many studies are not impressive. For example, it is not unusual for accuracy rates to fall at about 50 percent, although substantially higher and lower rates have been reported.

Attempts to distinguish brain-damaged individuals from individuals with purely psychiatric disturbance have met with mixed success, but in general, accuracy rates are lower than those achieved when comparing brain-damaged individuals to normals. Although some researchers have shown undoubted sophistication in work in this area, some of these studies, or the underlying rationale, could justifiably be considered naive. Individuals with psychiatric disturbance can show intellectual deficits, and among psychiatric patients there are undoubtedly a considerable percentage with CNS dysfunction. Any "clean" dichotomy between brain-damaged and psychiatric patients is thus a mistaken one, and one is left to question how these studies should come out: Does a clear separation between the two groups on neuropsychologic measures actually mean that these measures are committing many *false negative* errors in the psychiatric group? In some cases, however, it is helpful to know whether or not an individual has brain dysfunction.

A negative finding—a trustworthy demonstration that cognitive functioning is normal or that brain damage is not present—can be very useful, as well as reassuring to patients. On the other hand, a positive finding may be of little value. The most pressing questions, however, are often left unanswered: What is the impact on everyday functioning? Are intervention strategies available? What can be done to help the patient? What is the disease process that is present?

If the purpose of neuropsychologic assessment is limited to determining the presence or absence of brain damage alone, then the information derived from these tests, in most cases, is not being fully exploited. Neuropsychologic assessment is the best means available for precisely delineating and describing cognitive functioning in a comprehensive manner. The phrase *cognitive functioning*, rather than *organic dysfunction*, is used advisedly. In some cases, based on the cognitive profile, one may be able to draw relatively confident inferences about the presence or absence of brain damage and about localization. In many cases, however, especially if an initial assessment is being performed, one simply may not know the cause of the dysfunction. For example, the patient may present with a history of head injury, medication side effects, gross mood disorder, and a history of learning difficulties. With all of these potentially interacting factors, some of which may be transient and some of which may not, how often is it possible to make a definitive statement about what is causing what? However, knowing that dysfunction is present, describing it in detail, creating a baseline for future comparison, and drawing implications for patient management or treatment can be of great value. It is in the *description* of cognitive status and dysfunction that neuropsychologic assessment clearly has no peer. No matter the sophistication or thoroughness of the mental status examination performed, no matter what the EEG or CT scan shows, no matter how well one administers an intelligence test, a competently performed neuropsychologic assessment will add detail and depth of description.

The description of cognitive functioning produced by neuropsychologic assessment can be applied in a number of ways. First, the information may be used in treatment design and evaluation. For example, many cases of moderately severe memory disorder are not diagnosed prior to neuropsychologic assessment. Some of these patients have been receiving verbal individual psychotherapy, which must be of limited benefit because the patients cannot remember much from their sessions. There are also many cases in which patients with subtle language disorders that greatly impede oral comprehension are given complex verbal instructions by hospital staff or by family members, which result in poor compliance because of misunderstanding. In other cases, physicians explain complex medication schedules to patients with memory impairment. The result, of course, is likely to be noncompliance or, even worse, practices that endanger the patient's health. By knowing the patient's cognitive status in detail, the physician can make appropriate environmental and therapeutic adjustments. Within inpatient settings, staff may thus make it a point to simplify a patient's environment and provide frequent orienting information, a therapist may adjust the complexity of oral communications or decide to forego certain approaches entirely, or the family therapist may help family members better understand the patient's strengths and weaknesses and aid in the facilitation of effective communication.

Second, a detailed assessment of cognitive functions can help in the identification, specification, and evaluation of target symptoms. For example, suppose a patient has trouble on measures of continuous attention, and that the attentional difficulties interfere with performance on a wide variety of everyday tasks. If pharmacologic intervention is attempted, quantitative measures of attentional functions can be repeated once a therapeutic level of the drug has been established. To a great extent, these measures take the guesswork out of evaluating drug effects on the target symptom or symptoms, especially regarding functions, such as attention, that are hard to measure precisely without formal procedures. With a patient in the early stages of a dementing condition, one might try a pharmacologic intervention to improve memory functioning. Determination

of baseline neuropsychologic test performance for purposes of comparison of pretreatment and posttreatment functioning permits objective evaluation of the drug trial.

Neuropsychologic assessment can assist in determining the course of an illness affecting cognitive functioning over time and in this manner can assist in differential diagnosis. If a detailed baseline of cognitive functioning is established, retesting at a later date can provide much more exact information than would be available otherwise. Repeated neuropsychologic assessment may thus be used to follow the course of an individual who presents with equivocal cognitive complaints or findings that might or might not represent the early stages of a dementing condition. A steady downward curve in scores over time may provide the first hard evidence of a progressive disease process.

Variations in Approaches to Neuropsychologic Assessment

When one requests neuropsychologic consultation, the report that one receives varies with the psychologic consultant who performs the assessment and the particular procedures that are utilized. Four distinct approaches will be described.

The *quantitative* approach to neuropsychology emerged from a tradition sometimes referred to as "dustbowl empiricism." The intent was to develop measures sensitive to the cognitive and behavioral manifestations of brain dysfunction. Theoretical models were considered secondary. Empirical procedures were used to identify tests or test items that achieved maximal separation between brain-damaged and non-brain-damaged individuals, and among individuals with different forms of brain damage.

The Halstead-Reitan Battery

The prototypical, and arguably the most advanced, battery emerging from the quantitative approach is the Halstead-Reitan. Actually, there is no single Halstead-Reitan. Rather, the term encompasses three different batteries that are applied to individuals at different age levels. Each one of these batteries includes a number of tests, from which at least 26 variables are derived, plus an additional, rather gross screening test for language disorder and constructional disorder. Most practitioners will supplement the Halstead-Reitan with one of the Wechsler intelligence scales, and many practitioners add a number of further measures, such as measures to assess memory functions. For the adult version of the battery, one can compute an Impairment Index, based on 5 tests from which one derives 7 scores. The Impairment Index reflects the number of scores that fall within the impaired range. Typically, cutoffs are used to separate individuals into three groups: individuals likely to have brain damage, borderline cases, and individuals likely to be free of brain damage. As noted earlier, use of the Halstead-Reitan Impairment Index results in relatively high accuracy rates among certain patient groups. Excellent overall discussions and summaries of the battery are provided by Boll (1981) and by Reitan (1986).

One considerable strength of the Halstead-Reitan is that it provides precise, quantitative scores for all tests. As a result, it is relatively easy to compare the results of one patient with another, to compare different sets of results for one patient over time, and to conduct research on the battery. In fact, it is the most thoroughly researched battery in neuropsychology. Further, interpretation can be performed, in substantial part, by prespecified or standardized decision rules.

One obvious problem with Halstead-Reitan is that it does not adequately sample certain critical areas of cognitive functioning. For example, coverage of memory and higher-level reasoning is quite restricted. Another potential problem is tht the battery' is not tailored to particular referral questions or other case features. When the battery is not supplemented with other measures, every adult patient, for example, receives the identical set of tests. A 34-year-old referred to rule out brain damage will thus receive the same measures as a 71-year-old referred to obtain a more detailed understanding of memory dysfunction. A related problem is that very little information is available about the performance of special groups, such as the elderly, individuals of high intelligence, or individuals from disadvantaged sociocultural backgrounds. Most of the normative and validation studies have been conducted with individuals of middle age. It is thus unclear to what extent current empirically derived interpretive rules lose discriminating power with various special groups. Complex medical-psychiatric patients in particular have been insufficiently studied.

The Luria Approach

An approach to neuropsychologic assessment first described in detail by A. R. Luria stands in sharp contrast to the Halstead-Reitan and other quantitative approaches. Luria's approach emphasizes theory, observation, flexibility, and the clinical method, as opposed to quantification and standardization. Luria's approach is much too complicated to review in any detail here, and the interested reader should consult original sources (Luria, 1973, 1980).

Neuropsychologic assessment, as conducted from the Luria approach, is founded on a theory of brain-behavior relations. In essence, Luria's view is that, although specific brain areas are responsible for specific functions, virtually all meaningful cognitive activities are complex and require the integrated working of multiple brain areas. A

breakdown in any of the required components, therefore, can result in a breakdown
in the entire activity. For example, even a
simple activity, such as repeating a set of
digits, requires adequate comprehension of
the task, adequate auditory acuity and adequate auditory discrimination, the temporary storage of information, the transfer of
information to centers for motor encoding,
and so on. A deficiency in any one of these
functions, each of which has a corresponding or underlying brain area for its execu-
tion, can result in a disruption of the entire
activity. This disruption can appear the
same, superficially, regardless of which
particular component is deficient. For example, two patients who fail to repeat digits
correctly may make similar errors but do so
for completely different reasons.

Starting with this set of assumptions,
one first conducts a broad-based assessment to discover which, if any, complex
functions are disrupted. This is done primarily through a series of clinical tasks,
although some of the tasks may be fairly
structured and standardized. For example,
to assess various facets of memory, one
may use a set of tasks that covers the full
range of memory functions. If problems are
observed, the examiner proceeds to disen-
tangle, or isolate, the specific underlying
components that account for the manifest
difficulties. In the example of problems
with repeating digits, one would look at the
possible contributing factors one at a time.
If one hypothesized that the patient's failure might be due to difficulties in motor
encoding, one might simply have the patient read off a series of visually presented
digits. A failure to articulate these digits
properly would point toward motor encoding as one contributing factor. One proceeds in this manner, uncovering any general difficulties in cognitive functioning, and
then probing to determine underlying contributions or components. A great variety
of clinical tasks might be asked. In one
work, Luria (1980) describes scores, if not

hundreds, of such procedures. The ultimate
goal is the determination of the specific
areas of difficulty and their full range of
impact on cognitive or intellectual functioning.

One strength of the Luria approach is
its extreme flexibility in tailoring assessment to a patient's presentation and initial
performance. In fact, it is not unusual at all
for an examiner to literally invent procedures on the spot that allow information to
be obtained about specific questions raised
by ongoing results. Further, because assessment is based on a fairly well-devel-
oped theory of brain-behavior relationships, such innovations can be guided and
organized by theoretical postulates so that
they will not deteriorate into a shotgun
approach. Additionally, the derived information can be extremely rich and detailed
and is often related directly to everyday
functioning and remedial planning.

Among the potential shortcomings of
the Luria approach is that the usefulness of
accuracy of the assessment may be highly
dependent on the experience and skills of
the examiner. Although Luria may have
used this approach to great advantage, Luria was an exceptionally gifted individual.
Whether others, or how many others, can
achieve comparable results is uncertain. A
long and intensive period of training with
high-quality supervision is probably a minimal requirement for competency with the
approach.

The Lezak Approach

Lezak (1983) is a prominent advocate
of another approach to neuropsychologic
assessment, often referred to as the "flexible battery approach." Most neuropsychologists in practice utilize this approach to
assessment. The assessment method and
specific tests are tailored to the patient's
presenting characteristics and the nature of
the referral question. To the extent possible, however, standardized and validated
tests are used so that quantitative scores

can be derived. The examiner begins with a broad set of screening instruments, which are supplemented depending on the patient's presentation. Additions to the standard memory screen are made for a patient with an apparent decline in memory functioning and with subjective complaints about forgetfulness. Further, depending on the results of the initial screen, further testing of problematic areas is carried out. If standard, validated measures are not available, experimental, less-established tests are used. The reader should consult Lezak (1983) for a full description of the flexible battery approach.

Lezak provides a compelling rationale for the flexible battery approach, pointing out that it provides rich descriptive data that incorporate both qualitative and quantitative information and that it specifically addresses the question leading to the consultation. That many neuropsychologists use the flexible battery approach testifies to the positive perception of the method, but we currently do not know, or have not determined empirically, the extent to which these positive perceptions are truly warranted. There has been virtually no research on the flexible battery approach, and, in fact, it is fairly hard to imagine how many types of critical questions about it could even be subject to empirical test.

Process/Qualitative Approach

A final approach to neuropsychologic assessment is a process-oriented, or qualitative, approach, championed by Edith Kaplan. As described by Milberg, Hebben, and Kaplan (1986), this approach uses a core set of tests, but depending largely on the patient's presentation, additional tests are also used to attain greater clarity about specific problem areas and to cross-validate impressions or hypotheses derived from the core tests. Standard tests are commonly modified for use with cognitively impaired individuals, in order to provide more detailed information about the cognitive pro-

cesses underlying test performance. For example, after a test has been administered in standardized fashion, the same test might be repeated, allowing the patient extra time. Encouragement or cues might be provided to examine their effects upon performance and thereby achieve a greater in-depth understanding of the patient's disabilities and the potentially effective approaches to remediation and rehabilitation.

The process-qualitative approach is founded, in part, on traditions within psychology that have yielded noteworthy insights. For example, Jean Piaget, the famous developmentalist, became interested in the systematic patterns of reasoning underlying children's failures on standard test items. The approach also incorporates Werner's (1937) landmark work on cognitive development. This overall effort to incorporate findings from various areas of cognitive science and experimental neuropsychology predated, and in part created, the emerging emphasis on the cognitive neurosciences. As is the case with Luria's approach and the flexible battery approach, the process-qualitative approach has been subjected to little formal empirical testing. From this standpoint, the approach remains largely unproven, although it is often the procedure of choice in clinical settings.

Determination of Suitable Patients for Neuropsychologic Assessment and Procedures for Referral

Who should receive neuropsychologic assessment? Although virtually every patient seen by a psychiatrist deserves detailed mental status testing, not every patient is appropriate for neuropsychologic services. Referring patients on a routine basis is a disservice both to the patient and to the neuropsychologist. Aside from wasted time and expense, the patient may worry needlessly about the possibility of brain damage. Only patients with suspected or definite cognitive impairment for whom more exact detailed assessment is clinically relevant need to be referred.

Ideally the psychiatrist will use a sufficiently detailed and sensitive mental status examination or cognitive screening procedure to reliably rule out cognitive dysfunction. Unfortunately, typical items used on traditional mental status examinations, or by brief bedside screening tests, lack sensitivity, and even moderate deficits may go entirely undetected. For example, discrete right-hemisphere lesions that mainly affect contructional praxis are likely to be missed. A detailed review of bedside cognitive screening tests has been provided by Nelson, Fogel & Faust (1986).

Since bedside or office screening has many false negatives, the presenting problem and the history may indicate neuropsychologic assessment even if bedside screening shows no deficit. *Patients complaining of a decline in cognitive function almost always require neuropsychologic assessment.* For example, neuropsychologic assessment would be indicated for a patient with complaints of decreasing memory functions beyond normal changes with aging. A past history of injuries or diseases with significant CNS effects combined with a current behavioral problem is also a reason for referral. Patients with a history of moderate head injury, unexplained school failure, or an episode of encephalitis usually should be referred. Chronic drug or alcohol abuse is frequently associated with cognitive dysfunction; substance abusers often need neuropsychologic assessment to help plan therapy and rehabilitation. Patients with occupational exposure to toxic agents and current neuropsychiatric complaints should also be studied.

What findings on mental status examination should initiate referral? Detection of cognitive impairment on bedside mental status examination does not imply that a patient needs neuropsychologic assessment. If cognitive defects detected at the bedside are consistent with the patient's medical and psychiatric diagnoses and do not require further delineation or quantification for treatment planning, no further neuropsychologic testing is needed. Furthermore, patients should not be referred for neuropsychologic assessment when their status is rapidly fluctuating, as in drug withdrawal or delirium.

There is a right way and wrong way to make a referral to a neuropsychologist. The wrong way is not to provide any background information nor to specify in any way the questions of interest. As previously discussed, many neuropsychologists tailor assessment procedures to the features of the patient and to the referral question. Failure to specify the referral questions may thus place the neuropsychologist at a decided disadvantage. Further, if referral questions are stated explicitly, the neuropsychologist can alert the psychiatrist to potential circumstances that preclude satisfactory answers. A good referral might be something like the following: "68-year-old female, previously functioned very well in advanced executive position, but has shown dramatic decline in work performance over last year. Described by husband as very forgetful, overlooks important work details. Physical examination reveals several vegetative signs of depression and markedly depressed mood. Depression seems to have predated declining performance. Also scheduled for neurologic examination. Please provide baseline for future comparison, and impressions regarding dementia versus pseudodementia."

Identifying Appropriate Neuropsychologic Services

Currently, there are no restrictions on who can be called a neuropsychologist, although guidelines and regulations are likely to be forthcoming in the next few years. Some psychologists who indicate they offer neuropsychologic services may not specialize in this area. It is currently *not* unethical for them to do so. Formal fellowship training, publications in neuropsychology, and well-supervised experience distinguish the appropriately qualified neuropsychologist.

CONCLUSION

Neurologic and neuropsychologic investigations work best when used to test specific hypotheses. Further, soft data are most meaningful when they are corroborated by other data obtained independently. Even with adequate corroboration and the use of statistical criteria for abnormality of tests results, it may be difficult to establish a firm neuropsychiatric diagnosis on one single evaluation of a patient. The greatest resource of the clinician in this situation is reexamination of the patient at another time. Replicability of results after an interval supports their meaningfulness, and the presence or absence of progression may confirm or disconfirm a diagnostic hypothesis.

Even with the best testing procedures, psychiatric manifestations of organic illness may appear before tests of organic dysfunction turn positive. Reexamination after an interval sometimes reveals specific neurologic disease where it revealed nothing definite at the time of the psychiatric presentation. For this reason, it is important to avoid premature diagnostic closure. The psychiatrist should maintain an open mind about the etiology of the patient's illness and be prepared to reevaluate the patient neurologically should new symptoms develop or the treatment response be less than expected.

ACKNOWLEDGMENTS

Parts of Part I of this chapter were previously published as "Neurological Screening of Psychiatric Patients" in Extein I, Gold M (Eds) (1986). *Medical Mimics of Psychiatric Disorders.* Washington: APA Press. They are reprinted with the permission of the American Psychiatric Press, Inc.

REFERENCES

Ahokas A, Koskiniemi M-L, Vaheri A, (1985). Altered white cell count, protein concentration, and oligoclonal IgG bands in the cerebrospinal fluid of many patients with acute psychiatric disorders. *Neuropsychobiology*, *14*, 1–4.

Ajmone-Marsa C & Zivin LS (1970). Factors related to the occurrence of typical paroxysmal abnormalities in the EEG records of epileptic patients. *Epilepsia*, *11*, 361–381.

Alarcon RD & Thweatt RW. (1983). A case of subdural hematoma mimicking severe depression with conversion-like symptoms. *American Journal of Psychiatry*, *140*, 1360–1361.

Arne-bes MC, Calvet U, Thiberge M, (1982). Effects of sleep deprivation in an EEG study of epileptics. In MB Sterman, MN Shouse, P Passouant, (Eds), *Sleep and epilepsy*. New York: Academic Press.

Baker HL, Berquist TH, Kispert DB, (1985). Magnetic resonance imaging in a routine clinical setting. *Mayo Clinic Proceedings*, *60*(2), 75–90.

Baldessarini RJ, Cole JO, Davis JM, (1979). *Tardive dyskinesia* (Task Force Report 18, pp 177–199. Washington: American Psychiatric Assoc.

Ballenger CE, King DW, Gallagher BB. (1983). Partial complex status epilepticus. *Neurology*, *33*, 1545–1552.

Becker PM, Feussner JR, Mulrow CD, (1985). The role of lumbar puncture in the evaluation of dementia: The Durham Veterans Administration/Duke University Study. *Journal of the American Geriatrics Society*, *33*(6), 392–396.

Bentson J, Reza M, Winter J, (1978). Steroids and apparent cerebral atrophy on computed tomography scans. *Journal of Computer Assisted Tomography*, *2*, 16–23.

Blackwood DHR, St Clair DM, & Kutcher SP. (1986).

P300 event-related potential abnormalities in borderline personality disorder. *Biological Psychiatry*, *21*, 557–560.

Boll TJ. (1981). The Halstead-Reitan Neuropsychological Battery. In SB Filskov and TJ Boll (Eds), *Handbook of clinical neuropsychology* (pp 577–607). New York: John Wiley & Sons.

Borson S. (1982). Behcet's disease as a psychiatric disorder: A case report. *American Journal of Psychiatry*, *139* 1348–1349.

Brant-Zawadski M, Fein G, Van Dyke C, (1985). MR imaging of the aging brain: Patchy white-matter lesions and dementia. *American Journal of Neuroradiology*, *6*, 675–682.

Bresnahan B. (1982). CNS Lupus. *Clinics in Rheumatic Disease*, *8*, 183–195.

Brizer DA & Manning DW. (1982). Delirium induced by poisoning with anticholinergic agents. *American Journal of Psychiatry*, *139*, 1343–1344.

Cala LA, Jones B, Burnes P, (1983). Results of computerized tomography, psychometric testing, and dietary studies in social drinkers with emphasis on reversibility with abstinence. *Medical Journal of Australia*, *2*, 264.

Campbell DR, Skikne BS, & Cook JD. (1986). Cerebrospinal fluid ferritin levels in screening for meningism. *Archives of Neurology*, *43*(12), 1257–1263.

Caroscio JT, Kochwa S, Sacks H, (1986). Quantitative cerebrospinal fluid IgG measurements as a marker of disease activity in multiple sclerosis. *Archives of Neurology*, *43*(11), 1129–1137.

Celesia GG. (1986). EEG and event-related potentials in aging and dementia. *Journal of Clinical Neurophysiology*, *3*(2), 99–112.

Chiappa KH & Young RR. (1985). Evoked responses overused, underused, or misused? *Archives of Neurology*, *42*(1), 76–77.

Chu NS. (1985). Computed tomographic correlates of auditory brain stem responses in alcoholics. *Journal of Neurology, Neurosurgery, and Psychiatry*, *48*(4), 348–353.

Coben LA, Danziger W, & Storandt M. (1985). A longitudinal EEG study of mild senile dementia of the Alzheimer type: Changes at one year and at 2.5 years. *Electroencephalography and Clinical Neurophysiology 61*, 101–112.

Cornelius JR, Brenner RP, Soloff PH. (1986). EEG abnormalities in borderline personality disorder: Specific or non-specific. *Biological Psychiatry*, *21*, 977–980.

Cowdry RW, Pickar D, & Davies R. (1985–86). Symptoms and EEG findings in the borderline syndrome. *International Journal of Psychiatry in Medicine*, *15*(3), 201–211.

Cummings JL, Gosenfield LF, Houlihan JP, (1983). Neuropsychiatric disturbances associated with

the ideopathic calcification of the basal ganglia. *Biological Psychiatry*, *18*, 591–601.

D'Alessandro R, Benassi G, Cristina E, (1986). The prevalence of lingual-facial-buccal dyskinesias in the elderly. *Neurology*, *36*, 1350–1351.

Declerck AC, Sijben-Kiggen R, Wauquier A, (1982). Diagnosis of epilepsy with the aid of sleep methodology: Evaluation of 1,163 cases. In MB Sterman, MN Shouse, P Passouant (Eds), *Sleep and epilepsy*. New York: Academic Press.

DiChiro G. (1985). Magnetic resonance imaging: A time for assessment. *Mayo Clinic Proceedings*, *60* (2), 135–136.

Driver MV & McGillivray BB. (1982). Electroencephalography. In J Laidlaw, A Richens (Eds), *A textbook of epilepsy* (2nd ed). New York: Churchill Livingstone.

Drury I, Klass DW, Westmoreland BF, (1985). An acute syndrome with psychotic symptoms and EEG abnormality. *Neurology*, *35*(6), 911–4.

Duara R, Grady C, Haxby J, (1984) Human brain glucose utilization and cognitive function in relation to age. *Annals of Neurology*, *16*(6), 703–713.

Dubin WR, Weiss KJ, Zeccardi JA. (1983). Organic brain syndrome: A psychiatric imposter. *Journal of the American Medical Association*, *249*, 60–62.

Duffy FH (1985). The BEAM method of neurophysiological diagnosis. *Annals of the New York Academy of Sciences*, *457*, 19–34.

Ebersole JS & Bridgers SL. (1985). Direct comparison of 3- and 8-channel ambulatory cassette EEG with intensive inpatient monitoring. *Neurology 35*, 846–854.

Ebersole JS & Leroy RF. (1983). An evaluation of ambulatory, cassette EEG monitoring: 2. Detection of interictal abnormalities. *Neurology*, *33*(1), 8–18.

Ebner A, Haas JC, Lucking CH, (1986). Event-related brain potentials (P300) and neuropsychological deficit in patients with focal brain lesions. *Neuroscience Letters*, *64*, 330–334.

Elliott TR & Walsh FM. (1925). The Babinski or extensor form of plantar response in toxic states, apart from organic disease of the pyramidal tract or systems. *Lancet*, *1*, 65–68.

Engel J, Driver MV, & Falconer MA. (1975). Electrophysiological correlates of pathology and surgical results in temporal lobe epilepsy. *Brain*, *98*, 129.

Epstein BS, Epstein JA, Postel DM. (1971). Tumors of the spinal cord simulating psychiatric disorders. *Diseases of the Nervous System*, *32*, 742–743.

Evans DL, Edelsohn GA, Golden RN. (1983). Organic psychoses without anemia or spinal cord symptoms in patients with vitamin B_{12} deficiency. *American Journal of Psychiatry*, *140*, 218–221.

Fariello RG, Booker HE, Chun RWM, et al. (1983).

Reenactment of the triggering situations for the diagnosis of epilepsy. *Neurology*, 33, 878–884.

Farrell MJ. (1941). Influence of locomotion on the plantar reflex in normal and physically and mentally inferior persons. *Archives of Neurology*, 46, 22–230.

Folstein MF, Folstein SE, & McHugh PR. (1975). Mini-Mental State. *Journal of Psychiatric, Research*, 12, 189–198.

Fowler CJ & Harrison MJG. (1986). EEG changes in subcortical dementia: A study of 22 patients with Steele-Richardson-Olszewsky (SRO) Syndrome. *Electroencephalography and Clinical Neurophysiology*, 64, 301–303.

Frackowiak RSJ. (1986). An introduction to positron tomography and its application to clinical investigation. In MR Trimble (Ed), *New brain imaging techniques and psychopharmacology*. Oxford: Oxford University Press.

Friedland RP, Budinger TF, Brant-Zawadski M, (1984). The diagnosis of Alzheimer-type dementia: Positron emission tomography verus NMR. *Journal of the American Medical Association*, 252(19), 2750–2752.

Gabarski SS, Gabrielsen TO, & Gilman S. (1985). The initial diagnosis of multiple sclerosis: Clinical impact of magnetic resonance imaging. *Annals of Neurology*, 17, 469–474.

Gado MH & Press GA. (1986). Computed tomography in the diagnosis of dementia. *Geriatric Medicine Today*, 5(7), 47–73.

Gasser T, Bacher P, & Steinberg H. (1985). Test/retest reliability of spectral parameters of the EEG. *Electroencephalography and Clinical Neurophysiology*, 60(4), 312–319.

Gibb WRG. (1984). Current practice of diagnostic lumbar puncture. *British Medical Journal*, 289, 530.

Gilliland BC & Mannik M. (1983). Reiter's syndrome, psoriatic arthritis, arthritis associated with gastrointestinal diseases, and Behret's syndrome. In RG Petersdorf (Eds), *Harrison's principles of internal medicine* (10th ed). New York: McGraw-Hill, pp 1992–1994.

Griffith JF & Ch'ien LT. (1983). Herpes simplex virus encephalitis: Diagnostic and treatment considerations. *Medical Clinics of North America*, 67, 991–1008.

Griffith JF & Ch'ien LT. (1984). Viral infections of the central nervous system. In GJ Galasso, TC Merigan, RA Buchanan (Eds), *Antiviral agents and viral diseases of man*. New York: Raven Press.

Guarino JR. (1982). Auscultatory percussion of the head. *British Medical Journal of Clinical Research*, 284, 1075–1077.

Gumnit RJ. (1986). Intensive neurodiagnostic monitoring: Role in the treatment of seizures. *Neurology*, 36, 1340–1346.

Haggerty JG, Evans DL, & Prang EHA. (1986). Organic brain syndrome associated with marginal hypothyroidism. *American Jounal of Psychiatry*, 143(6), 785–786.

Hamilton NG, Frick RB, Takahashi T, et al. (1983). Psychiatric symptoms in cerebellar pathology. *American Journal of Psychiatry*, 140, 1322–1326.

Hammerstrom DC & Zimmer B. (1985). The role of lumbar puncture in the evaluation of dementia: The University of Pittsburgh Study. *Journal of the American Geriatrics Society*, 33(6), 397–400.

Harper CG, Giles M, & Finlay-Jones R. (1986). Clinical science in the Wernicke-Korsakoff complex role in a retrospective analysis of 131 cases diagnosed in necropsy. *Journal of Neurology, Neurosurgery, and Psychiatry*, 49, 341–345.

Haxby JV, Grady CL, Duara R, (1986). Neocortical metabolic abnormalities precede non-memory cognitive defects in early Alzheimer's-type dementia. *Archives of Neurology*, 43, 882–885.

Heinz E, Martinex J, & Hawnggeli A. (1977). Reversibility of cerebral atrophy in anorexia nervosa and Cushing's syndrome. *Journal of Computer Assisted Tomography*, 1, 415–418.

Howard JE & Dorfman LJ. (1986). Evoked potentials in hysteria and malingering. *Journal of Clinical Neurophysiology*, 3(1), 39–50.

Jacobs L & Glassman MD. (1980). Three primitive reflexes in normal adults. *Neurology*, 30, 184–188.

Jacobs L, Kinkel WR, Polachini I, & Kinkel RP. (1986). Correlations of nuclear magnetic resonance imaging, computerized tomography, and clinical profiles in multiple sclerosis. *Neurology*, 36, 27–34.

Jagust WJ, Friedland RP, & Budinger TF. (1985). PET with [18F] fluorodeoxyglucose differentiates normal pressure hydrocephalus from Alzheimer-type dementia. *Journal of Neurology, Neurosurgery, and Psychiatry*, 48(11), 1091–1096.

Jenkyn LR, Walsh DB, Culver CM, et al. (1977). Clinical signs of diffuse cerebral dysfunction. *Journal of Neurology, Neurosurgery, and Psychiatry*, 40, 956–966.

Kellner CHR, Davenport MSW, Post RM, et al. (1983). Rapidly cycling bipolar disorder in multiple sclerosis. *American Journal of Psychiatry*, 141, 112–113.

Kiloh LG, McComas AJ, Osselton JW, (1981). The values and limitations of electroencephalography. In *Clinical electroencephalography* (4th ed). London: Butterworths & Co.

Kraiuhin C, Gordon E, Meares R, (1986). Psychometrics vs ERPs in the diagnosis of dementia. *Journal of Gerontology*, 41(2), 154–162.

Kuhl DE, Phelps ME, Markham CH, (1982). Cerebral

metabolism and atrophy in Huntington's disease determined by [18]FDG and computed tomographic scan. *Annals of Neurology, 12,* 425–434.

Langfitt TW, Obrist WD, Alavi A, et al. (1986). CT, MRI, and PET in the study of brain trauma. *Journal of Neurosurgery, 64*(5), 760–767.

Laster DW, Penry JK, Moody DM, (1985). Chronic seizure disorders: Contribution of MR imaging when CT is normal. *American Journal of Neurological Research, 6,* 177–180.

Lee SH, Kieffer SA, & Montoya JH. (1983). Pitfalls and limitations of CT in neurodiagnosis. In SH Lee & KCVG Rao (Eds), *Cranial computed tomography.* New York: McGraw-Hill.

Lesser RP, Modic MT, Weinstein MA, (1986). Magnetic resonance imaging (1.5 Telsa) in patients with intractable seizures. *Archives of Neurology, 43,* 367–371.

Levin HS, Madison CF, Bailey CB, et al. (1983). Mutism after closed-head injury. *Archives of Neurology, 40,* 601–606.

Levin R, Leaton EM, & Lee SI. (1986). The value of nasopharyngeal recording in psychiatric patients. *Biological Psychiatry,* 21, 1236–1238.

Lezak MD. (1983). *Neuropsychological assessment.* (2nd ed). New York: Oxford University Press.

Luria AR. (1973). *The working brain* (B Haigh, Trans). New York: Basic Books.

Luria AR. (1980). *Higher cortical functions in man* (2nd ed, B Haigh, Trans). New York: Basic Books.

Margulis AR & Amparo E. (1985). Magnetic resonance imaging in clinical practice. *Postgraduate Medicine, 78*(5), 127–132.

Markand ON. (1984). Electroencephalography in diffuse encephalopathies. *Journal of Clinical Neurophysiology, 1*(4), 357–407.

Marks IM & Kettl PA. (1986). Neurological factors in obsessive-compulsive disorder. *British Journal of Psychiatry, 149,* 315–319.

Martin MJ. (1983). Brief review of organic diseases masquerading as functional illness. *Hospital and Community Psychiatry, 34,* 328–332.

Martin WRW. (1985). Positron emission tomography in movement disorders. *Canadian Journal of Neurological Sciences,* 12, 6–10.

Massey EW & Scherokman B. (1981). Soft neurologic signs. *Postgraduate Medicine,* 70, 66–67.

Mattis S. (1976). Mental status examination for organic mental syndromes in the elderly patient. In L Bellak & TE Karasu (Eds), *Geriatric psychiatry.* New York: Grune & Stratton.

Mayes, AR. (1986). Learning and memory disorders and their assessment. *Neuropsychologia, 24,* 25–39.

Maziere B, Comar D, & Maziere M. (1986). Pharmacokinetic studies using positron emission tomography. In MR Trimble (Ed), *New brain imaging techniques and psychopharmacology.* Oxford: Oxford University Press.

McEvoy JP & Lohr JB. (1984). Diazepam for catatonia. *American Journal of Psychiatry, 141,* 284–285.

McGinnis MR. (1985). Detection of fungi in cerebrospinal fluid. *American Journal of Medicine, 75,* 129–138.

Meary D, Snowden JS, Bowen DM, (1986). Neuropsychological syndromes in presenile dementia due to cerebral atrophy. *Journal of Neurology, Neurosurgery, and Psychiatry, 49,* 163–174.

Milberg WP, Hebben N, & Kaplan E. (1986). The Boston process approach to neuropsychological assessment. In I Grant & KA Adams (Eds), *Neuropsychological assessment and neuropschiatric disorders* (pp. 65–86). New York: Oxford University Press.

Munetz MR & Schulz SC. (1986). Screening for tardive dyskinesia. *Journal of Clinical Psychiatry, 47,* 75–77.

Naeser MA. (1985). Quantitative approaches to computerized tomography in behavioral neurology. In MM Mesulam (Ed), *Principles of behavioral neurology.* Philadelphia: FA David.

Nelson A, Fogel B, & Faust D. (1986). Bedside cognitive screening instruments: A critical assessment. *Journal of Nervous and Mental Disorders, 174*(2), 73–83.

Nolfe G & Giaquinto S. (1986). The EEG and the normal elderly: A contribution to the interpretation of aging and dementia. *Electroencephalography and Clinical Neurophysiology, 63,* 540–546.

Okuno T, Masatoshi I, Konishi Y, (1980). Cerebral atrophy following ACTH therapy. *Journal of Computer Assisted Tomograpy, 4,* 20–23.

Oommen KJ, Johnson PC, Ray, CG. (1982). Herpes simplex type II virus encephalitis presenting as psychosis. *American Journal of Medicine, 73*(3), 445–448.

Pandurangi AK, Dewan MJ, Boucher M, (1986). A comprehensive study of chronic schizophrenic patients: 2. Biological, neuropsychological, and clinical correlates of CT abnormality. *Acta Psychiatrica Scandinavica, 73*(2), 161–171.

Parasuraman R & Davies DR. (1984). *Varieties of attention.* New York: Academic Press.

Peroutka SJ. (1982). Hallucinations and delusions following a right temporoparietal occipital infarction. *Johns Hopkins Medical Journal, 151,* 181–185.

Petersdorf RG, Adams RD, Braunwald E, (1983). *Harrison's principles of internal medicine* (10th ed). New York: McGraw-Hill.

Peterson LG & Perl M. (1982). Psychiatric presentations of cancer. *Psychosomatics*, 23, 601–604.

Reitan RM. (1985). Relationships between measures of brain functions and general intelligence. *Journal of Clinical Psychology*, 41, 245–253.

Reitan RM. (1986). Theoretical and methodological bases of the Halstead-Reitan Neuropsychological Battery. In I Grant & KM Adams (Eds), *Neuropsychological assessment of neuropsychiatric disorders*, (pp 3–30) New York: Oxford University Press.

Reulen JPH, Sanders ACM, Hogerhuis LAH. (1983). Eye movement disorders in multiple sclerosis and optic neuritis. *Brain*, 106, 121–140.

Rimel RW & Tyson GW. (1979). The neurologic examination in patients with a central nervous system trauma. *Journal of Neurosurgical Nursing*, 11, 148–155.

Robins PV. (1983). Reversible dementia in the misdiagnosis of dementia: A review. *Hospital and Community Psychiatry*, 34, 830–835.

Rodnan GP & Schumacher HR (Eds). (1983). *Primer on the rheumatic diseases* (8th ed). Atlanta: Arthritis Foundation.

Sheldon JJ, Siddharthan R, Tobia J, (1985). Magnetic resonance imaging of multiple sclerosis: A comparison with clinical and CT examinations in 74 patients. *American Journal of Roentgenology*, 145(5), 957–964.

Shinar D, Gross CR, Mohr JP, (1985). Inter-observer variability in the assessment of neurological history and examination in the Stroke Data Bank. *Archives of Neurology*, 42(6), 557–565.

Shraberg D & D'Souza T. (1982). Coma vigil masquerading as psychiatric diagnosis. *Journal of Clinical Psychiatry*, 43, 375–376.

Sindic CJ, Kevers L, Chalon MP, et al. (1985). Monitoring and tentative diagnosis of herpetic encephalitis by protein analysis of cerebrospinal fluid. Particular relevance of the assays of ferritin and S-100. *Journal of Neurological Science*, 67(3), 359–369.

Sotaniemi KA (1983). Cerebral outcome after extracorporeal circulation. *Archives of Neurology*, 40, 75–77.

Spencer SS, Williamson PD, Bridger SL, (1985). Reliability and accuracy of localization by scalp ictal EEG. *Neurology*, 35(11), 1567–1575.

Sperling MR, Wilson G, Engel J, (1986). Magnetic resonance imaging in intractable partial epilepsy: Correlative studies. *Annals of Neurology*, 20, 57–62.

Stahl SM. (1985). Can CSF measures distinguish among schizophrenia, depression, movement disorders, and dementia? *Psychopharmology Bulletin*, 21(3), 396–399.

Stockard JJ & Iragui VJ. (1984). Clinically useful application of evoked potentials in adult neurology. *Journal of Clinical Neurophysiology*, 1(2), 159–202.

Strauss I & Keshner M. (1935). Mental symptoms in cases of tumor of the frontal lobe. *Archives of Neurologicy and Psychiatry*, 33, 986–1005.

Sudarsky L & Ronthal M. (1983). Gait disorders among elderly patients. *Archives of Neurology*, 40, 740–743.

Tarter, Hegedus AM, Van Thiel DH, & Schade RR. (1985). Portal-systemic encephalopathy: Neuropsychiatric manifestations. *International Journal of Psychiatry in Medicine*, 15(3), 265–275.

TerPogossian MM. (1985). PET, SPECT, and NMRI: Competing or complementary disciplines? *Journal of Nuclear Medicine*, 26(12), 1487–98.

Tippin J & Dunner FJ. (1981). Biparietal infarction in a patient with catatonia. *American Journal of Psychiatry*, 138, 1386–1287.

Trzepacz PT, Maue FR, Coffman G, (1986). Neuropsychiatric assessment of liver transplantation candidates: Delirium and other psychiatric disorders. *International Journal of Psychiatry in Medicine*, 16(2), 101–111.

Visser SL, Van Tilburg W, Hooijer C, (1985). Visual evoked potentials in senile dementia (Alzheimer type) and in non-organic behavior disorders in the elderly; comparison with EEG parameters. *Electroencephalography and Clinical Neurophysiology*, 60(2), 115–121.

Walker WR. (1982). Phenothiazine therapy in latent organic brain syndrome. *Psychosomatics*, 23, 962–968.

Warrington EK, James M, & Maciejewski C. (1986). The WAIS as a lateralizing and localizing diagnostic instrument: A study of 656 patients with unilateral cerebral lesions. *Neuropsychologia*, 24, 223–239.

Werner H. (1937). Process and achievement: A basic problem of education and developmental psychology. *Harvard Educational Review*, 7 350–368.

Wolfson LI & Katzman R. (1983). The neurologic consultation at age 80. In R Katzman, RD Terry (Eds). *The Neurology of Aging*. Philadelphia: FA David.

Wright BE & Henkind P. (1983). Aging changes and the eye. In R Katzman, RD Terry (Eds), *The Neurology of Aging*. Philadelphia: FA Davis.

Yik KY, Sullivan SN, & Troster M. (1982). Neuropsychiatric disturbance due to occult occlusion of the parietal vein. *Canadian Medical Association Journal*, 126, 50–52.

Zeitlhofer J, Brainin M, & Reisner T. (1984). Brain stem auditory evoked responses in tardive dyskinesia. *Journal of Neurology*, 231(5), 266–268.

Alan Stoudemire
Barry S. Fogel

4
Psychopharmacology in the Medically Ill

Medically ill patients may often benefit markedly from the use of psychopharmacologic agents. Implementation of psychoactive drug therapy in the medically ill, however, may be complicated for a number of reasons. Psychotropic drugs may interact with underlying medical illness, causing serious complications, as when tricyclic antidepressants exacerbate heart block. Metabolic abnormalities associated with physical illness may increase the chances of drug toxicity because of altered pharmacokinetics, as when lithium is used in patients with renal insufficiency. Since medical patients are likely to be taking other, nonpsychotropic medications, the likelihood of a clinically significant drug interaction is increased. Finally, the elderly medically ill patient is at high risk for adverse central nervous system (CNS) effects of psychotropic agents, particularly delirium. This chapter will review the basic psychopharmacologic principles that should be considered in using psychotropic agents in the medically ill. Individual specialty chapters in this volume will develop these psycho-

pharmacologic considerations in greater detail.

CYCLIC ANTIDEPRESSANTS

One of the primary concerns in using cyclic antidepressants (CyAD) in medically ill patients is the possible precipitation or exacerbation of cardiovascular complications. However, absolute cardiovascular contraindications to the use of CyAD are few, and outside of the known high-risk groups, the risks are small. For example, the Boston Collaborative Drug Surveillance Program found no evidence that tricyclics caused arrhythmias or sudden death (Boston Collaborative Drug Surveillance Program, 1972). While they are relatively safe when used appropriately, the CyAD may cause serious toxicity in excessive dosage and in deliberate overdosage.

Excessive fear of complications in patient groups not actually at high risk for severe cardiovascular complications may partially explain why seriously depressed medically ill patients may receive no antidepressant drug treatment or treatment at inadequate doses. In fact, the majority of patients with cardiovascular disease can safely be treated with CyAD if appropriate consideration is given to careful pretreatment evaluation and drug monitoring.

Cardiovascular Effects of Tricyclic Antidepressants

Standard tricyclic antidepressants such as imipramine and amitriptyline have quinidine-like effects on the electrocardiogram (ECG). They produce an increase in the PR interval, QRS duration, and QT_c time as well as T-wave flattening. Clinically significant lengthening of the PR, QRS, and QT intervals, may imply plasma levels above the normal range (RC Smith, Chojnacki, Hu, et al., 1980). Clinically relevant effects on conduction time at therapeutic dosage levels are observed primarily in patients with preexisting, usually advanced, conduction problems, such as atrioventricular (AV) nodal block. Even in patients with first-degree block quinidine-like actions of tricyclics at therapeutic doses may be minor and need not impede treatment. For example, a prospective study compared 150 depressed patients with normal ECGs and 41 depressed patients with first-degree AV and/or bundle branch block treated for depression with imipramine or nortriptyline. The likelihood of second-degree AV block developing during treatment was greater in patients with preexisting bundle branch block (defined as a QRS interval greater than .11 sec) than in patients with normal ECGs (9 percent versus 0.7 percent); more than 90 percent of patients with preexisting conduction disease, however, did not develop second-degree heart block (Roose, Glassman, Giardina, et al., 1987).

In patients with *pre-existing* bundle branch block (especially second-degree heart block), dissociative (third-degree) AV heart block may develop. If type I antiar-rhythmic medications (quinidine, disopyramide, procainamide) are concurrently being administered with tricyclics, additive effects on conduction may be observed (Levenson, 1985). Administration of these agents with tricyclics in patients with conduction disease may be hazardous. Frequent monitoring of drug levels and EKG's is a helpful precaution. The quinidine-like effect of imipramine can be sufficiently antiarrhythmic in some patients that the tricyclic alone may suffice to suppress premature ventricular contractions (AH Glassman & Bigger, 1981; Veith, 1982).

Right bundle branch block may be seen as part of underlying cardiovascular disease, but is not in itself a contraindication for CyAD treatment; also, left bundle branch block usually implies some degree of ischemic or hypertensive heart disease. When treating patients with these conduction defects, the psychiatrist and cardiologist should jointly establish a schedule for monitoring cardiac effects when CyAD treatment is to be pursued. In our experience, *asymptomatic* patients with right bundle branch block, isolated left anterior fascicular block, and left posterior fascicular block can be treated if dosages are increased gradually and ECGs obtained following each increase. Inpatient dosing is advisable.

Frail elderly patients and patients with *symptomatic* conduction defects should begin tricyclics in the hospital. Patients with bifascicular or trifascicular block are at high risk for bradyarrhythmias and Stokes-Adams attacks. These patients, and patients with chronic bifascicular block associated with syncopal attacks should not be treated with CyAD unless a pacemaker is implanted first.

Although asymptomatic first-degree heart block, right bundle branch block, and focal fascicular blocks are not absolute contraindications to tricyclics, these same defects contraindicate CyAD therapy if they produce syncopal attacks. When they do, patients usually require pacemaker insertion first if CyAD are to be used. The presence of symptoms is crucial.

Myocardial Infarction

In patients with uncomplicated myocardial infarction (MI), institution or reinstitution of cyclic antidepressant therapy is noncontroversial after a 6-week waiting period; in the absence of complications such as heart block or orthostatic hypotension CyAD can be begun sooner. If the depression is life threatening, however, early treatment may be justifiable. Data are lacking to determine a lower time limit for *re*starting tricyclics following uncomplicated myocardial infarction in patients who have previously done well on them. Dialogue between the psychiatrist and the cardiologist should address the patient's particular psychiatric and cardiac vulnerabilities. CyAD may have a mild negative inotropic effect that is usually clinically insignificant in stable congestive heart failure (CHF), but may destabilize marginally compensated patients. Patients with CHF or arrhythmias not yet stabilized by treatment therefore probably should not receive CyAD.

Prolonged QT Syndromes

As mentioned above, one of the quinidine-like effects CyAD on the electrocardiogram is a prolongation of the QT interval. Significant prolongation of the QT interval may be associated with an increased risk of ventricular tachycardia and ventricular fibrillation, particularly in patients with congenital or acquired heart disease. The QT interval ordinarily varies with heart rate, so that guidelines for CyAD use are best based on the *corrected* QT interval, QT_c, which is defined as the actual QT interval divided by the square root of the R-R interval. The upper limit of normal for QT_c is .42 seconds for men and .43 seconds for women (Lipman, Dunn, & Massie 1984).

Patients who have had myocardial infarction with persistently prolonged QT intervals are at relatively higher risk for subsequent fatal ventricular fibrillation. Since the standard tricyclics may further prolong the QT_c interval, ECGs following each dosage increase should be obtained if QT_c lengthening is a possibility. An upper bound for QT_c should be established in consultation with the cardiologist. We use a QTc of 0.45 second is used as a guideline. Despite these concerns, there are no empirical studies that report increased mortality or increased ventricular arrhythmias in post-MI patients treated with tricyclics (JM Smith & Baldessarini, 1980).

Other Effects on Cardiac Conduction

Individual CyAD may differ in their effects on cardiac conduction. One study found that the QRS interval tended to be prolonged by maprotiline but was *decreased* by doxepin (Ahles, Swirtsman, Halaris, et al., 1984). Furthermore, in this same report doxepin did not appear to suppress premature ventricular contractions (PVCs), suggesting it has weaker quinidine-like effects than imipramine (Ahles et al., 1984). Earlier reports of doxepin's superior safety margin in cardiac disease in studies such as this, however, have been appropriately criticized because doxepin blood levels may have been subtherapeutic (Burrows, 1977; Luchins, 1983).

Trazodone initially appeared not to promote cardiac arrhythmias in animals and in humans free of heart disease (Himmelhoch, 1981). Subsequent case reports, however, have described complete heart block (Rausch, 1984), aggravation of ventricular arrhythmias (D Janowsky, 1983), and development of first-degree heart block (Irwin & Spar, 1983). Cardiovascular complications from trazodone are nevertheless rare, even in overdoses (Richelson, 1984).

A recent report comparing trazodone, imipramine, and placebo in elderly depressed patients found no significant group differences in PR, QRS, and QT intervals (Hayes, 1983). Of 21 patients on imipramine, however, 5 developed tachycardia and 1 developed atrial fibrillation; 3 developed intraventricular conduction defects and 1 developed first-degree AV block. These events did not occur in the patients given trazodone or placebo. The relative cardiovascular safety of trazodone in the elderly is mitigated by the fact that trazodone may be heavily sedating in elderly patients, and by the perception by some authorities that its antidepressant potency is less than that of standard tricyclic agents (Rudorfer, Golden, & Potter, 1984).

Despite the safety of CyAD in the vast majority of patients without preexisting cardiac disease, malignant ventricular arrhythmias do occur rarely as a complication of CyAD treatment (Fowler, McCall, Chou, et al., 1976; Krikler & Curry, 1976). Two groups of patients at risk are patients with preexisting QT interval prolongation (congenital long QT syndrome) and patients who develop undue QT interval prolongation during antidepressant treatment (acquired QT syndrome) Flugelman, Tal, Pollack, et al., 1985). As noted above a QT_c of 0.45 second is regarded by some cardiologists as an acceptable upper limit of QT prolongation. We would recommend, however, the setting of a criterion for each individual case in consultation with a cardiologist. CyAD would be avoided or discontinued if the QT_c exceeded the selected criterion.

Therefore, in evaluating cardiac patients with depression, particularly patients with a history of cardiac arrhythmias, special attention should be given to considering whether or not a quinidine-like effect would aggravate heart block or increase vulnerability to ventricular tachycardia–ventricular fibrillation. Lengthening of the QT interval by a cyclic antidepressant could contribute to dysrhythmia, since if the QT interval corrected for rate (QT_c) is longer than 0.440 second, risk of ventricular tachycardia or ventricular fibrillation increases (Schwartz & Wolf, 1978). The toxic effects of tricyclics, however, on the QT interval in *inducing* such life-threatening arrhythmias have been documented primarily in overdose situations and not at therapeutic blood levels (Fricchione & Vlay, 1986).

Depressed patients with the Wolff-Parkinson-White (WPW) syndrome require special consideration in the use of cyclic antidepressants. The WPW syndrome is characterized by the presence of a short PR interval and widened QRS in individuals prone to paroxysmal tachycardia. The condition is caused by an accessory pathway between the atrium and ventricle that allows atrial impulses to prematurely activate the ventricular tissue, in effect short-circuiting the AV conduction system. Arrhythmias associated with WPW have been described as deriving from "circus movement"—that is, a reentrant tachycardia usually based on ventriculoatrial retrograde conduction over the accessory pathway and by antegrade conduction through the AV node. Electrocardiographic findings reveal a prolonged QRS duration, a shortened PR interval, and a delta wave (slowing of the upstroke component of the QRS complex).

In some patients with WPW, atrial flutter–fibrillation may occur. If quinidine-like drugs such as the cyclic antidepressants are administered, the atrial rate may slow during atrial fibrillation–flutter, to the extent that antegrade conduction via the anomalous accessory pathway will predominate, sometimes leading to ventricular tachycardia or ventricular fibrillation (Sellers, Campbell, Bashore et al, 1977).

WPW patients with a short (less than

0.270 seconds) refractory period are at higher risk for life-threatening ventricular tachycardia when atrial fibrillation occurs (Wellens & Durrer, 1974). Patients with the short refractory period can be identified by a special cardiology procedure known as the procainamide infusion test, in which patients with WPW are monitored with an ECG during an intravenous infusion of procainamide. If during this infusion the delta wave does not dissipate and the QRS duration shorten, it indicates the presence of a short refractory period and vulnerability to atrial fibrillation (Wellens, Braat, Brugado, et al, 1982). All patients with WPW should be evaluated by a cardiologist prior to treatment with a CyAD.

CyAD are relatively safe in patients with adequately treated cardiac heart failure unless patients have symptomatic orthostatic hypotension. In elderly patients (mean age 70) with evidence of preexisting left ventricular dysfunction, imipramine (mean daily dose 223 mg/day, mean plasma level 338 ng/ml) had little or no effect on cardiac ejection fraction as measured by first-pass radionuclide angiography (AH Glassman, Johnson, Giardina, et al., 1983). These findings are consistent with those of Veith et al. (1982) that demonstrate the safety of imipramine and doxepin in patients with chronic heart disease. In Veith's series, 23 of 24 patients had a history of myocardial infarction, and one-third had a history of coronary artery bypass. Recent reports indicate that nortriptyline also does not significantly affect ejection fraction in patients with stable congestive heart failure, and may be less likely than imipramine to induce orthostatic hypotension (see the following subsection) (Roose et al., 1986b). Nortriptyline would thus be a reasonable first choice of CyAD in a patient with treated CHF.

The implementation of a cyclic antidepressant following myocardial infarction will depend on a number of factors, including (a) residual conduction defects after MI;

(b) degree of unstable congestive heart failure; (c) presence of arrhythmias, particularly reentrant arrhythmias, and vulnerability to ventricular tachycardia and fibrillation; (d) degree of symptomatic orthostatic hypotension that could possibly exacerbate angina, increase the likelihood of further ischemic events, or cause syncope. These specific complicating factors are more important in determining if an antidepressant after MI is safe than the actual time elapsed since the infarction occurred. If no contraindications to CyAD exist, then doxepin or nortriptyline may be considered as first-line choices, with trazodone as an alternative, although its antidepressant potency has been questioned by some. Alprazolam may also be considered for milder depressive reactions in which anxiety is a prominent component of the patient's condition.

Orthostatic Hypotension

The cardiovascular effect of the CyAD most often leading to discontinuation of treatment is orthostatic hypotension. In the previously mentioned study by Glassman and associates (1983), almost half of the study patients had to discontinue the drug because of orthostatic hypotension. The investigators stated that the degree of orthostatic hypotension during tricyclic treatment could be predicted by the extent of pretreatment orthostatic hypotension (AH Glassman, Bigger, Giardina, et al., 1979). Other investigators, however, have not found consistent correlations between pretreatment orthostatic changes and changes observed during treatment (Neshkes, Gerner, Jarvik, et al., 1985; Thayssen, Bjerre, Kragh-Sorensen, et al., 1981; Jarvik, Read, Mintz, et al., 1983). Impairment of left ventricular function with or without hypotension is a significant risk factor for the development of tricyclic-induced orthostatic hypotension (AH Glassman et al., 1983). Bundle branch block may be another risk factor for orthostatic hypotension during treatment (Roose et al., 1986b).

Glassman and colleagues (1979) reported no consistent relationship between the daily dose or plasma level of imipramine and subsequent development of orthostatic hypotension. A similar lack of predictive correlation between plasma levels and subsequent orthostatic hypotension has also been observed with nortriptyline (RC Smith et al., 1980).

Nortriptyline may be less likely than imipramine to produce orthostatic hypotension at therapeutically equivalent dosages. Nortriptyline causes little orthostatic hypotension in patients with compensated left ventricular impairment and does not appear to significantly alter the ejection fraction when used at therapeutic serum levels. (Roose et al., 1986a). Doxepin has also been reported to be relatively unlikely to produce hypotension in patients with cardiovascular disease (Veith et al., 1982).

Even with nortriptyline or doxepin, there will be many patients who develop treatment-limiting orthostatic hypotension. In those without heart failure, volume expansion with salt tablets or fluorocortisone could be considered. For the patient with mild, stable CHF on diuretics, a carefully monitored reduction in diuretic therapy might be tried.

Anticholinergic Effects

With the possible exception of trazodone, all of the available CyAD have anticholinergic effects (Richelson, 1984; Hershey & Hales, 1984). Particularly in elderly patients, drugs with high muscarinic receptor affinity are relatively poorly tolerated, with common complications being constipation and anticholinergic delirium. In men with benign prostatic hypertrophy, urinary retention may be a major problem, necessitating surgical correction before

CyAD can be tolerated. In patients with diabetic gastroparesis, the anticholinergic side effects can exacerbate problems with delayed gastric motility. Precipitation of narrow-angle glaucoma "crises" may occur, although patients with narrow-angle glaucoma can be safely treated with CyAD if they have first been treated ophthalmologically. Open-angle glaucoma, which is more common than the narrow-angle type, is not exacerbated by tricyclics (Lieberman & Stoudemire, 1987).

In patients prone to the anticholinergic side effects, drugs with lower antimuscarinic properties should be chosen, such as desipramine, trazodone, and possibly maprotiline. Amitriptyline is the most anticholinergic antidepressant and should not be used in such patients. While the use of trazodone does not appear to produce pronounced anticholinergic effects, it may cause priapism or bladder outlet obstruction, and it frequently is excessively sedating in therapeutic doses (300–600 mg/day). Trazodone also has a very short half-life (4 hours) in comparison with more traditional antidepressants, though the therapeutic relevance of the short half-life is not established (Richelson, 1984). The relative side-effect profiles of the currently available antidepressants are presented in Table 4-1.

While the side effects of the cyclic antidepressants are of most frequent concern in elderly patients and patients with preexisting cardiac disease, a few other organ system illnesses may affect their use. The CyAD are metabolized in the liver, and, theoretically, their half-life could be increased in patients with liver disease. However, this hypothesis is poorly supported by data. In the absence of reliable data, however, it is reasonable to predict slower metabolism of CyAD in these patients and to reduce the standard CyAD dosing by two-thirds in patients with severe liver disease until stable drug levels can be obtained. Similar recommendations are made for patients on dialysis, even though

Table 4-1

Properties of Antidepressants

	Effect on Serotonin Reuptake	Effect on Norepinephrine Reuptake	Sedating Effect	Anti-cholinergic Effect	Orthostatic Effect	Dose Range§ (mg)
Amitriptyline*	+ + + +	+ +	+ + + +	+ + + +	+ + + +	75–300
Imipramine*	+ + + +	+ +	+ + +	+ + +	+ + + +	75–300
Nortriptyline	+ + +	+ + +	+ +	+ +	+	40–150
Protriptyline	+ + +	+ + + +	+	+ + +	+	10–60
Trazodone	+ + +	±	+ + +	±†	+ +	200–600
Desipramine	+ + +	+ + + +	+	+	+ +	75–300
Amoxapine‡	+ +	+ + +	+ +	+ +	+ +	75–600
Maprotiline	+	+ +	+ +	+	+ +	150–200
Doxepin	+ + +	+ +	+ + +	+ +	+ +	75–300
Trimipramine‡	+	+	+ +	+ +	+ +	50–300

Relative potencies (some ratings are approximated) based partly on affinities of these agents for brain receptors in competitive binding studies (Richelson E [1982]. Pharmacology of antidepressants in use in the United States, *Journal of Clinical Psychiatry, 43,* 4–11).

0 = none, + = slight, + + = moderate, + + + = marked, + + + + = pronounced, ± = indeterminant.

* Available in injectable form.

† Most in vivo and clinical studies report the absence of anticholinergic effects (or no difference from placebo). There have been case reports, however, of apparent anticholinergic effects.

‡ Amoxapine and trimipramine have dopamine receptor blocking activity.

§ Dose ranges are for treatment of major depression. Lower doses may be appropriate for other therapeutic uses.

tricyclics (and trazodone) are not dialyzed and are metabolized by the liver (Levy, 1985). In patients with asthma and chronic obstructive pulmonary disease, the anticholinergic properties of CyAD may increase drying of bronchial secretions. Of much more concern is the possibility of the precipitation of acute asthmatic attacks in asthmatic patients with tartrazine sensitivity, since certain antidepressants contain tartrazine as coloring component of FD & C yellow dye number 5. This coloring is present in doxepin HCl (25 mg), desipramine hydrochloride (25, 50, 75, and 100 mg), imipramine hydrochloride (100 mg and 125 mg), trazodone (50 mg), and in the MAO inhibitor pargyline hydrochloride (Thompson & Thompson, 1984).

Although the occurrence of seizures in tricyclic overdose has led to the clinical maxim that tricyclics lower seizure thresholds and should be used with caution in

patients with seizure disorders, these agents may actually have suppressant effects on some forms of seizure activity within their therapeutic dose ranges (Clifford, Rutherford, Hicks, et al., 1985). Vernier (1961) demonstrated that amitriptyline and imipramine were comparable to phenytoin as anticonvulsants in maximal electroshock seizures in mice. Similar results were observed with imipramine.

A recent study found that antidepressants actually reduce after-discharge duration of electrically kindled hippocampal seizures in rats (Clifford et al., 1985). Of the drugs studied, amitriptyline, imipramine, desipramine, and maprotiline reduced behavioral seizures, but behavioral seizures were not reduced by buproprion or trazodone. Another study, using a somewhat different animal model, showed proconvulsant effects for imipramine and amitriptyline, but anticonvulsant effects for protriptyline and trimipramine (Luchins, Oliver, & Wyatt, 1984). Not surprisingly, clinical effects of CyAD on seizure frequency in known epileptics are variable (Edwards, Long, Sedgwick, et al., 1986). The implication of these studies for the clinical treatment of depression in patients with seizure disorders is discussed in Chapter 24.

At present, there appears to be no contraindication to CyAD therapy for patients with seizures, provided that (a) adequate levels of anticonvulsant drugs are maintained, (b) seizures are controlled, and (c) the CyAD are discontinued if they exacerbate seizures in the particular patient despite maintenance of therapeutic anticonvulsant blood levels. For patients without seizures but with known brain damage, a pretreatment EEG is recommended. If the EEG shows definite paroxysmal features, an anticonvulsant such as phenytoin should be started prior to initiating CyAD therapy.

Special note, however, should be made that maprotiline has been associated much more than other available antidepressants with seizures, particularly with rapid loading and in doses above 200 mg/day. Bupropion at the time of this writing is being withheld from the U.S. market because of the propensity of the drug to cause seizures in doses above 350 mg/day. (Despite this drawback, the drug is reported to have a favorable cardiovascular side-effect profile [Rudorfer et al., 1984].)

A few final miscellaneous points regarding the CyAD may be noted. They will be further discussed in subsequent chapters. Amoxapine has the potential for extrapyramidal side effects because of dopamine receptor blocking activity and should be avoided in elderly patients prone to parkinsonism or in patients with preexisting Parkinson's disease. Tardive dyskinesia is a possibility with prolonged use. Nortriptyline and trazodone have received special study in stroke patients and have been found to be efficacious for poststroke depression (see Chapter 24), but their antide-

pressant effect in these patients is probably shared by all the CyAD (Lipsey, Robinson, Pearlson, et al., 1984). Because of its potent antihistaminic effects, doxepin may be the preferred drug in patients with peptic ulcer disease, gastritis, or skin allergy. Doxepin and trimipramine have actually been used as primary treatments of peptic ulcers in nondepressed patients (Hoff et al., 1981; Moshal & Kahn, 1981; Rees, Gilbert, & Katon, 1984). Antidepressants that primarily block serotonin reuptake may be preferred on theoretical grounds in depressed patients with Parkinson's disease, because of the findings of low 5-HIAA metabolites in the cerebrospinal fluid (CSF) of these patients (Mayeux, Stern, Williams, et al., 1986). No particular antidepressant, however, has established clinical superiority in the treatment of depression in Parkinson's disease. CyAD may be used in patients with myasthenia gravis, since it is the nicotinic, not the muscarinic, receptor that is affected in this disorder (Cohen-Cole & Stoudemire, 1987).

Drug Interactions

Cyclic antidepressants block the antihypertensive effects of guanethidine and reserpine and, to a lesser extent, clonidine. By contrast, CyAD *potentiate* the hypotensive effects of prazosin. The CyAD will inhibit the metabolism of anticoagulants, leading to increased prothrombin times. Cigarette smoking, oral contraceptives, alcohol, barbiturates, and phenytoin lower CyAD serum levels through hepatic enzyme induction. Disulfiram, antipsychotics, and methylphenidate may raise CyAD levels. CyAD block the reuptake of norepinephrine and thus may potentiate the *hyper*tensive effects of direct and indirect sympathomimetics. Cyclic antidepressants may also increase receptor sensitivity to catecholamine in patients on thyroid replacement (Blackwell & Schmidt, 1984).

Imipramine may increase phenytoin

levels. Phenytoin, in contrast, may lower nortriptyline levels by as much as 50 percent (Ayd, 1980), or decrease desipramine levels (Fogel & Haltzman, in press). When L-dopa is used to treat Parkinson's disease, CyAD may decrease absorption of L-dopa, leading to decreased effects (Hershey & Hales, 1984). Amoxapine may impair glucose tolerance in diabetics (Tollefson & Lesar, 1983). Further discussion of drug interactions may be found in this book's chapters on specific organ systems.

Cimetidine may raise tricyclic antidepressant levels substantially. Imipramine clearance is decreased by concurrent use of cimetidine, Tricyclic blood levels should be monitored carefully in patients on cimetidine and probably in those using ranitidine as well. Both drugs have been associated with inducing depression and perhaps should be avoided when possible in depressed patients. In any case, if depressed patients are treated with cimetidine and tricyclics, the tricyclic dose may need to be lowered to prevent toxicity (Abernethy & Todd, 1986).

Dosage and Plasma Levels

An essential principle for the safe use of antidepressant medication in elderly and medically ill patients is careful titration of dosage. Starting doses should be low (10 mg or 25 mg) in patients with orthostatic hypotension or with other predictable vulnerabilities to side effects. Doses may be increased every 2–4 days as tolerated. Assessment for expected side effects (e.g., hypotension or cardiac arrhythmia) should be carried out after each dosage increase.

Peak plasma levels for most antidepressants are reached 2–4 hours after dosage, and because of the long half-life of most of the standard antidepressants, dosage may be given once daily in the evening, which may facilitate both sleep induction and compliance. Trazodone should gener-

ally be given immediately after meals because it may be a gastric irritant, because it is better absorbed if given with food, and because it may cause dizziness if taken on an empty stomach. If a particular patient experiences severe sedation, however, q.H.S. dosage may be preferable despite these considerations.

Steady-state serum levels of a CyAD may not be reached for 5–14 days after a constant dose has been established. While the role of plasma levels of tricyclic antidepressants in the drug therapy of depression has not yet been definitively determined, the monitoring of tricyclic levels in medically ill and elderly patients is justified by the tremendous pharmacokinetic variability of these patients and by the numerous drug interactions to which they are subject.

Specifically, if toxic symptoms develop at a low dosage, a drug level may help determine whether the problem is due to pharmacokinetic mechanisms or to the patient's unusual sensitivity to side effects at therapeutic levels. We have seen patients develop tricyclic levels exceeding 300 ng/ml on dosages of 50 mg/day; some of these patients have satisfactory outcomes from tricyclic therapy at apparently homeopathic doses of 10–25 mg/day (JN Glassman, Dugas, & Tsuang, et al., 1985). The patient with little or no therapeutic effect from an apparently high dose of a tricyclic also deserves a blood level check. If the blood level is very low, a further dosage increase may be warranted. Knowledge of a low serum level may allay clinical and medicolegal concerns about prescribing apparently high doses of drugs for medically ill or elderly individuals.

The value of tricyclic blood levels is debated by many psychiatrists because of a relative lack of studies establishing therapeutic ranges (American Psychiatric Association [APA], 1985). Despite this lack of data, clinical laboratories offer "therapeutic ranges" that have a potential to mislead. A conservative approach is to check levels in the special situations just described, in which one is looking mainly for very high or very low levels. In these situations, interlaboratory variations are less relevant.

An additional use of tricyclic blood levels is to establish a ''therapeutic level'' for an individual patient who is already responding well to a tricyclic. This level may be used as a reference point if a patient subsequently relapses, and it may help detect problems with drug compliance or with pharmacokinetic interaction. A repeat level at a time of relapse helps determine the reason for the relapse. This strategy may be particularly helpful if the patient requires many other drugs for medical problems, with frequent changes in medical therapy that may affect tricyclic pharmacokinetics and thereby alter treatment response.

Regarding specific tricyclics, consensus on therapeutic levels is best for the secondary amine tricyclics nortriptyline and desipramine (APA, 1985). For the former, a therapeutic range of 50–150 ng/ml is suggested, with higher levels associated not only with more side effects, but also with poorer antidepressant effect. For desipramine, Nelson, Jatlow, Quenlan, et al. (1984) have shown that raising levels over 125 ng/ml may convert poor responders to good responders. Other authors have asserted that the therapeutic range of desipramine is 50–300 ng/ml (Boyer & Friedel, 1984). For the tertiary amines, amitriptyline, doxepin, and imipramine, there is less consensus. There is also the additional problem of active metabolites. Although laboratories may quote a therapeutic range for the sum of drug and active metabolite, the significance of drug-to-metabolite ratios for clinical response is largely unexplored.

In evaluating drug levels, the clinician should strive to obtain levels under uniform conditions. A standard procedure is to draw levels in the morning, approximately 12 hours after the last dose of medication.

In determining antidepressant serum levels and doses in elderly patients, desip-ramine and nortriptyline are the best studied. In depressed elderly patients the steady state and the half-life of desipramine appear to be approximately the same as in younger and middle-aged individuals (Antal, Lawson, Alderson et al., 1982; Cutler, Zavadil, Eisdorfer, et al., 1981; Cutler & Narang, 1984). Results for nortriptyline conflict as to whether or not half-lives are prolonged in the elderly. One report quotes an average therapeutic dose of 40 mg/day in elderly patients (Dawling, Crome, & Braithwaite, 1980), and another, 30 mg/day (Dawling, Crome, Heyer, et al., 1981). Imipramine tends to have a prolonged half-life in the elderly, thus requiring a reduction in dosage (Nies, Robinson, Friedman, et al., 1977).

A word of caution regarding dosages of antidepressants in elderly patients is in order. The antidepressants show large variance, as does the necessary dose to achieve a clinical remission of depression. While the dose of the antidepressant in elderly or medically ill patients may need to be handled with conservative titration and with monitoring for cardiovascular of EKG side effects, some elderly patients may tolerate and require doses of antidepressants equal to or even above those required by most healthy younger adults (Fogel, 1983).

NEUROLEPTICS

Selection of neuroleptic agents in medically ill and elderly patients is based on their side-effect profiles and potential drug interactions (Table 4-2). High-potency neuroleptic agents include haloperidol, thiothixene, fluphenazine, trifluoperazine, and perphenazine. These high-potency drugs are more likely to cause extrapyramidal side effects than low-potency neuroleptics such as chlorpromazine and thioridazine. On the other hand, the high-potency agents are much less likely to cause orthostatic hypotension and have lesser anticholinergic

Table 4-2
Side Effect Profiles and Dose Equivalents of Commonly Used Neuroleptics

Drug	Equivalent Dose (mg)	Dosage Forms	Side Effects			
			Sedative	Extrapyramidal	Hypotensive	Anticholinergic
Phenothiazines						
Chlorpromazine	100	t,i,c,s,r	+++	++	IM +++ oral ++	+++
Thioridazine	95	t,c,s	+++	+	++	++++
Mesoridazine	50	t,i,c	+++	+	++	+++
Fluphenazine	2	t,i,d,s,c	+	+++	+	+
Perphenazine	10	t,i,c	++	++	+	+
Trifluoperazine	5	t,i,c	+	+++	+	+
Butyrophenones						
Haloperidol	2	t,i,c,d	+	+++	+	+
Thioxanthenes						
Thiothixene	5	t,i,c	+ to ++	++	++	+
Dihydroindolone						
Molindone	10	t,c	++	+	0	+
Dibenzoxazepine						
Loxapine	15	t,i,c	+	++	+	++
Diphenylbutyl-piperidine						
Pimozide*	2	t	+	+	+	+
Clozapine[†]	50	t	+++	+	++	++++

0 = none, + = slight, ++ = moderate, +++ = marked, ++++ = pronounced

t = tablet or capsule, i = injectable, c = concentrate, s = suspension, r = rectal suppository, d = depot injection

* Pimozide may have a greater propensity for prolonging the QT interval than other neuroleptics

[†] Clozapine may become commercially available in the United States in late 1987.

Information in table extracted in part from:

Mason A & Granacher RP (1980). *Clinical handbook of antipsychotic drug therapy*. New York: Brunner/Mazel, pp. 19–108.

and

Baldessarini RJ (1978). Chemotherapy. In Nicholi AM (Ed.): *The Harvard Guide to Modern Psychiatry*. Cambridge: Harvard University Press, p. 390.

effects than chlorpromazine and thioridazine. Elderly patients in particular are prone to develop parkinsonian symptoms (rigidity, drooling, bradykinesia, resting tremor, masklike facies) from agents such as haloperidol and are at increased risk for tardive dyskinesia if treatment is prolonged (Smith & Baldessarini, 1980). All of the neuroleptic agents may cause extrapyramidal symptoms (acute dystonia, rigidity, parkinsonism), but thioridazine (and its injectable analogue mesoridazine) has the lowest incidence of extrapyramidal side effects. The primary limitation of chlorpromazine in elderly or medically ill patients is its tendency to cause orthostatic hypotension. Chlorpromazine also tends to be the most sedating neuroleptic and may also induce cholestatic jaundice and photosensitivity. Photosensitivity occurs in elderly patients treated with chlorpromazine with a frequency of about 3 percent.

Thioridazine has relatively strong anticholinergic properties. It should not be used in doses higher than 800 mg/day because of the danger of retinopathy at higher dosages. Of all the neuroleptics, thioridazine is most likely to produce male sexual dysfunction.

Clozapine, a neuroleptic without reports of tardive dyskinesia should be marketed in the United States by Sandoz sometime in late 1987 or 1988. The drug's major problem has been its association with agranulocytosis, and restrictions may be put on its use when it is approved for the United States market.

Although the neurologic, endocrine (galactorrhea), dermatologic, and hematologic (agranulocytosis) side effects of the neuroleptics are relatively well known, only recently has widespread attention been given to the relatively rare but severe side effects that include neuroleptic-induced catatonia (NIC) and neuroleptic malignant syndrome (NMS).

Neuroleptic induced catatonia is a profound catatonic state accompanied by severe, immobilizing muscle rigidity. It is most commonly seen with high-potency agents such as haloperidol. It is most effectively treated with amantadine, 100–200 mg/day, or possibly with L-dopa or bromocriptine (Stoudemire & Luther, 1984).

Neuroleptic malignant syndrome is a catastrophic reaction to neuroleptics that is characterized by hyperthermia, muscle rigidity, catatonic stupor, tachycardia, blood pressure instability, diaphoresis, and a plethora of extrapyramidal signs (Levenson, 1985). Creatinine phosphokinase (CPK) levels are elevated, even in the rare cases in which muscle rigidity is not a prominent part of the syndrome (Rogers & Stoudemire, in press). Muscle breakdown may lead to acute renal failure. The death rate, often from pulmonary and renal complications, may be as high as 20–25 percent in severe cases. The syndrome may last weeks after neuroleptics are discontinued.

Depot neuroleptics are associated with a long duration of symptoms. Agents with high dopamine blocking activity, such as fluphenazine and haloperidol, are associated with the majority of cases. Preexisting brain disease may be a risk factor. Episodes may be triggered by febrile illness and may occur in patients who have been on longstanding neuroleptic therapy (Addonizio, Susman, & Roth, 1986; Levinson and Simpson, 1986; Mann, Caroff, Bleier, et al., 1986).

Reports indicate that both intravenous dantrolene sodium (1.25–1.5 mg/kg) and oral dantrolene sodium (50 mg every 12 hours) may be effective in reversing NMS. Bromocriptine (a dopamine agonist) in oral doses of 2.5–10 mg every 8 hours is also claimed to be of help (Guze & Baxter, 1985). The most critical aspect of treatment, however, is recognition of the disorder and immediate cessation of neuroleptic agents (Harpe and Stoudemire, 1987). Vigorous supportive measures including hydration, pulmonary support, and cooling blankets are essential. Recognition is facilitated by regarding incipient or partial forms of NMS as worthy of immediate action. If a patient develops severe rigidity, delirium, and elevated CPK levels, one should not wait for fulminant hyperthermia to develop before instituting treatment with dantrolene or dopamine agonists (Fogel & Goldberg, 1985). NMS-like symptoms with only low-grade fever are not uncommon (Levinson and Simpson, 1986).

Physicians in general hospitals most frequently use neuroleptics for control of agitated, psychotic behavior in delirious patients. The most commonly used drug in this setting is haloperidol, and initial doses may be 2–5 mg (p.o. or i.m.) every 1–2 hours until adequate sedation is achieved. With frail or debilitated patients, 0.5–2 mg doses may be sufficient. Haloperidol may also be given by slow intravenous push (at about 1 mg/min). Thiothixene also may be used, with initial starting doses of 5–10 mg, and is also available in intramuscular and elixir form, with doses of 2–4 mg often effective in severely debilitated patients.

The use of chlorpromazine in the intensive care setting may be limited by its propensity to cause hypotension. In low doses (100 mg/day or less), however, it is generally well tolerated, and its sedative and antiemetic effects may be desirable. High-potency drugs are preferable for *severe* agitation, as dosage can be rapidly increased if necessary. Chlorpromazine is also available as a rectal suppository.

Some authorities feel that prophylactic and concurrent administration of agents such as diphenhydramine, benztropine, or trihexiphenidyl may decrease the chances that acute extrapyramidal symptoms (EPS) will develop. In acute episodes of EPS, 25–50 mg of diphenhydramine may be given intramuscularly or intravenously or, alternatively, 1–2 mg of benztropine intramuscularly or intravenously. Diphenhydramine may be continued in the dose of 25–50 mg orally three times a day; benztropine may be continued at 1–2 mg orally two or three times a day, and trihexiphenidyl may be continued at 2–5 mg orally three times a day. If anticholinergic effects are contraindicated and the sedative antihistaminic effects of diphenhydramine are undesirable, amantadine may be used. The usual dose is 100 mg twice a day. Elderly patients and those with renal impairment often require less, and some young patients may need up to 400 mg/day. Toxic delirium is usually the dose-limiting side effect; orthostatic hypertension occasionally develops. For those who tolerate it, amantadine may be the antiparkinson agent of choice because of its lack of anticholinergic effect. Unfortunately, it is not available in a parenteral form.

Neuroleptics may affect cardiac conduction, producing increased PR and QT intervals and flattened T-waves, but this is rarely clinically significant. As with the tricyclics, additive effects with type I antiarrhythmics may occur. Phenothiazines also may block the antihypertensive effect of guanethidine.

Neuroleptics may cause respiratory dyskinesias in patients with chronic obstructive pulmonary disease (COPD), resulting in puffing, grunting, snorting, and respiratory spasms. Neuroleptics may also increase the risk of respiratory depression in patients with acute CNS injuries and should be avoided in patients with acute head injuries (Hershey & Hales, 1984). Chlorpromazine may cause loss of glucose control in diabetic patients, particularly those treated with oral hypoglycemics.

Phenothiazine induced hyponatremia, often with acute neurological effects, has been observed particularly in elderly patients treated with neuroleptics and is probably mediated by increased levels of antidiuretic hormone (ADH) (Kimelman & Albert, 1984). Galactorrhea due to increased prolactin levels may also be observed in younger women. Symptomatic breast enlargement may precede spontaneous discharge, and in many cases milk is obtained only upon manual expression.

Phenothazines raise the levels of tricyclics and propranolol through competition for metabolic enzymes in the liver. Drugs that increase neuroleptic metabolism, thus lowering levels, include barbiturates, nonbarbiturate hypnotics, rifampin, griseofulvin, phenylbutazone, and carbamazepine (Blackwell and Schmidt, 1984). Drugs that will increase neuroleptic levels include chloramphenicol, disulfiram, MAO inhibitors, acetaminophen, and tricyclics. Neuroleptics antagonize the antiparkinsonian effects of L-dopa and bromocriptine. They can potentially increase the hypotensive effects of alpha-adrenergic blocking agents such as prazosin. Gel-type antacids that contain aluminum and magnesium ions may interfere with neuroleptic absorption from the gut (Hershey & Hales, 1984).

Hypotensive effects of neuroleptics are

potentiated by narcotics, epinephrine, and the anesthetics enflurane and isoflurane. Their sedative effects are additive with those of narcotics, CyAD, barbiturates, and other sedatives. On the other hand, synergistic effects on pain relief may be observed when these agents are used with narcotics. (See Chapter 16.) Hepatotoxicity and encephalopathy may be observed when neuroleptics are used with iproniazid (Blackwell & Schmidt, 1984). Similar problems may occur with other MAO inhibitors, including the antituberculosis drug isoniazid (Griffin & D'Arcy, 1984). The antihypertensive effects of guanethidine and clonidine may also be partially decreased by concurrent neuroleptic administration.

Alternatives to Neuroleptics in Managing Agitation

Although an appropriate choice of neuroleptic may avoid or minimize drug-specific side effects on blood, skin, liver, or blood pressure, the neurotoxicity of neuroleptics is shared by all drugs in the class. Dystonia, parkinsonism, tardive dyskinesia, hyperthermia and NMS are potential side effects of all neuroleptics, with the possible exception of clozapine. The problem of neurotoxicity of neuroleptics has led to a search for neuroleptic alternatives for the management of psychosis and agitated states. A number of such alternatives have been documented, although none have been as thoroughly studied in large well-controlled trials as the neuroleptics themselves. For most patients, low-dose high-potency neuroleptics are the standard treatment for acute agitation and psychosis. However, in patients who are intolerant of neuroleptics, or who are at especially high risk for neuroleptic neurotoxicity, alternatives may be preferable.

Even when there is no reasonable alternative to neuroleptics, it is prudent to minimize the dose and if necessary, augment the therapeutic effect of neuroleptics with other less-toxic agents, such as benzodiazepines. Even in schizophrenia, high doses of neuroleptics do not necessarily give better results than low doses, and they definitely cause more side effects (McEvoy 1986). Therefore, while further studies of alternatives to neuroleptics are in progress, we advise that alternative drug therapies be seriously considered in patients with a history of severe neuroleptic toxicity or with tardive dyskinesia. Other patients, who do tolerate neuroleptics, should have dosages minimized, and low-dose neuroleptics supplemented with non-neuroleptic adjuncts should be regarded as preferable to a high-dose neuroleptics for long-term use.

Neuroleptics are used in medical settings not only for the treatment of schizophrenia but also for the treatment of agitated states, including agitated delirium, dementia complicated by agitation, agitated depression, mania, and overwhelming anxiety. They are also used to treat impulsive violence in retarded or brain-damaged patients. This section will suggest alternative treatments for each of these patient groups.

In agitated delirium, the goal of drug therapy is to diminish agitation so that the patient can be easily managed while the underlying cause of the delirium is found and treated. Acutely, this can almost always be accomplished with a benzodiazepine-lorazepam, 1–2mgs orally or intramuscularly every hour until the patient is calm and slightly drowsy. Lorazepam, however, may cause anterograde amnesia when given in this manner. Elderly patients are at highest risk for developing confusion or amnesia from benzodiazepines. Benzodiazepines nevertheless may permit the performance of laboratory tests, radiographs, and physical examinations so that a diagnosis can be reached. Benzodiazepines are relatively contraindicated in patients with pulmonary disease who are at risk for retaining CO_2, and in patients with cirrhosis and other types of severe liver disease. In the latter groups of patients, benzodiazepines can precipitate an encephalopathic episode; the risk is considerably greater for agents metabolized by the liver. In virtually all other patients they are safer than neuroleptics. Specific risks avoided by using neuroleptic alternatives include hyperthermia, exacerbation of seizures, and acute dystonia. Benzodiazepines may be particularly useful in treating acute delirious agitation in patients with suspected NMS.

If it appears that the delirium will take several days to resolve, and the patient's agitation cannot be easily managed environmentally, a switch to a low-dose, high-potency neuroleptic is reasonable. In these subacute situations, high potency neuroleptics offer behavior control equal to or better than benzodiazepines, with less sedation and amnesia.

For severe agitated depression, electroconvulsive therapy (ECT) is the best therapeutic choice. If ECT is refused or is not available, benzodiazepines may suffice to manage all but the most severe depressive agitation. When neuroleptics are needed, we recommend low doses (no more than 300 mg chlorpromazine equivalents), and early use of antiparkinsonian medication if any extrapyramidal signs or symptoms develop. If high neuroleptic doses appear necessary, ECT is the safer and wiser choice.

For dementia complicated by agitation, neuroleptics are frequently used and frequently recommended, although the experimental support for their efficacy is limited (Helms, 1985) and it is well known that the elderly are at high risk for tardive dyskinesia (Kane & Smith, 1982). It is well worth the effort to find effective non-neuroleptic therapy for an agitated demented patient, as some form of neurotoxicity is highly likely to occur with long-term use of neuroleptics.

Alternatives may include trazodone (Simpson & Foster, 1986), beta blockers (Jenike, 1983; Petrie & Ban, 1981), and carbamazepine (Jenike, 1985). Although each of these drugs has its own risks and contraindications, it behooves the clinician to check the current state of the literature and plan a carefully monitored trial of a nonneuroleptic agent that is *not* contraindicated. If successful, the trial benefits the patient, and if unsuccessful, it provides further clinical and ethical justification for the use of neuroleptics.

Further alternatives exist if the demented person's agitation is due to a superimposed depression. In this situation antidepressant therapies such as tricyclics, MAOIs, or ECT may be helpful despite the presence of an underlying dementia. Since demented patients may not describe the cognitive elements of a major depression, vegetative signs and observed affect must guide the decision to try antidepressant therapy.

For mania, the generally recognized treatment of first choice is lithium. Not all patients respond to lithium, however, and lithium response may take as long as 2 weeks—too long if the mania is disrupting needed treatment for a concurrent surgical or medical condition. In these situations, standard practice is to combine lithium with a neuroleptic. When neuroleptics are contraindicated, ineffective, not tolerated, or refused, we find it helpful to combine lithium with an anticonvulsant antimanic drug—either carbamazepine or clonazepam. Both of these drugs have been reported to have antimanic efficacy (Chouinard, 1985; Chouinard, Young, & Annable, 1983; Post, 1986; Post and Uhde, 1985) and have the advantage of calming the patient rapidly.

Despite the increasingly widespread use of carbamazepine for the treatment of mania, there have been only a few well-controlled, randomized, double-blind trials of this drug compared with lithium (Lerer,

Moore, Meyendorff, et al., 1987; Placidi, Lenzi, Lazzerini, et al., 1986). Conservative clinicians will still prefer lithium as a first choice because of the better documentation of efficacy.

Clonazepam has been reported to reduce manic agitation in hours. Clonazepam can be given at the rate of 2 mg every 2 hours until the patient is calm; the total loading dose is then given each 24 hours on an every 8 hours schedule. The dosage is adjusted downward if the patient becomes excessively drowsy, and is tapered and discontinued once lithium or other antimanic therapy begins to take effect. The major side effects are sedation and ataxia; the only major contraindication is pulmonary disease with the risk of CO_2 retention. Controlled studies of its efficacy, however, are lacking.

Carbamazepine is begun at 200 mg every 12 hours in an acutely manic patient; it is increased every 2–3 days to obtain a blood level of 8–12 µg/dl. Sedation, ataxia, and diplopia are common acute side effects. The well-known hematologic and hepatic side effects are rare but require monitoring of blood counts and liver function tests at least weekly during the first month of treatment. We also find it useful to instruct patients and their families regarding the importance of a blood count if fever or systemic symptoms develop on carbamazepine therapy.

Overwhelming anxiety is sometimes treated with neuroleptics when it fails to respond to benzodiazepines. One alternative is to add a beta blocker to the benzodiazepine (Kathol, Russell, Slymen, et al., 1980; Ouslander, 1981). We have found this particularly useful if tachycardia and tremor are among the principal signs of the anxiety state. A second alternative is to substitute clonazepam for more conventional benzodiazepines. Finally, if the anxiety state is subacute or chronic, antidepressant therapy should be considered. An antidepressant trial is an obvious move if

panic attacks accompany the generalized anxiety; recent evidence suggests that antidepressants may help chronically anxious individuals even without panic attacks (Kahn, McNair, Lipman, et al, 1986).

Finally, alternatives to neuroleptics are available for patients with agitation or self-injurious behavior accompanying mental retardation and for patients with agitation following head injury. In both of these groups beta blockers have been shown to be helpful (Greendyke & Kanter, 1986; Greendyke, Kanter, Schuster, et al, 1986). Ratey, Mikkelsen, Smith et al, 1986; Yudofsky, 1981; Yudofsky, Stevens, Silver et al, 1984). One may begin with 40 mg a day of propranolol or nadolol and gradually increase until the resting pulse is approximately 60. Hypotension, bradycardia, and oversedation are the three limiting side effects. Once the patient is established on an adequate dose of a beta blocker, one might need to wait a month or more for maximum effects on behavior, so the drug trial should not be discontinued prematurely.

In these patients with brain damage, an EEG should always be obtained, and anticonvulsants should be tried if there are paroxysmal or epileptiform features on the EEG. Carbamazepine is the anticonvulsant of first choice because it has calming effects and is less likely than barbiturates to disinhibit impulsive behavior. In these situations, dialogue with a neurologist may be useful in arriving at an optimal drug choice.

MONOAMINE OXIDASE INHIBITORS

Monoamine oxidase inhibitors have increasingly been used as treatment for depression unresponsive tricyclics (Fawcett & Kravitz, 1985), and some evidence suggests they may be superior to tricyclics for atypical depression (DS Robinson, Nies, Ravaris, & Lamborn, 1973), agoraphobia (Sheehan, Ballenger, & Jacobsen, 1980), social phobia (Liebowitz, Fyer, Gorman, et al., 1986), panic attacks (Klein, 1985), bulimia (Pope, 1986), and depression in medically ill geriatric patients (Jenike, 1984). Case reports suggest that they may be valuable in obsessive/compulsive disorder (Jenike, Surman, Cassem, et al., 1983) and migraine (Anthony & Lance, 1969). Because MAOIs were in disfavor for several years, however, there is less literature on their safe use in complex medically ill patients than there is for tricyclics. Substantial clinical judgment must therefore be employed in balancing benefits and risks when these drugs are used.

The two most commonly prescribed MAOIs in this country are phenelzine and tranylcypromine. While these drugs probably are of equal efficacy, there are differences in side effects that are relevant to the medical setting. First, phenelzine is an irreversible inhibitor of monoamine oxidase, while tranylcypromine is a reversible inhibitor. When phenelzine is discontinued, it may take up to 2 weeks for normal levels of MAO activity to return. In contrast, MAO activity may return to normal within a few days following discontinuation of tranylcypromine (Gilman, Goodman, & Gilman, 1980). Tranylcypromine would thus be preferable in patients who might be facing urgent surgery, such as patients with visceral cancer.

Second, tranylcypromine usually is stimulating, while phenelzine may be sedating or stimulating. If insomnia develops or worsens on tranylcypromine, phenelzine could be substituted (see below for recommendations on switching MAOIs). While tranylcypromine usually should be given early in the day, some patients can take phenelzine in the evening without sleep disturbance.

Third, phenelzine is more likely to lead to weight gain or sexual dysfunction than tranylcypromine (Rabkin, Quitkin, Harrison, et al., 1984). In patients who are obese, or those, such as diabetics, who can poorly tolerate weight gain, tranylcypromine would be preferable. In patients in whom sexual dysfunction is an important clinical issue, the same choice would be made.

If a patient tolerates one MAOI poorly, another may be tried, but it is judicious to discontinue one drug and wait two weeks before beginning another. This precaution is taken because of hypertensive crises resulting when patients were switched from phenelzine to tranylcypromine without a drug-free period (Gelenberg, 1984).

The manufacturers of MAOIs recommend a dosage of 30 mg/day for tranylcypromine and 45 mg/day for phenelzine (*Physicians' Desk Reference*, 1986), but recent evidence suggests that these dosages often are inadequate and that higher doses are safe and more effective. Most clinicians actively using MAOIs would be comfortable with doses of up to 60 mg/day of tranylcypromine and up to 90 mg/day for phenelzine (Klein, Gittleman, Quitkin, et al., 1980). Some experts in mood disorders have resorted to even higher doses (Fawcett & Kravitz, 1985). When exceeding manufacturers' guidelines for dosage, it is essential to carefully discuss with the patient and family the reasons for the high dosages and to offer a balanced view of risks and potential benefits. This discussion should be documented. If effects of the MAOI therapy on the patient's medical illness or its treatment are of concern, the internist should be included in the decision.

The most feared complication of MAOI therapy is hypertensive crisis, which may be accompanied by cerebral hemorrhage (Klein, et al., 1980). The frequency of severe hypertensive syndromes has been estimated by Klein and his associates to be 0.3 percent, with the risk of death less than or equal to 0.001 percent. Insufficient evidence is available to know if preexisting cerebrovascular disease or hypertension increases the risk of hypertensive reactions with MAOIs.

Orthostatic hypotension occurs in 11–14 percent of patients with MAOIs (Rabkin et al, 1984); in this respect the MAOIs are comparable to imipramine (Georgotas et al, 1986). However, some patients who cannot tolerate tricyclics due to orthostatic hypotension may be able to tolerate tranylcypromine (Jenike, 1984). Orthostatic hypotension may be particularly problematic in patients with cerebrovascular disease or with osteoporosis. If MAOIs are essential to the patient's treatment, volume expansion (Rabkin, Quitkin, McGrath, et al., 1985) or coadministration of stimulants (Fawcett & Kravitz, 1985) may permit successful treatment. The latter strategy runs the risk of hypertension and should be done in hospital, with both medical consultation and psychopharmacologic consultation if the treating psychiatrist is unfamiliar with MAOIs. Apart from hypertensive crises and orthostatic hypotension, MAOIs are relatively safe in patients with cardiovascular disease. They may shorten the QT_c interval (Robinson, 1982), but this usually is not clinically relevant. MAOIs probably may thus be safely used in patients with heart block.

Many clinicians are unwilling to prescribe MAOIs because of concern that the dietary restrictions will be burdensome to the patient or that the patient will break the diet with disastrous results. Severe reactions to MAOIs are uncommon, however, even though patients do occasionally break their diets (Neil, Licata, May, et al., 1979; Pare, 1985). Dietary compliance can be greatly enhanced by keeping the restrictions simple, focusing on serious offenders like aged cheeses and not on questionable or infrequent offenders like bananas or avocados. Permitting moderate amounts of white wine or clear spirits may also facilitate compliance with the more essential restrictions.

Many prescribed drugs are contraindicated when MAOIs are being used; one should check for *current* evidence on inter-

actions before using MAOIs concurrently with any other drug. Some specific points bear mentioning:

1. Fatal reactions may occur when meperidine is given to patients on MAOIs. Meperidine should never be used in patients on MAOIs. Other narcotics, such as codeine, may be used; starting dosages should be half of the usual dose.
2. Indirect sympathomimetics are particularly dangerous in MAOI-treated patients (see the discussion following this list). If a sympathomimetic drug is needed to treat an asthmatic attack or intra-operative hypotension, a direct-acting agent should thus be selected.
3. MAOIs are probably compatible with general anesthesia, based on a recent retrospective report on 27 patients (El-Ganzouri, Ivankovich, Braverman, et al, 1985). Concern about rare interactions with anesthetics and pressors, however, makes it prudent to discontinue MAOIs one to two weeks before elective surgery. The waiting period with tranylcypromine probably can be shorter, because MAO activity is more rapidly restored after discontinuation of this drug, than after discontinuation of phenelzine. If anesthesia must be given for surgery or ECT while a patient is taking an MAO inhibitor, risks can be minimized by proper anesthetic technique. Specifically: a) direct-acting agents should be used if pressors are needed; b) phentolamine or nitroprusside can be used to manage hypertensive crises; c) since phenelzine may reduce cholinesterase activity, smaller doses of succinylcholine should be used to avoid prolonged apnea; d) since MAOIs potentiate the anticholinergic effect of atropine, smaller doses should be used; and e) droperidol should be avoided because it may lead to prolonged cardiorespiratory depression in

the MAOI-treated patient (EC Janowsky & DS Janowsky, 1985).

4. In patients with Parkinson's disease, the use of MAOIs and L-dopa may predispose to a hypertensive reaction (Jenike, 1984). Anticholinergic antiparkinsonian drugs are safe; bromocriptine and amantadine may be safe (severe adverse reactions have not been reported to our knowledge).

5. Asthmatics may receive MAOIs if they can be managed with steroids, cromolyn, and theophylline. If the need is compelling to use an MAO inhibitor with a metaproterenol inhaler, the patient should have test doses of the combination in a hospital setting.

6. MAOIs may interact with the new antianxiety agent buspirone to cause hypertensive reactions; thus, these two agents should not be used together.

Anticholinergic side effects of MAOIs are, in general, minimal, but dry mouth, constipation, and difficulty with achieving orgasm have been reported (Sheehan et al., 1980). A variety of other side effects have been described, including gastrointestinal distress, muscle twitching, hyperreflexia, "shocklike" sensations, generalized periodic edema, inappropriate antidiuretic hormone (ADH), weight gain, sleep disturbance, and carpal tunnel syndrome. The major serious side effects in addition to orthostatic hypotension are hypertensive reactions, hepatotoxicity, and potentiation of the side effects of other drugs (Sheehan & Claycomb, 1984; Sheehan, Claycomb, & Kouretas, 1980).

Hepatotoxicity may occur because of direct hepatocellular damage. The nonhydrazide MAOIs (e.g., tranylcypromine) are less associated with liver damage than hydrazide MAOIs (e.g., phenelzine). On the other hand, nonhydrazide MAOIs such as tranylcypromine may be more likely to cause hypertensive crises (Sheehan et al., 1980).

The *indirect*-acting sympathomimetic amines that work by displacing norepinephrine from storage sites carry the most risk of hypertensive effects. Indirect-acting sympathomimetic amines include cocaine, amphetamines, tyramine, methylphenidate, phenethylamine, metaraminol, ephedrine, and phenylpropanolamine. *Direct*-acting amines, such as epinephrine, norepinephrine, isoproterenol, and methoxamine, are theoretically safer but may also act partially by indirect mechanisms and should be avoided as well whenever possible. Dopamine, methyldopa, and L-dopa all may lead to hypertensive episodes when used concurrently with MAOIs. Agents that have both direct *and* indirect pressor effects are most hazardous; these include pseudoephedrine and metaraminol (Sheehan et al., 1980). Pseudoephedrine poses special problems because it is a popular ingredient in over-the-counter decongestants and cold remedies. Inquiry about over-the-counter medications is essential when a patient on MAOIs presents with severe hypertension.

Despite these potential problems, the authors have successfully used MAOIs together with albuterol (for asthma) and with bromocriptine (for parkinsonism). In both cases, the drugs used with MAOIs were direct agonists. Safe use of MAOIs in this setting requires frequent monitoring of blood pressure and pulse during institution of therapy and slow upward titration of MAOI dosage. It would be unwise to initiate even a direct catecholamine agonist on a patient who was already on a full therapeutic dose of MAOI.

Antihypertensive agents such as propranolol, alpha-methyldopa, guanethidine, and reserpine have been reported to lead to hypertensive crises with MAOIs. Individual patients treated by the authors, however, have done well on MAOIs together with beta blockers.

The anticholinergic drugs used in anesthesia may be potentiated with MAOIs; these include atropine and scopolamine.

MAOIs may lower blood sugar and potentiate hypoglycemic agents (Sheehan et al., 1980). MAOIs may have intrinsic anticoagulant effects and may potentiate other anticoagulants (DeNicola, Fumarola, & DeRinaldis, 1964; Williams, Griffin, & Perkins, 1975). Caffeine and other methylxanthine derivatives, such as theophylline and aminophylline, may have mild pressor effects when used with MAOIs. On occasion, this interaction may be used to treat orthostatic hypotension that would otherwise limit MAOI treatment. Specifically, a few cups of coffee or tea in the morning may be used to prevent hypotension (Pollack & Rosenbaum, 1987). In patients with asthma, agents with "pure" beta-2 agonist activity, such as albuterol, terbutaline, metaproterenol, and isoetherine, may be used safely.

In conclusion, MAOIs may be used in the setting of severe medical or surgical illness if proper precautions are taken. These should include the following:

1. Discuss in detail the risks, benefits, and alternatives to MAOI therapy with the patient, the family, and the internist.
2. Conduct a *current* literature review of drug interactions between the patient's current medical regimen and MAOIs.
3. Substitute medical drugs when necessary to reduce interaction risk, in collaboration with the medical physician.
4. Obtain psychopharmacologic consultation if unfamiliar with the use of MAOIs.
5. Instruct the patient and family in the dietary restrictions, with emphasis on the most common and most severe food–drug and drug–drug interactions. Published lists such as those in Tables 4–3 and 4–4, while they may differ in some details from our recommendations, are excellent tools for educating the patient. The lists can be modified to emphasize risks particular to individual patients or to remove precautions not relevant for particular patients. Specifically warn them about the risks of over-the-counter medications.
6. Start the drug in the hospital whenever there are major doubts about its safety.

LITHIUM CARBONATE

The primary consideration in the use of lithium in medically ill patients is the patient's renal function. Lithium is excreted by the kidney, and rates of excretion are affected by age and creatinine clearance. Before starting lithium, all patients need a routine assessment of renal function via measurement of serum electrolytes, BUN and creatinine, and a standard urinalysis. In patients with known or suspected kidney disease, 24-hour urine collections to determine baseline creatinine clearance should also be obtained. Lithium excretion is primarily determined by glomerular filtration rate (GFR) and proximal reabsorption. Lithium is filtered freely at the glomerulus; then approximately 55 percent of filtered lithium is reabsorbed in the proximal tubule (DePaulo, 1984), and a further 15 percent is reabsorbed in the descending loop. Hyponatremia increases the reabsorbed fraction of both sodium and lithium ions up to 95 percent, therefore decreasing clearance of lithium. Thiazide diuretics that act primarily at the distal tubule enhance proximal reabsorption of lithium because they deplete sodium, leading to enhanced proximal reabsorption of sodium and lithium. Loop diuretics such as furosemide appear to have less effect on lithium clearance, although they can deplete sodium as well. Potassium-sparing diuretics such as spironolactone and triamterene also may reduce lithium clearance, although they have been less well studied than other diuretics.

Medications such as acetazolamide, theophylline, and aminophylline, which act as diuretics by inhibiting proximal tubular reabsorption, increase lithium excretion moderately. Nonsteroidal anti-inflammatory drugs, including indomethacin, ibuprofen, phenylbutazone, and piroxicam, decrease renal lithium clearance and increase lithium levels (Rogers, 1985). Aspirin, however, has no effect on lithium clearance.

Patients on thiazide diuretics usually need approximately 50 percent less lithium to attain therapeutic levels, but there is considerable interindividual variation. Patients on diuretics should be loaded slowly, and lithium levels should be monitored at least twice a week during the initiation of therapy. Frequent monitoring of levels should be resumed for a few weeks after any change in diuretic dosage or in diet. Patients on diuretics and their families deserve especially detailed warnings about the early signs of lithium intoxication, and commercially available bracelets with imprinted medical warnings may be desirable.

Lithium is dialyzable. Therefore, lithium should be given to renal failure patients after dialysis, with the usual dose being 300 to 600 mg by mouth. The dose need not be repeated until after the next dialysis. Serum levels of lithium should be taken several hours after dialysis, since plasma levels may actually rise in the postdialysis period, when reequilibration with tissue stores occurs (Bennett, 1980). The dialyzability of lithium can be exploited to rapidly reduce lithium levels in life-threatening cases of lithium toxicity.

In virtually all patients on lithium, there is some loss of the kidney's ability to concentrate the urine. Occasionally, this leads to symptomatic polyuria and a diagnosis of diabetes insipidus. Even when it does not, a careful history reveals more frequent urination and larger urine volumes in most patients on lithium. Polyuria may disrupt work or sleep routines, and may aggravate incontinence in patients with impaired bladder control.

The mechanism of these changes is a direct toxic effect of lithium on the loop of Henle and the distal tubule. The effect is dose related. In some cases, losses of concentrating ability are irreversible.

When lithium-induced polyuria threatens to limit lithium treatment, there are several options open. First, thiazide diuretics may be employed, with suitable precautions, to enhance lithium reabsorption at the proximal tubule, thereby protecting the more distal nephron from high lithium concentrations (Forrest, Cohen, Torretti, et al., 1974; Lippman, Wagemaker, & Tuker, 1981; MacNeil Hanson-Nortey, Passhalis, et al., 1975). The total lithium dose is reduced by as much as 50 percent if this strategy is used.

A second option is the potassium-sparing diuretic amiloride, which has been reported helpful in ameliorating this side effect in a dose of 10–20 mg/day (Kosten and Forrest, 1986). In refractory cases, 50 mg/day of hydrochlorothiazide could be added. With or without adjunctive thiazide therapy, amiloride still could increase lithium levels, potentially leading to lithium toxicity. If amiloride is used alone, hyperkalemia is a risk; if used with hydrochlorothiazide, lithium dosage must be reduced.

Enalapril, an angiotensin converting enzyme inhibitor used the treatment of hypertension has been reported to have a toxic interaction with lithium. This may be due to enalapril-induced lithium retention. The two drugs should be used together with caution, if at all. (Douste-Blazy, Rostin, Livarek, et al, 1986).

Finally, once-daily lithium dosing can lead to reduced urine volume. A recent review suggests that the low trough levels of lithium produced by once-daily dosing may protect the kidney (Plenge & Mellerup, 1986). It is not yet known however, whether once-daily dosing is as effective in preventing episodes of mood disorder as more conventional schedules.

The issue of permanent kidney damage from therapeutic dosages of lithium is controversial (DePaulo, 1984). Lithium has been reported to cause focal atrophy and

Table 4-3
Dietary Restrictions for Patients Taking MAOIs (Avoid 1 day before and for 2
weeks after taking MAOIs)

Danger of Blood Pressure Rise

A. *Foods*

1.	***	All cheese
	***	All foods containing cheese, e.g., pizza, fondue, many Italian dishes and salad dressings
	SAFE	Fresh cottage cheese, cream cheese and yogurt are safe in moderate amounts
	**	Sour cream
2.	**	All fermented or aged foods, especially aged meats or aged fish, e.g., aged corned beef, salami, fermented sausage, pepperoni, summer sausage, pickled herring
3.	**	Liver (chicken, beef or pork)
	**	Liverwurst
4.	***	Broad bean *pods* (English bean pods, Chinese pea pods)
5.	**	Meat extracts or yeast extracts, e.g., Bovril or Marmite
	SAFE	Baked products raised with yeast, e.g., bread, are safe
	SAFE	Yeast is safe
6.	**	Spoiled fruit, e.g., spoiled bananas, pineapple, avocados, figs, raisins
	SAFE	Fresh fruits are safe

B. *Drinks*

1.	**	Red wine, sherry, vermouth, cognac
2.	**	Beer and ale
3.	SAFE	Other alcoholic drinks are permitted *in moderation*, e.g., gin, vodka, whiskey, white wine

C. *Drugs*

1.	***	Cold medications, e.g., Dristan, Contac
2.	***	Nasal decongestants and sinus medicine
3.	***	Asthma inhalants
	SAFE	Pure steroid asthma inhalants, e.g., Vanceril, are safe
4.	**	Allergy and hay fever medication
	SAFE	Pure antihistamines (chlorpheniramine, brompheniramine)
5.	***	Demerol
	SAFE	Other narcotics, e.g., codeine—use lower doses

6. ***	Amphetamines
**	Antiappetite (diet) medicine

7. **   a. Sympathomimetic amines—direct acting: e.g., epinephrine, isoproterenol, methoxamine, levarterenol (norepinephrine)

   ***   b. Indirect acting: amphetamines, methylphenidate, phenylpropanolamine, ephedrine, cyclopentamine, pseudoephedrine, tyramine

   ***   c. Direct & indirect acting: metaraminol, phenylephrine

8. **   a. Local anesthetics with epinephrine
  SAFE   b. Local anesthetics without epinephrine

9. **   Levodopa for parkinsonism
  **   Dopamine

10. Blood Sugar   Diabetics on insulin may have increased hypoglycemia requiring a decreased dose of insulin (otherwise safe)

11. B.P. (decreased)   Patients on hypotensive agents for high blood pressure may have more hypotension requiring a decrease in their use of hypotensive agent (otherwise safe)

The following foods have been rarely reported to cause hypertensive reactions with MAOIs. The evidence supporting these claims is weak and often based on a single isolated case. Warnings based on such evidence have been uncritically perpetuated especially in view of the large numbers of patients on MAOIs who ate these foods with no problem.

In practice a blanket prohibition of these foods seems unjustified, unless they are clearly spoiled or decayed, and except for specific patients in whom they have already caused symptoms.

Danger of B.P. Rise:

* Chocolate	* Colas	* Beet root (beets)	* Worcestershire sauce
* Anchovies	* Figs, raisins, dates	* Rhubarb	* Soy sauce
* Caviar	* Sauerkraut	* Curry powder	* Licorice
* Coffee	* Mushrooms	* Junket	* Snails

* Minimal Danger, ** Moderate Danger, *** Very Dangerous

Source: Reprinted with permission from Jenike MA (1987). Affective illness in elderly patients: Part II. *The Psychiatric Times IV* (3).

interstitial fibrosis, leading to a permanent decrease in renal function (Barrow, Davies, & Kincaid-Smith, 1978; Hestbech, Hansen, & Amdisen, 1977). The true incidence of clinically relevant renal changes is not known, though clinical experience suggest it is low. Patients with known renal disease deserve careful serial measurements of creatinine clearance, and reconsideration of lithium therapy if renal insufficiency is progressing.

Lithium-induced ECG changes include inversion and flattening of T-waves. Sinus node dysfunction and SA block have been described, as well as rare episodes of ventricular irritability even at therapeutic

Table 4-4
Instructions for Patients Taking MAO Inhibitors

While taking this medication:

1. Avoid all the food and drugs mentioned on the list. Be particularly careful to avoid those foods and drugs with two and three stars.

2. In general, all the foods you should avoid are decayed, fermented or aged in some way. Avoid any spoiled food even if it is not on the list.

3. If you get a cold or flu, you may use aspirin or Tylenol. For a cough, glycerin cough drops or PLAIN Robitussin may be used.

4. All laxatives or stool softeners for constipation may be used.

5. For infections, all antibiotics may be safely prescribed, e.g., penicillin, tetracycline, erythromycin.

6. Avoid all other medications without first checking with me. This includes any over-the-counter medicines bought without prescription, e.g., cold tablets, nose drops, cough medicine, diet pills.

7. Eating one of the restricted foods may cause a sudden elevation of your blood pressure. When this occurs, you get an explosive headache, particularly in the back of your head and temples. Your head and face will feel flushed and full, your heart may pound and you may perspire heavily and feel nauseated.

8. If you need medical or dental care while on this medication, show these restrictions and instructions to the doctor. Have the doctor call my office if he has any questions or needs further clarification or information.

9. Side effects such as postural lightheadedness, constipation, delay in urination, delay in ejaculation and orgasm, muscle twitching, sedation, fluid retension, insomnia and excess sweating are quite common.

    Many of these side effects lessen considerably after the third week.

10. Lightheadedness may occur following sudden changes in position. This can be avoided by getting up slowly. If tablets are taken with meals, this and the other side effects are lessened.

11. The medication is rarely effective in less than three weeks.

12. Care should be taken while operating any machinery or while driving, since some patients have episodes of sleepiness in the early phase of treatment.

13. Take the medication precisely as directed. Do not regulate the number of pills without first consulting with me.

14. In spite of the side effects and special dietary restrictions, your medication (an MAO inhibitor) is safe and effective when taken as directed.

15. If any special problems arise, call me at my office.

Source: Reprinted with permission from Jenike MA (1987). Affective illness in elderly patients: Part II. *The Psychiatric Times IV* (3).

levels (Mitchell & MacKenzie, 1982). Clinically significant cardiovascular side effects of lithium, however, are sufficiently rare that they are seldom relevant to drug choice, even in patients with cardiovascular disease. ECGs before and after initiation of lithium therapy are an appropriate precaution for patients with asymptomatic abnormalities of cardiac conduction or repolarization. In patients with symptomatic arrhythmias, appropriate monitoring during initiation of lithium therapy should be worked out in collaboration with a cardiologist.

Elderly patients and patients with cerebral disease are particularly susceptible to developing confusion and tremor even at therapeutic lithium levels. Since lower serum levels of lithium (0.6 to 1.0 mEq/l) may be effective in prophylaxis of manic episodes, the lower end of the range is recommended for elderly individuals and others susceptible to the neurological side effects of lithium (DePaulo, 1984). Maintenance doses of lithium for elderly patients usually are about 50 percent of the maintenance doses required in younger individuals. When lithium is used to potentiate tricyclics in elderly unipolar depressives, doses are even smaller. At times, doses as small as 150 mg a day may yield therapeutic effects, with much less likelihood of CNS toxicity (Kushnir, 1986).

Lithium may prolong neuromuscular blockade induced moderately by succinylcholine or pancuronium (Blackwell, 1984). So lithium therapy should usually be discontinued during ECT treatment. The aggravation of post-ECT confusion and amnesia by lithium in some patients is another possible reason to discontinue lithium during ECT.

Because lithium may induce hypothyroidism, patients should have baseline thyroid function tests including a thyroid-stimulating hormone (TSH) level. The TSH, repeated at quarterly intervals, is an excellent screen for lithium-induced hypothy-roidism in its early, asymptomatic stages. In patients with known hypothyroidism, lithium is safe provided adequate thyroid replacement is given. Patients with Hashimoto's disease may have fluctuating thyroid hormone levels; when they are treated with lithium, fluctuations may increase, because lithium may actually cause increases or decreases in thyroid antibody levels. TSH and T_4 levels are advisable whenever there is an unexplained change in physical or mental status in a patient with Hashimoto's disease who is taking lithium (Lazarus, 1986).

BENZODIAZEPINES

Two aspects of benzodiazepine (BZ) pharmacology are of special relevance to the use of BZ in medically ill and elderly patients; the first concerns pharmacokinetics and the second their potential for respiratory depression. The metabolism of benzodiazepines occurs in two separate pathways. Certain BZ undergo an oxidation reaction (Phase I) via the mixed-function oxidase system, whereas other BZ undergo conjugation reactions with glucuronic acid and/or glycine (see Table 4-5). Drugs metabolized by glucuronide conjugation (Phase II) have relatively short half-lives, accumulate less with multiple doses, reach steady-state levels shortly after initiation of therapy, and are more rapidly cleared after discontinuation of treatment. Drugs with long half-lives reach steady-state levels more slowly and are eliminated over a longer period of time if therapy is stopped. They may accumulate rapidly if given several times a day. Drugs with long half-lives can be given effectively on once-a-day schedules and are less likely than drugs with short half-lives to cause severe withdrawal symptoms if they are abruptly discontinued.

Benzodiazepines metabolized primarily by oxidation have longer half-lives in the

Table 4-5

Commonly Used Benzodiazepines

	Primary Route of Biotransformation	Elimination Half-Life
Diazepam (Valium)	oxidation	36–200
Flurazepam (Dalmane)	oxidation	50–120
Halazepam (Praxipam)	oxidation	36–200
Chlordiazepoxide (Librium)	oxidation	30–90
Alprazolam (Xanax)	oxidation	12–15
Triazolam (Halcion)	oxidation	3–5
Clorazepate (Tranxene)	oxidation	36–200
Prazepam (Centrax, Vestran)	oxidation	36–200
Midazolam (Versed)*	oxidation	2–4
Lorazepam (Ativan)	conjugation	10–20
Temazepam (Restoril)	conjugation	8–12
Oxazepam (Serax)	conjugation	8–12

* IM or IV route only

elderly. In contrast, BZ metabolized primarily by glucuronide conjugation, such as oxazepam and lorazepam, do not have prolonged half-lives in the elderly. Chlordiazepoxide, desmethyldiazepam, diazepam, and other BZ metabolized primarily by the oxidase system have significantly reduced clearance in aged patients. Accumulation of these agents is determined primarily by hepatic metabolic clearance, so it may also be affected by liver disease (Cutler & Narang, 1984).

Pharmacokinetic differences do not translate into superiority of one benzodiazepine over another in the elderly, since appropriate serum levels of even the longer-acting benzodiazepines may be attained by giving lower doses on a once-a-day schedule. The theoretical advantages of drugs such as oxazepam and lorazepam in the elderly have not been confirmed in controlled clinical studies (Greenblatt, Divoll, Abernathy, et al., 1983).

Elderly patients as a group are more vulnerable than younger patients to developing neuropsychologic impairment on standard therapeutic dosages (Cutler & Narang, 1984; Meyer, 1982). Adult benzo-

diazepine doses of the oxidase-metabolized drugs should be reduced by 50–75 percent in the elderly, and increases should be made in relatively smaller increments (Cutler & Narang, 1984).

Drugs that inhibit microsomal enzymes may cause elevations in benzodiazepine blood levels and prolong their half-life. Drugs that inhibit microsomal enzymes include cimetidine, disulfiram, alcohol, and isoniazid. Clinical relevance of this pharmacokinetic interaction has not been established, but additive neurotoxic effects of alcohol plus benzodiazepines on a pharmacodynamic basis are well known. Conversely, estrogens, cigarette smoking, methylxanthine derivatives, and rifampin can lower levels by enzyme induction. The apparent need of a heavy smoker for high doses of benzodiazepine may deserve investigation with a blood level to see if the problem is pharmacokinetic rather than addictive.

Certain BZ have been specifically marketed as sleep-inducing agents. These include flurazepam, temazepam, and triazolam. Flurazepam has long half-life, which may vary between 50 and 120 hours. This may be helpful if daytime anxiolytic effects are desired, but it may cause daytime neuropsychologic performance decrements, particularly in the elderly. Flurazepam may accumulate, leading to oversedation, ataxia, and falls. Temazepam, which is metabolized by glucuronide conjugation, is slowly absorbed, partially on account of its hard gelatin capsule. Triazolam has an "ultrashort" half-life of 3–5 hours. Although it appears to resolve the problem of daytime hangover, this drug has been associated with amnestic episodes, dissociative episodes, confusional states, and rebound insomnia. These effects are less likely to occur at the low dosage of 0.125 mg but should be carefully watched for even at low dosages.

Finally, lorazepam and midazolam have the distinction of being the only BZs that have reliable and predictable absorption following intramuscular injection. They may thus be used in patients unwilling or unable to take oral medication. Lorazepam has been used as a sedative, anxiolytic, antimanic, or neuroleptic potentiator. Its amnestic effects are a drawback, but they may be desirable when it is used for premedication prior to chemotherapy or invasive procedures.

Alprazolam, a triazolobenzodiazepine, has received attention as a potential antidepressant. Several controlled clinical trials have revealed antidepressant efficacy comparable to amitriptyline, imipramine, and doxepin (Feighner, 1983; Rickels, Feighner, & Smith, 1985). The generalizability of these results to medically ill depressives and to individuals with severe melancholic depression has not been established. Alprazolam thus, cannot be seen as a substitute for CyAD as a first-line treatment of depression. Alprazolam may produce physical dependency, profound rebound anxiety, and a withdrawal state not suppressible by diazepam (Zipursky, Baker, & Zimmer, 1985). Like CyAD, it can produce secondary hypomania in bipolar patients (Remick, 1985). Alprazolam may nevertheless prove to have some usefulness in mildly depressed individuals with prominent symptoms of anxiety who have underlying cardiac disease that contraindicates the use of cyclic antidepressants.

Oral benzodiazepines are remarkably safe drugs, even in overdosage, but the dangers of cardiorespiratory depression increase dramatically if other CNS depressants such as alcohol or barbiturates are taken concurrently (Prescott, 1983). Intravenous benzodiazepines, used for premedication and for treatment of status epilepticus, may cause apnea or hypotension, especially if infused too rapidly. Gross CNS disease, or concurrent use of other depressants such as barbiturates, significantly raises the risk of cardiorespiratory problems (Lake & Boyer, 1983).

Patients with moderate to severe chronic pulmonary disease are at risk for CO_2 retention even with oral benzodiazepines at relatively low doses. When long-acting BZ such as chlordiazepoxide are used, the respiratory depression gradually worsens as active metabolites accumulate. Baseline CO_2 levels as low as 43 mm Hg have been associated with significant benzodiazepine-induced retention (Model & Berry, 1974).

Pathophysiologically, the problem with BZ is that they reduce the ventilatory response to hypoxia (Lakshminarawan et al., 1976). Since the response to hypercapnia usually predominates, this effect only becomes relevant when hypercapnic drive is reduced, as in some cases of chronic bronchitis. In such patients, low-flow oxygen increases the respiratory depressant effects of BZ, as it further reduces the hypoxic drive.

"Pink puffers" without CO_2 retention may actually improve symptomatically with BZ (Mitchell-Heggs et al., 1980). Baseline blood gases are thus indispensable in deciding on the appropriateness of BZ therapy for the anxious patient with lung disease.

If BZ must be used in patients with lung disease, it follows from this discussion that short-acting agents are preferable. Blood gases should be rechecked following attainment of a steady state after each increment in dose. When in doubt, low doses of high-potency neuroleptics would offer a safer alternative for the short-term therapy of incapacitating anxiety.

PSYCHOSTIMULANTS IN THE MEDICALLY ILL

Psychostimulants such as methylphenidate and dextroamphetamine may have a place in the clinical management of some medically ill depressed patients (Jenike 1985; Kaufmann, Murray, & Cassem 1982; Katon, & Raskind 1980; Woods, 1986). Before discussing the possible indications for these drugs in the medical setting, it should be emphasized that the use of psychostimulants for the treatment of depression may be illegal in some states and that these drugs do not carry FDA approved indications for their use in the treatment of depression. Clinicians should be advised, therefore, to exert caution in their use by checking with the appropriate local medical authorities and carefully documenting the rationale for their use.

Psychostimulants have been used in a variety of ways in debilitated medical patients. Stimulants such as methylphenidate and dextroamphetamine have been most frequently used in depressed, retarded anergic, withdrawn elderly patients with debilitating medical illnesses. Another use has been as an adjuvant to narcotic analgesics in the treatment of chronic pain in cancer patients. Other studies have advocated their use in dementia patients with depression (Kaplitz, 1975) and in patients with neurological disease (particularly frontal lobe disease) (Kaufmann, Cassem & Murray, et al., 1984).

The dose range is between 10-40 mg/day for methylphenidate and 10-20 mg/day for dextroamphetamine. The half-life of dextroamphetamine is approximately 12 hours; methylphenidate has a much shorter half-life of about 2 hours. To prevent insomnia and nocturnal agitation, the drugs should be given early in the day with breakfast and at the noontime meal. A number of reports in the literature document activating responses with diminution of depression and social withdrawal soon after institution of psychostimulants (Kaufmann, Murray, & Cassem, 1982).

Despite the occasional reports of the effectiveness of psychostimulants in the medically ill depressed patients, a number of problems exist with their use that should cause physicians to exert caution. First, most of the reports of their efficacy have not addressed the long term effects of the use of these patients such as rebound depression following discontinuation, and their habituating potential. In fact, published reports of psychostimulants for depression in medical settings emphasize their limited, short-term use. Tricyclics would be instituted if longer-term antidepressant drug therapy were needed. Psychostimulants may cause anxiety, irritability, agitation, delirium, and paranoid psychoses. They may interact with a variety of medications including guanethidine (decreased antihypertensive effect); vasopressors (increased pressor effect); oral anticoagulants (increased prothrombin time with methylphenidate); anticonvulsants (increased levels of phenobarbital, phenytoin, and primidone); tricyclics (increased blood levels), and MAO inhibitors (hypertension crises) (Jenike, 1985).

An indication for the use of psychostimulants that is much less controversial is their use in cancer patients who are being treated with narcotics. Relative low doses of methylphenidate (10–20 mg/day) may effectively combat excessive sedation and act synergistically with the mood-enhancing effects of opiate analgesics. Since most of the patients treated in this manner have a limited life expectancy, the problems of rebound depression after discontinuation of the medications and the development of dependency are moot concerns. Clinicians interested in more extensive reviews regarding the use of psychostimulants in the treatment of depression and other psychiatric disorders are referred to recent comprehensive literature reviews (Chiarello & Cole, 1987).

REFERENCES

Abernethy D & Todd E (1986). Doxepin—cimetidine interaction: Increased doxepin bioavailability during cimetidine treatment. *Journal of Clinical Psychopharmacology, 6,* 8–12.

Addonizio G, Susman VL, & Roth SD (1986). Symptoms of neuroleptic malignant syndrome in 82 consecutive inpatients. *American Journal of Psychiatry, 143,* 1587–1590.

Ahles S, Swirtsman H, Halaris A, (1984). Comparative cardiac effects of maprotiline and doxepin in elderly depressed patients. *Journal of Clinical Psychiatry, 45,* 460–465.

American Psychiatric Association (1985). Task force report on antidepressant drug levels. *American Journal of Psychiatry, 142,* 155–162.

Antal EJ, Lawson IR, Alderson LM, et al. (1982). Estimating steady-state desipramine levels in noninstitutionalized elderly patients using single dose disposition parameters. *Journal of Clinical Psychopharmacology, 2,* 193–198.

Anthony M, Lance JW (1969). Monoamine oxidase inhibition in the treatment of migraine. *Archives of Neurology, 21,* 263–268.

Ayd FJ, Jr (1980). Selecting an antidepressant for epileptics and the seizure prone. *International Drug Therapy Letter, 15,* 7–8.

Baldessarini RJ (1980). Drugs and the treatment of psychiatric disorders. In AG Gilman, LS Goodman, & A Gilman (Eds), *The pharmacological basis of therapeutics.* New York: MacMillan, pp 427–430.

Barrow GD, Davies B & Kincaid-Smith P (1978). Unique tubular lesion after lithium. *Lancet, 1,* 1310–1313.

Bennett WM, Muther RS, Parker RA, (1980). Drug therapy in renal failure: Dosing guidelines for adults: Part II. Sedatives, hypnotics, and tranquilizers; cardiovascular antihypertensive, and diuretic agents; miscellaneous agents. *Annals of Internal Medicine, 93,* 286–325.

Blackwell B & Schmidt GL (1914). Drug interactions in psychopharmacology. *Psychiatric Clinics of North America, 7,* 625–637.

Boston Collaborative Drug Surveillance Program (1972). Adverse reactions to the tricyclic-antidepressant drugs. *Lancet, 1,* 529–531.

Boyer WF & Friedel RO (1984). Antidepressant and antipsychotic plasma levels. *Psychiatric Clinics of North America, 7,* 601–610.

Burrows GD, Vohra J, Dumovic P, (1977). TCA drugs in cardiac conduction. *Progress in Neuropsychopharmacology, 1*(3–4), 329–334.

Chiarello RJ & Cole JO, (1987). The use of psychostimulants in general psychiatry. A reconsideration. *Archives of General Psychiatry, 44,* 286–295.

Chouinard G (1985, September). *Use of clonazepam in the maintenance treatment of manic-depressive illness.* Paper presented at Fourth World Congress of Biological Psychiatry, Philadelphia.

Chouinard G, Young SN, & Annable L (1983). Antimanic effect of clonazepam. *Biological Psychiatry, 18,* 451–466.

Clifford DB, Rutherford JL, Hicks FG, (1985). Acute effects of antidepressants on hippocampal seizures. *Annals of Neurology, 18* (6), 692–697.

Cohen-Cole SA & Stoudemire A (1987). Major depression and physical illness: Special considerations in diagnosis and biological treatment. *Psychiatric Clinics of North America, 10,* 1–17.

Cutler NR & Narang PK (1984). Implications of dosing tricyclic antidepressants and benzodiazepines in geriatrics. *Psychiatric Clinics of North America, 7,* 845–861.

Cutler NR, Zavadil AP, III, Eisdorfer C, (1981). Concentrations of desipramine in elderly women are not elevated. *American Journal of Psychiatry, 138,* 1235–1237.

Dawling S, Crome P, Braithwaite RA (1980). Pharmacokinetics of single oral dose of nortriptyline in depressed elderly hospital patients and young healthy volunteers. *Clinical Pharmacokinetics, 5,* 394–401.

Dawling S, Crome P, Heyer EJ, et al. (1981). Nortriptyline therapy in elderly patients: Dosage prediction from plasma concentration at 24 hours after a single 50 mg dose. *British Journal of Psychiatry, 139,* 413–416.

deMontigny C (1985). Using lithium to enhance the efficacy of antidepressants. *Currents in Affective Illness, 4*, 5–9.

deMontigny C, Grunberg F, Mayer A, (1981). Lithium induces rapid relief of depression in antidepressant drug non-responders. *British Journal of Psychiatry, 138*, 252–256.

DeNicola P, Fumarola D, DeRinaldis P (1964). Beeinflussung der gerinnung shemmender wirkung der indirekten Antikoagulantient durch die MAO-inhibituren, *Thrombosis et Diathesis Haemorrhagica*, (Suppl) *12*, 125–127.

DePaulo JR (1984). Lithium. *Psychiatric Clinics of North America, 7*, 587–599.

Douste-Blazy PH, Rostin M, Livarek B, et al. (1986). Angiotensin converting enzyme inhibitors and lithium treatment. *Lancet, 1*, 1448.

Edwards JG, Long SK, Sedgwick EM, (1986). Antidepressants and convulsive seizures: Clinical electroencephalographic, and pharmacological aspects. *Clinical Neuropharmacology, 9*(4), 329–360.

El-Ganzouri AR, Ivankovich AD, Braverman B, & McCarthy R (1985). Monoamine oxidase inhibitors: Should they be discontinued pre-operatively? *Anesthesia and Analgesia, 64*, 592–596.

Fawcett J & Kravitz HM (1985). Treatment-refractory depression. In AF Schatzberg (Ed), *Common treatment problems in depression*. Washington DC: American Psychiatric Press.

Feighner JR, Aden SC, Fabre LF, (1983). Comparison of alprazolam, imipramine, and placebo in the treatment of depression. *Journal of the American Medical Association, 249*, 3057–3064.

Flugelman MY, Tal A, Pollack S, (1985). Psychotropic drugs and long QT syndromes: Case reports. *Journal of Clinical Psychiatry, 46*, 290–291.

Fogel BS (1983). Caution in the use of drugs in the elderly [Letter]. *New England Journal of Medicine, 308*, 1600.

Fogel BS & Goldberg RJ (1985). Neuroleptic malignant syndrome [Letter]. *New England Journal of Medicine, 313*, 1292.

Fogel B & Haltzman S (in press). Desipramine and phenytoin, a possible pharmacokinetic interaction. *Journal of Clinical Psychiatry*.

Forrest JN, Cohen AD, Torretti K, (1974). On the mechanism of lithium-induced diabetes insipidus in man and rat. *Journal of Clinical Investigation, 53*, 1115–1123.

Fowler NO, McCall D, Chou TC, (1976). Elctrocardiographic changes and cardiac arrhythmias in patients receiving psychotropic drugs. *American Journal of Cardiology, 37*, 223–230.

Fricchione GL & Vlay SC (1986). Psychiatric aspects of patients with malignant ventricular arrhythmias. *American Journal of Psychiatry, 143*(12), 1518–1526.

Gelenberg A (1984). Switching MAOIs. *Biological Therapies in Psychiatry, 7*(9), 33–36.

Georgotas A, McCue RE, Hapworth W, (1986). Comparative efficacy and safety of MAOIs versus TCAs in treating depression in the elderly. *Biological Psychiatry, 21*(12), 1155–1166.

Gilman AG, Goodman LS & Gilman A (1980). *The pharmacological basis of therapeutics*. New York: MacMillan.

Glassman AH & Bigger JT (1981). Cardiovascular effects of therapeutic doses of tricyclic antidepressants: A reveiw. *Archives of General Psychiatry, 38*, 815–820.

Glassman AH, Bigger JT, Giardian EV, (1979). Clinical characteristics of imipramine-induced orthostatic hypotension. *Lancet, 1*(8114), 468–472.

Glassman AH, Johnson LL, Giardina EV, (1983). The use of imipramine in depressed patients with congestive heart failure. *Journal of the American Medical Association*, JAMA, *250*, 1977–2001.

Glassman JN, Dugas JE, Tsuang MT, (1985). Idiosyncratic pharmacokinetics complicating treatment of major depression in an elderly woman. *Journal of Nervous and Mental Disease, 173*, 573–576.

Greenblatt DJ, Divoll M, Abernethy DR, (1983). Benzodiazepine kinetics: Implications for therapeutics and pharmacogeriatrics. *Drug Metabolism Review, 14*, 251–292.

Greendyke RM, & Kanter DR (1986). Therapeutic effects of pindolol on behavioral disturbances associated with organic brain disease: A double-blind study. *Journal of Clinical Psychiatry, 47*, 423–426.

Greendyke RM, Kanter DR, Schuster DB, (1986). Propranolol treatment of assaultive patient with organic brain disease: A double-blind crossover placebo-controlled study. *Nervous and Mental Disease, 174*, 290–294.

Griffin JP & D'Arcy PF (1984). *A manual of adverse drug interactions (3rd edition*, pp 30, 153, 312, 355). Bristol, England: JW Wright.

Guze BH & Baxter LR (1985). Current concepts: Neuroleptic malignant syndrome. *New England Journal of Medicine, 313*, 163–166.

Harpe C & Stoudemire A (1987). Aetiology and treatment of the neuroleptic malignant syndrome. *Medical Toxicology, 2*, 166–176.

Hayes RL, Serner RH, Fairbanks L, (1983). ECG findings in geriatric depressives given trazodone, placebo, or imipramine. *Journal of Clinical Psychiatry, 44*, 180–183.

Helms, PM (1985). Efficacy of antipsychotics in the treatment of the behavioral complications of dementia: A review of the literature. *Journal of the American Geriatrics Society, 33*(3), 206–209.

Hershey SC & Hales RE (1984). Psychopharmacologic approach to the medically ill patient. *Psychiatric Clinics of North America*, 7, 803–816.

Hestbech J, Hansen HE, & Amdisen A (1977). Chronic renal lesions following long-term treatment with lithium. *Kidney International*, 12, 205–213.

Himmelhoch JM (1981). Cardiovascular effects of trazodone in humans. *Journal of Clinical Psychopharmacology*, 1(Suppl.) 76–81.

Hoff GS, Ruud TE, Tornder M, (1981). Doxepin in the treatment of duodenal ulcer: An open clinical and endoscopic study comparing doxepin and cimetidine. *Scandinavian Journal of Gastroenterology*, 16, 1041–1042.

Irwin M & Spar JE (1983). Reversible cardiac conduction abnormality associated with trazodone administration [Letter]. *American Journal of Psychiatry*, 140, 945–946.

Janowsky D, Curtis G, Zisook S, (1983). Ventricular arrhythmias possibly aggravated by trazodone. *American Journal of Psychiatry*, 140, 796–797.

Janowsky EC & Janowsky DS (1985). What precautions should be taken if a patient on an MAOI is scheduled to undergo anesthesia? *Journal of Clinical Psychopharmacology*, 5, 128–129.

Jarvik LF, Read SL, Mintz J, (1983). Pretreatment orthostatic hypotension in geriatric depression: Prediction of response to imipramine and doxepin. *Journal of Clinical Psychopharmacology*, 3, 368–371.

Jenike MA (1983). Treatment of rage and violence in elderly patients with propranolol. *Geriatrics*, 38, 29–34.

Jenike MA (1984). The use of monoamine oxidase inhibitors in elderly depressed patients. *Journal of the American Geriatrics Society*, 1984, 32, 571–575.

Jenike MA (1985). *Handbook of geriatric psychopharmacology*. Littleton, PSG Publishing.

Jenike MA, Surman OS, Cassem NH, (1983). Monoamine oxidase inhibitors in obsessive/compulsive disorders. *Journal of Clinical Psychiatry*, 44, 131–132.

Kahn RJ, McNair DM, Lipman RS, (1986). Imipramine and chlordiazepoxide in depressive and anxiety disorders, II. *Archives of General Psychiatry*, 43, 79–85.

Kane JM & Smith JM (1982). Tardive dyskinesia. *Archives of General Psychiatry*, 39, 473.

Kaplitz SE (1975). Withdrawn, apathetic geriatric patients responsive to methylphenidate. *Journal of the American Geriatrics Society*, 23, 271–276.

Kathol RG, Russell N, Slymen DJ, (1980). Propranolol in chronic anxiety disorders. *Archives of General Psychiatry*, 37, 1361–1365.

Kaufmann MW, Cassem NH, Murray GB, et al.

(1984). Use of psychostimulants in medically ill patients with neurological disease and major depression. *Canadian Journal of Psychiatry*, 29, 46–49.

Kaufmann MW, Murray GB, Cassem NH (1982). Use of psychostimulants in medically ill depressed patients. *Psychosomatics*, 23, 817–819.

Kayton W, Raskind M (1980). Treatment of depression in the medically ill elderly with methylphenidate. *American Journal of Psychiatry*, 137, 963–965.

Kimelman N & Albert SG (1984). Phenothiazine-induced hyponatremia in the elderly. *Gerontology*, 30, 132–136.

Klein DF (1985). An update on panic disorders. *Currents in Affective Illness*, 4, 5–10.

Klein DF, Gittleman R, Quitkin F & Rifkin A (1980). *Diagnosis and drug treatment of psychiatric disorders: Adults and children* (2nd ed). Baltimore: Williams & Wilkins.

Kosten TR & Forrest JN (1986). Treatment of severe lithium-induced polyuria with amiloride. *American Journal of Psychiatry*, 143(12), 1563–1568.

Krikler DM & Curry POL (1976). Torsades de pointes, an atypical ventricular tachycardia. *British Heart Journal*, 38, 117–120.

Kushnir SL (1986). Lithium-antidepressant combinations in treatment of depressed, physically ill geriatric patients. *American Journal of Psychiatry*, 143(3), 378–379.

Lake CR & Boyer WF (1983). Psychopharmacology in the ICU. In B Chernow (ed), *The pharmacologic approach to the critically ill patient*. Baltimore: Williams & Wilkins.

Lakshminarawan S, Sahn SA, Hudson LD, (1976). Effects of diazepam on ventilatory responses. *Clinical Pharmacology and Therapeutics*, 20, 173–183.

Lazarus JH (1986). *Endocrine and metabolic effects of lithium*. New York: Plenum Medical Books Co., 99–117.

Lerer B, Moore N, Meyendorff, et al. (1987). Carbamazepine versus lithium in mania: A double-blind study. *Journal of Clinical Psychiatry*, 48(3), 89–93.

Levenson JL (1985). Neuroleptic malignant syndrome. *American Journal of Psychiatry*, 142, 1137–1145.

Levinson DF & Simpson GM (1986). Neuroleptic-induced extrapyramidal symptoms with fever. *Archives of General Psychiatry*, 43, 839–848.

Levy NB (1985). Use of psychotropics in patients with kidney failure. *Psychosomatics*, 26, 699–709.

Lieberman E & Stoudemire A (1987). The use of tricyclic antidepressants in patients with glaucoma. *Psychosomatics*. 28, 145–148.

Liebowitz MR, Fyer AJ, Gorman JM, (1986).

Phenelzine for social phobia. *Journal of Clinical Psychopharmacology*, *6*, 93–98.

Limpan BS, Dunn M, & Massie E (1984). *Clinical electrocardiography. 7th Edition.* Chicago: Year Book Medical Publishers.

Lippman S, Wagemaker H & Tuker D (1981). A practical approach to management of lithium concurrent with hyponatremia, diuretic therapy, and/or chronic renal failure. *Journal of Clinical Psychiatry*, *42*, 304–306.

Lipsey JR, Robinson RG, Pearlson GD, (1984). Nortriptyline treatment of post-stroke depression: A double blind study. *Lancet*, *1*(8372), 297–300.

Luchins DJ (1983). Review of clinical and animal studies comparing the cardiovascular effects of doxepin and other tricyclic antidepressants. *American Journal of Psychiatry*, *140*, 1006–1009.

Luchins DJ, Oliver AP & Wyatt RJ (1984). Seizures with antidepressants: An in vitro technique to assess relative risk. *Epilepsia 25*, 25–32.

Lumpkin J, Watanabe AS, Rumach BH, (1979). Phenothiazine induced ventricular tachycardia following acute overdose *Journal of the American College of Emergency Physicians*, *8*, 476–478.

MacNeil S, Hanson-Nortey E, Paschalis C, (1975). Diuretics during lithium therapy. *Lancet*, *1*, 1925–1926.

Mann SC, Caroff SN, Bleir HR, (1986). Lethal catatonia. *American Journal of Psychiatry*, *143*, 1374–1381.

Mason AS & Granacher RP (1986). *Clinical handbook of antipsychotic drug therapy.* New York: Brunner/Mazel.

Mayeux R, Stern Y, Williams JBW, (1986). Clinical and biochemical features of depression in Parkinson's disease. *American Journal of Psychiatry*, *143*, 756–759.

McEvoy JP (1986). The neuroleptic threshold as a marker of minimum effective neuroleptic dose. *Comprehensive Psychiatry*, *27*(4), 327–335.

Meyer BR (1982). Benzodiazepines in the elderly. *Medical Clinics of North America*, *66*, 1017–1035.

Mitchell JE & MacKenzie TB (1982). Cardiac effects of lithium therapy in man: A review *Journal of Clinical Psychiatry*, *43*, 47–51.

Mitchell-Heggs P, Murphy K, Minte K, (1980). Diazepam in the treatment of dyspnoea in the "pink puffer" syndrome. *Quarterly Journal of Medicine*, *49*, 9–20.

Modei DG & Berry DJ (1974). Effects of chlordiazepoxide in respiratory failure due to chronic bronchitis. *Lancet*, *2*, 869–870.

Moshal MG & Kahn F (1981). Trimipramine in the treatment of active duodenal ulceration. *Scandinavian Journal of Gastroenterology*, *16*, 295–298.

Neil JF, Licata SM, May SJ, (1979). Dietary noncompliance during treatment with tranylcypromine. *Journal of Clinical Psychiatry*, *40*, 33–37.

Nelson JC & Byck B (1982). Rapid response to lithium in phenelzine non-responders. *British Journal of Psychiatry*, *141*, 85–86.

Nelson JC, Jatlow PI, Quenlan DM, (1984). Subjective complaints during desipramine treatment. *Archives of General Psychiatry*, *41*, 55–59.

Neshkes RE, Gerner R, Jarvik LF, (1985). Orthostatic effect of imipramine and doxepin in depressed geriatric outpatients. *Journal of Clinical Psychopharmacology*, *5*, 102–106.

Nies A, Robinson DS, Friedman MJ, (1977). Relationship between age and tricyclic antidepressant plasma levels. *American Journal of Psychiatry*, *134*, 790–793.

Ouslander JG (1981). Drug therapy in the elderly. *Annals of Internal Medicine*, *94*, 711–722.

Care CME (1985). The present status of monoamine oxidase inhibitors. *British Journal of Psychiatry*, *146*, 576–584.

Petrie W & Ban TA (1981). Propranolol in organic agitation. *Lancet*, *1*, 324.

Physicians' desk reference (40th ed). (1986). Oraden, NJ: Medical Economics Co.

Pinder RM, Brogden RN, Swayer R, et al. (1976). Pimozide: A review of its pharmacological properties and therapeutic uses in psychiatry. *Drugs*, *12*(1), 1–40.

Placidi GF, Lenzi A, Lazzerini F, et al. (1986). The comparative efficacy and safety of carbamazepine versus lithium: A randomized, double-blind 3-year trial in 83 patients. *Journal of Clinical Psychiatry*, *47*(10), 490–494.

Plenge P & Mellerup T (1986). Lithium and the kidney: Is one daily dose better than two? *Comprehensive Psychiatry*, *27*, 336–342.

Pollack MH, Rosenbaum JF (1987). Management of antidepressant-induced side effects: A practical guide for the clinician. *Journal of Clinical Psychiatry*, *48(1)*, 3–8.

Pope, HG (1986). What we know about bulimia in 1986. *Currents in Affective Illness*, *5(7)*, 5–12.

Post RM (1986). Carbamazepine (Tegretol) and affective disorders. *Currents in Affective Illness*, *5(2)*, 5–10.

Post RM & Uhde TW (1985). Carbamazepine in bipolar illness *Psychopharmacology Bulletin*, *21(1)*, 10–17.

Prescott LF (1983). Safety of the benzodiazepines. In E Costa (Ed), *The benzodiazepines: From molecular biology to clinical practice* (pp 253–266). New York: Raven Press.

Rabkin J, Quitkin F, Harrison W, (1984). Adverse reactions to monoamine oxidase inhibitors: Part I. A comparative study. *Journal of Clinical Psychopharmacology*, *4*, 270–278.

Rabkin JG, Quitkin F, McGrath P, (1985). Adverse reactions to monoamine oxidase inhibitors: Part II. Treatment correlates and clinical management. *Journal of Clinical Psychopharmacology*, 5, 2–9.

Raskind M, Veith R, Barnes R, (1982). Cardiovascular and antidepressant effects of imipramine in the treatment of secondary depression in patients with ischemic heart disease. *American Journal of Psychiatry*, 139, 1114–1117.

Ratey JJ, Mikkelsen EJ, Smith GB, (1986). Beta-blockers in the severely and profoundly mentally retarded. *Journal of Clinical Psychopharmacology*, 6, 103–107.

Rausch JL, Pavlinac DM & Newman PE (1984). Complete heart block following a single dose of trazodone. *American Journal of Psychiatry*, 141, 1472–1473.

Rees RK, Gilbert DA, & Katon W (1984). Tricyclic antidepressant therapy for peptic ulcer disease. *Archives of Internal Medicine*, 144, 566–569.

Remick RA (1985). Alprazolam-induced manic switch [Letter to the editor]. *Journal of Clinical Psychiatry*, 46(9), 406–407.

Richelson E (1982). Pharmacology of antidepressants in use in the United States. *Journal of Clinical Psychiatry*, 43, 4–11.

Richelson E (1984). The newer antidepressants: Structures, pharmacokinetics, pharmacodynamics, and proposed mechanism of action. *Psychopharmacology Bulletin*, 20, 213–223.

Rickels K, Feighner JP & Smith WT (1985). Alprazolam, amitriptyline, doxepin, and placebo in the treatment of depression. *Archives of General Psychiatry*, 42, 134–141.

Robinson DS, Nies A, Corcelia J, (1982). Cardiovascular effects of phenelzine and amitriptyline in depressed outpatients. *Journal of Clinical Psychiatry*, 43, 8–15.

Robinson DS, Nies A, Ravaris L, & Lamborn (1973). A monoamine oxidase inhibitor, phenelzine, in the treatment of depressive/anxiety states. *Archives of General Psychiatry*, 29, 407–413.

Robinson RG, Lipsey JR, & Price TR (1985). Diagnosis and clinical management of post-stroke depression. *Psychosomatics*, 26, 769–778.

Rogers J & Stoudemire A (in press). Neuroleptic malignant syndrome in multiple sclerosis. *Psychosomatics*.

Rogers MP (1985). Rheumatoid arthritis: Psychiatric aspects and use of psychotropics. *Psychosomatics*, 26, 915–925.

Roose SP, Glassman AH, Giardina EV, (1986). Nortriptyline in depressed patients with left ventricular impairment. *Journal of the American Medical Association*, 256(23), 3253–3257.

Roose SP, Glassman AH, Giardina EGV, et al (1987). Tricyclic antidepressants in depressed patients with cardiac conduction disease. *Archives of General Psychiatry*, 44, 273–275.

Rudorfer MV, Golden RN & Potter WZ (1984). Second-generation antidepressants. *Psychiatric Clinics of North America*, 7, 519–534.

Schwartz P & Wolf S (1978). QT interval prolongation as predictor of sudden death in patients with myocardial infarction. *Circulation*, 57, 1074–1077.

Sellers TD, Jr, Campbell RWF, Bashore TM & Gallagher JJ (1977). Effects of procainamide and quinidine sulfate in the Wolff-Parkinson-White syndrome. *Circulation*, 55, 15–22.

Sheehan D, Ballenger J, & Jacobsen G (1980). Treatment of endogenous anxiety with phobic, hysterical, and hypochondriacal symptoms. *Archives of General Psychiatry*, 37, 51–59.

Sheehan DV & Claycomb JB (1984). The use of MAO inhibitors in clinical practice. In TC Manschreck & GB Murray (Eds), *Psychiatric medicine update* (pp 143–162). New York: Elsevier Science Publishing.

Sheehan DV, Claycomb JB & Kouretas N. (1980–81). Monoamine oxidase inhibitors: Prescription and patient management. *International Journal of Psychiatric Medicine*, 10, 99–121.

Simpson DM & Foster D (1986). Improvement in organically disturbed behavior with trazodone treatment. *Journal of Clinical Psychiatry*, 47, 191–193.

Smith JM & Baldessarini RJ (1980). Changes in prevalence, severity and recovery in tardive dyskinesia with age. *Archives of General Psychiatry*, 37, 1368–1373.

Smith RC, Chojnacki M, Hu R, (1980). Cardiovascular effects of therapeutic doses of tricyclic antidepressants: Importance of blood level monitoring. *Journal of Clinical Psychiatry*, 41, 57–63.

Stoudemire A, Luther J (1984). Neuroleptic-induced catatonia and neuroleptic malignant syndrome: Differential diagnosis and treatment. *International Journal of Psychiatry in Medicine*, 14, 57–63.

Thayssen P, Bjerre M, Kragh-Sorensen P (1981). Cardiovascular effects of imipramine and nortriptyline in elderly patients. *Psychopharmacology (Berlin)*, 74, 360–364.

Thompson WL & Thompson TL, II (1984). Treating depression in asthmatic patients. *Psychosomatics*, 25, 809–812.

Thompson TL, II, Moran MG, Nies AS, (1983). Psychotropic drug use in the elderly. *New England Journal of Medicine*, 308, 134–138, 194–199.

Tollefson G & Lesar T (1983). Nonketotic hyperglycemia associated with loxapine and amoxapine. *Journal of Clinical Psychiatry*, 44, 347–348.

Veith RC, Raskind MA, Caldwell JH, (1982). Cardiovascular effects of tricyclic antidepressants in depressed patients with chronic heart disease. *New England Journal of Medicine, 306*, 954–959.

Vernier VG (1961). The pharmacology of antidepressant agents. *Diseases of the Nervous System 22*, 507–513.

Wellens HJJ, Braat S, Brugada P, Gorgels APM & Bar FW (1982). Use of procainamide in patients with the Wolff-Parkinson-White syndrome to disclose a short refractory period of the accessory pathway. *American Journal of Cardiology, 50*, 1087–1089.

Wellens HJ & Durrer D (1974). Wolf-Parkinson-White syndrome and atrial fibrillation: Relation between refractory period of accessory pathway and ventricular rate during atrial fibrillation. *American Journal of Cardiology, 34*, 777–782.

Williams JRB, Griffin JP, Parkins A (1975). Effect of concomitantly administered drugs on the control of long term anticoagulant therapy. *Quarterly Journal of Medicine, 45*, 63–73

Woods SW (1986). Psychostimulant treatment of depressive disorders secondary to medical illness. *Journal of Clinical Psychiatry, 47*, 12–15.

Yudofsky S (1981). Propranolol in the treatment of rage and violent behavior in patients with chronic brain syndrome. *American Journal of Psychiatry, 138*, 218–230.

Yudofsky S, Stevens L, Silver J, (1984). Propranolol in the treatment of rage and violent behavior associated with Korsakoff's psychosis. *American Journal of Psychiatry, 141*, 114–115.

Zipursky RB, Baker RW, & Zimmer B (1985). Alprazolam withdrawal delirium unresponsive to diazepam: Case report. *Journal of Clinical Psychiatry, 46*(8), 344–345.

Richard D. Weiner
C. Edward Coffey

5

Electroconvulsive Therapy in the Medically Ill

Electroconvulsive therapy (ECT) is the application of a series of electrically induced seizures in order to produce a clinical remission in severe episodes of susceptible disorders. At present in the United States, ECT is administered each year to 30,000–80,000 individuals (American Psychiatric Association, 1978; Thompson, 1986), nearly all of whom suffer from major depressive disorder, schizophrenia, or mania (American Psychiatric Association, 1980).

The fact that ECT still remains a clinically viable treatment modality, after nearly 50 years and the development of literally dozens of psychopharmacologic alternatives, is in itself a testimonial to its therapeutic potency and also to its capacity to evolve over the years into a safer, if not a more acceptable, treatment modality. At intervals during this time period, panels of scholars have carefully considered the question of whether a role for ECT still exists in contemporary psychiatric practice. One of the most recent of these evaluations was undertaken in June 1985 by a National Institute of Mental Health (NIMH)/National Institutes of Health

(NIH) Consensus Development Panel (Consensus Conference, 1985). In agreement with virtually all previous such investigations, the panel concluded that ECT is, when properly administered, a safe and effective procedure for which there continues to be an established clinical need.

At present, ECT is typically not, at least in the United States, a "first-line" treatment. Its use is generally reserved for those who either have not responded to psychopharmacologic trials (see Chapter 4) or cannot tolerate such an attempt, whether for reasons of adverse effects or because of an urgent need for immediate relief (Fink, 1979; Weiner, 1979). In practice one frequently finds that such individuals are more severely ill not only from a psychiatric perspective, but from a medical standpoint as well. More and more often it is the elderly, frail, chronically physically ill patient who is considered for referral for ECT. In such a situation, the referring physician must be able to carefully evaluate the delicate balance of risks and benefits that represent the logical determinants of clinical choice. The presence of significant concurrent medical illness in these cases raises a number of salient questions, which must be addressed as part of this process: Is ECT truly indicated for the patient? Is it safe? Should the ECT procedure be modified in any way? It is to these issues, each of them becoming more commonplace as our population ages, that this chapter is directed. It is our hope that the reader (1) will arrive at a better understanding of whether and under what circumstances a medically ill patient should be referred for ECT and (2) will be better capable of achieving the safest and most effective ECT delivery possible under such circumstances.

CLINICAL INDICATIONS

ECT is chiefly used in the management of severe major depressive episodes, which represent around 5 out of every 6 ECT referrals in the United States (American Psychiatric Association, 1978). Nearly all of the remaining ECT referrals are for acute schizophrenic episodes, with mania running a distant third. In most cases it is easier as well as more "acceptable" to follow the psychopharmacologic management route initially, reserving the use of ECT for times when an adequate therapeutic response is not forthcoming. Another consideration is the presence of adverse drug effects, whose occurrence can sometimes abort even the most promising pharmacologic venture. A final factor in the decision to refer a patient for ECT is the rather substantial therapeutic delay that can be expected with drug management, especially in affective disorders. In some such cases, ECT might even be considered truly lifesaving (Roy-Byrne & Gerner, 1981). Regardless of the point at which ECT is chosen, however, it is important to recognize that the result of a successful course of ECT is reflected by a remission of the index episode, rather than by a cure of the underlying, typically recurrent, disor-

der. This distinction, true for psychopharmacologic treatment as well, is integral to an understanding of the role ECT plays in the longitudinal management of each case, and will be dealt with later, in the context of post-ECT continuation/maintenance therapy.

Depressive Disorders

ECT is extremely effective in major depressive episodes, especially in the presence of melancholia (Brandon et al., 1984; Gregory, Shawcross, & Gill, 1985). It is generally recognized that ECT is more effective in inducing a remission than antidepressant drugs (Scovern & Kilmann, 1980; Siris, Glassman, & Stetner, 1982), and also that ECT can exert a powerful therapeutic effect in drug nonresponders (Avery & Lubrano, 1979; Paul et al., 1981). The key issue in the efficacy of ECT in depressive disorders is diagnosis (see Chapter 2). With a "classic" presentation of melancholia, the likelihood of inducing a remission with ECT is at least 80 percent. The less "endogenous" the symptomatologic profile and the less pervasive the core affective disturbance, the lower the likelihood of a good response to ECT.

Although there have been many attempts to arrive at a successful means of predicting a positive ECT response in terms of more specific historical, demographic, and symptomatologic factors, these efforts have not met with success when applied across groups of patients from differing settings (Fink, 1979). One possible exception to this rule is the presence of delusions, which may actually represent a marker for endogenicity and which appears to be linked to a quite good response to ECT (Clinical Research Centre, 1984). Depressive illness other than major depressive episode, for example dysthymia, does not respond to ECT any better than to alternative approaches. Still, it is more important to recognize that patients with dysthymic disorder can develop a superimposed major depressive episode and may thereby be considered appropriate candidates for ECT.

It is of interest that the presence of concurrent medical illness has not been adequately investigated as a potential influence on ECT response. Indeed, such a study would be difficult to carry out. Not only does medical illness vary enormously in type, severity, and chronicity, but it also varies in the manner in which it interacts with the patient's psychiatric condition. In practice, medical illness often exerts an exacerbating, if not a causal effect. The linkage can be on either a functional or a biological basis. Particularly if the basis is biological, it is important to recognize that purely medical, rather than psychiatric, intervention may be indicated. Still, even if a major depressive episode began as a reaction to medical illness, it can, over time, become autonomous.

Schizophrenia

Although only an extremely small fraction of patients with schizophrenia are referred for ECT, this condition still most likely accounts for at least 10 percent of the total ECT population (American Psychiatric Association, 1978). Recent controlled investigations have shown once more that ECT is effective in schizophrenia (Brandon et al., 1985). In fact, in cases in which a distinct acute psychotic episode exists, the efficacy of ECT appears to be commensurate with neuroleptic treatment. Although a greater number of treatments may be required in such cases, the occurrence of affective or catatonic symptoms indicates the likelihood of a rapid recovery with ECT (Salzman, 1980; Small, 1985). Chronic schizophrenia, however, especially in the presence of predominantly "negative" symptomatology (see Chapter 27), is unfortunately associated with a very poor response to ECT, despite case reports of

dramatic recovery, which abound in the older literature.

Mania

The discovery of lithium's antimanic effects (see Chapter 4) rapidly led to a major decrease in referrals of manic patients for ECT. At present, the use of ECT in mania is largely reserved for those individuals who are refractory to or intolerant of psychopharmacologic alternatives (American Psychiatric Association, 1978; Fink, 1979). Although the relative efficacies of lithium and ECT have never been firmly established, the two appear roughly comparable (Small et al., 1986). Interestingly, a switch to hypomania or mania has been reported to occur in bipolar depressed patients during a course of ECT, much as with antidepressant drugs, although the incidence of this phenomenon is in question. In such a case, the ECT course can either be stopped, and antimanic medication initiated, or be continued on the basis of ECT's own antimanic properties.

Other Psychiatric Conditions

The use of ECT for functional disorders other than depression, schizophrenia, and mania is supported only on an anecdotal basis and represents a minuscule fraction of ECT referrals. There is no convincing evidence that ECT should be considered in the absence of the primary indications discussed earlier. In making this determination, however, the practitioner must also keep in mind that a major depressive episode may coexist with, and at times even be masked by, other intercurrent functional illnesses.

CONTRAINDICATIONS AND RISKS

One of the many controversies surrounding ECT concerns contraindications to its use. It is our belief that, instead of "absolute" contraindications to ECT, there exist a variety of situations characterized by the presence of significantly increased risk of death or serious morbidity. In such cases the clinical need for ECT must be particularly well established and documented. In addition, efforts must be made, where possible, to modify the ECT procedure to minimize the likelihood of adverse sequelae. Relative contraindications to ECT include the following conditions, all of which will be discussed later in this chapter: space-occupying intracerebral lesion, recent myocardial infarction, and leaky or otherwise unstable aneurysm.

The mortality associated with ECT is quite low, typically quoted at 1 in 10,000 patients (Fink, 1979). This figure is comparable to that corresponding to brief periods of anesthesia alone. At the same time, however, it must also be pointed out that advanced age, along with the presence of significant intercurrent medical disease, may substantially raise the risk of both death and serious morbidity. Major medical sequelae that can be produced by a course of ECT are uncommon (Frederiksen & d'Elia, 1979; Heshe & Roeder, 1976). The most frequent such events are severe delirium and prolonged cardiac arrhythmia. Less serious, and also more prevalent, adverse sequelae of ECT are transient cardiac arrhythmia, prolonged apnea, oral trauma, injury to dental structures, and mild to moderate levels of delirium. As will be described, modifications of ECT technique may prevent or at least ameliorate many of these events.

Adverse effects produced by ECT can be explained in terms of the medical physiology of induced seizures. Profound autonomic surges during and following the ictal discharge lead to systemic hypertension and abrupt transitions in cardiac rate and output (Perrin, 1961). The hypertension, in combination with an ictal loss in cerebrovascular autoregulation, results in a transient breakdown in the blood–brain barrier and an accompanying increase in intracere-bral pressure (Bolwig, Hertz, & Westergaard, 1977). The sudden increase in cardiac output, particularly in the presence of a preexisting impairment of myocardial blood supply, may precipitate significant myocardial ischemia (Deliyiannis, Eliakim, & Bellet, 1962).

In addition to vascular effects, the ictal discharge transiently disrupts neuronal metabolism, eliciting nonspecific encephalopathic changes in the electroencephalogram (Weiner, 1983), which build up over the treatment course and which are correlated with behavioral aspects of delirium, such as disorientation. Along with these global cerebral effects, certain areas of the brain, such as the hippocampus, are particularly sensitive to metabolic dysfunction and other pathophysiologic changes, and may account for the more specific form of cerebral impairment (i.e., amnesia) that is often present during and immediately following a course of ECT (Squire, 1986).

Alterations of cerebral function raise the possibility of pathologic changes in cerebral anatomy, a consideration that is particularly of concern given the complaints of severe and permanently altered cognitive function elicited from a small minority of ECT recipients (Breggin, 1979). A careful evaluation of the literature does not allow the conclusion that ECT is associated with a significant risk of "brain damage" per se (Kolbeinsson, Arnaldsson, Petursson, & Skulason, 1986; Weiner, 1984), although a subtle, persistent retrograde amnesia, at least for recent weeks and months prior to the ECT, can be present in some circumstances. As with many other of the adverse effects already described, this amnesia can be considerably attenuated by modifications in ECT technique.

ECT TECHNIQUE

A thorough medical evaluation is a necessary prerequisite to a determination of potential risks with ECT (Abramczuk &

Rose, 1979; Elliot, Linz, & Kane, 1982). The characteristics of this pre-ECT workup include a complete medical history and physical examination, with special attention to systems affected most by ECT: cardiac, CNS and pulmonary. Pertinent laboratory tests include serum electrolytes, chest X-ray, and electrocardiogram. Additional procedures are used selectively: for example, EEG, neuroradiologic, and neuropsychologic evaluation in patients in whom cerebral dysfunction is known or suspected (see Chapter 3). This category includes many elderly depressives as well as patients with depression and cognitive impairment.

Given the use of anesthesia with ECT, a preoperative anesthesia consultation is indicated, unless the treating psychiatrist is adequately trained in the relevant anesthetic and resuscitative skills required with ECT and risk factors are minimal. Because the medically ill patient often has heightened risk factors, it is important to ascertain in advance the ability of available medical resources to manage the occurrence of potential untoward events. Such resources include not only the individual providing anesthesia and the emergency equipment and supplies present in the ECT treatment area, but also the institutions's ability to provide immediate and appropriate emergency assistance if required. Patients with significant anesthetic risk, for example, should have a well-trained anesthesiologist in attendance at all treatments. For these reasons, seriously medically ill patients are best given ECT in a general rather than a psychiatric hospital setting. Provision of ECT in a surgical or recovery room suite provides the highest level of medical support for high-risk patients.

A final component of the pre-ECT workup, and one that is of great importance, is the informed consent procedure. Presently, ECT is nearly always a voluntary procedure, with the attainment of consent guided by a variety of clinical, ethical, and legal considerations (Parry, 1986; Roth-

man, 1986). Adequate informed consent must include the provision, in terms understandable to the patient, of data on the nature of the treatment, its likely benefits and risks, and whatever treatment alternatives exist in lieu of ECT. This information must be given in sufficient depth to allow a reasonable person to arrive at a decision whether or not to agree to the treatment, and the delivery of this information must be documented. Standardized patient information sheets are available for assistance in eliciting informed consent for ECT (American Psychiatric Association, 1978). Not inconsequentially, such tools also serve as documentation that the material was provided to the patient. Establishment of patient competency to provide consent for treatment varies from state to state. In general, some degree of understanding of the existence of the psychiatric illness, the nature of the treatment offered, and the likely consequences of treatment versus no treatment is required. In some jurisdictions a spouse or other clearly designated significant other may sign for a patient, but in other locations a formal judicial guardianship procedure is required. In the latter case, separate regulations concerning emergency provision of treatment to the incompetent patient usually exist.

Before the ECT treatments themselves are initiated, a decision must be made concerning the handling of the patient's medications during the treatment course. In addition to concerns about potential drug interactions with anesthetic agents, which will be discussed below, the evidence that psychotropic medications augment response when given concurrently with ECT is unproven, except for the use of neuroleptics in schizophrenics or other agitated psychotic individuals (Barkai, 1985; Siris, Glassman & Stetner, 1982; Smith, Surphlis, Gynther, & Shimkunas, 1967). Theoretically, neuroleptics with minimal autonomic effects, such as haloperidol, should be used in such cases, though no investigation of this issue has ever been carried out. Antidepressant agents (see Chapter 4) are generally discontinued prior to onset of ECT, though a prolonged drug-free period is probably not necessary either for cyclic antidepressants or for monoamine oxidase inhibitors (Azar & Lear, 1984; El-Ganzouri, Ivankovich, Braverman, & McCarthy, 1985; Freese, 1985). When stopping antidepressant drugs, one must keep in mind that an abrupt termination may be associated with withdrawal effects, including cardiac irritability (Raskin, 1984). Lithium should usually be discontinued prior to ECT because it may produce neurotoxic effects (Small, Kellams, & Milstein, 1980; Weiner, Whanger, Erwin, & Wilson, 1980), enhance the effects of muscle relaxants, and lessen the degree of therapeutic response. Sedative hypnotic agents, including L-tryptophan and particularly benzodiazepines, are also problematic in combination with ECT, as they decrease seizure duration or increase seizure threshold or do both (WA Price & Zimmer, 1985; Standish-Barry, Deacon, & Snaith, 1985). Should the patient experience extreme anxiety during the ECT course, modest doses of agents with low anticonvulsant properties (e.g., hydroxyzine) or short half-life (e.g., oxazepam or triazolam) can be administered.

All of the patient's nonpsychotropic medications should be reviewed prior to ECT, as well, and those not deemed presently indicated should be discontinued. A number of such agents may be associated with specific adverse effects during ECT. Anticonvulsant drugs can create obvious problems with inducing seizures, though, if clinically necessary, ECT can still be carried out with certain modifications (see the following section). Lidocaine also has a negative effect on seizure duration (Hood & Mecca, 1983; Ottosson, 1960), whereas agents with stimulant properties, for example, theophylline, may increase the risk of prolonged seizures, particularly with high blood levels (Peters, Wochos, & Peterson,

1984). Reserpine may be associated with cardiovascular collapse with ECT. Although most daily medications should be delayed until after the procedure on the day of each treatment, drugs that will exert a protective effect during ECT—for example, cardiac and antihypertensive medications—should be administered 2–3 hours prior to each treatment with minimal amounts of accompanying fluid. Also, insulin doses in diabetics receiving ECT should be structured to accommodate timing of meals on the ECT days.

ECT treatments typically are administered at a frequency of three a week on alternate days in the United States, although this pattern may occasionally be altered because of induced cerebral impairment (treatments decreased in frequency) or because of a particularly urgent need for a rapid response (treatments increased in frequency). One seizure is induced per ECT treatment, except in the case of an ECT modification called multiple-monitored ECT, in which several serial seizure inductions are elicited in each treatment session. This practice has not been adequately investigated and remains controversial (Abrams, 1985; Maletzky, 1981). Multiple-monitored ECT potentially offers the opportunity of a more rapid response with fewer periods of anesthesia, but at the cost of a greater number of induced seizures, a more intense autonomic activation, and greater post-ECT confusion. A lower number of treatment sessions makes multiple-monitored ECT theoretically attractive for cases requiring a significant amount of additional supportive services at the time of each treatment, for example, medical specialists, specialized monitoring capabilities, endotracheal intubation, or provision of ECT in the operating room area.

The number of ECT treatments administered is determined by clinical response. Once a plateau in the therapeutic effect has occurred (typically after 6–10 treatments for depression and mania), the ECT course may be stopped (Snaith, 1981). The number of treatments that should be given in the absence of a major therapeutic response is still open to debate, though many clinicians use a figure of 8–12 for depression and mania and 12–20 for schizophrenia, with the lower figures more applicable to the case of absolutely no response. Despite its initial appeal as a potential biological marker for establishing the presence of a treatment response (Papakostas, Fink, Lee, Irwin, & Johnson, 1981), the dexamethasone suppression test does not appear to be useful for this purpose (Coryell, 1986), probably because of the complex effect of the induced seizures upon the pituitary-adrenal axis.

As described earlier, anesthesia during ECT should be performed by an individual experienced in anesthetic inductions of this type, and readily able to initiate management of any potential adverse sequelae. The use of anticholinergic premedication with ECT remains in question (Regestein & Reich, 1985; Wyant & MacDonald, 1980), though the use of such agents will certainly act to prevent vagally mediated arrhythmias that occasionally occur at either seizure onset or seizure termination. This phenomenon is of particular concern in patients with baseline cardiac impairment and in those whose sympathetic response is deficient, that is, patients taking beta-blocking agents (Decina, Malitz, Sackeim, Holzer, & Yudofsky, 1984). The specific anticholinergic preparation administered is generally either atropine (0.6–1.0 mg) or glycopyrrolate (0.2–0.4 mg). The latter is sometimes preferred because it does not pass the blood–brain barrier (Mondimore, Damlouji, Folstein, & Tune, 1983) and appears, therefore, not to add to the postictal disorientation. Still, glycopyrrolate may be more likely to be associated with cardiac arrhythmia and with nausea occurring after the recovery period (Kramer, Allen, & Friedman, 1986). Theoretically, anticholinergic premedication could present a prob-

lem with certain groups of patients, for example, those with prostatic hypertrophy and other causes of urinary retention, those with constipation, and particularly those with acute closed-angle glaucoma, but, except in the last case, its use should not be considered contraindicated. Finally, if the patient is already taking medication with anticholinergic properties, further premedication may be unnecessary.

An increasing number of ECT centers in the United States are switching from thiopental as the anesthetic agent to methohexital, largely because of the latter's rapid action and lesser cardiac toxicity (Pitts, Desmarias, Stewart, & Schaberg, 1965). Still, care must be taken with the infusing of methohexital, which can cause tissue damage if infiltration occurs. The anesthetic dosage should be titrated to response. Too high a dose will make it more difficult to induce an adequate seizure and may prolong the postictal apnea. Too low a dose, on the other hand, may be associated with an autonomic arousal, or even a return to consciousness, during the time the relaxant agent is taking effect. In practice, an initial methohexital dose of 1 mg/kg is generally used.

Muscular relaxation with ECT is induced by the drug succinylcholine. Typical doses of 1 mg/kg usually result in a modified convulsion with only minor tonic-clonic movements, mainly apparent in the distal extremities. If the patient's medical condition indicates (see discussion later in chapter), more complete relaxation can be achieved with a higher dosage. Should the patient complain of muscle pain after the treatments, or should the succinylcholine-induced fasciculations be felt to be of potential danger—for example, in the case of an extremely fragile musculoskeletal system or an inability to tolerate the sudden rise in serum potassium associated with the procedure, pretreatment several minutes prior to anesthesia induction with curare (3–6 mg IV) can be carried out.

The metabolism of succinylcholine is somewhat variable (Packman, Meyer, & Verdun, 1978). Genetic deficiencies of the main metabolizing enzyme, pseudocholinesterase, though rare (Whittaker, 1980), can lead to extremely prolonged apnea. A personal or family history of suspicious postsurgical complications should alert the practitioner to the possibility of this phenomenon and suggest consideration of a pre-ECT pseudocholinesterase assay. In lieu of an actual enzyme assay, a small test dose can be administered at the time of the first treatment (Cass, Doolan, & Gutteridge, 1982). If an enzyme deficiency is indeed present, succinylcholine can still be used as the muscle relaxant with ECT, but in greatly reduced dosage (Shea & Pollard, 1978). Should the occurrence of this genetic variant not be predicted and a prolonged apnea take place, a unit of fresh cross-matched blood can be used to provide a source of exogenous enzyme. In addition to genetic enzyme deficiency states, succinylcholine metabolism can also be slowed by a variety of other conditions, including malnutrition, hepatic disease, certain antibiotics and cardiac medications (see below), and lithium (Packman, Meyer, & Verdun, 1978). Some practitioners have advocated the use of a pre-ECT enzyme assay in such cases and also in cases in which the occurrence of a prolonged apnea would be extremely risky, though this has not yet become established practice on a widespread basis. In any event, these factors should be taken into account in determining initial succinylcholine dosage.

At present, there is a wide spectrum of practices concerning stimulus electrode location with ECT (Weiner, 1986). The most widely used type of electrode placement, bilateral, involves the application of stimulus electrodes over both frontotemporal regions. An alternative form of electrode placement is unilateral nondominant (Lancaster, Steinert, & Frost, 1958). In unilateral nondominant ECT, the stimulus electrodes are both placed over the hemisphere presumed to be nondominant for speech. This type of placement is associated with considerably less severe and less persistent confusion and memory impairment (Squire, 1986; Weiner, Rogers, Davidson, & Squire, 1986). Unfortunately, there remains considerable controversy about the relative efficacy of these two types of electrode placement. Although many studies claim equal benefits (d'Elia & Rotama, 1975; Pettinati, Mathisen, Rosenberg, & Lynch, 1986), a significant minority report an advantage for bilateral ECT (Abrams, 1986). In addition, for patients with manic symptomatology, there is now some evidence of a specific therapeutic advantage in bilateral ECT (Small, Milstein, Klapper, et al., 1986).

At present, it is still unclear whether the observed therapeutic differences in depressed patients are based on an intrinsically lower potency for unilateral nondominant ECT or whether the discrepancies among the various findings are the result of nonoptimal ECT technique (Weiner & Coffey, 1986). In an attempt to provide at least some temporary guidance on this matter, it has been proposed that, unless a particularly urgent response is needed, patients start on unilateral nondominant ECT and then switch to bilateral ECT if an adequate response is not forthcoming after 6 treatments or so (Abrams & Fink, 1984). Still, the absence of evidence supporting such a switch (Stromgren, 1984) leads us to question the validity of such a practice. In this regard, we have postulated that a major factor in assuring an adequate clinical response to unilateral nondominant ECT is the use of electrode locations which allow maximal seizure generalization (Weiner and Coffey, 1986) and that this can be achieved in practice by a frontotemporal-to-high-centroparietal electrode configuration (d'Elia, 1970). This latter practice is also associated with a low incidence of missed seizures, a problem reported with other types of unilateral placement.

The nature and intensity of the electrical stimulus itself has been a further source of contention in the ECT literature. Present evidence seems to suggest that a low-energy, interrupted stimulus waveform, such as the brief pulse, is as effective as a standard, higher-energy stimuli such as the sine wave, while also being significantly less cerebrotoxic (Weiner, Rogers, Davidson, & Kahn, 1986; Weiner, Rogers, Davidson, & Squire, 1986). The situation is not, however, completely resolved, and some clinicians report that pulse stimuli, at least when combined with unilateral nondominant electrode placement, may not be as effective in eliciting therapeutic change (Price & McAllister, 1986). It is also recognized that the energy content of the stimulus waveform can be lowered to a point at which equivalent efficacy is clearly not present (Robin & De Tissera, 1982).

A final technique-related factor is the stimulus dosing strategy. The amount of electricity (measured either in charge [millicoulombs] or energy [watt-seconds or joules]) required to produce a seizure is the *seizure threshold*. This parameter varies enormously from patient to patient, being particularly high in the elderly. In addition to interpatient variability, the seizure threshold typically rises over a course of treatments, typically by 100 percent or even more. The choice of stimulus intensity parameters used in clinical practice has traditionally been somewhat arbitrary, with little scientific data available for assistance. Dosing strategies ranging from the use of barely suprathreshold stimuli to the use of maximum machine settings are in practice today (Weiner & Coffey, 1986). It is likely that a "moderate" dosage strategy is most justifiable at the present time, as barely suprathreshold stimuli may not be as therapeutically effective, at least for unilateral electrode placement (Malitz, Sackeim, Decina, Kanzler, & Kerr, 1986), and maximally suprathreshold stimuli appear to be more cerebrotoxic (Fink, 1979).

CLINICAL MANAGEMENT OF PATIENTS AFTER ECT

As already noted, when successful, ECT produces a therapeutic remission in the present episode of the patient's psychiatric illness; it does not cure the underlying disorder. Without continuation therapy, the likelihood of relapse is extremely high, running 30–65 percent in the first 12 months for major depressive disorder (Imlah, Ryan, & Harrington, 1965). Particularly since many relapses occur in the first few months, patients are typically begun on psychopharmacologic agents soon after the ECT course has been completed, and this treatment is continued, depending on the patient's clinical history, for at least 6 months. There is now convincing evidence that such therapy is effective in decreasing the incidence of relapse (Coppen, Abou-Saleh, Milln, et al., 1981; Imlah, Ryan & Harrington, 1965). Furthermore, it is likely that a prophylactic effect is present even when pharmacotherapy was not beneficial during the index episode. For patients who have a history of early relapse and are either intolerant of or do not respond to psychopharmacologic prophylaxis, maintenance ECT may be considered (Stevenson & Geoghegan, 1951), although, despite decades of clinical use, there have never been any controlled studies of its efficacy in preventing relapse.

THE USE OF ECT IN SPECIFIC MEDICAL CONDITIONS

ECT is now being used widely in medically ill patients (Regestein & Reich, 1985). Although the principles of ECT practice already outlined are relevant to patients with concurrent medical illness, there are at times increased risks, precautions, and indicated modifications of ECT technique that should be kept in mind. In rare cases, the presence of a specific medical condition may even be an indication, in itself, for consideration of ECT. To elucidate the use of ECT in the medically ill, the following sections will focus on those specific medical conditions for which there are data concerning ECT utilization. For purposes of consistency, a physiologic systems orientation will be used.

Central Nervous System

The diagnosis of dementia may be quite difficult in an elderly depressed patient, since cognitive dysfunction is often an accompanying feature of a depressive episode (see Chapter 6). This cognitive impairment is likely to be responsive to ECT (McAllister & Price, 1982; Snow & Wells, 1981). Even with a history of organic dementia, some degree of exacerbation by depression may exist, suggesting an improvement in cognitive status post-ECT in these patients as well. Still, other than largely anecdotal material, there is not much in the literature focusing on the use of ECT in patients with preexisting dementia (Dubovsky, 1986). From what little data exist, one gets the sense that, as long as a standard clinical indication for ECT is present, a beneficial clinical response can often be attained. At the same time, however, the presence of dementia may be associated with a greater degree of confusion and amnesia over the ECT course (Miller, Siris, & Gabriel, 1986). Should this occur, a common practice is to lower the frequency of the treatments. If not already in use, a switch to brief-pulse unilateral nondominant ECT may also be of help in such a situation (Daniel, Weiner, Crovitz, Strong, & Christenbury, 1983).

Especially in prior decades, ECT has been used in patients suffering from delirium of varying etiologies (Kramp & Bolwig, 1981). Interestingly, ECT appears to exert a specific antidelirium effect on underlying pathophysiologic mechanisms in at least some conditions, including delirium tremens (Kramp & Bolwig, 1981), typhoid catatonia (Breakey & Kala, 1977), CNS syphilis (Paulson, 1967), and phencyclidine psychosis (Rosen, Mukherjee, & Shinbach, 1984). Still, there is, again, the risk that the delirium may be exacerbated by the ECT. In any event, a careful neurologic and metabolic workup is always indicated in the evaluation of patients with delirium, since any of a large number of etiologies, including some for which ECT may be associated with considerable risk, may be present.

The existence of a space-occupying intracerebral lesion, such as a brain tumor (Maltble, Wingfield, Volow, et al., 1980) or a subdural hematoma (Paulson, 1967), is cause for particular concern. Probably because of the transient increases in cerebral blood flow and intracerebral pressure produced by the induced seizure, a significant fraction of patients with such lesions will experience neurologic sequelae, occasionally of an irreversible nature. Given the increased risks, use of ECT in this situation must be preceded by well-documented clinical justification. Along with a careful reconsideration of clinical indications, the practitioner should also endeavor to implement certain modifications of the ECT procedure, which, at least on theoretical grounds, might serve to decrease morbidity. These modifications include the addition of antihypertensive agents, steroids, and diuretics and the use of hyperventilation, all of which should act to attenuate the increase in intracranial pressure occurring during and immediately following the seizure.

ECT has often been used in patients with a history of cerebrovascular disease, including transient ischemic episodes, infarctions, and also cerebrovascular anomalies such as aneurysms and angiomata. This use may be either in cases in which the cerebrovascular and functional disorders are merely coexisting (Coffey, Hinkle, et al., 1987) or in cases in which psychiatric disturbance appears to secondary to the neurologic insult (Murray, Shea, & Conn, 1986). With regard to strokes, a variety of review sources suggest that it is prudent to wait a period of weeks to months following a cerebrovascular accident to allow healing to take place before proceeding with ECT (Dubovsky, 1986). This concern is based upon the reasonable theoretical assumptions that increased cerebrovascular fragility during the acute poststroke period might lead to adverse effects from the increased cerebral blood flow, breakdown of the blood–brain barrier, and increase in intracranial pressure that all generally accompany the induced seizure. Still, the absence of reports of adverse events following the use of ECT in such a setting suggest that if ECT is strongly indicated otherwise and if a significant wait is believed to be dangerous, the procedure may be carried out earlier in the recuperative period. In patients with ischemic cerebrovascular disease, the acute use of antihypertensive agents in conjunction with ECT may be harmful, whereas in those at risk for cerebral embolism or hemorrhage, such drugs may be of benefit (Husum, Vester-Andersen, Buchmann, & Bolwig, 1983). Increased muscular relaxation should be considered in patients prone to cerebral embolism, as it will likely decrease the chance of new emboli being dislodged during the procedure.

Because the typical rise in seizure threshold during a course of ECT is consistent with anticonvulsive properties, it is not surprising that ECT, in its early days, was evaluated as a treatment for epilepsy (Kalinowsky & Kennedy, 1943). Although benefits in the form of decreasing seizure frequency and the ability to abort status epilepticus were claimed, neurologists today prefer to consider only pharmacologic management of epilepsy. As with cerebrovascular disease, depressive or psychotic episodes in epileptics may or may not be related to the underlying seizure disorder. In either case, ECT appears to be of benefit in inducing a therapeutic response in the psychiatric episode. In most cases this can be accomplished without a subsequent increase in seizure frequency, although a small degree of risk for this eventuality, along with the theoretical possibility of triggering status epilepticus, may be present. The presence of anticonvulsant medication in epileptics receiving ECT can be problematic in that seizure threshold is usually elevated and seizure durations are usually abbreviated. If difficulties in producing adequate seizures ensue, careful attempts can be made to decrease anticonvulsant drug levels. This decrease may be easier to accomplish with carbamazepine because of its relatively short half-life. Alternatively, pharmacologic prolongation of the induced seizures can be considered. Mechanisms for prolongation include hyperventilation (Bergsholm, Gran, & Bleie, 1984), intravenous caffeine (Coffey, Weiner, Hinkle, et al., 1987; Shapira, Zohar, Newman, Drexler, & Belmaker, 1985), and a switch to ketamine anesthesia (Brewer, Davidson, & Hereward, 1972).

Patients with a history of brain injury, whether traumatic or secondary to surgery, are sometimes referred for ECT treatment. The few anecdotal reports dealing with such occurrences have not indicated the presence of adverse sequelae (Hsiao & Evans, 1984; Ruedrich, Chu, & Moore, 1983). Clinicians have generally been careful to avoid stimulation directly over or adjacent to a skull defect, in order to prevent high intracerebral current densities. In patients with indwelling ventricular shunts, it is important to establish the shunt patency prior to ECT (Coffey, Smith, Weiner, & Mossy, in press; Tsuang, Tidball, & Geller, 1979) because of the increased intracranial pressure associated with a shunt blockage.

A high incidence of depressive illness occurs in Parkinson's disease. A number of reports have established a significant degree of efficacy for ECT in such conditions (Ananth, Samra, & Kolwakis, 1979; Levy,

Savit, & Hodes, 1983; Young, Alexopoulos, & Shamoian, 1985). In general, the clinical improvement is associated with either a transient improvement or no change in the neurologic symptomatology. Such improvement, which is most likely related to an increased sensitivity of postsynaptic dopamine receptors, is particularly prominent in cases of the "on-off" syndrome of Parkinson's disease (Balldin et al., 1980). Interestingly, tardive dyskinesia may either worsen (Holcomb, Sternberg, & Heninger, 1983) or improve (Chacko & Root, 1983) with ECT, suggesting that the action of this treatment modality upon dopaminergic systems may be more complex than initially believed (Lerer, 1984).

In addition to the neurologic disorders mentioned above, ECT has a variable effect on psychiatric symptoms and neurologic status in patients with multiple sclerosis (Coffey, Weiner, McCall, & Hines, 1987; Karliner, 1978; Regestein & Reich, 1985). Whether this is related to the degree to which the psychiatric illness was preexisting is unclear. The use of ECT in myasthenia gravis is potentially hazardous unless appropriate modifications are made in the anesthetic technique. This is because of the sensitivity of myesthenic patients to muscle relaxant agents. Patients with incompletely treated cerebral or meningeal infections represent yet another increased-risk group for ECT (Paulson, 1967), as disruption of the blood–brain barrier and increased intracranial pressure may be present. The further transient breakdown in the blood–brain barrier at the time of ECT might raise the risk of a systemic spread of such an infection, though this has not been reported. Chronic pain syndrome not infrequently occurs in conjunction with severe depressive symptomatology (see Chapter 10). In this regard, there are some suggestive data that ECT may be of benefit for both conditions, often showing improvement in such cases (Mandel, 1975). Finally, there is some evidence that depressive illness itself can lead to focal neurologic findings in the apparent absence of organic disease. Successful treatment of such a depressive episode with ECT is accompanied by disappearance of the neurologic signs (Freeman, Galaburda, Cabal, & Geschwind, 1985).

Cardiovascular Disease

No somatic treatments for depressive disorders are without significant cardiovascular morbidity. As already noted, electrically induced seizures are associated with marked, though transient, increases in cardiac output, pulse, and blood pressure, along with a variety of generally short-duration disturbances in cardiac rhythm. Although no increase in cardiac enzymes typically occurs with ECT, even in the presence of a positive history of cardiac disease (Dec, Stern, & Welch, 1985), patients with such a history have been reported to have a significantly higher cardiac morbidity (Gerring & Shields, 1982; Lewis, Richardson, & Gahagan, 1955). In ischemic disease, some measure of protection from further anoxic changes during and shortly following the induced seizures can be gained through the use of preoxygenation (McKenna, Engle, Brooks, & Dalen, 1970) or nitroglycerine (either sublingually or transdermally) and sufficient muscular relaxation.

A history of myocardial infarction should not be considered a contraindication for ECT, though if the insult is recent or incompletely healed, the damaged myocardium is at risk for futher injury as a result of the marked cardiovascular fluctuations occurring with each seizure. The ideal waiting period for ECT following myocardial infarction is unknown and would appear to vary with the nature and extent of myocardial injury, the presence or absence of postinfarction angina, the stability of postinfarction arrhythmias, and the status of the blood supply to the surviving myocardium, as determined by nuclear medicine procedures or angiography. In a patient with life-threatening or profoundly disabling depression, a discussion among the psychiatrist, the cardiologist, and the anesthesiologist would be needed to balance the risk–benefit ratio of ECT in any given situation. For patients with uncomplicated myocardial infarction and no postinfarction angina, arrythmia, or heart failure, we would be comfortable in giving ECT 6 weeks after the myocardial infraction. As much as possible, pharmacologic blockade of relevant cardiac and vascular receptor sits can decrease the level of associated morbidity. Needless to say, ongoing cardiac medications should always be given on days of ECT unless otherwise contraindicated (see the discussion that follows).

Patients with preexisting ventricular ectopy or with bradycardia should be considered particularly prone to asystole or bradyarrhythmic-related ventricular contractions during both the onset of the seizure and the immediate postictal period, when parasympathetic tonus is greatest. The ongoing use of medications with cardiac rate-lowering properties, such as beta blockers, makes the need for adequate parasympathetic blockade even more important (Decina et al., 1984). In other cases, the greatest risk period for cardiac arrhythmias is during the seizure and the postictal period of arousal from anesthesia, when the sympathetic nervous system predominates and when tachycardia-related cardiac ischemia is most likely to occur. Beta-blocking agents can be useful in these instances (Weiner, Henschen, Dellasega, & Baker, 1979), though, again, adequate anticholinergic premedication should be given as well (London & Glass, 1985). Though the effect of an induced seizure upon a preexisting cardiac arrhythmia is not entirely predictable, adverse changes will most likely be mild and transient if adequate precautions are taken as outlined above. There have even been reports of

arrhythmias being "cured" with ECT (O'Leary, 1981), with such beneficial effects possibly related to a restabilization in autonomic tone following the acute ictal and postictal sympathetic and parasympathetic surges.

Antiarrhythmic medications can sometimes interfere with the ECT procedure. The greatest problems occur with lidocaine, which significantly attenuates seizure duration (Hood & Mecca, 1983; Ottosson, 1960). Theoretically, quinidine and, to a lesser degree, digitalis may prolong metabolism of succinylcholine (Packman et al., 1978), though use of these agents with ECT has not been reported to produce adverse clinical sequelae.

The presence of a cardiac pacemaker in a patient referred for ECT should be a source of relief rather than concern (Abiuso, Dunkleman, & Prober, 1978; Alexopoulos & Frances, 1980), as the regulation of cardiac rhythm during the ECT procedure exerts a protective effect. This effect also obviates the need for anticholinergic premedication. Because of the theoretical possibility of erroneous pacemaker triggering on the basis of either muscle fasciculations or muscle contractions, some sources have recommended that demand pacemakers be switched to a fixed mode prior to ECT, though this procedure may not be necessary for more recent devices. The only pacemaker situation that could be risky from an electrical safety standpoint is the rather rare use of an internal pacemaker unit with transcutaneous pacing electrodes.

Hypertension has frequently been stated as a risk factor for ECT, although an increased rate of complications has not been documented. It is thus not clear when additional antihypertensive agents should be utilized with ECT (Anton, Uy, & Redderson, 1977). In practice, it is probably best to think of antihypertensive agents as means of decreasing morbidity from other medical conditions—for example, aneurysms, intracerebral masses, and hypercoagulable states (see subsection on other medical disorders)—rather than from the direct effects of hypertensive disease itself. A wide spectrum of specific pharmacologic agents have been advocated for attentuating the rise in blood pressure with ECT, including nitroprusside (Regestein & Lind, 1980), diazoxide (Kraus & Remick, 1982), ganglionic blocking agents (Egbert, Wolfe, Melmed, Deas, & Mullin, 1959), beta blockers (Jones & Knight, 1981), and nitroglycerin (Lee, Erbguth, Stevens, & Sack, 1985), the last two types being indicated when a mild degree of attenuation is desired. When using these drugs, one must still realize that some degree of hypertension may be necessary during the induced seizure in order to provide the increased flow of oxygen and glucose required by the brain at this time. It is also likely that the systolic pressure required to deliver adequate cerebral perfusion in patients with ongoing hypertensive disease is higher than for those without this condition. Because of this situation, it is difficult to recommend optimum pressure levels to use as targets.

Endocrine Disorders and Metabolic Dysfunction

There has been much controversy over the use of ECT in patients with diabetes mellitus. There is a report that ECT lowers blood glucose levels in very mild diabetes (Fakhri, Fadhli, & El Rawi, 1980), but the initial high glucose levels may have been secondary to a depression-related stress effect. In individuals with more severe forms of diabetes, particularly those who are insulin dependent, ECT may transiently elevate blood glucose, requiring increased doses of antidiabetic agents (Finestone & Weiner, 1984). For this reason, blood glucose levels should be followed on a more frequent basis in patients at risk for such a response, with daily determinations necessary in some particularly brittle cases. Because of an ictally mediated hypothalmic

activation and associated potentiating effects on pituitary function, ECT has been advocated as a treatment for certain neuro-endocrine hypofunctional states, such as hypopituitarism (Ries & Bokan, 1979) and inappropriate antidiuretic hormone secretion (Brent & Chodroff, 1982).

Since hypothyroidism is often associated with depressive symptomatology, patients with this condition may occasionally find themselves referred for ECT, particularly if functional symptoms do not improve with replacement therapy or if an urgent clinical response is indicated. ECT can be carried out in such cases without difficulty (Garrett, 1985). Theoretically, hyperthyroidism is a cause for concern with ECT, because of the potential for provoking a "thyroid storm" via the transient massive sympathetic activation that occurs. In practice, however, this effect can be prevented by the use of beta-blocking agents. Asymptomatic mild hyperthyroid states, which may sometimes be secondary to stress-related effects associated with the depressive illness, can actually show improvement with ECT (Diaz-Cabal, Pearlman, & Kawecki, 1986).

The presence of a pheochromocytoma is a source of potential danger with ECT, and beta-blocking agents should be used in sufficient dosages to obviate the occurrence of a hypertensive crisis (Carr & Woods, 1985). Cortisol supplementation should be continued during ECT in patients with Addison's disease (Cumming & Kort, 1956). In fact, induced seizures appear to be associated with a transient increase in corticosteroid requirements, suggesting the need for additional supplementation prior to each treatment, for example, 100 mg IV hydrocortisone, in such cases. Patients on long-term steroid therapy should also receive hydrocortisone on the morning of ECT.

Patients with metabolic imbalances may sometimes present problems in ECT. Dehydration has been reported to be associated with elevated seizure threshold. In addition, there are anesthetic implications in the volume depletion that is, by definition, present in dehydrated individuals. Electrolyte imbalance tends not to be a great concern, except in the case of potassium imbalance, since both hypokalemia and hyperkalemia raise the risk or cardiac dysfunction with ECT. Cardiac risk is particularly worrisome with hyperkalemia, because a sudden rise in serum potassium is produced by both muscle fasciculations and ictal motor contractions. Patients with severe widespread burns, chronic immobilization, or spastic paralysis may experience a particularly high serum potassium level during ECT (Bali, 1975). The transient rise in serum potassium can be greatly diminished by the use of complete relaxation. This state may be induced by curare (3–6 mg IV), followed several minutes later by approximately 1.5–2 times the standard dose of succinylcholine. *Hypo*kalemia, on the other hand, creates a risk of prolonged paralysis and apnea after succinylcholine is administered. As for other metabolic disorders, the presence of porphyria should result in the consideration of nonbarbiturate anesthetic agents.

Other Medical Disorders

Because of the risk of dislodging emboli, thrombophlebitis used to be considered a relative contraindication for ECT. With the innovation of anticoagulants, however, this is no longer the case. The preferred agent for patients with hypercoagulable states is heparin, as its action can be readily reversed by protamine, its metabolism is not affected by anesthetic agents used with ECT, and it has a short half-life (Alexopoulos, Nasr, Young, Wikstrom, & Holzman, 1982; Loo, Cuche, & Benkelfat, 1985). Patients on warfarin should be switched to heparin. It is recommended that heparin be withheld for 6–8 hours prior to the treatment in order to

allow coagulability to stabilize. This effect can be monitored by partial thromboplastin time, which should be around 1–1.5 times control values by an hour before each ECT treatment (Alexopoulos et al., 1982). In addition to the adjustment of anticoagulant medication, augmented muscle relaxant dosages should be administered and the adjunctive use of antihypertensive drugs considered. With regard to platelet count, ECT has been administered without difficulty in both thrombocytopenic (Kardener, 1968) and thrombocythemic states (Hamilton & Walter-Ryan, 1986).

Very little has been written on the use of ECT in pulmonary disorders. Chronic obstructive pulmonary disease (COPD), which is rather prevalent in the age range of patients typically referred for ECT, is reflected clinically in decreased ventilatory capacity during the ECT procedure. Preoxygenation prior to each treatment may minimize potential for hypoxia in such cases. Patients with COPD or asthma are at relatively higher risk for bronchial spasm following ECT. For this reason, it is recommended that bronchodilators be continued, even though theophylline may increase the likelihood of prolonged seizures. Theophylline levels should be kept at 15 μg/ml or below, and other bronchodilators should be used if this is insufficient. The anesthesiologist should also be alerted to the possibility of prolonged seizures, so that diazepam will be on hand to deal with such an occurrence.

Before the days of muscular relaxation, patients with musculoskeletal disease or abnormalities were referred for ECT with great trepidation. Now, potential complications resulting from either ictal contractions or pre-ictal fasciculations can be prevented by providing a state of complete muscular relaxation (Coffey, Weiner, Kalayjian, & Christison, 1986). This effect can be achieved, as discussed above, with a combination of curare and increased succinylcholine dosage and can be monitored with the use of a peripheral nerve stimulator. The brief contraction of the jaw muscles that often occurs during the passage of the stimulus current varies in intensity and may be only partially modified by the muscle relaxant agent. Particularly with patients with poor dentition, dental fractures can occur unless a soft rubber mouthpiece, properly inserted, is used and the mandible and maxilla held in close apposition during the passage of the stimulus current (Faber, 1983). Patients with very loose or damaged teeth may require more specific dental protection or removal of involved teeth prior to beginning ECT. Although all patients receiving ECT should be instructed to void prior to the procedure, this instruction is more critical in individuals with urinary retention, where the rare occurrence of bladder rupture during the seizure is a possibility (Irving & Drayson, 1984).

Although ECT produces a transient increase in intraocular pressure of around 20 mm Hg (Epstein, Fagman, Bruce, & Abram, 1975), this change is generally of no clinical consequence, even in cases of chronic open-angle glaucoma (Nathan, Dowling, Peters, & Kreps, 1986). It is only with acute closed-angle glaucoma, a much rarer condition, that a significant ophthalmologic risk with ECT is present (Sibony, 1985). Cholinesterase inhibitors typically used in treating glaucoma, such as physostigmine and neostigmine, will prolong the effects of succinylcholine, but generally only to a mild degree, and thus they do not usually constitute a major problem with ECT. Organophosphorus anticholinesterases, such as echothiophate, on the other hand, have a much more profound and long-lasting effect on succinylcholine metabolism (Packman, Meyer, & Verdun, 1978).

In addition to anticholinesterases, a variety of other medications may interact in an adverse fashion with ECT. The ability of a number of pharmacologic agents to prolong the paralytic effects of succinylcholine has already been discussed. As noted, the use of a beta-blocking agent without adequate anticholinergic premedication can produce cardiac asystole (Decina, Malitz, Sackeim, et al., 1984). The anticonvulsive effect of sedative hypnotic agents, particularly benzodiazepines (Standish-Barry, Deacon, & Smith, 1985), has also been mentioned, as have the effects of other drugs that significantly shorten seizure duration, for example, lidocaine (Hood & Mecca, 1983) and L-tryptophan (Price & Zimmer, 1985). On the other hand, stimulants, such as theophylline (Peters, Wochos, & Peterson, 1984) and caffeine (Shapira, Zohar, Newman, et al., 1985), prolong the ictal period.

Malignant hyperthermia, a rare hypermetabolic state, is pharmacologically triggered on an idiosyncratic basis and presents with tachycardia, muscle spasms, acidosis, and anoxia. The most common offending agent is succinylcholine, though other anesthetic and even psychotropic drugs have been reported (Yacoub & Morrow, 1986). A personal and, given the inherited predisposition to this condition, family history of similar past presentations can alert the practitioner to a potential high-risk situation (Bidder, 1981). In such occurrences, a muscle biopsy will allow a definitive assessment. Prophylactic use of the muscle relaxant dantrolene, 1–2.5 mg/kg given intravenously at the time of each anesthesia induction, has been recommended if the condition is anticipated, though the effectiveness of such prophylaxis is not yet proven.

THE USE OF ECT IN PREGNANCY

ECT has been performed in many pregnant patients in all three trimesters of gestation without difficulties (Dorn, 1985; Remick & Maurice, 1978). Adequate oxygenation and muscular relaxation should always be assured in such cases. The addition of fetal monitoring, including, at times, real-time ultrasonography and uterine muscle dynamometry, should be considered where applicable, at least in high-risk cases (Wise, Ward, Townsend-Parchman, Gilstrap, & Hauth, 1984).

ECT IN THE ELDERLY

Elderly patients are at greater risk for adverse sequelae with *either* psychopharmacologic treatment or ECT (Gerring & Shields, 1982; Alexopoulos, Shamoian, Lucas, Weiser, & Berger, 1984). The question whether the increased risk is greater for one type of modality than for the other, however, remains unsettled, and a well-controlled study of this type would be difficult to carry out. Still, many sources report a subjective belief that ECT is in fact "safer" than drugs in this age group (Weiner, 1982). Medical morbidity with ECT in the elderly is most likely due to the presence of concurrent medical disease, particularly chronic cardiac dysfunction.

One potential problem in the provision of ECT for the elderly is the ability to induce seizures of sufficient duration. At times even maximum stimulus intensities may prove unsuccessful, although this failure is less likely with the higher maximum output provided by most contemporary ECT devices. As already mentioned, a variety of means exist to deal with this situation, should it occur. First, one should be certain that the dose of anesthetic agent is not greater than necessary. Second, stimulus should not be given until at least 2 minutes have elapsed following administration of the barbituarate anesthetic. Third, drugs with anticonvulsant effects should be discontinued whenever possible. Fourth, a stimulant agent such as caffeine can be used. Fifth, an anesthetic with minimal anticonvulsant properties, for example, ketamine, should be considered.

REFERENCES

Abiuso P, Dunkleman R, & Prober M (1978). Electroconvulsive therapy in patients with pacemakers. *Journal of the American Medical Association*, *240*, 2459–2460.

Abramczuk JA & Rose NM (1979). Preanesthetic assessment and prevention of post ECT morbidity. *British Journal of Psychiatry*, *134*, 582–587.

Abrams R (1985). Multiple-monitored ECT. *Convulsive Therapy*, *1*, 285–286.

Abrams R (1986). Is unilateral electroconvulsive therapy really the treatment of choice in endogenous depression? In S Malitz & HA Sackeim (Eds), *Annals of the New York Academy of Sciences*: *vol. 462 Electroconvulsive Therapy: Clinical and Basic Research Issues* (pp 50–55). New York: New York Academy of Sciences.

Abrams R & Fink M (1984). The present status of unilateral ECT: Some recommendations. *Journal of Affective Disorders*, *7*, 245–247.

Alexopoulos GS & Frances RJ (1980). ECT in cardiac patients with pacemakers. *American Journal of Psychiatry*, *137*, 1111–1112.

Alexopoulos GS, Nasr H, Young RC, et al. (1982). Electroconvulsive therapy in patients on anticoagulants. *Canadian Journal of Psychiatry*, *27*, 46–47.

Alexopoulos GS, Shamolan CJ, Lucas J, et al. (1984). Medical problems of geriatric psychiatric patients and younger controls during electroconvulsive therapy. *Journal of the American Geriatrics Society*, *32*, 651–654.

American Psychiatric Association (1978). *Electroconvulsive therapy* (Task Force Report No. 14). Washington, DC: American Psychiatric Association.

American Psychiatric Association (1987). *Diagnostic and statistical manual of mental disorders* (3rd ed, revised). Washington, DC: American Psychiatric Association.

Ananth J, Samra D, & Kolwakis T (1979). Amelioration of drug-induced parkinsonism by ECT. *American Journal of Psychiatry*, *136*, 1094.

Anton AH, Uy DS & Redderson CL (1977). Autonomic blockade and the cardiovascular catecholamine response to electroshock. *Anesthesia and Analgesia, 56*, 46–54.

Avery D & Lubrano A (1979). Depression treated with imipramine and ECT: The DeCarolis study reconsidered. *American Journal of Psychiatry, 136*, 549–562.

Azar I & Lear E (1984). Cardiovascular effects of electroconvulsive therapy in patients taking tricyclic antidepressants. *Anesthesia and Analgesia, 63*, 1139.

Bali IM (1975). The effect of modified electroconvulsive therapy on plasma potassium concentration. *British Journal of Anaesthesia, 47*, 398–401.

Balldin J, Eden S, Granerus AK, et al., (1980). Electroconvulsive therapy in Parkinsons's syndrome with "on-off" phenomenon. *Journal of Neural Transmission, 47*, 11–21.

Barkai AI (1985). combined electroconvulsive and drug therapy. *Comprehensive Therapy, 11*, 48–53.

Bergsholm P, Gran L, & Bleie H (1984). Seizure duration in unilateral electroconvulsive therapy: The effect of hypocapnia induced by hyperventilation and the effect of ventilation with oxygen. *Acta Psychiatrica Scandinavica, 69*, 121–128.

Bidder TG (1981). Electroconvulsive therapy in the medically ill patient. *Psychiatric Clinics of North America, 4*, 391–405.

Bolwig TG, Hertz MM, & Westergaard E (1977). Acute hypertension causing blood brain barrier breakdown in epileptic seizures. *Acta Neurologica Scandinavica, 56*, 335–342.

Brandon S, Cowley P, McDonald C, et al., (1984). Electroconvulsive therapy: Results in depressive illness from the Leicestershire trial. *British Medical Journal, 288*, 22–25.

Brandon S, Cowley P, McDonald C, et al. (1985). Leicester ECT trial: Results in schizophrenia. *British Journal of Psychiatry, 146*, 177–183.

Breakey WE & Kala AK (1977). Typhoid catatonia responsive to ECT. *British Medical Journal, 2*, 357–359.

Breggin PR (1979). *Electroshock: Its brain disabling effects*. New York: Springer-Verlag.

Brent RH & Chodroff C (1982). ECT as a possible treatment of SIADH: Case report. *Journal of Clinical Psychiatry, 43*, 73–74.

Brewer CL, Davidson JRT, & Hereward S (1972). Ketamine ("ketalar"): A safer anaesthetic for ECT. *British Journal of Psychiatry, 120*, 679–680.

Carr ME Jr & Woods J W (1985). Electroconvulsive therapy in a patient with unsuspected pheochromocytoma. *Southern Medical Journal, 78*, 613–615.

Cass NM, Doolan LA, & Gutteridge GA (1982). Repeated administration of suxamethonium in a patient with atypical plasma cholinesterase. *Anaesthesia and Intensive Care, 10*, 25–28.

Chacko RC & Root L (1983). ECT and tardive dyskinesia: Two cases and a review. *Journal of Clinical Psychiatry, 44*, 265–266.

Clinical Research Centre (1984). The Northwick Park ECT trial: Predictors of response to real and simulated ECT. *British Journal of Psychiatry, 144*, 227–237.

Coffey CE, Hinkle PE, Weiner RD, et al., (1987). Electroconvulsive therapy of depression in patients with white matter hyperintensity. *Biological Psychiatry, 22*, 629–636.

Coffey CE, Smith G, Weiner RD, & Moossy JJ (in press). Electroconvulsive therapy in a depressed patient with a functioning ventriculo-atrial shunt. *Convulsive Therapy*

Coffey CE, Weiner RD, Hinkle PE, et al., (1987). Augmentation of ECT seizures with caffeine. *Biological Psychiatry, 22*, 637–649.

Coffey CE, Weiner RD, Kalayjian R, & Christison C (1986). Electroconvulsive therapy in osteogenesis imperfecta: Issues of muscular relaxation. *Convulsive Therapy, 2*, 207–211.

Coffey CE, Weiner RD, McCall WV, & Hines ER (1987). Electroconvulsive therapy in multiple sclerosis: A brain magnetic resonance imaging study. *Convulsive Therapy, 3*, 137–144.

Consensus Conference (1985). Electroconvulsive therapy. *Journal of the American Medical Association, 254*, 2103–2108.

Coppen A, Abou-Saleh MT, Milln P, Bailey J, et al., (1981). Lithium continuation therapy following electroconvulsive therapy. *British Journal of Psychiatry, 139*, 284–287.

Coryell W (1986). Are serial dexamethasone suppression tests useful in electroconvulsive therapy? *Journal of Affective Disorders, 10*, 59–66.

Cumming J & Kord K (1956). Apparent reversal by cortisone of an electroconvulsive refractory state in a psychotic patient with Addison's disease. *Canadian Medical Association Journal, 74*, 291–292.

Daniel WF, Weiner RD, Crovitz HF, et al., (1983). ECT-induced delirium and further ECT: A case report. *American Journal of Psychiatry, 140*, 922–924.

Dec GW Jr, Stern TA, & Welch C (1985). The effects of electroconvulsive therapy on serial electrocardiograms and serum cardiac enzyme values: A prospective study of depressed hospitalized inpatients. *Journal of the American Medical Association, 253*, 2525–2529.

Decina P, Malitz S, Sackeim HA, et al., (1984). Cardiac arrest during ECT modified by beta-adrenergic blockage. *American Journal of Psychiatry, 141*, 298–300.

d'Elia G (1970). Unilateral ECT. *Acta Psychiatrica Scandinavica* (Suppl 215), 1–98.

d'Elia G & Raotma H (1975). Is unilateral ECT less effective than bilateral ECT? *British Journal of Psychiatry*, *126*, 83–89.

Dellyiannis S, Eliakim M, & Bellet S (1962). The electrocardiogram during electroconvulsive therapy as studied by radioelectrocardiography. *American Journal of Cardiology*, *10*, 187–192.

Diaz-Cabal R, Pearlman C, & Kawecki A (1986). Hyperthyroidism in a patient with agitated depression: Resolution after electroconvulsive therapy. *Journal of Clinical Psychiatry*, *47*, 322–323.

Dorn JB (1985). Electroconvulsive therapy with fetal monitoring in a bipolar pregnant patient. *Convulsive Therapy*, *1*, 217–221.

Dubovsky SL (1986). Using electroconvulsive therapy for patients with neurological disease. *Hospital and Community Psychiatry*, *37*, 819–824.

Egbert LD, Wolfe S, Melmed RM, et al., (1959). Reduction of cardiovascular stress during electroshock therapy by trimethaphan. *Journal of Clinical Experimental Psychopathology & Quarterly Review of Psychiatric Neurology*, *20*, 315–319.

El-Ganzouri AR, Ivankovich Ad, Braverman B, & McCarthy R (1985). Monoamine oxidase inhibitors: Should they be discontinued preoperatively? *Anesthesia and Analgesia*, *64*, 592–596.

Elliot JL, Linz DH, & Kane JA (1982). Electroconvulsive therapy: pretreatment medical evaluation. *Annals of Internal Medicine*, *142*, 979–981.

Epstein HM, Fagman W, Bruce DL, & Abram A (1975). Intraocular pressure changes during anesthesia for electroshock therapy. *Anesthesia and Analgesia*, *54*, 479–481.

Faber, R (1983). Dental fracture during ECT. *American Journal of Psychiatry*, *140*, 1255–1256.

Fakhri O, Fadhli AA, & El Rawi RM (1980). Effect of electroconvulsive therapy on diabetes mellitus. *Lancet*, *2*, 775–777.

Finestone DH & Weiner RD (1984). Effects of ECT on diabetes mellitus. An attempt to account for conflicting data. *Acta Psychiatrica Scandinavica*, *70*, 321–326.

Fink M (1979). *Convulsive therapy: Theory and Practice*. New York: Raven Press.

Frederiksen SO & d'Elia G (1979). Electroconvulsive therapy in Sweden. *British Journal of Psychiatry*, *134*, 283–287.

Freeman RL, Galaburda AM, Cabal RD, & Geschwind N (1985). The neurology of depression: Cognitive and behavioral deficits with focal findings in depression and resolution after electroconvulsive therapy. *Archives of Neurology*, *42*, 289–291.

Freese KJ (1985). Can patients safely undergo electroconvulsive therapy while receiving monoamine oxidase inhibitors? *Convulsive Therapy*, *1*, 190–194.

Garrett MD (1985). Use of ECT in a depressed hypothyroid patient. *Journal of Clinical Psychiatry*, *46*, 64–66.

Gerring JP & Shields HM (1982). The identification and management of patients with a high risk for cardiac arrhythmias during modified ECT. *Journal of Clinical Psychiatry*, *43*, 140–143.

Greenberg LB (1986). Electroconvulsive therapy in treating neuroleptic malignant syndrome. *Convulsive Therapy*, *2*, 61–62.

Gregory S, Shawcross CR, & Gill D (1985). The Nottingham ECT study: A double-blind comparison of bilateral, unilateral and simulated ECT in depressive illness. *British Journal of Psychiatry*, *146*, 520–524.

Hamilton RW & Walter-Ryan WG (1986). ECT and thrombocythemia. *American Journal of Psychiatry*, *143*, 258.

Heshe AJ & Roeder E (1976). Electroconvulsive therapy in Denmark. *British Journal of Psychiatry*, *128*, 241–245.

Holcomb HH, Sternberg DE, & Heninger GR (1983). Effects of electroconvulsive therapy on mood, parkinsonism, and tardive dyskinesia in a depressed patient: ECT and dopamine systems. *Biological Psychiatry*, *18*, 865–873.

Hood DA & Mecca RS (1983). Failure to initiate electroconvulsive seizures in a patient pretreated with lidocaine. *Anesthesiology*, *58*, 379–381.

Hsiao JK & Evans DL (1984). ECT in a depressed patient after craniotomy. *American Journal of Psychiatry*, *141*, 442–444.

Hughes JR (1986). ECT during and after the neuroleptic malignant syndrome: Case report. *Journal of Clinical Psychiatry*, *47*, 42–43.

Husum B, Vester-Andersen T, Buchmann G, & Bolwig TG (1983). Electroconvulsive therapy and intracranial aneurysm: Prevention of blood pressure elevation in a normotensive patient by hydralazine and propranolol. *Anaesthesia*, *38*, 1205–1207.

Imlah NW, Ryan E, & Harrington JA (1965). The influence of antidepressant drugs on the response to electroconvulsive therapy and on subsequent relapse rates. *Neuropsychopharmacology*, *4*, 483–442.

Irving AD & Drayson AM (1984). Bladder rupture during ECT. *British Journal of Psychiatry*, *144*, 670.

Jones RM & Knight PR (1981). Cardiovascular and hormonal responses to electroconvulsive therapy: Modification of an exaggerated response in an hypertensive patient by beta receptor blockade. *Anesthesia*, *36*, 795–799.

Kalinowsky LB & Kennedy F (1943). Observation in

electroshock therapy applied to problems of epilepsy. *Journal of Nervous and Mental Disorders*, *98*, 56–67.

Kardener SH (1968). EST in a patient with idiopathic thrombocytopenic purpura. *Diseases of the Nervous System*, *29*, 465–466.

Karliner W (1978). ECT for patients with CNS disease. *Psychosomatics 19*, 781–783.

Kolbeinsson H, Arnaldsson OS, Petursson H, & Skulason (1986). Computed tomographic scans in ECT-patients. *Acta Psychiatrica Scandinavica*, *73*, 28–32.

Kramer BA, Allen RE, & Friedman B (1986). Atropine and glycopyrrolate as ECT preanesthesia. *Journal of Clinical Psychiatry*, *47*, 199–200.

Kramp P & Bolwig TG (1981). Electroconvulsive therapy in acute delirious states. *Comprehensive Psychiatry*, *22*, 368–371.

Kraus RP & Remick RA (1982). Diazoxide in the management of severe hypertension after electroconvulsive therapy. *American Journal of Psychiatry*, *139*, 504–505.

Lancaster NP, Steinert RR, & Frost I (1958). Unilateral electroconvulsive therapy. *Journal of Mental Science*, *104*, 221–227.

Lee JT, Erbguth PH, Stevens WC, & Sack RL (1985). Modification of electroconvulsive therapy induced hypertension with nitroglycerin ointment. *Anesthesiology*, *62*, 793–796.

Lerer, B (1984). ECT and tardive dyskinesia. *Journal of Clinical Psychiatry*, *45*, 188.

Levy LA, Savit JM, & Hodes M (1983). Parkinsonism: Improvement by electroconvulsive therapy. *Archives of Physical and Medical Rehabilitation*, *64*, 432–433.

Lewis WH Jr, Richardson DJ, & Gahagan LH (1955). Cardiovascular disturbances and management in electrotherapy in psychiatric illness. *New England Journal of Medicine*, *252*, 1016–1020.

London SW & Glass DD (1985). Prevention of electroconvulsive therapy-induced dysrhythmias with atropine and propranolol. *Anesthesiology*, *62*, 819–822.

Loo H, Cuche H, & Benkelfat C (1985). Electroconvulsive therapy during anticoagulant therapy. *Convulsive Therapy*, *1*, 258–262.

Maletzky BM (1981). *Multiple-monitored electroconvulsive therapy*. Boca Raton, FL: CRC Press.

Malitz S, Sackeim HA, Decina P, et al., (1986). The efficacy of electroconvulsive therapy: Dose-response interactions with modality. In S Malitz & HA Sackeim (Eds): *Annals of the New York Academy of Sciences Vol. 462 Electroconvulsive Therapy: Clinical and Basic Research Issues* (pp 56–64). New York: New York Academy of Sciences.

Maltbie AA, Wingfield MS, Volow MR, et al., (1980).

Electroconvulsive therapy in the presence of brain tumor: Case reports and an evaluation of risk. *Journal of Nervous and Mental disorders*, *168*, 400–405.

Mandel MR (1975). Electroconvulsive therapy for chronic pain associated with depression. *American Journal of Psychiatry*, *132*, 632–636.

McAllister TW & Price TRP (1982). Severe depressive pseudodementia with and without dementia. *American Journal of Psychiatry*, *139*, 626–629.

McKenna G, Engle RP, Brooks H, & Dalen J (1970). Cardiac arrhythmias during electroshock therapy: Significance, prevention and treatment. *American Journal of Psychiatry*, *127*, 530–533.

Miller ME, Siris SG, & Gabriel AN (1986). Treatment delays in the course of electroconvulsive therapy. *Hospital and Community Psychiatry*, *37*, 825–827.

Mondimore FM, Damlouji N, Folstein MF, & Tune L (1983). Post-ECT confusional states associated with elevated serum anticholinergic levels. *American Journal of Psychiatry*, *140*, 930–931.

Murray GB, Shea V, & Conn DK (1986). Electroconvulsive therapy for poststroke depression. *Journal of Clinical Psychiatry*, *47*, 258–260.

Nathan RS, Dowling R, Peters JL, & Kreps A (1986). ECT and glaucoma. *Convulsive Therapy*, *2*, 132–133.

O'Leary J (1981). Cardiac effects of electroconvulsive therapy. *Anaesthesia and Intensive Care*, *9*, 400–401.

Ottosson JO (1960). Experimental studies on the mode of action of electroconvulsive therapy. *Acta Psychiatrica Neurologica Scandinavica*, *35* (Suppl 145), 1–141.

Packman M, Meyer MA, & Verdun RM (1978). Hazards of succinylcholine administration during electrotherapy. *Archives of General Psychiatry*, *35*, 1137–1141.

Papakostas Y, Fink M, Lee J, et al., (1981). Neuroendocrine measures in psychiatric patients: Course and outcome with ECT. *Psychiatry Research*, *4*, 55–64.

Parry J (1986). Legal parameters of informed consent for ECT administered to mentally disabled persons. *Psychopharmacology Bulletin*, *22*, 490–494.

Paul SM, Extein I, Calil HM, et al., (1981). Use of ECT with treatment-resistant depressed patients at the National Institute of Mental Health. *American Journal of Psychiatry*, *138*, 486–489.

Paulson GW (1967). Exacerbation of organic brain disease by electroconvulsive treatment. *North Carolina Medical Journal*, *28*, 328–331.

Pearlman CA (1986). Neuroleptic malignant syndrome: A review of the literature. *Journal of Clinical Psychopharmacology*, *6*, 257–273.

Perrin GM (1961). Cardio-vascular aspects of

electroshock therapy. *Acta Psychiatrica Neurologica Scandinavica*, *36*(Suppl 152), 1–44.

Peters SG, Wochos DN, & Peterson GC (1984). Status epilepticus complicating electroconvulsive therapy in the presence of theophylline. *Mayo Clinic Proceedings*, *59*, 568–570.

Pettinati HM, Mathisen KS, Rosenberg J, & Lynch JF (1986). Meta-analytical approach to reconciling discrepancies in efficacy between bilateral and unilateral electroconvulsive therapy. *Convulsive Therapy*, *2*, 7–17.

Pitts FN Jr, Desmarias GM, Stewart W, & Schaberg K (1965). Induction of anesthesia with methohexital and thiopental in electroconvulsive therapy. *New England Journal of Medicine*, *273*, 353–360.

Price TRP & McAllister TW (1986). Response of depressed patients to sequential unilateral nondominant brief-pulse and bilateral sinusoidal ECT. *Journal of Clinical Psychiatry*, *47*, 182–186.

Price WA & Zimmer B (1985). Effect of L-tryptophan on electroconvulsive therapy seizure time. *Journal of Nervous and Mental Disorders*, *175*, 636–638.

Raskin DE (1984). Dangers of monoamine oxidase inhibitors. *Journal of Clinical Psychopharmacology*, *4*, 238.

Regestein QR & Lind JF (1980). Management of electroconvulsive treatment in an elderly woman with severe hypertension and cardiac arrhythmias. *Comprehensive Psychiatry*, *21*, 288–291.

Regestein QR & Reich P (1985). Electroconvulsive therapy in patients at high risk for physical complications. *Convulsive Therapy*, *1*, 101–114.

Remick RA & Maurice Wl (1978). ECT in pregnancy. *American Journal of Psychiatry*, *135*, 761–762.

Ries R & Bokan J (1979). Electroconvulsive therapy following pituitary surgery. *Journal of Nervous and Mental Disorders*, *167*, 767–768.

Robin A & De Tissera S (1982). A double-blind controlled comparison of the therapeutic effects of low and high energy electroconvulsive therapies. *British Journal of Psychiatry*, *141*, 357–366.

Rosen AM, Mukherjee S, & Shinbach K (1984). The efficacy of ECT in phencyclidine-induced psychosis. *Journal of Clinical Psychiatry*, *45*, 220–222.

Rothman DJ (1986). ECT: The historical, social, and professional sources of the controversy. *Psychopharmacology Bulletin*, *22*, 459–463.

Roy-Byrne P & Gerner RH (1981). Legal restrictions on the use of ECT in California: Clinical impact on the incompetent patient. *Journal of Clinical Psychiatry*, *42*, 300–303.

Ruedrich SL, Chu CC, & Moore SL (1983). ECT for major depression in a patient with acute brain trauma. *American Journal of Psychiatry*, *140*, 928–929.

Salzman C (1980). The use of ECT in the treatment of schizophrenia. *American Journal of Psychiatry*, *137*, 1032–1041.

Scovern AW & Kilman PR (1980). Status of ECT: A review of the outcome literature. *Psychology Bulletin*, *87*, 260 303.

Shapira B, Zohar J, Newman M, et al., (1985). Potentiation of seizure length and clinical response to electroconvulsive therapy by caffeine pretreatment: A case report. *Convulsive Therapy*, *1*, 58–60.

Shea L & Pollard B (1978). E.C.T. for patients with prolonged response to suxamethonium. *Anaesthesia and Intensive Care*, *6*, 170.

Sibony PA (1985). ECT risks in glaucoma. *Convulsive Therapy*, *1*, 283–287.

Siris SG, Glassman AH, & Stetner F (1982). ECT and psychotropic medication in the treatment of depression and schizophrenia. In R Abrams & WB Essman (Eds), *Electroconvulsive therapy: Biological Foundations and clinical applications* (pp 91–111). New York: Spectrum Publications.

Small JG (1985). Efficacy of electroconvulsive therapy in schizophrenia, mania, and other disorders: 1. Schizophrenia. *Convulsive Therapy*, *1*, 263–270.

Small JG, Kellams JJ, & Milstein V (1980). Complications with electroconvulsive therapy combined with lithium. *Biological Psychiatry*, *15*, 103–112.

Small JG, Milstein V, Klapper MH, et al., (1986). Electroconvulsive therapy in the treatment of manic episodes. In S Malitz & HA Sackeim (Eds), *Annals of the New York Academy of Sciences*: *Vol. 462. Electroconvulsive therapy*: *Clinical and Basic Research Issues* (pp 37–49). New York: New York Academy of Sciences.

Smith K, Surphlis WRP, Gynther MD, & Shimkunas AM (1967). ECT-chlorpromazine and chlorpromazine compared in the treatment of schizophrenia. *Journal of Nervous and Mental Disorders*, *144*, 284–290.

Snaith RP (1981). How much ECT does the depressed patient need? In RL Palmer (Ed.), *Electroconvulsive therapy*: *An appraisal* (pp 61–64). Oxford: Oxford University Press.

Snow SS & Wells CE (1981). Case studies in neuropsychiatry: Diagnosis and treatment of coexistent dementia and depression. *Journal of Clinical Psychiatry*, *42*, 439–441.

Squire LR (1986). Memory functions as affected by electroconvulsive therapy. In S Malitz & HA Sackeim (Eds), *Annals of the New York Academy of Sciences*: *Vol. 462. Electroconvulsive therapy*: *Clinical and Basic Research Issues* (pp 307–314). New York: New York Academy of Sciences.

Standish-Barry HMAS, Deacon V, & Snaith RP (1985). The relationship of concurrent benzodiazepine administration to seizure duration in

ECT. *Acta Psychiatrica Scandinavica, 71*, 269–271.

Stevenson GH & Geoghegan JJ (1951). Prophylactic electroshock—a five-year study. *American Journal of Psychiatry, 107*, 743–748.

Stromgren LS (1984). Is bilateral ECT ever indicated? *Acta Psychiatrica Scandinavica, 69*, 484–490.

Thompson JW (1986). Utilization of ECT in U.S. psychiatric facilities, 1975 to 1980. *Psychopharmacology Bulletin, 22*, 463–465.

Tsuang MT, Tidball JS & Geller D (1979). ECT in a depressed patient with shunt in place for normal pressure hydrocephalus. *American Journal of Psychiatry, 136*, 1205–1206.

Weiner RD (1979). The psychiatric use of electrically induced seizures. *American Journal of Psychiatry, 136*, 1507–1517.

Weiner RD (1982). The role of ECT in the treatment of depression in the elderly. *Journal of the American Geriatrics Society, 30*, 710–712.

Weiner RD (1983). EEG related to electroconvulsive therapy. In JR Hughes & WP Wilson (Eds.), *EEG and evoked potentials in psychiatry and behavioral neurology* (pp 101–126). Boston: Butterworth Publishers.

Weiner RD (1984). Does ECT cause brain damage? *The Behavioral and Brain Sciences, 7*, 1–53. 1984.

Weiner RD (1986). Electrical dosage, stimulus parameters, and electrode placement. *Psychopharmacology Bulletin, 22*, 499–502.

Weiner RD & Coffey Ce (1986). Minimizing therapeutic differences between bilateral and unilateral nondominant ECT. *Convulsive Therapy, 2*, 261–265.

Weiner RD, Henschen GM, Dellasega M, & Baker JS (1979). Propranolol treatment of an ECT-related ventricular arrhythmia. *American Journal of Psychiatry, 136*, 1594–1595.

Weiner RD, Rogers HJ, Davidson JRT, & Kahn EM (1986). Effects of electroconvulsive therapy upon brain electrical activity. In S Malitz & HA Sackeim (Eds), *Annals of the New York Academy of Sciences: Vol. 462. Electroconvulsive Therapy: Clinical and Basic Research Issues* (pp 270–281). New York: New York Academy of Sciences.

Weiner RD, Rogers HJ, Davidson JRT, & Squire LR (1986). Effects of stimulus parameters on cognitive side effects. In S Malitz & HA Sackeim (Eds), *Annals of the New York Academy of Sciences: Vol. 462 Electroconvulsive Therapy: Clinical and Basic Research Issues* (pp 315–325). New York: New York Academy of Sciences.

Weiner RD, Whanger AD, Erwin CW, & Wilson WP (1980). Prolonged confusional state and EEG seizure activity following concurrent ECT and lithium use. *American Journal of Psychiatry, 137*, 1452–1453.

Whittaker M (1980). Plasma cholinesterase variants and the anaesthetist. *Anaesthesia, 35*, 174–197.

Wise MG, Ward SC, Townsend-Parchman W, et al., (1984). Case report of ECT during high-risk pregnancy. *American Journal of Psychiatry, 141*, 99–101.

Wyant GM & MacDonald WB (1980). The role of atropine in electroconvulsive therapy. *Anaesthesia and Intensive Care, 8*, 445–450.

Yacoub OF & Morrow DH (1986). Malignant hyperthermia and ECT. *American Journal of Psychiatry, 143*, 1027–1029.

Young RC, Alexopoulos GS, & Shamoian CA (1985). Dissociation of motor response from mood and cognition in a parkinsonian patient treated with ECT. *Biological Psychiatry, 20*, 566–569.

Andrew Edmund Slaby
Leah Oseas Cullen

6
Dementia and Delirium

DEMENTIA

Dementia is a chronic impairment of cognitive ability secondary to cerebral cortical or subcortical cellular dysfunction (Slaby, 1982, 1986). The prevalence of dementia is not precisely known. Estimates vary greatly depending on whether populations sampled include only individuals over 65, whether subjects are from the general community or from institutional populations, whether attempts have been made to differentiate subtypes of dementing illnesses, and whether standardized diagnostic criteria for dementia have been employed (Henderson, 1986). It has been estimated that dementia affects 10 percent of persons aged 65 years or older (Roca et al., 1984), with an annual incidence rate of 1 percent in the same age group (Henderson, 1986). It is significant to note that the prevalence of severe dementias increases dramatically in the institutionalized elderly: 15 percent in retirement communities, 30 percent in nursing homes, and 54 percent in state hospitals (Cummings & Benson, 1983). Delirium is also more frequent in hospitalized patients with multiple medical

problems and medications and is associated with poor prognosis and higher mortality than uncomplicated dementia (Lipowski, 1983; Rabins & Folstein, 1982; Trzepacz, Teague, & Lipowski, 1985). The frequency of delirium in terminally ill cancer patients may be as high as 85 percent (Massie, Holland, & Glass, 1983).

Dementia is not a diagnosis per se and requires a differential diagnosis. Dementia is not always irreversible. At least 20 percent of cases diagnosed as dementia are at least partially reversible (McCartney & Palmateer, 1985). The degree to which the dysfunction is reversible depends on the extent, character, and location of central nervous system damage and on the degree to which cognitive function is determined by psychiatric disorder rather than anatomic central nervous system (CNS) damage.

Clinical Description

Early signs of dementia include (Murray, 1987; Read, Small, & Jarvik, 1985; Waldinger, 1986): lack of initiative, increasing irritability, loss of interest in life activities, and problems learning new information or carrying out activities requiring original thought. The latter symptoms are most apparent in patients with artistic, intellectual, or creative jobs. Early memory is lost first, requiring repetition of instructions or information.

In the chronically medically ill, an early sign of dementia may be an impaired coping with the tasks of daily living that is due to a decline in cognitive capacity rather than solely to a decline in physical status. For example, a patient with compensated congestive heart failure may stop driving although the heart failure is no worse, or a type II diabetic who has been well controlled on self-administered insulin injections may suddenly begin making mistakes in self-care.

Early dementing processes are best detected through the systematic performance of serial mental status examinations supplemented by regular inquiry about activities of daily living such as the handling of personal finances, arrangement of transportation and driving, cooking, shopping, housework and chores, and communication with friends and relatives. Such inquiry enables the physician to detect changes that may be largely denied by patients themselves, and family interviews are critical to an assessment of the patient as well. Some clinicians prefer the use of formal scales, such as subtests of the Philadelphia Geriatric Center Multi-Level Assessment Instrument, as a guide to formal inquiry (Lawton, Moss, Fulcomer, et al., 1982).

Differential Diagnosis

The challenge in evaluating a patient with dementia is early identification and treatment of potentially treatable or reversible causes. Patients with clouding of consciousness or poor education frequently are mistakenly labeled as primarily demented, while the diagnosis of dementia tends to be

overlooked in younger individuals. In one study (Larson, Reifler, Featherstone, et al., 1984), 15 out of 83 outpatients designated as having irreversible dementias were found to have potentially reversible or at least partially treatable dementing processes, such as hypothyroidism, subdural hematoma, transient ischemic attacks, rheumatoid vasculitis, bipolar disorder, and drug toxicity. Decompensation in any organ system may cause or exacerbate cognitive dysfunction in the elderly (cardiovascular, renal, pulmonary, gastrointestinal, etc.). A complete list of the possibilities would comprise practically all medical illnesses with systemic effects affecting the CNS. More common problems, however, include B_{12} and folate deficiency, iron deficiency anemia, congestive heart failure, chronic obstructive pulmonary disease (COPD), Parkinson's disease, urinary tract infections, and dehydration. In a sample (Rubenstein, 1982) of 406 younger people with dementia, 10 percent were found to have multi-infarct dementia, 5.4 percent normal pressure hydrocephalus, and 3.7 percent resectable mass lesions.

The original concept of differentiation between treatable dementias and untreatable ones has given way to a newer system of classification. Estimates of so-called reversible dementias range from 10–30 percent of all dementing illnesses (Roca et al., 1984; Sloane, 1983). In addition, another 25–30 percent of patients may be partially treatable but not fully reversible dementing disorders (Sloane, 1983). The issue of "treatable dementia" is, therefore, better cast in terms of searching for any drug-induced, toxic, or metabolic disturbance that could be contributing to cognitive dysfunction in the patient, regardless of whether or not a primary underlying dementia is present.

Guidelines facilitating recognition of treatable or reversible cognitive dysfunction include (1) milder symptoms of relatively brief duration (Roca et al., 1984;

Freeman & Rudd, 1982) and (2) the presence of clouding of consciousness suggestive of delirium (Roca et al., 1984).

The list of potential causes of dementia is lengthy and may be found in standard textbooks of neurology, psychiatry, and internal medicine. Although the psychiatrist will generally refer a patient with a suspected dementia to a neurologist or internist for further diagnostic workup, the psychiatrist may be instrumental in finding potential aggravating factors in dementia that other specialists may overlook. For example, psychiatrists obtain detailed histories of drug, alcohol, and medication use and obtain collateral histories when drug toxicity or withdrawal states are suspected. Psychiatrists also are keenly aware of the central nervous system side effects of therapeutic medications in the medically ill, understand the pharmacodynamic and pharmacokinetic variability that comes with age, organ failure, and other disease states, and realize, as the internist may not, that central nervous system toxicities can occur even at therapeutic levels of certain medications.

Psychiatrists may also be instrumental in guiding nonpsychiatrists in diagnostic evaluation beyond the standard textbook dementia workup. For example, mild degrees of hypothyroidism may go undetected by the physician who orders only a T_4 and RT_3U in a patient who appears euthyroid by physical examination. The psychiatrist's index of suspicion, however, may guide the physician to order a thyroid-stimulating hormone (TSH) level. Elevated TSH levels almost always imply hypothyroidism, even when circulating levels of thyroid hormone are normal. The prevalence of this occurrence is 2–5 percent, especially in women over age 60, and may represent the earliest form of thyroid failure (Wilson & Jefferson, 1985). Cognitive impairment and other psychiatric symptoms often occur with hypothyroidism, despite the absence of other physical stigmata of thyroid disease. Standard textbooks do not as a rule, however, recommend obtaining TSH levels as part of their routine screening battery.

Psychiatrists may also be more aware of when drug levels are indicated in situations in which drug combinations may be additive or synergistic. Psychiatrists may also assist by putting together pieces of clinical history to promote more aggressive investigation of a particular diagnosis. For example, if a detailed history suggests the evolution of gait disturbance, urinary incontinence, and mild frontal lobe symptoms, in that order, the psychiatrist will encourage a thorough evaluation for hydrocephalus. Since routine CT scan findings may be equivocal for hydrocephalus, the psychiatrist's input helps decide whether a radioisotope cisternogram or a large-volume lumbar puncture should be carried out (Cummings & Benson, 1983).

Pseudodementia

"Pseudodementia" has been defined as intellectual impairment due to a primary nonorganic psychiatric disorder (Caine, 1981). Wells (1979) opined that pseudodemented individuals, unlike their demented counterparts, are aware of their cognitive deficit and complain of their cognitive losses, highlighting their failures. They exert little effort to perform simple tasks and demonstrate a strong sense of distress, often with pervasive affective changes. Behavior and test performance are inconsistent with severity of cognitive dysfunction. Nocturnal fluctuations are uncommon. Memory loss is equal for recent and remote memory with memory gaps for specific events or periods of time. The pseudodemented give more "don't know" answers to tests of intellect and memory, rather than the near-miss responses seen on cognitive examination of demented patients. Wells's observations may apply to a subgroup of patients, but they are not consistently helpful with more common patients, who have a *mixture* of organic and psychiatric causes for their cognitive impairment.

The term *pseudodementia* should probably be abandoned because individuals with so-called pseudodementia due to a psychiatric disorder almost never have symptoms that fit diagnostic criteria for true dementia. The cognitive deficits associated with depression usually take the form of attention, concentration, and mild memory problems *unless* there exists an underlying primary dementia, such as Alzheimer's disease, or some other neurologic cause of cognitive impairment.

Pragmatically, the diagnosis of depressive pseudodementia is made by a response to psychotropic medication or electroshock therapy. Since dementia and depression frequently occur together (Shraberg, 1978), however, improvement of symptoms with antidepressant treatment does not automatically imply that dementia is not present. Reevaluation following successful antidepressant treatment may reveal a persistence of cognitive impairment. Reifler (1986) has proposed a classification of mixed cognitive-affective disorders. Patients with *type I* mixed disturbance have depression with associated cognitive disturbance due to the depression alone, and patients with *type II* have both depression and dementia. Treatment of *type I* depression results in improvement of both mood and cognitive deficits, whereas treatment of *type II* depression results in improvement only of mood and vegetative symptoms. Cognitive problems remain in *type II* patients, suggesting the presence of two separate disorders. Reifler, Larson, and Hanley (1982) estimate the prevalence of coexistent depression and dementia at 19 percent in geriatric psychiatry clinics.

Physical and Neurologic Examination in Dementia

Physical examination provides clues to the underlying disorder. Many authors suggest that the physician looking for neurologic signs of dementia may find such primitive release signs as the snout and palmomental reflexes in adult patients with impaired higher cortical function. It should be noted, however, that the palmomental reflex may occur in up to 60 percent and the snout reflex in up to 33 percent of normal elderly volunteers, so the presence of primitive reflexes in elderly patients is not necessarily diagnostic (Wolfson & Katzman, 1983). With this in mind, it is important to be aware of the physical changes that occur with natural aging and to be able to differentiate such changes from pathologic processes. Furthermore, classic responses to acute disease may be masked in the elderly patient, so medical disease may present primarily as a confusional state. An elderly patient with an acute infection may not have an elevated white blood count or a fever but may become increasingly cognitively impaired (Wolfson & Katzman, 1983).

Parietal lobe dysfunction is suggested by aphasia, astereognosis, sensory extinction, difficulty in distinguishing weight and texture, and problems with two-point discrimination. Left hemispheric dysfunction is indicated by impairment of language and conceptualization. Right hemispheric lesions may produce neglect of the left side. The combination of agraphia, acalculia, finger agnosia, and right–left confusion (Gerstmann's syndrome) indicates a lesion of the angular and supramarginal gyri of the dominant hemisphere. Neglect of the left side seen in lesions of the right parietal lobe may be demonstrated by asking a patient to draw the face of a clock. The left side of the clock may be distorted or absent in the presence of right parietal lobe lesions.

The subtlety of impairment early in the course of a dementia cannot be overemphasized. Demented individuals with a greater premorbid repertoire of well-practiced skills will perform better on neuropsychologic assessment.

Changes in gait often accompany aging

and include problems with balance, as noted by problems with one-legged standing and tandem walking. Deterioration of gait leading to falls may provide important clues to the underlying pathology of dementing processes. Gait apraxia is a gait characterized by difficulty in initiating the act of walking, leading to slow, hesitating, and sliding steps, in which the patient's feet appear to stick to the floor (Wolfson & Katzman, 1983). This type of gait suggests bilateral frontal lobe dysfunction, as seen with bilateral frontal subdural hematomas, multiple infarcts, meningiomas, butterfly gliomas, or late-stage Alzheimer's disease. Gait apraxia with urinary incontinence in the presence of dementia indicates normal pressure hydrocephalus (Adams, Fisher, Hakim, et al., 1965). A shuffling, festinating gait accompanied by tremor, cogwheel rigidity, bradykinesia, and masklike facies suggests Parkinson's disease or drug-induced extrapyramidal dysfunction. A waddling gait may be due to proximal muscle weakness, as seen in hypothyroidism (Wolfson & Katzman, 1983). An ataxic gait with a dementing process may be due to multiple infarctions that include the cerebellum or its connections, or may be due to chronic alcoholism. Acute onset of a small-step gait accompanied by slowness, brisk reflexes, extensor plantar responses, dysarthria, dysphagia, and pathologic laughing or crying in a patient with a history of hypertension also suggests multi-infarct dementia (Hachinski, Lassen, & Marshall, 1974).

Other specific neurologic signs that may be of diagnostic significance in the dementing patient include (Kaufman, 1981)

1. Myoclonus, which can occur with Creutzfeldt-Jakob disease, postanoxic events, or myoclonic epilepsy and which complicates about 10 percent of Alzheimer's disease cases.
2. Asterixis, which can occur with hepatic encephalopathy, uremia, CO_2 retention, or hypoxia.
3. Chorea, which may suggest Huntington's chorea, Wilson's disease, or other disorders of the basal ganglia.
4. Peripheral neuropathy with dementia, which suggests Wernicke-Korsakoff syndrome, infectious processes such as tertiary syphilis, systemic vasculitis, heavy metal or organic solvent exposure, or the effect of such medications as isoniazid or phenytoin. If a patient presents with peripheral neuropathy that includes impaired vibratory and position sense in the lower extremities, B_{12} deficiency should be considered.
5. Extrapyramidal signs and dyskinesias that may occur independent of neuroleptics.

Careful monitoring of vital signs may assist in the differential diagnosis. Hypertension increases the likelihood of multi-infarct dementia. In the presence of rapid pulse with fever, it suggests sepsis or sedative hypnotic withdrawal (Goldfrank, Flomerbaum, Lewis, et al., 1982). Tachycardia in the cognitively impaired patient warrants rectal temperature, as many demented patients are unable to keep an oral thermometer under their tongue long enough to give an accurate reading.

Pupillary signs may also provide diagnostic clues: pupillary mydriasis may suggest anticholinergic drug side effects, and pupillary constriction may suggest opiate toxicity. The Argyll-Robertson pupil, which fails to react to light but constricts on accommodation, suggests tertiary syphilis (Victor & Adams, 1974).

Mental Status Examination

Symptoms seen with dementia, regardless of etiology, relate both to the location and extent of impaired brain function and to individual adaptation to it. Premorbid defenses and psychopathology, the sociocultural matrix, and concurrent medical illnesses are other contributing factors. Cognitive changes may be insidious in onset and proceed over months, as in the instance of Creutzfelt-Jakob syndrome, or years, as in cases of Alzheimer's disease. Changes persist, regardless of stress, although environmental factors exaggerate or diminish symptoms.

Consciousness is not impaired, except in advanced cases. *Memory disturbance, greater for recent events, is a cardinal feature.* This may be disregarded as "absent-mindedness" early in the course of a dementia. Careful mental status and neuropsychologic examinations should be performed to document the extent of changes and to provide a baseline on which to gauge progression of illness. Acquisition of new skills eventually becomes impossible; individuals become more dependent on earlier acquired skills to function.

Disorientation is a predictable outcome of progressive dementia, but it often occurs late in the course; its absence certainly does not rule out dementia. Disorientation to time occurs first, follwed by disorientation to place and person. Judgment becomes impaired, and a critical perspective is lost. Family and friends may be upset by sexual indiscretions and violations of norms of modesty. Judgment entails comprehension of data presented, weighing of alternatives, and selecting a course of action. Individuals with major monetary or administrative responsibilities are more likely to be diagnosed earlier than those with lesser responsibility or those whose lives have been characterized by routine. Mental status examinations should be tailored to an individual's unique status in life. A cook may be examined on details of recipes for various dishes, a stockbroker on market trends, and a cattle farmer on care of his livestock.

Affect is altered, and premorbid defenses may be exaggerated. Those who project may become paranoid; those who withdraw, schizoid. Those who use denial may take on a manic quality. The *catastrophic response*, a defense against conscious recognition of the cognitive deficit, is characterized by anxiety, anger, or even rage, despite initial amiability, when a person is confronted with a task he or she cannot perform.

Early in the course of a dementia, only one cognitive function may be impaired, and this impairment may be demonstrated only on neuropsychologic testing or in a very detailed mental status examination. A person may have good recent and remote memory and a full fund of knowledge and may be well oriented and exhibit good judgment but may have lost the ability to calculate, to name uncommon items, or to learn new skills. With time, however, more global deterioration will evolve.

Depression can occur alone and present as dementia or can accompany a dementiform process, enhancing its severity. Concrete thinking, paucity of associations, negativism, withdrawal, and memory impairment are symptoms of profound depression, as well as of dementia. The diagnosis of mood disorder is suggested by prior personal history or family history of depression and by other clinical signs of affective illness, such as the characteristic diurnal variation in mood, sleep disturbance, and changes in appetite and libido. Definitive diagnosis of depression as a complicating or primary etiologic factor, however, may not be confirmed until a response to antidepressant therapy occurs.

Performing serial mental status examinations, obtaining cumulative histories over several meetings, and making longitudinal clinical observations offer diagnostic advantages over any single evaluation. When the diagnosis or the etiology of the dementing process still remains unclear, serial examinations over several months will generally clarify the situation.

Electroencephalography

Bilateral slowing on the electroencephalogram (EEG) is seen with some *but not all* cases of degenerative brain disease; profound cognitive deficits have been reported with relatively little EEG abnormality (Slaby, 1986; Slaby & Wyatt, 1974). The EEG is nevertheless a useful tool in differentiating "pseudodementia" from dementia (Goodnick, 1985; Kiloh, 1961; Post, 1975; Wells, 1977, 1979), as approximately 70 percent of patients with "pseudodementia" have normal EEGs.

It should be noted that although definitely abnormal EEGs are not consistent with normal aging, 30–40 percent of normal persons over age 60 may show brief runs of irregular focal anterior temporal slowing in the delta-to-theta range, especially on the left, occasionally with some sharp components that appear maximally with drowsiness and that disappear with sleep. When present to a mild degree, these are not felt to be pathologic in this age group (Busse & Obrist, 1963).

Early EEG abnormalities often seen with senile dementia include a decrease in the frequency of the posterior rhythm and a decrease in the amplitude of background activity. As the dementia progresses, the EEG may show an increase in generalized slowing with a disappearance of fast activity. Such changes may lag behind the clinical picture of deterioration, although on a population basis the extent and presence of such changes is correlated with the degree of cognitive deterioration (Weiner, 1983).

Absence of cerebral dysrhythmia does not exclude true dementia. The EEG is often normal in early cases of such true dementias as Pick's disease (Mahendra, 1984a). In Huntington's disease, the EEG will show gradual flattening, which correlates with the degree of cortical atrophy, until only very low-voltage, irregular delta and theta activity is seen (Shista, Troupe,

Marszalek, et al., 1974). Other specific EEG patterns, such as the burst suppression pattern of paroxysmal sharp waves on a slow background may be pathognomic for Creutzfeldt-Jakob disease (Goto, Umegaki, & Suetsugu, 1976). Triphasic waves may be seen in hepatic encephalopathy, as well as in some heavy-metal poisonings and subacute encephalitis (Cummings & Benson, 1983; Lesse, Hoefer, & Austin, 1958). Finally, the presence of spike or sharp wave activity may indicate an epileptogenic focus suggestive of either an occult seizure disorder or a cerebral lesion due to tumor or infarction, which may indicate specific treatment. Patients with Alzheimer's disease, however, occasionally have seizures and slow focal electroencephalographic changes (Cummings & Benson, 1983).

Subtle abnormalities in background may be detected by the more sensitive computer-analyzed EEG. Furthermore, serial EEGs may be more helpful in detecting the changes of a dementing process than a single tracing. Serial EEGs complement serial neuropsychologic examination in the evaluation of suspected cases of dementia.

Computerized Tomography

Computerized tomography (CT) scans may assist in the diagnosis of focal brain lesions or hydrocephalus, or may show cortical atrophy that suggests a suspicion of Alzheimer's disease. Mild cortical atrophy and ventricular dilatation may, however, be found in older patients without a dementing process, and conversely, cerebral atrophy and ventricular dilatation can be minimal in true dementia (Tomlinson, Blessed, & Roth, 1968, 1970).

Brain weight decreases with normal aging, with associated anatomic changes, including widening sulci and ventricular enlargement; such changes are generally greater in patients with senile dementia than in normals of the same age. Ventricular dilatation correlates better than sulcal enlargement with the severity of the dementia (McGeer, 1986). Attempts have been made to quantify ventricular volume and shape, to measure age-corrected ventricle–brain ratios, and to measure gray–white discriminability, to permit differentiation of changes associated with normal aging from those due to senile dementia. At the time of this writing, such measurements are not routinely available, nor have their discriminating capabilities been confirmed (McGeer, 1986). Serial CT scans may offer another approach to tracking increasing ventricular size associated with progressive atrophy from advancing dementing illness (Brinkman & Largen, 1984).

The CT scan is excellent for the detection of intracranial masses and blood collections (subdural hematomas) within the cranium. Contrast enhancement will increase visibility of focal changes in most conditions, with the exception of static or degenerative processes, such as scarring from past trauma or old strokes (Cummings & Benson, 1983). In the detection of infarcts, the use of the CT scan can be problematic. If the infarct is large, it may be well visualized, but *smaller infarcts, such as the lacunar infarcts of multi-infarct dementia, may go undetected*. Most lesions must be at least one-half centimeter before they are visualized (Cummings & Benson, 1983). In addition, tissues after infarction may be isodense for up to 10 days before the infarct is demonstrated. Although contrast enhancement may overcome this problem (Ambrose, 1973), it is not always successful in doing so (Oldendorf, 1980). CT scans obtained 3 or more weeks after the insult provide greater yield (Cummings and Benson, 1983). Magnetic resonance imaging (MRI) will probably emerge as the most useful test for the detection of multiple small infarcts.

In hydrocephalus with blockage at the level of the temporal hiatus, CT scan findings include enlarged third and lateral ventricles, ballooning of the temporal horns, and obliteration of the cerebral sulci over the convexities (Gado & Press, 1986). When cerebrospinal fluid flow is blocked over the higher convexities, the sulci may enlarge, minimizing cerebral atrophy. In differentiating normal pressure hydrocephalus from the atrophy noted with Alzheimer's disease, enlargement of the temporal horns along with a pattern of periventricular lucency suggests the diagnosis of normal pressure hydrocephalus (Gado & Press, 1986). Radionuclide cisternography is used to distinguish between degenerative conditions and cerebrospinal fluid flow obstruction. Bilateral circumscribed atrophy is found in the frontotemporal regions on computed tomography (CT) scan in instances of Pick's disease.

The radiologic diagnosis of Huntington's disease is based on a quantitative measure of caudate atrophy (Gado & Press, 1986). This measure is the ratio of the length of the line connecting the two anterior corners of the frontal horn to the length of the bicaudate line measured between the medial borders of the two caudate nuclei. The mean ratio in normals is 2.48. In Huntington's disease, the mean is approximately 1.33. A ratio of less than 1.6 suggests Huntington's disease. Individuals with parkinsonian dementia have a normal ratio.

Normal pressure hydrocephalus is characterized by gait apraxia, urinary incontinence, and dementia (Adams, Fisher, Hakim, et al., 1965) and is generally differentiated from high pressure hydrocephalus by a normal opening pressure on lumbar puncture of less than 180 mm of water, and from Alzheimer's disease by a CT scan presentation of markedly enlarged ventricles with minimal cortical atrophy (Black, 1982). If, however, the cerebrospinal fluid flow is blocked at the higher convexities or the superior saggital sinus, then the cerebral sulci can enlarge and mimic cerebral atrophy (Gado & Press, 1986). In such cases, cisternography may be useful. In this technique, a radioactive material (usually indium) is injected into the cerebrospinal fluid via lumbar puncture. In normal people the isotope will rarely be detected in the ventricular system because of the one-way flow away from the ventricles (Cummings & Benson, 1983). The isotope will diffuse over the convexities of the brain, to be absorbed and disappear within 48 hours (Black, 1982). In normal pressure hydrocephalus, the isotope rapidly refluxes into the ventricles, with failed or delayed visualization over the convexities, even at 48–72 hours and as late as 96 hours (Tyler & Tyler, 1984). Large-volume lumbar puncture (the removal of 30–50 cc of cerebrospinal fluid), performed every 2–3 days, may also aid in the diagnosis by demonstration of an improved clinical picture with the cerebrospinal fluid removal (Tyler & Tyler, 1984). Although shunting of the cerebrospinal fluid has offered marked improvement in many patients, it has failed to improve others. Several studies have been done to determine prior to surgery which candidates will be helped most by shunting, and it appears that patients with the complete triad of gait disturbance, dementia, and incontinence do better than patients with dementia alone (Black, 1980). Jacobs, Conti, Kinkel, et al. (1976) felt that the presence of motor signs alone (i.e., gait dyspraxia alone or accompanied by extrapyramidal signs) augured a good response from ventriculoatrial shunting, whereas no reliable relationship to shunting outcome could be established from cisternography or radiographic evidence. Despite a large literature on various predictors of response to shunting, clinical criteria remain most helpful.

It has been suggested that CT scan diagnosis of normal pressure hydrocephalus (NPH) be based on evidence of (1) more than moderately dilated ventricles without evidence of ventricular obstruction, (2) obliteration of the cerebral sulci, (3) areas of periventricular low density, and (4) "rounding" of the frontal horns of the lateral ventricles (Vassilouthis, 1984). Patients who satisfied at least one of the first two clinical criteria in addition to showing CT scan evidence of dilated ventricles underwent ventriculoperitoneal shunting with a favorable response. CT findings may thus be confirmatory of the clinical diagnosis.

Regarding surgical therapy, better clinical results have been reported when low-pressure (as opposed to medium-pressure) shunts are employed (McQuarrie, Saint-Louis, & Scherer, 1984). The most frequently encountered complications of shunting are subdural hematomas, shunt malfunction, infection, and postoperative seizures (Black, 1980; Tyler & Tyler, 1984).

It should be remembered that many causes of dementing processes may not be visible on CT scan. Those include chronic meningitis, vasculitis, chronic alcohol abuse, multiple sclerosis, and toxic metabolic encephalopathies. We have observed that after a CT scan is found to be "negative," the diagnostic evaluation sometimes stops, and other causes of treatable dementia are not sought. Knowledge of the limitations of CT scanning should help prevent premature diagnostic closure.

Dexamethasone Suppression Test

The dexamethasone suppression test (DST) has been used to attempt to differentiate cases of depression with secondary cognitive impairment from true dementia (McAllister, Ferrell, Price, et al., 1982; McAllister & Price, 1985; Rudorfer & Clayton, 1981). Clinical usefulness, however, is only claimed in a case report. The DST is abnormal in many nondepressed patients. Specifically, the DST has been reported to fail to distinguish between depression and Alzheimer's disease (Spar & Gerner, 1982).

Nonsuppression rates are high for the dexamethasone suppression test in nondepressed elderly patients with organic disorders. Furthermore, this nonsuppression is not correlated with a past history of depression in the patient or family (McKeith, 1984). It has been further suggested that the 5 mg/dl cutoff for normality may not be relevant in the elderly. Retrospective studies of postdexamethasone cortisol concentrations in the elderly have shown that whereas elderly inpatients with major depressive disorders frequently show levels of 15 mg/dl or greater, elderly patients without major depressive disorder rarely attain such concentrations (Fogel & Satel, 1985; Fogel, Satel, & Levy, 1986). This finding suggests that higher cutoff criteria may be used to identify elderly depressives with significant pituitary-adrenal dysfunction and that they may help differentiate geriatric patients with depression from nondepressed chronically ill or demented patients.

Cerebrospinal Fluid Examination

Although many neurology texts suggest the routine use of lumbar puncture in the diagnostic workup of dementia, its clinical utility has been cast into doubt. Recent studies suggest that although complications from this procedure are infrequent, it is expensive, and the yield of useful diagnostic information is low (Hammerstrom & Zimmer, 1985). For this reason, cerebrospinal fluid evaluation is suggested for cases of dementia with rapid onset or progression, for cases of positive serology for syphilis, for patients under the age of 55, for suspected cases of viral encephalitis, and for patients with headache, meningeal signs, elevated white blood count, pulmonary infiltrates on chest X ray, or fever suggesting low-grade fungal meningitis (Hammerstrom & Zimmer, 1985).

Sodium Amytal Test

Sodium amytal may be used in the evaluation of pseudodementia. Specifically, it helps in diagnosing a psychiatric basis for cognitive symptoms in younger individuals

with suspected conversion or psychosis. A 5% solution (500 mg of amytal dissolved in 10 cc of sterile water) is administered at a rate no faster than 1 cc/min (50 mg/min) (Perry & Jacobs, 1982). Dosage is sufficient when yawning, slurred speech, or lateral nystagmus occurs. Dosage is then stopped and the patient is reevaluated. Pseudodemented patients may show improvement in memory and orientation and increased verbalization (Snow & Wells, 1981; Ward, Rowlett, & Burke, 1978; Wells, 1979). Patients with organic disease show no improvement or transient deterioration. False positive, false negative, and inconclusive results limit the test's usefulness (McAllister et al., 1982; Ward et al., 1978). In some instances, the difficulty appears due to faulty technique (e.g., injecting the drug too slowly or rapidly) or to the fact that patients' symptoms are due to malingering (Herman, 1938; Lambert & Rees, 1944; Ward et al., 1978).

The amytal test is likely to be most useful in differential diagnosis in young to middle-aged patients with atypical features in their cognitive disturbance. In the more typical elderly patient with coexistent depression and dementing or other neurologic illness, the amytal test usually is uninterpretable.

Other Diagnostic Tests (MRI and PET Scans)

Magnetic resonance imaging (MRI) and positron emission tomography (PET) are leading to improvements in detection of Alzheimer's disease and in differentiation of it from other dementing illnesses. MRI provides a more detailed picture of the brain tissues' physical properties than CT and, in particular, is more able to discriminate between white and gray matter than the CT scan (Friedland, Budinger, Brat-Zawadski, et al., 1984). In addition, it offers better definition of discrete brain lesions (McGeer, 1986). The MRI is superior to CT scan for the detection of infarcts, tumor edema, posterior fossa lesions, and the demyelination of multiple sclerosis (McGeer, 1986). For this reason, MRI has clear advantages over the CT scan in differentiating other causes of dementing illness, although the MR image is not specifically diagnostic for Alzheimer's disease. If the clinician had to choose one brain imaging procedure, it would be the MRI. MRI is expensive, however, and not readily available at all centers at the present time.

Positron emission tomography (PET) offers the greatest promise of providing new information regarding in vivo brain metabolism in patients with Alzheimer's disease (McGeer, 1986). The PET image is a map of brain glucose metabolism (through the use of isotope ^{18}F-fluoro-2-deoxy-D-glucose) or of cerebral blood flow and oxygen metabolism (through the use of oxygen 15) (Cutler, Duara, Creasey, et al., 1984; McGeer, 1986). Brain glucose metabolism by PET image does not appear to change significantly with age (Cutler et al., 1984; McGeer, 1986), offering a clear advantage over the use of the CT scan, which may show atrophy in healthy elderly. There is a marked reduction in local cerebral glucose metabolism in patients with dementia, although the patterns of cortical involvement are variable (Friedland et al., 1984; McGeer, 1986). In mild to moderate Alzheimer's dementia, memory deficits often precede reductions in brain glucose metabolism (Cutler et al., 1984). Patients with Alzheimer's or Pick's disease also have patterns of decreased cortical oxygen metabolism, which differentiate them from patients with other dementing illnesses (Cummings & Benson, 1983). Because the PET scanner requires the use of a cyclotron, it is available only at a few research centers. With time, however, the PET scanner may hold promise for the confirmation of early Alzheimer's dementia before any CT scan or MRI evidence of deterioration is noted.

Neuropsychologic Testing

Neuropsychologic testing is a valuable adjunct in the evaluation of the demented patient when the bedside mental status examination is equivocal. Documentation of specific cognitive deficits, quantification of the extent of impairment, and measurement of the rate of cognitive deterioration may be used not only to clarify the diagnosis, but also to develop management strategies and to measure response to treatment (Huppert & Tym, 1986). Neuropsychologic testing may also differentiate the cognitive changes associated with depression from those of Alzheimer's disease, by identifying such specific cortical signs as apraxia, aphasia, and acalculia. Neuropsychologic testing is also useful in disability evaluations and in gathering the necessary documentation for legal decisions regarding competency or guardianship. (Neuropsychologic assessment is discussed in detail in Chapter 3, by Fogel and Faust.)

Management

Rational inpatient and outpatient management of dementia entails development of a biopsychosocial formulation to direct management. Special adaptation of the plan is required when the patient is hospitalized acutely for medical or surgical illness. In such instances, the removal from a familiar environment, the effects of the medical illness, and the stresses of treatment aggravate problems that have been successfully managed prior to hospitalization. Effective treatment is based on (1) diagnosis of the primary illness, (2) diagnosis of concomitant psychiatric disorders, such as delirium, depression, mania, and psychosis, (3) diagnosis of medical or surgical illness, (4) assessment of auditory and visual impairment, (5) assessment of premorbid personality style, (6) measurement of the nature, extent, and progression of cognitive deficit, (7) evaluation of functions of adult daily living, including ability to care for self and sphincter control, (8) assessment of gait, stance, balance, and impairment of ambulation or movement, and (9) evaluation of social and family relationships and other significant community contacts (Mahendra, 1984; Roth, 1982). The Visiting Nurse Association or social agencies may provide direct assessment of patients' physical environment and nursing needs.

Environmental Strategies

Most demented patients can live at home in the early stages (Mahendra, 1984). Performance of daily activities may be better if memory is assisted by written daily reminders and better organization of daily routine. Placing a calendar (with large numbers and names of the days of the week), a large clock, and a night-light prominently in the patient's room and having the patient keep a memo book, a diary, or a pocket calendar to track daily events, appointments, and medications are helpful. Reading newspapers and regularly watching programs on television or listening to scheduled radio programs are organizing experiences that facilitate retention of current information. Familiar street routes should be used for short errands, and the patient should be accompanied by a list of what must be done.

Families frequently express a concern that their relatives with dementia may be harmful to themselves, others, or property because of lack of attention to stoves, heaters, and electrical appliances. Signs with large letters and repeated reminders accompanied by demonstrations of how to properly handle appliances facilitate remembering to turn on and off appliances and to lock and unlock windows and doors (Mahendra, 1984). Restriction of use of automobiles or street access too early in the course of a progressive dementia causes unnecessary limitations (Read et al., 1985). Identification bracelets, wallet cards, and labels sewn into the neckbands of clothing with

name and address assist patients in finding home.

Some hospital departments of occupational therapy have model rooms, including bathrooms and kitchens, to assess patients' abilities to get in and out of a bathtub and to use a stove. Tub guardrails, elevated toilet seats, bedside toilets (commodes), and hospital beds with siderails are aids to continued functioning at home for patients with impairment in gait, coordination, or strength. Durable powers of attorney and other transfers of legal authority, if required, should be established early in the course of illness to maximize patients' participation in the decision-making process. (See also Chapter 21, by Mills and Daniels.)

Caretakers and family must learn to accept patients' slower pace with patience, tact, and understanding, while supervising daily activities such as personal hygiene, dressing, and eating. Special attention must be paid to maintaining adequate nutrition, hydration, and exercise. Patients should be asked to perform only one task at a time and should be expected to attend to only one stimulus at a time (Read et al., 1985). Although this process takes more time, especially for nursing staff with multiple patient assignments, demented patients are confused by multiple requests or excessively complex information. Instructions and medical procedures should be explained in simple, nontechnical language. Repetition followed by written explanation enhances comprehension. Problems arise in medical and surgical services when time is not taken to explain procedures or tests to patients with dementia. This lack of explanation contributes to patients' feeling lost in the system. Care must be taken not to infantilize elderly demented patients, despite their increased dependency. For example, calling older people by their first names with whom one does not have a close personal relationship is inappropriate.

Adequate management requires social support from the family. Responsible family members should be advised of the diagnosis, the prognosis, and possible problems they may encounter because of patients' cognitive deficits. Where impairment impedes job performance or monetary transactions, friends, neighbors, and business associates should be advised to avert potential problems (Pearce, 1984). The patient's consent for such notifications should be obtained early in the course of the illness, if possible. Frequent but brief visits to homes of patients living alone by caretakers, friends, or neighbors minimizes likelihood of accidents and allows monitoring of patients for falls, malnutrition, dehydration, apathy, alcoholism, and self-neglect arising from loneliness and depression.

Coordinated care by social agencies, the Visiting Nurse Association, and mobile geriatric units from local mental health facilities helps maintain patients' physical and emotional health. Meals on Wheels, homemakers, and home health aides help in maintaining adequate living standards so that patients can remain safe in the home environment. In many communities, supervised apartments, day care centers, and day hospitals (Gilleard, Gilleard, & Whittick, 1984) provide necessary supervision, respite for working families, and important leisure and social activities, as well as occupational and physical therapy. Community resources are, however, frequently limited to provision of food, shelter, and custodial care for patients whose families are unable to adequately attend to the growing demands of increasingly dependent family members. Patients may, out of neglect, deteriorate and develop incontinence, emaciation, dehydration, bedsores, infections (e.g., pneumonia), contractures, and hip fractures, leading to further depression and immobility. Nursing homes and chronic care hospitals become primary care providers in end-stage disease.

Research suggests that the burden of care borne by families, rather than deterioration of patients' mental or physical capacity, is the leading factor in institutionalization (Ross & Kedward, 1977). Relocation of demented patients to custodial care settings can be disastrous, because demented patients have considerable difficulty learning to adapt to new environments (Borup, Gallego, & Hefferman, 1979, 1980). Patients become more agitated and confused, often requiring psychotropic medication for behavior management (Zarit & Zarit, 1984).

Role of the Psychiatrist

The psychiatrist, along with the psychiatric nurse clinical specialist and psychiatric social worker, can provide a unique role in the development of environmental management strategies for the patient and family, in addition to providing adequate diagnosis and proper medication management. For patients in the home setting, the psychiatric treatment team can educate family and caretakers about environmental manipulation that, when used in conjunction with appropriate medication, will improve the patient's performance and decrease the need for nursing home placement.

In the hospital and nursing home settings, the treatment team can apply environmental strategies similar to those used in the home, such as calendars, night-lights, primary nursing to increase familiarity with staff, written instructions to the patient in simple language regarding procedures and medications, and other daily reminders. Other techniques that have been employed successfully in the nursing home setting have included token economies, in which tokens to purchase privileges, food, candy, or clothing are given for desired behaviors; milieu therapy, with cash used as a reinforcer; and "reality orientation," with staff reinforcing orientation and current information in daily conversation. Hospital and nursing home staff must first be made aware of the patient's memory deficits, as they are often not obvious without formal testing, and frustrated staff may misconstrue non-compliance secondary to memory problems as passive-aggressive or uncooperative behavior. Staff may be instructed that verbal repetition or written instruction may be necessary to overcome the patient's impairment. Additionally, the treatment team can educate staff on the special psychologic issues of the demented patient, to aid in their developing management plans (Herst & Moulton, 1985). In the nursing home setting, this is particularly important, because although it has been estimated that over three quarters of the patients in skilled nursing homes have diagnosable psychiatric illness (Teeter, Garetz, Miller, et al., 1976), nursing home staff are often poorly educated regarding psychiatric diagnosis and treatment and are not comfortable around patients with psychologic disturbances. Optimal environments attend to consistency, structured daily living plans, and activities, with special attention to the patient's need for privacy and personal dignity. The liaison relationship that the psychiatrist and the multidisciplinary treatment team have with nursing home and hospital staff gives them a unique role in advocating for the demented patient while educating and providing support when staff are frustrated with these often taxing patients.

Family Therapy

Alzheimer's disease and other related disorders have a slow course that will produce cognitive, physical, and personality deterioration over the course of 10 years or more (O'Quin & McGraw, 1985). Although dementia may spare, in part, patients' full realization of what is occurring to them, it is a source of emotional suffering for the caregiver. For this reason, "caregiver burden" (O'Quin & McGraw, 1985) has become an important focus of attention. The most troublesome behaviors for caretakers to manage include aimless wandering (Arie,

1986)—often worse at night, with disruption of the caretaker's sleep (Sanford, 1975)—dependency, confusion, falls, rages, urinary incontinence, apathy, and sullen moods. Family members also find constant repetition of questions, findings of lost items, and frequent reorientation of the demented patient a source of constant frustration (Zarit, Reever, & Bach-Peterson, 1980). Although problems of memory loss and disorientation are the primary reason for families to seek help for demented patients, the major reason for institutionalization is not behavioral problems, but families' becoming overwhelmed by caretaking responsibilities. In three independent samples of caregivers of elderly mentally infirm attending or about to attend day hospital, prevalence levels of emotional distress varied from 57 to 73 percent with high General Health Questionnaire scores related to diagnosable psychiatric illness (Gilleard, Belford, Gilleard, et al., 1984). Caregivers are at risk for depression, chronic fatigue, insomnia, and appetite changes (Fiore, Becker, & Coppel, 1983; Rabins, Mace, & Lucas, 1982). The psychiatrist, therefore, may have a unique role in the alleviation of "caregiver burden" through the diagnosis and treatment of major depression or early dementia in the caretaker.

Formal family therapy can aid in reducing caregiver distress, enhance environmental management, and prevent elder abuse and premature institutionalization. Contextual family therapy (Boszormenyi-Nagy & Krasner, 1986), which addresses the issues of rights and obligations of family members to one another in the context of illness, may be helpful. Other useful techniques include educating families about Alzheimer's disease and related disorders, incorporating family participation in the behavioral management of the patient, individual counseling for the primary care provider, and multifamily support groups (Fuller, Ward, Evans, et al., 1979). Another experimental approach is supporter endurance training (SET) (Levine, Gendron, Dastoor, et al., 1984). SET is a cognitive-behavioral training program designed to teach anxiety reduction by using social skills training. Educational materials for the patient and family are also provided by the Alzheimer's Disease and Related Disorders Association (70 East Lake Street, Chicago, IL 60601; 1-800-621-0379 outside Illinois; in Illinois, 1-800-572-6037). In spite of these interventions, care providers still require respite, which may be provided through brief hospital admission, elder sitters who can be hired to allow family to catch up on sleep and household activities, and hospice care for terminally ill demented patients (Arie, 1986).

Individual Psychotherapy

Individual psychotherapy may be a viable treatment option for the mildly demented patient who still retains sufficient cognitive capacity to participate in this form of therapy. The psychotherapist should maintain a flexible therapeutic approach that makes allowances for (a) communication problems secondary to hearing deficits, mild aphasia, or primary languages other than English, (b) repetition to compensate for memory loss, (c) somatization by the patient as a resistance to further exploration, and (d) transference to the therapist, who may be viewed as a child or grandchild (Charatan, 1985; Goldberg & Cullen, 1986; Kroetsch & Shamoian, 1986).

Common issues in psychotherapy include dependency (Cohen, 1981), injury to self esteem secondary to loss of intellectual capacity, mourning of multiple "partial losses"—including loss of spouse, friends, and employment, diminishing physical function, and change in family role (Berezin, 1972; Goldberg & Cullen, 1986)—and realistic concerns regarding the future. Some advocate the use of "life review" therapy with the therapeutic use of reminiscence to repair wounds in self-esteem through the review of accomplishments, to resolve intrapsychic conflicts and help patients to come to terms with the meaning of their lives (Butler, 1963; Lewis & Butler, 1974). The skilled therapist must balance potential benefits of reminiscence against the possibility that review of the past may be met with regret for the life not lived, guilt, and greater sense of loss (Cohen, 1981). Because of the diminished capacity of the mildly demented patient to reason abstractly, interpretations and clarifications should be straightforward and simple. In supportive psychotherapy, the goal of better adaptation may be enhanced by engaging the family as collaborators or participants in the therapy, by using telephone interventions for reassurance, support, and advice, and by identifying the specific social, psychologic, or biologic problems that are most amenable to change and that, therefore, are most likely to respond to focused intervention (Kroetsch & Shamoian, 1986).

Nutrition

Demented patients neglect food, particularly if indigent or living alone. Vitamin deficiencies may be compounded by excess use of alcohol. Alcohol may be taken both to attempt to release depression and insomnia, or with unconscious or conscious self-destructive intent. Frequent weighings to determine food intake and monitoring of skin turgor and other signs of dehydration is necessary. Supplemental vitamins are recommended for all patients with dementia. Dysphagic patients require semisoft or soft diets. Tube feeding is needed if swallowing is markedly impaired.

Severe protein–calorie malnutrition predisposes the patient with senile dementia of Alzheimer's type to bedsores, impaired cellular and humoral immunity, and increased mortality rates (Johnson, 1985). Laboratory tests are available for the assessment of protein–calorie malnutrition and include serum albumin, total lymphocyte count, the creatinine height index (the ratio of 24-hour creatinine clearance to the patient's height in centimeters), and serum transferrin levels. These tests, however, are affected by aging, acute and chronic disease, infection, and anemia (Johnson, 1985). For this reason, although some suggest serum albumin and total lymphocyte counts be done to determine those patients with malnutrition at risk for bedsores, others suggest that protein–calorie malnutrition may be assessed by serial weights, with 10 percent loss of usual body weight indicating a malnourished state (Johnson, 1985). Formal nutrition support consultation should be obtained in patients with profound weight loss or decubiti.

Sensory Augmentation

Decreased sensory input stresses the demented patient. Eyeglasses of correct prescription and hearing aids facilitate functioning. Quiet, dark nights provoke anxiety and agitation (called "sundowning"). Night lamps calm patients and may help them stay oriented. When institutional placement is required, the presence of familiar objects, such as family photographs or bed lamps from home, facilitates functioning. Visits by friends and family members well known to a patient reduce paranoia and help maintain orientation.

Custodial Care

Institutionalization is often required in final stages of dementia. Friends and families require guidance in identifying when the time is right and where to place the patient. Financial concern, guilt, helplessness, and despair plague families as the demented approach death. Psychiatric intervention with families may help reduce excessive guilt and help family members grieve the loss of the demented patient.

Abuse of Elderly Patients

Abuse represents an extreme reaction to the burden of care (Rathbone-McCuan & Goodstein, 1985). The spectrum of abuse includes physical beatings, starvation, verbal abuse, overmedication, tying patients in bed or locking them in a room for excessive periods of time, withholding of basic care, and financial exploitation or theft of money and property (Rathbone-McCuan & Voyles, 1982). Physical, behavioral, social, and emotional clues, assisted by home visits, facilitate discovery of victimization. Clues include (Rathbone-McCuan & Goodstein, 1985) (1) rope, chain, cigarette, and iron burns or marks on the neck or extremities suggestive of being tied to bed, a chair, or the toilet; (2) unusual patterns of bruises and welts or lacerations on the back, legs, arms, or face, suggesting beatings by electric cords, hangers, and other objects; (3) scalp hemorrhage or bald patches on the scalp, suggestive of hair pulling; (4) frequent emergency room visits for fractures and injuries; (5) caretakers' indifference to seek medical attention for injuries; (6) excess fear of care providers, evinced by hypervigilance or moving away from the caretaker as if dodging a blow; and (7) excessive control or restriction by caregivers of out-of-home contact, such as preventing friends and relatives from seeing the patient, locking doors and phones, and not allowing the patient to go out of doors. Abusers may be under influence of drugs themselves and obsessed with losing control, thus justifying their overmedicating the patients under their care. Abusers commonly have histories of having been abused themselves. Anger may exist toward a debilitated parent because of unsatisfactory past parenting, as well as because of the current burden of care.

Some communities have departments of elderly affairs with teams to make home assessments and hospital-based protocols for abuse detection. Treatment involves de-escalation of the home situation through use of community resources, day care to increase outside contacts, and emergency hospitalization or institutionalization in extreme cases. Brief hospitalization is sometimes advocated to provide families respite and to de-escalate chaotic home situations (Arie, 1986).

Sleep Disturbance in Dementia

Sleep disturbance in the demented patient is a special problem that deserves careful evaluation. While dementing illness itself is associated with sleep difficulties, other factors of normal aging, medication, or concurrent disease may exacerbate the problem. With normal aging, total sleep time decreases, sleep latency increases, sleep is disturbed by more frequent awakenings, and decreased time is spent in sleep stages 3 and 4 (Thompson, Moran, & Nies, 1983a; Jenike, 1985). Sometimes educating the older patient that this is a normal occurrence of aging will improve sleep quality without the addition of medication. Other nonpharmacologic interventions include (Jenike, 1985) (1) the elimination of alcohol, caffeine, and cigarette smoking, (2) discouragement of daytime naps and provision of regularly scheduled activities to stave off lack of daytime stimulation and resultant boredom, (3) regular exercise, which should be encouraged when physically permissible but should be avoided in the evening when it may lead to problems with falling asleep, (4) regularly set times for going to bed and arising in the morning, (5) correction of urinary problems and restriction of evening fluid intake, which may help to decrease nighttime awakenings due to nocturia, (6) correction or maximal control of pain or itching, nocturnal dyspnea of congestive heart failure, respiratory problems, angina, or other chronic diseases associated with disturbed sleep.

The patient should also be evaluated for depression or superimposed delirium or psychosis with behavioral disturbance and nighttime agitation. Intractable insomnia may be treated with benzodiazepine sedative-hypnotic preparations. Barbiturates are not recommended, because of problems with paradoxical excitation and suppression of REM sleep, leading to rebound insomnia and nightmares. The elderly patient's increased sensitivity to barbiturates can also lead to overdosing (Thompson et al., 1982a; Kales & Kales, 1974). In addition, barbiturates are habituating (Kales & Kales, 1974).

Benzodiazepine pharmacokinetics vary widely. Long-acting agents such as diazepam, flurazepam, chlorazepate, and chlordiazepoxide have half-lives that may be as long as 90 hours in the elderly (see Chapter 4, by Stoudemire and Fogel); the half-life increases with aging because of decreased hepatic metabolism and increased volume of distribution (Thompson et al., 1983a). The long-acting benzodiazepines may accumulate and produce unwanted daytime sedation not immediately reversible with cessation of the drug. Diazepam can produce sedation up to 2 weeks after cessation in healthy elderly volunteers (Salzman, Shader, Greenblatt, et al., 1983). For these reasons, shorter-acting benzodiazepine sedative-hypnotics such as temazepam may be preferred, especially in patients with liver impairment, because they are not metabolized by the hepatic mixed-function oxidase system (Thompson et al., 1983a). Even short-acting benzodiazepines, such as lorazepam, oxazepam, and triazolam, may have problems, however, including retrograde and anterograde amnesia, rebound insomnia, and greater problems with withdrawal symptoms with the abrupt cessation of usage. In addition, both long- and short-acting benzodiazepines may worsen cognitive impairment in mild dementia and occasionally may produce delirium. Small doses for brief periods are generally recommended. Benzodiazepines will worsen sleep apnea, which occurs with relatively high prevalence in patients with dementia (Reynolds, Kupfer, Taska, et al., 1985).

Low doses of sedating antidepressants may be useful for elderly patients with insomnia, especially if depression or anxiety appears to be a primary determinant of insomnia. Doxepin, 25–50 mg, or trazodone, 50–100 mg (given after a light snack to improve absorption) may be used.

Other drugs used to treat insomnia, such as sedating antihistamines and chloral hydrate, deserve mention. Elderly patients are often prescribed 25–50 mg of diphenhydramine hydrochloride (Benadryl). Because of anticholinergic effects, however, especially in combination with other medication that the patient may be taking, such drugs may precipitate delirium or clinical deterioration in Alzheimer's disease patients, who already have impaired cholinergic systems. Chloral hydrate has been a safe and effective hypnotic with a short half-life (8 hours) and seldom is reported to produce delirium. Problems, however, with chloral hydrate include gastrointestinal (GI) discomfort and excessive flatus and hepatic enyzme induction, increasing the metabolic rate of drugs, including anticoagulants (Jenike, 1985). Chloral hydrate's metabolites may displace acidic drugs, such as diphenylhydantoin or warfarin from plasma proteins, producing transient increases in drug effect and shortening drug half-lives (Thompson et al., 1983a).

Psychopharmacotherapy

Psychopharmacologic agents are used in dementia primarily for behavior and symptom control (Maletta, 1985). Prior to use of medication for behavioral control, psychiatrists must ascertain if signs and symptoms observed are caused or exacerbated by concomitant medical illness or the medications used to treat it. If medication was used for a previous psychiatric disorder, was it effective? Did any adverse reac-

tions occur? Patients tend to be prescribed medication by several physicians. Psychiatrists thus need to ascertain *all* medications currently taken. The "bathroom cupboard test" (Miller, 1984) entails asking demented patients or their families to bring in all medication bottles in order to evaluate all possible drug interactions and side effects. Patients prescribed psychotropics are re-evaluated at frequent intervals to assess continued medication need and to avert such problems as tardive dyskinesia.

Administration of psychotropic drugs is commenced with relatively small initial doses that can reasonably be expected to be tolerated. They may be one-third to one-half the dose for younger, healthier adults. Dosage is gradually raised until symptoms are relieved or excessive side effects emerge (Mahendra, 1984). Upon achievement of symptom control, the minimum effective dose is prescribed. After patients are symptom free for a week or two, the dose is tapered downward until the least amount required to prevent symptom exacerbation is defined. This may be as little as one-third of the original therapeutic dose (Thompson et al., 1983a, 1983b).

Neuroleptics for Agitation in Patients with Dementia

Antipsychotic medication is indicated for aggression, hostility, assaultiveness, restlessness, agitation, and hyperactivity, with or without such evidence of psychosis as delusions, hallucinations, and paranoia. Family members should be aware that antipsychotic medication will not reverse intellectual deterioration (Maletta, 1985). Furthermore, trials of neuroleptics for agitation should be a maximum of several weeks, for three reasons. First, there is no evidence that they are of long-term benefit for patients with dementia. Second, the risks of neurologic side effects are significant. Third, agitation in many patients with dementia is transient and is a response to medical illness or environmental change.

An attempt to withdraw neuroleptics, therefore, should be made as soon as the medical, social, or environmental precipitant has been identified and corrected.

Selection of antipsychotic medication depends on disease state, history of previous exposure and response to a particular drug, and side effects of the drug (Maletta, 1985). Some psychiatrists favor thioridazine for agitated elderly patients because of its low incidence of extrapyramidal side effects when given in divided doses ranging from 50 to 300 mg per day (Mahendra, 1984c). Others contend that Alzheimer patients have problems with decreased acetylcholine and that, therefore, it is illogical to use highly anticholinergic drugs, which further decrease cholinergic transmission (Maletta, 1985). Even mildly demented patients can develop central anticholinergic problems in the absence of peripheral anticholinergic signs. Because anticholinergic side effects for thioridazine increase with advancing dosages, patients who require more than 100 mg of thioridazine to control psychotic processes should be switched to high-potency neuroleptics, although these agents do present a greater likelihood of parkinsonian side effects, which will have to be controlled. Patients given high-potency neuroleptics should be started on a prophylactic antiparkinsonian agent. Amantadine hydrochloride, at dosages of 100 mg orally twice a day, is preferred over benzotropine or trihexyphenidyl (Artane) for this purpose, because of amantadine's lack of anticholinergic effects. Haloperidol is given in doses of 0.5–1 mg at bedtime or twice a day and thiothixene in doses of 2–4 mg at bedtime or twice a day, with a gradual increase in dose over several days until a response occurs or limiting side effects develop. Drug choice is determined by the prescriber's preference, as well as the specific side effects of the neuroleptic. Thiothixene is as efficacious as haloperidol and may have fewer extrapyramidal side effects. Although both loxapine and thioridazine are equally effective for management of anxiety, excitement, emotional lability, and uncooperativeness in disturbed, demented patients, a greater incidence of sedation and extrapyramidal symptoms may occur with loxapine, and more problems with orthostatic hypotension occur with thioridazine (Barnes, Veith, Okimoto, et al., 1982).

Sedating neuroleptics may help agitated patients with difficulty falling asleep. In some patients, however, sedation increases confusion and disorientation, actually aggravating agitation. Administration of sedating neuroleptics with hypnotics, analgesics, and antihistaminics further depresses CNS function (Salzman, 1982). Orthostatic hypotension is a serious side effect. It predisposes to falls, resulting in fractures, to stroke, and to myocardial infarction. Vulnerability to falls is increased in patients with cervical osteoarthritis, patients with low cardiac output, and patients concomitantly on cyclic antidepressants (Salzman, 1982). Risk is reduced by using higher-potency neuroleptics with less alpha-adrenergic blocking activity (e.g., haloperidol, thiothixene, or molindone), concurrent use of supportive stockings, and practice in rising slowly from the recumbent position (particularly at night).

Extrapyramidal side effects (e.g., akathisia) may be confused with mounting agitation and emergence of psychosis, resulting in an increase rather than a decrease in dosage. Akinesia may be misdiagnosed as depression, leading to use of antidepressants or electroconvulsive therapy (ECT). Both side effects are best managed by neuroleptic dose reduction or a switch to neuroleptics with fewer extrapyramidal side effects. Jaundice, pigmentary retinopathy, and agranulocytosis are rare side effects of phenothiazines. Incidence of these is greatest in elderly white women (Thompson et al., 1983b).

Fear exists that certain neuroleptics, especially thioridazine, may aggravate cognitive dysfunction. An open cross-over study, however, comparing efficacy and side effects of haloperidol and thioridazine in the management of behavioral symptoms in Alzheimer patients indicated that thioridazine, up to 75 mg a day for 2 weeks, did not affect intellectual function (C Steele, Lukas, & Tune, 1986).

A trend exists in the psychopharmacotherapy of the demented to reduce neuroleptic dose by addition or substitution of benzodiazepines, such as lorazepam and clonazepam. These are both used for control of acute psychotic agitation in delirium and manic states. Caution must be used to prevent oversedation—more common with clonazepam—and paradoxical aggressive responses (Van Praag, 1977). Well-controlled studies of this approach are lacking, but it should be considered in patients who cannot tolerate neuroleptics.

Psychostimulants

Interest has been renewed in psychostimulant use for depression with dementia. Katon and Raskind (1980) report significant antidepressant effect compared with placebo when methylphenidate is used in elderly apathetic withdrawn patients. Insomnia is avoided by administration of 5 mg in the morning and again at midday. Rapid therapeutic response in comparison with tricyclics is a decided advantage. Adverse reactions include insomnia, anorexia, palpitations, and hypertensive crises when used in combination with antidepressants (Thompson et al., 1983b). Ventricular arrhythmias may be precipitated, although the incidence of this side effect is undetermined. Methylphenidate inhibits hepatic microsomal enzymes, affecting metabolism of other drugs. Psychostimulants may be useful in depressed, demented patients when medical conditions, intolerance of anticholinergic side effects, or patient and family preference militate against use of ECT or tricyclics. Paranoia, overt psycho-

sis, rapid tolerance, euphoriant effects, and abuse rarely occur with small doses in this population. (See also Chapter 4 by Stoudemire and Fogel.)

Hydergine

A number of drugs have been advocated for treating the *cognitive deterioration* associated with senile dementia of the Alzheimer's type. The drug ergoloid mesylates (Hydergine) has been most widely studied and has been safely used over the last 30 years (Jenike, 1985). Hydergine is given in dosages averaging 3–6 mg a day but has been given in doses as high as 12 mg without serious side effects. Hydergine has shown the most promise with improvements reported in mood, dizziness, locomotion, and self-care (Kopelman and Lishman, 1986; Yesavage, Tinklenberg, Hollister, et al., 1979) and some reports of improved memory and orientation. The most significant improvement, however, appears to be in lifting depression (Jenike, 1985). The studies supporting Hydergine's efficacy are limited, and some patients are reported to improve only if a trial of 3–6 months is attempted. If no effect is achieved by the end of 6 months, then the trial should be discontinued (Jenike, 1985). A dose of 2 mg three times a day is recommended if it is tolerated, as some patients respond to 6 mg/day but do not respond to 3 mg/day. *Mildly* demented patients with less than major depression are most likely to benefit.

Clear, simple instructions on how medication is to be taken should be provided. Family, friends, or attendants are required to administer medication in advanced stages of dementia. Failure to monitor drug intake may result in drug automatism, in which a patient in a semitoxic state repeats dosages and becomes confused and sedated. In the extreme, such behavior can lead to death by unintentional overdose.

Referral for Experimental Therapies

A number of experimental therapies for Alzheimer's disease are under investigation. Many are based on efforts to enhance cholinergic transmission; others try to improve cerebral metabolism. A superb recent review of experimental treatments is *Treatment Development Strategies for Alzheimer's Disease*, edited by Crook, Bartus, Ferris, et al. (1986). Patients with mild to moderate Alzheimer's disease may be considered for referral to a research center if they are motivated and their expectations are realistically moderate. Patients with Alzheimer's disease should not be referred to clinical research centers when they have deteriorated severely and all other interventions for cognitive and behavioral management have failed. The patients who are most likely to benefit from referral are relatively young patients with memory loss who are otherwise in good physical health and do not yet have severe problems with basic activities of daily living. Experimental therapies have the greatest likelihood of benefiting patients early in the course of the disease (Jenike, 1985).

Multi-Infarct Dementia

The second leading cause of dementia, multi-infarct dementia, generally is distinguishable from Alzheimer's disease by its suddenness of onset, stepwise deterioration of intellectual functioning (Waldinger, 1986), and greater association with hypertension and cardiac disease, including a history of myocardial infarction, angina, and congestive heart failure (Tresch, Folstein, Rabins, et al., 1985). A history of diabetes is common. Depression and neurologic abnormalities, such as asymmetric reflexes, dysarthria, gait abnormalities, limb spasticity, and focal deficits secondary to stroke, are also seen (Read et al., 1985). Personality is often preserved until late (Sloane, 1983), although depression is common. The male-female ratio of incidence of multi-infarct dementia is 2:1. Onset is earlier than for Alzheimer's (Sloane, 1983). While CT scan evidence of multi-infarct dementia is more commonly found, more than 50 percent with the disease do not have positive tomography (Sloane, 1983). If available, MRI should be obtained in patients with suspected multi-infarct dementia because of its superiority to CT in detecting small infarcts (McGeer, 1986).

Treatment focuses on blood pressure control and reduction of stroke risk by management of transient ischemic attacks and cardiac conditions increasing stroke incidence, such as cardiomyopathies, chronic left heart failure, aortic valve disease, a trial myxoma, rheumatic heart disease, and subacute bacterial endocarditis, as well as complications of prosthetic heart valve insertion. Control of other stroke risk factors, such as diabetes, smoking, and the hyperlipidemias, is also important (Mahendra, 1984).

Reduction of blood pressure should be undertaken cautiously. Patients with arteriosclerotic disease may require higher baseline blood pressures to perfuse their brains. Longitudinal studies of hypertensive patients with multi-infarct dementia suggest that systolic blood pressure be maintained in a high normal range (135–150 mm Hg) to improve cognition and to prevent clinical deterioration associated with blood pressure reduction below this range. Multi-infarct demented normotensive patients have the greatest cognitive improvement with smoking cessation (Meyer, Judd, Tawakina, et al., 1986).

Aside from aspirin use to reduce platelet-induced hypercoagulation to prevent ischemic attacks (Marcus, 1977) and anticoagulant use by patients with prosthetic valve replacement, use of anticoagulants is not indicated, as they increase morbidity due to hemorrhage. Carotid endarterectomy may be beneficial to patients with carotid stenosis, which is detected by ultrasound studies or by digital subtraction angiography.

Often, primary care physicians become less aggressive about the prevention of future strokes and controlling stroke risk factors when dementia and psychiatric complications supervene. The psychiatrist has a crucial role in reiterating to primary care providers that multi-infarct dementia, unlike Alzheimer's dementia, has a better course when such risk factors are properly attended to (Meyer et al., 1986).

Psychogeriatric Units

Psychogeriatric units exist in psychiatric, geriatric, and general hospitals to provide a multidisciplinary approach to care, early diagnosis and intervention for psychiatric and medical illness, proper coordination of social services and community resources, and avoidance of crisis hospitalizations (Jeff & Roth, 1969). Their focus is rehabilitation and maintenance of demented patients' remaining functions. Psychogeriatric units also differ from custodial care facilities in their emphasis on developing controlled and safe environments in the community, tailored to individual patient needs and care provider supports.

Forensic Issues and Competency

Need for power of attorney, guardianship, and conservatorship and concerns regarding testamentary capacity and competency are legal issues in all instances of dementia. If dementia is diagnosed early and deterioration is spotty, patients may be able to make some decisions regarding the distribution of assets upon their death and the selection of a guardian to handle their affairs later in their course. Individuals who live with a fantasy of eternal good health are sometimes struck down with wills absent or so dated that property and money

remain tied up in litigation for years after death while care providers attempt to recoup the cost of care. Families should be advised early in the course of illness to seek legal help in protecting the rights and property of patients while providing access to funds for care required.

The psychiatrist plays a dual role in the legal management of the patient with dementia. First, the psychiatrist can assess the patient's degree of cognitive impairment and the effects that this impairment has on the patient's judgment and decision-making capacity with regard to person and property. Second, the psychiatrist can intervene with the patient and the family to work out a mutually agreeable legal mechanism to protect the patient's rights. This is often done with the psychiatrist acting as direct liaison with an attorney.

Competency is a complex concept whose legal standard varies from state to state. The presence of a dementing illness does not automatically make the patient incompetent, nor does involuntary commitment of such a patient to a psychiatric facility imply incompetence. Competence in a demented patient is also not an all-or-nothing phenomenon (Baker, 1986; Beis, 1984b). To be declared incompetent "under the Uniform Probate Code, an individual must show a clear lack of understanding and inability to communicate" (Baker, 1986). A comprehensive assessment of competence includes interviews with the patient, the family or other significant care providers, and medical treatment staff, as well as a review of previous medical records. In addition to the patient's mental status and clinical state, accuracy of historical data given by the patient, the ability of the patient to understand and accurately recall information that is provided to him or her, the patient's views of his or her illness, the patient's rationale for decisions made, and any prior history of incompetent refusal should be noted. Serial mental status examinations should be performed and may

be supplemented by repeated neuropsychologic testing to demonstrate the stability or
progression over time (Baker, 1986; Gutheil
& Bursztajn, 1986). It also is important to
document areas of preserved functional capacity (Gutheil & Bursztajn, 1986). In subtle cases, second opinions by psychiatrists
not directly involved with the clinical management of the case should be sought.

The psychiatrist in the hospital setting
frequently is asked to make statements regarding a patient's competence in matters
regarding refusal of hospitalization or refusal of medical treatment. In general, if an
elderly demented patient with impaired
cognition and judgment agrees to hospitalization, the next of kin should be made
aware of this situation, although this is not
a legal issue unless comprehension is severely limited. Many states permit the next
of kin to give consent for hospitalization
(Baker, 1986).

Involuntary hospitalization may also
be permitted either on the principle of
parens patriae ("parent of the country"),
by which the state lends its power to hospitalize patients on the basis of inability to
care for and make decisions regarding their
own physical needs, or by the "police-
power principle" of a patient's being a
danger to self or others (Baker, 1986; Beis,
1984). Some states, however, have tried to
exclude a dementing illness as a basis for
involuntary commitment (Baker, 1986). In
evaluating refusal for medical treatment,
documentation includes the patient's rationale for refusal, his or her cognitive capacity, and an assessment for the presence of
depression or psychosis (Baker, 1986). In
cases of terminally ill demented patients
where a "living will" has been previously
made, physicians ethically may withhold
treatment that would serve only to prolong
the dying process. Artificial feeding is included in the 13 living wills laws passed in
1985 (Baker, 1986). The procedures and
interpretation of such laws, however, vary
from state to state.

In cases where the dementing illness
appears to be unrelenting and irreversible,
then the psychiatrist may be asked to assess the patient for guardianship or
conservatorship. The psychiatrist must be
familiar with state laws, which may include
as criteria for incompetence documentation
of specifically observed behaviors, such as
proof of inability to care for self or inability
to make appropriate judgments regarding
the management of financial affairs. In
some states, the psychiatrist must also document evidence of socially unacceptable
behavior, such as gambling, excessive drug
and alcohol abuse, "idleness," or "de-
bauchery" (Beis, 1984). The psychiatrist
should also be aware that guardianship and
conservatorship definitions may overlap in
some states, but in general, where the
states conform to the Uniform Probate
Code, guardianship refers to control over
person and may permit the guardian to
make decisions regarding hospitalization,
medical treatment, and where a patient may
live, such as a nursing home. In a
conservatorship, the conservator manages
the patient's financial affairs and property
with or without management of the person
as well (Baker, 1986). In addition, many
states will grant limited guardianship, ap-
pointing a guardian only "to the extent
necessitated by the individual's actual mental, physical, and adaptive limitations"
(Beis, 1984). Attainment of durable power
of attorney by the spouse or family early in
the course of dementia obviates the need
for lengthy, expensive guardianship proceedings and should be an early recommendation to all patients with Alzheimer's disease and their families. It should be
emphasized that the family should obtain
durable, as opposed to nondurable, power
of attorney, because nondurable power of
attorney becomes invalid if the grantor becomes mentally incompetent, whereas durable power of attorney will be upheld. (See
Chapter 21, by Mills and Daniels.)

DELIRIUM

Delirium (also called acute confusional state, toxic psychosis, acute organic brain syndrome with psychosis, toxic-metabolic encephalopathy, acute brain syndrome, and acute cerebral insufficiency) (Ellison, 1984; Engel & Romano, 1959; *Psychogeriatrics*, 1972) represents the behavioral response to widespread disturbances in cerebral metabolism (Strub, 1982). It is characterized by confusion, disorientation, short-term memory defects, and fluctuating states of arousal. Autonomic and other neurologic signs appear with visual and tactile hallucinations (Crump, Pellegrini, Lippmann, et al., 1984). Characteristically, symptoms are global, appear abruptly, and are of relatively brief duration (usually less than one month).

It has been estimated that 33 percent of hospitalized medically ill patients have serious cognitive impairments (Knight & Folstein, 1977), with delirium occurring in as many as 85 percent of terminally ill cancer patients (Massie et al., 1983). Delirium carries prognostic significance for patients. It is associated with a high incidence of morbidity, mortality, and dementia if unrecognized and untreated (Guze & Cantwell, 1964; Ibe & Kitchen, 1983).

Death rates for delirious patients exceed rates for demented, depressed, and cognitively intact controls at index admission and at one-year follow-up (Rabins & Folstein, 1982). Delirious patients have a greater incidence of diffusely slow EEGs, hyperthermia, lower mean blood pressures, and tachycardia than the comparison groups. Fatality rates of the delirious are twice those of control groups matched for age, race, sex, ward status, and medical diagnosis, indicating that medical diagnosis alone does not explain findings (Guze & Daengsurisri, 1967). Delirium suggests a more serious form of medical illness and at times is a harbinger of death. A review (Black, Wanack, & Winokur, 1985) of 543 delirious patients indicated that they, particularly if under 40, are predisposed to early death when compared with controls. Risk is greatest in the first two years of follow-up, with higher risk of death from heart disease and cancer in women and from pneumonia and influenza in men. Forty percent of elderly demented patients die soon after developing delirium (Post, 1965). One-fourth of patients with delirium referred for psychiatric consultation in the study by Trzepacz et al. (1985) died within six months of consultation, with two-thirds of those dying during the index admission. Weddington, Muelling, and Moosa (1982) report a 33 percent 3-month mortality rate for delirious hospital patients referred for psychiatric consultation.

Delirium (Lipowski, 1967, 1983) mimics other psychiatric disturbances and misleads physicians by depressive, paranoid, schizophrenic, phobic, and hysterical symptoms. Agitation, belligerence, and bizarre behavior or depressed, stuporous, or apathetic behavior may occur in the same patient, depending on the time the patient is evaluated (Dubin, Weiss, & Zeccardi, 1983).

Psychosocial stress precipitates medical, as well as psychiatric, illness, and the two can occur concurrently, with overt signs of delirium discounted because symptoms are attributed to the psychiatric disorder (Daniel and Rabin, 1985). Physical examinations of patients with lupus cerebritis, hypothyroidism, hypoglycemia, and phenobarbital toxicity may be indistinguishable from those with nonorganic psychiatric disorders. Clues suggesting medical illness include onset after age 40 with no prior psychiatric history and the occurrence of cardinal features of delirium (viz., rapid onset in the elderly, global cognitive impairment, fluctuating levels of consciousness, disturbance of the sleep/wake cycle, disorientation, worsening of psychosis at night, tremors, pathologic reflexes, and visual/tactile/olfactory hallucinations) that are rarely seen with functional psychosis alone. In one survey (Trzepacz et al., 1985) of general hospital psychiatric consultations resulting in the diagnosis of delirium, 67 percent were referred because of occurrence of psychiatric symptoms. Thirty-five percent of these were referred for affective symptoms: depression, suicidal ideation, and tearfulness. The majority of the patients were perceived as manipulative or "a nuisance" by referring staff. Of 100 hospitalized cancer patients referred for depression in another study (Levine, Silberfarb, & Lipowski, 1978), 65 percent ultimately were diagnosed as having an organic mental syndrome. Of course, organic etiology does not obviate need for protection against self-injurious behavior. It is estimated that 7 percent of delirious patients in a general hospital make suicide attempts or other self-injurious acts (Wolff & Curran, 1935).

Delirium is confused with dementia, as well as with depression, because it is often superimposed on dementia (Lipowski, 1983). Symptoms of dementia may remain after delirium has cleared (Gallant, 1985). Patients presenting with acute, as opposed to insidious, onset of change in mental status and fluctuating levels of consciousness should be evaluated for delirium, with appropriate correction of underlying medical problems.

Clinical Description

Clouding of consciousness, fluctuating over the course of a day, is the hallmark of delirium (F Adams, 1984; Lipowski, 1967; Murray, 1987; Strub, 1982). Onset of symptoms is usually acute. Insomnia, nightmares, intermittent nighttime disorientation, and anxiety often appear first, progressing gradually to full-blown delirium. Review of nursing progress notes will often document transient fluctuations of symptoms in suspected instances.

Symptoms are worse at night. Agitated behavior and visual hallucinations are more likely at night. At one moment, patients appear combative and suspicious, shouting obscenities. At another, they are stuporous, mumble incoherently, pick at clothing, and drift off to sleep in midsentence. The picture alternates with periods of relative lucidity. Medical care is compromised by the patient's suspicion of staff, medication, and medical procedures, and by accidental or intentional disconnection of catheters, intravenous lines, and tubes (F Adams, 1984). Associated features include purposeless movements of arms and legs and multifocal myoclonus. Tremor is often present (Ellison, 1984). Other neurologic signs are relatively uncommon in the absence of a primary CNS cause of delirium. Asterixis, a motor disturbance marked by intermittent lapses of a sustained posture, such as flapping movements of hyperextended hands, accompanies hepatic encephalopathy and some other metabolic states.

It should be noted that the mildly delirious patient may present differently from the patient with a full-blown delirium. In the mildly delirious patient, abnormalities of mood and demanding or nuisance behaviors are often prominent. If cognitive disturbances are not tested for in these patients, they are often overlooked or misdiagnosed as "functional."

Differential Diagnosis

Older people are at the greatest risk for delirium (Wells & Duncan, 1980), but the very young are also predisposed. Mortality ranges from 7–12 percent (Daniel and Rabin, 1985), due to underlying illness. Preexisting brain disease; drug and alcohol addiction; chronic hepatic, renal, cardiac, and pulmonary dysfunction; and organ failure are other risk factors (McEvoy, 1981; Wells & Duncan, 1980). Elderly patients display more cognitive accompaniments of neurologic and metabolic problems than younger patients. Common physical illnesses leading to delirium are pneumonia, cancer, urinary tract infection, hyponatremia, dehydration, congestive heart failure, uremia, and stroke (Lipowski, 1983).

Visceral illness can produce a delirium with no abnormalities in routine blood tests. In these cases, patients are often referred to psychiatrists for the evaluation of "functional illness" because of mental status changes that are not explained by abnormal laboratory data. It is then the task of the psychiatrist to refocus the primary care physician's attention back on the possibility that there may still exist undiagnosed physical disease. Alcohol intoxication and withdrawal are common causes of delirium in young populations, and CNS effects of polypharmacy are common in the elderly. Drugs contribute to delirium in young and old equally (Cassem & Hackett, 1987; Trzepacz et al., 1985). Of the many drugs that have been cited in causing delirium, a few commonly occurring medications are worth noting.

1. Narcotic analgesics may produce agitated delirium. Meperidine, in particular, has been noted to produce delirium, including tremor, seizures, and multifocal myoclonus (Foley, 1982). This complication has been reported to be secondary to the accumulation of meperidine's active metabolite, normeperidine, with repeated (particularly intravenous) dosing, and it appears to be more common in patients with renal insufficiency. Often, substitution of a different narcotic analgesic will eliminate the problem. Another narcotic analgesic that has psychotomimetic properties is pentazocine. The psychotomimetic effect of this narcotic is noted with higher doses of the drug and therefore limits its usefulness for patients with severe or chronic pain (Foley, 1982). In addition to this, pentazocine is a narcotic with agonist–antagonist properties and therefore can precipitate an acute withdrawal state in a patient who was previously receiving chronic narcotic agonists of the morphine type (Foley, 1982). For this reason, care must be taken in switching a patient from other morphine-type narcotics to Talwin; this problem is often overlooked by primary care physicians (Foley, 1985).

2. Blood levels of medication can suggest toxicity for such agents as anticonvulsants, digoxin, theophylline, lithium, and tricyclics. It is, however, important to note that, particularly in the elderly, delirium may occur with digitalis and quinidine at serum levels well within the normal limits of most clinical laboratories. Although psychotoxicity generally is dose-dependent, the threshold for toxicity varies from individual to individual. Even more importantly, CNS toxicity may precede signs of EKG or GI disturbance; digitalis has been noted to be associated with formed visual hallucinations that may precede electrocardiographic clues that such intoxication is occurring (Volpe & Soave, 1979).

3. Confusion and delirium may occur with propranolol, especially in the elderly. This drug has been noted to produce depression or visual hallucinations, as well as toxic confusional states (Paykel, Fleminger, & Watson, 1982; Gershon, Goldstein, Moss, et al., 1979). Although neurotoxic reactions to propranolol have been most often reported with large doses, the CNS side effects also can occur in low or therapeutic dose ranges (i.e., less than 160 mg a day) (Remick, O'Kane, & Sparling, 1981). Substitution of a water-soluble beta blocker such as atenolol or nadolol sometimes solves the problem.

4. Another class of medication not often considered as a cause of delirium is the antibiotics. Central nervous sys-

tem toxicity and delirium have been seen with high-dose intravenous penicillin. In addition to hallucinations, other neurotoxic effects include generalized seizures, myoclonus, and hyperreflexia. These effects are more common in patients with renal insufficiency (Snavely & Hodges, 1984). Cephalosporins also may produce central nervous system toxicity, including reversible encephalopathy, particularly in patients with renal failure. Psychiatric symptoms have also been noted with chloramphenicol, although the occurrence of the symptoms is infrequent, even with prolonged use. Neurotoxic reactions have also been seen from the aminoglycoside class of medication, including gentamicin and tobramycin, and with metronidazole (McCartney, Hatley, & Kessler, 1982; Snavely & Hodges, 1984).

5. Anticonvulsants can produce delirium; this usually occurs at high serum levels. Paradoxical excitation has, however, occurred with barbiturates even within the normal therapeutic range (Penry & Newmark, 1979), particularly in individuals with preexisting brain damage or mental retardation. Concurrent administration of drugs, including chloramphenicol, sulfamethoxazole, phenylbutazone, and disulfiram may inhibit the metabolism of phenytoin, increasing the risk of delirium (Delgado-Escueta, Treimen, & Walsh, 1983). Phenytoin levels have also been reported to be elevated by the concurrent administration of estrogen-containing oral contraceptives, phenothiazines, and warfarin anticoagulants (Rivinus, 1982).

6. Cimetidine may produce neuropsychiatric side effects, including auditory and visual hallucinations, agitation, paranoia, disorientation, and stupor, as well as depression and anxiety states (Weddington et al., 1982). Central nervous system problems from cimetidine are seen more commonly in the very young, the elderly, and patients with cirrhosis or uremia (Strum, 1984). In addition, cimetidine interference with drug metabolism, from its interaction with the hepatic microsomal enzyme system, has been shown to slow the metabolism of a number of drugs, including the benzodiazepines and the oral tricyclic antidepressants, including doxepin, imipramine, and nortriptyline (Abernethy and Todd, 1986). Often, when such a reaction occurs, the psychiatrist will switch the patient to ranitidine as there have been some reports of reduction in problems with CNS side effects by switching agents. Ranitidine, however, has been reported to reduce hepatic blood flow by 20–40 percent (Goff, Garber, & Jenike, 1985; McCarthy, 1983), thus leading to a potential for retarded metabolism of other drugs. Ranitidine may also cause depression (Billings & Stein, 1986), and it has been shown to interfere with the metabolism of a number of drugs, including acetaminophen, benzodiazepines, nifedipine, metoprolol, and warfarin (McCarthy, 1983; Rubin, 1984).

7. Antihypertensives can precipitate delirium. Although it is more common for the diuretics to produce delirium via electrolyte disturbances, other antihypertensives, such as reserpine and methyldopa, can cause delirium by direct action on the central nervous system (Paykel et al., 1982). If there is a sudden alteration of mental status in a patient who is receiving diuretics, electrolyte levels, including calcium, should be checked.

8. Mental status changes have also been noted with nonsteroidal anti-inflam-

matory agents. Psychotic reactions have been reported with sulindac, indomethacin, tolmetin, and naproxen ("Drugs That Cause Psychiatric Symptoms," 1981; Kruis & Barger, 1980; Sotsky & Tossell, 1984; TE Steele & Morton, 1986). Mental status changes are dose dependent. With salicylates, blood levels in the toxic range are associated with major psychiatric side effects. Levels are particularly helpful because the pharmacokinetics of salicylates are highly variable between individuals.

9. Caffeine may produce a delirium. CNS toxic effects of caffeine have appeared in some individuals with ingestion of doses as small as 50 mg of caffeine a day. One gram of caffeine (8–10 cups of coffee or five 200-mg over-the-counter caffeine tablets) may be sufficient to produce frank delirium (Goldfrank, Lewis, Melinek, et al., 1981; Stillner, Popkin, & Pierce, 1978). The exact incidence of caffeine delirium is, however, unknown at this time.

10. Theophylline, which is used in patients with asthma and COPD, may also cause a delirium that is dependent upon serum level and is unusual at levels within the therapeutic range. For this reason, plasma concentrations should be carefully monitored. Coarse tremor in conjunction with a delirious state suggests theophylline toxicity in patients on this drug (Park, 1986).

11. Corticosteroids very frequently cause mental status changes ranging from delirious psychosis to mania to depression. The reaction has been more commonly recorded in females than in males. A prior history of psychiatric illness does not necessarily predispose the patient to the development of toxic delirium from corticosteroids. In addition, although steroid-induced delirium usually has been reported with higher dosages (i.e., 40 mg of prednisone or more), one study suggests that neither the dosage nor the duration of treatment appears to affect the time of onset, the severity, the type of mental disturbance, or the duration of mental disturbance in patients receiving corticosteroids (Ling, Perry, & Tsuang, 1981). Steroid-induced delirium usually responds to dosage reduction or drug cessation. For patients in whom corticosteroids must be used, lithium may prevent steroid-related psychosis (Goggans, Weisberg, & Koran, 1983); others have found low-dose neuroleptics helpful.

12. Polypharmacy, especially with drugs having anticholinergic side effects, contributes to delirium in the elderly (Bernstein, 1979; Blazer, Federspiel, Ray, et al., 1983; Lipowski, 1983).

"Pseudodelirium"

Differentiation of delirium from primary psychiatric disorders presenting with features of delirium is not always easy (Golodny, 1979). Cognitive impairment of delirious proportions may be a manifestation of schizophrenia or bipolar illness alone, but patients with a history of recurrent episodes of psychiatric illness may also have a superimposed delirium due to a coexistent medical problem. If the current disorder is phenomenologically unlike past episodes, the patient definitely requires a medical evaluation for causes of delirium. Pseudodelirium accompanies mania (Bond, 1980), schizophrenia, depression, paranoid disorders, atypical and brief reactive psychoses (Lipowski, 1983), and hysteria (Wells & Duncan, 1980). Delirious mania is identified (Bond, 1980) by acute onset, irritability, insomnia, emotional withdrawal, other hypomanic and manic symptoms, personal or family history of affective illness, and responsivity to treatment for mania. Fluctuating levels of consciousness and visual hallucinations are rare with schizophrenia. Schizophrenics' hallucinations tend to be auditory (Wells & Duncan, 1980), and despite schizophrenics' marked disorganization of thought, they usually maintain attention to and awareness of the examiner. The generalized cognitive and memory impairment seen with delirium is not found with schizophrenia. Schizophrenics rarely are disoriented. When they age, their disorientation is bizarre and remote in content. Familiar situations and surroundings appear unfamiliar to the schizophrenic, while delirious patients more often mistake the unusual for the familiar. When paranoid, the delirious perceive danger for all. Schizophrenics personalize danger. Flat, distant affect is absent in people with delirium, whose affect tends to be labile, intense, and transient. Nocturnal worsening of symptoms characteristic of delirium may be absent in schizophrenics, who often sleep well despite symptomatic exacerbation on arousal. Finally, schizophrenics do not have the multifocal myoclonus and bilateral asterixis felt to be pathognomic of diffuse CNS dysfunction.

Orientation and cognitive functioning usually remain intact in hysteria (Wells & Duncan, 1980), and asterixis, myoclonus, and usually hallucinations are absent. Hallucinations, when they occur, generally carry an air of drama. Impairment of cognition and orientation, if present, is inconsistent with what is known of organic dysfunction. A hysterical person may be disoriented to person but not to place or time. This is rarely true in delirium. Cognitive dysfunction in hysteria is out of keeping with the patient's level of alertness and responsivity to examiner and environment.

Laboratory tests may be abnormal in delirium because of primary psychiatric illness. T_4 can be transiently elevated in acute delirious mania. Creatinine phosphokinase (CPK) may be mildly elevated in schizophrenics. Major elevation in a treated schizophrenic, however, suggests neuroleptic malignant syndrome.

History

The patient and collateral sources, including the primary physician, primary nurse, family, and significant friends and neighbors, provide the history of delirium. For hospitalized patients, chart review often reveals previous episodes of "confusion" in relation to specific drugs or procedures. It is often more helpful to review medications directly from the nurse's medication record rather than from the order sheet, as this will aid in detecting transcription or administration errors and will document the use of PRN, or as-needed, medication. Nursing notes document episodes of transient fluctuations in mental status, nighttime disorientation, agitation, or insomnia, giving clues to etiology. An underlying medical disorder is suggested by transient visual hallucinations and illusions (Hall, Popkin, DeVaul, et al., 1978). Hospital discharge summaries also provide important information regarding previous medical problems, hospital course, and discharge medications, as well as a record of previous psychiatric consultations. Family and collateral sources provide data on past psychiatric history and information on drug or alcohol abuse or dependence, which the patient may deny.

Vital sign changes, such as fever, hypotension, and elevation of blood pressure and pulse, reported in current hospital records provide leads to identification of withdrawal states, hypertensive encephalopathy, thyroid abnormalities, and sepsis.

Oral temperatures are often misleading, as the delirious patient may not be able to keep the thermometer in the mouth; rectal temperatures are therefore preferred. Furthermore, elderly patients may have severe inflammation or serious infection without fever or leukocytosis (Blass & Plum, 1983). Even relatively mild infections, such as lower urinary tract infections, may be sufficient to produce delirium in the elderly (Blass & Plum, 1983).

Patients with recent surgery have records of anesthesia that record anesthetic agents used, blood loss and replacement, hypoxia, cardiac arrhythmias, and blood pressure fluctuations (Murray, 1987). Prolonged hypoxia or hypotension are particularly relevant to prolonged postoperative delirium.

Physical Examination

Complete physical examination including vital signs is necessary when seeking an etiology of delirium. Particular attention is paid to the head and neck regions and the tympanic membranes. Deep tendon reflexes and plantar reflexes are tested, and meningeal signs are sought. Asterixis is elicited by hyperextending the wrist and spreading the fingers while observing for flapping or subtle, abnormal, irregular jerking movements. Multifocal myoclonus is most often observed in muscles of the face and shoulders. Gentle massage of the lids over the closed eyes or placement of a blank, white sheet of paper a few inches in front of the open eye sometimes evokes vivid visual images in a delirious patient.

Patients are observed for attention and spontaneous movement. Do patients attend to examiners, or do they stare off into space and startle easily? Are they alert to the calling of their names, only to drift off to sleep (F Adams, 1984)? Do patients speak to themselves and stare at the ceiling or windows as if communicating with an unseen stimulus? Do patients mumble incoherently, pick at their clothes, or grasp unseen objects in the air? Are myoclonic movements present?

Does calling patients' names alert them when they appear stuporous or is painful stimulation required? Is left-right orientation preserved, both on self and on the examiner (F Adams, 1984)? Is speech coherent and logical or pressured, soft, or slurred? Are patients dysphasic or circumlocutory? Are thoughts goal directed, and is conversation relevant to the current situation, or is there a paucity of spontaneous speech? If a patient is respirator dependent or if vocal cords are absent or paralyzed, written responses can be used. Is handwriting legible or does it show signs of tremor? Do patients print or use cursive writing? Are spelling and syntax correct, or is there evidence of perseveration by repetition of letters or words? In metabolically induced cognitive dysfunction, handwriting is disproportionately more impaired than speech (Adams, 1984).

Mental Status Examination

Formal mental status examination should be performed, including evaluation of mood and affect; level of consciousness; motor behavior; rate, pressure, and rhythm of speech; grammar and syntax; perceptual disturbances, including hallucinations and illusions; delusions and psychotic thinking; memory (immediate, recent, and remote); attention and concentration; abstraction; ability to name objects, both on visual confrontation and from description; writing; reading; calculations; visual-spatial orientation; orientation to person, place, and time; ability to perform commands on verbal and visual instruction; grasp of the current situation; thought content; and judgment.

Formal examination provides clues to diagnosis and establishes a baseline for repeated testing to enable detection of improvement or deterioration. A number of formal mental status examinations, though not specific for delirium, are available. These include the Mini-Mental Status Examination (Folstein, Folstein, & McHugh, 1975) and the Cognitive Capacity Screening Examination (Jacobs, Bernhard, Delgado, et al., 1977).

The major value of the structured instruments, such as the Mini-Mental State and the Cognitive Capacity Screening Examination, is that they can be repeated over time by the primary care physician or even by nonphysician staff in order to document either improvement or deterioration of the patient's mental status. Reexamination of the patient at intervals often yields more diagnostic information than even the most detailed examination at one point in time. *It should be noted, however, that these structured instruments often are insensitive to the milder forms of delirium.* In such cases, mild delirium is better diagnosed by careful bedside testing of attention and concentration, by having the patient write sentences to dictation or draw a clock, and by observing the performance of other multistep activities upon verbal and visual instruction.

In delirium, visuospatial skills can be assessed by having the patient copy a geometric figure or by having the patient draw a clock face with hands set to a specific time, such as 10 minutes after 11. Some common tests, such as proverb interpretation, naming of presidents, serial sevens, or spelling the word "world" backward, all of which are often part of routine mental status examination, are without proven value if given in isolation (F Adams, 1984). A sufficiently extensive examination is necessary for diagnostic confidence.

Clinical Laboratory Examinations

Laboratory tests are ordered with attention to specific suspected etiologic agents. In addition to complete blood count (CBC) and differential, electrolytes, blood urea nitrogen (BUN), creatinine, fasting blood glucose, arterial blood gases, serum ammonia level, erythrocyte sedimentation rate, VDRL, thyroid and liver function studies, urine and serum toxicology screens, and lumbar puncture may be indicated (Murray, 1987).

Lumbar puncture is not a first-line test in patients with a change in mental status. It should be performed only after thorough clinical evaluation and serious consideration of the values and hazards of performing such a procedure (Fishman, 1980). It is

an emergency procedure in patients who have an acute mental status change in which fungal or bacterial meningitis is suspected, and it is a serious consideration in patients with fever of unknown origin. Lumbar puncture is occasionally used in patients with suspected acute subarachnoid hemorrhage, although the CT scan detects this problem in most cases. CSF examination also helps in the evaluation of encephalitides, neurosyphilis, and unexplained seizures (Fishman, 1980).

Electroencephalography, EKG, and CT scan with and without contrast are helpful in diagnosing the presence of delirium and its cause. If a CT scan without contrast is negative and there is concern regarding the presence of a mass lesion or new stroke, which is remaining initially isodense on CT scan, it may be better visualized with the use of contrast.

It is not necessary to perform a CT scan on every patient with delirium, as toxic metabolic disorders are the most common cause and the diagnosis of such disorders may be readily confirmed by laboratory tests or history in most cases. In the presence of any physical sign of increased intracranial pressure, however, such as the presence of papilledema, signs of meningeal irritation, a history of recent head trauma or headache, focal neurologic findings, or coma, a CT scan is indicated early in the workup. Eventually, however, any prolonged, undiagnosed delirium deserves a CT scan.

Electroencephalography

In the differential diagnosis of delirium, special attention is accorded the EEG. Slowing of background activity with mixed spikes and sharp waves is seen with hyperactive delirious patients. Those who are quiet usually show slow background activity. Periodic high-amplitude sharp waves are seen in herpes simplex encephalitis, triphasic waves in hepatic encephalopathy, and paroxysmal slow waves in dialysis encephalopathy. Computer-analyzed EEG may reveal changes correlating with the hallucinatory syndrome and withdrawal seen with acute termination of heavy alcohol use (Spehn and Stemmler, 1985), though routine EEG may be read as normal.

Abnormal EEGs do not rule out coexistent psychiatric and medical illness; conversely, certain deliria, such as delirium tremens or alcohol withdrawal delirium, do not present with slowing on routine EEG (Allahyari, Deisenhammer, & Weiser, 1976; Lipowski, 1967; Weiner, 1983). Most patients with delirium, however, do have generalized diffuse background slowing, and the degree of slowing is correlated with the degree of cognitive impairment (Lipowski, 1967). Electroencephalography may not be as useful in the differential diagnosis of dementia from delirium because generalized slowing may occur in primary degenerative dementia. A decrease in generalized background slowing, correlated with behavioral improvement (Romano & Engel, 1944) seen on serial EEGs, serves to differentiate suspected dementia from delirium (Lipowski, 1983).

Behavioral abnormalities parallel levels of CNS abnormality in delirium (Weiner, 1983). Slowing of the posterior alpha rhythm is found early in delirium. Subsequent changes, in order of progression, are generalized delta slowing, decrease in EEG level of reactivity, and, finally, loss of fast (alpha and beta) activity, concomitant with diffuse, very slow (delta) activity. Moderate behavioral impairment is seen with fluctuating amounts of frontal, intermittent, rhythmic delta activity superimposed upon a slow background. Low-voltage, irregular delta activity with suppresion-burst activity occurs with coma (Weiner, 1983). Further discussion of the EEG can be found in Chapter 3, by Fogel and Faust.

Alpha waves (8–12 Hz) and faster beta waves (greater than 13 Hz) are predominant in EEGs of normal adults in the awake state. Prominent theta waves (4–7 Hz) and delta waves (less than 4 Hz) are abnormal in an awake patient. Specific abnormalities characterize certain disease states. Hepatic encephalopathy and renal and pulmonary failure may produce bilateral synchronous triphasic waves (Weiner, 1983). Occasional triphasic waves and frontal, intermittent, rhythmic delta activity is seen with moderate to severe hypercalcemia. Excess fast beta waves, especially in the frontocentral areas, are seen in states of barbiturate and benzodiazepine intoxication; a milder accentuation of beta occurs even at therapeutic levels of these drugs. Anoxic brain injury may be accompanied by suppression-burst activity. State-dependent EEG changes facilitate diagnosis of comatose patients where history is not readily available.

Toxic Screens

Toxic screens are often helpful in acute mental status changes, particularly in the young where there is a possibility of drug or alcohol abuse, and especially in the absence of previous psychiatric history. Toxic screens for specific drugs, such as digoxin, phenytoin, theophylline, anticonvulsants, barbiturates, lithium, and other psychotropic medications, may be useful in determining their role in the production of a delirious state. There may be major variations in sensitivity and accuracy among laboratories, however. In the elderly, toxicity may take place within the therapeutic range of many drugs, and for patients on multiple drugs, toxicities may be additive, although each drug alone may be in the therapeutic range. Multiple drugs with anticholinergic effects may produce postoperative delirium, which is associated with excessive cholinergic receptor binding by cholingeric antagonists in the plasma (Tune, Holland, Folstein, et al., 1981).

Management

Management of delirium is contingent on correction of underlying medical problems and on treating agitation by environmental manipulation and medication. Patients are placed in safe, structured settings with limited sensory input. Private rooms, adequate lighting, and removal of monitors or equipment to areas outside patients' rooms or to nursing stations serves this end. One-to-one nursing or the companionship of family members reduces patients' anxiety, reorients them to familiar persons, and prevents wandering away and accidents. Misinterpretations are corrected at the time they are voiced. Orientation is facilitated by well-placed calendars and wall clocks. Treatment plans are simple and repeatedly explained, allowing for memory limitations (Lazarus & Hagens, 1968; Massie et al., 1983; Waldinger, 1986). The basis of delirium should be explained to frightened family and friends of patients, who fear that the patient is "going crazy" or will be chronically psychotic.

The incidence of postoperative and post-myocardial-infarction delirium has been decreased by preoperative psychiatric interviews conducted two to three days prior to surgery (Kornfeld, Heller, Frank, et al., 1974; Lazarus & Haens, 1968). Recommendations are then made to nursing staff and attending physicians based on the patients' concepts of their illness, the treatment and prognosis, their personality style and past psychiatric history, and their current life situation and stressors (Lazarus & Hagens, 1968). Maintenance of adequate sleep is encouraged (Lazarus & Hagens, 1968; Parker & Hodge, 1967). Mobility is allowed within reasonable limits. Patients respond best to movement to a side room or general medical unit with family members in attendance for long periods of time to approximate a nearly normal environment (Parker & Hodge, 1967).

Psychopharmacotherapy

There is no established drug of choice for the management of agitation in delirious patients (F Adams, 1984). Some prefer benzodiazepines; others, neuroleptics. Of the benzodiazepines, diazepam is avoided because of its long half-life, poor intramuscular (IM) absorption, and problems with tissue depot accumulation (F Adams, 1984). Lorazepam given in 1-to-2-mg increments orally or intramuscularly every hour until low-level sedation is achieved, is a better alternative, because it is reliably absorbed by the IM route and does not require hepatic metabolism. Lorazepam, however, may cause anterograde amnesia. Benzodiazepines as a group are relatively contraindicated in patients with respiratory compromise who are at risk for CO_2 retention. Benzodiazepines *raise* seizure threshold, unlike neuroleptics, and do not carry the risk of extrapyramidal side effects.

Of neuroleptics, low potency phenothiazines are considered least preferable because of their potential for hypotension secondary to alpha-adrenergic antagonism (F Adams, 1984). Haloperidol and thiothixine are preferred because of ease of administration and relative lack of cardiac, pulmonary, and hemodynamic side effects. They are employed at low doses, 0.5–2 mg orally or intramuscularly every 30–60 minutes. When given intravenously, haloperidol is administered at 1 mg/min (Massie et al., 1983). No extrapyramidal, cardiac, pulmonary, or hypotensive side effects were noted in a series of over 1,000 patients with advanced malignancy (some of whom were on dopamine drugs to sustain blood pressure) treated with intravenous haloperidol and lorazepam (F Adams, 1984).

One procedure for the rapid intravenous treatment of agitation entails initial administration of 3 mg of haloperidol and 0.5–1 mg of lorazepam, given in less than 1 minute each (F Adams, 1984). If no response is seen in 30 minutes, the dose is increased to 5 mg of haloperidol and 0.5–2 mg of lorazepam. If in another 30 minutes there is no response, another 10 mg of haloperidol and 0.5–10 mg of lorazepam is given until sedation is obtained. No further medication is given until restlessness recurs. If symptoms reemerge in 4 hours, the patient is provided a dose every 4 hours for the next 12–18 hours, after which time lorazepam is stopped and haloperidol dosing intervals are lengthened to allow the patient to awaken. Intravenous haloperidol does not carry specific FDA approval and therefore may require hospital approval and proper consent. Another approach to intravenous haloperidol is discussed by Goldstein in Chapter 18.

In treating the agitated, delirious patient, the psychiatrist should always be suspicious of the possibility of *neuroleptic malignant syndrome* (NMS) in those patients who deteriorate when treated with neuroleptics. The incidence of NMS has been estimated to be 0.5–1 percent of those patients who receive neuroleptics; it carries a high mortality rate, 14 percent in patients receiving oral neuroleptics and 38 percent in patients receiving intramuscular neuroleptics (Mueller, 1985). (Treated mortality probably is lower.) It is more common with depot and high-potency neuroleptics and can occur with drug combinations, specifically lithium carbonate and haloperidol (Smego & Durack, 1982). The most typical laboratory abnormalities are an elevated serum CPK, an elevated white blood count, and an elevated urine myoglobin. CPK levels appear to correlate with intensity of the neuroleptic malignant syndrome; therefore, it has been suggested that serial CPKs be used to follow the course of the syndrome (Harpe & Stoudemire, 1987). Some authors suggest that there are patients who appear to have an atypical form of NMS, without the classic signs of fever or muscular rigidity; others suggest that the neuroleptic malignant syndrome is actually a misnomer and probably represents a spectrum that

includes (1) patients with medical problems that may cause fever, accompanied by severe extrapyramidal symptoms, (2) patients with medical problems unlikely to cause fever, with severe extrapyramidal symptoms, and (3) patients who present with the neuroleptic-induced syndrome in the absence of any other medical disorder (DF Levinson & Simpson, 1986). In other cases, authors report incomplete episodes that may be *forme fruste* of an NMS, heralding the possibilities of future episodes (DF Levinson & Simpson, 1986). This distinction is important, as neuroleptic malignant syndrome must be differentiated from catatonic functional disorders, as well as other infectious, vascular, neoplastic, or toxic-metabolic disease (Smego & Durack, 1982).

NMS must be differentiated from viral encephalitis, tetanus, bacterial and fungal meningitis, heat stroke (secondary to neuroleptics), tetany due to hypocalcemia, hyperthryoidism, severe forms of Parkinson's disease, malignant hyperthermia, and other allergic drug reactions (Caroff, 1980; JL Levinson, 1985). Fever in the presence of a neuroleptic should not be automatically ascribed to the use of the neuroleptic; concomitant medical illness should be sought. Any extrapyramidal disorder should be treated promptly, as well as hyperthermia and dehydration. Patients who develop severe extrapyramidal symptoms with immobility, rigidity, and impaired cognition, whether fever is present or not, should be treated vigorously for their extrapyramidal symptoms. It has been recommended that in moderate cases the neuroleptic dosage be reduced and regular dosages of anticholinergic drugs or amantadine be instituted, or increased if the patient is already on them. If the patient appears to have akinesia, inability to speak or eat, or has respiratory problems, and if these symptoms do not respond immediately to the administration of antiparkinsonian agents, then neuroleptics should be discontinued with the institution of more vigorous therapies, including dantrolene sodium or bromocriptine or both. These drugs should be given for at least 8–12 days following clinical improvement, as the cessation of the drug may cause a relapse (DF Levinson & Simpson, 1986). With oral neuroleptic cessation alone, NMS may last 5–10 days after cessation of therapy; with depot neuroleptics, NMS may persist for as long as a month (Caroff, 1980). (The editors have seen occasional cases persist for two months, one of which was associated with very high oral dosages of haloperidol.)

Forensic Issues

There are far fewer legal issues involved in care of individuals with delirium than in dementia, in which problems regarding testamentary capacity, right to treatment, right to refuse treatment, commitment, and guardianship arise. Delirium usually is a medical emergency. The patient, therefore, can usually be treated without informed consent, under the common law doctrine of implied consent (Fogel, Mills, & Landen, 1986). This doctrine states that in a true medical emergency, a temporarily incompetent person can be treated "as a reasonable person would choose to be treated." In urgent situations, the doctrine of implied consent often can be extended if measures are taken to safeguard patients' interests, including involving family members in treatment decisions, obtaining second opinions, and seeking administrative consultation. A temporary guardian is necessary if time permits and if the medical risks and alternatives are nontrivial. In any case, careful documentation is required. Ethical and existential questions arising regarding quality of life and concern for limitation of supportive and resuscitative efforts in the late stages of dementia are not of concern in instances of delirium, unless the patient is suffering from a terminal medical illness.

REFERENCES

Abernethy D & Todd E (1986). Doxepin-cimetidine interaction: Increase doxepin bioavailability during cimetidine treatment. *Journal of Clinical Psychopharmacology, 6*, 8–12.

Adams F (1984). Neuropsychiatric evaluation and treatment of delirium in the critically ill cancer patient. *Cancer Bulletin, 36*(3), 156–160.

Adams RD, Fisher CM, Hakim S, et al. (1965). Symptomatic occult hydrocephalus with "normal" cerebrospinal fluid pressure: A treatable syndrome. *New England Journal of Medicine, 273*, 117–126.

Allahyari H, Deisenhammer E, & Weiser G (1976). EEG examination during delirium tremens. *Psychiatric Clinics* (Basel), *9*, 21–31.

Ambrose J (1973). Computerized transverse axial scanning (tomography): 2. Clinical application. *British Journal of Radiology, 46*, 1023–1047.

Arie T (1986). Management of dementia: A review. *British Medical Bulletin, 42*(1):91–96.

Baker FM (1986). Legal issues affecting the older patient. *Hospital and Community Psychiatry,* 37(11), 1091–1093.

Barnes RE, Veith R, Okimoto J, et al. (1982). Efficacy of antipsychotic medications in behaviorally disturbed dementia patients. *American Journal of Psychiatry, 139*(9), 1170–1174.

Beis EB (1984). *Mental health and the law*. Rockville, MD: Aspen Publications.

Berezin MA (1972). Psychodynamic considerations of aging and the aged: An overview. *American Journal of Psychiatry, 128*, 33–41.

Bernstein JG (1979). Antipsychotic drugs in the general hospital: Uses and cautions. *Psychosomatics, 20*(5), 335–347.

Billings RF & Stein MD (1986). Depression associated with ranitidine *American Journal of Psychiatry, 143*(7), 915–916.

Black DW, Wanack G & Winokur G (1985). The Iowa record-linkage study II: Excess mortality among patients with organic mental disorders. *Archives of General Psychiatry, 42*, 78–81.

Black PM (1980). Idiopathic normal pressure hydrocephalus: Results of shunting in 62 patients. *Journal of Neurosurgery, 52, 371–377.

Black PM (1982). Normal pressure hydrocephalus: Current understanding of diagnostic tests and shunting. Postgraduate Medicine, 71(2) 57–67.

Blass JP & Plum (1983). Metabolic encephalopathies in older adults. In R Katzman & R Terry (Eds), The neurology of aging (chap 9, pp 189–220). Philadelphia: FA Davis.

Blazer DG, Federspiel CF, Ray WA, et al. (1983). The risk of anticholinergic toxicity in the elderly: A study of prescribing practices in two populations. Journal of Gerontology, 38, 31–35.

Bond TC (1980). Recognition of acute delirious mania. Archives of General Psychiatry, 37, 553–554.

Borup JH, Gallego D, & Hefferman P (1979). Relocation and its effects on mortality. Gerontologist, 19, 135–140.

Borup JH, Gallego D, & Hefferman P (1980). Relocation and its effect on health functionings and mortality. Gerontologist, 20, 468–479.

Boszormenyi-Nagy I & Krasner B (1986). Between give and take: A clinical guide to contextual therapy. New York: Brunner/Mazel.

Brinkman SD & Largen JW (1984). Changes in brain ventricular size with repeated CT scans in suspected Alzheimer's disease. American Journal of Psychiatry, 141, 81–83.

Busse EW & Obrist WD (1963). Significance of focal electroencaphalographic changes in the elderly. Postgraduate Medicine, 34 179–182.

Butler RN (1963). The life review: An interpretation of reminiscence in the aged. Psychiatry, 26, 65–76.

Caine ED (1981). Pseudodementia: Current concepts and future directions. Archives of General Psychiatry, 38, 1359–1364.

Caroff SN (1980). The neuroleptic malignant syndrome. Journal of Clinical Psychiatry, 41, 79–83.

Cassem NH & Hacket TP (1987). The setting of intensive care. In NH Cassem & TP Hacket (Eds), Massachusetts General Hospital handbook of general psychiatry, (2nd ed, chap 18, pp 353–379). Littleton, MA: PSG Publishing.

Cavenar JO, Maltbie AA, & Austin L (1979). Depression simulating organic brain disease. American Journal of Psychiatry, 136, 895–900.

Charatan FB (1985). Depression and the elderly: diagnosis and treatment. Psychiatric Annals, 15(5), 313–316.

Cohen GD (1981). Perspectives on psychotherapy with the elderly. American Journal of Psychiatry, 138(3), 347–350.

Crook T, Bartus R, Ferris S, et al. (1986). Treatment development strategies for Alzheimer's disease. Madison, CT: Mark Powley Associates.

Crump GL, Pellegrini AJ, Lippmann S, et al. (1984). Diagnosing delirium in acute mental disturbance.

Journal of the Kentucky Medical Association, 22, 168–169.

Cummings JL & Benson DF (1983). Dementia: A clinical approach Boston: Butterworths.

Cutler NR, Duara R, Creasey H, et al. (1984). Brain imaging: Aging and dementia. Annals of Internal Medicine, 101, 355–369.

Daniel DG & Rabin PL (1985). Disguises of delirium. Southern Medical Journal, 78, 666–671.

Delgado-Escueta AV, Treiman DM, & Walsh GO (1983). The treatable epilepsies (2nd of 2 parts), New England Journal of Medicine, 308(26), 1576–1579.

Drugs that cause psychiatric symptoms (1981, February 5). Medical Letter on Drugs and Therapeutics, 23(3), 9–12.

Dubin WR, Weiss KJ, & Zeccardi JA (1983). Organic brain syndrome—the psychiatric imposter. Journal of the American Medical Association, 249(1), 60–62.

Ellison JM (1984). DSM-III and the diagnosis of organic mental disorders. Annals of Emergency Medicine, 13, 521–528.

Engel GL & Romano J (1959). Delirium: A syndrome of cerebral insufficiency. Journal of Chronic Diseases, 9, 260–277.

Fiore J, Becker J, & Coppel DB (1983). Social network interactions: A buffer or a stressor. American Journal of Community Psychology, 11, 423–439.

Fishman RA (1980). Clinical examination of cerebrospinal fluid. In Cerebrospinal fluid in diseases of the nervous system (chap 5, pp 141–167). Philadelphia: WB Saunders.

Fogel BS, Mills MJ, & Landen JE (1986). Legal aspects of the treatment of delirium. Hospital and Community Psychiatry, 37, 154–158.

Fogel BS & Satel SL (1985). Age, medical illness and the DST in depressed general hospital inpatients. Journal of Clinical Psychiatry, 46(3), 95–97.

Fogel BS, Satel SL, & Levy S (1985). Occurrence of high concentrations of post-dexamethasone cortisol in elderly psychiatric inpatients. Psychiatry Research, 15, 85–90.

Foley KM (1982). The practical use of narcotic analgesics. Medical Clinics of North America, 66(5), 1091–1104.

Foley KM (1985). The treatment of cancer pain. New England Journal of Medicine, 313(2), 84–95.

Folstein MF, Folstein SE, & McHugh PR (1975). Mini-Mental State, a practical method for grading the cognitive state of patients for the clinician. Journal of Psychiatric Research, 12, 189–198.

Freeman FR & Rudd SM (1982). Clinical features that predict potentially reversible progressive intellectual deterioration. Journal of the American Geriatric Society, 30, 449–451.

Friedland RP, Budinger TR, Brat-Zawadski M, et al.

(1984). The diagnosis of Alzheimer's-type dementia: A preliminary comparison of positron emission tomography and proton magnetic resonance. *Journal of the American Medical Association*, *252*(19), 2750–2752.

Fuller J, Ward E, Evans A, et al. (1979). Dementia: Supportive groups for relatives. *British Medical Journal*, *1*, 1684.

Gado MH & Press GA (1986). Computed tomography in the diagnosis of dementia. *Geriatric Medicine Today*, *5*(7), 47–73.

Gallant DM (1985). Differential diagnosis of confusion in the geriatric patient. *Geriatric Medicine Today*, *4*(4), 72–81.

Gershon ES, Goldstein RE, Moss AJ, et al. (1979). Psychosis with ordinary doses of propranolol. *Annals of Internal Medicine*, *90*(6), 938–939.

Gilleard CJ, Gilleard E, & Whittick JE (1984). Impact of psychogeriatric day hospital care on the patient's family. *British Journal of Psychiatry*, *145*, 487–492.

Gilleard CJ, Belford H, Gilleard E, et al. (1984). Emotional distress amongst the supporters of the elderly mentally infirm. *British Journal of Psychiatry*, *145*, 172–177.

Goff DC, Garber HJ, & Jenike MA (1985). Partial resolution of ranitidine-associated delirium with physostigmine: case report. *Journal of Clinical Psychiatry*, *46*, 400–401.

Goggans FC, Weisberg LJ, & Koran LM (1983). Lithium prophylaxis of prednisone psychosis: A case report. *Journal of Clinical Psychiatry*, *44*, 111–112.

Goldberg RJ & Cullen LO (1986). Depression in geriatric cancer patients: Guide to assessment and treatment. *The Hospice Journal*, *2*(2), 79–98.

Goldfrank L, Flomerbaum N, Lewis N, et al. (1982, January). Withdrawal? *Hospital Physician*, pp 12–36.

Goldfrank L, Lewis N, Melinek M, et al. (1981). Caffeine. *Hospital Physician*, *11*, 42–59.

Golodny R (1979). Pseudodelirium. *Medical Journal of Australia*, *1*, 630.

Goodnick PJ (1985). Pseudodementia. *Geriatric Medicine Today*, *4*(10), 31–40.

Goto K, Umegaki H, & Suetsugu M (1976). Electroencephalographic and clinicopathological studies in Creutzffeldt-Jakob syndrome. *Journal of Neurology, Neurosurgery and Psychiatry*, *39*, 931–940.

Gutheil TG & Bursztajn H (1986). Clinician's guidelines for assessing and presenting subtle forms of patient incompetence in legal settings. *American Journal of Psychiatry*, *143*(8), 1020–1023.

Guze SB & Cantwell DP (1964). The prognosis in "organic brain" syndromes. *American Journal of Psychiatry*, *120*, 878–881.

Guze SB & Daengsurisri S (1967). Organic brain syndromes prognostic significance in general medical patients. *Archives of General Psychiatry*, *17*, 365–366.

Hachinski VC, Lassen NA, & Marshall J (1974, July 27). Multi-infarct dementia, a cause of mental deterioration in the elderly. *Lancet*, pp 207–209.

Hall RCW, Popkin MA, DeVaul RA, et al. (1978). Physical illness presenting as psychiatric disease. *Archives of General Psychiatry*, *35*, 1315–1320.

Hammerstrom DC & Zimmer B (1985). The role of lumbar puncture in the evaluation of dementia: The University of Pittsburgh study. *Journal of the American Geriatric Society*, *33*(6), 397–400.

Harpe C & Stoudemire A (1987). Aetiology and the treatment of neuroleptic malignant syndrome. *Medical Toxicology*, *2*, 166–176.

Henderson AS (1986). The epidemiology of Alzheimer's disease. *British Medical Bulletin*, *42*(1), 3–10.

Herman M (1938). The use of intravenous sodium amytal in psychogenic amnesia states. *Psychiatry Quarterly*, *12*, 738.

Herst L & Moulton P (1985). Psychiatry in the nursing home. *Psychiatric Clinics of North America*, *8*(3), 551–561.

Huppert FA & Tym E (1986). Clinical and neuropsychological assessment of dementia. *British Medical Bulletin*, *42*(1), 11–18.

Ibe O & Kitchen AD (1983). Differentiation of delirium from dementia [Letter to the editor]. *Journal of the American Medical Association*, *250*(11), 1393–1394.

Jacobs JW, Bernhard MR, Delgado A, et al. (1977). Screening for organic mental syndromes in the medically ill. *Annals of Internal Medicine*, *86*, 40–46.

Jacobs L, Conti D, Kinkel WR, et al. (1976). "Normal pressure" hydrocephalus relationship of clinical and radiographic findings to improvement following shunt surgery. *Journal of the American Medical Association*, *235*(5), 510–512.

Jeff O & Roth M (1969, October). The new psychogeriatric unit at Newcastle General Hospital. *Occupational Therapy*, pp 21.

Jenike MA (1985). *Handbook of Geriatric Psychopharmacology*. Littleton, MA: PSG Publishing.

Johnson J. (1985). Nutrition as a factor of mortality in senile dementia of the Alzheimer's type. *Psychiatric Annals*, *15*(5), 323–330.

Kales A & Kales JD (1974). Sleep disorders: Recent findings in the diagnosis and treatment of disturbed sleep. *New England Journal of Medicine*, *280*, 487–499.

Katon W & Raskind M (1980). Treatment of depression in the medically ill elderly with methylphenidate. *American Journal of Psychiatry 137*, 963–965.

Kaufman DM (1981). *Clinical neurology for psychiatrists*. Orlando: Grune & Stratton.

Kiloh LG (1961). Pseudodementia. *Acta Psychiatrica Scandinavica, 37,* 336–361.

Knights EB & Folstein MF (1977). Unsuspected emotional and cognitive disturbance in medical patients. *Annals of Internal Medicine, 87*(6), 723–724.

Kopelman MD & Lishman WA (1986). Pharmacological treatments of dementia (noncholinergic). *British Medical Bulletin, 42*(1), 101–105.

Kornfeld DS, Heller SS, Frank KA, et al. (1974). Personality and psychological factors in postcardiotomy delirium. *Archives of General Psychiatry, 31,* 249–253.

Kroetsch P & Shamoian CA (1986). Psychotherapy for the elderly. *Medical Aspects of Human Sexuality, 20*(3), 62–65.

Kruis R & Barger R (1980). Paranoid psychosis with sulindac [Letter to the editor]. *Journal of the American Medical Association, 243*(14), 1420.

Lambert C & Rees WL (1944). Intravenous barbiturates in the treatment of hysteria. *British Medical Journal, 11,* 70.

Larson EB, Reifler BV, Featherstone, HJ, et al. (1984). Dementia in elderly outpatients: A prospective study. *Annals of Internal Medicine, 100,* 417–423.

Lawton MP, Moss M, Fulcomer M, et al. (1982). A research and service oriented multilevel assessment instrument. *Journal of Gerontology, 37,* 91–99.

Lazarus HR & Hagens JH (1968). Prevention of psychosis following open heart surgery. *American Journal of Psychiatry, 124*(9), 76–81.

Lesse S, Hoefer PFA, & Austin JH (1958). The electroencephalogram in diffuse encephalopathies. *Archives of Neurological Psychiatry 79,* 359–375.

Levine PM, Silberfarb PM, & Lipowski ZJ (1978). Mental disorders in cancer patients: A study of 100 psychiatric referrals. *Cancer, 42,* 1385–1391.

Levine NB, Gendron, CE, Dastoor DP, et al. (1984). Existential issues in the management of the demented elderly patient. *American Journal of Psychiatry, 38*(2), 215–223.

Levinson JL (1985). Neuroleptic malignant syndrome. *American Journal of Psychiatry, 142*(10), 1137–1145.

Levinson DF & Simpson GM (1986). Neuroleptic-induced extrapyramidal symptoms with fever: Heterogeneity of the "Neuroleptic Malignant Syndrome." *Archives of General Psychiatry, 43,* 839–848.

Lewis MI & Butler RN (1974). Life review therapy. *Geriatrics, 29,* 165–173.

Ling, MHM, Perry PJ & Tsuang MT (1981). Side-effects of corticosteroid therapy: Psychiatric aspects. *Archives of General Psychiatry, 38,* 471–477.

Lipowski ZJ (1967). Delirium, clouding of consciousness and confusion. *Journal of Nervous and Mental Disorders, 145,* 227–255.

Lipowski ZJ (1983). Transient cognitive disorders (delirium, acute confusional states) in the elderly. *American Journal of Psychiatry, 140*(11), 1426–1436.

Mahendra B (1984). *Dementia. A survey of the syndrome of dementia.* Lancaster, England: MTP Press.

Maletta GJ (1985). Medication to modify at home behavior of Alzheimer's patients. *Geriatrics, 40*(12), 31–42.

Marcus AJ (1977). Aspirin and thromboembolism—a possible dilemma. *New England Journal of Medicine, 297,* 1284–1285.

Massie M, Holland J, & Glass E (1983). Delirium in terminally ill cancer patients. *American Journal of Psychiatry, 140,* 1048–1050.

McAllister TW, Ferrell RB, Price TRP, et al. (1982). The dexamethasone suppression test in two patients with severe pseudodementia. *American Journal of Psychiatry, 139,* 479–481.

McAllister TW & Price TRP (1985). Severe depressive pseudodementia with and without dementia. *American Journal of Psychiatry, 139*(5), 626–629.

McCarthy DM (1983). Ranitidine or cimetidine. *Annals of Internal Medicine, 99*(4), 551–553.

McCarthy JR & Palmateer LM (1985). Assessment of cognitive deficit in geriatric patients: A study of physician behavior. *Journal of the American Geriatric Society, 33,* 467–471.

McCartney CF, Hatley LH & Kessler JM (1982). Possible tobramycin delirium. *Journal of the American Medical Association, 247*(9), 1319.

McEvoy JP (1981). Organic brain syndromes. *Annals of Internal Medicine, 95,* 212–220.

McGeer PL (1986). Brain imaging in Alzheimer's disease. *British Medical Bulletin, 42*(1), 24–28.

McKeith J (1984). Clinical use of the DST in a psychogeriatric population. *British Journal of Psychiatry, 145,* 389–393.

McQuarrie IG, Saint-Louis L, & Scherer PB (1984). Treatment of normal pressure hydrocephalus with low versus medium pressure cerebrospinal fluid shunts. *Neurosurgery, 15,* 484–488.

Meyer JS, Judd BW, Tawakina T, et al. (1986). Improved cognition after control of risk factors for multi-infarct dementia. *Journal of the American Medical Association, 256*(16), 2203–2209.

Miller E (1984). Psychological aspects of dementia. In JHS Pearce (Ed), *Dementia: A clinical approach.* (chap 10, pp 1135–1531). Boston: Blackwell Scientific Publications.

Mueller PS (1985). Neuroleptic malignant syndrome. *Psychosomatics*, *26*, 654–662.

Murray GB (1987). Confusion, delirium and dementia. In TP Hacket & NH Cassem (Eds), *Massachusetts General Hospital handbook of general hospital psychiatry*, (2nd ed, chap 6, pp 84–115). Littleton, MA. PSG Publishing.

Oldendorf WH (1980). *The quest for an image of the brain*. New York: Raven Press.

O'Quin J & McGraw KO (1985). The burdened caregiver: An overview. In TJ Hutton & AD Kenny (Eds), *Senile dementia of the Alzheimer type: Proceedings of the Fifth Tarbox Symposium* (pp 65–75). New York: Alan R Liss.

Park GD (1986). Rheumatic diseases. In R Spector (Ed), *The scientific basis of clinical pharmacology: Principles and examples* (chap 20, p 360). Boston: Little, Brown & Co.

Parker DL & Hodge JR (1967). Delirium in a coronary care unit. *Journal of the American Medical Association*, *201*(9), 132–133.

Paykel ES, Fleminger R & Watson JP (1982). Psychiatric side-effects of antihypertensive drugs other than reserpine. *Journal of Clinical Psychopharmacology*, *2*(1), 14–39.

Pearce JMS (1984). Management. In *Dementia: A clinical approach* (chap 11, pp 154–165). Boston: Blackwell Scientific Publications.

Penry JK & Newmark ME (1979). The use of antiepileptic drugs. *Annals of Internal Medicine*, *90*, 207–218.

Perry JC & Jacobs D (1982). Overview: Clinical applications of the amytal interview in psychiatric emergency settings. *American Journal of Psychiatry 139*, 552–559.

Post F (1965) *Clinical psychiatry of late life*. Oxford: Pergamon Press.

Post F (1975) Dementia, depression and pseudodementia. In DF Benson & D Blumer (Eds), *Psychiatric aspects of neurologic diseases*. New York: Grune & Stratton.

Psychogeriatrics (1972). (World Health Organization Technical Report 507). Geneva: World Health Organization.

Rabins P, Mace N, & Lucas M (1982). The impact of dementia on the family. *Journal of the American Medical Association*, *248*, 333–335.

Rabins PV & Folstein MF (1982). Delirium and dementia: Diagnostic criteria and fatality rates. *British Journal of Psychiatry*. *140*, 149–153.

Rathbone-McCuan E & Voyles B (1982). Case detection of abused parents. *American Journal of Psychiatry*, *139*, 189–192.

Rathbone-McCuan E & Goodstein RK (1985). Elder abuse: Clinical considerations. *Psychiatric Annals*, *15*(5), 331–339.

Read SL, Small GW, & Jarvik LF (1985). Dementia syndrome. In RE Hales & AJ Frances (Eds), *Psychiatry update: The American Psychiatric Association annual review* (Vol. 4, chap 11, pp 211–226). Washington, DC: APA Press.

Reifler BV (1986). Mixed cognitive-affective disturbances in the elderly: A new classification. *Journal of Clinical Psychiatry*, *47*, 354–356.

Reifler B, Larson E, & Hanley R (1982). Coexistence of cognitive impairment and depression in geriatric outpatients. *American Journal of Psychiatry*, *139*(5), 623–626.

Remick RA, O'Kane J, & Sparling TG (1981). A case report of toxic psychosis with low-dose propranolol therapy. *American Journal of Psychiatry*, *138*(6), 850–851.

Reynolds CF, III, Kupfer DJ, Taska LS, et al. (1985). Sleep apnea in Alzheimer's dementia: Correlation with mental deterioration. *Journal of Clinical Psychiatry*, *46*, 257–261.

Rivinus TM (1982). Psychiatric effects of the anticonvulsants regimens. *Journal of Clinical Psychopharmacology*, *2*(3), 165–192.

Roca RP, Klein LE, Kirby SM, et al. (1984). Recognition of dementia among medical patients. *Archives of Internal Medicine*, *144*, 73–75.

Ross HE & Kedward HB (1977). Psychogeriatric hospital admissions from the community and institutions. *Journal of Gerontology*, *32*, 420–427.

Roth M (1982). Perspectives in the diagnosis of senile and presenile dementia of Alzheimer's type. In M Sarner (Ed), *Advanced Medicine* (Vol. 18). London: Royal College of Physicians.

Rubin CE (1984). Cimetidine and ranitidine [Letter to the editor]. *Journal of the American Medical Association*, *251*, 2211–2212.

Rudorfer MV & Clayton PJ (1981). Depression, dementia and dexamethasone suppression [Letter to the editor]. *American Journal of Psychiatry*, *138*, 701.

Salzman C (1982). A primer on geriatric psychopharmacology. *American Journal of Psychiatry*, *139*, 67–74.

Salzman C, Shader RI, Greenblatt DJ, et al. (1983). Long versus short half-life benzodiazepines in the elderly: Kinetics and clinical effects of diazepam and oxazepam. *Archives of General Psychiatry*, *40*, 293–297.

Sanford JRA (1975). Tolerance of debility in elderly dependents by supporters at home. *British Medical Journal*, *3*, 471–473.

Shista SK, Troupe A, Marszalek KS, et al. (1974). Huntington's chorea: An electroencephalographic and psychometric study. *Electroencephalography and Clinical Neurophysiology*, *36*, 387–393.

Shraberg D (1978). The myth of pseudodementia: Depression and the aging brain. *American Journal of Psychiatry*, *135*, 601–603.

Slaby AE (1982). Dementia. In AJ Giannine (Ed), *Neurologic, neurogenic, and neuropsychiatric disorders*. Garden City, NY: Medical Examination Publishing.

Slaby AE Dementia. In LI Sederer (Ed), *Inpatient psychiatry: Diagnosis and treatment* (2nd ed, pp 150–170). Baltimore: Williams & Wilkins.

Slaby AE & Wyatt RJ (1974). *Dementia in the presenium*. Springfield, IL: Charles C Thomas.

Sloane RB (1983). Organic mental disorders. In L Grinspoon (Ed), *Psychiatric update: The American Psychiatric Association annual review* (Vol. 2, chap 8, pp 106–118). Washington, DC: APA Press.

Smego RA & Durack DT (1982). The neuroleptic malignant syndrome. *Annals of Internal Medicine, 142*, 1183–1185.

Snavely SR & Hodges GR (1984). The neurotoxicity of antibacterial agents. *Annals of Internal Medicine, 101*, 92–104.

Snow SS & Wells CE (1981). Case studies in neuropsychiatry: Diagnosis and treatment of coexistent dementia and depression. *Journal of Clinical Psychiatry, 42*(11), 439–441.

Sotsky SM & Tossell JW (1984). Tometin induction of mania. *Psychosomatics, 25*(8), 626–628.

Spar JE & Gerner R (1982). Does the dexamethasone test distinguish dementia from depression? *American Journal of Psychiatry, 139*, 283–290.

Spehn W & Stemmler G (1985). Post-alcoholic diseases: Diagnostic relevance of computerized EEG. *Electroencephalography and Clinical Neurophysiology, 60*, 106–114.

Steele C, Lucas M, & Tune L (1986). Haloperidol versus thioridazine in the treatment of behavioral symptoms in senile dementia of the Alzheimer's type: Preliminary findings. *Journal of Clinical Psychiatry, 47*, 310–312.

Steele TE & Morton WA (1986). Salicylate-induced delirium. *Psychosomatics, 27*(6), 455–456.

Stillner V, Popkin MK, & Pierce CM (1978). Caffeine-induced delirium during prolonged competitive stress. *American Journal of Psychiatry, 135*(7), 855–856.

Strub RL (1982). Acute confusional state. In FD Benson & D Blumen (Eds), *Psychiatric aspects of neurologic disease* (Vol. 2, chap 1). New York: Grune & Stratton.

Strum WB (1984). Cimetidine and ranitidine. *Journal of the American Medical Association, 251*(17), 2212.

Teeter RB, Garetz FK, Miller WR, et al. (1976). Psychiatric disturbances of aged patients in skilled nursing homes. *American Journal of Psychiatry, 133*(12), 1430–1434.

Thompson TL, Moran MG, & Nies AS (1983a). Psychotropic drug use in the elderly (1st of 2 parts). *New England Journal of Medicine, 308*, 134–138.

Thompson TL, Moran MG, & Nies AS (1983b). Psychotropic drug use in the elderly (2nd of 2 parts). *New England Journal of Medicine, 308*, 194–199.

Tomlinson BE, Blessed G, & Roth M (1968). Observations on the brain of nondemented old people. *Journal of Neurological Science, 7*, 331–356.

Tomlinson BE, Blessed G, & Roth M (1970). Observations on the brains of demented old people. *Journal of Neurological Science, 11*, 205–242.

Tresch DD, Folstein MF, Rabins PV, et al (1985). Prevalence and significance of cardiovascular disease and hypertension in elderly patients with dementia and depression. *Journal of the American Geriatric Society 33*(8), 530–537.

Trzepacz PT, Teague GB, & Lipowski ZJ (1985). Delirium and other organic mental disorders in a general hospital. *General Hospital Psychiatry, 7*, 101–106.

Tune, LE, Holland A, Folstein MF, et al. (1981, September 26). Association of postoperative delirium with raised serum levels of anticholinergic drugs. *Lancet*, pp 651–652.

Tyler KL & Tyler HR (1984). Differentiating organic dementia. *Geriatrics, 39*(3), 38–52.

Van Praag HM (1977). Psychotropic drugs in the aged. *Comprehensive Psychiatry, 18*, 429–442.

Vassilouthis J (1984). The syndrome of normal pressure hydrocephalus. *Journal of Neurosurgery, 61*, 501–509.

Victor M & Adams RD (1974). Common disturbances of vision, ocular movement, and hearing. In MM Wintrobe, GW Thron, RD Adams, et al. (Eds), *Harrison's principles of internal medicine* (7th ed, pp 100–110). New York: McGraw-Hill.

Volpe BT & Soave R (1979). Formed visual hallucinations and digitalis toxicity. *Annals of Internal Medicine, 91*(6), 865.

Ward NG, Rowlett DB, & Burke P (1978). Sodium amylobarbitone in the differential diagnosis of confusion. *American Journal of Psychiatry, 135*(1), 75–83.

Weddington WW, Muelling AE, & Moosa HH (1982). Adverse neuropsychiatric reactions to cimetidine. *Psychosomatics, 23*(1), 49–53.

Weiner RD (1983). EEG in organic brain syndrome. In JR Hughes & WP Wilson (Eds), *EEG and evoked potential in psychiatry and behavioral neurology* (pp 1–24). Boston: Butterworths.

Wells CE (1977). Dementia: Definition and description. In CE Wells (Ed), *Contemporary neurology series: Dementia* (2nd ed, pp 1–14). Philadelphia: FA Davis.

Wells CE (1979). Pseudodementia. *American Journal of Psychiatry*, *136*, 895–900.

Wells CE & Duncan GW (1980). Delirium. In *Neurology for psychiatrists*. Philadelphia: FA Davis.

Wilson WH & Jefferson JW (1985). Thyroid disease, behavior, and psychopharmacology. *Psychosomatics*, *26*(6), 481–492.

Wolff HG & Curran D (1935). Nature of delirium and allied states: The dysergastic reaction. *Archives of Neurology and Psychiatry*, pp 1175–1215.

Wolfson LI & Katzman R (1983). The neurological consultation at age 80. In R Katzman & RD Terry (Eds), *The neurology of aging* (pp 221–224). Philadelphia: FA Davis.

Yesavage JA, Tinklenberg JR, Hollister LE, et al. (1979). Vasodilators in senile dementias: A review of the literature. *Archives of General Psychiatry*, *36*, 220–223.

Zarit S, Reever K, & Bach-Peterson J (1980). Relative of the impaired elderly: Correlates of feelings of burden. *Gerontologist*, *20*, 649–655.

Zarit SH & Zarit JM (1984). Psychological approaches to families of the elderly. In MG Eisenberg, LC Sutkin, & MA Jansen (Eds), *Chronic illness and disability through the life span: Effects on self and family* (chap 13, pp 269–288). New York: Springer Publishing.

Richard J. Goldberg

7
Anxiety in the Medically Ill

The evaluation of anxiety in the medical or surgical patient requires a biopsychosocial approach (Goldberg, 1982). What the consultee or patient labels as anxiety may turn out to be a manifestation of delirium, a primary anxiety disorder, a symptom of some other psychiatric diagnosis, or an adjustment reaction determined by the meaning of the patient's experience. Even in situations where the explanation for the patient's anxiety seems patently obvious, the clinician must regard anxiety as a non-specific indicator of some potential problem requiring differential diagnosis. It is always an error to dismiss anxiety by saying, "Wouldn't you be anxious if you were in the same situation as that patient?" Instead, the clinician should proceed with an evaluation that includes attention to possible underlying biologic causes, concurrent psychiatric disorders, and psychologic and social systems dynamics. These dimensions are not mutually exclusive, but rather form complementary dimensions of the patient's experience.

This chapter presents an approach to the evaluation of anxiety in medical pa-

tients that addresses three sequential dimensions. First, the clinician should look for the possibility of an underlying medical basis for the anxiety, since if this is present, the rest of the evaluation may need to be deferred until the underlying medical abnormality is corrected. For example, it would not make sense to begin speculating about the psychologic basis of anxiety if the patient were hyperthyroid or undergoing substance withdrawal. The primary intervention in such situations would be to correct the underlying medical disorder, re-evaluate the patient, and proceed with the evaluation if the anxiety persisted.

The second step in this evaluation involves obtaining a complete past personal and psychiatric history along with a psychiatric review of systems, to determine if the patient's anxiety is part of some underlying psychiatric disorder, such as panic disorder, affective disorder, or borderline personality disorder. If so, the intervention consists of addressing that primary psychiatric disorder, of which the anxiety may be one of the presenting symptoms.

The third stage in the evaluation, if the

PRINCIPLES OF MEDICAL PSYCHIATRY
ISBN 0-8089-1883-4

177

problem is not solved by this time, involves assessing whether the anxiety represents a psychologic adjustment response. In such instances, the intervention consists of some form of psychotherapy to help provide insight, reassurance, information, or reorganization of the system of care to match the perceived needs of the patient.

This systematic approach assures that the clinician will not fall into the trap of prematurely assuming the patient's anxiety represents only an adjustment reaction. At the same time, it also assures that the patient will be treated as a person, since even the patient with a clear medical basis for anxiety may also have some psychologic concerns or behavioral factors to that need to be addressed.

MEDICAL DISORDERS THAT PRESENT AS ANXIETY: ORGANIC ANXIETY SYNDROMES

Medical disorders may produce anxiety directly or indirectly. Some medical disorders have specific effects on neurotransmitter systems or on neuroanatomic sites associated directly with the production of anxiety. Examples of such direct causes are tumors of the temporal lobe (Dietch, 1984) or hyperthyroidism (Hall, 1983). Many medical disorders produce anxiety more nonspecifically, however, by causing delirium. The cognitive blurring associated with delirium, which impairs the patient's ability to organize experience, especially when coupled with a stressful physical or emotional situation, creates an experience of anxiety.

Medical disorders that can present with anxiety as a prominent symptom include the following:

1. Angina pectoris
2. Cardiac arrhythmias
3. Hyperthyroidism
4. Hyperventilation
5. Hypocalcemia

6. Hypoglycemia
7. Hypoxia
8. Mitral valve prolapse syndrome
9. Opiate withdrawal
10. Pheochromocytoma
11. Postconcussion syndrome
12. Sedative withdrawal
13. Stimulants
14. Sympathomimetic toxicity
15. Temporal and frontal lobe (partial; complex) seizures
16. Xanthine toxicity

Toxic and Withdrawal Effects of Drugs

The toxic and withdrawal effects of drugs are a prevalent cause of anxiety in medical patients (Abramowitz, 1984). The clinician should compile a comprehensive list of all substances inhaled, ingested, or injected by the patient over the previous month. If there is any doubt about what drugs the patient has been taking, a toxicology screen should be ordered. Such screening is especially useful when the patient is suspected of surreptitious drug use. A drug history should include inquiry about over-the-counter medications, items from health food stores, occupational exposures, and borrowed medications. If there is uncertainty about whether any of the substances can cause anxiety, a drug information service should be consulted.

Caffeine

Caffeine is one of the most widely used psychotropic drugs in the United States (Abelson & Fishburne, 1976), found in many beverages and drug combinations. The approximate amount of caffeine in a cup of coffee is 150 mg. Although individual sensitivity varies, symptoms of caffeinism, which may occur at doses of only 200 mg, are identical to the classical description of an anxiety episode (Victor, Lubersky, Greden, 1981). Caffeine modifies catecholamine levels, inhibits phosphodiesterase breakdown of cyclic AMP in the central nervous system, and sensitizes central catecholamine receptors, particularly for dopamine (Waldeck, 1975). Caffeine may precipitate an actual panic attack in patients with that underlying diagnosis (Charney, Heninger, & Jatlow, 1985). In chronic users, caffeine abstinence should also be considered as a possible source of intermittent anxiety (White et al, 1980).

Cocaine

The United States is in the midst of a cocaine use epidemic, with the wide availability of "crack," a form of cocaine that is readily smoked, leading to higher and more intense effects, including hyperpyrexia, seizures, and ventricular arrhythmias (Abramowicz, 1986a). Symptoms of anxiety, irritability, tremulousness, fatigue, or depression may appear soon after the initial euphoriant effects (Resnic, Kestenbaum, Schwartz, 1976). Cocaine has been reported to induce panic attacks in susceptible individuals and to actually precipitate panic disorder, which continues autonomously even after the cocaine use is discontinued (Aronson & Craig, 1986). Detectable amounts of cocaine are found in the urine or plasma only for a few hours after use, though one of the metabolites, benzoylecgonine, may be detected in a urine sample for as long as 48 hours after use (Wilkerson et al, 1980). There is evidence that the ability of laboratories to accurately detect cocaine (and other substances) varies widely (Hansen, Caudill, & Boone, 1985).

Alcohol

It is estimated that 30–50 percent of hospitalized medical patients have a problem that is in some way related to alcohol use (Moore, 1985), and alcohol withdrawal (Lerner & Fallon, 1985) is a frequent etiology for agitation and anxiety. Minor abstinence syndrome, which has its modal onset about 24 hours after cessation of drinking, presents with anxiety and tremulousness (the "shakes" and insomnia) and is a self-limited syndrome resolving over several days. While the patient with minor abstinence syndrome may have discomfort and complain of anxiety, the major concern for the physician is whether or not such symptoms are the harbinger of alcohol withdrawal delirium (also known as delirium tremens), which has a modal onset 72 hours following cessation or significant reduction of drinking but may occur as early as 24 hours or up to 7 days later. In the patient with major abstinence, anxiety and tremulousness are accompanied by symptoms of autonomic arousal, including tachycardia, mydriasis, diaphoresis, and increased temperature. The constellation of these classic symptoms of "DTs" should be considered a serious medical problem and requires supervised medical management (Sellers & Kalant, 1976). Because of the association of Wernicke-Korsakoff syndrome with alcohol use (Reuler, Girard, & Cooney, 1985), such patients should always be given thiamine. The syndrome of major abstinence from alcohol may be duplicated by withdrawal from any central nervous system (CNS) sedative. The time of onset and the severity of the withdrawal symptoms are related to the half-life of the sedative in question. Drugs with short half-lives have more rapid onset of major abstinence and more severe withdrawal symptoms, often including seizures. The classic signs and symptoms of sedative withdrawal may be masked by the concurrent use of other medications. For example, mydriasis may be absent if the patient is on narcotics, and tachycardia may be masked by use of beta blockers. The sudden onset of extreme anxiety (with delirium), fever, and tachycardia in a hospitalized patient several days after admission should be considered probable alcohol withdrawal. The treatment of alcohol withdrawal is covered in chapter 10.

Neuroleptics

Akathisia, a common side effect of neuroleptics, presents as a sense of internal restlessness often described as anxiety. It is estimated that as many as 40–50 percent of patients on neuroleptics (and other dopamine-receptor blockers, such as metaclopramide) have akathisia (Ratey & Salzman, 1984). Akathisia may be treated by lowering the neuroleptic dose or by adding anticholinergic agents or beta blockers (Ratey, Sorgi, & Polakoffs, 1985).

Opiate Withdrawal

Narcotic abstinence is always accompanied by anxiety. In the hospital setting, patients may be undergoing narcotic withdrawal because they are addicted prior to admission and no longer have access to narcotics, or because of iatrogenic causes such as the abrupt lowering of dose often seen on surgical services. Iatrogenic withdrawal may occur when patients are changed from parenteral to oral narcotics without consideration of differences in oral/parenteral ratios. The patient who has just had a change in narcotic orders is therefore likely to be anxious because of increased pain due to inadequate medication or to withdrawal effects.

Other Drugs

Alpha adrenergic stimulants, which are used in over-the-counter decongestants, include phenylpropanolamine, ephedrine, phenylephrine, and pseudoephedrine. These agents are closely related to amphetamines and can produce symptoms of anxiety, restlessness, irritability, and insomnia (Weiner, 1980).

Bronchodilators, which chemically resemble the catecholamines, include isoetharine, isoproterenol, epinephrine, metaproterenol, and albuterol. These drugs have peripheral effects that include increased heart rate, elevated blood pressure, and elevated lactate levels, all of which can contribute to feelings of anxiety. Systemic effects, reported even with metered-dose inhalers (Harris, 1985), include symptoms of anxiety, restlessness, nervousness, tremor, irritability, insomnia, and emotional lability.

Theophylline is a methylxanthine related chemically to caffeine and is capable of producing powerful cardiovascular effects, with tachycardia, along with nervousness and anxiety states (Jacobs, Senior, & Kessler, 1976).

Calcium channel blockers, including verapamil, nifedipine, and diltiazem, all have been reported to produce neuropsychiatric symptoms, which include anxiety, tremulousness, jitteriness, and sleep disturbance (Bela & Raftery, 1980: Muller & Chahine, 1981; Rickenberger, Psystowsky, Heger, et al., 1980; Singh, Ellrodt, & Peter, 1978).

Other drugs reported to produce anxiety as a side effect (Abramowitz, 1984) include: amphetamines and similar anorexic agents, antihistamines, baclofen, cycloserine, indomethacin, oxymetazoline, and quinacrine.

Other Medical Disorders

Hypoglycemia

Endogenously produced profound hypoglycemia may occur secondary to insulinoma. Wide and abrupt fluctuations in plasma insulin levels may lead to anxiety and panic states, including symptoms of depersonalization and sympathetic autonomic discharge (Marks & Rose, 1965). Other secondary sequelae may include angina, seizures, focal neurologic signs, or unconsciousness. With insulinoma, relief by eating is not regularly reported. Between attacks, the patient feels well and functions in a normal manner. The clinical picture of insulinoma may also result from excessive exogenous insulin or oral hypoglycemic use that is iatrogenic, inadvertent, or purposeful. Hypoglycemia may also occur secondary to a number of drugs, including salicylates, antihistamines, monoamine oxidase inhibitors, propranolol, phenylbutazone, alcohol, phenytoin, and estrogens.

Reactive (postprandial) hypoglycemia occurs 3–4 hours after eating, with symptoms resulting from an exaggerated and asynchronous physiologic response to carbohydrate ingestion. An impairment of insulin regulation interferes with the switching off of the hepatic uptake of glucose, which normally occurs several hours after a meal. A-cell (pancreatic) glucagon deficiency has recently been demonstrated to be a factor in some cases of adult reactive hypoglycemia (Foa et al, 1980). Clinically significant hypoglycemia is associated with a variety of neuroendocrine responses, including increased serum cortisol, along with such symptoms as sympathetic autonomic arousal, anxiety, irritability, sweating, tremulousness, and tachycardia. Episodes of reactive hypoglycemia do not show the progression in frequency or severity that is characteristic of insulinoma (Freinkel & Metzger, 1969). When reactive hypoglycemia is suspected on the basis of characteristic symptoms, the appropriate diagnostic evaluation is a properly performed 5-hour glucose tolerance test (GTT) (Anderson & Lev-Ran, 1985). Anxious patients often feel that hypoglycemia accounts for their symptoms; however, there is scant documentation of psychiatric symptoms as a direct consequence of low blood sugar (Kwentus, Achilles, & Goyer, 1982; Leggett & Favazza, 1978; Zivin, 1970).

In a population of patients identified as having a clinical picture of postprandial hypoglycemia, a significant percentage have another diagnosis (Fabrykant, 1955). Of 9 patients with panic disorder given a standard glucose tolerance test, 7 developed symptomatic hypoglycemia but not panic attacks (Uhde, Vittone, & Post, 1984). Patients who have had gastrectomy, gastrojejunostomy, or vagotomy and pyloroplasty have a much higher incidence of reactive hypoglycemia than normals (Breurer, Moses, Hagan, et al., 1972; Cameron, Ellis, McGill, et al., 1969; Hafken, Leichter, & Reich, 1975; Wiznitzer, Chapira, Stadler, et al. 1974), with high insulin levels about one-half hour after feeding.

Complex Partial Seizures

Anxiety is the most common ictal emotion associated with temporal lobe epilepsy (Weil, 1959). Anxiety as a feature of temporal lobe epilepsy may be more readily identified when it occurs in the context of other classical features of complex partial seizures (such as autonomic symptoms, motor automatisms, perceptual distortions, or disturbances in the subjective sense of reality), which occur in a variety of circumstances for no apparent reason, and last for several minutes. In addition, the likelihood of complex partial seizures is increased if the patient has a history of head injury, febrile convulsions in childhood, birth trauma, personal or family history of seizures, or history of encephalitis.

The characteristic abnormality in temporal lobe seizures is the anterior temporal spike focus; however, in the waking state at least one-half of patients have normal EEGs (Gibbs & Gibbs, 1982). A sleep record does increase the percentage of abnormal EEGs in epileptic patients, although the percentage of false negatives remains about 30–40 percent. The value of nasopharyngeal leads is uncertain, though the use of continuous ambulatory EEG monitoring (Kristensen & Sendrup, 1978; Lieb, Walsh, Babb, et al. 1976) can increase the diagnostic yield (see ch. 4). Because of the high incidence of false negatives, the EEG is not a definitive test, and the diagnosis of temporal lobe seizure disorder often must be made on clinical grounds and tested by an empiric trial of carbamazepine.

Angina Pectoris

Patients may experience episodes of dyspnea and palpitations accompanied by only mild chest discomfort and seem to be experiencing an episode of anxiety rather than angina. When such episodes are precipitated by exercise or emotional stress, angina should be considered and cardiac evaluation considered, especially in patients over 40 or those with a cardiac history.

Cardiac Arrhythmias

Cardiac arrhythmias may produce palpitations, dyspnea, and light-headedness, which can be mistaken for an episode of anxiety. For this reason, pulse regularity should always be checked during an episode of anxiety. If the diagnosis of arrhythmia is suspected, Holter monitoring may be helpful in confirming the diagnosis. For those patients with arrhythmias, a host of medical conditions that are also associated with anxiety symptoms need to be considered, such as hyperthyroidism, caffeinism, and nicotine abuse (Lynch, Paskewitz, Gimbel, et al., 1977).

Recurrent Pulmonary Emboli

Recurrent pulmonary emboli may present as repeated episodes of acute anxiety associated with hyperventilation and dyspnea (Ferrer, 1968). Arterial blood gases may reveal decreased oxygen during an episode, though the confirmatory test of most use is the ventilation-prefusion lung scan. This diagnosis should be considered in those patients who have some predisposition, such as hyperviscosity, prolonged bed rest, peripheral venous thrombosis, or recent pelvic surgery.

Hyperthyroidism

Hyperthyroidism usually presents with symptoms of nervousness, palpitations, diaphoresis, heat intolerance, and diarrhea. Signs include tachycardia, tremor, weight loss, and hot moist skin. The combination of T4 and T3 uptake (to correct for protein binding abnormalities) will provide accurate diagnosis in most cases of hyperthyroidism. About 10 percent of cases of hyperthyroidism are accounted for by T3 thyrotoxicosis for which the T4 and T3 uptake are normal. For those cases, a T3RIA is necessary. The development of more sensitive assays (now available in selected centers) for thyroid-stimulating hormone (TSH) may allow hyperthyroidism to be distinguished on the basis of a low TSH value (Cobb, Lamberton, & Jackson, 1984). MacCrimmon, Wallace, Goldberg, et al. (1979) compared the MMPI scores of hyperthyroid patients with those of normal subjects and found that the hyperthyroid patients produced a typical "neurotic" pattern, which returned to normal after successful treatment of the hyperthyroidism.

Pheochromocytoma

Pheochromocytoma is a rare disorder involving catecholamine secretion by a tumor of the renal medulla. The output of catecholamines may be episodic or continuous, producing acute or chronic symptoms of anxiety, often accompanied by headache and flushing (Lishman, 1978). Hypertension is usually present during acute episodes and 60–80 percent of patients have sustained hypertension. The most accurate diagnostic test for detection involves plasma catecholamine assay (Bravo, Tarazi, Gifford, et al., 1979). In one study of 17 patients with active pheochromocytoma (Starkman, Zelnik, Nesse, et al., 1985), none experienced the severe apprehension or fear characteristic of panic attacks. One patient received a diagnosis of possible panic disorder, 2 met criteria for generalized anxiety disorder, and 2 met criteria for major depressive episode. Therefore, there does not appear to be a strict and predictable relationship between the presence of catecholamine-secreting tumors and severe anxiety.

Hypoparathyroidism

Hypoparathyroidism may present with a wide range of psychiatric disorders including anxiety as the primary symptom in about 20 percent of the cases (Denko & Kaelbling, 1962). Hypoparathyroidism should be suspected in patients who have had thyroid surgery, because of the possibility of inadvertant damage to the parathyroids. It should also be considered in patients with hypocalcemia and hyperphosphatemia in the presence of normal renal function. Parathormone assays will usually be depressed.

Mitral Valve Prolapse

Although some studies have shown that patients with panic disorders have a higher incidence of mitral valve prolapse (MVP) than psychiatrically normal people (Gorman, Fyer, Gliklich, et al., 1981; Kantor, Zitrin, & Zeldis, 1980; Pariser, Pinta, & Jones, 1978; Venkatesh, Pauls, Crowe, et al., 1980), other studies fail to document this increased prevalence (Kathol, Noyes, Slymen, et al., 1980; Shear, Devereux, Dramer-Fox, et al., 1984), possibly because of differences in the stringency of criteria used for the diagnosis of MVP. About half of patients with MVP at some time complain of palpitations, but continuous cardiac monitoring of such patients often reveals no relationship between the complaint of palpitations and any form of cardiac rhythm disturbance (Devereux, Perloff, Reichek, et al., 1976). Furthermore, a study of the prevalence of anxiety disorder in patients with MVP found no differences between patients and controls, casting further doubt on the etiologic role of MVP in panic attacks (Mazza, Martin, Spacavento, et al., 1986). While there continues to be support for some relationship between MVP and panic attacks (Liberthson, Sheehan, King, et al., 1986), there is no evidence that MVP causes panic attacks.

Hyperventilation Syndrome

Hyperventilation syndrome (HVS) has an estimated prevalence of 10 percent in a general medical clinic (Rice, 1950), 5.8 percent in a gastroenterology practice (McKell & Sullivan, 1947), and 5 percent in a neurology clinic practice (Pincus & Tucker, 1985). Anxiety is a cardinal symptom along with a variety of other medical symptoms, including faintness and visual disturbances, nausea, vertigo, headache, palpitations, dyspnea, diaphoresis, and parathesias. The diagnosis of HVS can be made on the basis of the patient's response to overbreathing (breathing by mouth for up to 3 minutes or until dizzy). If the symptoms in question are entirely reproduced, without an alternative explanation by physical examination, medical history, or laboratory tests, the diagnosis can be established.

Hyperventilation leads to excessive elimination of CO_2, acute respiratory alkalosis, and cerebral artery constriction. In 240 seconds of overbreathing, cerebral blood flow can be reduced by 40 percent (Plum & Posner, 1972). This reduction is the cause of the EEG slowing that often accompanies hyperventilation (Gotoh, Meyer, & Takagi, 1965). Muscular tension is heightened by a decreased ionization of calcium associated with the increase in pH (Neill & Hattenhauer, 1975). Hyperventilation also causes increased coronary artery resistance and may result in chest discomfort that is difficult to distinguish from angina pectoris (Evans & Lum, 1977), along with nonspecific downward depression of the ST segment and T wave flattening (Christensen, 1946). Unlike ischemic ST changes, those caused by hyperventilation usually appear early during exercise and tend to disappear as exercise continues (McHenry, Cogan, Elliott, et al., 1970).

Postconcussion Syndrome

Cerebral concussion is classically regarded as a disorder that produces no irreversible anatomic lesions. Clinically, concussion results in an instantaneous diminution of function or loss of consciousness followed by rapid and complete recovery. The episode may be surrounded by a sphere of amnesia that rapidly shrinks to a finite minimum, including about one-tenth of the total as retrograde amnesia (Parkinson, 1977). For most patients, the symptoms abate after a few weeks to a few months. It has been estimated, however, that 20 percent of head injuries involving no demonstrable damage lead to a syndrome involving medically unexplained symptoms, with anxiety as one of the most frequent disabling symptoms (Leigh, 1979). The postconcussion syndrome typically consists of anxiety, impairment of sleep and appetite, irritability, lightheadedness, headaches, and poor concentration.

Symptoms that follow concussion may be a direct result of neuronal damage (Oppenheimer, 1968) and alteration of cerebral blood flow, resulting in regional and generalized abnormalities correlating with the presence of psychologic symptoms (AR Taylor & Bell, 1966) and impaired information processing (Gronwall & Wrightson, 1974). Mild head trauma may also lead to an increase in catecholamines (Wortsman, Burns, Van Beek, et al., 1980).

Non-specific Medical Causes

Many medical disorders may be associated with a broad array of psychiatric symptoms, which may include anxiety as a nonspecific reaction to delirium, though not as a prominent feature. Such disorders include Cushing's Syndrome (Lishman, 1978), hypomagnesemia (Hall and Joffe, 1973), hyponatremia (Gehi, Rosenthal, Fizette, et al. 1981), renal failure (Marshall, 1979), and other electrolyte imbalance (Webb & Gehi, 1981).

CONCURRENT PSYCHIATRIC DISORDERS IN MEDICAL PATIENTS

The second step in evaluating the presentation of anxiety in a medical or surgical patient is to evaluate for the possibility of underlying psychiatric disorder. The clinician should inquire about previous personal and family psychiatric history. It may turn out, for example, that the patient has a generalized anxiety disorder that is really no different now in the hospital from the way it was for years prior to hospitalization. The patient's anxiety may represent the incipient personality disorganization associated with relapsing schizophrenia or borderline personality. Anxiety may be a significant component of a mood disorder. The clinician should inquire specifically about panic attacks, since panic disorder often presents with physical symptoms (Sheehan, 1982). Those patients with agoraphobia may have special difficulty being contained in the hospital environment. The patient's anxiety may represent a form of homosexual panic in those patients vulnerable to this response, who become anxious from the forced intimacy of the hospital setting. Somatoform disorder may present as continuous anxiety focused on physical symptoms. Finally, dementia may impair a patient's coping responses and thereby lead to anxiety.

It is not enough to determine that the patient has no "formal" psychiatric history in terms of actually seeing a psychiatrist. Patients should be asked whether they have had any symptoms, whether or not they have seen a psychiatrist.

PSYCHOSOCIAL ISSUES AND ANXIETY IN MEDICAL PATIENTS

No evaluation of the anxious medical patient is complete without an inquiry into the psychosocial dimensions of the patient's experience. The psychosocial dimension encompasses the intrapsychic meanings that patients attach to experiences and their behaviorally conditioned responses. These dimensions are not to be evaluated as an alternative to the biomedical diagnostic approach but rather as a complementary aspect in every consultation. The fact that a patient has increased autonomic arousal as a result of hyperthyroidism does not mean that the consultant should neglect the patient as a person and ignore the meaning of being ill and its contribution to the patient's distress.

A patient's anxiety may represent fear of an obvious physical threat, but in the realm of intrapsychic meaning, anxiety is accounted for not by obvious events, but rather by private mental associations of which the person may not be fully aware. It may not be the visible situation itself that is important to understanding the patient's anxiety, but the meaning of the situation to the individual. It is because situations have private and often distorted meanings for people that we see patients who have anxiety that appears to be out of proportion to any ostensible danger.

As medical therapies become more complex and patients survive in life-threatening situations for extended periods of time, issues involving the emotional consequences of illness and its treatment become more prominent. Although physicians often assume that the distress associated with illness is accounted for by the physical morbidity, it is now appreciated that a significant component of the distress associated with cancer, for example, is due to issues involving psychosocial adjustment (Goldberg & Cullen, 1985). In dealing with medically ill patients, clinicians should be aware of, and be prepared to help address, the major psychologic issues that are known to be commonly associated with anxiety in that group of patients. The identification of a psychologic component of anxiety does not imply that psychologic

treatment is always going to provide an effective answer for such patients. It is often therapeutic, however, simply to help the patient identify emotional problem areas that are being transferred into symptoms and to help contain the anxiety by putting it into words. The following sections are a discussion of five major psychological areas worth reviewing in terms of understanding potential psychologic sources of anxiety.

Alienation

Social support plays an important role in maintaining mental and physical health. Fears of abandonment and isolation can be even more important to patients than fear associated with the disease itself or of death. The isolation and the loss of social acceptability that befall patients with chronic illnesses often create anxiety over potential abandonment. Even well-meaning friends, family, or employers withdraw because they do not know what to talk about or because they feel guilt or anger toward the patient.

The physician should identify the patient's major social supports and assess the extent to which they remain involved or have become alienated as a result of the patient's illness. Even if they remain involved, the patient may have fears of losing their support. The physician should look to the spouse (or other key support) as an important ally in preventing the anxiety associated with alienation. Whenever possible, the physician should meet with patient and key support person together, since such situations provide an opportunity to observe their interaction and facilitate better sharing and communication. The physician should tactfully bring out into the open issues that remain hidden between the two, for example, fear that the spouse will leave because of being overwhelmed by potential caretaking responsibilities. It is sometimes overlooked that the patient's supports are under tremendous strain owing to emotional demands and new responsibilities, which may include managing the family, coordinating finances, and even providing primary care for the patient. Helping the spouse become a more effective support may be an important therapeutic measure for the patient whose anxiety arises from a fear of abandonment. The patient's intrapsychic concern about abandonment is sometimes best dealt with by a concrete intervention, such as arranging homemaker or visiting nurse assistance.

As diseases progress, patients may become anxious because of a growing sense of distance from the physician. Patients nearing the end of an intensive treatment program are noted to experience an increase in anxiety rather than a sense of relief (Mastrovito, 1972; Peck & Boland, 1977). Such feelings may be accounted for partly by the cumulative physical side effects of treatment but are also related to the anticipated loss of close physician or nursing support. After an intensive stay in the intensive care unit, patients may respond to the news of transfer to a regular medical unit with anxiety rather than relief, fearing that the detachment will jeopardize their survival. Physicians may have a tendency to withdraw from patients seen as terminal because of the sense that, medically, there is little left to do. Patients notice decreased therapeutic zeal in magnified fashion, and panicky feelings can be triggered by a decreasing frequency in hospital rounds, which is interpreted as a sign of abandonment. Maintenance of regular contact and communication of concern are valuable positive interventions although to the action-oriented physician such visits may seem like doing very little. The continued availability of the physician to provide ongoing support for the patient can be a crucial element in counteracting some of the impersonality involved in the highly technical therapies offered to patients. Alienation is, of course, a special risk for

any patient with imparied sensory and communicative abilities, which may result from being intubated or suffering an aphasia due to stroke.

Loss of Control

While loss of control is inherent in all illness, it varies in importance for individual patients. For the adolescent, this issue may be magnified, since control represents both a developmental task as well as a treatment issue. For many patients, the role reversal necessitated by becoming dependent on others may be the crucial factor underlying anxiety symptoms. Such patients may attempt to reduce anxiety by reasserting control through maladaptive anger and noncompliance. These patients should therefore be given appropriate opportunities to exercise some form of control over their therapy and environment. A classic example involves the controlling personality whose anxiety leads to attempts to sign out of the coronary care unit. The underlying issue often involves the patient's sense of loss of physical and social control. A sense of panic may occur in the chronic dialysis patient who cannot tolerate the dependence on machines and the continued erosions of autonomy necessitated by physician visits, blood tests, and dietary restrictions. Such patients can resume some sense of control by learning behavioral methods of relaxation, helping keep a record of their medications, or even selecting a vein that can be used to start an IV. The consultant must be creative in identifying areas where the patient can exercise some choice in control without jeopardizing medical treatment. Intellectual mastery is another means of reasserting control over alien and powerful therapeutic forces for some patients. Sharing information about diagnosis should therefore be considered an important means of allowing the patient to resume control and actually may reduce anxiety in patients, though physicians often worry that patients may become more upset by hearing about their diagnosis.

Physical Damage

Threatened or real loss of bodily integrity or a body part can trigger profound anxiety, along with insomnia, anorexia, and difficulty in concentrating. Patients who view themselves as less than whole may withdraw from relationships because of anxiety over rejection. Before surgery, patients can become panicked and often feel they have a poor chance of survival (Bard & Sutherland, 1977). It is always important to explore what patients have heard from others about the procedure they are awaiting, since misconceptions can arise from stories of a friend or relative who did poorly with a similar situation (Baudry & Weiner, 1968). Preoperative review of potential misconceptions may even decrease certain surgical complications (Egbert, Batlit, Welch, et al., 1964).

The anxious patient should not be dismissed with well-intentioned remarks such as "Relax and you'll soon get over it," which ignore the anxiety-provoking issues, such as concerns about bodily damage and mortality. Affect may need to be addressed in dealing with anxious patients, who may ask, for example, "Am I going to be all right?" There is a tendency to prematurely reassure the person rather than to continue to explore difficult feelings. Patients may seem very concerned about symptoms that seem insignificant. Such minor hypochondriacal symptoms should not be simply dismissed. The attitude of the interviewer must convey a sense of interest in understanding what is concerning the person. If given the chance, most patients with minor complaints will relate their private reasons for concern if they feel the interviewer is interested in listening. Some preoperative anxiety, however, appears to be helpful, since it stimulates realistic planning. Patients who are extraordinarily calm may be

masking fears that place them at higher risk for not coping with later inevitable events (Sutherland, Orback, Duk, et al., 1977).

The problem of coping with physical loss such as amputation is mostly determined by the private meaning the loss has for the individual. The physician should not make assumptions and should not project his or her own responses onto the situation. Instead, the patient should be prompted to reveal his or her own private issues with such questions as "What was it like for you to hear about needing surgery?" or "What sort of difficulties are you having at home now?" or "What has been the most difficult part of your treatment to adust to?"

Physical loss, scarring, or disfigurement can lead to new feelings of anxiety helplessness. The young man who suffers a therapeutic amputation may respond to the anxiety over his perceived loss of manhood by masturbating in front of nurses. Successful management of such anxiety-induced behavior involves recognizing and helping the patient share his emotional reactions to the loss. Further, anxiety over loss of mobility, impaired self-care, role function, or sexual problems can be concretely addressed using rehabilitative and counseling resources.

Death

The issue of dying may or may not be brought up directly by the patient; it may emerge instead through some related symptoms of anxiety. As long as patients with life-threatening illness function adaptively, elements of denial play an important role in continued function (Dimsdale & Hackett, 1982). The natural course of progressive illness, however, usually challenges the patient to slowly adjust denial mechanisms to the emerging medical reality (Weismen, 1979). Recurrence of disease often erodes initial optimism and creates a situation in which the patient for the first time deals with issues of dying. Signs of physician willingness to engage the patient on these issues are important in allaying fears, which otherwise remain insulated from the rest of the world. Dealing in some way with their own sense of mortality probably is important for clinicians to be effective in dealing with patients' anxiety about death.

PHARMACOLOGIC MANAGEMENT

Benzodiazepines

Benzodiazepines are by far the most widely used antianxiety agents. The best indication for using benzodiazepines is when a psychologic cause of the anxiety can be identified and is expected to be of time-limited duration, as in the case of the patient awaiting a cardiac catheterization who becomes increasingly anxious in anticipation. Benzodiazepines are also helpful in treating primary anxiety disorders and adjunctively for patients with organic anxiety syndromes. The following sections address the specific issues of benzodiazepine use in the medically ill.

Pharmacokinetics

All the benzodiazepines are well absorbed orally and reach peak blood levels after a single dose in times varying from 2–6 hours. The differences in time to reach peak plasma level largely reflect differences in gastrointestinal absorption. As metabolites reach a steady state, however, initial differences due to absorption and distribution disappear, and differences due to metabolism become prominent.

The bewildering metabolic fate of various benzodiazepines may be simplified by appreciating that they fall into two classes—long acting and short acting (see Table 7-1). Lorazepam and oxazepam, as examples of short-acting agents, have no active metabolites, do not depend on the liver for metabolism, and are quickly inac-

tivated by conjugative transformation. With relatively short half-lives, these drugs are most suited for use when prolonged sedation is undesirable. Because there are no active metabolites, these drugs tend not to accumulate with repeated administration but require twice-a-day or three-times-a-day administration. The long acting benzodiazepines, such as diazepam and chlordiazepoxide, share common oxidative metabolic pathways in the liver, with half-lives ranging to more than 100 hours.

On the basis of their pharmacokinetics, these medications may be prescribed on a once-a-day schedule. Nevertheless, most patients feel more comfortable psychologically with divided daily doses. Repeated use of long-acting benzodiazepines may lead to accumulation, with potential impairment of cognitive and motor performance. Drug accumulation is a special risk to be kept in mind with the long-acting agents, especially for older patients and those with liver impairment (Greenblatt, Allen, Harmatz, et al., 1980; Hoyumpa, 1978). It is not uncommon, for example, to see a 66-year-old anxious, hypertensive patient who has become confused and depressed following several weeks of treatment with diazepam, 5 mg three times a day and flurazepam, 30 mg once a day. It is also important to realize that while chlordiazepoxide, diazepam, and lorazepam are available in injectable form, chlordiazepoxide (Greenblatt, Shader, Koch-Weser, et al., 1974) and diazepam (Greenblatt & Koch-Weser, 1976) are poorly and unpredictably absorbed from intramuscular (IM) sites, whereas lorazepam and midazolam have the distinct property of prompt and reliable IM absorption (Greenblatt, Divoll, Harmatz, et al., 1982). Despite the long half-lives and accumulation of active substances, chronic use of these drugs usually does not lead to oversedation. The sedative and antianxiety effects of benzodiazepines appear to be distinct, and as a steady state is reached, the CNS seems to adapt to the

Table 7-1

Pharmacokinetic Summary Comparison of Benzodiazepines

Drug Given	Half-Life	Active Metabolites	Half-Life Metabolities
Alprazolam	12–15	alphahydroxyalprazolam	6
Chlordiazepoxide	7–28	desmethylchlordiazepoxide	5–30
		demoxepam	14–95
		desmethyldiazepam	25–200
		oxazepam	6–8
Clonazepam	18–56		
Clorazepate	*	desmethyldiazepam	25–200
		oxazepam	6–8
Diazepam	20–50	desmethyldiazepam	25–200
		oxazepam	6–8
Flurazepam	2–3	n-desalkylflurazepam	32–100
Lorazepam	10–24	none	
Midazolam	1–12†		
Oxazepam	3–24	none	
Prazepam	*	desmethyldiazepam	25–200
		oxazepam	6–8
Temazepam	7–14	none	
Triazolam	2.3	none	

* Unmetabolized drug is inactive. † Pharmacologic effect correlates poorly with blood level; sedative effects are terminated largely by redistribution of drug rather than elimination.

nonspecific sedative effects (Johnson & Chernik, 1982).

Drug Interactions

Benzodiazepines have relatively few significant adverse drug interactions. Their major drug interaction, augmentation of other CNS depressants, can be controlled by adjusting dosage downward. There are a few reports of benzodiazepines increasing diphenylhydantoin levels (Vajda, Prineas, Lovell, 1971) and decreasing prothrombin times for patients on coumadin (PJ Taylor, 1967). Concomitant use of cimetidine alters the pharmacokinetics of diazepam but with-

out clinically relevant effects (Greenblatt, Abernethy, Morse, et al., 1984). It has been reported that diazepam increases digoxin binding to plasma proteins, resulting in increased digoxin blood levels (Castillo-Ferrando, Garci & Carmona, 1980). Long-term use of low-dose estrogen-containing oral contraceptives greatly increases the elimination half-life of diazepam (Abernathy, Greenblatt, Divoll, et al., 1982). There is a recent report that erythromycin significantly inhibits the metabolism of triazolam (Phillips, Antal, Smith, 1986). Because absorption of benzodiazepines may be impaired under conditions of high pH (over

7.4), antacid preparations should not be given concomitantly. In fact, since the conversion of clorazepate to an active substance depends on its conversion in acidic medium, alkaline pH in the stomach will create a situation in which no active drug is available. Concurrent use of anticholinergic agents, which delay gastric emptying, also may impair bioavailability and the lipophilic nature of diazepam may lead to malabsorption in the presence of mineral oil.

Side Effects

Overall, the benzodiazepines have little toxicity and few consistent unwanted effects. The most common adverse effects of the benzodiazepines involve CNS depression: muscle weakness, ataxia, dysarthria, vertigo, somnolence, and confusion. These side effects can be a major problem for the medically ill patient, however, who may be weak from prolonged bed rest or already impaired by other CNS illness.

There is some question whether or not benzodiazepines, in some people, release hostility and rage reactions (Karch, 1979). Such instances may represent a type of disinhibition phenomenon. In addition to the release of hostility, diazepam may have a paradoxical stimulating effect in some patients (Hall & Jaffe, 1972); in others, it may produce or increase depressive symptomatology (Ryan, Merrill, Scott, et al., 1968). Van der Kropf (1979) reported finding depersonalization, anxiety, and paranoia in subjects with chronic insomnia treated with triazolam. Large doses of benzodiazepines produce only minor changes in cardiovascular function even in patients with underlying cardiac disease (Rao, Sherbaniuk, Prasad, et al., 1973). In patients without pulmonary disease, changes in tidal volume and response to elevated Pco_2 are barely detectable (Lakshminarayan, Sahn, Hudson, et al., 1976). In a single-blind study, 25 mg of diazepam per day actually improved the breathlessness of patients with chronic airflow obstruction associated with emphysema (Mitchells-Heggs, Murphy, Minty, et al., 1980). The respiratory depressant effects of benzodiazepines appear to be most marked in patients with CO_2 retention. Benzodiazepines should not be given to patients who may be retaining CO_2 before checking an arterial blood gas. Anxious carbon dioxide retainers may be treated with low-dose neuroleptics, which do not alter respiratory drive. Intravenous benzodiazepines given concurrently with parenteral narcotics produce significant respiratory depression of a greater degree than is found with the opiate alone, especially in patients with some pulmonary impairment (Cohen, Finn, & Steen, 1969).

Clinicians should keep in mind that the benzodiazepines may be associated with the development of amnesia lasting for several hours after the dose. Lorazepam, but not diazepam or clorazepate, has been demonstrated to have a dose-dependent effect on memory assessed by word-recall testing (Healey, Pickens, Meisch, et al., 1983; Scharf, Khosla, Brocker, et al., 1984), though intravenous diazepam does impair recall memory (Wolkowitz, Weingartner, Thompson; et al., 1987). This effect may be an advantage when these drugs are used prior to surgery, but may be a problem in other situations and may augment already-present memory impairment.

Toxicity

Benzodiazepines are the most benign of all psychoactive drugs with respect to the danger of overdose. In the medical literature there have been fewer than a dozen suicides by diazepam ingestion alone (Finkel, McCloskey, & Goodman, 1979). In fact, recovery has been reported from overdoses up to 1400 mg of diazepam and 6000 mg of chlordiazepoxide. Such high doses produce obtundation and rarely coma. Benzodiazepines are, however, often used in combination with other sedative drugs and ethanol in fatal overdoses.

Withdrawal

Withdrawal from large doses of benzodiazepines resembles barbiturate withdrawal. Symptoms may include anxiety, insomnia, dizziness, headache, anorexia, hypotension, hyperthermia, neuromuscular irritability, tinnitus, blurred vision, shakiness, and psychosis. Higher doses taken over longer durations create a greater risk of moderate to severe withdrawal (Hollister, Motzenbecker, & Degan, 1961). There are reports of abstinence phenomena beginning at 5–7 days and lasting for 16 days after abrupt cessation of usual therapeutic doses of diazepam (Pevnik, Jasinski, & Haertzen, 1978; Winokur, Rickels, Greenblatt, et al., 1980) and of seizures occuring in association with the discontinuation of moderate doses of lorazepam (DelaFuenta, Rosenbaum, Martin, et al., 1980) and triazolam (Tien & Gujavarty, 1985). One advantage of long-acting benzodiazepines is that they tend to self-taper if discontinued. Long-term use of diazepam will produce a withdrawal syndrome lasting up to 4 weeks when tapered (Busto, Sellers, Naranjo, et al, 1986). Although abrupt discontinuation of long-acting benzodiazepines is usually not dangerous, it can lead to a persistent state of heightened anxiety. It is therefore, unlikely that there will be medically significant withdrawal symptoms for patients discontinued from long-acting benzodiazepines even at moderately high doses. The short-acting benzodiazepines are associated with a greater prevalence and severity of withdrawal reactions, because their plasma concentrations decline more rapidly following discontinuation. Withdrawal symptoms can be minimized by tapering rather than abruptly discontinuing the drug. During withdrawal, autonomic symptoms can be relieved by a beta-adrenergic blocker

(Abernethy, Greenblatt, & Shader, 1981). It should be kept in mind that withdrawal symptoms from alprazolam may not be fully covered by other benzodiazepines (Zipursky, Baker, & Zimmer, 1985).

Use during Pregnancy

Benzodiazepine use during the first trimester of pregnancy has been suspected of causing an increased risk of cleft palate (Calabrese & Gulledge, 1985). Their use late in pregnancy or during nursing has been associated with "floppy infant syndrome" (Gilberg, 1977), and there are two case reports—one of severe congenital malfunction possibly associated with use of the clorazepate dipotassium in the first trimester (Patel & Patel, 1980) and the other of intrauterine growth retardation and possible withdrawal symptoms in a neonate exposed to diazepam during several months of gestation (Backes & Cadero, 1980). Such cases serve to heighten awareness and concern for the judicious use of medication during pregnancy.

Midazolam

Midazolam is a new parenteral benzodiazepine recently marketed in the United States for intravenous sedation for short diagnostic or endoscopic procedures and sedation associated with general anesthesia. Midazolam is three to four times as potent as diazepam. It is highly lipid-soluble and readily crosses the blood–brain barrier, resulting in extremely rapid onset of action. It is metabolized by the liver, mainly by microsomal oxidation, with an elimination half-life of 1–4 hours. Its onset of action is within 15 minutes, reaching peak activity within 30 minutes, with a duration of action lasting 1–2 hours. One advantage over diazepam is that it is formulated in an aqueous solution; therefore, it does not cause local irritation after intramuscular or intravenous injection.

Like other benzodiazepines, midazolam can cause respiratory depression and lead to apnea, especially when combined with narcotics. Hypotension has also been reported. Anterograde amnesia may persist for 1 or 2 hours after injection; therefore, postoperative patients need to be given instructions in writing. The approximate dose used for intravenous sedation for a diagnostic procedure is an initial dose of 1 or 2 mgs, up to 0.15 mg/kg. Dose should be reduced in patients on concomitant narcotics (Abramowicz, 1986b).

Buspirone

Buspirone is a recently introduced, nonbenzodiazepine anxiolytic approved for the treatment of anxiety. Its mechanism of action is unknown, though it has been found to bind to serotonin and presynaptic dopamine receptors but not to benzodiazepine receptors or to affect gamma amino butyric acid (GABA) (AS Eison & Temple, 1986; MS Eison & AS Eison, 1984). It does not induce catalepsy in animals and, in fact, reverses neuroleptic-induced catalepsy. Since it does not induce catalepsy, it is thought that buspirone is unlikely to have any extrapyramidal or tardive dyskinesia liability; however, its long-term effects in this area are not fully known. In doses over 30 mg/day, buspirone can lead to increased plasma prolactin levels. Unlike the benzodiazepines, buspirone lacks muscle relaxant, anticonvulsant, and hypnotic activity. Buspirone does not block the withdrawal syndrome associated with CNS sedatives or benzodiazepines (Schweizer & Rickels, 1986). Buspirone should not be used with MAO inhibitors since hypertensive reactions may occur.

Pharmacokinetics

Buspirone is rapidly and completely absorbed from the gastrointestinal tract, with extensive first-pass hepatic metabolism. Taking the drug with food appears to decrease its rate of absorption and its first-pass metabolism, making more drug available. Peak plasma level is reached in about one hour. Average elimination half-life is 2.5 hours. About 65 percent is eliminated by the kidneys, mostly in a metabolized form; 35 percent has fecal elimination. There is little information available about the effects of liver or renal impairment on drug effects. Buspirone has one active (hydroxylated) metabolite with a half-life of about 4.8 hours. The parent drug is 95 percent protein bound, with one known potentially significant drug interaction—it may displace digoxin (Goa & Ward, 1986), leading to increased risk of toxicity.

Side Effects

The major side effects include dizziness, headache, and nervousness. Buspirone is notably less sedative than the benzodiazepines, which is one of its primary advantages (Cohn & Wilcox, 1986; Newton, Marunycz, Alderdice, et al. 1986). In fact, buspirone causes no more drowsiness than placebo and does not impair psychomotor performance skills, such as driving. There have been no deaths reported as a result of buspirone overdose, out of more than 375 cases. Major sequelae of overdose have included nausea and vomiting, dizziness, drowsiness, and miosis. No withdrawal syndrome has been reported following the abrupt discontinuation of its use.

Buspirone has a low abuse potential (Griffith, Jasinski, & McKinney, 1986), lacking euphoric properties and actually having some dysphoric properties with repeated, excessive use. This property, coupled with the fact that it does not potentiate the sedative effects of alcohol (or other CNS sedatives), seems to make buspirone a good drug for the treatment of anxiety in alcoholic patients (Kastenholz & Crismon, 1984; Meyer, 1986).

Clinical Use

Buspirone is equipotent to diazepam and has been demonstrated to have comparable clinical anxiolytic efficacy (Cohn, Bowden, Fisher, et al. 1986; Rickels, Weisman, Norstad, et al. 1982; Schuckit, 1984). The recommended initial dose is 5 mg three times a day, adjusted by 5 mg/day increments every 2–3 days as needed, up to a maximum of 60 mg/day. It is not cross-tolerant with other CNS sedatives (including the benzodiazepines). The best candidates for buspirone, therefore, are those patients not already on benzodiazepines. It is important to be aware that since there are few sedative effects and since the anxiolytic effects of buspirone may take several weeks to occur, the patient may not notice any drug effects for a while and may, therefore, become prematurely discouraged about the potential effectiveness of this medication. Buspirone is not useful as an as-needed medication and must be given regularly to maximize its therapeutic effects. An additional issue, the significance of which is yet to be determined, is that some patients who have been on benzodiazepines appear not to report comparable anxiolytic benefit from buspirone.

Beta-Adrenergic Blocking Agents

Autonomic symptoms associated with anxiety (such as palpitations and tremulousness) are mediated by beta-adrenergic sympathetic activity. Because beta-adrenergic blocking agents can antagonize these symptoms at the target organ, there has been considerable interest in the anxiolytic use of these agents since the first demonstration of such activity (Granville-Grossman & Turner, 1966). Consistent with the assumption that propranolol is a peripherally active agent, its usefulness has been promoted for patients whose major manifestations of anxiety are somatic rather than psychic (Tyrer & Lader, 1974). Propranolol has also, however, been noted to abolish subjective symptoms of nervousness, restlessness, and tension (Kathol et al., 1980).

It has been suggested that propranolol has a unique role for patients in situations of acute situational distress, such as public performance anxiety, in which the psychomotor intellectual impairment produced by benzodiazepines is not desirable. Forty milligrams of propranolol given 90 minutes before performance was shown to have a positive effect in decreasing performance anxiety in a group of musicians (James, Pearson, Griffith, et al, 1978).

Evaluation of the effectiveness of beta blockers in anxiety has become more complex with the recognition that these agents (especially propranolol) enter the central nervous system and may produce direct neurologic and behavioral effects. Evidence of a central nervous system effect is revealed by neuropsychiatric side effects, which include insomnia, hallucinations, and depression (Fraser & Carr. 1976; Greenblatt & Koch-Weser, 1973). Although weakness and depression are the most common neuropsychiatric symptoms associated with propranolol, patients may also have vivid nightmares, hypnogogic hallucinations, or toxic psychosis, even at relatively low doses (Gershon, Goldstein, Moss, et al., 1979). Such mental changes tend to reverse within 48 hours after discontinuation of propranolol. Nadolol and atenolol are beta blockers that do not cross the blood–brain barrier to any significant extent but also seem to improve some components of anxiety. It may be, therefore, that the central effects are exerted by some kind of neurohumoral feedback to the CNS rather than by a direct action.

Issues in Prescribing

Propranolol is almost completely absorbed following oral administration. It undergoes extensive first-pass metabolism in the liver, and variation in this component results in as much as 20-fold variability in plasma concentration among individuals on comparable doses. The half-life is initially about three hours, and it may increase to four hours during chronic use. It is 90–95 percent bound to plasma protein, which also may contribute to its variabilities in plasma concentrations. Propranolol is almost completely metabolized in the liver before urinary excretion. Nadolol is poorly absorbed from the GI tract (Dreyfuss, Griffith, Singhvi, et al., 1979) and is excreted largely by the kidney in unchanged form (Frishman, 1981). The elimination half-life is 14–24 hours, increasing dramatically in patients with renal dysfunction. Contraindications to the use of betablockers include bradycardia, atrioventricular block, and congestive heart failure. Because of its effects on bronchial smooth muscle and interference with glycogenolysis during hypoglycemia, beta blockers are contraindicated in patients with bronchospastic or chronic obstructive pulmonary disease. They should be used cautiously in diabetics because they can mask clinical signs of hypoglycemia.

Beta-receptor blockade has little effect on the normal heart at rest, though there is some decrease in heart rate, cardiac output, and blood pressure. During exercise and anxiety, however, sympathetic responses may be significantly blocked. Maximum exercise tolerance may therefore be decreased in otherwise normal patients. Serious cardiac depression is uncommon, but heart failure may develop slowly or suddenly, especially if the heart is compromised by intrinsic disease or by other drugs, such as digitalis.

Other Anxiolytics

Neuroleptics have been commonly used for the treatment of anxiety, more so in the past than in the present, largely because of concerns about extrapyramidal symptoms and tardive dyskinesia and more

specific thinking about psychopharmacologic practice. Whenever possible, it is preferable to use benzodiazepines as anxiolytics, though there are certain situations in which neuroleptics can be effectively used, especially for short periods of time when the risk of tardive dyskinesia is not an issue (Rickels, 1983). These situations include anxiety in patients with CO_2 retention, in whom suppression of the hypoxic respiratory drive by benzodiazepines should be avoided; patients whose anxiety represents an incipient psychotic disorganization, such as some borderline personality-disordered patients under stress; schizophrenic patients; patients with organic anxiety syndrome with disorganized cognition or behavior (such as the severely anxious patient with racing thoughts precipitated by steroids); and patients with anxiety in the context of significant delirium (in whom further cortical suppression by benzodiazepines may exacerbate the delirium). There does not appear to be any evidence of superior antianxiety effects of any specific neuroleptics, though the phenothiazine neuroleptics have been demonstrated to have some moderate anxiolytic properties (Fann, Lake, & Majors, 1974).

Antihistamines such as hydroxyzine and diphenhydramine are sometimes prescribed to treat anxiety. The have no specific anxiolytic properties (except in doses so high that marked sedation occurs [Rickels, Gordon, Zamostien, et al., 1970]), though patients may feel less anxious on them because of the sedative effects. There is little rational to support their use, since they have a number of unwanted side effects, such as anticholinergic properties, especially if used in repeated doses. Diphenhydramine is less effective than benzodiazepines for sleep induction (Rickels, Morris, Newman, et al., 1983). The only situation involving anxiety in which they might have a special use would be when anxiety is the accompaniment of an allergic response, for which their antihistaminic properties are the primary value.

Finally, antidepressant drugs have been noted to be of value in the treatment of anxiety. For many years, the tricyclics and MAO inhibitors have been recommended for the treatment of panic attacks (Klein, 1982; Pohl, Berchou, & Rainey, 1982; Sheehan, Ballenger, & Jacobsen, 1980; Zitrin, Klein, & Woerner, 1978). Both groups of drugs are also effective in patients with mixed anxiety and depression (Paykel, Rowman, Parker; et al., 1982; Rickels, Csanalosi, Chung, et al, 1974), especially in so-called atypical depressions, which are characterized by high levels of anxiety (Robinson, Nies, Ravaris, et al., 1973). There is also the possibility that the tricyclics may be effective in the treatment of some patients with chronic anxiety alone (Lipman, Covi, Downing, et al., 1981). In a double-blind, placebo-controlled study of the treatment of anxiety (even eliminating patients with panic-phobic syndromes) with imipramine, chlordiazepoxide, or placebo, antianxiety effects of imipramine were superior to those of the others by the second treatment week, becoming clearly more significant thereafter, independent of baseline levels of depression and anxiety (Kahn, McNair, Lipman, et al., 1986).

SELF-REGULATION METHODS

A variety of self-regulation treatment methods are available to address anxiety as well as to counteract the lost sense of self-control that may contribute to it. It is now well established that in a relatively brief period of time most patients can be taught techniques that induce relaxation. These techniques should be considered appropriate in the following anxiety situations:

1. For patients with generalized anxiety
2. As a component of a desensitization therapy for specific anxiety-producing

situations, such as phobias or fear of a medical procedure (see Chapter 6)
3. When stress seems to be a major factor in initiating or maintaining other medical symptoms (e.g., tension headaches or hyperventilation)

Muscle Relaxation Therapies

People are intuitively aware that muscle relaxation is in some way associated with anxiety reduction. Unfortunately, many people are either unaware of chronically tensed muscles or are unable to relax even when they become aware of their problem. Learning to specifically sense and control muscle tension is a widely utilized and effective method for anxiety reduction. The Jacobson method of progressive relaxation depends on systematically tensing and relaxing muscle groups starting with the feet and eventually involving the entire body (Jacobson, 1938). Of course, it is important to discuss the intent of the procedure with the patient beforehand and to elicit any specific questions, misconceptions, or concerns the patient might have. A comfortable, quiet setting without interruptions is important. Although tape-recorded or printed instructions can be used, the initial session with the physician can be an important factor in establishing a positive alliance for future work. There seem to be few contraindications to the use of relaxation methods. People with organic mental disorders may have difficulty maintaining attention, and psychotic patients are unable to control intrusive thoughts. Muscle relaxation procedures may be more successful in introverted than in extroverted personality types (Stoudenmire, 1972). Furthermore, while participating in biofeedback, some extroverted patients have actually shown an increase in anxiety, along with dysphoric symptoms such as fear of losing control (Leboeuf, 1977). The homeliness and simplicity of relaxation training should not mislead people to underestimate its potential usefulness (Wilson, 1981), since relaxation training has been shown to be superior to nonspecific therapy in the reduction of anxiety.

Electromyographic Biofeedback

The Jacobson method was devised to induce relaxation by heightening awareness of muscle tension. Electromyographic biofeedback (EMG-BF) goes one step further by providing the person with precise information about the electrical potentials of selected muscle groups. If muscular relaxation helps to decrease anxiety, then it would be expected that EMG-BF would facilitate this process. EMG-biofeedback treatment of anxiety usually selects the frontalis muscle for monitoring, the frontalis EMG level being regarded as an index of overall physiologic arousal. It is conveniently accessible for electrode placement and has been considered one of the most difficult muscles in the body to relax voluntarily. Others have suggested that the biceps brachialis is the most effective muscle to monitor to produce general muscle relaxation (deVries, Burke, Hopper, 1977). Using data that show no correlation between EMG reductions and decreased anxiety levels, (Raskin, Bali, & Peeke (1980) have challenged the assumption that a profound degree of muscle relaxation is necessary for achieving anxiety relief when using self-regulatory therapies.

Meditation Techniques and the Relaxation Response

Meditation has been shown to produce a physiologic state of restful alertness that is different from sleeping or walking (Wallace, 1970). Physiologic findings during meditation are generally opposite to those encountered in an anxiety patient. With experienced meditators, reported physiologic changes during meditation include decreased oxygen consumption, CO_2 elimination, respiratory rate, and minute ventilation with no change in respiratory quotient. After reviewing a range of meditative practices, Herbert Benson concluded that within the apparent multiplicity of practices resided common features that could serve as the basis for a nonsectarian form of practice capable of inducing a state he called the *relaxation response* (Benson, Beary, & Carol, 1974). The technique for eliciting the relaxation response consists of four basic elements:

1. *A mental device*: There needs to be some constant stimulus, for example, a sound, a word (such as "one"), or a phrase repeated silently or audibly. Fixed gazing at an object is a suitable alternative. The purpose of this procedure is to focus attention away from the continuous flow of sensory distractions and intellectual preoccupations.

2. *A passive attitude*: During the aural or visual practice, distracting thoughts are to be disregarded. One should not be concerned with performance standards. When lapses are recognized, the practitioner should patiently return to the mental device without self-criticism or concern about success or failure.

3. *Decreased muscle tone*: The subject should be in a comfortable position to minimize any muscular strain or tension.

4. *A quiet environment*: A quiet environment with decreased stimuli should be chosen. A quiet room where there is no concern about unexpected interruptions is usually suitable. Most techniques instruct the practitioner to close the eyes.

The relaxation response has achieved wide popular recognition and in many places is emerging as part of the armamentarium of the primary care physician as a technique to manage anxiety and a wide array of stress-related disorders (Goldberg, 1982).

THE INTEGRATED TREATMENT OF ANXIETY

This chapter has presented an approach to the diagnosis and treatment of anxiety addressing both the biologic and psychosocial dimensions. The following case demonstrated the integration of these factors in a medically ill, anxious patient.

Case example. Mrs. T. was a 60-year-old married woman with a long history of chronic obstructive pulmonary disease (COPD). She had been on nasal oxygen 24 hours a day for the previous four years and now had evidence of cor pulmonale. She had been on theophylline spansules, 300 mg twice a day; prednisone, 15 mg every other day; and flurazepam, 15 mg once a day. Over the past month, her emotional condition had deteriorated despite any changes in objective measurements of her medical condition. She had been increasingly agitated and because of marked anxiety regarding a number of somatic symptoms had been making repeated calls to her physician. For example, she reported that trying to insert her nasal cannula had become impossible because she became nervous and tremulous. She had been preoccupied with a fear of "hemorrhaging" since she had had a small amount of nasal bleeding from drying of her nasal mucosa. Reassurance alone did not decrease her anxiety level.

Biologic Factors

Chronic hypoxic insults. While most COPD patients apparently adjust to long-term changes in blood gases without developing gross psychiatric symptoms, ongoing hypoxic insults can contribute to cumulative cortical neuronal damage, eventually leading to an organic mental disorder. This woman had no previous psychiatric history and had coped well with a number of significant problems in the past. Many patients with a life-threatening illness continue to cope well until they become handicapped by brain dysfunction, which disrupts their cognitive organization and modulation of affect. An electroencephalogram showed diffuse slowing consistent with a mild to moderate encephalopathy.

Medications. Theophylline may produce physiologic states that mimic anxiety. In addition, patients on steroids may report such symptoms as confusion, anxiety, and insomnia, all of which were reported by this patient. Caffeine also can augment anxiety status. Once it was discovered, the patient was asked to decrease her consumption of 8 cups of coffee daily, a habit she had developed because she was at home with nothing to do. A theophylline level was in the borderline toxic range; therefore, her dose was decreased. Despite strong suspicions that steroids were related to some of her symptoms, it was not clinically possible to alter her steroid dose at this time.

Psychosocial Factors

Marital issue. An interview with the patient and husband revealed a significant problem. Having had the experience of a brother dying of emphysema, the husband himself was quite anxious about his wife's symptoms. He was concerned that his wife would become totally dependent on him for care and reacted to this by ignoring some of her realistic dependency needs, denying the extent of her medical problems, and deemphasizing the severity of her agitation and anxiety symptoms. He seemed unable to bring himself to recognize her plight for fear of being overwhelmed. With help from the social services department, arrangements were made for a home health aide to assist the husband in home care tasks. In this case, concrete assistance helped the husband feel less overwhelmed. In follow-up sessions, he was then able to voice some of his genuine concern for his wife.

Patient's fear of abandonment. The patient's perception of her husband's withdrawal increased her fears of abandonment. As she spoke about her illness experience, it became clear that her "problem" in inserting her nasal cannula was partly a "demonstration" of helplessness meant to assure her husband's continuing involvement in her daily care. The patient seemed entirely unaware of any such intent. Her anxious and helpless behavior increased the stress on her husband, leading to his withdrawal and an eventual management crisis. Clarification of this chain of events, along with her husband's reassurance, helped to break the vicious cycle in the relationship that had prompted and reinforced her anxiety.

The Role of Psychotropic Medication

Useful participation in therapy depends on the patient's ability to listen to, comprehend, and organize thinking about complicated issues. This patient's organicity was a hindrance to such participation. Institution of low-dose neuroleptic medication (in this case, 2 mg of haloperidol in the morning and at bedtime) helped to reduce her anxiety significantly and facilitate her collaboration in the treatment process. Benzodiazepines were avoided for two reasons: (1) increased risk of respiratory depression and (2) augmentation of CNS depression, which could worsen her organic mental disorder. Bedtime flurazepam was therefore also discontinued.

Summary

Management of this patient's anxiety required an assessment of biologic as well as family system and psychologic issues. A successful intervention required a coordinated plan involving medication adjustment, recognition of her fear of abandonment, provision of concrete social services, and meetings with the couple to alter their maladaptive interaction.

REFERENCES

Abelson HI & Fishburne PM (1976). *Nonmedical use of psychoactive substances: 1975–76.* Princeton, NJ: Response Analysis Corporation.

Abernethy DR, Greenblatt DJ, Divoll M, et al. (1982). Impairment of diazepam metabolism by low dose estrogen-containing oral-contraceptive steroids. *New England Journal of Medicine, 306,* 791–792.

Abernethy DR, Greenblatt DJ, & Shader RI (1981). Treatment of diazepam withdrawal syndrome with propranolol. *Annals of Internal Medicine, 94,* 354–355. 1981.

Abramowicz M (1984). Drugs that cause psychiatric symptoms. *Medical Letter, 26,* 75–78.

Abramowicz M (1986a). Crack. *Medical Letter, 28,* 69–70.

Abramowicz M (Ed) (1986b). Midazolam. *Medical Letter, 28*(719), 73–76.

Anderson RW & Lev-Ran A (1985). Hypoglycemia: The standard and the fiction. *Psychosomatics, 26,* 38–47.

Aronson TA & Craig TJ (1986). Cocaine precipitation of panic disorder. *American Journal of Psychiatry, 143,* 643–645.

Backes CR & Cadero L (1980). Withdrawal symptoms in the neonate from presumptive intrauterine exposure to diazepam: Report of a case. *Journal of American Osteopathic Association, 79,* 584–585.

Bard M & Sutherland AM (1977). Adaptation to radical mastecomy. In *The Psychological Impact of Cancer* (pp 55–71). New York: American Cancer Society.

Baudry F & Weiner A (1968). Preoperative preparation of the surgical patient. *Surgery*, *63*, 885–889.

Bela SV & Raftery EB (1980). The role of verapamil in chronic stable angina: A controlled study with computerized multistage treadmill exercise. *Lancet*, *1*, 841–844.

Benson H, Beary JF, & Carol MP (1974). The relaxation response. *Psychiatry*, *37*, 37–46.

Bravo EL, Tarazi RC, Gifford RW, et al. (1979), Circulating and urinary catecholamines in pheochromocytoma. *New England Journal of Medicine*, *301*, 682–686.

Breurer RI, Moses H, Hagen TC, et al. (1972). Gastric operations and glucose homeostasis. *Gastroenterology*, *62*, 1109–1119.

Busto U, Sellers EM, Naranjo CA, et al. (1986). Withdrawal reaction after long-term therapeutic use of benzodiazepines. *New England Journal of Medicine*, *315*(14), 854–859.

Calabrese JR & Gulledge AD (1985). Psychotropics during pregnancy and lactation: A review. *Psychosomatics*, *26*, 413–426.

Cameron AJ, Ellis JP, McGill JI, et al. (1969). Insulin response to carbohydrate ingestion after gastric surgery with special reference to hypoglycemia. *Gut*, *10*, 825–830.

Castillo-Ferrando JR, Garci M, & Carmona J (1980). Digoxin levels and diazepam. *Lancet*, *2*, 368.

Charney DS, Heninger GR, & Jatlow PI (1985). Increased anxiogenic effects of caffeine in panic disorders. *Archives of General Psychiatry*, *423*(3), 233–243.

Christensen B (1946). Studies on hyperventilation: II. Electrocardiographic changes in normal man during voluntary hyperventilation. *Journal of Clinical Investigation*, *24*, 880.

Cobb WE, Lamberton P, & Jackson IMD (1984). Use of a rapid, sensitive immunoradiometric assay for thyrotropin to distinguish normal from hyperthyroid subjects. *Clinical Chemistry*, *30*, 1558–1560.

Cohen RB, Finn H, & Steen SM (1969). Effect of diazepam and meperidine, alone and in combination, on the respiratory response to carbon dioxide. *Anesthia and Analgesia*, *48*, 353–355.

Cohn JB, Bowden CL, Fisher JG, et al. (1986). Double-blind comparison of buspirone and clorazepate in anxious outpatients. *American Journal of Medicine*, *80*(Suppl 3B), 10–16.

Cohn JB & Wilcox CS (1986). Low-sedation potential of buspirone compared with alprazolam and lorazepam in the treatment of anxious patients: A double-blind study. *Journal of Clinical Psychiatry*, *47*(8), 409–412.

De La Fuenta JR, Rosenbaum AH, Martin HR, et al. (1980). Lorazepam-related withdrawal seizures. *Mayo Clinic Proceedings 55*, 190–192.

Denko JD & Kaelbling R (1962). The psychiatric aspects of hypoparathyroidism. *Acta Psychiatrica Scandinavica*, *38*(Suppl 164), 1–70.

Devereux RB, Perloff JK, Reichek N, et al. (1976). Mitral valve prolapse. *Circulation*, *54*, 3–14.

DeVries HA, Burke RK, Hopper RT, et al. (1977). Efficacy of EMG biofeedback in relaxation training: A controlled study. *American Journal of Physiology and Medicine*, *56*(2), 75–81.

Dietch JT (1984). Cerebral tumor presenting with panic attacks. *Psychosomatics*, *25*, 861–863.

Dimsdale JE & Hackett TP (1982). Effect of denial on cardiac health and psychological assessment. *American Journal of Psychiatry*, *139*, 1477–1480.

Dreyfuss J, Griffith DL, Singhvi SM, et al. (1979). Pharmacokinetics of nadolol, a beta-receptor antagonist: Administration of therapeutic single and multiple-dosage regimens to hypertensive patients. *Journal of Clinical Pharmacology*, *19*, 712–720.

Egbert LD, Battit GE, Welch CE, et al. (1964). Reduction of post-operative pain by encouragement and instruction of patients: A study of doctor-patient rapport. *New England Journal of Medicine*, *270*, 825–827.

Eison AS & Temple DL, Jr (1986). Buspirone: Review of its pharmacology and current perspectives on its mechanism of action. *American Journal of Medicine*, 80(Suppl 3B) 1–9.

Eison MS & Eison AS (1984). Buspirone as a midbrain modulator: Anxiolysis unrelated to traditional benzodiazepine mechanisms. *Drug Development Research*, *4*, 109–119.

Evans DW & Lum LC (1977). Hyperventilation: An important cause of pseudoangina. *Lancet*, *1*, 155–157.

Fabrykant M (1953). The problem of functional hyperinsulinism or functional hypoglycemia attributed to nervous causes: laboratory and clinical correlations. *Metabolism*, *4*(6), 469–479.

Fann WE, Lake RC, & Majors LF (1974). Thioridazine in neurotic, anxious, and depressed patients. *Psychosomatics*, *15*, 117–121.

Ferrer M (1968). Mistaken psychiatric referral of occult serious cardiovascular disease. *Archives of General Psychiatry*, *18*, 112–113.

Finkel BS, McCloskey KL & Goodman LS (1979). Diazepam and drug-associated deaths. *Journal of the American Medical Association*, *242*, 429–434.

Foa PP, et al. (1980). Reactive hypoglycemia and A-cell ("pancreatic") glucagon deficiency in the adult. *Journal of the American Medical Association*, *244*, 2281–2285.

Fraser HS & Carr AC (1976). Propranolol psychosis. *British Journal of Psychiatry*, *129*, 508–509.

Freinkel N & Metzger BE (1969). Oral glucose tolerance curve and hypoglycemias in the fed state. *New England Journal of Medicine*, *280*, 820–828.

Frishman WH (1981) Nadolol: A new β-adrenoceptor

antagonist. *New England Journal of Medicine*, *305*, 678–682.

Gehi MM, Rosenthal RH, Fizette NB, et al. (1981). Psychiatric manifestations of hyponatremia. *Psychosomatics*, 22, 739–743.

Gershon ES, Goldstein RE, Moss AJ, et al. (1979). Psychosis with ordinary doses of propranolol. *Annals of Internal Medicine*, *90*, 938–940.

Gibbs FA & Gibbs EC (1952). *Atlas of electroencephalography* (Vol. 2). Cambridge, MA: Addison-Wesley.

Gilberg C (1977) "Floppy infant syndrome" and maternal diazepam. *Lancet*, *2*, 224.

Goa KL & Ward A (1986). Buspirone: A preliminary review of its pharmacological properties and therapeutic efficacy as an anxiolytic. *Drugs*, *32*, 114–129.

Goldberg RJ (1982). *Anxiety: A guide to biobehavioral diagnosis and therapy for physicians and mental health clinicians.* New York: Free Press.

Goldberg RJ (1982). Anxiety reduction by self-regulation: Theory, practice and evaluation. *Annals of Internal Medicine*, *96*, 483–487.

Goldberg RJ & Cullen LO (1985). Factors important to psychosocial adjustment to cancer: A review of the evidence. *Social Science and Medicine*, *20*, 803–807.

Gorman JM, Fyer AJ, Gliklich J, et al. (1981). Mitral valve prolapse and panic disorders: Effect of imipramine. In DF Klein & JG Rabkin (Eds), *Anxiety: New research and changing concepts.* New York: Raven Press.

Gotoh F, Meyer JS & Takagi Y (1965). Cerebral effects of hyperventilation in man. *Archives of Neurology*, *12*, 410.

Granville-Grossman KL & Turner P (1966). The effect of propranolol on anxiety. *Lancet*, *1*, 788–790.

Greenblatt DJ, Abernethy DR, Morse DS, et al. (1984). Clinical importance of the interaction of diazepam and cimetidine. *New England Journal of Medicine*, *310*, 1639–1643.

Greenblatt DJ, Allen MD, Harmatz MJ, et al. (1980). Diazepam disposition determinants. *Clinical Pharmacological Therapy*, *27*, 301–312.

Greenblatt DJ, Divoll M, Harmatz JS, et al. (1982). Pharmacokinetic comparison of sublingual lorazepam with intravenous, intramuscular and oral lorazepam. *Journal of Pharmaceutical Science*, *71*, 248–252.

Greenblatt DJ & Koch-Weser J (1973). Adverse reactions to propranolol in hospitalized medical patients: A report from the Boston Collaborative Drug Surveillance Program. *American Heart Journal*, *86*, 478–484.

Greenblatt DJ & Koch-Weser J (1976). Intramuscular injection of drugs. *New England Journal of Medicine*, *295*, 542–546.

Greenblatt DJ, Shader RI, Koch-Weser J, et al. (1974). Slow absorption of intramuscular chlordiazepoxide. *New England Journal of Medicine*, *291*, 1116–1118.

Griffith JD, Jasinski DR, & McKinney GR (1986). Investigation of the abuse liability of buspirone in alcohol-dependent patients. *American Journal of Medicine 80*(Suppl 3B), 30–35.

Gronwall D & Wrightson P (1974). Delayed recovery of intellectual function after minor head injury. *Lancet*, *2*, 605–609.

Hafken L, Leichter S, & Reich T (1975). Organic brain dysfunction as a possible consequence of postgastrectomy hypoglycemia. *American Journal of Psychiatry*, *132*, 1321–1324.

Hall RCW (1983) Psychiatric effects on thyroid hormone disturbance. *Psychosomatics 24*, 7–18.

Hall RCW & Joffe JR (1972). Aberrant response to diazepam: A new syndrome. *American Journal of Psychiatry*, *126*, 738–742.

Hall RCW & Joffe JR (1973). Hypomagnesemia: Physical and psychiatric symptoms. *Journal of the American Medical Association*, *224*, 1749–1751.

Hansen HJ, Caudill SP, & Boone J (1985). Crisis in drug testing: Results of a CDC blind study. *Journal of the American Medical Association*, 253(16), 2282–2387.

Harris MC (1958). The use and abuse of pocket nebulizers in the treatment of asthma. *Postgraduate Medicine*, *23*(2), 170–173.

Healey M, Pickens R, Meisch R, et al. (1983). Effects of clorazepate, diazepam, lorazepam, and placebo on human memory. *Journal of Clinical Psychiatry*, *44*(12), 436–439.

Hollister LE, Motzenbecker FP, & Degan RO (1961). Withdrawal reactions from chlordiazepoxide (Librium) *Psychopharmacologia*, *2*, 63–68.

Hoyumpa AM (1978). Disposition and elimination of minor tranquilizers in the aged and in patients with liver disease. *Southern Medical Journal*, *71*, 23–28.

Jacobs MA, Senior RM, & Kessler G (1976). Clinical experience with theophylline: Relationship between dosage, serum concentration, and toxicity. *Journal of the American Medical Association*, *235*, 1983–1986.

Jacobson E (1938). *Progressive relaxation* (2nd ed). Chicago, University Press.

James IM, Pearson RM, Griffith DNW, et al. (1978). Reducing the somatic manifestations of anxiety by beta-blockage: A study of stage fright. *Journal of Psychosomatic Research*, *22*, 327–337.

Johnson LC & Chernik DA (1982). Sedative-hypnotics and human performance. *Psychopharmacology*, *76*, 101–113.

Kahn RJ, McNair DM, Lipman RS, et al. (1986). Imipramine and chlordiazepoxide in depressive and anxiety disorders: II. Efficacy in anxious outpatients. *Archives of General Psychiatry*, *43*, 79–85.

Kantor JS, Zitrin CM, & Zeldis SM (1980). Mitral valve prolapse syndrome in agoraphobic patients. *American Journal of Psychiatry*, *137*; 467–469.

Karch FE (1979). Rage reaction associated with clorazepate dipotassium. *Annals of Internal Medicine 91*, 61–62.

Kastenholz KV & Crismon ML (1984). Buspirone, a novel nonbenzodiazepine anxiolytic. *Clinical Pharmacy*, *3*, 600–607.

Kathol RG, Noyes R, Jr, Slymen DJ, et al. (1980). Propranolol in chronic anxiety disorders: A controlled study. *Archives of General Psychiatry*, *37*, 1361–1365.

Klein DF (1982). Medication in the treatment of panic attacks and phobic states. *Psychopharmacology Bulletin*, *18*, 85–90.

Kristensen O & Sendrup EH (1978). Sphenoidal electrodes. *Acta Neurologica Scandinavica*, *58*, 157–166.

Kwentus JA, Achilles JT, & Goyer PF (1982). Hypoglycemia: Etiologic and psychosomatic aspects of diagnosis. *Postgraduate Medicine*, *71*, 99–104.

Lakshminarayan MD, Sahn SA, Hudson LD, et al. (1976). Effect of diazepam on ventilatory responses. *Clinical Pharmacological Therapy*, *20*, 178–183.

Leboeuf A (1977). The effects of EMG feedback training on state anxiety in introverts and extroverts. *Journal of Clinical Psychology*, *33*, 251–253.

Leggett J & Favazza AR (1978). Hypoglycemia: An overview. *Journal of Clinical Psychiatry*, *39*, 51–57.

Leigh D (1979). Psychiatric aspects of head injury. *Psychiatry Digest*, *40*, 21–32.

Lerner WD & Fallon HJ (1985). The alcohol withdrawal syndrome. *New England Journal of Medicine*, *313*, 951–952.

Liberthson R, Sheehan DV, King ME, et al. (1986). The prevalence of mitral valve prolapse in patients with panic disorders. *American Journal of Psychiatry*, *143*, 511–515.

Lieb JP, Walsh GO, Babb TL, et al. (1976). A comparison of EEG seizure patterns recorded with surface and depth electrodes in patients with temporal lobe epilepsy. *Epilepsia*, *17*, 137–160.

Lipman RS, Covi L, Downing RW, et al. (1981). Pharmacotherapy of anxiety and depression. *Psychopharmacology Bulletin 17*, 91–103.

Lishman WA (1978). Endocrine disorders and metabolic disorders. In *Organic psychiatry* (pp 595–672). London: Blackwell.

Lynch JJ, Paskewitz DA, Gimbel KS, et al. (1977). Psychological aspects of cardiac arrhythmia. *American Heart Journal*, *93*, 645–657.

MacCrimmon DJ, Wallace JE, Goldberg WM, et al. (1979). Emotional disturbance and cognitive deficits in hyperthyroidism. *Psychosomatic Medicine 41*, 331–340.

Marks V & Rose FC (1965). *Hypoglycemia*. Philadelphia: FA Davis.

Marshall JR (1979). Neuropsychiatric aspects of renal failure. *Journal of Clinical Psychiatry*, *40*, 81–85.

Mastrovito RC (1972). Symposium: Emotional considerations in cancer and stroke. *New York State Journal of Medicine*, *72*, 2874–2877.

Mazza DL, Martin D, Spacavento L, et al. (1986). Prevalence of anxiety disorders in patients with mitral valve prolapse. *American Journal of Psychiatry*, *143*, 349–352.

McHenry PL, Cogan OJ, Elliott WC, et al (1970). False-positive ECG response to exercise secondary to hyperventilation: Cineangiographic correlation. *American Heart Journal*, *79*, 683–687.

McKell TE & Sullivan AJ (1947). The hyperventilation syndrome in gastroenterology. *Gastroenterology*, *9*, 6–16.

Meyer RE (1986). Anxiolytics and the alcoholic patient. *Journal of Studies on Alcohol*, *47*(4), 269–273.

Mitchells-Heggs P, Murphy K, Minty K, et al. (1980). Diazepam in the treatment of dyspnea in the "pink puffer" syndrome. *Quarterly Journal of Medicine*, *49*, 9–20.

Moore RA (1985). The prevalence of alcoholism in medical and surgical patients. In MA Schuckit & AE Slaby (Eds), *Alcohol patterns and problems* (chap 8). New Brunswick, NJ: Rutgers University Press.

Mueller HS & Chahine RA (1981). Interim report of multicenter double-blind placebo-controlled studies of nifedipine in chronic stable angina. *American Journal of Medicine*, *71*, 645–657.

Neill WA & Hattenhauer M (1975). Impairment of myocardial O_2 supply due to hyperventilation. *Circulation*, *52*, 854–858.

Newton RE, Marunycz JD, Alderdice MT, et al. (1986). Review of the side-effect profile of buspirone. *American Journal of Medicine 80*(Suppl 3B), 17–21.

Oppenheimer RD (1968). Microscopic lesions in the brain following head injury. *Neurology Neurosurgery and Psychiatry 3*, 299–306.

Pariser SF, Pinta ER & Jones BA (1978). Mitral valve prolapse syndrome and anxiety neurosis/panic disorder. *American Journal of Psychiatry*, *135*, 246–247.

Parkinson D (1977). Concussion. *Mayo Clinic Proceedings*, *52*, 492–496.

Patel DA & Patel AR (1980). Clorazepate and congenital malformations. *Journal of the American Medical Association, 244,* 135–136.

Paykel ES, Rowman PR, Parker RR, et al. (1982). Response to phenelzine and amitriptyline in subtypes of outpatient depression. *Archives of General Psychiatry, 39,* 1041–1049.

Peck A & Boland J (1977). Emotional reactions to radiation treatment. *Cancer, 40,* 180–184.

Pevnick JS, Jasinski DR & Haertzen CA (1978). Abrupt withdrawal from therapeutically administered diazepam. *Archives of General Psychiatry, 35,* 995–998.

Phillips JP, Antal EJ & Smith RB (1986). A pharmacokinetic drug interaction between erythromycin and triazolam. *Journal of Clinical Psychopharmacology, 6*(5), 297–302.

Pincus JH & Tucker GJ (1985). *Behavioral neurology.* (3rd ed.) New York: Oxford University Press.

Plum F & Posner JB (1972). *Diagnosis of stupor and coma* (2nd ed). Contemporary Neurology Series. Philadelphia: FA Davis.

Pohl R, Berchou R, & Rainey JM (1982). Tricyclic antidepressants and monoamine oxidase inhibitors in the treatment of agoraphobia. *Journal of Clinical Psychopharmacology, 2,* 399–407.

Rao S, Sherbaniuk RW, Prasad K, et al. (1973). Cardiopulmonary effects of diazepam. *Clinical Pharmacological Therapy, 14,* 182–189.

Raskin M, Bali LR, & Peeke HV (1980). Muscle biofeedback and transcendental meditation. *Archives of General Psychiatry 37,* 93–97.

Ratey JJ & Salzman C (1984). Recognizing and managing akathisia. *Hospital and Community Psychiatry, 35,* 975–977.

Ratey JJ, Sorgi P, & Polakoffs (1985). Nadolol as a treatment for akathisia. *American Journal of Psychiatry, 142,* 640–642.

Resnick RB, Kestenbaum RS & Schwartz LK (1976). Acute systemic effects of cocaine in man: A controlled study by intranasal and intravenous routes. *Science, 195,* 696–698.

Reuler JB, Girard DE, & Cooney TG (1985). Wernicke's encephalopathy. *New England Journal of Medicine, 312,* 1035–1039.

Rice RL (1950). Symptom patterns of the hyperventilation syndrome. *American Journal of Medicine, 8,* 691–700.

Rickels K (1983). Nonbenzodiazepine anxiolytics: Clinical usefulness. *Journal of Clinical Psychiatry, 44*(11), Sec 2, 38–43.

Rickels K, Csanalosi I, Chung HR, et al. (1974). Amitriptyline in anxious-depressed outpatients: A controlled study. *American Journal of Psychiatry, 131,* 25–30.

Rickels K, Gordon PE, Zamostien BB, et al. (1970). Hydroxyzine and chlordiazepoxide in anxious neurotic outpatients: A collaborative controlled study. *Comprehensive Psychiatry, 11,* 457–474.

Rickels K, Morris RJ, Newman H, et al. (1983). Diphenhydramine in insomniac family practice patients: A double-blind study. *Journal of Clinical Pharmacology, 23,* 235–242.

Rickels K, Weisman K, Norstad N, et al. (1982). Buspirone and diazepam in anxiety: A controlled study. *Journal of Clinical Psychiatry, 43*(12), Sec 2, 81–86.

Rinkenberger RL, Psystowsky EN, Heger JJ, et al. (1980). Effect of intravenous and chronic orgal verapamil administration in patients with supraventricular arrhythmias. *Circulation, 62,* 996, 1010.

Robinson DS, Nies A, Ravaris CL, et al. (1973). The monoamine oxidase inhibitor, phenelzine, in the treatment of depressive-anxiety states: A controlled clinical trial. *Archives of General Psychiatry, 29,* 407–413.

Ryan HF, Merrill FB, Scott GE, et al. (1968). Increase in suicidal thoughts and tendencies: Association with diazepam therapy. *Journal of the American Medical Association, 203,* 1137–1139.

Scharf MB, Khosla N, Brocker N, et al. (1984). Differential amnestic properties of short- and long-acting benzodiazepines. *Journal of Clinical Psychiatry, 45*(2), 51–53.

Schuckit MA (1984). Clinical studies of buspirone. *Psychopathology, 17*(Suppl 3), 61–68.

Schweizer E & Rickels K (1986). Failure of buspirone to manage benzodiazepine withdrawal. *American Journal of Psychiatry, 143,* 1590–1592.

Sellers EM & Kalant H (1976). Alcohol intoxication and withdrawal. *New England Journal of Medicine, 294,* 757–762.

Shear MK, Devereux RB, Dramer-Fox R, et al. (1987). Panic patients with a low prevalence of mitral valve prolapse. *American Journal of Psychiatry, 141,* 302–303.

Shearer RM & Bowres IT (1985). Tardive akathisia and agitation depression during MTC therapy. *Acta Psychiatrica Scandinavica, 70*(5), 428–431.

Sheehan DV (1982). Panic attacks and phobias. *New England Journal of Medicine, 307,* 156–158.

Sheehan DV, Ballenger J, & Jacobsen G (1980). Treatment of endogenous anxiety with phobic, hysterical, and hypochondriacal symptoms. *Archives of General Psychiatry, 37,* 51–59.

Singh BN, Ellrodt G, & Peter CT (1978). Verapamil: A review of its pharmacological properties and therapeutic use. *Drugs, 15,* 169–197.

Starkman MN, Zelnik TC, Nesse RM, et al. (1985). Anxiety in patients with pheochromocytomas. *Archives of Internal Medicine, 145*(2), 248–252.

Stoudenmire J (1972). Effects of muscle relaxation training on state and trait anxiety in introverts and extroverts. *Journal of Personality and Social Psychology*, *24*, 273–275.

Sutherland AM, Orbach CE, Duk RB, et al. (1977). Adaptation to the dry colostomy; Preliminary report and summary of findings. In *The Psychological Impact of Cancer* (pp 1–16). New York: American Cancer Society.

Taylor AR & Bell TK (1966). Slowing of cerebral circulation after concussional head injury: A controlled trial. *Lancet*, 2, 178–180.

Taylor PJ (1967). Hemorrhage while on anticoagulant therapy precipitated by drug interaction. *Arizona Medicine*, *24*, 697–699.

Tien AY & Gujavarty KS (1985). Seizure following withdrawal from triazolam [Letter to the editor]. *American Journal of Psychiatry*, *142*(12), 1516–1517.

Tyrer PJ & Lader MH (1974). Response to propranolol and diazepam in somatic anxiety. *British Medical Journal*, 2, 14–16.

Uhde TW, Vittone BJ & Post RM (1984). Glucose tolerance testing in panic disorder. *American Journal of Psychiatry*, *141*(11), 1461–1463.

Vajda FJE, Prineas RJ & Lovell RPH (1971). Interaction between phenytoin and the benzodiazepines. *British Medical Journal*, 1, 346.

Van der Kropf C (1979). Reactions to triazolam. *Lancet*, 2, 526.

Venkatesh A, Pauls DL, Crowe R, et al. (1980). Mitral valve prolapse in anxiety neurosis (panic disorder). *American Heart Journal*, *100*, 302–305.

Victor BS, Lubetsky M, & Greden JF (1981). Somatic manifestations of caffeinism. *Journal of Clinical Psychiatry*, *42*, 185–188.

Waldeck B (1975). Effect of caffeine on locomotor activity in central catecholamine mechanisms: A study with special reference to drug interaction. *Acta Pharmacentica Toxilogica 36*, 1–23.

Wallace RK (1970). Physiological effects of transcendental meditation. *Science*, *167*, 1751–1754.

Webb WL & Gehi M (1981). Electrolyte and fluid imbalance: Neuropsychiatric manifestations. *Psychosomatics*, *22*, 199–203.

Weil AA (1959). Ictal emotions occurring in temporal lobe dysfunction. *Archives of Neurology*, *1*, 87–97.

Weiner N (1980). Norephedrine, ephedrine, and sympathomimetic amines. In AG Goodman, LS Goodman, A Gilman (eds), *Pharmacological basis of therapeutics* (p 163). New York: Macmillan.

Weisman A (1979). *Coping with cancer* New York: McGraw-Hill.

White BC, et al. (1980). Anxiety and muscle tension as consequences of caffeine withdrawal. *Science*, *209*, 1547–1548.

Wilkerson et al. (1980). Intranasal and oral cocaine kinetics. *Clinical Pharmacology and Therapeutics*, *27*, 386–394.

Wilson JF (1981). Behavioral preparation for surgery: Benefit or harm? *Journal of Behavioral Medicine*, *4*, 79–102.

Winokur A, Rickels K, Greenblatt DJ, et al. (1980). Withdrawal reaction from long-term low-dosage administration of diazepam. *Archives of General Psychiatry*, *37*, 101–105.

Wiznitzer T, Chapira N, Stadler J, et al. (1974). Late hypoglycemia in patients following vagotomy and pyloroplasty. *International Surgery 59*, 229–232.

Wolkowitz OM, Weingartner H, Thompson K, et al. (1987). Diazepam-induced amnesia: A neuropharmacological model of an ''organic amnestic syndrome''. *American Journal of Psychiatry*, *144*, 25–29.

Wortsman J, Burns G, Van Beek Al, et al. (1980). Hyperadrenergic state after trauma to the neuroaxis. *Journal of American Medical Association*, *243*, 1459–1460.

Zipursky RB, Baker RW, & Zimmer B (1985). Alprazolam withdrawal delirium unresponsive to diazepam: Case report. *Journal of Clinical Psychiatry*, *46*(8), 344–345.

Zitrin CM, Klein DF, & Woerner MG (1978). Behavior therapy, supportive psychotherapy, imipramine, and phobias. *Archives of General Psychiatry*, *35* 307–316.

Zivin I (1970). The neurological and psychiatric aspects of hypoglycemia. *Diseases of the Nervous System*, *31*, 604–607.

Charles V. Ford
G. Richard Smith, Jr.

8
Somatoform Disorders, Factitious Disorders, and Disability Syndromes

Patients who present with somatoform disorders are among the most difficult patients to treat. By definition they have psychic problems that have been translated into somatic symptoms. The first task is thus to rule out physical disease as the cause of the presenting symptoms. It is likely, however, even when physical disease can be eliminated as the etiology for the symptoms, that the patient will resist any implication that the problems are of psychologic etiology. The reasons for this resistance are multiple and include (but are not limited to) the use of the symptom as a defense against conscious awareness of psychic conflicts, religious or cultural interpretations of disease processes, economic considerations, and the fact that some psychiatric disorders do produce physiologic dysfunction (Ford, 1986). When confronted with the diagnosis "no physical disease found," many of these somatizers will deny all possibility of a psychiatric disorder and will seek further medical care from another source, hoping for a diagnosis that is more acceptable. The

capacity to be therapeutically effective with these patients is often dependent upon the skill of the physician to "package" the diagnosis and recommended treatment program within the personal philosophic and psychologic constructs of the patient. This skill requires an understanding of the patient's needs and the language with which such patients communicate their distress.

DIAGNOSIS

The "official" somatoform disorders, as determined by the *Diagnostic and Statistical Manual of Mental Disorders* (DSM-III-R) (American Psychiatric Association, 1987), are conversion disorder, somatization disorder, hypochondriasis, somatoform pain disorder, and body dysmorphic disorder. Although not officially considered somatoform disorders, factitious disorders, malingering, and disability syndromes are closely related phenomenologically and can be considered in a general way to be "somatizing disorders"

PRINCIPLES OF MEDICAL PSYCHIATRY
ISBN 0-8089-1883-4

205

(Ford, 1983). They will thus also be included in this chapter because of their many commonalities with the somatoform disorders.

It is of importance to note that, in the viewpoint expressed in this chapter, the various somatizing disorders do not fit tightly into the discrete diagnostic categories that are didactically described. There is considerable overlap among them, and diagnostic boundaries then to become blurred in the everyday practice of medicine (RC Smith, 1985). Furthermore, the process of somatization does *not* require an absence of physical disease! One frequently encounters an admixture of somatization with medical disease. This concept cannot be overemphasized because too many physicians have found themselves trapped by the either-or approach. It is stressed instead, that what exist are different styles of illness behavior and that rather than searching for discrete diagnostic entities, the clinician should determine patterns of illness behavior. (See also Chapter 1.)

The foregoing is not intended to reflect diagnostic nihilism, nor to set up excuses for imprecise diagnostic efforts. Rather, what is implied is that there is a need for a more sophisticated evaluation than merely fitting symptoms into arbitrary lists of diagnostic criteria. The clinician must ask such questions as these: What is the evidence of abnormal illness behavior? Is there objective evidence of a disease process? Is the patient 's subjective sense of suffering and disability (the illness) proportional to the disease process? Does the patient's illness help resolve life problems? Do the phenomenological features of the patient and the presentation of symptoms fit one of the somatizing disorders? Do the physical symptoms express an underlying psychiatric disorder?

With regard to the last issue, a significantly high percentage of somatizing patients, even those who appear to meet the diagnostic criteria for one of the somatoform disorders, have instead an underlying psychiatric disorder. Poorly differentiated physical symptoms are a frequently presentation of depression (Lesse, 1980). Estimates suggest that only 25–50 percent of patients who have major depression are so diagnosed and treated by physicians who see them for a wide variety of physical complaints (Katon, 1982). Patients who have been diagnosed as having "somatization disorder" may also have underlying (or concurrent) psychiatric disorders, such as panic disorder (Sheehan & Sheehan, 1982a, 1982b) or major depression (Liskow, Othmer, Penick, et al. 1986). These two disorders are important to recognize because specific and effective treatment interventions are available. Thus, both physical diseases and other psychiatric disorders must be differentiated from the somatizing disorders, but to add confusion to the diagnostic picture, they may coexist.

GENERAL TREATMENT PRINCIPLES FOR SOMATIZATION

Before proceeding to discuss the specific somatoform disorders and their treatment it is useful to consider several general principles that are applicable across diagnostic lines.

The first and cardinal rule is that *invasive diagnostic and therapeutic procedures should be initiated only on the basis of objective evidence of pathophysiologic dysfunction, not solely on subjective complaints*. The unfortunate tendency to expose these patients to increasingly complex, potentially dangerous, and expensive diagnostic procedures not only places them at risk for iatrogenic complications, but also tends to reinforce the somatization. The possibility of somatization should be considered *before* every esoteric organic possibility has been ruled out.

Second, after a diagnosis of somatization has been established, *it is important that the primary physician remain involved in the treatment plan, even if formal psychiatric intervention is undertaken.* A continuing relationship implies that the patient's symptoms have been redefined in their meaning in the disease process but that the patient's distress (illness) has not been discounted.

Third, *arguing with a patient about the reality of a physical symptom is not only fruitless—it is antitherapeutic in that it denies the personal experience of the patient.* Somatoform pain is no less painful for the patient than pain from a known organic disease. The therapeutic approach is to help the patient understand the symptom within a different context, for example, to get the hypochondriac to recognize fatigue as a symptom of "stress" rather than to interpret it as probable cancer.

Each of the major syndromes of somatization will be discussed separately with regard to specific issues of differential diagnosis and treatment intervention.

Although the process of somatization is usually associated with individuals with more primitive levels of personality organization and defensive structures, it should be noted that relatively higher-functioning individuals may somatize at times of extreme stress or regression or during a period of intercurrent affective disorder. The choice between supportive psychotherapy and anxiety-provoking, insight-oriented psychotherapy for these higher-functioning patients should be based on an assessment of the patient's current level of ego functioning and an evaluation of the patient's ability to tolerate the regression associated with the anxiety-provoking intensive psychotherapy. For further details, please see Chapter 1, by Green.

SOMATIZING DISORDERS

Hypochondriasis

Hypochondriacs are characterized by their obsessive fear of disease. They repeatedly return to their physicians with a variety of concerns, often interpreting them as indicative of serious disease. Patients with hypochondriasis often seek medical care because they are concerned or anxious about having a specific *disease*, rather than because they are troubled by a specific symptom. Though they may present with a symptom, it often becomes apparent that they are anxious about a certain diagnosis. This concern is in contrast to the patient who is only troubled by a symptom or a pain, as in the situation of the patient who manifests somatization disorder. Usually patients with hypochondriasis can be reassured only temporarily that the symptom is not a reflection of serious organic pathology. The psychiatric literature is replete with articles about hypochondriasis and formulations and observations about the disorder. Several of these are important to note. Schmale (1969) postulates that hypochondriacs have secondarily focused their anxiety on bodily functions as a defense against acting out a forbidden wish. This is a type of displacement of the need for intrapsychic control to an attempt to control a bodily function. Other psychodynamic theories propose that hypochondriasis is a defense against low self-esteem (Sullivan, 1953), while others see it as a defense against guilt or innate badness (Engel, 1959; Lipsitt, 1970). More recent formulations note that their self-esteem is shaky and that they are very vulnerable to feeling incomplete (Adler, 1981). Barsky and Klerman (1983) have suggested a new term, "amplifying somatic style," to describe those patients who scrupulously monitor bodily function, scrutinize trivial symptoms, and attribute them to physical disease.

Hypochondriacs are a heterogeneous group, requiring careful assessment and individualized therapeutic interventions. One group is comprised of individuals who demonstrate *transient hypochondriacal symptoms* in response to acute life stressors. Examples of such stressors include a proposed change of residence for an elderly person; an industrial accident, and a life-threatening illness, such as a myocardial infarction. Transient hypochondriasis can be differentiated from primary or characterologic hypochondriasis by the syndrome's relatively short duration (months rather than years), and from major depression by a relative lack of vegetative symptoms. The treatment of transient hypochondriasis comprises education regarding the benign nature of the symptom, combined with psychotherapy, formal or informal, according to the patient's motivation and level of ego function. When the hypochondriasis is associated with life stresses, sometimes environmental manipulation may be useful (e.g., increasing the social contacts of a lonely elderly person).

Hypochondriacal symptoms may be the presentation of *somatized depression* (Katon, Kleinman, Rosen, 1982a, 1982b). Some individuals with major depression differentially focus on their physical symptoms with little awareness of any mood change. (See Chapter 2 by Cohen-Cole and Harpe.) Elderly patients may be especially liable to somatize depression (Fogel & Fretwell, 1985). As a part of the depressive phenomenon, they interpret every symptom in the most pessimistic fashion. Depressed patients can be differentiated from those with primary hypochondriasis by a shorter duration of symptoms, a positive personal or family history of affective disorder, and, most important, physiologic symptoms of depression, including sleep disturbance, anhedonia, change in appetite, decreased libido, and impaired concentration. Though the patient may try to explain these symptoms as secondary to the physical problems, this rationalization should not dissuade the physician from treating the depression. The treatment is the same as that for other symptomatic expressions of major depression, with the possible exception that monoamine oxidase inhibitors (MAOIs) might be considered as a specific treatment before cyclic antidepressants are tried, since MAOIs are well tolerated by

somatically preoccupied patient because their side effects are less likely to overlap with patients' presenting complaints. There is no conclusive evidence, however, that MAOIs are more efficacious for this particular patient population (Davidson, Miller, Turnbull, et al. 1982).

Primary hypochondriacs are those patients who have exhibited preoccupation with their bodily symptoms all or most of their lives. In this sense the disorder can be considered to be a characterological. These patients usually come from childhood homes in which there was preoccupation with illness because of chronic disease in a family member or because of hypochondriacal concerns of one or both parents. The childhood home was frequently without emotional warmth except when someone was ill. The patients themselves are often emotionally constricted and have difficulty in communicating to others except through physical complaints (Ford, 1983; Kenyon, 1965; Pilowsky, 1970).

As mentioned earlier in discussing personality assessment in the patient with somatization, a careful assessment of the patient's level of object relations, development, and defensive style is important for selecting the appropriateness of adjunctive psychotherapy in the treatment of a patient with hypochondriasis. Patients with hypochondriacal symptoms may be dependent individuals who use somatic symptoms as a primary means of forming a meaningful interpersonal relationship with the physician, who functions as a transference object (parent figure). Other patients with hypochondriacal symptoms may be obsessional, paranoid, passive-aggressive, or borderline personalities. Assessment of the patient's basic personality organization and defensive style is important for treatment planning as well. For example, a passive-dependent personality could be predicted to be more likely to respond to support and reassurance and to comply with therapy than patients with passive-aggressive, paranoid, or borderline personalities.

Treatment strategies for passive-dependent hypochondriacal patients have emphasized the need for an ongoing relationship with a physician and scheduled office visits that are *not* dependent upon the development of new symptoms. Through subtle behavior techniques the physician can attend differentially to comments made by the patient in reference to emotional or interpersonal issues instead of the physical complaints (Ford, 1983; Lipsitt, 1970; Wahl, 1964). Obsessional, paranoid, or borderline patients with hypochondriacal symptoms may not respond well to reassurance and manipulation: they may respond better to formal supportive psychotherapy, if they respond to anything.

The response to psychotherapy for hypochondriasis has not, in general, been impressive. Kellner (1964, 1982) has reported a favorable response, however, with improvement still demonstrable at a 2-year follow-up, using techniques that included repeated reassurance, explanations, multiple physical examinations, and suggestions. The personality structures of Kellner's patients have not been specified in detail.

Group therapy may be a cost-effective therapeutic adjuvant for hypochondriacal patients (Ford, 1984), but this therapeutic modality may require the more specialized services offered by a large medical center or health maintenance organization. One such setting is the medical care offered for military dependents.

Monosymptomatic hypochondriasis is a term that has been used to describe a rare and bizarre, yet fascinating, group of disorders in which patients present with what amount to delusional beliefs about their bodies (Bishop, 1980). For this reason, these disorders might be best conceptualized as belonging primarily to the diagnostic group of paranoid disorders. Patients with body dysmorphic disorder believe that there is something wrong with their appearance and repetitively seek consultation from physicians, especially plastic surgeons, in their desire to have these defects corrected. The defects are usually not perceptible to others, or are so minor as to be inconsequential. Patients with *delusions of bromosis* believe that they emit an odor that is offensive to other persons. They, in addition to dousing themselves with aromatics, also repetitively seek medical consulation to treat this imagined symptom. *Delusions of parasitosis* is a symptom in which patients believe that they have been infested with worms or some other form of parasite. These patients return to their physicians time and time again, demanding treatment for a nonexistent disease.

Patients with monosymptomatic hypochondriasis are notoriously difficult to manage. They almost always refuse psychiatric consultation and treatment and usually refuse to accept a treatment from any physician that includes psychotropic medications. Some of these patients, however, are exhibiting a "somatic delusion" as a symptom of psychotic depression. This group of patients probably has the best prognosis if they will accept treatment (Hopkinson, 1973). The other patients, as already mentioned, probably suffer from variants of true paranoia. Pimozide has been reported to be markedly effective for this group of syndromes (Munro, 1978), although further research to confirm its efficacy is needed. Tranylcipromine was reported to be effective in one case (Jenike, 1984).

Conversion Disorders

Conversion phenomena are the prototypical somatoform symptoms. They have been described throughout the medical literature for literally thousands of years (Veith, 1965) but remain much debated and controversial as to their very existence (A Lewis, 1975; Slater, 1965), as well as to their etiology. Modern phenomenologic research suggests that they are very common symptoms. Farley, Woodruff, and Guze (1968) found that 1 of 3 postpartum women in their study had experienced at least one conversion symptom. Although DSM-IIIR lists conversion disorder as a specific diagnostic entity, Ford & Folks (1985) have taken the position that these phenomena should be regarded as *symptoms* rather than as a discrete disorder. The analogy is fever, now considered a symptom, not a diagnostic entity as was believed in premodern medicine.

A review of the phenomenology of conversion suggests that there is frequently an underlying psychiatric disorder associated with the symptom. Commonly these disorders are acute adjustment disorders (in which the symptom is used as a coping mechanism), depression, and schizophrenia (Ziegler, Imsoden, & Meyer, 1960). Conversion symptoms are so common that some argue that they must occur as a simple, albeit striking, defense mechanism in a wide range of patients. (Schmale, 1969).

By definition, most conversion symptoms have a pseudoneurologic quality; pain syndromes have now been split off into a separate category (somatoform pain disorder) (Bishop & Torch, 1979). The most frequent symptoms include paralysis, anesthesia, movement disorders, or sensory changes, such as tunnel vision. The differentiation of conversion symptoms from neurologic disease is often very difficult because they appear to occur more frequently when there is underlying neurologic disease (Caplan & Nadelson, 1980; Merskey & Buhrich, 1975) or a history of head trauma.

Except for a few refractory symptoms that are often referred to tertiary care hospitals, most conversion symptoms are transient. They may remit spontaneously or respond to a wide variety of therapeutic interventions, such as suggestive therapies (including hypnosis), psychotherapy, or environmental manipulation (Folks, Ford, & Regan, 1984). Often the key element in the

therapeutic approach is to allow the patient the opportunity to discard the symptom in a face-saving manner. The evaluation of every conversion symptom demands a careful search for an underlying physical or psychotic disorder (Slater, 1965). Unfortunately, a significant number (perhaps 25 percent) of patients who have persistent "conversion" symptoms will later develop an organic disease that, in retrospect, will explain the original symptoms (Watson & Buranen, 1979). The precise diagnosis of conversion versus neurologic disease, thus remains problematic. When major depression is identified as a concurrent disorder, it must be treated. Patients with conversion disorder thus require both a meticulous neurologic assessment (see Chapter 4) and a specific interview to evaluate the possibility of an affective disorder.

Symptoms that are persistent may represent poorly understood organic disease (e.g., certain dystonias previously believed to be due to conversion are now known to have a neurophysiologic organic etiology [Roth, 1980]). Other persistent symptoms are perpetuated by positive reinforcers in the environment, such as family attention or financial benefits from disability. Patients who have persistent symptoms often require intensive diagnostic and therapeutic interventions, including inpatient psychiatric hopsitalization utilizing behavior modification techniques, to extinguish this form of abnormal illness behavior.

Somatization Disorder (Briquet's Syndrome)

The diagnostic term *somatization disorder* is the latest attempt to define the historical concept of "hysteria" (Hyler & Spitzer, 1978). The DSM-III-R diagnostic criteria are, in general, based on the careful phenomenologic research of Guze and colleagues (Guze, 1983) on Briquet's syndrome (or hysteria), a disorder consisting of a chronic, recurrent pattern of multiple somatic (and psychiatric) symptoms beginning before age 30 and associated with multiple hospitalizations and surgical operations. Although somatization disorder is generally regarded as a disorder of women, there have been reports of its existence in men (GR Smith, Monson, & Livingston, 1985). There is a significant correlation of this disorder with antisocial behavior and substance abuse, although these features are not part of the diagnostic criteria. Conservative prevalence estimates range from 0.1 to 0.4 percent for community populations (Robins, Helzer, Weissman, et al., 1984; Swartz, Blazer, George, et al. 1986; Weissman, Myers, & Harding, 1978).

Whether there may be an organic predisposition to somatization remains an interesting speculation. One unconfirmed report suggests a genetic contribution in that a disproportionate number of women with the disorder have type A blood (Rinieris, Stefanis, Lykouras, 1978). Another study reports cerebral dysfunction as determined by neuropsychologic testing (Flor-Henry, Fromm-Auch, Tapper, et al., 1981). Yet another study purports that these patients demonstrate a difference from control subjects in auditory evoked potential responses (Gordon, Kraiuhin, & Meares, 1986). These investigators interpret this finding as a suggestion that somatization disorder is associated with an impaired ability to filter out meaningless afferent stimuli.

Women with somatization disorder often come from chaotic childhood families where instability (e.g., divorce), alcoholism, and sexual abuse were relatively common. Frequently they have had premature, and unsuccessful, excursions into sexual behavior, and marriage, and often they have married alcoholics. The childhood pattern of a chaotic home life has thus been continued. Patients with somatization disorder often present with dramatic physical symptoms that create a sense of urgency in their physicians, probably the reason for the multiple surgical operations, which in

retrospect are usually for questionable indications. There may also be psychiatric symptoms, such as anxiety, depression, or suicidal gestures. Often these patients are impulsive and have problems of substance abuse, especially of analgesics and minor tranquilizers.

The multiplicity of these patients' symptoms may mimic systemic diseases that present with numerous poorly defined physical complaints. Conversely, patients with these diseases may have symptoms misinterpreted as being psychologic in etiology when in fact there is an organic basis or substrate. Examples of physical diseases that must be differentiated from somatization disorders include systemic lupus erythematosis (Hall, Stickney, & Gardner, 1981), systemic mastocytosis (Lewis, 1982), polycystic ovary disease (Orenstein & Raskind, 1983), endometriosis, and dysmenorrhea. A careful workup for physical disease, keeping these and other multisystem diseases in mind, is a necessary component of comprehensive treatment and diagnosis.

From the foregoing it is obvious that the management of these patients is difficult and often very expensive (GR Smith, Monson, & Ray, 1986b). Comorbid psychiatric disorders, particularly panic attacks (Sheehan & Sheehan, 1982a, 1982b), schizophrenia, and major depression (Liskow, Othmer, Penick, et al., 1986), must be considered in taking the history. A caveat, however, is that these patients overendorse all symptoms as a part of their histrionic style, so the physician needs to be suspect of poorly described symptoms and careful not to suggest new or different symptoms to the patient.

A careful psychiatric examination should be undertaken to diagnose these comorbid conditions. A severe, chronic psychotic disorder, such as schizophrenia, if present, should probably be seen as the primary disorder, with somatization disorder seen as a secondary diagnosis. The management, hence, would be first of the schizophrenia, then of the somatization disorder. A patient with somatization disorder and schizophrenia will most likely have the course of a patient with schizophrenia (deteriorating, decreased capacity for and social interactions, etc.), whereas the somatization disorder patient without schizophrenia will have a relatively stable course. Fortunately, the comorbidity of schizophrenia and somatization disorder is not high, ranging from 5 to 8 percent with only one study reporting a high 27 percent (Liskow, Othmer, Penick, et al., 1986). Our unpublished data show that 5 percent of a sample of somatization disorder patients from a primary care clinic also had schizophrenia.

Although somatization disorder is listed in DSM-III-R as an Axis I disorder, for management and treatment purposes it is better conceptualized as an Axis II problem (characterological), in which the patients use somatic symptoms as coping mechanisms during times of stress in their lives. Such a reconceptualization takes into account the patients impulsivity, their susceptability to medication abuse, and the general disorganization of their lives.

From the foregoing it is possible to develop a treatment plan that emphasizes coordinated care by the primary physician, frequent scheduled appointments, and avoidance of medications and procedures except when clearly indicated. Supportive psychotherapy, when available and accepted by the patient, as well as structured assistance with the patient's multiple and genuine life stressors can be helpful. The medical care costs for these patients can be significantly reduced by the implementation of these basic principles of management (GR Smith, Monson, & Ray, 1986b).

This treatment plan emphasizes the management of a chronic disorder rather than proposing a therapeutic intervention that permanently changes behavior. There is little experience that indicates efficiency

of treatment plans that emphasize permanent change. A promising yet-to-be confirmed report (Valko, 1976) indicated that group therapy that emphasized education of behavioral patterns and group confrontation of the use of somatization to deal with life stresses reduce the frequency of both somatic and psychiatric symptoms.

Although somatization disorder is sometimes lumped together with hypochondriasis, as if the two were equivalent, it is important to make certain key distinctions and to take these differences into account in treatment planning. As a rule, hypochondriacs are obsessive, fearful of disease, and emotionally constricted. On the contrary, patients with somatization disorder are dramatic and overly emotional and utilize physical symptoms as a way in which to manipulate the environment. Treatment techniques for the somatization disorder patient need to discourage emotionality and should facilitate alternative coping strategies that employ problem-solving tactics in place of the dramatic use of bodily symptoms (Murphy, 1982).

Somatoform Pain Disorders

The history of this diagnostic entity is that it was originally considered a part of the conversion reaction phenomenon but was split off in DSM-III to become "psychogenic pain disorder" and is now being redefined as "somatoform pain disorder" for DSM-III-R. All pain has a psychogenic component in that the perception of pain is highly influenced by psychologic states such as anxiety. Conversely, most patients who have pain syndromes have at least a nidus of organic dysfunction that may serve to generate some peripheral "painful" stimuli. Most pain syndromes thus contain some component of both organic and psychic influences.

Pain is best viewed from a systems theory perspective (Ford, 1983). The pain may represent an acute strain in the system (e.g., it may signal the emergence of depression or interpersonal conflicts) or, when present for a long time, may serve to maintain the system in a homeostatic manner (e.g., it may determine patterns of behavior within a family or be associated with the maintenance of disability payments). These issues, as well as the evaluation and treatment of somatoform disorders, are reviewed in depth by Stoudemire and Sandhu (1987).

Because of the importance of pain as a symptom throughout all of medicine, it will be dealt with separately in Chapters 16, by Goldberg, Sokol, & Cullen, in Chapter 17, by Houpt.

FACTITIOUS DISORDERS

Factitious illness is that in which patients surreptitiously produces the symptoms themselves. The possibilities for the simulation of disease are almost endless, as demonstrated by the extensive literature in this area. A typical factitious behavior would be the production of fever by self-inoculation of fecal material. As bizarre as such behavior may seem, the majority of patients with factitious illness are neither psychotic nor cognitively impaired. Factitious illness appears to be phenomenologically related to somatization disorder and is probably a more extreme form of abnormal illness behavior along a continuum, of which the other end consists of exaggeration or amplification of somatic symptoms (Nadelson, 1979). Patients with factitious disorders almost always have associated severe personality disorders, usually of the borderline or antisocial type. Because of the severity of the character pathology and these patients' need to deceive (pathologic lying is also a common associated finding), effective treatment is exceptionally difficult; there are few reported successes.

The therapeutic approach to the patient with factitious disease begins with the confrontation of the patient with the physician's knowledge of the behavior. This can be done in a supportive manner that conveys the physician's concern for the patient and willingness to be helpful but at the same time indicates that the behavior is not acceptable and that the illness needs to be redefined as to a behavioral problem instead of a physical illness (Hollender & Hersh, 1970). An offer of help can then be made. When confronted, some patients never admit the factitious nature of their symptoms but stop the behavior, and a few accept a referral to a psychiatrist, but many—perhaps most—merely change physicians or locales, and continue the same deceptive game (Abram & Hollender, 1974). Ethical conflicts arise concerning the propriety of conveying diagnostic information to the new physician without the patient's consent. (Ford & Abernethy, 1981). For those patients who do accept psychiatric treatment, the techniques of psychotherapy are those that would be appropriate for treatment of borderline personalities (Stone, 1977).

Occasionally a patient who displays factitious illness behavior will have an underlying depression. These patients have a better prognosis because depression is a treatable disorder. The case reported by Earle (1986) of a woman with factitious self-inflicted skin lesions had an excellent response to phenelzine.

MALINGERING

Although the motivation of factitious illness is believed to be determined by intrapsychic or interpersonal reasons, the motivation for malingering, by definition, is for some external gain. For example, patients malinger to obtain disability or compensation payments or to avoid conscription into military service.

Malingering is frequently viewed as sociopathic misbehavior (and it is, as is all factitious behavior), but a careful analysis of these patients suggests that it may be far more complex than it appears on the surface. Conscious misbehavior may be motivated by unconscious factors (Schneck, 1970). Such a statement is not an excuse for misbehavior but rather a signal that the skilled clinician should look beyond the presenting symptom for other problems.

Malingering is different from conversion primarily in the *degree* to which the symptom is being consciously produced. In actuality, conversion and malingering are on a continuum. Malingering can serve (as does conversion) as a mask for a more severe underlying problem (Ford, 1983).

When malingering is diagnosed (and, according to Szasz [1956], the "diagnosis" is actually an accusation), then "treatment" can proceed by a variety of means. At times the symptoms may represent overt fraud, and in those situations it is probably best handled by the appropriate legal authorities (Robertson, 1978). At other times, when the difference from conversion is less distinct, then suggestions to the effect that the etiology of the symptom is known and that improvement is expected will effect remarkable "therapeutic" benefit (Kramer, LaPiana, & Appleton, 1979). This may be more effective if done in a face-saving manner for the patient rather than by direct confrontation.

DISABILITY SYNDROMES

Among the most difficult patients to manage, and very expensive to the government or insurance companies, are those who as a result of an injury or disease fail to regain function as productive members of society. Their "disability" continues even when there is no evidence, or minimal evidence, of the persistence of any objective physical findings.

These patients continue to complain of a variety of physical symptoms, especially pain, and no medical intervention proves helpful. The problem of disability is not merely a medical issue, because it is determined by a wide variety of issues, including social, political, and economic factors, in addition to a variety of intrapsychic and interpersonal issues.

The first task in management of a disability syndrome is an accurate diagnosis. What factors are keeping this person from perceiving himself or herself as able to work? To arrive at a meaningful diagnostic formulation it is often necessary to have an extremely wide data base, information that is often out of the purview of the usual medical history. For example: What are the regulations concerning the disability payments? What was the nature of the patient's relationships with employers and supervisors at the time of the accident or illness? What does the spouse want with regard to the patient's employment? Is an attorney or union steward making recommendations or suggestions to the patient with regard to the report of symptoms?

The foregoing highlights the complexity of the issues but should not be interpreted as indicating the futility of attempting to develop an accurate diagnosis. There are several disorders for which a careful interview will establish the diagnosis and for which there are effective treatment interventions. These include major depression, posttraumatic stress disorder, and transient hypochondriacal states. Other syndromes more refractory to therapeutic interventions include the "justice neurosis" (Ramsay, 1939) and the "Humpty Dumpty" syndrome (Ford, 1978).

Treatment of major depression in these patients is the same as for primary major depressives. The treatment of posttraumatic stress disorder involves multiple modalities. Psychotherapy is indicated because the accident or illness has precipitated a crisis. The person may be searching for "a meaning to life" or be faced with the fragility of health and life for the first time. Phobias are common, and the person may be fearful of certain places or activities that reactivate memories of the accident (Berger, 1975). Medical psychotherapy, behavior modification techniques, and psychotropic medications are helpful for these symptoms. A variety of medications, including benzodiazepines, propranolol, and lithium carbonate, have been used, with inconsistent results, to treat these symptoms (Van der Kolk, 1983). Two drugs, however—phenelzine (Hogben, Cornfield, 1981) and imipramine (Burstein, 1984)—may be more specifically efficacious. In the experience of the authors, minor tranquilizers are most efficacious for posttraumatic stress disorder during the period immediately following an acute trauma (days to weeks), when symptoms of acute anxiety predominate. Antidepressant medications, particularly phenelzine, are most useful for prolonged or delayed posttraumatic stress disorders, when symptoms more characteristic of depression are predominant. Transient hypochondriacs in disabled patients is treated with medical psychotherapy as described previously.

With patients for whom the disability represents a "systems problem" in the family, a therapeutic intervention that includes family members may be necessary. For example, a wife who has learned new independence during a husband's illness may be reluctant to give it up and may therefore subtly (and perhaps unconsciously) encourage his continued somatic complaints and perceived disability (Bursten & D'Esopo, 1965). More difficult to treat but not uncommon is the working mother whose disability payments allow her to be at home and yet continue to have an income (Better, Fine, Simison, et al. 1979). Such a situation is a powerful disincentive to return to work.

Readers interested in more extended reviews of the somatoform disorders and associated syndromes are referred to the following references: Barsky & Klerman, 1983; Engel, 1959; Ford, 1983; Ford & Folks, 1985; Nadelson, 1979; Stoudemire, in press; and Stoudemire and Sandhu, 1987.

REFERENCES

Abram HS & Hollender MH (1974). Factitious blood disease. *Southern Medical Journal, 67,* 691–696.

Adler G (1981). The physician and the hypochondriacal patient. *New England Journal of Medicine, 304,* 1394–1396.

American Psychiatric Association (1987). *Diagnostic and statistical manual of mental disorders* (3rd ed revised). Washington, DC.

Barsky AJ & Klerman GL (1983). Hypochondriasis, bodily complaints, and somatic styles. *American Journal of Psychiatry, 140,* 273–283.

Berger JC (1975). Some psychological aspects of industrial injury. *Illinois Medical Journal, 147,* 364–365.

Better SR, Fine PR & Simison D, et al. (1979). Disability benefits as disincentives to rehabilitation. *Milbank Memorial Fund Quarterly: Health and Society, 57,* 412–427.

Bishop ER (1980). Monosymptomatic hypochondriasis. *Psychosomatics, 21,* 731–741.

Bishop ER & Torch EM (1979). Dividing "hysteria": A preliminary investigation of conversion disorder and psycholagia. *Journal of Nervous and Mental Disorders, 167,* 348–356.

Burstein A (1984). Treatment of post traumatic stress disorder with imipramine. *Psychosomatics, 25,* 681–687.

Bursten B & D'Esopo R (1965). The obligation to remain sick. *Archives of General Psychiatry, 12,* 402–407.

Caplan LR & Nadelson T (1980). Multiple sclerosis and hysteria: Lessons learned from their association. *Journal of the American Medical Association, 243,* 2418–2421.

Davidson JRT, Miller RD, Turnbull CD, et al. (1982). Atypical depression. *Archives of General Psychiatry, 39,* 527–534.

Earle J (1986). Factitious skin disease. *General Hospital Psychiatry, 8,* 448–450.

Engel GC (1959). "Psychogenic" pain and the pain prone patient. *American Journal of Medicine, 26,* 899–918.

Farley J, Woodruff RA, & Guze SB (1968). The prevalence of hysteria and conversion symptoms.

British Journal of Psychiatry, 114, 1121–1125.

Flor-Henry P, Fromm-Auch D, Tapper M, et al. (1981). A neuropsychological study of the stable syndrome of hysteria. *Biologic Psychiatry, 16*, 601–626.

Fogel BS & Fretwell M (1985). Reclassification of depression in the medically ill elderly. *Journal of the American Geriatrics Society, 33*(6), 446–448.

Folks DG, Ford CV, & Regan WM (1984). Conversion symptoms in a general hospital. *Psychomatics, 25*, 285–295.

Ford CV (1978). A type of disability neurosis: The "Humpty Dumpty syndrome" *International Journal of Psychiatry in Medicine, 81*, 2815–294.

Ford, CV (1983). *The somatizing disorders: Illness as a way of life.* New York: Elsevier.

Ford CV (1984). Somatizing disorders. In HB Roback (Ed), *Helping patients and their families cope with medical problems* (pp 35–59). San Francisco: Jossey-Bass.

Ford CV (1986). The somatizing disorders. *Psychosomatics, 27*, 327–337.

Ford CV & Abernethy V (1981). Factitious illness: A multidisciplinary consideration of ethical issues. *General Hospital Psychiatry, 3*, 329–336.

Ford CV & Folks DG (1985). Conversion disorders: An overview. *Psychosomatics, 26*, 371–383.

Gordon E, Kraiuhin C, Meares R, et al. (1986). Auditory evoked response potentials in somatization disorder. *Journal of Psychiatric Research, 20*, 237–248.

Guze SB (1983). Studies in hysteria. *Canadian Journal of Psychiatry, 28*, 434–437.

Hall RCW, Stickney SK & Gardner ER (1981). Psychiatric symptoms in patients with systemic lupus erythematosis. *Psychosomatics, 22*, 15–24.

Hogben GL & Cornfield RB (1981). Treatment of traumatic war neurosis with phenelzine. *Archives of General Psychiatry, 38*, 440–445.

Hollender MH & Hersh SP (1970). Impossible consultation made possible. *Archives of General Psychiatry, 23*, 343–345.

Hopkinson G (1973). The psychiatric syndrome of infestation. *Psychiatric Clinics, 6*, 330–345.

Hyler SE & Spitzer RL (1978). Hysteria split asunder. *American Journal of Psychiatry, 135*, 1500–1504.

Jenike M (1984). Successful treatment of dysmorphobia with tranylcipromine. *American Journal of Psychiatry, 141*, 1463–1464.

Katon W (1982). Depression: Somatic symptoms and medical disorders in primary care. *Comprehensive Psychiatry, 23*, 274–287.

Katon W, Kleinman A, & Rosen G (1982a). Depression and somatization: A review (Part 1). *American Journal of Medicine 72*, 127–135.

Katon W, Kleinman A, & Rosen G (1982b). Depres-

sion and somatization: A review (Part 2). *American Journal of Medicine, 72*, 241–247.

Kellner R (1964). Prognosis of treated hypochondriasis. *Acta Psychiatrica Scandinavica, 67*, 69–79.

Kellner R (1982). Psychotherapeutic strategies in hypochondriasis: A clinical study. *American Journal of Psychotherapy, 36*, 146–157.

Kenyon FE (1965). Hypochondriasis: A survey of some historical, clinical and social aspects. *British Journal of Medical Psychology, 38*, 117–133.

Kramer KK, LaPiana FG, & Appleton B (1979). Ocular malingering and hysteria: Diagnosis and management. *Survey of Opthalmology, 24*, 89–96.

Lesse S (1980). Masked depression—the ubiquitous but unappreciated syndrome. *Psychiatry Journal of the University of Ottawa, 5*, 268–273.

Lewis A (1975). The survival of hysteria. *Psychological Medicine, 5*, 9–12.

Lewis RA (1982). Mastocytosis. In JB Wyngaarden & LH Smith (Eds), *Cecil Textbook of Medicine* 16th ed, pp 1819–1820). Philadelphia: WB Saunders.

Lipsitt DR (1970). Medical and psychological characteristics of "crocks". *Psychiatry in Medicine, 1*, 15–25.

Liskow B, Othmer E, Penick C, et al. (1986). Is Briquet's syndrome a heterogenous disorder? *American Journal of Psychiatry, 143*, 626–629.

Merskey H & Buhrich NA (1975). Hysteria and organic brain disease. *British Journal of Medical Psychology, 48*, 359–366.

Munro A (1978). Monosymptomatic hypochondriacal psychosis: A diagnostic entity which may respond to pimozide. *Canadian Psychiatric Association Journal, 23*, 497–500.

Murphy GE (1982). The clinical management of hysteria. *Journal of the American Medical Association, 247*, 2559–2564.

Nadelson T (1979). The Munchausen spectrum (1979). *General Hospital Psychiatry, 1*, 11–17.

Orenstein H & Raskind MA (1983). Polycystic ovary disease in two patients with Briquet's disorder. *American Journal of Psychiatry, 140*, 1202–1204.

Pilowsky I (1970). Primary and secondary hypochondriasis. *Acta Psychiatrica Scandinavica, 47*, 484–509.

Ramsay J (1939). Nervous disorder after injury: Review of 400 cases. *British Medical Journal, 2*, 385–390.

Rinieris PM, Stefanis CN, Lykouras EP, et al. (1978). Hysteria and ABO blood types. *American Journal of Psychiatry, 135*, 1106–1107.

Robertson AJ (1978). Malingering, occupational medicine and the law. *Lancet, 2*, 828–831.

Robins LN, Helzer JE, & Weissman MW et al. (1984). Lifetime prevalence of specific psychiatric disorders in three sites. *Archives of General Psychiatry, 41*, 949–958.

Roth N (1980). Torsion dystonia, conversion hysteria, and occupational cramps. *Comprehensive Psychiatry, 21*, 292–301.

Schmale AH (1969). Somatic expressions and consequences of conversion reactions. *New York State Medical Journal, 69*, 1878–1884.

Schneck JM (1970). Pseudomalingering and Leonid Andreyeus' "The Dilemma"? *Psychiatric Questions, 44*, 49–54.

Sheehan DV & Sheehan KH (1982a). The classification of anxiety and hysterical states: 1. Historical review and empirical delineation. *Journal of Clinical Psychopharmacology, 2*, 235–244.

Sheehan DV & Sheehan KH (1982b). The classification of anxiety and hysterical states: 2. Toward a more heuristic classification. *Journal of Clinical Psychopharmacology, 2*, 386–393.

Slater E (1965). Diagnosis of hysteria. *British Medical Journal, 1*, 1395–1399.

Smith GR, Monson RA, & Livingston RL (1985). Somatization disorders in men. *General Hospital Psychiatry, 7*, 4–8.

Smith GR, Monson RA, & Ray DC (1986a). Patients with multiple unexplained symptoms: Their characteristics, functional health, and health care utilization. *Archives of Internal Medicine, 146*, 69–72.

Smith GR, Monson RA, & Ray DC (1986b). Psychiatric consultation in somatization disorder: A randomized controlled in somatization disorder: A randomized controlled study. *New England Journal of Medicine, 314*, 1407–1413.

Smith, RC (1985). A clinical approach to the somatizing patient. *Journal of Family Practice, 21*, 294–301.

Stone MH (1977). Factitious illness: Psychological findings and treatment recommendations. *Bulletin of the Menninger Clinic, 3*, 239–254.

Stoudemire A (in press). Somatoform disorders, factitious disorders and malingering, in J Talbott, R Hales, & S Yudofsky (eds.) *Textbook of Psychiatry*. Washington DC: American Psychiatric Press.

Stoudemire A & Sandhu J (1987). Psychogenic/idiopathic pain syndromes. *General Hospital Psychiatry, 9*, 79–86.

Sullivan HS (1953). *The interpersonal theory of psychiatry*. New York: WW Norton & Co.

Swartz M, Blazer D, George L, et al. (1986). Somatization disorder in a community population. *American Journal of Psychiatry, 143*, 1403–1408.

Szsaz TS (1956). Malingering: "Diagnosis" or social condemnation. *Archives of Neurological Psychiatry, 76*, 432–443.

Valko, RJ (1976). Group therapy for patients with hysteria (Briquet's disorder). *Diseases of the Nervous System, 37*, 484–487.

Van der Kolk BA (1983). Pharmacological issues in posttraumatic stress disorder. *Hospital and Community Psychiatry, 34*, 683–684.

Veith I (1965). *Hysteria: The history of a disease*. Chicago: University of Chicago Press.

Wahl, CW (1964). Psychodynamics of the hypochondriacal patient. In *New Dimensions in Psychosomatic Medicine* (pp 201–214). Boston: Little, Brown.

Watson CG & Buranen C (1979). The frequency and identification of false positive conversion reactions. *Journal of Nervous and Mental Disease, 167*, 243–247.

Weissman, MM, Myers JK, & Harding PS (1978). Psychiatric disorders in a U.S. urban community: 1975–1976. *American Journal of Psychiatry, 135*, 459–462.

Whitlock F (1967). The aetiology of hysteria. *Acta Psychiatrica Scandanavia, 43*, 144–162.

Ziegler F, Imsoden J, & Meyer E (1960). Contemporary conversion reactions: A clinical study. *American Journal of Psychiatry, 116*, 901–909.

Lucy Davidson

9
Suicide and Violence in the Medical Setting

No form of treatment is effective with a dead patient.
R. S. Mintz

Violence, whether self-inflicted (suicidal) or interpersonal, assails our therapeutic efforts. Intentional destructiveness by patients can exact a high toll in injury and death. The destructive patient endangers more than the immediate physical well-being of himself or others. Even if only a trivial physical injury occurs, the therapeutic collaboration among patient, physician, and other health care professionals is disrupted. The patient may break off treatment precipitously, or the physician may unconsciously retaliate in ways that drive the patient away. Witnessing or hearing about the violence may exacerbate other patients' illnesses. Confidence in the physician's ability to heal and protect may suffer. Medical staff who have been the object of an assault may be psychologically disabled by it and may have extraordinary difficulty caring for other patients or recovering from their own physical injuries. A patient's suicide or suicide attempt exposes the physician's own fears of inadequacy. When these conflicts are rekindled, ability to appropriately attend to patient needs suffers.

The prospect of malpractice litigation for physician liability can be debilitating in itself.

Physicians clearly are motivated to prevent violence and these harmful sequelae. Moreover, the opportunity for physician–patient contact should make suicide and interpersonal violence in the medical setting especially preventable. Even with the desire to "never do harm to anyone" and the opportunity to forestall destructive behavior, often very little effective prevention occurs. This chapter will identify characteristics of patients at high risk for violence and situations in the medical setting in which violence is likely to occur and will describe techniques for interviewing, stabilization, and support to reduce the likelihood of violence. Frequently psychiatric consultation is initiated because of violent or potentially violent confrontation. The intervention and prevention activities discussed are designed to restore the patient and staff to a therapeutic relationship as rapidly as possible. Although self-directed and interpersonal vio-

PRINCIPLES OF MEDICAL PSYCHIATRY
ISBN 0-8089-1883-4

219

lence are closely related, they will be discussed separately, beginning with suicide.

SUICIDAL PATIENTS

Assessing the Suicidal Patient

A suicide is a self-inflicted, intentional death. A suicide attempt is a nonlethal self-inflicted act that has as its intended purpose death or the appearance of willingness to die.

How does the psychiatrist assess suicide potential? As Bakwin (1957) said, "the sole approach to the . . . suicide problem lies in recognizing beforehand the susceptible individuals and in their proper management." Four general categories of data are weighed in assessing suicidality: (1) personal risk factors, (2) environmental and situational factors, (3) psychodynamic meaning, and (4) information from the mental status examination.

Epidemiology and Risk Factors

Suicide has become the eighth leading cause of death among Americans and the second leading cause among youth. Epidemiologic data help to profile high-risk groups. White males have the highest rates of any race or sex group and account for 70 percent of all suicide deaths in the United States. Suicide rates decrease in the following order among race and sex groups: white males (70 percent), white females (22 percent), black and other males (6 percent), and black and other females (2 percent). Some tribes of native Americans have astoundingly high suicide rates, but rates vary markedly among tribes. The ratio of male to female suicides is about 3:1 overall, increasing to 5:1 for youth (Centers for Disease Control, 1985).

The proportion of suicides among youth 15–24 years old has increased in the last three decades while decreasing among older adults. Male suicide rates are now bimodally distributed, with peaks in the young adult years and in old age. Rates for females peak in midlife. The lifetime suicide risk among persons with mood disorders, schizophrenia, or substance abuse is increased. The lifetime risk is estimated at 10 percent for schizophrenics and at 15 percent for persons with mood disorders (Miles, 1977). Among affectively disordered patients, those who commit suicide show these differentiating clinical features: hopelessness, loss of pleasure or interest, and loss of reactivity. Patients who complete suicide have fewer preceding episodes of affective disorder than affectively disordered patients who have not committed suicide (Fawcett, Scheftner, Clark, et al., 1987). This suggests that suicide may occur fairly early in the course of the disease for persons with mood disorders.

In contrast to the situation for patients with mood disorders, suicide is a relatively late complication of alcoholism (Rob-ins, 1981). One of the few long-term follow-up studies of alcoholics is that of Ojesjo (1981), who found that 12 percent of alcoholics committed suicide. Medical examiner data show that nearly 20 percent of suicides are alcohol abusers and 25 percent of suicides have a positive blood alcohol concentration at death (Riddick & Luke, 1978).

Alcoholics who committed suicide have been compared with living alcoholics, highlighting factors that increased the alcoholics' susceptibility to suicide. More of the alcoholic suicides were divorced or widowed. A history of previous suicide attempts was obtained for 67 percent of the alcoholic suicides versus 10 percent of the controls. When compared with nonalcoholic suicides, more alcoholic suicides had made an overt suicide threat, and more had seen a psychiatrist or other doctor in the week before death (Barraclough, Bunch, Nelson, et al., 1974).

Of alcoholic patients with bipolar disorder, 80 percent had attempted suicide versus 13 percent of nonalcoholic bipolar patients (Johnson & Hunt, 1979). Of persons admitted for alcoholism treatment, 27 percent had made a previous suicide attempt, and 12 percent had current suicidal ideation (Beck, Steer, & McElroy, 1982). In another series, 15 percent of alcoholics who died from all causes had a history of suicide attempt (Choi, 1975).

We tend to think of the typical suicide as a depressed, elderly white male who abuses alcohol, is in poor health, and has experienced a recent emotional loss. Risk factors for adult suicides may not, however, be prototypes for youth suicides. Depression, while still an important risk factor, is less common among youth suicides. Youth suicides are often impulsive acts, and the suicidal youth often fits into the diagnostic spectrum of conduct disorders.

A family history of suicide increases risk, both genetically and through role modeling (Egeland & Sussex, 1985). Persons who have ever attempted suicide are also at increased risk. Married persons are less susceptible to suicide than are the never-married, widowed, or divorced. Suicides are more common in urban than rural areas, and rates vary by region of the country. Rates peak in the western United States. Gunshot is the most frequent method of suicide in this country for men and women of all ages, providing an immediately lethal means (Centers for Disease Control, 1985). Though one cannot dismiss the possibility of suicide in a 30-year-old, married black woman simply because she doesn't fit the epidemiologic profile of the high-risk patient, the patient who is at risk epidemiologically should be seen as at risk clinically.

Environmental and Situational Factors

Environmental and situational factors offer clues to suicidal intent. Most suicidal persons express their intent to die either directly or indirectly. The myth of "talkers" versus "doers" provides false reassurance at the expense of lives. Suicidal persons may tell others, "You'd be better off without me," or, "It just doesn't seem worth it." The term *suicide threat* connotes manipulation and histrionic confrontation. The threat may, however, be a very matter-of-fact conclusion, "I'm going to kill myself."

More indirect indications of intent to die include expressions of hopelessness and intolerable pain (physical or emotional). Patients may give away cherished possessions or put things in order and make wills at a time out of context for their life situation and medical prognosis. They may rehearse fatal behavior in a tentative way, imagining what it would be like to hang or suffocate themselves. They may contact significant people to say last good-byes (CDC, 1986).

Some time periods are high-risk periods for suicide. The recovery period from a major depression or schizophrenic break juxtaposes increasing energy and organization to carry out a fatal act with increasing insight and despair over the effects of illness. Bereavement is also a period of heightened risk, especially if the decedent committed suicide. The term *suicide contagion* has been used to describe a series of suicides in which one death appears to influence another, probably through identification and modeling. Reported clusters of such suicides, especially among youth, have received widespread media attention recently. The time period surrounding an ongoing cluster of these suicides or around intense media attention to a real or fictional suicide story constitutes a high-risk period for suceptible individuals (Davidson & Gould, in press).

Family and other social supports may be a protective factor, and their absence may be an indication of increasing isolation, alienation, and withdrawal leading to suicide. Self-destructive feelings are transient, and even completed suicides represent a fatal outcome of an ambivalent state.

The availability of social supports may provide auxiliary emotional resources to bridge the time period of intense suicidality.

The family interview complements the patient interview in the management of the suicidal patient. The depressed stroke patient who has 11 children and adult grandchildren who arrive promptly for a family conference is less at risk than the blind man whose seething wife drops him off for hospitalization because she is worried he might hurt himself with the gun she does not know how to hide. Families can provide the information patients edit from their interviews with the doctor. Willing family members can also store and administer medications, remove dangerous materials from the household, transport patients to appointments, and convey by their interest and involvement that the patient's situation is not hopeless.

More disturbed families may communicate that the patient is expendable. The patient may have already exhausted the family's resources, and the family may present him to the hospital to be relieved of their burden. Even well-meaning families have unrealistic expectations of psychiatric treatment. The patient and family may benefit from plain talk about the time course of psychiatric treatment and its limitations in affecting behavior. This gentle disillusionment is particularly relevant for the chronically suicidal patient's family, who wishes that the psychiatrist could assume responsibility for the patient's life.

Psychodynamic Factors

In considering psychodynamic factors, the psychiatrist examines the meaning of suicide in the light of the patient's ego strengths, patterns of defense, and fantasies. No single paradigm accurately reconstructs the psychic function of suicidal impulses and behavior for all patients. Nonetheless, loss is a predominant theme. Loss may be either tangible (the death of a pet) or intangible (a blow to self-esteem). The loss may be actual or threatened. Understanding the immediate loss in its genetic context, the patient's defensive strategies in coping with loss, and the function of loss in the patient's fantasies is useful in determining probable outcomes for the patient and possible interventions. A suicide attempt and its sequelae may, in effect, make some restoration or restitution for loss, and this can be a major determinant in assessing what's next for the patient.

Classically, suicide is viewed as retroflexed rage—taking revenge on an internalized bad object (Menninger, 1933). The suicide may be an effort to punish significant others or to express hostility that would be socially prohibited towards others. Some suicides and attempts are most usefully viewed as a cry for help. Persons, for example, who cannot tolerate dependency needs or cannot express needs for affection may enact these needs self-destructively. Other people can never be totally responsible for preventing a patient's suicide, and whatever intervention is planned must reestablish the patient's internal impulse control. Understanding the psychic meaning of suicide for the particular patient is central in this transition.

The Mental Status Examination

The mental status exam identifies the psychotic patient whose reality testing is impaired, perhaps even to the extent of responding to self-destructive command hallucinations or delusions. Typically, though, data from the mental status exam are used to assess more subtle impairments of insight and judgment. A patient may present a rational, intellectualized discourse on the logic of committing suicide or the reasons he would never commit suicide. The patient's conclusions, however, may reflect as much impairment of insight and judgment as a schizophrenic's disordered thinking. Ability to establish rapport with the interviewer also contributes to the psychiatrist's impression that the patient could contact the physician if feeling overwhelmed by suicidal impulses, avail himself of proffered supports, or keep a follow-up appointment. Clinical judgment about the presence of treatable psychiatric illnesses, such as depression, that predispose to suicide is grounded in the mental status exam as well as the history. Murphy has documented the physicians' errors of omission in neglecting to examine the patient for depression (Murphy, 1975).

The Chronically Suicidal Patient

Chronic self-destructiveness and suicidality occur among patients with borderline personality organization, whose day-to-day functioning is frequently impulsive and whose dramatic attempts to control others may be enacted with lethal props. Kernberg (1984) points out that the risk of suicide is high throughout an episode of affective illness for these patients, instead of being specifically heightened during the recovery stage, as in patients with an Axis I disorder only. "Patients who simultaneously display general impulsivity, dishonesty, chronic self-mutilating tendencies, alcohol and/or drug abuse, and a profound interpersonal aloofness or emotional unavailability may develop suicidal behavior at any time" (Kernberg, 1984).

Clinical management of these patients includes immediate hospitalization when a major affective illness or psychotic syndrome is superimposed. Psychopharmacologic or electroconvulsive treatment is imperative. The patient's bland denial of suicidal intent and indifferent or devaluing attitude toward the therapist heightens the risk of suicide; the patient's communication is dishonest, either consciously or through splitting and denial. Kernberg's (1984) treatment recommendations include the following:

1. Confronting patients with their behavior patterns and their effect on others
2. Refusing to carry out treatment under circumstances that would cripple it, such as the patient's refusing integral components (medication, family involvement, regular sessions)
3. Continuing open and direct communication, which does not ignore the angry and manipulative aspects of the patient's life-style and through which the therapist's interpretations consistently explore suicidality
4. Diagnosing and controlling secondary gains of suicidal behavior, especially as the patient may attempt to dominate and control the family and the therapist
5. Communicating to the patient that the therapist "would feel sad but not responsible if the patient killed himself and that his life would not be significantly affected by such an event" (Kernberg, 1984)
6. Communicating the patient's chronic suicide risk to the family and realistically limiting the therapist's role in changing such behavior

Suicidal Patients in the Emergency Room and on the Medical-Surgical Ward

The most pressing consideration in the evaluation of the suicidal patient in the emergency room is to protect the patient from immediate self-harm. The patient should not be left alone, even momentarily, until the interviewer is convinced that the patient is not immediately suicidal (Bassuk, 1984). The interviewing area should not offer any easily accessible means of suicide, such as breakable windows, cigarette lighters, cleaning or pharmaceutical supplies, electric cords and window sashes, curtain or closet rods, or plastic trash can liners (Litman & Farberow, 1970).

In the emergency evaluation, the psychiatrist should not ask abruptly, "Are you suicidal?" Patients who feel that things are hopeless, wish they were dead, and yet have no concrete plan may answer no, precluding a thorough assessment of their suicidal ideation. They don't see themselves as suicidal because they aren't planning an immediate attempt. General inquiries such as, "How bad do you feel?" allow a natural progression to questions about hopelessness, wishing to be dead, wishing to harm oneself, wishing to die, and any details of plans and opportunities (Sletten & Barton, 1979). If the interviewer proceeds in an empathic, nonjudgmental way, the patient is more likely to be able to confide details of suicidal thoughts or plans. This approach provides data for the psychiatrist's clinical judgment instead of asking the patient to render a summary judgment of his suicidality.

Patient characteristics that make outpatient management reasonable are evidence of satisfactory impulse control, absence of psychosis or intoxication, absence of a specific plan and readily accessible means, presence of social supports, and ability to establish rapport with the interviewer. If the suicidal patient is not being admitted, the interviewer should set a definite follow-up appointment with some treatment provider. Nonspecific treatment referrals to the county mental health clinic or instructions to contact a psychiatrist are ineffectual. Calling the patient back to check those arrangements increases the likelihood of compliance.

Among those at increased risk of suicide in the hospital are patients admitted for injuries sustained in attempted suicide. The percentage of suicide attempters who kill themselves while hospitalized for their attempt is 0.2 percent (Glickman, 1980). Hospital policy usually provides that a psychiatrist be called to evaluate persons seen in the emergency room or admitted for intentional self-inflicted injuries. Determining whether the attempter should be discharged

to outpatient care or transferred to the psychiatry service when medically cleared is often a pressing decision.

A request to see a recently extubated self-poisoning patient, who is demanding to go home and whose doctor needs an intensive care unit (ICU) bed for the next admission forces the issue. If the patient is no longer appropriate for the medical-surgical service and the psychiatric evaluation cannot yet be thorough enough to determine present suicidality, then psychiatric hospitalization is imperative. A patient who has ingested a large dose of a long-half-life drug, such as diazepam, may be stable metabolically and out of danger of respiratory depression long before the drug's psychotropic effects have dissipated. The massive anxiety that precipitated the attempt may thus be masked. A period of psychiatric hospitalization for evaluation also allows time to meet with family members and significant others to provide a more reliable assessment of the patient's support systems.

Attempters who survive construct a rationale for their actions (Kiev, 1975). The physician who uncritically accepts this post hoc construction may mistakenly trivialize the attempt, consider it a "gesture," and dismiss serious suicidal behavior. The survivor's embarrassed denial of suicidal intent cannot be taken in lieu of a more thoughtful assessment of suicidality. Understanding the meaning of the attempt in its intrapsychic and interpersonal contexts provides a much sounder basis for assessing the patient's capacity to survive as an outpatient. In many instances this assessment may not be possible in the time and milieu available on the medical-surgical ward.

For some patients, transfer to the psychiatric service may be therapeutic in indirect ways. The transfer may convey the seriousness of the patient's actions to the patient and family in ways that underscore the need for continued treatment or that mobilize support systems. Patients may channel their rage toward the transferring physician or staff so that the vector of that rage is redirected from self-destructive injury to verbally expressed anger toward an external object.

Many suicide attempters have been in some form of psychotherapy. Inpatient psychiatric hospitalization may be indicated to evaluate that therapy, its possible role in precipitating the suicide attempt, and the configuration of therapies best suited to the patient's needs after discharge. The apparent attractiveness of discharging patients directly from the medical-surgical ward because they have ongoing psychiatric treatment to go back to is specious. The patient in therapy who has acted out self-destructive impulses has at least temporarily exceeded the patient–therapist capacity for working on those impulses. Analyzing these limitations of the patient, the therapist, and their interaction while the patient is hospitalized can allow the therapy to be restructured or permit different therapeutic arrangements to be made.

Some facilities offer the option of admitting suicidal patients to a medical-psychiatric unit, which allows more intensive psychiatric intervention than consultation can generally provide. Patients most appropriately managed on the medical-psychiatric unit are motivated for inpatient treatment and combine an organic physical disorder needing attention with a treatable Axis I disorder. Patients with severe personality disorders tend to do poorly on the medical-psychiatric unit because the milieu usually is not set up to control their limit testing and acting out.

With intensely suicidal patients, no environmental arrangements are sufficient deterrents. The patient must be under constant observation, even while toileting. Although environmental controls alone cannot prevent suicide, attention to these details reduces risk. The physician may leave orders for "suicide precautions," yet the patient may be receiving antibiotics in a glass bottle piggybacked to intravenous fluids or be lying in arm's reach of a glass window. The trash can may have a plastic liner suitable for asphyxiation. The meal tray may arrive with cutlery. The patient's roommate may have betadine, bandage scissors, shampoo, cologne, and a cigarette lighter on the beside table. The patient may cheek his medications and stockpile a lethal dose.

Aggressive diagnosis and treatment of underlying psychiatric disorders, environmental safety, and constant observation are the keys to managing the suicidal patient in the general hospital. Electroconvulsive therapy is the treatment of choice for the severely depressed and imminently suicidal patient. Necessary medications can be given in elixir form or by injection, both to ensure that the patient takes them and to prevent stockpiling.

The psychiatric unit generally provides an architecturally safer environment, with Plexiglas windows, break-away curtain rods, and locked storage of sharp and toxic materials. Hanging is nonetheless an almost universally available method of suicide. It does not require suspension from a high place, only kneeling and leaning forward with any sort of ligature around the neck. Even on the psychiatric unit, the imminently suicidal patient, open to employing any accessible lethal means, requires constant, one-to-one nursing.

Less intensive suicide prevention measures work on the basis of restricting access to immediately lethal methods and providing frequent staff contact to serve as auxiliary ego controls and to frequently reassess the patient's condition. This arrangement conveys that the hospital takes the patient's suicidal ideation seriously and will assist the patient in controlling his suicidal impulses. It assumes that the patient is ambivalent enough about killing himself to collaborate in these arrangements.

Treatment of the Suicidal Outpatient

Most persons with suicidal ideation are treated as outpatients. Pharmacotherapy of their underlying psychiatric disorders, though, may involve medications, such as tricyclic antidepressants, that are a readily lethal means of suicide. Amitriptyline is the most frequently ingested medication in suicide by overdose. Limiting tricyclics to 1200 mg total in a nonrefillable precription may help reduce deaths from antidepressant overdose. Limiting the prescription size should not be confused with limiting the dose. Homeopathic doses of tricyclics prescribed by overly tentative physicians increase the risk of suicide by leaving the patient's depression pharmacologically untreated. Sedative-hypnotic and anxiolytic drugs can also be lethal, especially combined with alcohol. Diazepam is the third most frequently ingested medication in suicide by overdose (Davidson, 1985).

The shift from barbiturate prescribing to more specific treatment of depression with antidepressants was associated with a steady decline in overdose suicide rates (Whitlock, 1975). The household pharmacy can be reduced by treating affective disorders and psychoses specifically, rather than with various sedative-hypnotics and anxiolytics, and by recommending disposal of old medications. A reliable family member can administer medications, and frequent office visits should be scheduled to assess patient response and suicidality. Outpatient electroconvulsive therapy or injectable neuroleptics are options when outpatient drug treatment appears to put the patient at excessive risk of lethal overdose.

Other Medical-Surgical Patients at High Risk

Cancer patients are regarded as a group at higher risk for suicide. Although patients hear the diagnosis cancer as less of a death knell now than it was in the past, cancer is still fearfully associated with pain, disfigurement, and loss of function. In the vulnerable patient, any of these may precipitate suicide. The physician's impression that it is normal to be depressed if one has cancer ("Well, I'd be depressed too if I had . . . ") may leave treatment-responsive major depression untreated and thereby increase the likelihood of suicide (see also Chapters 2 and 23).

The risk of suicide among cancer patients has been calculated from the Finnish Cancer Registry. Suicide was 1.3 times higher among male and 1.9 times higher among female cancer patients than in the general population. Patients with nonlocalized cancers had twice the risk of suicide as those with localized cancers, and gastrointestinal cancer patients had the highest relative risk. Those patients who underwent traditional surgical or radiation therapy were not at increased risk of suicide, but the suicide risk among patients receiving other or no specific treatment was significantly elevated (Louhivuori & Hakama, 1979). This latter group included patients receiving steroid therapy as well as those who committed suicide before any treatment could be initiated.

These findings are consistent with the hypothesis that cancer patients with better prognoses may be less likely to commit suicide. Even terminally ill cancer patients, however, have been reported *not* to wish to die unless they are also clinically depressed (Brown, Henteleff, Barakat, et al., 1986). Being suicidal or wishing for an early death was associated with the presence of clinical depression in the patients studied, not with the severity of their physical illness, since all were terminally ill, were aware of their prognosis, and had severe pain, disfigurement, or disability. Feeling suicidal is thus not inevitably part of the natural course of terminal illness.

Retrospectively comparing cancer patients who have committed suicide with nonsuicidal hospital controls highlights some of the situational variables that may cue the physician to suicidality besides depression (Farberow, Shneidman, & Leonard, 1963). The suicidal patients had been overly involved in their treatment, with behaviors perceived as controlling, complaining, and demanding. They were less tolerant of pain and more likely to feel that their physical and emotional resources were depleted. These needy and insistent patients may exhaust the responsiveness of their caregivers. Yet, such patients are acutely sensitive to withdrawal of contact or interest by others. Transfer to a private room to die exemplifies the type of environmental change that may be perceived as rejection and culminate in suicide.

Farberow, Shneidman, and Leonard (1970) emphasized the power of suicidal intent over physical frailty or motor limitations. The patient's deteriorating behavioral patterns or more overt suicidal communications have to be taken seriously and not discounted because of the patient's debilitated physical state. In their series, one partially paralyzed patient was immobilized in a Stryker frame and still committed suicide by self-immolation after dousing himself with lighter fluid. Clearly, when suicidal intent is strong, one cannot assume that physical limitations will prevent a suicide attempt.

The insistent, complaining, and controlling cancer patients who committed suicide were in a treatment setting that radically opposed their lifelong character structures. Once such potentially suicidal patients are identified, therapy may be initiated that (1) treats underlying depression or other concurrent psychiatric disorder, (2) reestablishes social and emotional supports, and (3) reestablishes the patient's sense of control. For some terminal patients, psychotherapy provides an arena for actively confronting the personal psychic meaning of their cancer and thus reestablishing emotional potency despite physical deterioration (Leigh, 1974). The psychia-

trist's acknowledgment that suicide remains an option for the patient, although not condoning it or accepting it as "rational," may help some patients regain their feelings of autonomy sufficiently to work toward other goals. Reestablishing purpose for oneself takes many forms; for example, one has been that of educating the doctor about the feelings and experiences of approaching death.

Hemodialysis patients are another high-risk group for suicide because of the characteristics of their illness. Their suicide rates are extraordinarily high. Including those whose suicide is effected by discontinuation of dialysis or intentionally fatal breaches of the treatment regimen, rates are up to 400 times that of the general population (Abram, Moore, & Westervelt, 1971; Haenel, Brunner, & Battegay, 1980). About 5 percent of dialysis patients commit suicide. Suicidal behavior is more common among patients attending dialysis centers than those on home dialysis.

Reasons for suicide among these patients are legion. The quality of life on dialysis is significantly impaired. Losses associated with this change in physical health are major threats, such as job loss and social isolation (Dorpat, Anderson, & Ripley, 1968). The loss in transplant failure may even exceed that in initiating dialysis and precipitate severe depression. As with the suicidal cancer patient, the chronic hemodialysis patient may act as though the locus of control were primarily external (Goldstein & Reznikoff, 1971). Death is an ever-present possibility. Those for whom the fearfulness and anxiety attendant to death are intolerable may defend against death through reaction formation and, paradoxically, commit suicide (Dorpat, Anderson, & Ripley, 1968). Ready access to lethal methods also contributes to the dialysis patient's likelihood of suicide. Disconnecting a shunt, severing the arteriovenous fistula, or inducing hyperkalemia through food binges are quite common. These methods particular to dialysis may also express the patient's conflict symbolically.

The dialysis patient without psychologic problems attendant to the illness is so rare that recommendations for suicide prevention in this special population emphasize the need for universal, ongoing psychologic support (Abram, Moore, & Westervelt, 1971; Haenel, Brunner, & Battegay, 1980). Although crises occur at nodal points in dialysis treatment, the severity of ongoing stresses for this patient population is so great that attempts to initiate treatment amidst crises are much less likely to succeed. Lethal impulses are too readily enacted, and the sum of previous losses rekindled by the current crisis may be too overwhelming (see Chapter 27).

Other medical-surgical patients at high risk for suicide are those in alcohol withdrawal delirium (delirium tremens), particularly if they are inadequately sedated (Kellner, Best, Roberts, et al., 1985). Additionally, patients with severe personality disorders may make suicide attempts when the organic basis of their medical symptoms is challenged (Reich & Kelly, 1976). Patients with respiratory diseases have also been reported to be overrepresented among hospital suicides (Baker, 1984). Whether their relative anoxia, progressive incapacity, or some other factor accounts for their increased suicide risk is unknown. Ongoing evaluation of medical-surgical patients' emotional status can detect potentially suicidal patients who did not suggest psychiatric concern on admission but have developed intense reactions to pain, unbridled fears of death, or clouded consciousness impairing reason (Pollack, 1957).

Countertransference to the Suicidal Patient

Acutely and chronically suicidal patients mobilize countertransference responses that can exacerbate their self-destructiveness. The frustration, peril, and feelings of helplessness their treatment can entail can evoke hatred in the therapist. This countertransference hatred is projected and then felt as dread that the patient will commit suicide (Maltsberger & Buie, 1974).

A psychiatrist's self-image as a physician is challenged by suicidal patients who do not respond to therapeutic interventions. If feelings of personal worth are attached to the ability to cure, rather than the ability to exercise one's best professional skills, the psychiatrist will feel increasingly unhappy and inadequate in working with suicidal patients (Maltsberger & Buie, 1974). The patient's sadism fuels lethal behavior when the patient perceives that the therapist has established an image as a "model of omnipotent goodness" (Zee, 1972).

VIOLENT PATIENTS

Homicide is the 11th leading cause of death for Americans and *the* leading cause for blacks 15–34 years old. Nearly half of all homicide victims knew the perpetrator, with 33 percent of homicides involving friends and acquaintances and 16 percent being within families. Firearms are the weapons used in 64 percent of all homicides. Most homicide victims are males (76 percent), and a disproportionate percentage (44 percent) are black or members of other minority groups. In 1980, 1.6 million incidents of aggravated assault were reported, and at least 355,500 victims were hospitalized. Males 20–24 years old are at highest risk of victimization. Interpersonal violence is associated with other mental health concerns; battered women are at higher risk of alcoholism and attempted suicide (Rosenberg & Mercy, 1985).

Interpersonal violence is a major public health problem. The perpetrators of violence outside the hospital have illnesses and injuries that make them our patients, too. Hospitalization is always stressful and represents a setting in which physical and verbal assaults may erupt.

Interpersonal Violence in the Medical-Surgical Setting

Instances of interpersonal violence among hospitalized medical and surgical patients are relatively uncommon but of great consequence. Like self-destructive patients, those who are violent towards others are overrepresented in certain diagnostic groups and in particular clinical contexts. Most typical is the male substance-abusing patient admitted for a complication of his drug use, such as cellulitis or endocarditis. This patient chafes at hospital rules, has escalating demands for pain medication, and loses control of his violent impulses. When violent patients were compared with nonviolent controls, the violent patients had longer hospital stays. The most likely time for violence to erupt was between seven P.M. and seven A.M. Prior documented threats were uncommon, but patients who later became violent had been perceived as uncooperative (Ochitill & Krieger, 1982).

To maintain his dependency, the drug abuser must be a rule breaker; so the usual hospital rules and regulations represent major sources of conflict. The hospital is an alien environment, and particular difficulties may arise at the end of visiting hours when the substance abuser does not want his friends to leave. Challenging the reality of the patient's pain can provoke violence. Substance abusers are often undermedicated for pain, especially if the physician assumes that a maintenance dose of methadone will block pain or that the half-life of pain medication for these patients will be as long as for nonabusers. Drugs are the way the patient treats his emotional problems, and the hospital situation exacerbates his problems while preventing access to his

usual remedy. Avoiding unnecessary confrontation and maintaining a sufficient pain-control regimen reduces the likelihood of violence among substance abusers (see Chapter 11).

Patients may be precipitously violent during confusional states. Regulating sensory stimuli, treating the underlying medical condition, and preserving sleep are helpful. Organic or brain-injured patients may increasingly rely on one or two staff members to organize tasks of daily living and attend to their needs. When those caregivers are away for extended periods or busy with others, patients can feel increasingly anxious and helpless, leading to fight–flight responses (Armstrong, 1978). Delirium from acute alcohol withdrawal is a medical condition that may be unsuspected in the surgical patient. The postoperative course begins benignly, but increasing agitation and irritability later explode in violence. Among general hospital patients, those with identified psychiatric disorders are infrequently violent. This may reflect the benefit of psychiatric consultation usually requested early in the hospital stay.

Hospitalization affords little privacy. Diagnostic procedures and room arrangements put patients physically closer to others than many would choose to be. Kinzel (1970) has identified a "body-buffer zone," which is the unpeopled space around oneself perceived necessary for emotional safety. This perimeter is larger for violent persons and is configured with greater distance behind than in front. The paranoid male, fearful of homosexual assault, may develop unbearable anxiety in crowded hospital situations and may explode violently.

Hospital boredom may also be intolerable to those character-disordered patients who feel empty when they are unstimulated. Verbal explosions, assaults, and self-destructive behaviors are pathologic responses that disperse the emptiness and reestablish a sense of reality (Kalogerakis, 1971).

Emergency Evaluation of and Response to Interpersonal Violence

Patients who present with fears of becoming violent require immediate evaluation. Many physicians are reluctant to take a history that inquires specifically about violence and available weapons. Hesitation in approaching the potentially violent patient may be assuaged if one's perspective is that "patients who experience violent impulses desperately want help in curbing such urges. Violent patients are terrified of losing control and welcome therapeutic efforts that restore a sense of control and prevent them from acting on their urges" (Lion & Pasternack, 1973).

The patient who is pacing in the waiting room or sitting on the edge of the chair gripping the armrests, who is hypervigilant and easily startled, and who cannot respond to a quiet offer of food or the invitation to talk requires immediate external controls (Lion, Bach-y-Rita, & Ervin, 1969). If the patient will take medication by mouth, anxiolytics or oral-concentrate neuroleptics should be given. Injections create their own problems with fears of homosexual penetration or bodily assault. When necessary, though, intramuscular neuroleptics, lorazepam or amobarbital sodium, rapidly help the patient shift away from fight–flight responses.

Medicating the Violent Patient

Rapid tranquilization requires close observation of the patient so that the medication can be titrated to an appropriate end point. Patients whose extreme agitation is relieved as quickly as possible without somnolence are less likely to feel that they have been chemically abused. Obtunding the patient is not the same as relieving anxiety and agitation sufficiently for the patient to talk, rest, or sleep. Most cases of psychotic agitation and paranoid intoxication, such as with PCP, cocaine, or amphetamines, respond to neuroleptics, for example, haloperidol, 5–10 mg oral concentrate or intramuscular injection every 30 minutes. Chlorpromazine, 50–100 mg, has been widely used but is more sedating and more likely to be dose-limited by orthostatic hypotension. Alternatives for patients with a history or symptoms of neuroleptic malignant syndrome or other contraindications to neuroleptics are lorazepam, 1–2 mg orally or intramuscularly every 30 minutes, or amobarbital sodium, 250 mg intramuscularly.

Specific medications are useful for those intoxications or withdrawals that present with agitation, irritability, and combativeness (see Chapter 10 for details).

Interviewing the Potentially Violent Patient

The interviewer should sit closest to, but never blocking, the exit. Other staff or security personnel within view, but not menacingly close, can feel protective to the patient and the physician. An interview room that is free of distractions and yet not isolated is most conducive to a productive interview.

The interview should begin with neutral questions rather than a direct opening inquiry about the precipitants for the patient's presentation. As the interview progresses, the physician does need to broach the particulars of the patient's impulses, past actions, immediate plans, and opportunity to carry out these plans. The psychiatrist may acknowledge the patient's anger and also indicate that the patient can be assisted in controlling violent urges. One goal of the interview is to "convert physical agitation and belligerence into verbal catharsis" (Lion, 1985).

As the interview progresses, the patient may produce a weapon. The physician can offer to have the weapon stored, indicating that the patient may have brought it to the hospital to be relieved of the possibility of losing control and using it. The patient should be instructed to lay the weapon down and told that the physician will then take it. Attempting to take a gun directly from the patient may reflexively cause the patient to pull the trigger.

If the decision is made to hospitalize the patient, it should be presented as a nonnegotiable event, but with thoughtful conveyance of its purpose. Patients who appear resistant to hospitalization are frequently relieved by it. Those who one believes might adamantly resist should be informed of hospitalization at the moment of transfer, to prevent escalating anxiety and loss of control during their wait. Sufficient staff should be assembled so that it is indisputably clear that the staff represent an overwhelming force and that resistance would be futile.

Advance planning for the rare instance in which forcible restraint is necessary encompasses policy and logistical decisions. Included are designations of permissible techniques, appropriate circumstances, and the chain of command. Controlling imminent violence is not the time for participatory democracy. Established guidelines should specify who will decide on the necessity of restraint, who will direct the staff in implementation, and what roles will be filled in carrying out this decision. A reporting system for events in which forcible restraint is necessary and an internal review process for examining what transpired in each instance are part of the unit plan.

On the hospital ward, the individual staff member may need to decide whether to intercede immediately with a violent patient before other help can arrive. Damage to property can usually wait; our obligation to intercede in violence directed toward other patients is more imperative. As reinforcements arrive, someone should be assigned to move other patients out of the area. Sufficient staff and unarmed security personnel should be assembled to

convey to even the irrational patient that resistance is impossible. The patient should be told clearly what to do, for example, to lie face down on the bed. Violent patients should be told that restraint is to prevent them from injuring themselves or others and to allow time for them to regain control of their impulses and that it will be discontinued as they are able to do that. Efforts to direct both the staff and the patient away from viewing restraint as retaliation or punishment make subsequent therapeutic interactions much easier.

Five staff members are the minimum necessary to restrain a patient—one to control each limb and one the head. Agitated patients can bang their heads and may bite. Grasping limbs close to the sockets reduces the likelihood of fracture or dislocation (Penningroth, 1975). Rapid-acting neuroleptic or anxiolytic medication is administered immediately, barring some rare contravening metabolic situation. Persons in three- or four-point restraints need to be in constant staff view. The immobilized patient's potential for aspiration, asphyxiation, and other hazards makes 15-minute checks useful for discovering the body while it is still warm, but not for preserving life.

ETHICAL AND LEGAL CONCERNS

Treatment of suicidal or violent patients raises ethical and legal concerns including involuntary hospitalization and nonconsensual treatment, confidentiality, and the protection of potential victims. The psychiatrist assesses the risk of danger to the patient or to others, and the assessment that the risk is substantial and that it is due to a mental disorder usually constitutes the legal basis for commitment. In some instances, the patient willing to be hospitalized but too psychotic to understand the nature of his treatment contract may be better served by the review and documentation processes of involuntary hospitalization (Skodol, 1984).

No matter how compelling the likelihood of injury, violence per se is not synonymous with psychiatric disorder (Skodol, 1984). When the bases of the patient's violence are social or environmental, not psychiatric, the evaluating psychiatrist should say so and decline custodial responsibility for those to whom no treatment can be offered. In assessing potential for violence, the psychiatrist relies on the patient's past history of violence, his current level of functioning, and the risk that accrues if the patient belongs diagnostically to a group with a significantly higher likelihood of violence. The ability of mental health professionals to predict individual violence over the long term does not exceed 50 percent, however, and is even less reliable in the short term (National Academy of Sciences, 1978). How risk was assessed should be carefully documented, along with a consultative opinion from another professional in less clear-cut cases.

Tarasoff v. Board of Regents (1976) illuminated the issue of injured third parties in forensic psychiatry (Dix, 1985). The psychiatrist's ethical duty to exercise reasonable professional care in identifying patients who pose substantial risk of harming others extends to exercising reasonable professional care in protecting those at risk. Warning those at risk is one way, but not the only way, to exercise that professional responsibility. Continuing the treatment itself may constitute reasonable professional care, but should warning individuals or notifying law enforcement authorities be necessary, information will be disclosed that the patient revealed in confidence. At a minimum, the psychiatrist must inform the patient of the need to disclose confidential information and must tell the patient what information will be disclosed to whom (Dix, 1985).

Nonconsensual treatment of suicidal or interpersonally violent patients may require increasingly intrusive interventions, including restraint, seclusion, and involuntary medication. Their justification rests on the determination that the risk of serious harm is substantial and imminent and that less intrusive methods have not been or are not likely to be effective. Periodic room searches or personal searches may be necessary if the patient appears to be secreting potentially lethal items. Detailing the behavior or condition that necessitated the treatment, the way the treatment decision was reached, the persons notified, and the outcomes of periodic reassessment to determine the patient's well-being and need for continued intervention will minimize the risk of litigation (Dix, 1985; Fogel, Mills, & Landen, 1986).

TREATMENT ISSUES FOR VIOLENT PATIENTS

More long-range treatments of violence are based on establishing the etiology of the patient's violent behavior. Outbursts resulting from temporal lobe epilepsy have a different therapeutic approach than violence as a reaction formation to feelings of passivity and weakness. The patient should be taught to recognize premonitory signs and physical sensations of impending violence. For example, pathologic intoxication may encompass a repetitive sequence of loosening inhibitions with alcohol, projection of closeness as a homosexual advance, autonomic nervous system responses to that, and assault. The patient certainly need not share the psychiatrist's psychodynamic formulation but can learn to recognize repetitive situational factors and proprioceptive responses. Patients are also taught to verbalize anger rather than handling it behaviorally and are taught assertiveness, which can reduce the buildup of anger. Working with patients so that they can elaborate fantasies of the probable consequences of their acts is designed to interpose insight and judgment between impulse and action.

Countertransference responses to violent patients are prominent. Denial is most typical. It leads the psychiatrist to miss taking a history of violence: criminal history, driving history, weapons ownership, and history of injury to others. In the extreme, there is identification with the aggressor. Inappropriate attempts may be made to foster a positive transference; if this is based on avoiding discussion of aggressive impulses, it will not reduce the patient's potential for violence. Violent patients can make the physician feel angry and helpless. These feelings lead to preoccupying fantasies that the patient will do something heinous for which the physician will be held responsible. The physician's anger toward such frustrating patients may be projected as excessive fears and ruminations about the patient's dangerousness and likelihood of assaulting the physician. The patient's patricidal or infanticidal impulses may touch similar unconscious impulses in the physician and generate the same sort of obsessive ruminations about the patient's dangerousness. Withdrawal from violent patients by physician and staff removes the patients from therapeutic human contact and actually increases the chance of violence. It conveys to patients the sense that they are truly uncontrollable (Lion & Pasternack, 1973; Lion, Madden, & Christopher, 1976).

SUMMARY

Neither suicide nor interpersonal violence constitutes a psychiatric diagnosis. Both are behavioral outcomes of complex social, emotional, biochemical, and environmental factors. The psychiatrist can, however, have a major role in reducing the likelihood of these destructive acts among medical and surgical patients. This role includes

1. Carefully assessing each patient's potential for suicide and interpersonal violence
2. Recognizing high-risk patients through their personal and situational risk factors, through diagnosis, and through psychodynamic factors
3. Incorporating environmental controls, family supports, and protective staffing
4. Aggressively treating underlying psychiatric disorders

REFERENCES

Abram HS, Moore GL, & Westervelt FB (1971). Suicidal behavior in chronic dialysis patients. *American Journal of Psychiatry*, *127*, 1199–1204.

Armstrong B (1978). Handling the violent patient in the hospital. *Hospital and Community Psychiatry*, *29*, 463–467.

Baker JE (1984). Monotoring of suicidal behavior among patients in the VA health care system. *Psychiatric Annals*, *14*, 272–275.

Bakwin H (1957). Suicide in children and adolescents. *Journal of Pediatrics*, *50*, 749–769.

Barraclough B, Bunch J, Nelson B, et al. (1974). A hundred cases of suicide: Clinical aspects. *British Journal of Psychiatry*, *125*, 355–373.

Bassuk EL (1984). Emergency care of suicidal patients. In EL Bassuk & AW Birk (Eds), *Emergency psychiatry: Concepts, methods, and practices*. New York: Plenum Press.

Beck AT, Steer RA, & McElroy MG (1982). Relationships of hopelessness, depression, and previous suicide attempts to suicidal ideation in alcoholics. *Journal of Studies of Alcohol*, *43*, 1042–1046.

Brown JH, Henteleff P, Barakat S, et al. (1986). Is it normal for terminally ill patients to desire death? *American Journal of Psychiatry*, *143*, 208–211.

Centers for Disease Control (1985). *Suicide surveillance*. Atlanta, GA.

Centers for Disease Control & Working Group (1986).

234   Davidson

Operational criteria for the classification of suicide. Atlanta, GA.

Choi SY (1975). Death in young alcoholics. *Journal of Studies of Alcohol, 36,* 1224–1229.

Davidson L & Gould MS (in press). Contagion as a risk factor for youth suicide. *Department of Health and Human Services.*

Dix GE (1985). Legal and ethical issues in the treatment and handling of violent behavior. In LH Roth (Ed), *Clinical treatment of the violent person.* Rockville, MD: National Institute of Mental Health.

Dorpat TL, Anderson WF, & Ripley HS (1968). The relationship of physical illness to suicide. In HL Resnik (Ed), *Suicidal behaviors: Diagnosis and management.*

Dubin WR & Stolberg R (1981). *Emergency psychiatry for the house officer.* New York: SP Medical & Scientific Books.

Egeland JA & Sussex JN (1985). Suicide and family loading for affective disorders. *Journal of the American Medical Association, 254,* 915–918.

Farberow NL, Shneidman ES, & Leonard CV (1963). Suicide among general medical and surgical hospital patients with malignant neoplasms. *Department of Medicine and Surgery Medical Bulletin, Veterans Administration, 9,* 1–11.

Farberow NL, Shneidman ES, & Leonard CV (1970). Suicide among patients with malignant neoplasms. In ES Shneidman, NL Farberow & RE Litman (Eds), *The psychology of suicide.* New York: Science House.

Fawcett J, Scheftner W, Clark D, et al. (1987). Clinical predictors of suicide in patients with major affective disorders: A controlled prospective study. *American Journal of Psychiatry, 144,* 35–40.

Fogel BS, Mills MJ, & Landen JE (1986). Legal aspects of the treatment of delirium. *Hospital and Community Psychiatry, 37,* 154–158.

Glickman LS (1980). *Psychiatric consultation in the general hospital.* New York: Marcel Dekker.

Goldstein AM & Rezinikoff M (1971). Suicide in chronic hemodialysis patients from an external locus of control framework. *American Journal of Psychiatry, 127,* 1204–1207.

Haenel T, Brunner F, & Battegay R (1980). Renal dialysis and suicide: Occurrence in Switzerland and in Europe. *Comprehensive Psychiatry, 21,* 140–145.

Johnson GF & Hunt G (1979). Suicidal behavior in bipolar manic-depressive patients and their families. *Comprehensive Psychiatry, 20,* 159–164.

Kalogerakis MG (1971). The assaultive psychiatric patient. *Psychiatric Quarterly, 45,* 372–381.

Kellher CH, Best CL, Roberts JM, et al. (1985). Self-destructive behavior in hospitalized medical and surgical patients. *Psychiatric Clinics of North America, 8,* 279–289.

Kernberg OK (1984). *Severe personality disorders: Psychotherapeutic strategies.* New Haven: Yale University Press.

Kiev A (1975). Psychotherapeutic strategies in the management of depressed and suicidal patients. *American Journal of Psychotherapy, 29,* 345–354.

Kinzel AF (1970). Body-buffer zone in violent prisoners. *American Journal of Psychiatry, 127,* 99–104.

Leigh H (1974). Psychotherapy of a suicidal, terminal cancer patient. *International Journal of Psychiatry in Medicine, 5,* 173–182.

Lion JR (1985). Clinical assessment of violent patients. In LH Roth (Ed), *Clinical treatment of the violent person.* Rockville, MD: National Institute of Mental Health.

Lion JR, Bach-y-Rita G, & Ervin FR (1969). Violent patients in the emergency room. *American Journal of Psychiatry, 125,* 120–125.

Lion JR, Madden DJ, & Christopher RL (1976). A violence clinic: Three year's experience. *American Journal of Psychiatry, 133,* 432–435.

Lion JR & Pasternack SA (1973). Countertransference reactions to violent patients. *American Journal of Psychiatry, 130,* 207–210.

Litman RE & Fareberow NL (1970). Suicide prevention in hospitals. In ES Shneidman, NL Farberow & RE Litman (Eds), *The psychology of suicide.* New York: Science House.

Louhivuori KA & Hakama M (1979). Risk of suicide among cancer patients. *American Journal of Epidemiology, 109,* 59–65.

Maltsberger JT & Buie D (1974). Countertransference hate in the treatment of suicidal patients. *Archives of General Psychiatry, 30,* 625–633.

Mental health and behavioral sciences service program guide: *Management of the violent and suicidal patient* (1983). Department of Medicine and Surgery Manual M-2, Part X, G-15. Washington, D.C.: Veterans Administration.

Menninger KA (1933). Psychoanalytic aspects of suicide. *International Journal of Psychoanalysis, 14,* 376–390.

Miles CP (1977). Conditions predisposing to suicide: A review. *Journal of Nervous and Mental Disorders, 164,* 231–246.

Mintz RS (1971). Basic considerations in the psychotherapy of the depressed suicidal patient. *American Journal of Psychotherapy, 25,* 56–73.

Murphy GE (1975). The physician's responsibility for suicide: II. Errors of omission. *Annals of Internal Medicine, 82,* 305–309.

Murphy GE (1983). On suicide prediction and prevention. *Archives of General Psychiatry, 40,* 343–344.

National Academy of Sciences (1978). *Deterrence and incapacitation: Estimating the effects of criminal sanctions on crime rates*. Washington, DC: Author.

Ochitill HN & Krieger M (1982). Violent behavior among hospitalized medical and surgical patients. *Southern Medical Journal, 75*, 151–155.

Ojesjo L (1981). Long term outcome in alcohol abuse and alcoholism among males in the Lundby general population, Sweden. *British Journal of Addiction, 76*, 391–400.

Penningroth PE (1975). Control of violence in a mental health setting. *American Journal of Nursing, 75*, 606–609.

Pollack S (1957). Suicide in general hospital. In ES Shneidman & NL Farberow (Eds), *Clues to suicide*. New York: McGraw-Hill.

Reich P & Kelley MJ (1976). Suicide attempts by hospitalized medical and surgical patients. *New England Journal of Medicine, 294*, 298–301.

Riddick L & Luke JL (1978). Alcohol-associated deaths in the District of Columbia—a postmortem study. *Journal of Forensic Sciences, 23*, 493–502.

Robins E (1981). *The final months*. New York: Oxford University Press.

Rosenberg ML & Mercy JA (1985). Homicide and assaultive violence. In ML Rosenberg (Ed), *Surgeon general's workshop on violence and public health source book*. Atlanta, GA: CDC.

Skodol AE (1984). Emergency management of potentially violent patients. In EL Bassuk & AW Birk (Eds), *Emergency psychiatry: Concepts, methods, and practices*. New York: Plenum Press.

Sletten IW & Barton JL (1979). Suicidal patients in the emergency room: A guide for evaluation and disposition. *Hospital and Community Psychiatry, 30*, 407–411.

Whitlock FA (1975). Suicide in Brisbane, 1956–1973: The drug-death epidemic. *Medical Journal of Australia, 1*, 737–743.

Zee H (1972). Blindspots in recognizing serious suicidal intentions. *Bulletin of the Menninger Clinic, 36*, 551–555.

Robert M. Swift

10
Alcohol and Drug Abuse in the Medical Setting

The alcohol- or drug-abusing patient presents a particular challenge to the physician who treats medically ill patients. In such patients the presence of chemical dependency may be etiologically related to their presenting medical or surgical problems, or its presence may complicate the medical and surgical treatment of other illnesses.

It is estimated that up to one-third of patients presenting at a general hospital, and at least as many patients in an ambulatory setting, are habitual users of psychotropic substances. In spite of the prevalence of psychoactive substance use among patients, physicians are ill-prepared to identify substance use and substance dependence and to treat substance abuse in their patients. The source of these deficiencies are multiple and include poor training and negative attitudes toward substance abusers (Clark, 1981; Holden, 1985).

Treatment of substance abuse and dependence requires knowledge about therapies for the acute management of intoxicated or withdrawing patients, and knowledge about options for long-term treatment and rehabilitation. This chapter will provide basic information on the identification and acute treatment of substance abuse and dependence in medical patients.

CRITERIA FOR THE DIAGNOSIS OF SUBSTANCE ABUSE

The description of substance use disorders is complicated by ambiguity of meaning in the words used to describe substance abuse. In particular, the words tolerance, dependence, withdrawal, and addiction are often confused; therefore, some definitions are in order. *Tolerance* is a pharmacologic effect implying that a larger dose of a drug is necessary to achieve the same effect. *Withdrawal* describes a physiologic state that follows cessation or reduction in amount of drug used. *Dependence* describes either a condition in which a withdrawal state follows cessation of substance use, or a syndrome of clinically significant symptoms that indicate loss of control and continued substance use despite adverse consequences. *Addiction* is a word that is frequently confused with dependence. Addic-

PRINCIPLES OF MEDICAL PSYCHIATRY
ISBN 0-8089-1883-4

237

238 Swift

tion describes a repertoire of behaviors, usually not sanctioned, that maintain drug use.

Formal diagnosis of substance use disorders has been instituted by the American Psychiatric Association in its Diagnostic and Statistical Manual of Mental Disorders (DSM-III R). Eleven distinct classes of substances are designated: alcohol, barbiturates or similarly acting sedatives or hypnotics, amphetamines or similarly acting sympathomimetics, opioids, cannabis, cocaine, phencyclidine or similarly acting arylcyclohexylamines, hallucinogens, nicotine, caffeine, and inhalants.

Psychoactive substance dependence is defined by the presence of at least three of the following, persisting for at least one month or occurring repeatedly over a longer period.

1. The substance is taken in larger amounts over a longer period of time than intended.
2. There is a persistent desire or one or more unsuccessful efforts to cut down on control substance use.
3. A great deal of time is spent in getting the substance, taking the substance, or recovering from its effects.
4. There are intoxication or withdrawal symptoms during major role obligations or when substance use is hazardous.
5. Social, occupational, or recreational activities are reduced or given up because of substance use.
6. Substance use continues despite knowledge of social, occupational, psychological, or physical problems.
7. Presence of marked tolerance to the substance.
8. Occurrence of characteristic withdrawal symptoms (may not apply to cannabis or hallucinogens).

The diagnostic criteria just described have undergone review and modification as presented in DSM-III-R. The major

changes from the DSM-III classification are the modification of the abuse designation to a residual category and a broadening of the concept of dependence to include any significant regular use of a psychoactive substance. Thus most cases defined as abuse under the DSM-III are now defined as dependence under the DSM-III-R.

EVALUATING SUBSTANCE USE IN PATIENTS

Although some patients may present with substance use or its sequelae as a chief complaint, many patients present with other medical or surgical problems and later reveal a substance use disorder through physical or laboratory findings or incidental discovery.

For a variety of reasons, many patients who use psychoactive substances are reluctant to report the full extent of their drug and alcohol use to physicians or other health care providers. Sometimes patients even deny the extent of their substance use to themselves. Patients and their family members often go to great lengths to deny the extent of problems with substance use.

Obviously, patients who are experiencing an altered mental status due to intoxication or withdrawal from a psychoactive substance may be incapable of providing an accurate history. In situations in which the patient is unable or unwilling to give a history of substance use, it is important to obtain additional history from family or acquaintances of the patient. It is also helpful to examine pill bottles or other medications in the patient's possession.

In the process of obtaining information about the patient's alcohol and drug use, most clinicians routinely ask quantity and frequency questions about psychoactive substances, such as "How much?" and "How often?" Unfortunately, these questions have been demonstrated to be notoriously unreliable in their sensitivity for detecting substance abuse. A more effective interview method focuses on whether the patient has experienced negative consequences from use of psychoactive substances, has poor control of use, or has received criticism from others about his substance use. In the case of alcohol, several formalized interviews exist that are well validated in their ability to discriminate alcoholism. The most reliable screen, with sensitivity of 90–98 percent, is the Michigan Alcohol Screening Test (MAST), a 25-item scale that identifies abnormal drinking through its social and behavioral consequences (Selzer, 1971). A shortened 10-item test, the Brief MAST, has been shown to have similar efficacy in the diagnosis of alcoholism. The CAGE questionaire (Ewing, 1984), is a simple, 4-item test with high sensitivity. It uses the letters C-A-G-E as a mnemonic device for the questions about alcohol use. An affirmative answer on more than one of the following questions is considered a basis for suspicion of alcohol abuse:

1. Have you ever felt the need to *c*ut down on drinking?
2. Have you ever felt *a*nnoyed by criticisms of drinking?
3. Have you ever had *g*uilty feelings about drinking?
4. Have you ever taken a morning *e*ye-opener?

Although less documentation exists regarding the optimal interview for the assessment of the drug-abusing patient, the same considerations apply: it is more effective to ask about the behavioral consequences of drug abuse than about quantity and frequence of use.

The physical examination of the patient provides important information about the presence of substance abuse and its medical complications. The presence of signs of repeated trauma, especially to the head, strongly suggests substance abuse (Skinner, Holt, Schuller, et al., 1984).

Other physical stigmata of substance abuse include track marks of intravenous drug abuse, a necrotic nasal septum from cocaine abuse, peripheral neuropathy from solvent inhalation, and signs of liver disease from alcoholism or needle-acquired hepatitis B. A mental status examination should also be performed on each patient to assess the current level of cognitive and neurologic impairment and to assess possible psychiatric disorders, such as mood disorders, anxiety disorders, or personality disorders, all of which are known to coexist frequently with substance abuse disorders. Cognitive mental status testing should be particularly detailed, because alcohol and drug abusers may have significant deficits in memory, concentration, and abstract reasoning, yet pass simple bedside tests of orientation, calculation, and immediate memory.

Abnormal results on laboratory testing provide an important adjunct for confirming the diagnosis of substance abuse but are not highly reliable or specific. A recent British study compared the use of questionnaires and abnormal laboratory testing results for the detection of alcoholism. Laboratory tests such as mean corpuscular volume (MCV) and liver function tests such as SGOT and GGT were found to be relatively poor discriminators of alcohol abuse (Bernadt, Taylor, Mumford, et al., 1982). Serum and urine toxicologic screens may also be unreliable and are affected by many factors, including methods of sample collection and accuracy of the laboratory (Hansen, Caudhill, & Boone, 1985).

TREATMENT

General Considerations

The treatment of the substance-abusing patient comprises several components. The primary task of the physician is to establish an effective therapeutic relationship. Physicians should assess their own attitudes toward substance abuse in order to avoid negative countertransference reactions. In the context of this relationship, the physician should conduct a detailed alcohol and drug history, conduct an appropriate physical examination, order and interpret necessary laboratory tests, engage the patient and family in appropriate short-term and long-term substance abuse treatment, and manage the acute and long-term consequences of substance abuse.

During short-term treatment, goals include cessation of substance use and the establishment of a substance-free state. If necessary, pharmacologically assisted detoxification occurs, as well as management of medical and psychiatric problems. In the long-term phase of treatment, the patient undergoes a process of rehabilitation and reestablishment of a viable drug-free lifestyle. Although the processes need not be distinct and separate, detoxification and rehabilitation frequently occur in different locations and are managed by personnel with different professional identities and different theoretical orientations. Detoxification usually is considered a medical process and occurs within a medical setting, whereas rehabilitation is more likely to occur within a nonmedical environment.

Most patients presenting for treatment do so in the context of a family structure that is also experiencing dysfunction. It is important for the clinician to be aware of dysfunctional family dynamics and the denial, defensiveness, and hostility often present in family members. Family members need education as well as emotional and social support. Organizations such as Al-Anon and Alateen also may provide meaningful education and support for spouses and family members. It is important to involve family members in the patient's treatment as much as possible, as well as to recommend treatment for other family members when appropriate.

The Alcoholic

It is estimated that 7–10 percent of adult Americans have alcoholism, defined as a "repetitive, but inconsistent and sometimes unpredictable loss of control of drinking which produces symptoms of serious dysfunction or disability" (Clark, 1981). Alcoholism is believed to be involved in 20–50 percent of hospital admissions, yet is diagnosed in fewer than 5 percent of the cases (Holden, 1985; Lewis & Gordon, 1983). In an AMA-sponsored poll of physicians, 71 percent felt they were either not competent enough or were too ambivalent to correctly treat alcoholic patients (Kennedy, 1975).

As mentioned earlier, treatment of the alcoholic patient is composed of two phases: detoxification and rehabilitation. Patients who present intoxicated with ethanol may show a continuum of behavioral effects, ranging from coma to a hyperactive state with affective lability. Ingestions of large amounts of alcohol may be fatal, and the toxicity of ethanol is increased in the presence of other sedative drugs. Patients may present to a facility with uncomplicated alcohol intoxication; however, many patients present intoxicated in the context of other medical or psychiatric problems. Alcohol use is highly correlated with suicidal or homicidal behavior and accidental injury (Goodwin, 1967; Waller & Turkel, 1966). Chronic alcohol use is a frequent cause of dementia and may produce hallucinosis, paranoia, or amnestic syndrome (Korsakoff's psychosis). Treatment of alcohol intoxication is essentially supportive and consists of maintaining physiologic homeostasis through support of vital functions as needed.

The withdrawal syndrome that follows the cessation of chronic alcohol administration is a complex physiologic process that results from increased neuronal activity in the central and peripheral nervous systems. The consequences of this process may be minimal or may include autonomic hyper-activity, seizures, delirium, and general physiologic dysregulation (Gross, Lewis, & Hastey, 1974). Treatment of this syndrome, when severe, requires acute medical treatment. Historically, the need for medical intervention in alcohol detoxification followed from observations that withdrawal from alcohol and other sedative-hypnotic drugs was associated with a significant morbidity and mortality. Studies done prior to the 1930s suggested that the mortality of untreated alcohol withdrawal was as high as 50 percent, although current sources quote mortality figures of 5–15 percent (Lewis & Gomolin, 1981). More recent studies suggest that approximately 5 percent of alcohol-dependent individuals undergoing detoxification will develop severe withdrawal delirium (delirium tremens) and, of those, approximately 10–15 percent will die. For those patients who do not develop delirium tremens, detoxification still may be associated with a variety of serious medical complications, including seizures, pneumonia or other infections, myocardial infarction, cardiac arrhythmias, and electrolyte disturbances, and less serious physiologic derangements, including hypertension, tachycardia, tremors, agitation, and insomnia (McIntosh, 1982). Alcoholics are often malnourished, and often have coexisting medical problems that require intervention. The clinician should be aware that signs and symptoms of withdrawal may obscure an underlying illness. For example, fever and change in mental status associated with withdrawal may coexist with an infection of the central nervous system, and a lumbar puncture may be required for diagnosis. Treatment of physiologic abnormalities, hydration, nutritional support, and pharmacologic therapy for the increased activity of the nervous system (Sellers & Kalant, 1976).

Patients undergoing acute alcohol treatment should always be medicated with thiamine and other B-vitamin supplements to prevent the development of the Wernicke-Korsakoff syndrome. This condition is characterized by ocular disturbances (nystagmus and sixth-nerve ophthalmoplegia), ataxia, and mental status changes and is primarily due to deficency of thiamine. Its presence should be considered a medical emergency, as delay in treatment diminishes the probability of reversibility. Given that the Wernicke-Korsakoff syndrome is underdiagnosed, *all* patients presenting with even a suspicion of alcoholism should be treated with intramuscular or intravenous thiamine as soon as possible. Although low doses of thiamine probably are effective, most patients receive 50–100 mg intramuscular thiamine daily for 3 days to ensure proper dosing. In patients with florid neurologic symptoms or signs, saving minutes may be critical, and thiamine should be administered immediately. Alcoholics also are frequently hypomagnesemic. Magnesium levels should be obtained and deficits replaced with intramuscular magnesium sulfate.

Physical dependence on alcohol and vulnerability to the withdrawal syndrome are due to compensatory central nervous system (CNS) changes in response to a chronically administered depressant substance (ethanol). It has long been known that readministration of such depressant substances markedly attenuates the signs and symptoms of withdrawal and greatly decreases the medical morbidity and mortality. Historically, a wide variety of pharmacologic agents have been noted to reduce the signs and symptoms of the withdrawal syndrome, including chloral derivatives, paraldehyde, barbiturates, antihistamines, neuroleptics, antidepressants, lithium, adrenergic blocking agents, and benzodiazepines (Golbert, Sanz, Rose, et al., 1967; Palestine & Alatorre, 1976; Sellers, Cooper, Zilm, et al., 1976). Indeed, almost any depressant substance may have efficacy. Today, benzodiazepine derivatives are the treatment of choice, and their efficacy is well established by double-blind controlled studies (Sellers, Narango, Harrison, et al., 1983). Benzodiazepines are superior to other agents because of their low toxicity and their anticonvulsant effects.

Recent studies on the physiology of alcohol dependence and withdrawal suggest that the central nervous system effects of alcohol may be mediated through modification of inhibitory brain mechanisms involving the inhibitory neurotransmitter gamma amino butyric acid (GABA). Alcohol has been shown to modify the binding of GABA to its receptors and to augment the electrophysiologic and behavioral effects of GABA in animals (Hunt, 1983). Alcohol also appears to have effects on the binding of other sedative drugs to the chloride channel, presumably by dissolving in the membrane and altering its fluidity (Seeman, 1972; Skolnick, Moncada, Barker, et al., 1981). The existence of a common mechanism for the actions of alcohol and sedative-hypnotic drugs accounts for the observed cross-tolerance between drugs of different chemical classes and for the efficacy of benzodiazepines and sedative-hypnotics in the treatment of the alcohol withdrawal syndrome.

Recently, the widespread use of pharmacologic agents in the detoxification from alcohol has been called into question. A variety of alcohol-treatment facilities have been experimenting with "social setting detoxification," a nondrug method. This procedure is usually performed outside a medical environment, and it relies on the extensive use of peer and group support. This method seems to be effective in reducing withdrawal signs and symptoms without an increased incidence of medical complications. There have been some questions about the possible bias in selection of healthier patients for detoxification in these nonmedical settings. Shaw, Kolesar, Sellers, et al. (1981) have demonstrated, however, that even within a medical setting, a

significant number of patients respond to "supportive care" and do not require pharmacologic intervention. In a double-blind study comparing parenteral diazepam treatment with placebo, over half of patients receiving a placebo injection responded with a marked attenuation of withdrawal symptoms within 5 hours (Sellers et al., 1983). Whitfield, Thompson, Lamb, et al. (1978) have reported on large numbers of patients who were successfully detoxified from alcohol without the use of psychotropic drugs.

The available evidence thus, suggests that many, and perhaps even most, alcohol-dependent individuals may be detoxified without the use of sedatives or other psychotropic drugs. There also exists, however, a subgroup of patients who apparently do require careful monitoring and pharmacologic treatment during the withdrawal process. Although it is established that a previous history of delirium tremens or seizures may predict subsequent episodes, little data exist for the clinician to predict which alcohol-dependent patients have an absolute requirement of pharmacologic treatment. The existence of such predictive data would not only be important for providing optimal clinical care for patients, but would also have impact on the cost of care, as those patients who do not require drug administration within a hospital setting could be detoxified out of hospital at lower cost.

For those patients who do require pharmacotherapy, benzodiazepines are the mainstay of treatment because of their low toxicity and anticonvulsant effects. A variety of methods have been described for titrating medication dosage to symptoms. The benzodiazepine-loading method appears to have utility in a wide variety of patients (Sellers et al., 1983). The advantages of this method include matching the dose of medication to an individual patient's tolerance and the avoidance of cumulative pharmacokinetics. During this procedure, patients are administered an initial oral or intravenous dose of a long-half-life benzodiazepine (10–20 mg diazepam or 50–100 mg chlordiazepoxide), which is then repeated every hour until the patient is sedated, develops nystagmus, or has a signficiant decrease in withdrawal signs and symptoms.

The vast majority of patients treated in this manner respond within several hours with a marked reduction in signs and symptoms. Many patients require no additional medication for the duration of their detoxification, presumably because of the long half-life of the drugs. Occasionally, patients may require additional doses of medication after several days, to suppress emergent symptoms. During the period of benzodiazepine loading, patients must be closely observed to avoid undermedication or overmedication. In particular, close attention must be paid to patients with respiratory disease, cardiovascular disease, or hepatic disease. In patients receiving adrenergic blocking drugs, some signs of withdrawal, such as hypertension, tachycardia, and tremor, may be obscured.

Other pharmacologic agents, such as beta-adrenergic blocking drugs, anticonvulsants, and antipsychotics, are often administered along with benzodiazepines to control specific target symptoms. Beta blocker drugs, such as propranolol and atenolol, have been found useful as primary agents in the treatment of alcohol withdrawal (Sellers & Kalant, 1976). Their efficacy, however, is primarily in the reduction of peripheral autonomic signs of withdrawal, and less in the reduction of the central nervous system signs, such as delirium. Adrenergic blocking drugs are particularly useful for controlling tachycardia and hypertension in patients with coronary disease.

Considerable controversy exists around the use of anticonvulsant medications to control withdrawal seizures. Single seizures do not require anticonvulsant treatment; for patients with multiple seizures during withdrawal, or those who have a chronic seizure disorder, anticonvulsants such as phenytoin may be useful. Given that many alcoholics are noncompliant in treatment, however, the erratic use of anticonvulsants on an outpatient basis may actually worsen a seizure problem (Hillbom & Hjelm-Jager, 1984). Neuroleptics, such as haloperidol, are useful for the treatment of hallucinosis and paranoid symptoms.

During and after detoxification, many alcoholic patients appear to suffer from major depression. A large proportion of these mood disorders are directly related to alcohol and resolve within 4 weeks of detoxification. Major depressive symptoms persisting beyond this time should be treated with antidepressants or electroconvulsive therapy (ECT). Patients previously known to have recurrent mood disorders may be treated immediately after detoxification if mood symptoms are severe.

Long-Term Treatment

The goals of long-term treatment include maintaining a state of abstinence from alcohol, with psychologic, family, and social interventions to maintain this recovery. This is best administered within the context of a comprehensive treatment program, which usually begins after discharge from the acute care hospital. Nevertheless, there are some aspects of long-term treatment that may be initiated during an acute hospital stay.

Alcoholics Anonymous (AA) is an independent organization founded by a physician alcoholic in 1939. Its only goal is to help individuals maintain a state of total abstinence from alcohol and other addictive substances, through group and individual interactions between alcoholics at various stages of recovery. Most clinicians agree that self-help programs such as AA are helpful, but there is a paucity of objective outcome data on the efficacy of such groups (Emrick, 1974). Nevertheless, self-help groups certainly are useful for certain indi-

viduals, and most detoxification and rehabilitation programs encourage liberal attendance at AA meetings by their patients.
Many general hospitals are used as meeting
sites by local AA groups, and medical and
surgical inpatients may easily attend these
meetings.

Disulfiram is an inhibitor of the enzyme acetaldehyde dehydrogenase and is
used as an adjunct treatment in selected
alcoholics. If alcohol is consumed in the
presence of this drug, the toxic metabolite
acetaldehyde accumulates, producing tachycardia, flushing of skin, dyspnea, nausea, and vomiting. The presence of this
unpleasant reaction is thought to provide a
deterrent to the consumption of alcohol
(Keventus & Major, 1979). Many alcoholics find disulfiram therapy to be a useful
adjunct to treatment, although it is not
extremely effective on a large-scale basis.
Those patients who are to be started on
disulfiram should be counseled about the
dangers of alcohol use; even the small
amounts of alcohol present in some prepared foods, shaving lotion, mouthwashes,
or over-the-counter medications may be
sufficient to produce a disulfiram reaction.
A usual dose of disulfiram is 250–500 mg
once daily. Disulfiram may have interactions with other medications, notably
phenytoin, and baseline and serial liver
function tests should be performed during
therapy. It is relatively contraindicated in
patients with preexisting liver disease. It
may retard the metabolism of phenytoin, so
phenytoin levels should be followed closely
after disulfiram is begun. Disulfiram may
also prolong prothrombin time in patients
receiving anticoagulants.

The Abuser of
Barbiturates or Other
Sedative-Hypnotics

Sedative medications are a major
source of adverse drug interactions and
drug emergencies, including overdose
(Gottschalk, McGuire, Heiser, et al., 1979).

Yet, they are among the most prescribed
drugs and are routinely used for their
anxiolytic and hypnotic effects. Medications in this group include barbiturates,
benzodiazepines, chloral derivatives, eth-
chlorvynol, glutethimide, meprobamate,
and methaqualone. Patients may obtain
such medications illicitly from the street, or
by prescription from physicians who may
be unwittingly contributing to an abuse or
dependence problem.

As is the case with alcohol, the effects
of other sedative-hypnotic drugs may also
be mediated through interactions with
GABA. In the case of benzodiazepines,
there exist neuronal binding sites for these
drugs, which have many of the properties
of neurotransmitter receptors. The benzodiazepine binding site appears to be linked
to the GABA receptor in both location and
function. Binding of a benzodiazepine to its
binding site appears to facilitate binding of
GABA to its receptors and augments
GABA neurotransmission (Hunt, 1983).
Barbiturates and certain other sedative-hypnotic drugs also appear to influence
GABA systems through effects on chloride
hyperpolarizing currents (MacDonald &
Schultz, 1981). There also appear to be
discrete binding sites for barbituratelike
drugs closely associated with the chloride
channel and GABA receptor (Seeman,
1972).

As with alcohol treatment, treatment
of the sedative abuser occurs in two stages,
detoxification and long-term rehabilitation.
As with alcohol, the withdrawal syndrome
that follows cessation of sedative drug use
may be severe, including seizures, cardiac
arrhythmias, and death. The need for
detoxification depends upon the duration
and amount of sedative drug abuse, which
can be estimated by means of a
pentobarbital challenge test (Wesson &
Smith, 1975; Wikler, 1968). Pentobarbital,
200 mg, is administered orally, and the
patient is observed 1 hour later. The patient's condition after the test dose will
range from unaffected to asleep. If the

patient develops drowsiness or nystagmus on a 200-mg dose, the patient is not barbiturate dependent. If 200 mg has no effect, the dose should be repeated hourly until nystagmus or drowsiness develop. The total dosage administered by this end point approximates the patient's daily barbiturate habit and may be used as a starting point for detoxification. The barbiturate dose should be tapered over 10 days, with a reduction of approximately 10 percent each day.

Long-term treatments should be tailored to the patient but may include residential drug-free programs and self-help groups such as AA or Narcotics Anonymous (NA).

The Opioid Abuser

Opioid abuse and dependence remains a significant sociologic and medical problem in the United States, with an estimated opioid addict population of approximately 500,000. These patients are frequent users of medical and surgical services because of the multiple medical sequelae of intravenous drug use and its associated life-style.

Current diagnostic criteria for opioid abuse (DSM-III-R) require the presence of a pattern of pathologic use, an inability to stop use, frequent intoxication or overdose, with impairments in social or occupational functioning, and a duration of at least one month. Requirements for a diagnosis of opioid dependence are the presence of tolerance or of opioid withdrawal.

Opiate drugs have a variety of physiologic effects on a number of organ systems. Their action is due to stimulation of receptors for endogenous hormones, enkephalins, endorphins, and dynorphins. Recent evidence suggests that there exist at least four distinct opioid receptors, which are designated by the Greek letters mu, kappa, sigma, and delta (Jaffe & Martin, 1985). Drugs that act primarily through mu-receptor effects include heroin, morphine, and methadone; such drugs produce analgesia, euphoria, and respiratory depression.

Drugs that appear to be mediated through the kappa-receptor include the so-called mixed agonist-antagonists butorphenol and pentazocine, which produce analgesia but less respiratory depression. The sigma-receptor appears identical with the receptor for the hallucinogenic drug phencyclidine. The delta-receptor appears to bind endogenous opioid peptides. At high doses, opioid drugs lose their receptor specificity and may have agonist or antagonist properties at multiple receptor subtypes.

Opiate overdose is a life-threatening emergency and should be suspected in any patient who presents with coma and respiratory suppression. Although miotic pupils are usually present, they are nondiagnostic and may not appear with ingestion of mixed agonist-antagonists. Other effects of intoxication include hypotension, seizures, and pulmonary edema. Treatment of suspected overdosage includes emergency support of respiration and cardiovascular functions. Parenteral adminstration of the opioid antagonist naloxone, 0.4–0.8 mg, is of both diagnostic and therapeutic value (Martin, 1976). Although naloxone will rapidly reverse the effects of opioids, including coma and respiratory suppression, it does not reverse central nervous system depression caused by other drugs, such as alcohol or sedative-hypnotics. Naloxone will precipitate withdrawal in any patient who is dependent on opioids, causing the patient whose life was just saved to be most ungrateful.

The opioid withdrawal syndrome is unpleasant but rarely life threatening. It is characterized by the presence of increased sympathetic nervous system activity, coupled with gastrointestinal symptoms of nausea, vomiting, cramps, and diarrhea. Patients may also report myalgias and arthralgias. There is increased restlessness, increased anxiety, insomnia, and an intense craving for opioids. Treatment of withdrawal consists of readministration of an opioid drug and gradual detoxification to minimize withdrawal signs and symptoms.

Many opioid-dependent patients are detoxified during their hospital stay, as current federal law allows narcotic maintenance with methadone only under the auspices of an approved methadone maintenance program. As most methadone programs have waiting lists of days to weeks before new patients can be accepted, an in-hospital detoxification is frequently performed. In addition, some patients may request detoxification while in the hospital.

Most in-hospital opioid detoxifications are performed by substituting methadone for the abused opioid and then gradually decreasing the dose of methadone over a period of up to 21 days, as specified by federal law (Fultz & Senay, 1975). Although a gradually decreasing dose of any opioid could be used for detoxifications, in practice, methadone is preferable because of its long half-life and once-daily oral administration. Initially, patients should be given 10–20 mg of methadone orally every 2–4 hours until withdrawal symptoms are suppressed. The total daily dose received is typically 20–40 mg for heroin addicts. This dose is then decreased by approximately 10 percent daily. For those patients who are unable to receive oral medications, the same dose of intramuscular methadone may be administered twice daily in divided doses.

Recently, several studies have reported that the alpha-2-adrenergic agonist clonidine hydrochloride suppresses many of the autonomic signs and symptoms of opioid withdrawal. Clonidine is thought to act as presynaptic noradrenergic nerve endings in the locus ceruleus of the brain, and it blocks the adrenergic discharge produced by opioid withdrawal (Aghajanian, 1978; Gold, Redmond, & Kleber, 1979). Clonidine has been reported to be effective in suppressing opioid withdrawal following discontinuation of opioids in dependent patients (Charney, Sternberg, Kleber, et al.,

1981; Gold, Pottash, Sweeney, et al., 1980; Washton & Resnick, 1981).

Clonidine detoxification is performed as follows: On the day prior to beginning clonidine, the usual dose of opioid is received. On day 1, the opioid is stopped completely, and clonidine is given instead, at a dose of 0.1 mg each 8 hours. From day 2 to day 4 the dose of clonidine is gradually increased to suppress withdrawal signs and symptoms, without allowing blood pressure to decrease below 80 mm systolic and 60 mm diastolic. For most patients a dose of 0.6–1.2 mg of clonidine is required by day 4, but the dose will depend upon the quantity of opioid used. This dose is continued until day 7 for patients using short-acting opioids, such as heroin, morphine, or meperidine, and until day 10–12 for those using longer-acting methadone. The dose of clonidine is then reduced by 0.2–0.3 mg a day until discontinued.

Clonidine detoxification has been performed in an outpatient setting without significant morbidity. Outpatients should be monitored closely, however, and blood pressure should be determined at least once daily.

Withdrawal symptoms that are not significantly ameliorated by clonidine include drug craving, insomnia, and arthralgias and myalgias. Insomnia is best treated with a short-acting hypnotic such as chloral hydrate. Muscle and joint pains may respond to acetaminophen or an anti-inflammatory agent such as ibuprofen. Clonidine may cause orthostatic hypotension, and patients should be cautioned to stand up slowly and to lie down if they become dizzy or lightheaded. Clonidine causes sedation, and the patient should be advised to avoid activities that require alertness, such as driving. The drug should be used with caution in patients with hypotension and those receiving other antihypertensive medications. Most patients also describe dry mouth, which may be annoying but is otherwise harmless.

Methadone Maintenance

Since its introduction in 1965, methadone maintenance has become a major modality of long-term treatment of opioid abuse and dependence (Dole & Nyswander, 1965). Currently, over 85,000 individuals are maintained on methadone in the United States. Because of diminished state and federal funding, the number of patients that can be accommodated in methadone maintenance programs has not increased to satisfy demand. Many programs have long waiting lists, with waiting periods of several months. It is thus not usually possible for a patient who is abusing opioids to be directly referred to a methadone program for treatment. Patients who are pregnant, however, or who have significant problems, such as renal failure, heart disease, or acquired immune deficiency syndrome (AIDS), are considered by some programs to be medical emergencies and may be accepted directly without a waiting period.

Patients who are members of methadone maintenance programs may have their usual daily dose of methadone continued in the hospital should they be hospitalized. It is important, however, to maintain frequent communication with the methadone program, particularly in regard to changes in methadone dosage. If pain medication is indicated, patients should receive additional short-to-intermediate-acting opioids, such as meperidine or oxycodone in addition to their usual dose of methadone, rather than have an increased dose of methadone. The use of narcotic analgesics other than methadone keeps separate the concept of opioids for analgesia and opioids for maintenance and does not change the dose of methadone as determined by the methadone maintenance program. Because methadone has made these patients tolerant of the effects of opioids, additional pain medication may be required over and above that required by most patients. Mixed agonist-antagonist drugs such as pentazocine and butorphanol should be avoided, as they will produce withdrawal in opioid-dependent individuals.

Alternatives to methadone maintenance include the use of opioid-antagonist therapy with naltrexone. Naltrexone is a long-acting, orally active opioid antagonist that, when taken regularly, entirely blocks the euphoric, analgesic, and sedative properties of opioids (Resnick, Schuyten-Resnick, & Washton, 1980). Naltrexone is administered either daily at a dose of 50 mg or three times weekly at doses of 100 mg, 100 mg, and 150 mg. The drug appears to be most effective in highly motivated individuals with good social supports, and appears less helpful for heroin addicts. Although naltrexone may be prescribed by any physician, it is most effective when part of comprehensive rehabilitative efforts.

A variety of nonpharmacologic and behavioral treatment modalities have been shown to be efficacious in the treatment of the opioid abuser. Programs may differ in their lengths of stay, their intensity, and their theoretical orientation. Long-term residential treatment may be most useful for the chronic opioid abuser who requires a change in life-style with vocational and psychologic rehabilitation (Bale, Zarcone, Van Stone, et al., 1984).

The Abuser of Cocaine and Other Stimulants

The use of cocaine has undergone a dramatic increase in the last two decades. The Haight-Ashbury Clinic reported a rise in cocaine use from less than 1 percent of patients in 1970 to greater than 6 percent in 1982 (Gay, 1982). During the mid-1970s the pattern of cocaine use changed from intranasal "snorting" of cocaine powder to smoking or intravenous injection of the more potent cocaine "freebase." Freebase cocaine is now widely available in a product called "crack," which is extremely potent, relatively inexpensive, and easily distributed. Crack is self-administered by smoking, usually by adding a small piece to a burning cigarette and inhaling the vapor. Because crack is so inexpensive and freely available, it has greatly increased the pool of cocaine users.

Cocaine has three major physiologic effects:

1. It is a local anesthetic of high potency, the only naturally occurring local anesthetic. It blocks the initiation and propagation of nerve impulses by affecting the sodium conductance of nerve cell membranes (Seeman, 1972).
2. It is a potent sympathomimetic agent that potentiates the actions of catecholamines in the autonomic nervous system, producing tachycardia and hypertension. It is a potent vasoconstrictor.
3. It is a potent stimulant of the central nervous system, potentiating the action of the central catecholamine neurotransmitters norepinephrine and dopamine. Its effects include increased arousal, euphoria, excitement, and motor activation. This may progress to agitation, irritability, apprehension, and paranoia at high doses.

Cocaine intoxication is characterized by elation, euphoria, excitement, pressured speech, restlessness, stereotyped movements, and bruxism. Physiologic signs of sympathetic stimulation are present, including tachycardia, mydriasis, and sweating. With chronic use, paranoia, suspiciousness, and frank psychotic symptoms may occur. Overdosage of cocaine produces hyperpyrexia, hyperreflexia, and seizures, which may progress to coma and respiratory arrest. Propranolol and haloperidol administration have been reported as useful in overdosage (Rappolt, Gay, & Inaba, 1977).

The plasma half-life of cocaine following oral, nasal, or intravenous administration is approximately 1–2 hours, which correlates with its behavioral effects (Van Dyke, Jatlow, Ungerer, et al., 1978). Along with the decline in plasma levels, most users experience a period of dysphoria, or "crash," which often leads to additional cocaine use within a short period. The dysphoria of the crash is intensified and prolonged following repeated use.

The optimal treatment of the chronic cocaine user is still not established. Although cessation of cocaine use is not followed by a physiologic withdrawal syndrome of the magnitude of that seen with opioids or alcohol, the dysphoria, depression, and drug craving that follow chronic cocaine use are often intense and make abstinence difficult. Psychotherapy, group therapy, and behavior modification have been found useful in maintaining abstinence (Rounsaville, Gawin, & Kleber, 1985). Recently, a variety of pharmacologic agents have shown promise as adjunct treatments. Several reports have shown efficacy of antidepressant agents such as imipramine, desipramine, lithium, or trazodone in reducing cocaine craving and usage (Gawin & Kleber, 1984; Rosecan, 1983; Tennant & Rawson, 1983). The doses of medication used were similar to those used for antidepressant therapy. The postsynaptic dopamine agonist bromocriptine may also have usefulness in cocaine treatment, as it appears to block cocaine craving (Dackis & Gold, 1985).

Intoxication with other sympathomimetic agents, such as amphetamines, methylphenidate, and other stimulants, may produce a clinical picture similar to that of cocaine intoxication, including sympathetic and behavioral hyperactivity. An "amphetamine psychosis," with manifestations of agitation, paranoia, delusions, and hallucinosis, may follow chronic use of these drugs (Ellinwood, 1969). Antipsychotic medication such as haloperidol is useful in the treatment of stimulant psychoses; however, such patients may frequently require psychiatric hospitalization. Severe hypertension is seen in overdose and may be treated with alpha-adrenergic blockade.

Chronic users of amphetamines engage in a pattern of use similar to that of chronic cocaine users. Escalating doses of the drug are administered for a period of several days, followed by a period of abstinence. Although a classic withdrawal syndrome with physiologic dysfunction does not follow abstinence, marked dysphoria, fatigue, and restlessness may occur. In the chronic user, it is important to consider whether an underlying psychiatric disorder exists, and psychiatric evaluation and treatment may be necessary.

The use of over-the-counter sympathomimetic amines, such as ephedrine and phenylpropanolamine, as stimulants has increased dramatically in the past decade (Dietz, 1981). Signs of intoxication are similar to those for amphetamines, although there tends to be less CNS stimulation. Hypertensive crises have resulted from the use of these drugs.

Hallucinogens

A wide variety of drugs may be used for their hallucinogenic or psychotomimetic effects. These include psychedelics, such as lysergic acid diethylamide (LSD), mescaline, psilocybin, and dimethyltryptamine (DMT); hallucinogenic amphetamines, such as methylenedioxyamphetamine (MDA) and methylenedioxymethamphetamine (MDMA, or "ecstasy"); phencyclidine (PCP) and similarly acting arylcyclohexylamines; and anticholinergics, such as scopolamine. All are capable of causing a state of intoxication characterized by hallucinosis, affective changes, and delusional states.

PCP intoxication has several definitive features: Patient often presents with violence, directed either at self or at others.

Eye signs, including vertical and horizontal nystagmus, are often present, and myoclonus and ataxia are frequent. Autonomic instability, with hypertension and tachycardia, is the rule.

The differential diagnosis of hallucinogen-induced psychosis includes schizophrenia, bipolar disorder, delusional disorder, as well as non-substance induced organic mental disorders and ingestions of toxin, not used as hallucinogens. Psychoses, including those that are drug induced, may produce an analgesic state, and the clinician needs to be aware of any coexisting medical problems, such as injuries or abdominal pain, which may be obscured. Treatment of the psychotic state includes supportive measures to prevent patients from harming themselves or others, maintenance of cardiovascular and respiratory functions, and amelioration of agitation and psychotic symptoms. In many cases, agitation and psychosis respond to decreased sensory stimulation and verbal reassurance; however, patients usually require sedation with benzodiazepines or high-potency neuroleptics. Severe tachycardia and hypertension, if present, can be treated with propranolol. Most cases of hallucinogen intoxication are short-lived (several hours), although prolonged drug-induced psychoses may occur. Prolongation is particularly common with use of PCP, which may produce a prolonged psychosis lasting 2–7 days (Walker, Yesavage, & Tinklenberg, 1981). In addition, it is believed that hallucinogenic drug use may precipitate psychotic illnesses in certain individuals predisposed to the development of such illnesses (Bowers & Swigar, 1983). If psychosis persists beyond 2 weeks after hallucinogen ingestion, it should be regarded as another primary psychiatric illness.

REFERENCES

Aghajanian GK (1978). Tolerance of locus ceruleus neurons to morphine and suppression of withdrawal response by clonidine. *Nature, 276,* 186–188.

Bale RN, Zarcone VP, Van Stone WW, et al. (1984). Three therapeutic communities: A prospective controlled study of narcotic addiction treatment process and follow up results. *Archives of General Psychiatry, 41,* 185–191.

Bernadt MW, Taylor C, Mumford J, et al. (1982). Comparison of questionnaire and laboratory tests in the detection of excessive drinking and alcoholism. *Lancet, 1,* 325–328.

Bowers MB & Swigar ME (1983). Vulnerability to psychosis associated with hallucinogen use. *Psychiatry Research, 9,* 91–97.

Charney DS, Sternberg DE, Kleber HD, et al. (1981). Clinical use of clonidine in abrupt withdrawal from methadone. *Archives of General Psychiatry, 38,* 1273–1278.

Clark WD (1981). Alcoholism: Blocks to diagnosis and treatment. *American Journal of Medicine, 71,* 275–285.

Costa E & Guidotti A (1979). Molecular mechanisms in the receptor action of benzodiazepines. *Annual Review of Pharmacology and Toxicology, 19,* 531–45.

Dackis CA & Gold M (1985). Bromocriptine as treatment of cocaine abuse. *Lancet, 1,* 1151.

Dietz AJ (1981). Amphetamine-like reactions to phenylpropanolamine. *Journal of the American Medical Association, 245,* 601–602.

Dole VP & Nyswander M (1965). A medical treatment for diacetylmorphine (heroin) addiction: Clinical trial with methadone hydrochloride. *Journal of the American Medical Association, 193,* 646–650.

Ellinwood EH (1969). Amphetamine psychosis: A multidimensional process. *Seminars in Psychiatry, 1,* 208–226.

Emrick C (1974). A review of psychologically oriented treatment of alcoholism. *Quarterly Journal of Studies on Alcohol, 38,* 1004–1031.

Ewing JA (1984). Detecting alcoholism: The CAGE questionaire. *Journal of the American Medical Association, 252,* 1905–1907.

Fultz JM, Jr, & Senay EC (1975). Guidelines for the management of hospitalized narcotics addicts. *Annals of Internal Medicine, 82,* 815–818.

Gawin FH & Kleber HD (1984). Cocaine abuse treatment: Open trial with desipramine and lithium carbonate. *Archives of General Psychiatry, 41,* 903–909.

Gay GR (1982). Clinical management of acute and chronic cocaine poisoning. *Annals of Emergency Medicine, 11,* 562–572.

Golbert TM, Sanz CJ, Rose HD, et al. (1967). Comparative evaluation of treatments of alcohol withdrawal syndromes. *Journal of the American Medical Association, 201,* 113–116.

Gold MS, Pottash AC, Sweeney DR, et al. (1980). Opiate withdrawal using clonidine: A safe, effective, and rapid nonopiate treatment. *Journal of the American Medical Association, 243*(4), 343–346.

Gold MS, Redmond DE, Jr, & Kleber HD (1979). Noradrenergic hyperactivity in opiate withdrawal suppressed by clonidine. *American Journal of Psychiatry 136,* 100–102.

Goodwin DW (1967). Alcohol in homicide and suicide. *Quarterly Journal of Studies on Alcohol, 28,* 517–528.

Gottschalk L, McGuire F, Heiser J, et al. (1979). *Drug abuse deaths in nine cities: A survey report* (NIDA Research Monograph No. 29). Washington, DC: U.S. Government Printing Office.

Gross M, Lewis E, & Hastey J (1974). Acute alcohol withdrawal syndrome. In B Kissin & H. Begleiter (Eds), *The biology of alcoholism* (Vol 3). New York: Plenum Press.

Hansen HJ, Caudhill SP, Boone DJ (1985). Crisis in drug testing: Results of the CDC blind study. *Journal of the American Medical Association, 253,* 2382–7.

Harvey SC (1980). Hypnotics and sedatives. In AG Gilman, LS Goodman, & A Gilman (Eds), *The Pharmacological basis of theraputics* (6th ed). New York: Macmillan.

Hillbom ME & Hjelm-Jager M (1984). Should alcohol withdrawal seizures be treated with anti-epileptic drugs? *Acta Neurologica Scandinavica, 69,* 39–42.

Holden C (1985). The neglected disease in medical education. *Science, 229,* 741–742.

Hunt WA (1983). The effect of ethanol on GABAergic transmission. *Neuroscience and Biobehavioral Reviews 7,* 87–95.

Institute of Drug Abuse (1981). *National survey on drug abuse.* Rockville, MD: Author.

Jaffe JH & Martin WR (1985). Opioid analgesics and antagonists. In AG Gilman, LS Goodman, TW Rall, et al. (Eds), *The Pharmacological Basis of Therapeutics* (7th ed). New York: Macmillan.

Kennedy W (1975). Chemical dependency: A treatable disease. *Ohio State Medical Journal, 71,* 77–79.

Keventus J & Major LF (1979). Disulfiram in the treatment of alcoholism. *Quarterly Journal of Studies on Alcohol, 40,* 428–446.

Lewis DC & Gomolin IH (1981). *Emergency treatment of drug and alcohol intoxication and withdrawal* (Medical Monograph II). Providence, RI: Brown University Program in Alcoholism and Drug Abuse.

Lewis D & Gordon A (1983). Alcoholism and the general hospital: The Roger Williams intervention program. *Bulletin of the New York Academy of Medicine, 59,* 181–197.

Martin WR (1976). Naloxone. *Annals of Internal Medicine, 85,* 765–768.

McIntosh I (1982). Alcohol-related disabilities in general hospital patients: A critical assessment of the evidence. *International Journal of Addictions, 17,* 609–639.

Palestine ML & Alatorre E (1976). Control of acute alcoholic withdrawal symptoms: A comparative study of haloperidol and chlordiazepoxide. *Current Therapy Research, 20,* 289–299.

Rappolt RT, Gay GR & Inaba D (1977). Propranolol: A specific antagonist to cocaine. *Clinical Toxicology, 10,* 265–271.

Resnick RB, Schuyten-Resnick E, & Washton AM (1980). Assessment of narcotic antagonists in the treatment of opioid dependence. *Annual Reveiw of Pharmacology and Toxicology, 20,* 463–474.

Rosecan JS (1983). The psychopharmacologic treatment of cocaine addiction [Abstract]. Seventh World Congress of Psychiatry, Vienna.

Rounsaville BJ, Gawin FH, & Kleber HD (1985). Interpersonal psychotherapy adapted for ambulatory cocaine users. *American Journal of Drug and Alcohol Abuse, 11,* 171.

Schulz DW & Macdonald RL (1981). Barbiturate enhancement of GABA-mediated inhibition and activation of chloride channel conductance: Correlation with anticonvulsant and anesthetic actions. *Brain Research, 209,* 177–88.

Seeman P (1972). Membrane effects of anesthetics and tranquilizers. *Pharmacology Review, 24,* 583–655.

Sellers EM, Cooper SD, Zilm DH, et al. (1976). Lithium treatment during alcoholic withdrawal. *Clinical Pharmacology and Therapeutics 20,* 199–206.

Sellers EM & Kalant H (1976). Drug therapy: Alcohol intoxication and withdrawal. *New England Journal of Medicine, 294,* 757–52.

Sellers EM, Narango CA, Harrison M, et al. (1983). Diazepam loading: Simplified treatment for alcohol withdrawal. *Clinical Pharmacological Therapy, 6,* 822.

Selzer ML (1971). The Michigan alcoholism screening test: The quest for a new diagnostic instrument. *American Journal of Psychiatry, 127,* 89–84.

Shaw JM, Kolesar GS, Sellers EM, et al. (1981). Development of optimal treatment tactics for alcohol withdrawal: Assessment and effectiveness of supportive care. *Journal of Clinical Psychopharmacology, 1,* 382–387.

Skinner HA, Holt S, Schuller R, et al. (1984). Identification of alcohol abuse using laboratory tests and a history of trauma. *Annals of Internal Medicine, 101,* 847–851.

Skolnick P, Moncada V, Barker J, et al. (1981). Pentobarbital: Dual action to increase brain benzodiazepine receptor affinity. *Science, 211,* 1448–50.

Tennant FS & Rawson RA (1983). Cocaine and amphetamine dependence treated with desipramine. In L Harris (Ed), *Problems of drug dependence* (Monograph Series 43, pp 351–355). Rockville, MD: National Institute on Drug Abuse.

Van Dyke C, Jatlow P, Ungerer J, et al. (1978). Oral cocaine: plasma concentration and central effects. *Science, 200,* 211–213.

Walker S, Yesavage JA, Tinklenberg JR (1981). Acute phencyclidine (PCP) intoxication: Quantitative urine levels and clinical management. *American Journal of Psychiatry, 138,* 674–5.

Waller JA & Turkel HW (1966). Alcoholism in traffic deaths. *New England Journal of Medicine, 275,* 532–536.

Washton, AM & Resnick RB (1981). Clonidine for opiate detoxification: Outpatient clinical trials. *Journal of Clinical Psychiatry, 43,* 39–41.

Wesson DR & Smith DE (1975). A new method for the treatment of barbiturate dependence. *Journal of the American Medical Association, 231,* 294–295.

Whitfield CL, Thompson G, Lamb A, et al. (1978). Detoxification of 1024 alcoholic patients without psychoactive drugs. *Journal of the American Medical Association, 239,* 1409–1410.

Wikler A (1968). Diagnosis and treatment of drug dependence of the barbiturate type. *American Journal of Psychiatry, 125,* 758–765.

Willow M & Johnston GAR (1981). Dual action of pentobarbitone on GABA binding: Role of binding site integrity. *Journal of Neurochemistry, 37,* 1291–94.

Woo E & Greenblatt DJ (1979). Massive benzodiazepine requirements during acute alcohol withdrawal. *American Journal of Psychiatry, 136,* 821–823.

Barry S. Fogel
Carol Martin

11
Personality Disorders in the Medical Setting

General hospital psychiatrists have long been interested in the impact of personality traits on adherence to medical treatment recommendations. The classic article of Kahana and Bibring (1964), known to most psychiatric consultants, describes proto-types of different personality styles, (hysterical, compulsive, etc.) and indicates how treatment instructions can be adapted to the patient's personality to promote treatment adherence. Since that article appeared, the diagnosis of personality disorders has been operationalized in DSM-III-R, a hierarchy of defense mechanisms has been empirically validated (Vaillant, 1986), the epidemiology of personality disorders has been studied in a variety of medical settings, and the overlap of Axis I and Axis II has become better appreciated. Further, techniques for circumventing resistance such as reframing and paradoxical intention, introduced by family therapists, have entered the mainstream of psychiatric practice.

This chapter discusses the core ideas of managing patients with personality disorders in the medical setting, emphasizing newer concepts of diagnosis, and presents guidelines for individualized management strategies. The first part of the chapter deals with epidemiology and principles of descriptive and psychodynamic personality diagnosis. The second part presents specific management strategies and suggests how they may be selected based on personality diagnosis. The third part of the chapter deals with the use of medications in patients with personality disorders. The chapter concludes with the discussion of liaison issues, counter-transference, special issues of the elderly, and legal considerations. The chapter presupposes knowledge of DSM-III-R, as well as of the hierarchy of defense mechanisms originally outlined by Anna Freud (1946) and recently elaborated and validated by Vaillant (1986).

HOW PERSONALITY DISORDERS PRESENT IN MEDICAL SETTINGS

In medical settings, patients with personality disorders are brought to the attention of the psychiatrist because (1) they

PRINCIPLES OF MEDICAL PSYCHIATRY
ISBN 0-8089-1883-4

display angry, manipulative, or self-destructive behavior; (2) they adhere poorly to treatment recommendations; (3) they evoke frustration and anger in their caretakers; (4) they develop severe anxiety, depression, or intractable physical complaints; or (5) they present with concurrent alcohol and drug abuse problems.

PREVALENCE

About 1 in 10 Americans has a personality disorder (Merikangas & Weissman, 1986). Since patients with personality disorders are more likely to seek medical and psychiatric help than patients without them, these disorders are highly prevalent among patients who see psychiatrists in general hospitals. In one series of patients presenting to a general hospital psychiatry service, 36 percent had personality disorders according to DSM-III Axis II criteria (Koenigsberg, Kaplan, Gilmore, et al., 1985). In this same series, patients with alcohol abuse disorders had a 46 percent rate of concurrent personality disorder, and patients with nonalcohol substance abuse had a 61 percent rate. In another study of narcotic addicts, 65 percent had personality disorders (Khantzian & Treece, 1985).

Patients with maladaptive personality traits falling short of Axis II diagnoses also are commonly encountered in medical-psychiatric populations. For example, among 609 patients at a general hospital-based psychiatry outpatient clinic, 51 percent had personality disorders, an additional 13 percent "almost met" DSM-III criteria, and another 24 percent had maladaptive traits listed among DSM-III Axis II criteria (Kass, Skodol, Charles, et al., 1985). The patients with maladaptive traits falling short of DSM-III criteria might well reveal these traits under the stress of medical illness or hospitalization, or in the context of the physician-patient relationship.

PROBLEMS IN DIAGNOSTIC ASSESSMENT

The diagnosis of personality disorders in the medical setting is beset by both theoretical and practical problems. Theoretical issues include distinguishing normality from pathology; choosing a categorical, dimensional, or prototypical diagnostic system (Frances, 1982; Livesley, 1985, 1986); and the question of whether cultural and sex biases may unduly influence diagnostic schemes (Kaplan, 1983; Presly & Walton, 1973). Furthermore, some DSM-III-R categories, such as borderline and schizotypal, may overlap significantly with each other (George & Soloff, 1986). Practical issues in accurate diagnosis include difficulties in obtaining an accurate history from severely ill patients, confounding effects of stress, and the hospital environment, which may facilitate regressive behavior. Acute and chronic pain, in particular, may exacerbate maladaptive personality traits (Bellissimo & Tunks, 1984). For these reasons, firm diagnoses of personality disorder should not be recorded in a patient's chart unless there is adequate historical evidence of *persistent* maladaptive traits antedating the current episode of medical illness. Such information often can be obtained from past psychiatric records, from discussions with significant others, and from other physicians.

Diagnostic reliability for personality disorders varies widely, and depends on the adequacy of the data base as well as how prototypical the patient is for a particular personality syndrome. For example, investigations using structured diagnostic interviews of patients and informants obtained kappa coefficients for inter-rater agreement of .70 or higher for histrionic, borderline, and dependent personalities (Stangl, Pfohl, Zimmerman, et al., 1985). In contrast, when three psychiatrists compared personality diagnoses obtained in everyday clinical settings, the *maximum* kappa coefficient was .49, for antisocial personality, and all other diagnoses were even less reliable (Mellsop, Varghese, Joshua, et al., 1982).

In gathering data regarding personality diagnoses, information from informants other than the patient is essential. This is easily gathered in hospital settings, as nurses offer a ready source of information about behavior, and visiting family and friends can be approached for additional historical data. For example, in one series of patients evaluated with a structured interview for personality disorders, diagnoses were changed in 20 percent of cases after further information was obtained from the structured interview of an informant. Inter-rater reliability, however, was not adversely affected by the additional information (Zimmerman, Pfohl, Stangl, et al., 1986).

Descriptive versus Psychodynamic Perspectives

Although a categorical diagnostic system such as DSM-III-R is helpful for epidemiologic study and clinical research, it has drawbacks that may be particularly evident in medical settings. Under the stress of severe medical illness, trauma, or surgery, individuals may transiently display regressive, primitive, "lower-level" defenses typical of borderline personalities although they lack the long-standing history of impaired function necessary for a formal DSM-III-R diagnosis of borderline personality disorder. In this situation, recognition and management of primitive ego defenses are essential, while a firm decision about categorical diagnosis is not. Severe stress and the regressive situation of the hospital may bring out paranoid behavior in ordinarily schizoid or obsessional individuals or induce typically borderline behavior in previously high-functioning histrionic or nar-

cissistic characters. Under other, less stressful circumstances, these same inividuals may not have baseline traits that are sufficient to warrant a formal Axis II diagnosis. Elderly patients with maladaptive traits or defenses of subsyndromal proportions may exhibit extreme denial, projection, and somatization in the context of dementia, delirium, or depression.

When a patient's history permits an Axis II diagnosis, the assignment of a diagnostic category may be helpful in anticipating management difficulties and in choosing therapeutic strategies. In the following sections, strategies for managing patients with personality disorders are presented and are matched to specific DSM-III-R disorders. In applying these strategies, however, descriptive diagnosis should be combined with an assessment of ego defenses and object relations in an effort to place the patient on a continuum of adaptive personality functioning. If a patient whose history suggests compulsive personality is currently utilizing paranoid defenses, management strategies for paranoid personalities would thus be appropriate. Likewise, if an ordinarily histrionic individual is able to mobilize higher-level defenses in response to the challenge of illness, management strategies should take the apparent improvement into account.

These intervention strategies are presented contrasting patients with predominantly "higher" or "lower" level of ego defenses and object relations. These therapeutic strategies apply both to patients with maladaptive personality traits of syndromal proportions and to patients with no psychiatric formal diagnosis who regress to more maladaptive defenses under the acute stress of medical illness, surgery, or trauma. The hierarchical classification of defense mechanisms as *higher level* (healthy or neurotic) or *lower level* (borderline or psychotic) is described in detail by Vaillant (1986).

Bedside Assessment

When evaluating problematic patients with suspected personality disorders several issues deserve emphasis in the initial interviews:

1. What is the patient's view of the problem? Is there a legitimate, practical issue that could defuse the problem? Is there a misunderstanding between the patient and the medical staff that needs clarification?
2. Are there practical, negotiable issues compounded by emotional conflicts? Could the practical problem be resolved if emotional conflicts were identified and separated from the practical issues?
3. Is there evidence of intercurrent delirium, dementia, psychosis, or major mood disorder? Is the patient under the influence of prescribed medications, alcohol, or illicit drugs?
4. What is the patient's perception of the physician-patient relationship and of the patient's role in the treatment?
5. Who has the more relevant personality problem—the patient or a member of the medical or nursing staff?

When information from the interview, collateral sources, professional caretakers, and the medical record is synthesized, a tentative personality diagnosis may then be possible, as well as a concise statement of the behavioral problem needing resolution. Specific strategies can be employed to address behavioral problems according to the patient's personality type while concurrent problems on Axis I receive appropriate pharmacologic or psychotherapeutic attention or both.

Concurrent Axis I and Axis II Diagnoses

Reciprocal relationships of Axis I and Axis II have received increased attention in the psychiatric literature. For example,

problems on Axis I may make a definitive Axis II diagnosis difficult, whereas the presence of personality disorder may alter the prognosis and treatment strategy for an Axis I disorder (Hyler & Frances, 1985). There is also a frequent concurrence of alcohol and drug abuse with personality disorders. Brief reactive psychosis is associated with borderline personality, as are episodes of major mood disorders (Gunderson & Elliott, 1985; Perry, 1985). Patients with all types of personality disorders are especially likely to develop adjustment disorders in reaction to stress, including the stress of acute medical illness.

Identification of superimposed major depression is of particular importance because the mood disorder may in itself exacerbate maladaptive personality traits (Hirschfeld, Klerman, Clayton, et al., 1983). A patient who appears dependent or histrionic before antidepressant treatment might be seen as within normal limits after recovery. In addition, a significant subgroup of borderline personalities may represent variants of mood disorders ("subaffective disorders") that respond to antidepressants. High premorbid functioning prior to stress-induced onset of an apparent borderline personality may predict a good response to somatic antidepressant treatment (Novac, 1986).

Organic Factors

Organic mental disorders may exacerbate personality traits to syndromal proportions in the context of medical illness. For example, pernicious anemia and lupus have been observed to exacerbate paranoid traits, and hypothyroidism to increase dependent behavior. Exacerbations of personality disorder traits in diabetes mellitus by nocturnal hypoglycemia have also been reported (Krahn & Mackenzie, 1984). Untreated temporal lobe epilepsy can produce idiosyncratic experiences suggesting schizotypal personality, or inappropriate rages mimicking those of borderline personality. Passive-aggressive phenomena may be produced by right-hemisphere lesions, causing denial and inattention. Organic mental disorders may also cause disinhibited behavior, magnifying latent problematic personality traits.

Adolescents and adults with attention deficit disorders (ADD) may display angry, impulsive, and uncooperative behavior in the hospital environment because of the combination of overstimulation and enforced passivity. Patients with borderline personality are particularly likely to suffer from concurrent ADD, with one study showing a prevalence rate of 25.5 percent (Andrulonis, Glueck, Stroebel, et al., 1982). When historical evidence or neurologic findings support a diagnosis of ADD, stimulant drug therapy for this disorder may improve the patient's adaptation to his physical illness. When stimulants are contraindicated and the need for behavior control is acute, thioridazine in low doses may be effective, and is less likely than high-potency neuroleptics to produce restlessness and akathisia in ADD patients.

Diagnostic Pointers

We assume that the reader is familiar with the DSM-III-R classification of personality disorders and with the ways in which patients with particular personality disorders are likely to show problematic behavior in medical settings. When the presence of a personality disorder or maladaptive personality traits impedes medical treatment, the specific personality diagnosis may assist in selecting management strategies but must be supplemented by a current assessment of defensive style and level of object relations development. This assessment is most important for individuals with narcissistic, histrionic, dependent, and passive-aggressive traits, who may have varying levels of personality organization. For example, histrionic or "hysteri-

cal" patients with relatively good impulse control and a more mature defensive structure require different management from lower-level, impulsive histrionic patients with narcissistic or borderline features (Kernberg, 1986). Diagnostic points to be remembered include the following:

1. Antisocial personalities, diagnosed on the basis of history, should always be presumed to have poorly developed defenses, even if they appear to be functioning at a higher level on a single cross-sectional assessment.

2. The formal diagnosis of borderline personality disorder by DSM-III-R criteria is less important for medical-psychiatric management than the identification of the patient as one with poor-quality object relations and a tendency to use the defenses of splitting and projective identification. Patients with a history of incest, multiple personality, factitious illness, or multiple suicide attempts are highly likely to have a borderline personality oranization (Barnard & Hirsch, 1985; Benner & Joscelyne, 1984; Task Force of American Psychiatric Association, 1980).

3. Passive-aggressive and dependent personalities may have either higher-level or lower-level defensive structures and object relations. More primitive passive-aggressive patients may passively attempt to sabotage medical treatment as an expression of rage against the physician, who serves as a transference figure. By contrast, the more neurotic passive-aggressive patient may primarily have conflicts over control and autonomy or may be identifying with a passive parent. Management should be in accord with the patient's defensive style and specific emotional conflicts.

4. Schizoid and avoidant personalities may be difficult to distinguish on a single cross-sectional assessment. Both, however, fear extreme closeness

and may fear being controlled by others. The enforced intimacy of medical settings and the attendant loss of control lead to anxiety, which is expressed according to the patient's defensive style.

MANAGEMENT STRATEGIES

Based on data from the patient interview and from collateral sources, the psychiatrist can develop a tentative personality diagnosis that comprises both an assignment of an Axis II diagnosis and if possible, an assessment of current defensive operations and the quality of the patient's object relations. Axis I problems and organic aggravating factors are also diagnosed, and their treatment is initiated as appropriate. The psychiatrist then must develop a short-term management strategy that permits medical treatment with a minimum of interference from the patient's maladaptive personality traits.

An individualized strategy is developed by combining strategies, most of which have a long history in the literature of psychiatric consultation (Groves, 1978). One group of strategies is particularly appropriate for patients with lower-level defenses and poor-quality object relations, and is especially useful for patients with borderline personality organization or antisocial personalities. A second group of strategies is useful for patients with higher-level defenses and better object relations. These basic strategies will be described in detail in the following subsections. The choice of strategy is summarized in Table 11-1.

Table 11-1
Match Diagnosis and Intervention Strategies

Level of Defenses and Object Relations	Diagnosis	Interventions
Low	Borderline Antisocial Paranoid	Giving a sense of control Being consistent Taking the "one-down" position Limit setting Antisplitting maneuvers
Lower	Schizoid Avoidant	Straightforward, matter-of-fact relationship; avoiding excessive closeness
Variable	Narcissistic Passive-aggressive	If lower-level, borderline strategies If higher-level, strategic reframing
	Histrionic Dependent "Hysterical"	If lower-level, borderline strategies If higher-level, personal leverage or strategic reframing
Higher	Compulsive Maladaptive traits of subsyndromal proportions	Strategic reframing

Strategies for Managing Patients with Lower-Level Defenses

In managing a patient with lower-level defenses, the physician must not assume, a priori, a trusting relationship or the patient's capacity to be consistent. Consistency and appropriateness must be provided by the physician, who must not be unduly moved by pleas, demands, manipulations, or threats or be personally affronted by the patient's mistrust.

Because patients with lower-level defenses may react dramatically to disappointment, it is all-important to clarify treatment expectations. The patient's understanding of the implicit therapeutic contract between physician and patient should be explored, and the goals and limits of the patient's medical treatment should be made clear at the outset. Sanity and healing on everyone's part can be maximized by frequently reorienting the patient, other physicians, nursing staff, and family toward the basic, circumscribed treatment contract. Whenever possible, this implicit contract should be stated in the patient's own words. Management strategies useful for patients with lower-level defenses involve giving patients a sense of control, being consistent, taking the "one-down" position, limit setting, and preventing and managing splitting of staff.

Giving a Sense of Control to the Patient

Giving a sense of control is maximizing the appropriate influence the patient has over the treatment situation. For outpatients, the physician may let the patient decide within reasonable limits a schedule of visits or let the patient choose a specific medication if there is more than one acceptable alternative. For inpatients, the physician may let the patient decide when to take certain medication, when to go to physical therapy, or what the exact discharge date

will be (Kahana & Bibring, 1964; Staleniam & Youngs, 1974). Giving a sense of control is aided by recalling that the physician is responsible for good professional judgment and advice but is not responsible for the patient's decision to follow the advice (Strain, 1978).

Being Consistent

Being consistent means minimizing changes in plan and personnel, thus reducing opportunities for confusion or misunderstanding. Consistency is facilitated by using the minimum number of drugs and orders. Being consistent is made easier for everyone concerned by having written instructions and plans and by allowing patients to restate the plans in their own words. When several caretakers are involved, this strategy means carefully coordinating the efforts of all caretakers, using written communications whenever possible, and sharing the agreements with the patient. The use of written instructions and plans is of documented value in improving compliance in all patients (Hayes, Taylor & Sackett, 1979) but is especially important for patients with lower-level defenses (Hall, 1977). Numerous papers have described "treatment contracts" and principles for writing them (McEnany & Tescher, 1985; O'Brien, Caldwell, & Transea, 1985).

Taking the "One-Down" Position

Taking the "one-down" position means realistically recognizing one's limitations in affecting another person's behavior and approaching the patient with genuine and appropriate humility. This approach, more an attitude than a technique, forestalls many potential control struggles with personality-disordered patients (David, 1979; Ellard, 1977; Schwartz, 1979; Strain, 1978; Watzlawick, Weakland, & Fisch, 1974).

For example, an elderly man with a ventricular arrhythmia was noncompliant with hospitalization because of mistrust of his doctors' motives. The working diagnosis was paranoid personality. The strategies selected were taking the one-down position and giving control. The patient was told that the physician could not and would not force him to stay in the hospital and that the physician did not expect him to believe his medical diagnosis. The physician wished to give him the opportunity to learn for himself whether medication could prevent him from having further fainting spells. The patient could do this on an outpatient basis, just as soon as a few tests were done. Furthermore, if the patient liked, he could have his wife check all medications before giving them to him to take. The patient accepted this arrangement, and in the next 48 hours was stabilized on an antiarrhythmic drug. He was then discharged from the hospital and at follow-up was continuing to take his antiarrhythmic drugs.

Limit Setting

Limit setting is the trump card, to be played if a patient is seriously impeding treatment or is endangering someone (Strain, 1978). For outpatients, such problematic behavior often involves abuse of prescribed drugs (Sternbach, 1974). For inpatients, it includes deliberately pulling out IV lines, smoking in a room with oxygen, screaming all night in a room full of very sick patients, and other extreme behavior.

In the inpatient case, all involved caretakers are told of the problem and decide together what limits will be set. The patient is told *without anger* which behaviors are unacceptable *in this hospital*. If limits are set angrily, the patient will respond more to the anger than to the limit. Kahana and Bibring (1964) warn, "Great care should be exercised not to introduce limits as if they were an expression of impatience or punitiveness." Reference to "this hospital" restricts the control struggle to the hospital rather than to the whole world. In the outpatient case, the patient is told that the behavior is unacceptable *within that physician's practice*. The patient is told that the

physician will not continue treating the patient or prescribing medication if the behavior continues. (Appropriate alternative sources of care would, of course, be explored with the patient to forestall charges of abandonment.)

In the variation called sympathetic limit setting, the physician adds that there must be good reasons for the patient's behavior *but* the behavior is unacceptable (Lipp, 1977). In either type of limit setting, the inpatient is told that discharge (termination of the treatment contract) is inevitable if the unacceptable behavior continues. If involuntary psychiatric treatment is indicated, a request for temporary certification is completed, and the patient is referred to an appropriate psychiatric facility. If the patient is too medically unstable for such a referral, control of destructive behavior is maintained with neuroleptics, special observation, or restraints until the patient's physical condition permits either discharge or referral to a secure mental health facility.

Limit setting, though often essential for treating patients with lower-level defenses, such as borderline personalities, can have negative effects on patients with higher-level defenses and should be used with them only when other methods have failed. One authority on the treatment of personality disorders has stated, "Consistency and limit setting are equally as important as benignness, availability, and good intentions. When each demand of the patient was met with yielding or bending of the rules, as with demanding, angry, overtly hostile patients in an effort to keep them from 'exploding,' the result was greater loss of control, (and) even more demanding behavior" (Hall, 1977).

Preventing and Managing Staff Splitting

Patients with borderline personality organization frequently employ *splitting* as a defense (Stoudemire & Thompson, 1982). The important people in their world are divided into "good" and "bad" objects, the former loved and idealized, the latter hated and devalued. In a medical setting, the patient with borderline personality organization may induce among different physicians and staff intense differences in attitude and feeling toward the patient so that they are split into two factions with strongly held opposing views regarding the patient's diagnosis and treatment. Issues frequently disputed include pain management, the need for psychotropic medication, the validity of the patient's physical complaints, and the limits that should be set on the patient's behavior.

Splitting of physicians and other staff may arise in three ways. First, the patient may manipulate some caretakers into a particular viewpoint while others, unaffected by the manipulation, disagree and may view the patient negatively as "manipulative." Second, caretakers may have differing countertransference reactions to the patient's behavior. Some may respond with sympathy and protectiveness while others respond with anger and annoyance. Third, the patient may actually show different affect or behavior with different caretakers because of different transferences, thereby inducing conflicting opinions in the absence of any deliberate manipulation.

However splitting arises, it may impede optimal care of the patient. Consequences of splitting may include inconsistent care, inappropriate medication, and staff inefficiency due to intrastaff conflict. Therefore, when splitting of caretakers occurs, "antisplitting maneuvers" are required.

The basic antisplitting maneuver is the network meeting. All physicians and staff involved in the patient's care are brought together in one room. The psychiatrist identifies the problem of splitting and initially encourages ventilation of feelings and disagreements. The psychiatrist then points out that these feelings and disagreements are *induced by the patient's behavior* and that they provide valuable information *about the patient*. The psychiatrist may

then explain that the patient must be treated with the utmost consistency. A rational treatment plan must be agreed upon and carried out, regardless of the patient's varying reactions to different caretakers and despite any attempts made at manipulation. The psychiatrist works with the staff to develop a consensus on an appropriate care plan, and this plan is written down. The psychiatrist or the primary medical physician then informs the patient of the meeting and reviews the key points of the care plan with the patient. Depending on the patient's level of function, it is sometimes reasonable to invite the patient into the staff meeting to hear the consensus directly.

Meetings of involved physicians and staff may be required periodically if the patient's length of stay in the hospital is relatively long. Splitting that arises concerning one issue may be resolved, but another issue may arise a few days later.

The most common error in network meetings to combat splitting is the failure to include an important caretaker. When this happens, those who have attended the meeting and those who have not may wind up on opposite sides of a split. If several physicians are regularly involved in the patient's care, all must be present. If nurses on day and evening shifts are split, both shifts must be represented at the meeting.

Splitting may occur in outpatient settings when patients with borderline personality organization see multiple physicians for their various medical problems. They seek opinions from each physician, attending especially to any differences or discrepancies among physicians' opinions. These perceptions may lead to noncompliance or to the patient's devaluing one physician while idealizing the other.

The psychiatrist can counteract this splitting by bringing together the physicians most involved in the patient's care, writing or telephoning those more peripherally involved, and developing a consensus among all physicians regarding the patient's diagnosis and appropriate treatment. If consensus is not possible, the basis of differences of opinion is clarified. Then the psychiatrist and the primary medical physician meet with the patient and review the information together. Family members may be included in the conference if they are higher-functioning than the patient.

When confronted with antisplitting measures, some patients become extremely anxious or enraged. Some defect from treatment. Others remain in treatment but may require short-term neuroleptics to contain the anxiety that emerges when the splitting defense is effectively confronted. Despite these problems, antisplitting maneuvers probably are safer for the patient than ignoring the problem, because significant caretaker splitting may lead to errors in physician or nursing judgment that increase the risk of a poor medical outcome.

Constructing a Management Strategy for Patients with Lower-Level Defenses

For patients with lower-level defenses, begin by clarifying expectations, being consistent, giving a sense of control, and taking the "one-down" position. Even if there is a past history of inappropriate behavior in the medical setting, there usually is no need to set limits until the patient acts or threatens to act destructively. Then limit setting can be done, sympathetically in the case of borderline and antisocial patients and matter-of-factly with paranoid and schizotypal patients. Sympathetic limit setting should not be used with paranoid, avoidant, and schizotypal patients, because sympathy may arouse further anxiety by instilling a sense of closeness (Braff, 1981; McGrath, 1978). If sympathetic limit setting is ineffective with a borderline or antisocial patient, one should proceed with matter-of-fact limit setting. Limits framed so that they save face for the patient are often embraced gratefully by patients with lower-level narcissistic personalities. When staff splitting

occurs, antisplitting maneuvers should be instituted.

Strategies for Patients with "Higher-Level" Defenses

Strategies for patients with higher-level defenses and object relations development presuppose a reasonable degree of trust and consistency and attempt to use these patients' personality styles and personal issues as leverage to help them comply with prescribed therapeutic interventions. Strategies for higher level personalities include use of strategic reframing statements and personal leverage.

Strategic Reframing

Strategic reframing means presenting medical instructions in language that is most consistent with the patient's characteristic coping style and personal issues or framing medical instructions in a manner designed to discourage subversion of the treatment plan by the patient's maladaptive defenses. The former can be called *positive reframing*, and the latter may be called *paradoxical reframing. These types of verbal approaches play into a patient's defenses and narcissism rather than confronting them.*

Positive reframing. After giving a narcissistic patient medical instructions, one might say, "Many patients would have difficulty with these instructions. Only a special person could really follow this regimen as it was intended" (Lipp, 1977). The medical need for compliance is expressed in language appealing to the patient's sense of entitlement to special treatment. A compulsive patient might be asked to carry out an instruction because "it will save you time and money." In this case, compliance is linked to the patient's concern with efficiency.

Paradoxical reframing. Disabled patients with dependent personalities might be given a detailed plan for a gradual return to normal activity and be told that it would be difficult for them to carry out and that they could probably do it only by having weekly visits with the psychiatrist for support. Even then, if they did succeed, it would be largely due to their own perseverance in the face of a frightening situation. The psychiatrist would see them, however, only if they did comply with rehabilitative activities. Dependent patients with a lack of self-confidence are thus offered a situation in which they will get all the credit if they succeed but no blame if they fail. Also, the personal need to depend on others is linked with rehabilitation, through the psychiatrist's offer of weekly support. Further, noncompliance is linked with the threatened loss of a dependent relationship.

Paradoxical intention, or prescribing the symptom, is a special type of strategic reframing. This controversial technique is anecdotally effective in patients with compulsive and passive-aggressive traits but may be risky in borderline patients, whose humorless reception of paradoxical requests may lead to regression or acting out (Greenberg & Pies, 1983).

Positive reframing statements may emphasize illness as an occasion for personal growth or the mastery of illness as a route to greater independence. These types of statements are particularly appealing to individuals with higher-level defenses who have sympathy for the ideas of humanistic psychology and the concept of the physician and patient as peers. Strategic reframing statements preferably use the patient's own language and focus on the patient's individual concerns. The process of creating reframing statements is similar to that used in developing hypnotic suggestions and self-hypnotic routines and may be combined with formal trance procedures by clinicians with sufficient expertise in hypnosis. Applications of self-induced trance in medical settings are described by Spiegel and Spiegel (1978).

Personal Leverage

Using personal leverage means motivating the patient with poor self-esteem by relating medically therapeutic behavior to an important personal relationship. The source of leverage may be the primary physician, a nurse, a consultant, a house officer, or a family member. Personal leverage may involve suggestions, direct orders, recommendations (Balint, 1957), reassurance, or handwritten instructions (Hayes et al., 1979). Typical statements are as follows:

1. "As your personal physician, I recommend X." (Kahana et al, 1964)
2. "I really believe that someone like you could handle this procedure just fine."
3. "Dr. Z., our eminent consultant, has reviewed your case and recommends Y."
4. "Do it for your children."

In some cases, having a personally influential person talk to the patient about the medical treatment or personal problem is most helpful. For instance, a spouse might be invited by the doctor to help explain a procedure to the patient, assuming that the spouse has previously been shown to be positively influential toward the patient's overall health.

Personal leverage may be useful with dependent, histrionic, and higher-level narcissistic patients, especially if the source of the personal leverage is someone who is currently in a stable positive relationship with the patient (Hall, 1977). Personal leverage is usually not effective with compulsive patients, who tend to mistrust personal appeals and are much more comfortable with a rational, factually oriented approach.

Appeals to religious or philosophical beliefs, subcultural expectations, and other transpersonal concerns are variants of personal leverage that can be extraordinarily effective if the clinician has sufficient understanding of the patient's cultural milieu and belief system.

Considerations in Choice of Strategy

For patients with higher-level personality disorders, the psychiatric interview determines the personal issue underlying the patient's noncompliance or emotional difficulty. The doctor then attempts to describe the proposed treatment in a way that addresses the personal issue. Frequently occuring personal issues are mentioned in the personality disorder descriptions; however, it is always best if a specific personal issue can be identified during the initial consultation.

For patients who avoid intimacy, whether they be schizoid, avoidant, schizotypal, or paranoid, it is useful for the physician to adopt a neutral, predictable, matter-of-fact style. In inpatient settings, where other caretakers are involved with patients, the psychiatrist might recommend that they do the same. This will avoid the anxiety that these patients experience when confronted with excessive intimacy (McGrath, 1978). By reducing their anxiety, it may diminish the intensity of other troublesome traits.

Medication

Use of Psychotropic Medications

The use of psychotropic medications to treat concurrent Axis I diagnoses is well-established and is recommended in virtually all cases. More controversial is the use of medication to improve Axis II personality disorders occurring alone. The issues are reviewed in the 1986 American Psychiatric Association Annual Review (Liebowitz, Stone, & Turkat, 1986). Neuroleptics may be helpful for borderline and schizotypal patients (Goldberg, Schulz, Schulz, et al., 1986; Gunderson, 1986;

Soloff, George, Nathan, et al., 1986). Monoamine oxidase inhibitors may be useful for patients with histrionic, avoidant, dependent, passive-aggressive, and narcissistic personalities if multiple "neurotic" symptoms, such as fears, compulsions, anxiety, and depression, are present (Klar & Siever, 1984). Clomipramine, yet to be marketed in the U.S., may help compulsive personalities, particularly if they have concurrent obsessive-compulsive disorder. Beta blockers and benzodiazepines may be useful in personality disorders in which excessive anxiety is hypothesized as an aggravating factor (Liebowitz et al., 1986).

Pragmatic psychiatrists often employ neuroleptics in treating borderline, schizotypal, and parnoid individuals who decompensate in medical settings. When disrupted behavior or distorted thinking preclude the patient's cooperation with medically necessary treatment, the risk–benefit ratio for low-dose neuroleptics is high. Relatively low doses minimize the risk of severe extrapyramidal symptoms, and seem to be effective in patients without concurrent schizophrenia. The use of benzodiazepines to treat anxiety in patients with personality disorders is more problematic because of these drugs' ability to destabilize impulsive behavior and to induce dependency.

Short-acting benzodiazepines, because of their tendency to cause rebound anxiety, may exacerbate drug-seeking behavior in patients with personality disorders. A preferred benzodiazepine may therefore be a longer-acting agent such as clorazepate, given twice a day in a relatively low dose, without as-needed (p.r.n.) doses. In patients with severe autonomic accompaniments of anxiety, beta blockers may be used alone or in combination with low-dose benzodiazepines. Of course, the medical contraindications to beta blockers, such as asthma, should be ruled out.

As noted above, stimulants may be valuable in patients whose personality disorder coexists with ADD. At low doses, they can be safe in patients with quite severe medical illness. It is recommended that their use be avoided, however, in patients with a strong history of antisocial acts or drug abuse unless the patient has already been assessed and is under treatment for ADD.

Use of Analgesics

Although many physicians do not regard analgesics as psychotropics, analgesics may profoundly affect behavior and mood, and their use may be especially problematic in patients with personality disorders. The association of pain with regressive behavior has already been noted. Although analgesic management is covered in Chapters 16 and 17, a few special points are worth emphasizing here.

Acute, organically based pain should always be adequately treated, though preferably not with p.r.n. schedules. Concerns about dependency can be addressed later, after the acute medical situation is resolved. Inadequate analgesia can provoke severe acting out in patients with lower-level personality disorders.

Only one physician should be responsible for prescribing analgesia, especially for patients with lower-level disorders. That physician should reevaluate the dosage schedule frequently. For most patients, medication should be given at regularly scheduled intervals and *not* p.r.n. Regular dose schedules permit patients to have autonomy without reinforcing pain complaints, if they offer medications at specific times rather than on demand but permit patients the option of refusing or delaying doses or of choosing a smaller dose. Such schedules also permit nursing staff to withhold or delay medication if a patient is oversedated.

Pentazocine and meperidine both may produce excitement and hallucinations; patients with severe personality disorders may be at greater risk for overt display of psychotoxicity. These agents should usually be avoided.

Psychodynamics of Prescribing

In patients with personality disorders, it is especially worthwhile to determine the psychologic meaning of medication to the patient. Medication compliance and medication abuse are frequent and can often be understood in terms of difficulties with impulse control, idiosyncratic ideas about medication, personal issues related to medication taking, or problems in the physician-patient relationship. A compulsive personality might focus excessively on the expense of medication while subconsciously resenting the loss of control implied in "depending" on a drug. A borderline personality might oppose discontinuation of a medication, despite medically unacceptable side effects, because the pill is a consistent anchoring point in a fragmented inner world (Adelman, 1985). Many problems can be avoided by *prospective* discussion of feelings about medication before initiating treatment and by prediction of the individual patient's confounding issues. The psychologic management strategies applied above can then be applied when making the prescription.

LIAISON ISSUES AND PSYCHIATRIC PRIMARY CARE

Patients with lower-level defenses and poor object relations are particularly likely to produce anger in caretakers; the consequence of their splitting defenses is the polarization of staff. For these patients, psychiatric consultation rarely helps unless the reactions of attending physicians and nursing staff are addressed explicitly. Attention to the consultee, liaison work with nursing staff, and ongoing availability of the consultant are needed to forestall crises. Weekend and holiday coverage for the consultant must be arranged to promote maximum consistency of advice given to the caretakers.

In dealing with caretakers, the consultant should permit ventilation of anger and disagreement and then emphasize that these reactions provide *diagnostic information* about the patient (Gallop, 1985; Groves, 1975). The consultant should help caretakers "cool down" so that the basic principles of being consistent, giving a sense of control, and setting limits without anger can be emphasized. Further details are offered in the earlier section Preventing and Managing Staff Splitting.

Often suggestion of a pharmacologic intervention, such as recommending low-dose neuroleptics for the patient, permits a face-saving reappraisal of the patient by the staff. If the patient can be viewed as "stabilized" by an external agent, anger over the patient's past behavior can be rationalized. These pharmacologic interventions must not be carried out *solely* for their effect on staff, but should be indicated by the patient's diagnosis and behavior.

Sometimes consultation, even with liaison and follow-up, is insufficient to contain the self-destructive, disruptive, or noncompliant behavior of the medically ill patient with a severe personality disorder. At other times, as with some pain patients, personality problems can prevent proper diagnosis and management in a purely medical setting. In these situations primary care of the patient by the psychiatrist may facilitate resolution of the problem. When this arrangement is chosen, all orders are written by the psychiatrist, who sees the patient daily and uses medical specialists as consultants. At hospitals where there is a medical-psychiatric unit, the patient may usually be transferred there. Psychiatric primary care can greatly improve consistency of management, because it puts the psychiatrist at the front-line position of deciding whether particular physical complaints need medical intervention or should be dealt with as somatic expressions of

psychiatric disorder (Fogel & Goldberg, 1983–84).

Psychiatric primary care is unsuitable if the medical problem is extremely unstable medically; in such a case concurrent care is better. Medical-psychiatric units may do better at *containing* the behavior of personality-disordered patients than they do at *changing* their maladaptive defenses; longer-stay, milieu-oriented units may be more suited for promoting enduring behavioral change. Patients with severe personality disorders and active medical illness, therefore, should usually be stabilized on a medical ward or medical-psychiatric unit and then transferred to a conventional psychiatric unit if milieu-oriented inpatient treatment is still needed after medical stabilization.

Psychiatric primary care at times may be suitable for long-term outpatient treatment. The patient's coping with the chronic illness and health care system can be used as a focus for psychotherapeutic exploration and behavioral change. (See Chapter 1 by Green for details of medical psychotherapy.)

Countertransference Reactions

Countertransference reactions to patients with personality disorders comprise a wide range of possibilities, including hate, anger, desire to avoid or abandon the patient, personal attraction, overprotectiveness, and taking sides with the patient against family members or other professional caretakers. The detection of countertransference reactions may be more difficult when they are defended against with reaction formation. For example, compulsive overconcern or excessive inclusiveness in a medical workup may be a defense against an unacceptable desire to avoid the patient.

In consultation-liaison work, the psychiatric consultant must tactfully assist the patient's professional caretakers in understanding their countertransference, learning to see it as information about the patient rather than an implication of their inadequacy.

In medical-psychiatric settings, the focus shifts to maintaining a clear awareness of countertransference issues despite the intense distractions offered by the patient's medical care. On medical-psychiatric units, psychiatrists and nurses may lose sight of countertransference issues that would not escape their notice in a strictly psychiatric setting. In fact, experience with psychiatric primary care in medical-psychiatric settings is an excellent way for a psychiatrist to build empathy for medical consultees.

Special Issues in the Elderly

Longitudinal studies suggest that personality traits are stable into old age (Costa & McCrae, 1980; McCrae, Costa, & Arenberg, 1980). Personality disorders endure into old age, although they may be less commonly diagnosed because the Axis I diagnoses of depression, dementia, and delirium occupy the foreground in geriatric psychiatry. Elderly medical patients' personality problems cannot be ignored, because they disrupt medical treatment just as they do in younger patients. Therapists of the elderly (Kernberg, 1986) suggest that elderly patients with some forms of personality disorder may be as responsive to psychotherapeutic treatment as younger patients.

Once a personality disorder is recognized, the same management techniques may be applied to elderly patients as to younger patients. There are, however, some differences in emphasis. Because of the high prevalence of organic mental disorders in the elderly, the search for aggravating organic factors must be aggressive and should always include adequate testing

of cognition and laboratory evaluation for toxic and metabolic factors.

Age prejudice may lead to insensitivity to elderly patients' personality problems, while oversolicitousness may lead to an underutilization of confrontation and limit setting. Psychiatrists must carefully examine their own attitudes toward the elderly as well as the attitudes of the caretakers seeking consultation. The presence of positive and negative biases toward elderly patients must be sought and gently explored with consultees. For example, many clinicians believe that elderly patients are more hypochondriacal than younger patients, but systematic studies of the issue do not support this view (Costa & McCrae, 1985). Elderly neurotics, like young neurotics, exaggerate physical problems. The greater number of complaints in the elderly is related to a higher prevalence of true somatic disease.

LEGAL ISSUES

Patients with lower-level personality disorders, having unstable object relations, may rapidly turn against their physicians because of disappointment or disagreement. If there has been an error of judgment or an unexpectedly poor medical outcome, the patient may sue the physician or may threaten litigation with manipulative intent. Lawyers, not understanding the dynamics of borderline personality, may with good intentions pursue patient claims that are based more on near-psychotic transference than on reality (Gutheil, 1985).

In the consultation-liaison setting, the psychiatrist is usually called after the physician-patient relationship has begun to deteriorate and threats have been made. While interventions with patient and caretakers are made to "cool down" the situation, the attending physician should be asked to obtain a second opinion on the medical management and to thoroughly document the reasons for all medical judgments made to date (Schwarcz & Halaris, 1984). The psychiatrist reviews with the attending physician the alternatives of discharging the patient or transferring the patient's care to another doctor. The psychiatrist then explores the patient's feelings toward the attending physician and explicitly discusses alternative treatment options. This discussion is documented thoroughly. The patient's responsibility for subsequent treatment choices is thus established. Limits can then be set if necessary, because alternatives have already been worked out that would not constitute abandonment of the patient.

Occasionally, the psychiatrist will have the opportunity for primary prevention. If a patient with a borderline or antisocial personality is idealizing a doctor, the psychiatrist can advise the doctor to review the treatment contract with the patient, to gently disillusion the patient about the idealized traits ascribed, to scrupulously document consent discussions, to obtain second opinions, and to use the language of humble collaboration rather than the language of rescue. With repeated consultations, consultees will learn to recognize and forestall dangerous levels of idealization.

When the psychiatrist is the primary caretaker of a patient with combined medical illness and personality disorder, a special issue arises around termination of treatment and discharge planning, because physical symptoms, rather than suicide threats, may be the currency of manipulation. The psychiatrist is at risk for medical malpractice if he minimizes the patient's physical complaints and an untoward medical outcome is the result. In this situation, we recommend that the psychiatrist call in a medical specialist to examine the patient and share responsibility for the decision that discharge is reasonable. Then responsible limit setting can be employed despite threats of litigation.

REFERENCES

Adelman SA (1985). Pills as transitional objects: A dynamic understanding of the use of medication in psychotherapy. *Psychiatry*, *48*, 246–253.

Andrulonis PA, Glueck BC, Stroebel CF, et al. (1982). Borderline personality subcategories. *Journal of Nervous and Mental Disorders*, *170*, 670–679.

Balint M (1957). *The doctor, his patient and illness*. New York: International Universities Press.

Barnard C & Hirsch C (1985). Borderline personality and victims of incest. *Psychological Reports*, *57*, 715–718.

Bellissimo A & Tunks E (1984). *Chronic pain: The psychotherapeutic spectrum* (pp 1–18). New York: Praeger.

Benner DG & Joscelyne B (1984). Multiple personality as a borderline disorder. *Journal of Nervous and Mental Disorders*, *172*, 98–104.

Braff DL (1981). Impaired speed of information processing in non-medicated schizotypal patients. *Schizophrenia Bulletin*, *7*, 499–508.

Costa PT & McCrae RR (1980). Still stable after all these years: Personality as a key to some issues in adulthood and old age. In Baites PB, Brim OC

(eds): *Life-Span Development and Behavior* (Vol 3). New York: Academic Press.

Costa PT & McCrae RR (1985). Hypochondriasis, neuroticism, and aging: When are somatic complaints unfounded? *American Psychologist*, *40*, 19–28.

David DS (1979). Humility and the physician. *Journal of Chronic Diseases*, *32*, 541–542.

Ellard J (1977). How to deal with personality disorders. *Modern Medicine in Asia*, *13*, 28–33.

Fogel BS & Goldberg RJ (1983–84). Beyond liaison: A future role for psychiatry in medicine. *International Journal of Psychiatry in Medicine*, *13*, 185–192.

Frances A (1982). Categorical and dimensional systems of personality diagnosis: A comparison. *Comprehensive Psychiatry*, *23*, 516–527.

Freud A (1946). *The ego and the mechanisms of defense*. New York: International Universities Press.

Gallop R (1985). The patient is splitting: Everyone knows and nothing changes. *Journal of Psychosocial Nursing*, *23*, 6–10.

George A & Soloff PH (1986). Schizotypal symptoms in patients with borderline personality disorders. *American Journal of Psychiatry*, *143*, 212–215.

Goldberg SC, Schulz SC, Schulz PM, et al. (1986). Borderline and schizotypal personality disorders treated with low-dose thiothixene vs. placebo. *Archives of General Psychiatry*, *43*, 680–686.

Greenberg RP & Pies R (1983). Is paradoxical intention risk-free? A review and case report. *Journal of Clinical Psychiatry*, *44*, 66–69.

Groves JE (1975). Management of the borderline patient on a medical or surgical ward: The psychiatric consultant's rule. *International Journal of Psychiatry in Medicine*, *32*, 178–183.

Groves JE (1978). Taking care of the hateful patient. *New England Journal of Medicine*, *298*, 883–887.

Gunderson JG (1986). Pharmacotherapy for patients with borderline personality disorder. *Archives of General Psychiatry*, *43*, 698–699.

Gunderson JG & Elliott GR (1985). The interface between borderline personality disorder and affective disorder. *American Journal of Psychiatry*, *142*, 277–288.

Gutheil TG (1985). Medicolegal pitfalls in the treatment of borderline patients. *American Journal of Psychiatry*, *142*, 9–14.

Hall A (1977). The psychotherapy of character disorder. *Australian and New Zealand Journal of Psychiatry*, *11*, 175–178.

Hayes B, Taylor D, & Sackett D (eds) (1979). *Compliance in health care* (pp 63–77). Baltimore: Johns Hopkins University Press.

Hirschfeld RMA, Klerman GL, Clayton PJ, et al. (1983). Assessing personality: Effects of the depressive state on trait measurement. *American Journal of Psychiatry*, *140*, 695–699.

Hyler SE & Frances A (1985). Clinical implications of Axis I–Axis II interactions. *Comprehensive Psychiatry*, *26*, 345–351.

Kahana RJ & Bibring GL (1964). Personality types in medical management. In NE Zinberg (Ed), *Psychiatry and medical practice in a general hospital* (pp 108–123). New York: International Universities Press.

Kaplan M (1983, July). A woman's view of DSM-III. *American Psychologist*, 786–792.

Kass F, Skodol AE, Charles E, et al. (1985). Scaled ratings of DSM-III personality disorders. *American Journal of Psychiatry*, *142*, 627–630.

Kernberg OF (1986). *Severe personality disorders: Psychotherapeutic strategies*. New Haven: Yale University Press.

Khantzian EJ & Treece C (1985). DSM-III psychiatric diagnosis of narcotic addicts. *Archives of General Psychiatry*, *42*, 1067–1071.

Klar H & Siever LJ (1984). The psychopharmacologic treatment of personality disorders. *Psychiatric Clinics of North America*, *7*, 791–801.

Koenigsberg HW, Kaplan RD, Gilmore MM, et al. (1985). The relationship between syndrome and personality disorder in DSM-III: Experience with 2,462 patients. *American Journal of Psychiatry*, *142*, 207–212.

Krahn DD & Mackenzie TB (1984). Organic personality syndrome caused by insulin-related nocturnal hypoglycemia. *Psychosomatics*, *25*, 711–712.

Liebowitz MR, Stone MH, & Turkat ID (1986). Treatment of personality disorders. In AI Frances & RE Hales (Eds), *American Psychiatric Association Annual Review (Vol 5*, pp 356–393) Washington, DC: APA Press.

Lipp MR (1977). *Respectful treatment: The human side of medical care* (pp 108–123). Hagerstown, MD: Medical Dept, Harper & Row.

Livesley WJ (1985). The classification of personality disorder: I. The choice of category concept. *Canadian Journal of Psychiatry*, *30*, 353–358.

Livesley WJ (1986). Trait and behavioral prototypes of personality disorder. *American Journal of Psychiatry*, *143*, 728–732.

McCrae RR, Costa PT, & Arenberg D (1980). Constancy of adult personality structure in males: Longitudinal cross-sectional and times-of-measurement analyses. *Journal of Gerontology*, *35*, 877–883.

McEnany GW & Tescher BE (1985). Contracting for care: One nursing approach to the hospitalized borderline patient. *Journal of Psychosocial Nursing*, *23*, 11–18.

McGrath WB (1978). The paranoid personality. *Arizona Medicine*, *35*, 604.

Mellsop G, Varghese F, Joshua S, et al. (1982). The reliability of Axis II of DSM-III. *American Journal of Psychiatry*, *139*, 1360–1361.

Merikangas KR & Weissman MM (1986). Epidemiology of DSM-III Axis II personality disorders. In AJ Frances & RE Hales (Eds), *American Psychiatric Association Annual Review* (Vol 5, pp 258–278). Washington, DC: APA Press.

Novac A (1986). The pseudoborderline syndrome: A proposal based on case studies. *Journal of Nervous and Mental Disease*, *174*, 84–91.

O'Brien P, Caldwell C, & Transea G (1985). Destroyers: Written treatment contracts can help cure self-destructive behaviors of the borderline patient. *Journal of Psychosocial Nursing*, *23*, 19–23.

Perry JC (1985). Depression in borderline personality disorder: Lifetime prevalence at interview and longitudinal course of symptoms. *American Journal of Psychiatry*, *142*, 15–21.

Presly AS & Walton JH (1973). Dimensions of abnormal personality. *British Journal of Psychiatry*, *122*, 269–276.

Schwarcz G & Halaris A (1984). Identifying and managing borderline personality patients. *American Family Physician*, *29*, 203–208.

Schwartz DA (1979). The suicidal character. *Psychiatry Quarterly*, *51*, 64–70.

Soloff PH, George A, Nathan RS, et al. (1986). Progress in pharmacotherapy of borderline disorders. *Archives of General Psychiatry*, *43*, 691–697.

Spiegel H & Spiegel D (1978). *Trance and treatment*. New York: Basic Books.

Staleniam MN & Youngs DD (1974). Psychiatric consultation with patients who refuse medical care. *International Journal of Psychiatry in Medicine*, *5*, 115–123.

Stangl D, Pfohl B, Zimmerman M, et al. (1985). A structured interview for the DSM-III personality disorders: A preliminary report. *Archives of General Psychiatry*, *42*, 591–596.

Sternbach RA (1974). *Pain patients: Traits and treatment*. New York: Academic Press.

Stoudemire A & Thompson T (1982). The borderline personality in the medical setting. *Annals of Internal Medicine*, *96*, 76–79.

Strain JJ (1978). *Psychological interventions in medical practice*. New York: Appleton-Century-Crofts.

Task Force on Nomenclature and Statistics of the American Psychiatric Association (1980). *Diagnostic and Statistical Manual of Mental Disorders* (3rd ed). Washington, DC: American Psychiatric Association.

Vaillant GE (Ed) (1986). *Empirical studies of ego mechanisms of defense*. Washington, DC: American Psychiatric Press.

Watzlawick P, Weakland JH, & Fisch R (1974). *Change: Principles of problem formation and problem resolution*. New York: WW Norton.

Zimmerman M, Pfohl B, Stangl D, et al. (1986). Assessment of DSM-III personality disorders: The importance of interviewing an informant. *Journal of Clinical Psychiatry*, *47*, 261–263.

Quentin R. Regestein

12
Sleep Disorders in the Medically Ill

EPIDEMIOLOGY

In medical patients, the more severe the symptoms, the less the sleep. Those with cardiovascular, neurologic, and musculoskeletal problems may be particularly affected (Johns, Egan, Gay, et al, 1970). In the elderly, who have increased chances of being medical patients, there is also decreased total sleep time, increased insomnia, and sleep apnea (Ancoli-Israel, Kripke, Mason, et al., 1981; Bixler, Kales, Jacoby, et al., 1984; Bixler, Scharf, Soldatos, et al., 1979; Carskadon, Harvey, Duke, et al., 1980; Johns, Egan, Gay, et al., 1970; Karacan, Thornby, Anch, et al., 1976; Lugaresi, Cirignotta, Coccagna, et al., 1980; Williams, Karacan, & Hursch, 1974). The sleep of medical inpatients is further disrupted by the consequences of acute illness and of hospital routines. For example, 38 percent of hospital inpatients in one teaching hospital took sleeping pills on one randomly chosen weekday, in addition to the minor tranquilizers taken by 20 percent of them (Salzman, 1981). This compares with 3 percent of adults in epidemiologic surveys reporting use of prescription hypnotics within the previous year (Mellinger, Balter, & Uhlenhuth, 1985).

PHYSIOLOGY

Sleep is part of a 24-hour sleep-wake rhythm governed by two bodily clocks (Moore-Ede, Sulzman, & Fuller, 1982). These "internal clocks" coordinate daily oscillations of all physiologic functions in a way that is controlled, economical, and adjusted to the individual's ecologic niche (Aschoff, 1964; Wever, 1975 a,b,c). The clocks obtain their timing information primarily from the light-dark cycle, although social schedule may be a stronger timing influence in man (Wever, 1970), except in less socially oriented individuals, such as those with chronic schizophrenia (R Morgan, Mirors, & Waterhouse, 1980). Mealtimes, if regular, also provide timing information. When timing influences or sensitivity to them are weak or inconstant, endogenous, longer-than-24-hour cycles emerge, causing slower physiologic rhythms. Conditions such as winter light in northern latitudes, social isolation, or lack of timed work obligations will foster this departure from 24-hour rhythms and may be reflected in progressively later bedtimes and arising times. The temporal coordination among physiologic systems becomes less secure under these circumstances, and "internal desynchrony," the breaking apart of usual synchronous relationships among sleep, body temperature, hormonal, and electrophysiologic parameters, may occur. Under isolation, for instance, one subject had a 33.2-hour sleep-wake cycle but a 24.9-hour body temperature cycle (Hauri, 1982). Desynchrony may also occur in normal circumstances (Czeisler, Allan, Strogatz, et al., 1986). Such desynchrony is more likely in elderly (Wever, 1975c) and neurotic (Lund, 1974) individuals, and may be associated with work inefficiency (Czeisler, Moore-Ede, & Coleman, 1982) and depression (Wehr, Wirz-Justice, Goodwin, et al, 1979). The increased prevalence of depression and suicide at more polar latitudes, known since the 19th century, may be due in part to the shorter periods of daylight there. Various drugs delay or advance circadian phases, including steroids, caffeine, alcohol, and benzodiazepines (Moore-Ede et al., 1982; Seidel, Roth, Roehrs, et al., 1984).

Of the two basic types of sleep, non-rapid-eye-movement (NREM) sleep is a continuous spectrum from light to deep sleep. By definition, it is composed of polygraphic sleep stages 1 through 4 (Rechtschaffen & Kales, 1968), which are characterized by increasingly slow EEG waves. Slow wave sleep occurs early in the night, increases disproportionately after sleep deprivation, preempts REM sleep during restricted sleep regimens, and is increased in association with states of increased metabolism such as exercise, increased body temperature, high normal thyroid indices, and hyperthyroidism (Baekeland & Lasky, 1966; Bunnell & Horvath, 1985; Dunleavy,

Oswald, Brom, et al., 1974; Hobson, 1968; Horne, 1980; Horne & Reid, 1984; Johns, Masterton, Paddle-Ledinek, et al., 1975; Oswald, 1980). Growth hormone is secreted mostly during stage 4 sleep (Parker, Sassin, Mace, et al., 1969). Some have postulated that slow-wave (deep) sleep is necessary for body restitution (Hartmann, 1973) or to enforce the idleness needed for restitution (Horne, 1980).

In contrast to NREM sleep, rapid-eye-movement (REM) sleep manifests more signs of arousal, such as electroencephalographic (EEG) fast waves, continual eye movements, dreams, increased oxygen consumption, and increased blood pressure (Brebbia & Altschuler, 1965; Hartmann, 1973; Khatri & Freis, 1969; Littler, Honour, Carter, et al., 1975; Snyder, 1971). Variability in heart rate and blood pressure increase, 50 percent in REM compared with NREM sleep (Snyder, Hobson, Morrison, et al., 1964). This increased variability may relate to the increase in both cardiac arrhythmias (Regestein, et al., 1987) and angina attacks (Murao, Harumi, Katayama, et al., 1972) during REM sleep. Ulcer patients may secrete more gastric acid during REM sleep (Armstrong, Burnap, Jacobson, et al., 1965).

Sleep may have evolved to conserve energy or to keep individuals within their own ecologic time niche (Allison Twyver, 1970), and is regulated at basic hindbrain levels. Serotonergic neurons in the raphe nuclei and in the preoptic area of the hypothalamus are necessary for normal sleep. Stimulation of the nucleus of the tractus solitarius, which receives vagal afferents, synchronizes forebrain EEG rhythms and causes decreased arousal, suggesting one possible mechanism for postprandial drowsiness. The suprachiasmic nuclei of the hypothalamus receive information about light directly from the retina and regulate circadian rhythms (Moore-Ede, 1982). An oscillating, reciprocally inhibiting pair of pontine cell groups, the cholinergic gigantotegmental field cells of the mesencephalon and the noradrenergic locus coeruleus, may time the cycle between NREM and REM sleep (Hobson, 1983). Disease processes that involve centers in the brain stem may increase specific sleep stages (Hobson, 1975) or abolish sleep (Fischer-Perroudon, Mouret, & Jouvet, 1974). Recently, however, sleep has been conceived more as deriving ultimately from multiple cortical and subcortical mechanisms (Kelly, 1985; McGinty, Drucker-Colin, Morrison, et al., 1985) that exert an influence on brain stem structures and are in turn affected by them.

Neurochemically, serotonergic neurons seem responsible for the initiation of NREM sleep and the priming of REM sleep, and some adrenergic neurons play a role in cortical arousal and REM sleep (Jouvet, 1974). Clinically, this translates into increased sleep when the dietary serotonin precursor, L-tryptophan, is administered (Hartmann, 1974) and insomnia as a frequent side-effect of methysergide, an antiserotonergic drug. There is an inverse relationship between the amount of REM sleep present and levels of brain catecholamines (Hartmann, 1973) as affected by mood states and catecholamine-affecting drugs. Raising CNS levels of acetylcholine by physostigmine injections increases arousal; that is, during slow-wave sleep such injections cause REM, and during REM they cause wakefulness (Sitaram, Wyatt, Dawson, et al., 1976).

COMMON SLEEP DISORDERS

Some sleep disorders, such as narcolepsy or sleep apnea, provide major reasons for medical or surgical intervention, but more commonly, a sleep disorder, for example, insomnia, will complicate the clinical status of a superimposed medical problem, or such problems as steroid treatments, rheumatoid arthritis, or renal dialysis will lead to disorder without sleep. Factors predisposing to disordered sleep will be discussed in the following subsections as a background for understanding the relationships between them and common medical problems.

The classification of sleep disorders has recently moved from specific clinical syndromes (Association of Sleep Disorders Centers, 1979) to more general classes (American Psychiatric Association, 1987). The major subheadings are now *dyssomnias*, that is, poor sleep quality, and *parasomnias*, that is, conditions provoked by sleep. The uncovering of common mechanisms—for example, between obstructive and central sleep apnea (e.g., Sanders, 1984; Sanders, Rogers, & Pennock, 1985)—has suggested that sleep problems should be thought of in terms of both symptoms and mechanisms; similar pathologic processes may underlie insomnia in one patient but hypersomnia in another. The following discussion will thus enumerate sleep disturbances that present as complaints of insufficient night sleep, daytime sleepiness, or behavioral problems during sleep, or as complaints from others about the patient's behavior during sleep.

Dyssomnias

Insomnia is a complaint of too little sleep. It usually results from a combination of predispositions and direct causes. The most common predispositions are the use of CNS-acting drugs, advancing age, schedule irregularities, and hyperarousal. More direct causes include various psychiatric, neurologic, and endocrine conditions, irritating symptoms of any disease and rarer primary sleep disorders. Hypersomnia means abnormally large amounts of sleep, often associated with excessive daytime sleepiness. Excessively sleepy patients develop low standards for wakefulness and often fail to seek help for sleepiness until others consider their continual dozing pathological, or an accident caused by sleepiness occurs.

Drug Effects

The most common offenders are caffeine, alcohol, and nicotine. Caffeine is consumed by over 80 percent of the adult population (Dews, 1982). It has a 12–20-hour duration of action (Hollingsworth, 1912), lessens sleep quality (Brezinova, 1974), and increases next-morning drowsiness (Goldstein, Kaizer, & Whitby, 1969). It increases symptoms in hospital patients (Victor, Lubetsky, & Greden, 1981) and may worsen their psychologic symptoms (Charney, Heninger, & Jaflow, 1985; Neil, Himmelhoch, Mallinger, et al., 1978). Coffee, tea, chocolate, and caffeine-containing medications should therefore be discontinued in insomnia patients. The caffeine withdrawal syndrome may last months and entail a significant loss of energy and initiative; overt depression may occur.

Alcohol ingestion lessens sleep quality. After only one drink in the evening, some patients will awaken in the middle of the night, often with a feeling of excess warmth or palpitations. This may be due to increased adrenergic activity, as suggested by increased cerebrospinal fluid 6–14 hours after alcohol ingestion (Borg, Krande, & Sedval, 1981). Increasing alcohol intake causes decreased sleep quality until at the extreme of severe alcoholism there is "fragmented" sleep, with frequent awakenings and shifts among sleep stages (Mello & Mendelson, 1970; Pokorny, 1978). Years after alcohol withdrawal alcoholics continue to suffer diminished sleep quality (Adamson & Burdick, 1973).

Nicotine is a stimulant (Henningfield, 1974), which partly accounts for its addicting and appetite-suppressing properties. Smokers take longer to fall asleep at night than nonsmokers, but may improve their sleep within a week after quitting (Soldatos, Kales, Scharf, et al., 1980). Daily sleep length diminishes with increased use of tobacco (Palmer & Harrison, 1983).

Of these common drugs, caffeine and alcohol usually are discontinued by the motivated insomnia patient, but nicotine retains a more tenacious hold on the patient, having an addiction profile and a recidivism rate paralleling that of heroin (Henningfield, 1984). Nicotine chewing gum reportedly increased the abstinence rate of patients in a smoking cessation clinic (Hialmarson, 1984), and clonidine may suppress cigarette craving during the withdrawal period (Glassman, Jackson, Walsh, et al., 1984). Further discussion of smoking cessation may be found in Chapter 15, by Abrams.

Some over-the-counter drugs aggravate insomnia, especially nasal decongestants and appetite-suppressants. Over-the-counter sleeping pills basically are placebo medications (Mendelson, 1980); their anticholinergic effects actually may diminish sleep quality in the elderly.

Of the prescription medications, catecholamine blockers, antibronchospastic agents, stimulating antidepressants, and antiarrhythmia drugs all commonly disrupt sleep. Methyldopa (Smirk, 1963), propranolol (Petrie, Maffucci, & Woosley, 1982), xanthine derivatives, and beta agonists are frequent offenders, and thyroid hormone, contraceptives, and methysergide deserve suspicion in individual cases. Use of diuretics commonly underlies restless-legs syndrome, a motor disorder that may disrupt sleep. Antibiotics that interfere with protein synthesis and that enter the nervous system (e.g., tetracyclines) may reduce deep sleep (Nonaka, Nakazawa, & Kotorii, 1983).

The shorter acting benzodiazepines, especially triazolam, may cause nocturnal agitation (Regestein & Reich, 1985), early morning insomnia (Kales, Soldatos, Bixler, et al., 1983), and next-day anxiety (K Morgan & Oswald, 1982), presumably by provoking a rapidly appearing withdrawal syndrome.

Given the panoply of drug effects on sleep, any use of CNS-acting drugs should be considered a possible factor in aggravating insomnia. The clinical dilemma between therapeutic and unwanted effects sometimes can be resolved by switching to peripherally acting drugs. For example, in the case of antihypertensives, an ACE inhibitor can be substituted for propranolol. In the insomniac asthmatic patient, careful titration of drug doses to minimal effective levels and the use of shorter-acting agents toward evening may lessen insomnia.

Age Effects

Sleep normally becomes lighter and more disrupted with aging. From the neonatal period through senescence, it takes progressively longer to fall asleep, there are an increasing number of nocturnal wakenings, and there is decreasing deep sleep (Williams, et al., 1974). The 30-year-old, for instance, obtains less than one-half the stage 4 sleep obtained by the 20-year-old (Gaillard, 1978). The decline of sleep parallels the decline of cerebral functioning with age as measured by cognitive functioning (Prinz, 1977), and cerebral blood flow (Prinz, Obrist, & Wang, 1975). Since behavioral and neurologic intactness covary in old people (Tomlinson, Blessed, & Roth, 1970), and since dementia amplifies the sleep deficits of aging (Reynolds, Kupfer, Taska, et al., 1985a), it would seem that the usual diminution of sleep with age derives from the normal progressive neuronal and dendritic loss (Brody & Vijayashankar, 1977). This structural decline with age, combined with waning biologic clock functioning (Wever, 1975c), predisposes older people to sleep disorders. It is not age per se, however, but state of health, that determines sleep quality. Almost any physiologic measurement shows wider variance with age (Comfort, 1968). For instance, sleep correlates with intellectual intactness

much more than with age (Prinz, 1977), and sleep apnea is found much more in random samples than in samples of *healthy* elderly (Ancoli-Isreal et al., 1981; Reynolds, Kupfer, Taska, et al., 1985a). A reduction in ventilation rate, however, and an increase in disturbed breathing during sleep have been noted even in normal aging subjects (Bliwise, Seidel, Greenblatt, et al., 1984; Krieger, Mangin, & Kurtz, 1980).

The psychologic regression that may accompany old age, the absence of timed work obligations, and a passive attitude toward controlling one's own habits both promote insomnia and lessen adherence to insomnia treatments (Regestein, 1980). Studies indicate that many aged individuals sleep 9.5 hours during a 12-hour daily in-bed time (Stramba-Badiale, Ceretti, & Forni, 1979; Webb & Swinburne, 1971), a practice likely to lessen the refreshment of sleep, since prolonged in-bed times may be detrimental to overall sleep quality. For instance, healthy experimental subjects tested in the afternoon on vigilance and performance tasks did worse after they were allowed to sleep late than when they arose after a more usual length of sleep (Taub, Globus, Phoebus, et al., 1971).

Schedule Effects

The entrainment of a 24-hour sleep-wake rhythm requires arising at the same clock time daily (Webb & Agnew, 1974). Over a quarter of U.S. workers work outside the usual daytime work schedules, however, out of synchrony with the daylight-night cycle, many of them on rotating shifts (Czeisler et al., 1982). Night workers sleep worse than others (Tepas, Stock, Maltese, et al., 1982), possibly because their off-work hours are less organized (Kripke, Cook, & Lewis, 1971). Some individuals without timed work obligations keep highly erratic schedules (Regestein, 1982) or else sleep progressively later until they come into conflict with daytime obligations. Such progressively later sleeping reflects the underlying longer-than-24-hour circadian rhythm found in individuals deprived of physiologic timing signals (e.g. periodic bright light and regular mealtimes). Among the elderly, an opposite tendency, toward increasingly earlier sleep schedules, is found (Tune, 1968), probably reflecting the shortening of the underlying endogenous circadian rhythm that occurs with age. (Weitzman, Moline, Czeisler, et al., 1982). Habitual late sleeping in the morning also predisposes to depression (Globus, 1969; Wehr et al., 1979).

Hyperarousal

Arousal is that state in which focused thought and sustained productive efforts occur. It is more than simple wakefulness. The arousal profile of an individual is related to neurophysiologic properties, such as the percentage of EEG alpha rhythm manifest under standard conditions (Gray, 1967) or the electrocortical responsiveness to stimuli (Tecce, 1971), and is expressed in particular behavioral tendencies (Eysenck, 1972). For instance, high-arousal individuals ordinarily have lower sensory thresholds and more prolonged duration of responses (Mangan, 1972), qualities likely to keep them up at night and to turn stress into insomnia (Healy, Kales, Monroe, et al., 1981). It is the intensity rather than the distress of stimuli that causes insomnia in the hyperaroused individual. Pleasurable but intense events in an evening will thus lengthen the time needed to fall asleep. For instance, watching exciting television dramas in the evening reportedly worsens sleep (Saletu, Gruenberger, & Anderer, 1983). Autonomic indices of arousal during the night also differ in poor sleepers, who show higher body temperatures, more body movements, more phasic vasoconstrictions, and higher skin resistances (Monroe, 1967). The rapidity with which the higher arousal individual forms conditioned connections may worsen the insomnia, once it starts, through the formation of a learned association between going to bed and not falling asleep (Hauri & Fisher, 1986).

Psychopathology

Although some attribute most insomnia to psychopathology (Sweetwood, Grant, Gerst, et al., 1980; Tan, Kales, Kales, et al., 1984) and others do not (Carskadon, Dement, Mifler, et al., 1976; Zorick, Roth, Hartze, et al., 1981), it may be that both insomnia and psychopathology result from some common factor (Hauri, 1979). In one series of hospitalized patients requiring psychiatric consultation, 80 percent had disturbed sleep (Berlin, Litovitz, Diaz, et al., 1984). Many insomnia patients have a common profile of psychologic traits. They describe themselves as thoughtful, conscientious, worried anticipators (Regestein, Hallett, Mufson, et al., 1985) who are more nervous, strained, brooding, and hopeless and who often feel anxious rather than sleepy at bedtime (JD Kales, A Kales, Bixler, et al., 1984). The sleep polygraphic findings of *primary insomniacs*—persons with insomnia of no obvious cause—resemble those of anxiety patients (Reynolds, Taska, Sewitch, et al., 1984). Unlike affective disorders or dementia, this pattern may be present when the cause of insomnia is relatively covert and the daytime functioning of the patient is relatively intact. It is unlikely that psychopathology per se causes insomnia, since some severe psychopathology, for example, that found in personality disorder or schizophrenia, causes little insomnia if unassociated with sleep-disrupting habits.

Hospitalization

Patients hospitalized with acute medical problems are likely to suffer noise, frequent disturbance, somatic symptoms, psychologic distress, enforced sleeping positions, casts or drainage tubes, polypharmacy, and a lessened distinction between night and day, any of which may lessen sleep. Even patients who sleep well in hospital may crave more sleep (Cumming, 1984). Sleep probably promotes healing (Adam & Oswald, 1984), whereas partial sleep deprivation, in addition to its commonly experienced psychologic consequences, also worsens somatic symptoms (Moldofsky & Scarisbrick, 1976). Despite the salutory effects of sleep, however, medical care apparently necessitates allowing the most seriously ill patients the least amount of sleep. Studies have revealed that intensive care unit patients average about five interruptions per hour during the calmest night hours (Dlin, Rosen, Dickstein, et al., 1971) and less total sleep than they do on other wards (Broughton & Baron, 1978). Elective surgery patients average less than 6 hours sleep before as well as after surgery (Ellis & Dudley, 1976; Murphy, Bentley, Ellis, et al., 1977). After open-heart surgery, sleep may become light, fragmented, and short, and result in as little as 1–4 hours on the first postoperative day (Johns, Large, Masterton, et al., 1974). Since such subtleties as the view from the patient's window may influence surgical convalescence (Ulrich, 1984), gross disruption of sleep probably does as well, although systematic confirmation of this effect has yet to be made.

Special Medical Problems

Various medical problems predictably worsen sleep via fever, discomfort, drug effects, and so forth. The sleep consequences of given medical problems vary widely. The subjective nature of insomnia (Regestein & Reich, 1978), the small amount of sleep that suffices for some people (HS Jones & Oswald, 1968), and the admixture of psychologic regression during illness all complicate complaints of sleeplessness. Many people with medical reasons for insomnia actually sleep well, and one must therefore consider preexisting tendencies before attributing insomnia entirely to the medical problem at hand.

Breathing disorders. Sleep decreases the ventilatory response (Cherniak, 1981) and thus predisposes to disordered breathing. The recumbent position itself increases the work of breathing (Anch, Remmers, & Bunce, 1982) and thus may aggravate any breathing disorder. Many other impediments may amplify the potential difficulty of breathing during sleep, thus damaging sleep quality (Roehrs, Conway, Wittig, et al., 1985). Nasal blockage forces mouth breathing, which impairs sleep quality (Olsen, Kern, & Westbrook, 1981), and impedes breathing during sleep, occasionally to the extent of apnea and death (Wynne, Block, & Boysen, 1980). Sleep apnea sometimes may be reversed simply by repair of nasal septal deviation (Heimer, Scharf, Lieberman, et al., 1983). The normal dilatation of the upper airway during inspiration may be impaired by topical nasal anesthesia (Oomen, Abu-osba, & Thach, 1982) or by sedatives, especially alcohol (Taasan, Block, Bayser, et al., 1981). Structural or functional impairment anywhere along the respiratory tract makes disturbed breathing during sleep more likely. The narrowing of the airway by obesity, large adenoids or tonsils, enlarged soft palate or uvula, patulous pharyngeal mucosa, micrognathia, macroglossia, or the thickened tissues of acromegaly thus all increase the risk of apnea (Fairbanks, 1984; Orr, 1983), as may the narrower glottis of women (Haponik, Bleecker, Allen, et al., 1981). The impairment of ventilatory control mechanisms in state of hypoxia, hypercapnia, or slowed circulation time also increase the risk of sleep apnea (Cherniack, 1981; Chada, Birch, & Sackner, 1985). Combinations of structural abnormalities and functional dysregulation often occur. For instance, brisk inspiratory efforts, possibly driven by hypoxemia, may be made against a compromised upper airway, thus generating a deep negative interthoracic pressure that sucks the hypopharynx closed, thereby obstructing breathing. (Remmers, de Groot,

Sauerland, et al., 1978). This negative pressure also diminishes cardiac output by reducing left ventricular filling and stroke volume (Tolle, Judy, Yu, et al., 1983). In the presence of any further heart failure, this may delay feedback information about carbon dioxide levels to central chemoreceptors, setting up ventilatory drive overshoot and thus risking further periodic breathing. Since airway compromise and impaired ventilatory control mechanisms damage sleep quality, patients with chronic lung disease sleep poorly, especially when there is significant hypoxia during wakefulness (Wynne et al., 1980). Prolonged oxygen desaturation during sleep may lead to gasping and prompt awakening, although patients who breathe poorly during sleep and complain of insomnia reportedly have less desaturation than those who complain of excess sleepiness (Roehrs et al., 1985).

Although sleep apnea has been specifically connected with insomnia in some patients, (Guilleminault, Eldridge, Dement, et al., 1973), it may also present as hypersomnia (see below). The presence of a breathing disorder clearly worsens sleep quality, but the means by which it causes complaints of insomnia or hypersomnia in given patients are not entirely clear (Orr, 1983). There are asymptomatic normal and obese subjects with sleep apnea (Block, 1979; Cook, Huse, Roudebush, et al., 1982), which suggests that breathing disorder does not explain complaints related to poor sleep quality. Presumably, nervous and psychologic factors are interposed between poor sleep quality of any cause and complaints about it. For instance, frequent, brief, unremembered nocturnal arousals may induce next-day sleepiness unaccompanied by complaints of insufficient sleep.

Snoring. Snoring results from a high-frequency opening and closing of the oropharynx (Sauerland & Harper, 1976). It is augmented by compromise of the upper airway from any structural narrowing or flaccidity and is associated with obesity, hypertension, and heart and lung disease (Norton & Dunn, 1985). It increases with age (Lugaresi et al., 1980). It is worsened by states of severe exhaustion and the use of alcohol (Issa Sullivan, 1984; Scrima, Broudy, & Cohn, 1982) and other sedatives. Sleep apnea becomes likely with loud snoring (Lugaresi, Coccagna, Farneti, et al., 1979), although a third of loud snores had no sleep apnea in one series (Miles & Simmons, 1984). Previously considered a benign inconvenience, snoring remains relatively little investigated even among inpatients, in whom it is easily detected.

Obesity. Obesity increases the risk of breathing disorder during sleep due to increased upper airway resistance (Anch et al., 1982), possibly from increased bogginess of mucosa in the supine position and fat deposition at the tongue base. The inefficiency of a broad, flat diaphragm and the resistance of abdominal fat may account for the diminished ventilatory response found with obesity (Lopata Onal, 1982). The presence of sleep apnea, in turn, contributes to the diurnal obesity-hypoventilation syndrome (JB Jones, Wilhoit, Findley, et al., 1985). A "night eating syndrome," composed of much eating after the evening meal, insomnia, and morning anorexia, is reportedly frequent in the obese (Stunkard, Grace, Wolff, 1955).

Cardiovascular disorder. Coronary artery disease is associated with breathing impairment during sleep, even in the absence of symptomatic lung disease (Olazabal, Miller, Cook, et al., 1982). The mechanism of this impairment is unclear. Patients with angina may have painful episodes that awaken them, especially from dreaming or REM sleep (Murao et al., 1972; Nowlin, Troyer. Collins, et al., 1965), possibly as a consequence of episodically increased heart rate (Quyyami, Mockus,

Wright, et al., 1984), but such patients sleep worse than their pain episodes alone would explain (Karacan, Williams, & Taylor, 1969). When oxygen desaturation occurs during sleep in coronary artery disease the myocardial blood flow requirement may be similar to those of maximal exercise (Shepard, Schweitzer, Keller, et al., 1984), predisposing toward anginal pain. Chronic hypoxia during sleep may also induce pulmonary hypertension (Coccagna & Lugaresi, 1978), leading to right-sided heart failure (Hall, 1986; Sullivan Issa, 1980).

In studies of the hypertensive male population, about 30 percent have manifested undiagnosed sleep apnea (Fletcher, DeBehnke, Lovoi, et al., 1985; JD Kales et al., 1984), whereas 50 percent of those with sleep apnea have reportedly had moderate hypertension (Guilleminault & Dement, 1978). This likely explains the association found between snoring and hypertension (Lugaresi et al., 1980). Sleep generally lessens the frequency and grade of cardiac arrhythmias (Lown, Tykocinski, Garfeir, et al., 1973; Regestein, deSilva, Lown, et al., 1981). Where chronic hypoxia shifts individuals to the sharply falling slope of the oxygen–hemoglobin dissociation curve, lessened ventilation during sleep may cause profound oxygen desaturation (Fleetham & Kryger, 1981), at which time ventricular ectopy may emerge (Shepard, Garrison, Grither, et al., 1985). A bradycardia–tachycardia pattern is frequently found during episodes of sleep-impaired breathing, although any type of cardiac arrhythmia may emerge (Tilkian, Guilleminault, Schroeder, et al., 1977).

Because of the association of sleep apnea with cardiac arrhythmia, readers of sensational articles in the lay press occasionally insist on immediate consultation for snoring spouses. Sleep breathing problems are common and chronic and are associated with high-grade ventricular arrhythmia only in a small minority of cases, often those with other risk factors such as massive obesity and hypertension.

Endocrine-metabolic factors. Exercise increases slow-wave (deep) sleep, more in physically fit than less fit individuals (Horne & Moore, 1985; Trinder, Stevenson, Paxton, et al., 1982; Walker, Floyd, Fein, et al., 1978). The mechanism may be metabolic, due to raised body temperature (Bunnell & Horvath, 1985; Horne & Staff, 1983) and consequently increased metabolism, (Oswald, 1980). Increased thyroid indices and hyperthyroidism are also associated with more (Dunleavy et al., 1974; Johns et al., 1975) and hypothyroidism with less (A Kales, Henser, Jacobson, et al., 1967) deep sleep. Clinically, however, hyperthyroidism may cause severe insomnia (Regestein, 1982). Fever induces broken sleep in some patients and prolonged sleep in others. Sleep itself decreases cerebral glucose metabolic rate, according to preliminary positron-emission tomography, except increases of cerebral metabolism were noted in conjunction with nightmares (Heiss, Dawlik, Herholz, et al., 1985).

The autonomic neuropathy of diabetes mellitus increases the risk of sleep apnea, presumably by interference with muscular responses of the pharyngeal airway (Guilleminault, Briskin, Greenfield, et al., 1981; Rees, Cochrane, Prior, et al., 1981) In two insulin-dependent diabetic patients seen at first hand, obstructive sleep apnea was atypically unaffected subjectively or objectively by surgical revision of the upper airway.

Androgens presumably cause the increase in sleepiness after puberty (Carskadon et al., 1980), as well as the arousal differences found between the sexes in adulthood (Broverman, Klaiber, Lobayashi, 1968). The large preponderance of men, for example, 15:1 in a typical series (Guilleminault & Dement, 1978), suggests that androgenic hormones also play an etiological role in obstructive sleep apnea. For instance, exogenous androgen administration has reportedly induced obstructive sleep apnea in a woman (Johnson, Anch, & Remmers, 1984) though this is not typical (Millman, 1985).

Exogenous growth hormone (GH) administration during sleep in normal subjects as well as in patients with acromegaly has resulted in much-decreased deep sleep, possibly because of a GH–deep sleep feedback mechanism (Carlson, Gillin, Gorden, et al., 1972; Mendelson, Slater, Gold, et al., 1980b). Acromegaly further increases the risk of obstructive sleep apnea, possibly because of thickened pharyngeal tissues (Cadieux, Kales, Santen, et al., 1982).

Menopause carries a high risk of sleep disturbance, even among questionnaire respondents who have been screened for psychopathology (Ballinger, 1976; Lauritzen, 1976). This may be due to estrogen lack in many patients, since it may be remedied by replacement estrogen (Campbell, 1976; Thompson & Oswald, 1977). In normal premenstrual women, however, menstrual fluctuations in estrogen level have little effect on sleep (Billiard & Passonant, 1974).

Other endocrinologic conditions may affect nervous system functioning to provoke a variety of arousal-related syndromes including sleep disturbance, for example, the premenstrual state (Abraham, 1983; Rubinow & Roy-Byrne, 1984), which may cause insomnia or hypersomnia (Billiard, Guilleminault & Dement, 1975; Endicott, Halbreigh Schacht, et al., 1981), and Cushing's syndrome (Regestein, Rose, & Williams, 1972; Starkman, Schteingart, Schork, 1981). A covarying time course of the condition and the sleep disturbance supports an etiologic relationship.

Neurologic conditions. Although sleep is most directly regulated by the nervous system, neurologic disorders disturb sleep surprisingly less than might be expected compared with breathing or endo-crine disorders, except when sleep regulating centers are directly affected. For instance, extensive pontine infarctions may occur without much polygraphic sleep abnormality (Markand & Dyken, 1976; Marquardsen & Harvald, 1964), although bilateral lesions of the midpontine tegmentum may show severe sleep abnormalities. Often neurologic conditions impair sleep through indirect effects, as breathing problems associated with parkinsonian rigidity, refusal to follow good sleep habits in the mildly demented, or enforced inactivity with irregular napping in the motorically disabled.

The polygraphic abnormalities of sleep in various neurologic diseases may not be highly relevant to the clinical status of the individual patient, and may be highly variable. For instance, Mouret (1975), who found slower sleep onset, less deep sleep, and increased blephorospasms during REM sleep in Parkinson's disease patients, writes that there is an "absence of clear and constant alterations of sleep patterns in this disease." Others have reported frequent sleep abnormalities in parkinsonism, including longer sleep onset, more wakefulness during sleep and less sleep spindle activity (A Kales, Ansel, Markham, et al., 1971; Puca, Bricolo, & Turella, 1973). The sleep disturbances correlate with clinical symptoms (Schneider, Maxion, Ziegler, et al., 1974); the rest tremor disappears during sleep (Stern, Roffwarg, & Duvoisir, 1968).

A marked heterogeneity of effects on sleep is also found in seizure disorders. Surveyed epilepsy patients report poor sleep quality and excessive daytime sleepiness (Ruiz-Primo, Coria, & Torres, 1985). Sleepwalking and night terrors, normally rare in adults, were reported with some frequency (Hoeppner, Garron, & Cartwright, 1984). Partial rather than generalized seizure disorders had more disturbed sleep. Epilepsy patients have lighter than normal polygraphically recorded sleep patterns (Declerck, Wanguier, Sijben-kiggen, et al., 1982), whereas temporal lobe epilepsy in particular shows frequent stage shifts and numerous awakenings (Baldy-Moulinier, 1982). Insomnia and nightmare problems have been observed in association with temporal lobe epilepsy and temporal lobe dysfunction, sometimes with frequent brief awakenings throughout laboratory sleep recordings. Such problems are probably not caused by anticonvulsant medications, which have indeed occasionally relieved such problems, although these agents exert various minor direct effects on sleep (Johnson, 1982).

Posttraumatic coma may ablate normal sleep polygraphic patterns; this is a poor prognostic sign (Bergamasco, Bergamini, Doriguzzi, et al., 1968). Even lesser degrees of head trauma without coma may lead to excessive daytime sleepiness. Whiplash has been associated with subsequent sleep apnea (Guilleminault, Faull, Miles, et al., 1983). Among a group of college students, even a history of birth trauma was associated with subsequent minor sleep problems (Coren & Searelman, 1985). Brain tumors may disrupt normal sleep EEG patterns with delta activity in which amplitude and regularity of rhythm during sleep may differ between cerebral and posterior fossa lesions (DD Daly, 1968; Ohgami, 1973). Thalamotomy lesions may cause ipsilateral alterations in sleep recordings (Jurko, Orlando, & Webster, 1971).

Impairments of cortical functioning consistently alter sleep patterns, but in a variety of ways. In mental retardation, for instance, total sleep time reportedly increases in Down's syndrome but decreases in aminoacidurias and idiopathic mental retardation (Petre-Quadens & Jouvet, 1967). REM sleep in particular is diminished by the last two conditions but increased in Prader-Willi syndrome, which involves hypothalamic dysfunction (Vela-Bueno, Kales Soldatos, et al., 1984). Sleep quality is much impaired by dementia in general (Feinberg, Koresko, & Heller, 1967; Prinz,

Peskind, Vitaliano, et al., 1982; Reynolds, Kupfer, Taska, et al., 1985a) and specifically by Jacob-Creutzfelt disease (Vitrey, Huquet, & Dollfus, 1970). The diminished arousal of senility presumably impairs the integration of ventilatory function and the reflex response to airway obstruction. Of 80 mostly middle-aged sleep apnea patients, however, 24 percent showed psychometric evidence of "mild to severe impairment of brain functioning" (A Kales, Cadieux, Shaw, et al., 1984). At this point, therefore, it seems likely that brain disease may cause or aggravate sleep apnea and that the latter impairs arousal functions. A disconnection between dreaming and verbalizing occurs in lobotomizing patients, who either fail to recall dreams upon being awakened from REM sleep or else remember the feeling of dreaming but not the dream content (A Jus, K Jus, Villanerve, et al., 1972).

Less devastating neurologic syndromes may also alter sleep quality. Migraine headache awakens the patient from REM sleep and may lead to excessive sleeping in the recovery phase, which distinguishes it in some cases from tension headache, which may occur after a period of wakefulness (Blau, 1982; Dexter & Weitzman, 1970). The aberrant catecholamine hypersensitivity found with prolapsed mitral valve syndrome may induce lighter sleep and middle-of-the-night waking episodes with anxiety, sweating, and tachycardia (Clark, Boudoulas, Schaal, et al., 1980), often confused with psychogenic insomnia.

Pregnancy. First-trimester pregnancy often causes increased sleep and sleepiness, sometimes enough to reverse an insomnia problem, presumably from the augmented levels of progesterone, which has mild sedating properties. In the third trimester, however, urinary frequency, movements of the unborn, and possibly interference with accustomed sleeping positions combine to lessen the quality of sleep. REM and stage 4 sleep lessen and wakefulness increases. These abnormalities may persist postpartum and possibly exacerbate postpartum emotional disturbances (Karacan & Williams, 1970). Further disturbances may arise from night sweating, which has reportedly been observed in a majority of normal obstetrical patients (Lea & Aber, 1985).

Gastrointestinal problems. Recumbency provokes the pain of hiatus hernia. Remarkably, experimental infusions of weak hydrochloric acid via a nasal-esophageal catheter, which are indistinguishable from water infusions by the awake subject, provoke arousals during sleep (Orr, Robinson, & Johnson, 1984), with greater frequency in the esophagitis patient. This suggests a mechanism for awakening that is unassociated with pain and thus unappreciated by the patient.

The secretion of gastric acid falls during sleep (Stacher, Presslich, & Starker, 1975). Increased secretion of gastric acid during REM sleep, mentioned previously, may characterize some patients (Armstrong et al., 1965) but not others (Orr, Hall, Stahl, et al., 1976). Nevertheless, gastric acid pain may disturb sleep, sometimes as a rebound hypersecretion effect from use of antacids, or possibly from the inhibition of esophageal clearing by sedatives (Orr, Robinson, & Randall, 1985).

The awakenings necessitated by irritative conditions of the large bowel and frequent urges to defecate worsen sleep much more if falling back to sleep is prolonged by additional sleep problems. The sleep of hepatic-failure patients is often short, light, and disrupted (Bergonzi, Bianci, Mazza, et al., 1978; Kurtz, Zenglein, Imler, et al., 1972) and worsens with worsening hepatic status. False neurotransmitters resulting from enzymes produced by gut bacteria and normally destroyed by the liver may be shunted into the circulation and thence to the brain, where they presumably interfere with neural function. This mechanism may also explain the occasional neurally intact patient whose sleep lessens after porto-caval shunt.

Miscellaneous medical problems. In general, symptoms of medical problems, such as pain, itch, or dypsnea, or the effects of treatments, such as use of CNS-acting drugs, may worsen sleep. In the acutely ill patient who previously obtained restful sleep, a covarying time course between the illness and the sleep problem supports a causal correction. In the chronically ill patient, the relationship between a medical problem and a sleep problem may be less clear.

Fibrositis syndrome patients have worse pain and mood symptoms when they obtain less stage 4 sleep (Moldofsky & Lue, 1980), and experimental stage 4 sleep deprivation of normal subjects also resulted in fibrositislike symptoms (Moldofsky & Scarisbrick, 1976). Poor sleep quality likely diminishes tolerance of most other disease symptoms. There is some evidence, for instance, that sleep quality is diminished in osteoarthritis patients who complain about morning joint pain and stiffness compared with those who do not (Moldofsky, Lue, & Saskin, 1986).

Chronic uremic patients show less deep sleep, less REM sleep, and many myoclonic jerks; they are all diminished but not abolished by hemodialysis (Passouant, Cadilhac, Baldy-Moulinier, et al., 1970). Sleep is worse after a chronic hemodialysis session, possibly because of direct effects of the hemodialysis but partly because of the schedule shifts and other encumbrances of the method (RJ Daly & Hassall, 1970).

Irritative symptoms of prostatism compel nocturia, but an associated problem with sleep results not from the nocturia per se, but form an inability to return to sleep within a tolerable interval. Occasionally, bladder training may increase the urinary volume at which the urinary urge supervenes, lessening nocturia disruptions.

Sensory impressions of the external world direct attention away from internal states (Hernandez-Peon, 1966). After the lights go out at bedtime, internal sensations may thus intensify, worsening disease symptoms. This especially augments itch and pain. Chronic itch delays sleep onset and disrupts sleep. Patients with pruritus, when visually and polygraphically monitored, show scratching during all stages of sleep, and diminished deep sleep (Brown & Kalucy, 1975; Savin, Peterson, & Oswald, 1973). Table 12-1 summarizes the most common causes of disturbed sleep in medical-surgical patients.

Idiopathic Disorders of Impaired Wakefulness

Medical problems tend to provoke lethargy rather than sleepiness. The ill patient dozes more out of default because of lassitude than because of an active supervening of sleep. In narcolepsy and idiopathic hypersomnia, however, sleep preempts all other activity. In narcolepsy, REM sleep supervenes, involving part or all of the REM state, including sleep, hallucinations or dreams, and bilateral paresis. In idiopathic hypersomnia, polygraphically normal sleep persistently occurs in multiple naps during the day or prolonged sleep at night (more than 10 hours). Individual presentations of narcolepsy vary from cases with one sleep attack daily to those with frequent 5–15-minute sleep attacks, cataplexy (i.e., brief bilateral paresis precipitated by sudden emotion or surprise), visual hallucinations at sleep onset, and sleep paralysis. Other narcolepsy features include disrupted nocturnal sleep, nocturnal automatic behavior, and diminution of social and occupational competence (Broughton, Ghanem, Hishikawa, et al., 1981). Idiopathic hypersomnia differs in having sleep attacks that may last hours rather than minutes, undisrupted nocturnal sleep, and neither cataplexy nor hallucinations (Roth, 1980). About half the patients have "sleep drunkenness," a severe inability to function upon first awakening mornings. This contrasts sharply with narcolepsy patients, who tend to function best on first arising.

Both conditions are associated with depression. Narcolepsy may also be associated with a higher incidence of multiple sclerosis (Poirier, Montplaisir, Duquette, et al., 1986) and may be acquired following head trauma or other CNS damage (Mitler, Shafor, Sobera, et al., 1986).

Narcolepsy and idiopathic hypersomnia most often begin before age 35 and remain present daily thereafter. This permanent state distinguished them from effect of acute medical illnesses.

EVALUATION AND TREATMENT

The Sleep History

The sleep pattern should be described, including regularity of bedtimes, untoward behavior during sleep (e.g., twitching, loud snoring, gasping, struggling, walking, night terrors, bed-wetting), bad dreams or nightmare, timing of any night wakings, and associated phenomena, such as palpitations, emotional arousal associated with anxiety, hot flashes, sweating, or other symptoms. The regularity of rising times and sleep patterns should be documented with a month's sleep chart of bed and arising times in cases of chronic insomnia. This may serve for baseline comparisons after treatment efforts are made. Patients with obstructive sleep apnea may have symptoms upon first awakening that include headache, extremely dry mouth, and grogginess, accompanied often by nasal blockage or a sense of sinus fullness. Dysphoria in the morning occurs in some depressive states. Grogginess on awaken-

Table 12-1

Common Causes of Sleep Disorders in Medical and Surgical Patients

1. Insomnia (complaint of poor sleep quality)
    External influences
        nursing care
        commotion on intensive units
        enforced sleeping positions, attached equipment
    Nervous system causes
        hyperarousal
        arousal-inducing psychopathology
        cortical impairments
        specific lesions of sleep control mechanisms
        acute trauma
        catecholamine hypersensitivity (prolapsed mitral valve syndrome)
        seizure disorders
        CNS-acting drugs
    Timing system disorder
        irregular sleep schedule
        systematic and progressive delay or advance of sleep
        insufficient timing information
        insufficient sensitivity to timing information
    Breathing disorder
        airway obstruction, upper or lower respiratory tract
        pulmonary disease with hypercapnia or hypoxia
        heart failure with slowed circulation time
        constricted mechanics of breathing
            obesity
            muscle disease
            parkinsonism
        diminished ventilatory response
    Metabolic factors
        increased cerebral metabolism
        thyroid abnormalities
        corticosteroid abnormalities
        diabetic neuropathy with airway function disturbance
        premenstrual and menopausal factors
    Gastrointestinal problems
        effects of large meal
        hiatus hernia and esophageal acid reflux
        peptic ulcer pain
        nocturnal symptoms of bowel disease
    Other problems
        nocturnal disturbance from any cause (e.g., pain, itch, dyspnea, nocturia)
        renal dialysis
        liver disease

2. Hypersomnia (complaint of excessive daytime sleepiness)
        idiopathic sleep disorder (narcolepsy, idiopathic hypersomnia)
        postencephalitic syndromes
        fever or increased cerebral metabolic rate (some patients)
        drugs
        states of severe lethargy and debilitation
        severe CNS disorder (e.g., toxic, vascular, traumatic)
        breathing disorders
        metabolic disorders
        poor nocturnal sleep quality from any medical or surgical cause

ing is worsened by heavy use of caffeine, delayed sleep phase syndrome, or generally poor sleep quality. Excessive daytime sleepiness is provoked especially by monotonous situations such as turnpike driving, meetings, and evening television watching. Hyperarousal is more likely in careful, organized, thoughtful, introspective people. Psychopathology and drug use are evaluated in the diagnostic interview. Childhood onset of insomnia suggests neurologic dysfunction (Hauri & Olmstead, 1980; Regestein & Reich, 1983).

The patient's story may neglect sleep difficulties found prior to the onset of any medical condition. Although some insomnia patients with psychopathology may deny psychologic causes for their insomnia (Kales & Kales, 1984), others may self-diagnose themselves as distress-prone neurotics bound to suffer irremediable sleep problems. Many excessively sleepy patients develop low standards for wakefulness, deny any impairment, and are pushed into medical consultation by relatives.

The patient's bed partner may provide information about snoring, twitching, and other behavioral signs of sleep disorder and may also augment information about the nature of the sleep problem and its effect on the patient's daytime functioning.

Narcolepsy may be diagnosed by history alone or in conjunction with treatment response (Regestein, Reich, & Mufson, 1983). Cataplexy is virtually pathogomonic, but an unrelenting pattern of brief sleep attacks, frequent sleepiness, poor school or work performance, and self-management with preventive naps and careful use of caffeine or over-the-counter stimulants strongly suggests narcolepsy. Some families have several diagnosed narcoleptic or unusually sleep-prone individuals.

The diagnosis of idiopathic hypersomnia rests primarily on a history of prolonged nocturnal sleep and obligatory daytime naps, with a sleepiness tendency from youth and sleep drunkenness.

In nocturnal myoclonus a 1–3-second muscle twitch, usually in the legs, appears every 20–30 seconds during sleep. This is sometimes an incidental polygraphic findings that increases in incidence with age (Roehrs, Zorick, Sicklesteel, et al., 1983). Alterations of central neurotransmitter levels may underlie this condition (Vardi, Glaubman, Rabey, et al., 1978).

Objective Evaluation of Sleep Disorder

In cases of insomnia, measuring the time it takes the patient to fall asleep—the *sleep latency*—and the proportion of in-bed time slept—the *sleep efficiency*—provides most of the therapeutically useful information. One night's sleep is one data point in the continuing sleep/wake cycle. The exact polygraphic stages of sleep are poorly correlated across nights (Moses, Lubin, Naitoh, et al., 1972) and rarely provide much therapeutic information. Insomnia is a subjective complaint, poorly understood through laboratory monitoring (Regestein & Reich, 1978). In one series of 150 insomnia patients, for instance, laboratory sleep monitoring neither specifically nor sensitively identified insomnia patients (Bixler, Kales, Kales, et al., 1986).

Considering the difficulties with laboratory monitoring, a month's chart of sleep is the best measure of insomnia. Bedtimes, waking times, and estimated sleep during the night may be charted with a horizontal line on a date–hour matrix such as that used in Figure 12-1. Relevant information, such as episodes of awakening with gasping or palpitations, drug use, and medical symptom ratings, can be recorded for each date. Appendix A, following this chapter on pages 303–305, provides a sample charted sleeping diary log, as well as blank sleep charts that may be copied for office use. Such records correlate with laboratory monitoring results (Lewis, 1969) and provide a baseline comparison by which to judge treatment outcome. Portable wrist-motion recorders permit long-term, inexpensive, and accurate ambulatory monitoring (Kripke, Mullaney, Messin, et al., 1978) and may be combined with continuous ambulatory body temperature data to demonstrate circadian desynchrony.

Hospital and nursing home inpatients may be monitored by an hourly 5-second nurse observation of whether the patient is asleep or awake (e.g., Webb & Swinburne, 1971). Patterns such as early night insomnia, fitful sleep, and daytime napping may be noted, while snoring and breathing disorder and various sleep behavioral problems may be detected for further investigation. Normal temperature will peak in late afternoon and be lowest in the early morning, an hour or two prior to normal arising times.

Breathing disorder during sleep may be investigated with ambulatory devices that record wrist motion, breathing, and electrocardiogram. Ambulatory electroencephalo-gram is possible but technically more difficult because of its relatively low signal voltage. Continual light densitometry of earlobe or finger measures blood oxygen saturation, thus providing a key estimate of sleep breathing disorder, and is best done in hospital at the time of this writing. In cases of mild obstructive apnea in the absence of cardiovascular complications and sever sleepiness, ambulatory monitoring may be sufficient and convenient, but in more severe cases of sleep breathing disorder, quantitative sleep laboratory assessment of apnea episodes, oxygen desaturation, and grade of cardiac arrhythmias permits sound judgement regarding surgery and other treatments.

The level of daytime alertness provides a test of nocturnal sleep quality. Sustained attention tasks are most sensitive to impaired sleep (Wilkinson, 1965). A continuous performance test in which the subject decides each second whether to respond to a visual stimulus (Rosvold, Mirsky, Sarason, et al., 1956) sensitively reflects poor sleep quality. Patients with chronic sleep problems may follow their daytime functions by regularly recording results of convenient arousal test, such as performance in computer games, exercise performance, or grip strength, measured against the patient's own baseline.

The multiple sleep latency test (MSLT) consists of four or five daytime trials to estimate polygraphically recorded time to sleep onset (sleep latency) (Richardson, Carskadon, Flagg, et al., 1978). It measures sleepiness rather than arousal. Of the primary sleep disorders, narcolepsy yields an average sleep latency of 5 minutes or less, and idiopathic hypersomnia shows an average sleep latency of 8 or 9 minutes. Sleep-onset REM periods may be elicited by this test and are found in states of central catecholamine depletion (e.g., with use of certain antihypertensive drugs, stimulant withdrawal, narcolepsy, or severe mood disorder). The MSLT should be used to

Brigham Hospital

For Addressograph Plate

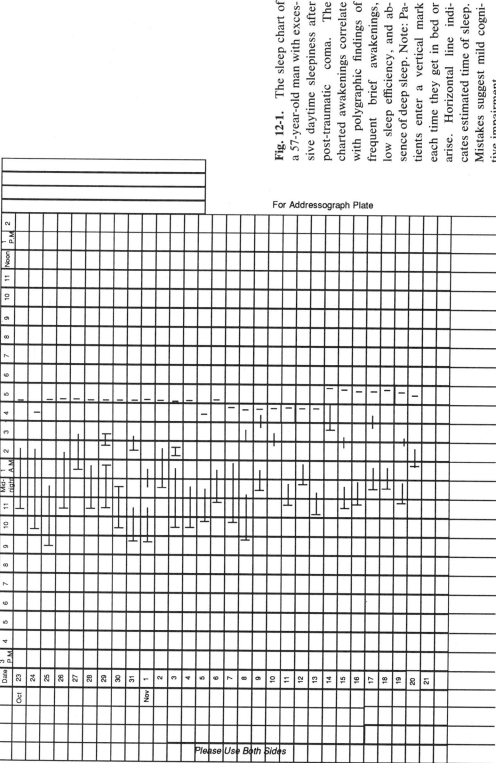

Fig. 12-1. The sleep chart of a 57-year-old man with excessive daytime sleepiness after post-traumatic coma. The charted awakenings correlate with polygraphic findings of frequent brief awakenings, low sleep efficiency, and absence of deep sleep. Note: Patients enter a vertical mark each time they get in bed or arise. Horizontal line indicates estimated time of sleep. Mistakes suggest mild cognitive impairment.

Please Use Both Sides

12020

Form 12-08 (176)

confirm narcolepsy where the diagnosis is unclear, for example, in the absence of cataplexy, but false negative results (Regestein et al., 1983) make this test unable to rule out narcolepsy.

A leukocyte antigen, DR-2, is reportedly present in almost all patients with narcolepsy and may help distinguish this condition from other hypersomnias (Mitler et al., 1986; Montplaisir, Poirer, DeCary, et al., 1986).

Improving Sleep Quality

Sleep disorders in the medical patient may be relieved by reversing the patient's preexisting predispositions to poor sleep, treating the medical illness, and ameliorating its nocturnal symptoms if total cure is not possible.

Drugs

Withdrawal from caffeine and alcohol is easily done in the motivated patient. Nicotine withdrawal requires careful distinction between the low-dose smoker with fluctuating blood nicotine levels, who may quit abruptly, and the high-dose smoker who almost always requires gradual withdrawal and a sophisticated multimodality treatment approach. When recreational drugs worsen sleep disorder, appropriate psychiatric intervention fosters abstinence. Therapeutic dilemmas may arise when prescription drugs cause insomnia. Revised drug regimens are usually possible, however, as already noted.

Age

Among the aged, a helpless passivity is often part of a psychologically regressed picture that involves demands of hypnotic drugs, coupled with a refusal to keep sleep charts, discontinue naps and sleep-disrupting drugs, maintain regular rising times, and adhere to medical treatment regimens. The sleep disorder often represents a confluence of disease manifestations and a lack of raison d'être. Since insomnia in the elderly is often attributed to "a mixture of medical, psychological, social and developmental factors" (Institute of Medicine, 1979), it is often deemed poorly treatable. In fact, physicians overestimate the social problems of the elderly (Branch, 1977), and good sleep habits are essentially mechanical, simple, cheap, and thus easy to institute for the motivated elderly.

The elderly are prescribed roughly double their proportionate amount of hypnotic drugs (Mellinger et al., 1985). This reflects, in part, their more continuous rather than intermittent use of such agents. Hypnotics, however, have disadvantages in elderly patients. The gut absorption of such agents is slower in elderly because of decreased gastric acid, absorptive area, gut blood flow, and enzyme transport system function (Salzman, 1979). For instance, chlordiazepoxide has an absorption half-life of 20 minutes in the elderly, compared with 5 minutes in others (Shader, Greenblatt, Harmatz, et al., 1977). Rapidity of action is necessary in the relief of bedtime insomnia, however, and patients prefer rapid-acting drugs (Hollister, 1978), so slow absorption may cause demands for a "better" pill. Drug excretion is also slowed, for example, from a half-life for diazepam of 20 hours at age 20 to about 90 hours at age 80 (Klotz, 1975). This slower drug metabolism and excretion in the elderly may lead to drug accumulation enough to cause severe psychologic or neurologic disturbance (Learoyd, 1972). One cannot generalize, however. Although longer-acting hypnotics are sometimes incriminated as causing next-day sedation in the elderly (Fillingim, 1982), the source of such information is often short-term studies that insufficiently reflect actual use. Next-day functioning after long-term use of such agents may actually show improved function on some measures, such as mental arithmetic tests (Bliwise, Seidel, et al., 1984).

The total dose of the drug may be more

important than pharmacokinetics in determining next-day hypnotic drug effects (Johnson & Chernik, 1982). After long-term use of hypnotics in a geriatric nursing home population, next-day differences among hypnotics of different classes were small, with barbiturates inducing slightly better ratings than benzodiazepines in "motility" and "continence" (Berg, Dehlin, Falkheden, et al., 1977). The hypnotic drug literature consists mostly of short-term studies of small populations of normal volunteers (see Johnson & Chernik, 1982; Williams & Karacan, 1976), and thus provides an inadequate guide for use of hypnotic agents in the elderly. Into this dearth of information sometimes steps confident opinion, for example, the decrying of hypnotics that diminish REM sleep or have long elimination half-lives, or of virtually any use of hypnotics (Orr, Altschuler, & Stahl, 1982), particularly chronic use (Kripke, 1985; Williams, 1980). The disadvantages of drug treatment must be balanced, however, against those of chronic sleep deprivation (Adam, 1979).

Hypnotics in the elderly should be prescribed only after obtaining regular charted sleep schedules, remedying nocturnal disease symptoms and specific sleep problems, and optimizing prescribed drug regimens. In general, drug tolerance may be prevented by restricting hypnotic drugs to intermittent use. Inability to withdraw the patient from reliance on hypnotics after several months warrants further illumination of the unremedied sleep problem.

For the working elderly person or the retired elderly without nervous system impairment, diazepam is rapidly absorbed and thus rapid in onset. Oxazepam and temazepam are intermediate-acting benzodiazepines whose slowness of onset may be reversed by using the powder taken out of the gel capsule. Chloral hydrate is much less expensive and comes in syrup form for those who have difficulty swallowing pills. For dependable patients, barbiturates may

be useful and pose fewer amnestic effects (Bixler, Scharf, Leo, et al., 1975).

For the elderly with mild cognitive impairment, lorazepam should be avoided because of its relatively larger amnestic effects (Roth, 1980; Scharf, Khosla, Brocker, et al., 1984). Flurazepam may cause next-day effects on memory (Bixler, et al., 1979) and motility (Crowley & Hydinger-Macdonald, 1979), although its longer action may also shorten rather than lengthen sleep latency on withdrawal nights (Bliwise, Seidel, et al., 1985). It is therefore more likely to foster intermittent drug use by the patient than are shorter-acting agents, which become a nightly habit.

For the geriatric outpatient with obvious cognitive deficits, hypnotic drugs become more perilous, but a careful empirical approach, using a family member to dispense medication and rating prescription benefit by sleep chart outcome, remains possible. Oxazepam or temazepam are perhaps the safest agents to use in such cases.

Almost half of institutionalized elderly are prescribed hypnotics (Marttila, Hammel, Alexander, et al., 1977). Some of this might presumably be avoided at the cost of analyzing each individuals sleep problem. In one hospital, staff education and delayed evening drug rounds reduced hypnotic doses per patient by almost half (Sheerin, 1972). The mildly sedative actions of antihistamines are occasionally prescribed for insomnia in the elderly, but this induces more sleepiness than sleep (Roehrs, Tietz, Zorich, et al., 1984). For chronically institutionalized and supervised elderly, where abuse and overdose is unlikely, the list of possible hypnotics is long, but hypnotic treatment should be coupled with good sleep habits, the avoidance of prolonged in-bed times, naps, and sleep-disrupting drugs. Almost any hypnotic agent may be chosen to titrate against quantified observations of sleep quality and daytime functioning. Individual variation may be more salient than the research averages described above, and even wine served with supper, despite the previously mentioned lessening of sleep by alcohol, has reportedly improved sleep of geriatric patients (Mishara & Kastenbaum, 1974). The complexities in cases of the medically ill, insomniac elderly must be considered individually (Regestein, 1984).

Scheduling Problems

Scheduling problems involve a departure from the ideal of arising at a regular clock time daily after an in-bed time of fixed length. Irregular rising times can usually be made regular. A systematic delay of bedtimes and wake times often found in "night people," the *delayed-sleep-phase syndrome*, is often amplified in patients taking caffeine, xanthine drugs, nicotine, beta agonists, or other long-acting stimulants. It may be remedied by a gradual progression of wake times forward around the clock (Czeisler, Richardson, & Coleman, 1981) in 2- or 3-hour daily delays, in keeping with the delaying tendency of the bodily clocks. Advances to earlier bedtimes, in extremely small steps (e.g., 5 minutes a day) can also accomplish the resetting of sleep time to earlier hours (Regestein, 1976). This obviates diurnal sleeping periods but takes several weeks to accomplish. In cases of evening or night work, patients must sleep the same clock hours on vacation days to maintain regular circadian rhythms. Rotating shifts should be changed as infrequently as possible and toward later time periods, that is, evenings to night rather than to days, again in keeping with the delaying tendency of the bodily clocks.

Hyperarousal

Hyperarousal is likely when sleep is delayed after bedtime but subsequently uninterrupted. It may be relieved by arousal-lowering routines instituted 2 or 3 hours prior to bedtime. Television watching may decrease sleep quality and impair next-day performance (Saletu et al., 1983) and

should be avoided, along with stimulating activities. Meditation and muscle relaxation procedures (Kales & Kales, 1984), hot water soaks (Bunnell & Horvath, 1985), and a predictable, relaxing evening routine are all useful remedies. Evening exercise has reportedly induced brief wakeful periods early in the night (Baekeland & Lasky, 1966). Practically, this does not occur in all hyperarousal insomniac patients, but for those so affected, exercise earlier in the day improves subsequent sleep. Hypnotic drugs may be used intermittently if arousing evening activity is unavoidable.

Psychopathology

Where sleeping pills are deemed indicated in anxious patients, the longer-acting agents, such as flurazepam, diazepam, desmethyldiazepam or phenobarbital, may provide next-day therapeutic sedation. L-tryptophan is an essential amino acid with measurable hypnotic effects (Hartmann & Spinweber, 1979), especially useful as a first hypnotic medication for patients who dislike "drugs." It exerts near-maximal effect after 1–2 g taken at bedtime (Hartmann, Cravens, & List, 1974). Patients requiring antidepressants may take one that is sedating at bedtime or else take more stimulating agents, such as tranylcypromine, protriptyline, and desipramine, earlier in the day to avoid aggravating insomnia. Alprazolam may provide both hypnotic and antidepressant actions in some patients (Feighner, 1984). In potentially suicidal patients prescribed a sedative, benzodazepines have proved relatively safe in acute overdose (Greenblatt, Allen, Noel, et al., 1977), provided they are not taken concurrently with alcohol or other sedatives.

Triazolam is better avoided in patients with significant psychopathology, since its rapid elimination time provokes a mini-withdrawal syndrome manifested by early morning insomnia (A Kales et al., 1983), next day anxiety (Morgan & Oswald, 1982), nocturnal agitated and amnestic episodes, or insidous types of agitation mimicking common presentations of anxiety (Poitras, 1980; Regestein & Reich, 1985).

Occasionally antidepressants remedy insomnia in patients who are not apparently depressed. The neurotransmitter systems affected by these agents regulate many functions, such as mood, pain, or biologic clocks, that affect sleep. Patients thus helped, however, often have occult depressions (Ware, 1983).

Hospitalization

Hypnotic drugs are routinely prescribed "as needed" for hospital inpatients, and constitute the major treatment for disordered sleep. In one study of medical-surgical inpatients in a university referral hospital, 38 percent were given a hypnotic medication, and of these, over half also took diazepam or another sleep medication (Salzman, 1981). Many patients are discharged on hypnotic drugs and continue to take them, so about 20 percent of drug dependency cases begin after hypnotic drugs were first prescribed in hospital (Clift, 1975).

The environments of tertiary care hospitals interfere with optimal management of sleep disturbance. However, staff may try to promote dark, quiet nights and brightly lit days, withholding of sedative-hypnotics from daytime nappers, discontinuation of caffeine and nicotine, substitution of radio for evening television, evening hot tub bath, relaxation exercises or back rubs, the relief of nocturnal disease symptoms such as itch, pain, or dypsnea, the delay of evening sedation rounds, and waiting until the patient requests a hypnotic rather than leaving "as needed" hypnotics at the patient's bedside.

Medical Problems

In addition to controlling the lung and cardiovascular diseases that induce disturbances in breathing and sleep quality, breathing during sleep may be assisted by continuous positive airway pressure devices (Sanders, 1984; Sullivan & Issa, 1980). Raising the inspired air pressure 5–10 cm of water may quickly reverse snoring and sleep breathing disorder. Low-flow nasal oxygen may help in some cases where airway obstruction is not major (Martin et al, 1982). Surgical removal of upper airway obstruction, for instance, deviation of the nasal septum (Heimer et al., 1983) or jaw–tongue retrusion (Spire, Kuo, & Campbell, 1983) as well as other thickened or redundant tissues (Fujita, Conway, Sicklested, et al., 1985; Simmons, Guilleminault, & Miles, 1984) relieves snoring and sleep apnea. Where sleep-disordered breathing causes oxygen desaturation, with severe hypertension, high-grade arrhythmias, or unsafe degrees of daytime sleepiness, tracheostomy may induce rapid relief (Guilleminault & Cummiskey, 1982), although there are psychologic difficulties that must be addressed in almost all cases of ambulatory tracheostomy and a careful home tracheostomy care routine must be developed (Dye, 1983). Weight reduction surgery has also been used to relieve obstructive sleep apnea (Peiser, Lavie, Ovnat, at al., 1984). Although medroxyprogesterone, which stimulates respiration, or protriptyline, which limits REM sleep, drys the airway, and provides mild stimulation, may alleviate sleep apnea (Brownell, West, Sweatman, et al., 1982; Hensley, Sanders, & Strohl, 1980), such treatments rarely provide uncomplicated long-term relief.

When sleep is disordered at the menopause, it may be ameliorated by replacement estrogen (Campbell, 1976). Sleep quality is improved (Thompson & Oswald, 1977), and insomnia relief is associated with shorter sleep latencies (Regestein et al., 1981).

The treatment of narcolepsy requires continual record keeping, empirical sleep and nap scheduling, physician support, and various drugs. A regimen of stimulants and antidepressants must be empirically fashioned (Regestein et al., 1983). Stimulant drug abusers feigning narcolepsy are rare but easy to spot by their relative lack of concern or sincerity, inconsistent history, lack of family confirmation, and history of difficulties associated with commissions rather than omissions of behavior. Perhaps because of specific arousal abnormalities, narcolepsy patients themselves do not sustain much euphoric effect from stimulants and do not tend to abuse such drugs. Idiopathic hypersomnia is treated similarly to myoclonus narcolepsy.

Nocturnal myoclonus should be treated only if there is a clearly demonstrable connection between it and diminished sleep quality. A number of muscle relaxing drugs, such as chlorazepate, diazepam, and baclofen, have been tried with variable results.

Sleep Hygiene

A number of nonspecific treatments, summarized as *sleep hygiene*, are frequently offered to patients with insomnia problems of all varieties (Hauri, 1985). They are as follows:

1. Rising at a regular clock time daily.
2. Limitation of total daily in-bed time to usual amount prior to sleep disturbance.
3. Discontinuation of CNS-acting drugs, such as caffeine, alcohol, nicotine, nasal decongestants, beta blockers, and beta agonists.
4. Regular mealtimes, with a relatively small meal at night and avoidance of after-supper eating. Small bedtime snacks help some but worsen sleep in others.
5. A regular, predictable evening routine. Overstimulating television should be avoided in favor of radio or relaxed reading.
6. Regular daytime exercise as appropriate for age and physical coordination. Evening exercise has variable effects.

7. Daytimes of purposeful activity or arousing involvement.
8. Evening relaxation routines, such as meditation techniques, progressive muscle relaxation, and hot tub soaks.

Many patients will claim regular arising times but forget weekend irregularities, Unemployment is a large factor in irregular wake times. These approximate guidelines are inapplicable to some patients. Some, for instance, are made rather uncomfortable by body-temperature-raising tub soaks; others, also made uncomfortable, nevertheless continue them because they sleep better.

Where the recumbent position of sleep worsens hiatus hernia pain or elicits the reflex wakening induced by mild acid in the esophagus, raising the head of the bed on blocks and using extra pillows may grant relief. Nocturnal peptic ulcer pain may be suppressed by bedtime administration of a histamine blocker such as ranitidine, although doxepin has reportedly resolved ulcers previously unresponsive to histamine blockers alone (Mangla & Pereira, 1982), presumably because of its powerful anticholinergic, antihistaminic, and possibly REM-suppressing effects. Trimipramine has been similarly used.

The nocturia associated with prostatism is too rarely treated with bladder training. Progressively increasing the interval between the urge to urinate and urination—for example, with 20-minute increments each week to perhaps a 100-minute interval—plus subsequent morning fluid loading and evening fluid restriction will raise the threshold against the urinary reflex and in many cases relieve nocturia.

The properties of specific sedative-hypnotic drugs render them less likely to cause side effects in some disease states, more likely in others. Oxazepam (Schuil, Wilkinson, & Johnson, 1971) and temazepam excretion is not slowed in liver disease. For those with renal impairments, hexobarbital is rapidly excreted. Chloral hydrate may aggravate symptoms of stomach irritation and affect the metabolism of anticoagulants (Mendelson, 1980). Patients using antacids may have delayed absorption of benzodiazepines (Shader, Georgotus, Greenblatt, et al., 1978), as will those taking pills after

meals. For patients taking major tranquilizers or antidepressants, a sedating agent taken near bedtime might substitute for hypnotic medication. Seizure disorder patients may take their phenobarbital, clonazepam, or other sedating anticonvulsant near bedtime.

REFERENCES

Abraham GE (1983). Nutritional factors in the etiology of the premenstrual tension syndromes. *Journal of Reproductive Medicine, 28*, 446–464.

Adam K (1979). Do drugs alter the restorative value of sleep? In P. Passouant & I Oswald (Eds), *Pharmacology of states of alertness* pp 105–111. New York: Pergamon Press.

Adam K & Oswald I (1984). Sleep promotes healing. *British Medical Journal, 2*, 1400–1401.

Adamson J & Burdick JA (1973). Sleep of dry alcoholic. *Archives of General Psychiatry, 28*, 146–149.

Allison T & Twyver H (1970). The evolution of sleep. *Natural History, 79*, 56–65.

American Psychiatric Association (1987). *Diagnostic and statistical manual of mental disorders* (3rd ed, rev). Washington, DC: Author.

Anch AM, Remmers JE, & Bunce H (1982). Supraglottic airway resistance in normal subjects and patients with obstructive sleep apnea. *Journal of Applied Physiology, 53*, 1158–1163.

Ancoli-Israel S, Kripke DF, Mason W, et al. (1981). Sleep apnea and nocturnal myoclonus in a senior population. *Sleep 4*, 349–58.

Armstrong RH, Burnap DB, Jacobson A, et al. (1965). Dreams and gastric secretions in duodenal ulcer patients. *The New Physician, 14*, 241–243.

Aschoff J (1964). Survival value of diurnal rhythms. In OG Edholm (Ed), *The biology of survival* (pp 79–98). London: Academic Press.

Association of Sleep Disorders Centers (1979). Diagnostic classification of sleep and arousal disorders. *Sleep, 2*, 1–137.

Baekeland F & Lasky R (1966). Exercise and sleep patterns in college athletes. *Perceptual and Motor Skills, 23*, 1203–1207.

Baldy-Moulinier M (1982). Temporal lobe epilepsy and sleep organization. In (Eds), MB Sterman & MN Shouse. *Sleep and epilepsy* (pp 329–337). New York: Academic Press.

Ballinger CB (1976). Subjective sleep disturbance at the menopause. *Journal of Psychosomatic Research, 20*, 509–513.

Berg S, Dehlin O, Falkheden T, et al. (1977). Long term study of hypnotic medication in geriatric

patients. *Scandinavian Journal of Social Medicine*, Suppl 14, 85–96.

Bergamasco B, Bergamini L, Doriguzzi T, et al. (1968). EEG sleep patterns as a prognostic criterion in post-traumatic coma. *Electroencephalography and Clinicalogy, Neurophysiol. 24*, 374–377.

Bergonzi P, Bianci A, Mazza S, et al. (1978). Night sleep organization in patients with severe hepatic failure. *European Neurology, 17*, 271–275.

Berlin RM, Litovitz GL, Diaz M, et al. (1984). Sleep disorders on a psychiatric consultation service. *American Journal of Psychiatry, 141*, 582–584.

Billiard M, Guilleminault C, & Dement WL (1975). A menstruation-linked periodic hypersomnia. *Neurology, 25*, 436–443.

Billiard M & Passouant P (1974). Sexual hormones and sleep in women. *Review of Electroencephalographic et de Neurolophysiologic. Clinique 4*, 89–106.

Bixler EO, Kales A, Jacoby JA, et al. (1984). Nocturnal sleep and wakefulness: Effects of age and sex in normal sleepers. *International Journal of Neuroscience, 23*, 33–42.

Bixler EO, Kales A, Kales J, et al. (1986). Insomnia: Validation of sleep laboratory criteria. American Psychiatric Association Meeting, Washington, DC: APA. *New Research Papers Abstracts*; p 71.

Bixler EO, Scharf MF, Leo L, et al. (1975). Hypnotic drugs and performance. In F Kagan, T Harwood, K Rickels, et al. (Eds), *Hypnotics*, (pp. 175–196). New York: Spectrum.

Bixler EO, Scharf MB, Soldatos C, et al. (1979). Effects of hypnotic drugs on memory. *Life Sci 25*, 1379–1388.

Blau JN (1982). Resolution of migraine attacks: Sleep and the recovery phase. *Journal of Neurology, Neurosurgery, & Psychiatry, 43*, 223–226.

Bliwise D, Seidel W, Greenblatt DJ, et al. (1984). Nighttime and daytime efficacy of flurazepam and oxazepam in chronic insomnia. *American Journal of Psychiatry, 141*, 191–195.

Block AJ (1979). Sleep apnea, hypopnea and oxygen desaturation in normal subjects. *New England Journal of Medicine, 300*, 513–517.

Borg S, Krande H, & Sedval G (1981). Central norepinephrine metabolism during alcohol intoxification in addicts and healthy volunteers. *Science, 213*, 1135–1137.

Branch LG (1977). Updating the needs of Massachusetts elderly. *New England Journal of Medicine, 297*, 838–840.

Brebbia DR & Altschuler KZ (1965). Oxygen consumption rate and electroencephalographic stage of sleep. *Science, 150*, 1621–1623.

Brezinova V (1974). Effect of caffeine on sleep: EEG study in late middle age. *British Journal of Clinical Pharmacology, 1*, 203–208.

Brody H & Vijayashankar N (1977). Anatomical changes in the nervous system. In CE Finch and L Hayflick (Eds), *Handbook of the biology of aging*, (pp 241–261). New York: Van Nostrand Reinhold.

Broughton R & Baron R (1978). Sleep patterns in the intensive car unit and the ward after acute myocardial infarction. *Electroencephalography and Clinical Neurophysiology, 45*, 348–360.

Broughton R, Ghanem Q, Hishikawa Y, et al. (1981). The socioeconomic and related life effects in 180 patients with narcolepsy from North America, Asia, and Europe compared to matched controls. In I Karacan (Ed), *Psychophysiological aspects of sleep*. Park Ridge, NJ: Nays.

Broverman DM, Klaiber EL, & Kobayashi V (1968). Roles of activation and inhibition in sex differences in cognitive abilities. *Psychological Review, 75*, 23–50.

Brown DG & Kalucy RS (1975). Correlation of neurophysiological and personality data in sleep scratching. *Proceedings of the Royal Society of Medicine, 68*, 530–32.

Brownell LG, West P, Sweatman P, et al. (1982). Protriptyline in obstructive sleep apnea. *New England Journal of Medicine, 307*, 1037–1042.

Bunnell DE & Horvath SM (1985). Effects of body heating during sleep interruption. *Sleep, 8*, 274–282.

Cadieux RJ, Kales A, Santen RJ, et al. (1982). Endoscopic findings in sleep apnea associated with acromegaly. *Journal of Clinical Endocrinology and Metabolism, 55*, 18–22.

Campbell S (1976). Double blind psychometric studies on the effect of natural estrogens on post-menopausal women. In S Campbell (Ed), *The management of menopause and post-menopausal years* (pp 149–158). London: University Park Press.

Carlson HE, Gillin JC, Gorden P, et al. (1972). Absence of sleep-related growth hormone peaks in aged normal subjects and in acromegaly. *Journal of Clinical Endocrinology and Metabolism, 34*, 1102.

Carskadon MA, Dement W, Mifler M, et al. (1976). Self-reports versus sleep laboratory findings in 122 drug-free subjects with complaints of chronic insomnia. *American Journal of Psychiatry, 133*, 1382–1388.

Carskadon MA, Harvey K, Duke P, et al. (1980). Pubertal changes in daytime sleepiness. *Sleep, 2*, 453–460.

Chada TS, Birch S, & Sackner MD (1985). Periodic breathing triggered by hypoxia in normal aware adults. *Chest, 88*, 16–23.

Charney DS, Heninger GR, & Jaflow PI (1985). Increased anxiogenic effects of caffeine in panic disorders. *Archives of General Psychiatry, 42*, 233–243.

Cherniack NS (1981). Respiratory dysrhythmias during sleep. *New England Journal of Medicine, 305*(6), 325–330.

Clark RW, Boudoulas H, Schaal SF, et al. (1980). Adrenergic hyperactivity and cardiac abnormality in primary disorders of sleep. *Neurology, 30*, 113–119.

Clift AD (1975). Dependence on hypnotic drugs in general practice. In AD Clift (Ed), *Sleep disturbance and hypnotic drug dependence* (pp 71–95). Amsterdam: Excerpta Medica.

Coccagna G & Lugaresi E (1978). Arterial blood gases and pulmonary and systematic arterial pressure during sleep in chronic obstructive pulmonary disease. *Sleep, 1*, 117–124.

Comfort A (1968). Physiology, homeostasis and ageing. *Gerontologia, 14*, 224–234.

Cook DB, Huse J, Roudebush C, et al. (1982). Asymptomatic sleep hypoventilation in morbid obesity. *Chest, 82*, 236.

Coren S & Searleman A (1985). Birth stress and self-reported sleep difficulty. *Sleep, 8*, 222–226.

Crowley TJ, Hydinger-Macdonald M (1979). Bedtime flurazepam and the human circadian rhythm of spontaneous motility. *Psychopharmacology (Berlin) 62* (2), 157–161.

Cumming G (1984). Sleep promotion, hospital practice, and recovery from illness. *Medical Hypotheses, 15*, 31–37.

Czeisler CA, Allan JS, Strogatz SH, et al. (1986). Bright light resets the human circadian pacemaker independent of the timing of the sleep-wake cycle. *Science, 233*, 667–671.

Czeisler CA, Moore-Ede MC, & Coleman RM (1982). Rotating shift work schedules that disrupt sleep are improved by applying circadian principles. *Science, 217*, 460–463.

Czeisler CA, Richardson GS, & Coleman RM (1981). Chronotherapy: Resetting the circadian clocks of patients with delayed sleep phase insomnia. *Sleep, 4*, 1–21.

Daly DD (1968). The effect of sleep upon the

electroencephalogram in patients with brain tumors. *Electroencephalography and Clinical Neurophysiology, 25*, 521–529.

Daly RJ & Hassall C (1970). Reported sleep in maintenance hemodyalisis. *British Medical Journal, 2*, 508–509.

Declerck AC, Wanguier A, Sijben-kiggen R, et al. (1982). A normative study of sleep in different forms of epilepsy. In MB Sterman & MN Shouse (Eds), *Sleep and epilepsy* (pp 329–337). New York: Academic Press.

Dews PB (1982). Caffeine. *Annual Review of Nutrition, 2*, 323–341.

Dexter & JD Weitzman ED (1970). The relationship of nocturnal headaches to sleep stage patterns. *Neurology, 20*, 513–518.

Dlin BM, Rosen H, Dickstein K, et al. (1971). The problems of sleep and rest in the intensive care unit. *Psychosomatics 12*(3), 155–163.

Dunleavy DLF, Oswald I, Brom P, et al. (1974). Hyperthyroidism, sleep and growth hormone. *Electroencephalography and Clinical Neurophysiology, 36*, 259–263.

Dye JP, (1983). Living with a tracheostomy for sleep apnea. *New England Journal of Medicine, 308*, 1167–1168.

Ekbom, KA (1960). Restless legs syndrome. *Neurology* (1981). *10*, 868–8732.

Ellis BW & Dudley HAF (1976). Some aspects of sleep research in surgical stress. *Psychosomatic Research, 20*, 303–308.

Endicott J, Halbreigh U, Schacht S, et al. (1981). Premenstrual changes and affective disorders. *Psychosomatic Medicine, 43*, 519–529.

Eysenck HJ (1972). Human typology, higher nervous activity, and factor analysis. In VD Nebylitsyn & JA Gray (Eds), *Biological bases of individual behavior* (pp 165–181). New York: Academic Press.

Fairbanks DN (1984). Snoring: Surgical vs nonsurgical management. *Laryngoscope, 94*, 1188–1192.

Feighner JP (1984). Open label study of alprazolam in severely depressed inpatients. *Journal of Clinical Psychiatry, 44*, 332–334.

Feinberg I, Koresko R, & Heller N (1967). EEG sleep patterns as a function of normal and pathological aging in man. *Journal of Psychiatric Research, 5*, 107–144.

Fillingim JM (1982). Double-blind evaluation of temazepam, flurazepam and placebo in geriatric insomniacs. *Clinical Therapy, 4*, 369–380.

Fischer-Perroudon C, Mouret J, & Jouvet M (1974). On a case of agrypnia (4 months without sleep) in the course of Morvan's disease. *Electroencephalography and Clinical Neurophysiology, 36*, 1–18.

Fisher JE & Baldessarini RJ (1971). False neurotransmitters and hepatic failure. *Lancet, 2*, 75–79.

Fleetham JA & Kryger MH (1981). Sleep disorders in chronic airflow obstruction. *Medical Clinics of North America, 65*, 549.

Fletcher E, DeBehnke R, Lovoi S, et al. (1985). Undiagnosed sleep apnea in patients with essential hypertension. *Annals of Internal Medicine, 103*, 190–195.

Fujita S, Conway W, Sicklested J, et al. (1985). Evaluation of the effectiveness of uvulopalatopharyngoplasty. *Laryngoscope, 95*, 70–74.

Gaillard JM (1978). Chronic primary insomnia: possible physiopathological involvement of slow wave sleep efficiency. *Sleep, 1*, 133–147.

Glassman A, Jackson WK, Walsh BT, et al. (1984). Cigarette craving, smoking withdrawal and clonidine. *Science, 126*, 864–866.

Globus GG (1969). A syndrome associated with sleeping late. *Psychosomatic Medicine, 31*, 528–535.

Goldstein A, Kaizer S, & Whitby O (1969). Psychotropic effects of caffeine in man: IV. Quantitative and qualitative differences associated with habituation to coffee. *Clinical Pharmacological Therapy, 10*, 489–497.

Gray JA (1967). Strength of the nervous system, introversion-extroversion, conditionability and arousal. *Behavior Research and Therapy, 5*, 151–169.

Greenblatt DI, Allen MD, Noel BJ, et al. (1977). Acute overdose with Benzodiazepine derivatives. *Clinical Pharmacological Therapy, 21*, 497–514.

Guilleminault C, Briskin JG, Greenfield M, et al. (1981). The impact of autonomic nervous system dysfunction on breathing during sleep. *Sleep, 4*, 263–278.

Guilleminault & C Cummiskey J (1982). Progressive improvement of apnea index and ventilatory response to CO_2 after tracheostomy in obstructive sleep apnea syndrome. *American Review of Respiratory Disease, 126*, 14–20.

Guilleminault C & Dement WC (1978). Sleep apnea syndromes and related disorders. In RC William & I Karacan (Eds), *Sleep disorders, diagnosis and treatment* (pp 9–28). New York: Wiley.

Guilleminault HC, Eldridge FL, Dement WC, et al. (1973). Insomnia with sleep apnea: A new syndrome. *Science, 181*, 856.

Guilleminault C, Faull KF, Miles L, et al. (1983). Posttraumatic excessive daytime sleepiness: A review of 20 patients. *Neurology, 33*, 1584–1589.

Halberg F (1960). The 24 hour scale: A time dimension of adaptive functional organization. *Perspective in Biological Medicine, 3*, 491–527.

Hall JB (1986). The cardiopulmonary failure of sleep-disordered breathing. *Journal of the American Medical Association, 255*, 930–933.

Haponik EF, Bleecker ER, Allen RP, et al. (1981). Abnormal inspiratory flow-volume curves in patients with sleep-disordered breathing *American Review of Respiratory Disease, 124*, 571–574.

Hartmann EL (1973). *The functions of sleep* (p 94). New Haven: Yale University Press.

Hartmann EL (1974). Hypnotic effects of L-tryptophan. *Archives of General Psychiatry, 31*, 394–397.

Hartmann EL, Cravens J, & List S (1974). Hypnotic effects of L-tryptophan. *Archives of General Psychiatry, 31*, 394–397.

Hartmann E & Spinweber CL (1979). Sleep induction by L-trytophan. *Journal of Nervous and Mental Disorders, 167*, 497–499.

Hauri P (1979). What can insomniacs teach us about the functions of sleep? In M Drucker-Colin, MF Shkurowich, & MB Sterman (Eds), *The functions of sleep* (pp 251–227). New York: Academic Press.

Hauri P (1982). *The sleep disorders* (p 11). Kalamazoo, MI: Upjohn.

Hauri P (1985). Primary sleep disorders and insomnia. In TL Riley (Ed), *Clinical aspects of sleep and sleep disturbance* (pp 81–112). Boston: Butterworth.

Hauri P & Fisher J (1986). Persistent Psychophysiologic (Learned) Insomnia. *Sleep, 9*, 38–53.

Hauri P &Olmstead F (1980). Childhood-onset insomnia. *Sleep, 3*, 59–65.

Healey ES, Kales A, Monroe LJ, et al. (1981). Onset of insomnia: Role of life-stress. *Psychosomatic Medicine, 43*, 439–451.

Heimer D, Scharf SM, Lieberman A, et al. (1983). Sleep apnea syndrome treated by repair of deviated nasal septum. *Chest, 84*, 184–185.

Heiss WD, Dawlik G, Herholz K, et al. (1985). Regional cerebral glucose metabolism in man during wakefulness, sleep and dreaming. *Brain Research, 327*, 362–366.

Henningfield JE (1984) Pharmacologic basis and treatment of cigarette smoking. *Journal of Clinical Psychiatry, 45*(12, Sec 2), 24–34.

Hensley MJ, Sanders MH, & Strohl TP (1980). Methoxyprogesterone treatment of obstructive sleep apnea. *Sleep, 3*, 441–446.

Hernandez-Peon R (1966). Physiological mechanisms of attention. In R Russell (Ed), *Frontiers of physiological psychology* (pp 121–144). New York: Academic Press.

Hialmarson AI (1984). Effect of nicotine chewing gum in smoking cessation. *Journal of the American Medical Association, 252*, 2835–2838.

Hobson JA (1968). Sleep after exercise. *Science, 162*, 1503–1505.

Hobson JA (1975). Dreaming sleep attack, and desynchronized sleep enhancement: Report of a case of brain stem signs. *Archives of General Psychiatry, 32*, 1421–1424.

Hobson JA (1983). Sleep: Order and disorder. *Behavioral Biology in Medicine, 1*, 1–36.

Hoeppner JB, Garron DC, & Cartwright RD (1984). Self-reported sleep disorder symptoms in epilepsy. *Epilepsia, 25*, 434–437.

Hollingsworth HL (1912). The influence of caffeine on mental and motor efficiency. *Archives of Psychology, 20*, 1–166.

Hollister LE (1978). *Clinical pharmacology of psychotheraputic drugs* (pp 25–28). New York: Churchill-Livingston.

Horne JA (1980). Sleep and body restitution. *Experientia, 36*, 11–13.

Horne JA & Moore J (1985). Sleep EEG effects of exercise with an additional body cooling. *Electroencephalography and Clinical Neurophysiology, 60*, 33–38.

Horne JA & Reid AJ (1984). Night-time sleep EEG changes following body heating in a warm bath. *Electroencephalography and Clinical Neurophysiology, 60*, 154–157.

Horne JA & Shackell BS (1985, July 8–13). Heating induced SWS rise—decays with interim wakefulness, inhibited by aspirin. Sleep Research Society Meeting, Seattle.

Horne JA & Staff, LHE (1983). Exercise and sleep: Body-heating effects. *Sleep, 6*, 36–46.

Institute of Medicine (1979). *Sleeping pills, insomnia and medical practice* (p 121). Washington, DC: National Academy of Sciences.

Issa FG & Sullivan CF (1984). Upper airway closing pressures in snorers. *Journal of Applied Physiology: Respiratory, Environmental and Exercise Physiology, 57*, 528–535.

Johns MW, Egan P, Gay TJA, et al. (1970). Sleep habits and symptoms in male medical and surgical patients. *British Medical Journal, 2*, 509–512.

Johns MW, Large AA, Masterton JP. et al. (1974). Sleep and delirium after open heart surgery. *British Journal of Surgery, 61*, 377–381.

Johns MW, Masterton JP, Paddle-Ledinek JE, et al. (1975). Variations in thyroid function and sleep in healthy young men. *Clinical Science and Molecular Medicine, 49*, 629–632.

Johnson LC (1982). Effects of anti-convulsant medication on sleep. In MB Sterman & M Shonse (Eds), *Sleep and epilepsy* (pp 381–394). New York: Academic Press.

Johnson LC & Chernik DA (1982). Sedative-hypnotics and human performance. *Psychopharmacology, 76*, 101–113.

Johnson LC & McLeod WL (1973). Sleep and awake behavior during gradual sleep reduction. *Perceptual Motor Skills, 36*, 87–97.

Johnson MW, Anch AM, Remmers JE (1984). Induction of the obstructive sleep apnea syndrome in a woman by exogenous androgen administration. *American Review of Respiratory Diseases 128*, 1023–1025.

Jones HS & Oswald I (1968). Two cases of healthy insomnia. *Electroencephalography and Clinical Neurophysiology, 24*, 378–380.

Jones JB, Wilhoit SC, Findley LJ, et al. (1985). Oxyhemoglobin saturation during sleep in subjects with and without the obesity hypoventilation syndrome. *Chest, 88*, 9–15.

Jouvet M (1974). The role of monoaminergic neurons in the regulation and function of sleep. In O Petre-Quadens & J Schlag (Eds), *Basic sleep mechanisms*. New York: Academic Press.

Jurko MF, Orlando J, & Webster CL (1971). Disordered sleep patterns following thalamotomy. *Clinical Electroencephalography, 2*, 213–217.

Jus A, Jus K, Villanerve P, et al. (1972). Absence of dream recall in lobotomized patients. *Lancet, 1*, 955–956.

Kales A, Ansel RD, Markham CH, et al. (1971). Sleep in patients with Parkinson's disease and normal subjects prior to and following levo-dopa administration. *Clinical Pharmacological Therapy, 12*, 397–406.

Kales A, Cadieux R, Shaw L, et al. (1984). Sleep apnea in a hypertensive population. *Lancet, 2*, 1005–1008.

Kales A, Henser G, Jacobson A, et al. (1967). All night sleep studies in hyperthyroid patients before and after treatment. *Journal of Clinical Endocrinology, 27*, 1593–1599.

Kales A, & Kales JD (1984). *Evaluation and treatment of insomnia*. New York: Oxford University Press.

Kales A, Soldatos CR, Bixler EO, et al. (1983). Early morning insomnia with rapidly eliminated benzodiazepines. *Science, 220*, 95–97.

Kales JD, Kales A, Bixler EO, Soldatos CR, et al. (1984). Biopsychobehavioral correlates of insomnia: V. Clinical characteristics and behavioral correlates. *American Journal of Psychiatry, 141*, 1371–1375.

Karacan I, Thornby JI, Anch M, et al. (1976). Prevalence of sleep disturbance in a primary urban Florida county. *Social Science and Medicine, 10*, 239–244.

Karacan I & Williams RL (1970). Current advances in theory and practice relating to post partum syndromes. *Psychiatric Medicine, 1*, 307–328.

Karacan I, Williams RL, & Taylor WJ (1969). Sleep characteristics of patients with angina pectoris. *Psychosomatics, 10*, 280–284.

Kelly DD (1985). Sleep and dreaming. In ER Kandel & JH Schwartz (Eds), *Principles of neural science* (pp 648–657). New York: Elsevier.

Khatri IM & Freis ED (1969). Hemodynamic changes during sleep in hypertensive patients. *Circulation, 39*, 785–790.

Klotz U (1975). Effects of age and liver disease on disposition and elimination of diazepam in adult man. *Journal of Clinical Investigations, 55*, 347–359.

Krieger J, Mangin P, & Kurtz D (1980). Respiratory changes in the course of sleep in the normal aged subject. *Review of Electroencephalography and Neurophysiology, 10*, 177–185.

Kripke DF (1985). Chronic hypnotic use: The neglected problem. In WP Koella, E. Ruether, H Schultz (Eds), *Sleep '84* (pp 338–340). Stuttgart, Germany: Gustave Fischer.

Kripke DF, Cook B, & Lewis OF (1971). Sleep of night workers: EEG recordings. *Psychophysiology, 7*, 377–384.

Kripke DF, Mullaney DJ, Messin S, et al. (1978). Wrist actigraphic measures of sleep and rhythm. *Electroencephalography and Clinical Neurophysiology, 44*, 674–676.

Kurtz D, Zenglein JP, Imler M, et al. (1972). Study of night sleep in the course of port-caval encephalopathy. *Electroencephalography and Clinical Neurophysiology, 33*, 167–178.

Lauritzen CR (1976). Female climacteric syndrome: Significance, problems and treatment. *Acta Obstetrica et Gyneocologica Scandinavica*, Suppl 51, 48–61.

Lea MJ Aber RC (1985). Descriptive epidemiology of night sweats upon admission to a university hospital. *Southern Medical Journal, 78*, 1065–1067.

Learoyd BM (1972). Psychotropic drugs and the elderly patient. *Medical Journal of Australia, 1*, 1131–1133.

Lewis SA (1969). Subjective estimates of sleep: An EEG evaluation. *British Journal of Psychology, 60*, 203–208.

Lipowski ZJ (1980). *Delirium* (p 161.) Springfield, IL: CC Thomas.

Littler WA, Honour AJ, Carter RD, et al. (1975). Sleep and blood pressure. *British Medical Journal, 3*, 346–348.

Lopata M & Onal E (1982). Mass loading, sleep apnea and the pathogenesis of obesity hypoventilation. *American Review of Respiratory Disease, 126*, 640–645.

Lown B, Tykocinski M, Garfein A, et al. (1973). Sleep and ventricular premature beats. *Circulation, 48*, 691–701.

Lugaresi E, Cirignotta F, Coccagna C, et al. (1980). Some epidemiological data on snoring and cardiocirculatory disturbances *Sleep, 3*, 221–224.

Lugaresi E, Coccagna G, Farneti P, et al. (1979). Snoring, *Electroencephalography and Clinical Neurophysiology, 39*, 59–64.

Lund R (1974). Personality factors and desynchronization of circadian rhythms. *Psychosomatic Medicine, 36*, 224–228.

Mangan GL (1972). The relationship of strength-sensitivity of the visual system to extraversion. In VD Nebylitsyn, JA Gray (Eds), *Biological bases of individual behavior* New York: Academic Press. (pp 254–261).

Mangla JC & Pereira M (1982). Tricyclic anti-depressants in the treatment of peptic ulcer disease. *Archives of Internal Medicine, 142*, 273–275.

Marquardsen J & Harvald B (1964). The electroencephalogram in acute vascular lesions of the brain stem and the cerebellum. *Acta Neurologica Scandinavica, 40*, 58–68.

Markand ON & Dyken ML (1976). Sleep abnormalities in patients with brain stem lesions. *Neurology, 26*, 769–776.

Martin RJ, Sanders MH, Gray BA, et al. (1982). Acute and long-term ventilatory effects of hyperoxia in the adult sleep apnea syndrome. *American Review of Respiratory Disease, 125*, 175.

Marttila JK, Hammel RJ, Alexander B, et al. (1977). Potential untoward effects of long-term use of flurazepam in geriatric patients. *Journal of the American Pharmacological Association, 17*, 692–695.

McGinty DJ, Drucker-Colin R, Morrison A, et al. (Eds). (1985). *Brain mechanisms of sleep*. New York: Raven Press.

Mellinger GD, Balter MB, & Uhlenhuth EH (1985). Insomnia and its treatment. Archives of General Psychiatry, 42, 225–232.

Mello NK & Mendelson JH (1970). Behavioral studies of sleep pattern in alcoholics during intoxication and withdrawal. *Journal of Pharmacology and Experimental Therapeutics* 175, 94–112, 1970.

Mendelson WB (1980). *The use and misuse of sleeping pills*. New York: Plenum.

Mendelson WB, Slater S, Gold P, Gillin JC (1980). The effect of growth hormone administration on human sleep: A dose response study. *Biological Psychiatry, 15*, 613–618.

Miles LE & Simmons FB (1984). Evaluation of 198 patients with loud and disruptive snoring. *Sleep Research, 13*, 154.

Millman RP (1985). Sleep apnea in hemodialysis patients: The lack of testosterone effect. *Nephron, 40*, 407–410.

Mishara BL & Kastenbaum R (1974). Wine in treatment of long-term geriatric patients in mental institutions. *Journal of the American Geriatrics Society, 22*, 88–94.

Mitler MM, Shafor R, Sobera M, et al. (1986). Human leucocyte antigen (HLA) studies in excessive somnolence: Narcolepsy versus sleep apnea. *Sleep Research, 15*, 148.

Moldolfsky H, & Lue FA (1980). The relationship of alpha and delta EEG frequencies to pain and mood in fibrositis patients treated with chlorpromazine and L-trytophan. *Electroencephalography and Clinical Neurophysiology, 50*, 71–80.

Moldolfsky H, Lue FA, & Saskin P (1986). Sleep and morning pain in primary osteoarthritis. *Sleep Research, 15*, 198.

Moldolfsky H & Scarisbrick P (1976). Induction of neurasthenic musculoskeletal pain syndrome by selective sleep stage deprivation. *Psychosomatic Medicine, 38*, 35–44.

Monroe LJ (1967). Psychological and physiological differences between good and poor sleepers. *Journal of Abnormal Psychology, 72*, 255–264.

Montplaisir J, Poirer G, DéCary F, et al. (1986). Association between HLA antigens and different types of hypersomnia. *Journal of the American Medical Association, 255*(17), 2295–2296.

Moore-Ede M, Sulzman FM, & Fuller CA (1982). *The clocks that time us*. Cambridge: Harvard University Press.

Morgan K & Oswald I (1982). Anxiety caused by a short-life hypnotic. *British Medical Journal, 284*, 942.

Morgan R, Mirors DS, & Waterhouse JM (1980). Does light rather than social factors synchronize the temperature rhythm of psychiatric patients? *Chronobiologia, 7*, 331–335.

Mouret J (1975). Differences in sleep in patients with Parkinson's disease. *Electroencephalography and Clinical Neurophysiology, 38*, 653–657.

Moses J, Lubin A, Naitoh P, et al. (1972). Reliability of sleep measures. *Psychophysiology, 9*, 78–82.

Murao S, Harumi K, Katayama S, et al. (1972). All night polygraphic studies of nocturnal angina pectoris. *Japanese Heart Journal, 13*, 295–306.

Murphy F, Bentley S, Ellis BW, et al. (1977). Sleep deprivation in patients undergoing operation: A factor in the stress of surgery. *British Medical Journal, 2*, 1521–1527.

Neil JF, Himmelhoch JM, Mallinger PG, et al. (1978). Caffeinism complicating hypersomnia depressive episodes. *Comprehensive Psychiatry, 19*, 377–385.

Nakazawa Y Kotorii T (1983). Effects of antibiotics, minocycline and ampicillin of human sleep. *Brain Research, 288*, 253–259.

Nonaka K, Nakazawa Y, Kotorii T (1983). Effects of antibiotics, minocycline and ampicillin, on human sleep. *Brain Research* 288 (1–2), 253–259.

Norton PG & Dunn V (1985). Snoring as a risk factor for disease: An epidemiological survey. *British Medical Journal, 291*, 630–632.

Nowlin JB, Troyer WG, Collins WS, et al. (1965). The association of nocturnal angina pectoris with dreaming. *Annals of Internal Medicine, 63*, 1040–1046.

Ohgami S (1973). Change of delta activity during rapid eye movement sleep in patients with brain tumor.

Electroencephalography and Clinical Neuro-physiology, 34, 153–162.

Olazabal JR, Miller MJ, Cook WR, et al. (1982). Disordered breathing and hypoxia during sleep in coronary artery disease. *Chest, 82*, 548–551.

Olsen KD, Kern EB, & Westbrook PR. (1981). Sleep and breathing disturbance secondary to nasal obstruction. *Otolaryngology and Head and Neck Surgery, 89*, 804–810.

Oomen MP, Abu-osba YK, & Thach BT (1982). Genioglossus muscle responses to upper airway pressure changes: Afferent pathways. *Journal of Applied Physiology: Respiratory, Environmental and Exercise Physiology, 52*, 445–450.

Orr WC (1983). Sleep related breathing disorders. *Chest, 84*, 475–479.

Orr W, Altschuler K, & Stahl M (1982). *Managing sleep complaints* (p 67). Chicago: Year Book Publishers.

Orr WC, Hall WH, Stahl ML, et al. (1976). Sleep patterns and gastric acid asecretions in ulcer disease. *Archives of Internal Medicine, 136*, 655–660.

Orr WC, Robinson MG, Johnson LF (1984). Responses to esophageal stimulation during sleep in normals and patients with severe esophagitis. *Sleep Research, 13*, 180.

Orr WC, Robinson MG, & Randall OH (1985). Arousal responses to endogenous stimulation during sleep. *Sleep Research 14*, 51.

Oswald I (1980). Sleep as a restorative process. *Progressive Brain Research, 53*, 279–288.

Palmer CD & Harrison GA (1983). Sleep latency and lifestyle in Oxfordshire villages. *Annals of Human Biology, 10*, 417–428.

Parker DC, Sassin JF, Mace JW, et al. (1969). Human growth hormone release during sleep. *Clinical Endocrinology and Metabolism, 29*, 871–877.

Passouant P, Cadilhac J, Baldy-Moulinier M, et al. (1970). Study of nocturnal sleep in chronic uremics undergoing an extrarenal dialysis. *Electroencephalography and Clinical Neurophysiology, 29*, 441–449.

Peiser J, Lavie P, Ovnat A, et al. (1984). Sleep apnea syndrome in the morbidly obese as an indication for weight reduction surgery. *Annals of Surgery, 199*, 112–115.

Petre-Quadens O & Jouvet M (1967). Sleep in the mentally retarded. *Journal of Neurological Science, 4*, 354–357.

Petrie WM, Maffucci RJ, & Woosley RC (1982). Propranolol and depression. *American Journal of Psychiatry, 139*, 92–93.

Poirier G, Montplaisir J, Duquette P, et al. (1986). Narcoleptic symptoms, HLA and MSLT data in multiple sclerosis. *Sleep Research, 15*, 156.

Poitras R (1980). On episodes of anterograde amnesia associated with use of triazolam. *L'Union Médicale du Canada 109*, 427–429.

Pokorny AD (1978). Sleep disturbances, alcohol, and alcoholism: A review. In RL Williams & I Karacan (Eds), *Sleep disorders, diagnosis and treatment* (pp 233–260). New York: Wiley.

Prinz PN (1977). Sleep patterns in the healthy aged: Relationship with intellectual functioning. *Journal of Gerontology, 32*, 179–186.

Prinz PN, Obrist W, & Wang H (1975). Sleep patterns in healthy elderly subjects: Individual differences as related to other neurobiological variables. *Sleep Research, 4*, 132.

Prinz P, Reskind E, Vitaliano P, et al. (1982). Changes in the sleep and waking EEG's of nondemented and demented elderly subjects. *Journal of the American Geriatrics Society, 30*, 86–93.

Puca FM, Bricolo A, & Turella G (1973). Effect of L-dopa or amantadine therapy on sleep spindles in parkinsonism. *Electroencephalography and Clinical Neurophysiology, 35*, 327–330.

Quuyumi A, Mockus LJ, Wright CA, et al. (1984). Mechanisms of nocturnal angina pectoris. *Lancet, 1*, 1207–1209.

Rechtschaffer A & Kales A (Eds) (1968). *A manual of standardized terminology, techniques and scoring system for sleep stages of human subject.* Los Angeles: Brain Information Service, Brain Research Institute, UCLA.

Rees PJ, Cochrane GM, Prior JG, et al. (1981). Sleep apnea in diabetic patients with autonomic neuropathy. *Journal of the Royal Society of Medicine, 74*, 192–195.

Regestein QR (1976). Treating insomnia: A practical guide for managing sleeplessness, circa 1975. *Comprehensive Psychiatry, 17*, 517–26.

Regestein QR (1980). Sleep and insomnia in the elderly. *Journal of Geriatric Psychiatry, 13*, 153–171.

Regestein QR (1982). Diagnosis and treatment of chronic insomnia. In R Gallon (Ed), *Psychosomatic approach to illness* (p 132). New York: Elsevier-North Holland.

Regestein QR (1984). Treatment of insomnia in the elderly. In C Salzman (Ed), *Clinical geriatric pharmacology* (pp 149–170). New York: McGraw-Hill.

Regestein QR (1987). Relationships between psychological factors and cardiac rhythm and electrical disturbances. *Comprehensive Psychiatry, 16*, 137–48.

Regestein Q, DeSilva R, & Lown B (1981). Cardiac ventricular ectopic activity increases during REM sleep. *Sleep Research, 10*, 58.

Regestein Q, Hallett M, Mufson M, et al. (1985). A hyperarousal scale. *Sleep Research, 14*, 135.

Regestein QR & Reich P (1978). Current problems in the diagnosis and treatment of chronic insomnia.

Perspectives in Biology and Medicine 21, 232–239.

Regestein QR & Reich P (1983). Incapacitating childhood-onset insomnia. *Comprehensive Psychiatry*, *24*, 244–248.

Regestein QR & Reich P (1985). Agitation observed during treatment with newer hypnotic drugs. *Journal of Clinical Psychiatry*, *46*, 280–283.

Regestein QR, Reich P, & Mufson MJ (1983). Narcolepsy: An initial clinical response. *Journal of Clinical Psychiatry*, *44*, 166–172.

Regestein QR, Rose LI, & Williams GH (1972). Psychopathology in Cushing's syndrome. *Archive of Internal Medicine*, *130*, 114–117.

Regestein QR, Schiff I, Tulchinski D, et al. (1981). Relationships among estrogen-induced psychophysiological changes in hypogonadal women. *Psychosomatic Medicine*, *43*, 147–155.

Remmers JE, deGroot WJ, Sauerland EK, et al. (1978). Pathogenesis of upper airway occlusion during sleep. J. Appl. Physiol; Respirat. Environ. Exercise Physiol. *Journal of Applied Physiology: Respiratory, Environmental and Exercise Physiology*, *44*, 931–938.

Reynolds CF, Kupfer DJ, Hoch CC, et al. (1985). Pills for the elderly: Are they ever justified? *Psychiatry*, *46*(2, Sec 2), 9–12.

Reynolds CF, Kupfer DJ, Taksa LS, et al. (1985a). EEG sleep in elderly depressed, demented and healthy subjects. *Biological Psychiatry*, *20*, 431–442.

Reynolds CF, Kupfer DJ, Taska LS, et al. (1985b). Sleep of healthy seniors: A revisit. *Sleep*, *8*, 20–29.

Reynolds CF, Taska LS, Sewitch DE, et al. (1984). Persistent psychophysiologic insomnia: Preliminary research diagnostic criteria and EEG sleep data. *American Journal of Psychiatry*, *141*, 804–805.

Richardson GS, Carskadon MA, Flagg W, et al. (1978). Excessive daytime sleepiness in man: Multiple sleep latency measurement of narcoleptic and control subjects. *Electroencephalography and Clinical Neurophysiology*, *45*, 621–627.

Roehrs T, Conway W, Wittig R, et al. (1985). Sleep-wake complaints in patients with sleep-related respiratory disturbances. *American Review of Respiratory Disease*, *132*, 520–523.

Roehrs TA, Tietz EI, Zorick FJ, et al. (1984). Daytime sleepiness and anti-histamines. *Sleep*, *7*, 137–141.

Roehrs T, Zorick MD, Sicklesteel J, et al. (1983). Age-related sleep-wake disorders at a sleep disorder center. *Journal of the American Geriatrics Society*, *31*, 364–370.

Rosvold HD, Mirsky AF, Sarason I, et al. (1956). A continuous performance test of brain damage. *Journal of Consulting Psychology*, *20*, 343–350.

Roth B (1980). *Narcolepsy and hypersomnia*. Base, Switzerland: S Karger.

Roth T, Hartse KM, Saab PG, et al. (1980). The effects of flurazepam, lorazepam, and triazolam on sleep and memory. *Psychopharmacology*, *70*, 231–237.

Rubinow DR & Roy-Byrne P (1984). Premenstrual syndromes: Overview from a methodologic perspective. *American Journal of Psychiatry*, *141*, 163–172.

Ruiz-Primo ME, Coria S, & Torres O (1985). Prevalence of subjctive sleep disorders in poorly controlled chronic epileptics. *Sleep Research*, *14*, 243.

Sack DA (1985). Potentiation of anti-depressant medications by phase advance of the sleep-wake cycle. *American Journal of Psychiatry*, *142*, 606–608.

Saletu B, Gruenberger, & J Anderer P (1983). Evening television and sleep. *Medizinlische Welt*, *34*, 866–870.

Salzman C (1979). Update on geriatric psychopharmacology. *Geriatrics*, *34*, 87–90.

Salzman C (1981). Psychotropic drug use and polypharmacy in a general hospital. *General Hospital Psychiatry*, *3*, 1–9.

Sanders MH, (1984). Nasal CPAP effect on patterns of sleep apnea. *Chest*, *86*, 839–844.

Sanders MH, Rogers RM, Pennock BE (1985). Prolonged expiratory phase in sleep apnea. *American Review of Respiratory Disease*, *131*, 401–408.

Sauerland EK & Harper RM (1976). The human tongue during sleep: Electromyographic activity of the genioglossus muscle. *Experimental Neurology*, *51*, 160–170.

Savin JA, Peterson WD, & Oswald I (1973). Scratching during sleep. *Lancet*, *2*, 296–297.

Scharf MB, Khosla N, Brocker N, et al. (1984). Differential amnestic properties of short and long-acting benzodiasepines. *Journal of Clinical Psychiatry*, *45*, 51–53.

Schneider E, Maxion H, Ziegler B, et al. (1974). The relationship between sleep and Parkinson's disease and its alteration by L-dopa. *Journal of Neurology*, *207*, 95–108.

Schuil HJ, Wilkinson GR, & Johnson R (1971). Normal disposition of oxyepam in acute hepatitis and cirrhosis. *Annals of Internal Medicine*, *84*, 420–425.

Scrima L, Broudy, KN, Cohn MA (1982). Increased severity of obstructive sleep apnea after bedtime alcohol ingestion: Diagnostic potential and proposed mechanism of action. *Sleep*, *5*, 318–328.

Seidel WF, Roth T, Roehrs T, et al. (1984). Treatment of a 12-hour shift of sleep schedule with benzodiazepines. *Science*, *224*, 1262–1264.

Shader RI, Georgotus A, Greenblatt DL, et al. (1978). Impaired desmethyldiazepam from chlorazepate by magnesium aluminum hydroxide. *Clinical Pharmacological Therapy, 24*, 308–315.

Shader RI, Greenblatt DJ, Harmatz JS, et al. (1977). Absorption and disposition of chlordiazepoxide in young and elderly male volunteers. *Journal of Clinical Pharmacology, 17*, 709–718.

Sheerin E (1972). A programme which led to a reduction in night sedation at a major hospital. *Medical Journal of Australia, 2*, 678–681.

Shepard JW, Garrison MN, Grither DA, et al. (1985). Relationship of ventricular ectopy to oxyhemoglobin saturation in patients with obstructive sleep apnea. *Chest, 88*, 335–340.

Shepard JW, Schweitzer PK, Keller CA, et al. (1984). Myocardial stress: Exercise versus sleep in patients with chronic obstructive lung disease. *Chest, 86*, 366–374.

Simmons FB, Guilleminault C, & Miles CE (1984). A surgical treatment for snoring and obstructive sleep apnea. *Western Journal of Medicine, 140*, 43–46.

Sitaram N, Wyatt RJ, Dawson S, et al. (1976). REM sleep induction by physostigmine infusion during sleep. *Science, 191*, 1281–1283.

Smirk H (1963). Hypotensive action of methyldopa. *British Medical Journal, 1*, 146–151.

Snyder F (1971). The physiology of dreaming. *Behavioral Science, 16*, 31–43.

Snyder F, Hobson JA, Morrison DF, et al. (1964). Changes in respiration, heart rate, and systolic blood pressure in human sleep. *Journal of Applied Physiology, 19*, 417–422.

Soldatos CR, Kales JD, Scharf MB, et al. (1980). Cigarette smoking associated with sleep difficulty. *Science, 207*, 551–553.

Spire JP, Kuo N, & Campbell N (1983). Maxillo-facial surgical approach: An introduction and review of mandibular advancement. *Bulletin of European Physiopathology and Respiration, 19*, 604–606.

Stacher G, Presslich B, & Starker H (1975). Gastric acid secretion and sleep stages during natural night sleep. *Gastroenterology, 68*, 1449–1455.

Starkman MN, Schteingart DE, & Schork MA (1981). Depressed mood and other psychiatric manifestations of Cushing's syndrome: Relationship to hormone levels. *Psychosomatic Medicine, 43*, 3–18.

Stern M. Roffwarg H, & Duvoisir R (1968). The parkinsonian tremor in sleep. *Journal of Nervous and Mental Disorders, 147*, 202–210.

Stramba-Badiale M, Ceretti A, & Forni G (1979). Aspects of sleep in the aged and very aged (long-lived) subject. *Minerva Medicina 70*, 2551–2554, 1979.

Stunkard A, Grace W, & Wolff H (1955). The night eating syndrome. *American Journal of Medicine, 19*, 78–86.

Sullivan C & Issa F (1980). Pathophysiological mechanisms in obstructive sleep apnea. *Sleep, 3*, 235–246.

Sweetwood H, Grant I, Gerst MS, et al. (1980). Sleep disorder over time: Psychiatric correlates among males. *British Journal of Psychiatry, 136*, 456–462.

Taasen VC, Block AJ, Bayser PG, et al. (1981). Alcohol increases sleep apnea and oxygen desaturation in asymptomatic men. *American Journal of Medicine, 71*, 240–245.

Tan T, Kales J, Kales A, et al. (1984). Biopsychobehavioral correlates of insomnia: IV. Diagnosis based on DMS-III. *American Journal of Psychiatry, 141*, 357–362.

Taub JM, Globus GG, Phoebus E, et al. (1971). Extended sleep and performance. *Nature, 233*, 142–143.

Tecce JJ (1971). Contingent negative variation and individual differences. *Archives of General Psychiatry, 24*, 1–16.

Tepas DL, Stock CG, Maltese JW, et al. (1982). Reported sleep of shift workers: A preliminary report. *Sleep Research, 7*, 313.

Thompson J & Oswald I (1977). Effect of oestrogen on the sleep, mood, and anxiety of menopausal women. *British Medical Journal, 2*, 1317–1319.

Tilkian A, Guilleminault C, Schroeder JS, et al. (1977). Sleep induced apnea syndrome. *American Journal of Medicine, 63*, 343–358.

Tolle FA, Judy WV, Yu PL, et al. (1983). Reduced stroke volume related to pleural pressure in obstructive sleep apnea. *Journal of Applied Physiology: Respiratory, Environmental and Exercise Physiology, 55*, 1718–1724.

Tomlinson BE, Blessed G, & Roth M (1970). Observations of the brains of demented old people. *Journal of Neurological Science, 11*, 205–242.

Trinder J, Stevenson J, Paxton SJ, et al. (1982). Physical fitness, exercise and REM sleep cycle length. *Psychophysiology, 19*, 89–93.

Tune GS (1968). Sleep and wakefulness in normal human adults. *British Medical Journal, 2*, 269–271.

Ulrich RS (1984) View through a window may influence recovery from surgery. *Science, 224*, 420–421.

Vardi J, Glaubman H, Rabey JM, et al. (1978). Myoclonic attacks induced by L-dopa and bromocryptine in Parkinson patients. *Journal of Neurology, 218*, 35–42.

Vela-Bueno A, Kales A, Soldatos C, et al. (1984). Sleep in the Prader-Willi syndrome. *Archives of Neurology, 41*, 294–296.

Victor BS, Lubetsky M, & Greden JF (1981). Somatic manifestations of caffeinism. *Journal of Clinical Psychiatry, 42*, 185–188.

Vitrey JM, Huquet P, & Dollfus D (1970) Recording of

two sleep records in the course of Jacob-Creutzfelt's disease. *Revue Neurologique, 122*, 528–529.

Walker JM, Floyd TC, Fein G, et al. (1978). Effects of exercise on sleep. *Journal of Applied Physiology: Respiratory, Environmental and Exercise Physiology, 44*, 945–951.

Ware JC (1983). Tricyclic anti-depressants in the treatment of insomnia. *Journal of Clinical Psychiatry, 44*(9, Sec 2), 25–28.

Webb WB & Agnew HW (1974). Regularity in the control of the free-running sleep-wakefulness rhythm. *Aerospace Medicine, 45*, 701–704.

Webb WB & Swinburne H (1971). An observational study of the sleep of the aged. *Perceptual and Motor Skills, 32*, 895–898.

Wehr TA, Wirz-Justice A, Goodwin FK, et al. (1979). Phase advance of the circadian sleep-wake cycle as an anti-depressant. *Science, 206*, 710–713.

Weitzman ED, Moline ML, Czeisler CA, et al. (1982). Chronobiology of aging: Temperature sleep-wake rhythms and entertainment. *Neurobiology of Aging, 3*, 299–309.

Wever R (1970). On the Zeitgeber strength of a light/dark cycle for circadian periodicity in man. *Pfluengers Archives, 321*, 133–142.

Wever RA (1975b). Autonomous circadian rhythms in man. *Naturwissenschaften, 62*, 443–444.

Wever R (1975a). The circadian multi-oscillator system of man. *European Journal of Chronobiology, 3*, 19–55.

Wever R (1975c). The meaning of circadian periodicity for old people. *Verhandlungen der Deutsche Gesellschaft Pathologie 59*, 160–180.

Wever RA (1979). *The circadian system of man: Results of experiment under temporal isolation.* New York: Springer.

Wilkinson RT (1965). Sleep Deprivation. In OG Edholm & AL Bacharach (Eds), *The physiology of human survival* (pp 399–429). New York: Academic Press.

Williams RL (1980). Sleeping-pill insomnia. *Journal of Clinical Psychiatry, 41*, 153–154.

Williams RL & Karacan I (1976). *Pharmacology of sleep* (p 142). New York: Wiley.

Williams RL, Karacan I, & Hursch CJ (1974). *Electroencephalography (EEG) of human sleep: Clinical applications.* New York: Wiley.

Wynne JW, Block AJ, & Boysen PG (1980). Oxygen desaturation in sleep: Sleep apnea and COPD. *Hospital Practice, 15*(10), 77–85.

Zorick F, Roth T, Hartze K, et al. (1981). Evaluation and diagnosis of resistant insomnia. *American Journal of Psychiatry, 138*, 769–773.

APPENDIX A: SLEEP DIARY LOG

Directions: Complete your SLEEP DIARY LOG on the other side of this sheet. Write all time in hours and minutes. For example, "CLOCK TIME INTO BED" asks for the time when you first got into bed, "CLOCK TIME TRY SLEEP" asks for the time when you first began trying to sleep, and "MINUTES BEFORE SLEEP" asks how long it took you to get to sleep once you really wanted to sleep. This means you should estimate the time in minutes from "CLOCK TIME TRY SLEEP" to the clock time you actually did fall asleep. Mark with a dark line all the times you are asleep including naps. Mark the times you eat with an "M" for a normal meal and an "S" for a snack. Show the times you took sleeping pills or tranquilizers with a "P" and the times you took other drugs such as diet pills or pep pills with a "D." Show the times you exercise with an "X." Try and write in all events or activities that may have influenced the time and quality of your sleep. You should begin your LOG on Sunday at 6 P.M. and finish the LOG one week later. Try to keep this form by your bed and try to make your entries at least twice a day such as in the morning and evening. If you awaken with an alarm clock, put an "A" at the end of your sleep period graph.

NAME   John Doe

WEEK BEGINNING   May   6   , 1956

Time axis: PM 6 7 8 9 10 11 | MIDNIGHT 12 1 2 3 4 5 6 7 8 | AM 9 10 11 | NOON 12 1 2 3 | PM 4 5

Day 1 (SUNDAY–MONDAY)

CLOCK TIME INTO BED	9:20
CLOCK TIME TRY SLEEP	11:00
MINUTES BEFORE SLEEP	20
SLEEP PERIOD GRAPH	M, napped in chair, SUNDAY–MONDAY, AM, S, X (4), X (5)
CLOCK TIME FINAL WAKE	7:30
CLOCK TIME OUT OF BED	8:00

Day 2 (MONDAY–TUESDAY)

Row	Entries
CLOCK TIME INTO BED	11:00
CLOCK TIME TRY SLEEP	11:30
MINUTES BEFORE SLEEP	30
SLEEP PERIOD GRAPH	M, alcohol, MONDAY–TUESDAY, S, M, 1, S (3), X (4), X (5)
CLOCK TIME FINAL WAKE	8:30, 2:10
CLOCK TIME OUT OF BED	9:00, 2:15

Day 3 (TUESDAY–WEDNESDAY)

CLOCK TIME INTO BED	10:30, 1:00
CLOCK TIME TRY SLEEP	10:30, 1:00
MINUTES BEFORE SLEEP	60, 1
SLEEP PERIOD GRAPH	M, heavy food, TUESDAY–WEDNESDAY, sick, S, D, X (4)
CLOCK TIME FINAL WAKE	9:00
CLOCK TIME OUT OF BED	9:00

Appendix A continues

303

NAME _____

WEEK BEGINNING _____, 19___

M = normal meal   P = sleeping pill or tranquilizer
S = snack   D = other drug such as diet pill
A = alarm   X = exercise

PM   MIDNIGHT   AM   NOON   PM

6 7 8 9 10 11 12 1 2 3 4 5 6 7 8 9 10 11 12 1 2 3 4 5

SUNDAY MONDAY

CLOCK TIME INTO BED
CLOCK TIME TRY SLEEP
MINUTES BEFORE SLEEP
SLEEP PERIOD GRAPH
CLOCK TIME FINAL WAKE
CLOCK TIME OUT OF BED

MONDAY TUESDAY

CLOCK TIME INTO BED
CLOCK TIME TRY SLEEP
MINUTES BEFORE SLEEP
SLEEP PERIOD GRAPH
CLOCK TIME FINAL WAKE
CLOCK TIME OUT OF BED

TUESDAY WEDNESDAY

CLOCK TIME INTO BED
CLOCK TIME TRY SLEEP
MINUTES BEFORE SLEEP
SLEEP PERIOD GRAPH
CLOCK TIME FINAL WAKE
CLOCK TIME OUT OF BED

304

CLOCK TIME INTO BED
CLOCK TIME TRY SLEEP
MINUTES BEFORE SLEEP
SLEEP PERIOD GRAPH
CLOCK TIME FINAL WAKE
CLOCK TIME OUT OF BED

WEDNESDAY THURSDAY

CLOCK TIME INTO BED
CLOCK TIME TRY SLEEP
MINUTES BEFORE SLEEP
SLEEP PERIOD GRAPH
CLOCK TIME FINAL WAKE
CLOCK TIME OUT OF BED

THURSDAY FRIDAY

CLOCK TIME INTO BED
CLOCK TIME TRY SLEEP
MINUTES BEFORE SLEEP
SLEEP PERIOD GRAPH
CLOCK TIME FINAL WAKE
CLOCK TIME OUT OF BED

FRIDAY SATURDAY

CLOCK TIME INTO BED
CLOCK TIME TRY SLEEP
MINUTES BEFORE SLEEP
SLEEP PERIOD GRAPH
CLOCK TIME FINAL WAKE
CLOCK TIME OUT OF BED

SATURDAY SUNDAY

6 7 8 9 10 11 12 1 2 3 4 5 6 7 8 9 10 11 12 1 2 3 4 5
PM   MIDNIGHT   AM   NOON   PM

Peter J. Fagan
Chester W. Schmidt, Jr.

13
Sexual Dysfunction in the Medically Ill

In recent years the sexual functioning of the medical patient has been recognized as an integral part of the patient's psychosocial adjustment to the illness. Reports on the effects on sexual functioning of specific diseases and conditions, such as diabetes (Jensen, 1985), multiple sclerosis (Barrett, 1982), coronary artery bypass surgery (Papadopoulos, Shelly, Piccolo, et al., 1986), and diseases of the reproductive organs (Stoudemire, Techman, & Graham, 1985; Wise, 1985), reflect a growing concern about the sexual lives of patients. In addition to the effects of the medical or surgical conditions themselves, pharmacologic agents may cause sexual dysfunction in patients and thereby hinder compliance with vital drug regimens.

Psychiatrists are thus beginning to receive more consultation requests in which the referring question concerns the sexual life of the patient. Even without this referring question, complete psychiatric evaluation of a medical or surgical patient should include the assessment of the sexual functioning of the patient.

This chapter first will provide a methodologic guide for the psychiatrist who is evaluating the sexual functioning of a medical or surgical patient. The major diagnostic questions and procedures that make up the sexual evaluation of the medical or surgical patient will be discussed. For more exhaustive descriptions of specific sexual problems of major illnesses and surgical procedures, the reader is referred to texts and reviews on sexual medicine (Kolodny, Masters, & Johnson, 1979; Wise & Schmidt, 1985). Sexual aspects of surgery are also addressed in Chapter 19 of this book, by Riether & Stoudemire. This chapter will also suggest treatment approaches for sexual dysfunction in the medical patient. While repeating what is available elsewhere in terms of general sexual therapy (Kaplan, 1981; Masters & Johnson, 1970; Meyer, Schmidt & Wise, 1983), an attempt will be made to adopt some of the therapeutic techniques and therapeutic approaches generally utilized to the special needs and limitations of the medical patient.

Although a conscious attempt will be made to discuss issues of sexuality for both

PRINCIPLES OF MEDICAL PSYCHIATRY
ISBN 0-8089-1883-4

men and women patients, the chapter reflects the bias in currently available research (and therefore knowledge) favoring men. The source of this bias is unknown, but it may relate to the ready availability of measurement for penile tumescence, or to men's greater tendency to complain about overt sexual dysfunction.

ELABORATION OF THE SEXUAL PROBLEM

The first task in the assessment of sexual functioning is to define the problem as clearly as possible. This is not always easy. Patients and physicians can collude in settling for a vague description. "I can't stay hard long enough" and "Sex with him is unenjoyable for me" are not definitive statements of the sexual dysfunction.

The Disorder and the Sexual Response Pattern

A direct way to obtain a behavioral description of a sexual dysfunction is to ask patients to describe their most recent attempt at sexual intercourse. One then compares this to the four-stage human sexual response cycle originally described by Masters and Johnson (1966) and amplified by Kaplan (1979) to include a stage of desire, the psychohormonal baseline from which the sexual response cycle ensues. The resultant five-stage sexual cycle of (1) desire, (2) excitement, (3) plateau, (4) orgasm, and (5) resolution provides a framework for the criteria for psychosexual dysfunctions in DSM-III-R. Figure 13-1 displays the commonly observed physiologic arousal patterns of the female and male sexual response cycles (Kolodny, Masters, & Johnson, 1979). The major difference be-

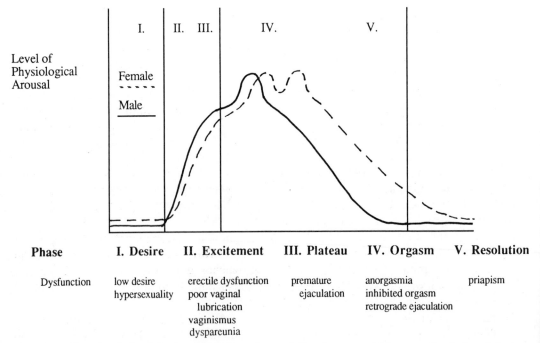

Fig. 13-1. Levels of physiologic arousal in males and females engaged in sexual activity. Adapted from Kolodny RC, Masters WH, & Johnson VE (1979). *Textbook of sexual medicine.* Boston: Little, Brown and Co.

tween male and female sexual response is that females are much more likely to be capable of multiple orgasms.

Disorders of Desire

Disorders of desire (libido) are expressed as a loss of interest in sexual activity. A disorder of sexual desire is usually a global decrease in cognitive, emotional, and physiologic readiness to initiate or respond to sexual overtures. Sexual fantasy life is practically nonexistent. The patient usually is able to describe a previous time when sexual interest and activity were greater. The distress shown about the loss of desire ranges from slight to great, but most often the patient will express a certain lack of interest in efforts to alter the level of sexual desire. In the setting of illness, malaise, pain, fatigue, and depression can lower sexual desire. On rare occasions the condition may be longstanding; when such is the case, the consultation is usually initiated by a dissatisfied partner. In such chronic conditions, the low sexual desire is usually ego-syntonic.

Disorders of sexual desire do not imply the inability to function sexually. Neurologic and endocrine disorders, as well as temporal lobe epilepsy or a pituitary adenoma, can selectively affect libido while leaving physical functioning intact. Patients on antihypertensive drugs report decreased libido and frequency despite apparent erectile competency.

Given an adequate amount of stimulation to the genital area, the resultant vasocongestion may cause erection or vaginal lubrication sufficient for satisfying coitus. Hypothetically, genital stimulation produces reflexogenic (sacral) arousal. This is processed cortically and subcortically, further augmenting the psychogenic arousal and intensifying erection or vaginal lubrication.

Sexual desire disorders can also be caused by interpersonal or psychosocial factors. In medical patients, reaction to the effects of the illness in the relationship (e.g., spouse as patient *and* partner) may contribute to decreased sexual desire. A recent study of diabetes and female sexuality (Schreiner-Engel, Schiavi, Vietorisz, et al., 1985) reported that diabetic women had relatively little impairment in sexual responses but were significantly lower than matched controls in sexual desire, psychosexual functioning, and satisfaction with their primary relationships.

The medical patient, with acquired cortical or subcortical dysfunction may present with a sexual desire problem such as gender dysphoria, hypersexuality, transvestism, or other paraphilias of acute onset apparently coinciding with the medical illness.

Disorders of Excitement

Disorders of excitement (arousal) denote a partial or complete failure to attain erection or the vaginal lubrication–swelling response following adequate sexual stimulation. For men there is insufficient vasocongestive reaction to permit the engorgement of the two cylindrical corpora cavernosa in the shaft of the penis and of the corpus spongiosum, which enlarges the glans penis. In women similar insufficient vasocongestion is manifested by limited (or no) vaginal lubrication and by absence of swelling in the labia majora.

In healthy men the self-report of firm, lasting morning erections (corroborated by spouse if possible) and the presence of turgid noncoital erections are the two most important items in the sexual history indicative of adequate physiologic erectile capability (Segraves, Schoenberg, & Ivanoff, 1983). There are not always, however, sufficient data for determining the etiology of erectile dysfunction among some groups of medically ill men. Certain sexual behaviors may occur so infrequently in some subgroups, such as masturbation attempts in older diabetic males, that the history alone is not sufficient for diagnosis. In addition, in some conditions, such as diabetes, hyper-prolactinemia, or decreased serum testosterone, men may be impotent with their spouses but because of the strong stimulus of an extramarital partner may be able to function adequately (Abel, Becker, Cunningham-Rather, et al., 1982; Schwartz, Bauman, & Kolodny, 1981; Segraves, 1982).

Dyspareunia and *vaginismus* are sexual dysfunctions that impede coitus despite the presence of an otherwise normal sexual response pattern. Dyspareunia in either sex is recurrent and persistent genital pain. In women it should be distinguished from pain caused by lack of lubrication (disorder of excitement). Vaginismus is the *involuntary* spasmodic contraction of the musculature around the vaginal outlet and of the outer third of the vaginal barrel. It is a reflex phenomenon comparable to the blink of an eye at an approaching object. Vaginismus renders penile penetration impossible whereas dyspareunia does not.

Disorders of Orgasm

Disorders of orgasm include premature ejaculation and inhibited orgasm in both sexes. Premature ejaculation occurs before the individual wishes it, because of recurrent absence of reasonable voluntary control in sexual activity. Viewed in this way, premature ejaculation may also be considered a disorder of the plateau phase. There is insufficient control of the plateau arousal prior to the stage of ejaculatory inevitability reached in the late plateau phase. As the disorder of premature ejaculation becomes more problematic to the partner, the orgasmic pleasure accompanying ejaculation often correspondingly decreases to minimal levels.

Inhibited orgasm is marked by a delay or absence of orgasm following a normal sexual excitement phase that is adequate in focus, intensity, and duration. Primary (lifelong) anorgasmia is found in both sexes, although it is extremely rare in men.

In men, orgasm with normal pleasurable sensations may occur without ejaculation, as in the retrograde ejaculation caused by sphincter muscle neuropathy, thioridazine treatment, or as a sequel of postorectomy. In women, orgasm may occur with noncoital clitoral stimulation alone. If this response pattern has been lifelong, such women should not be judged a priori to be abnormal or dysfunctional in their orgasmic response (Alzate, 1985; Derogatis, Fagan, Schmidt, et al., 1986).

The history of morning or noncoital erections does not imply normal orgasmic function. Patients on beta blockers or monoamine oxidase inhibitors may have drug-induced orgasmic dysfunction despite normal morning erections.

Disorders of Resolution

Disorders of resolution are those in which the anatomic and physiologic processes of the excitement and plateau phases are not reversed within a normal time period. A refractory period follows ejaculation, during which further ejaculation is impossible although partial or full erection may be maintained. This refractory period lengthens with age, and some men become distressed that "something is wrong" because they cannot have coitus as frequently during a night as when they were younger. The condition of *priapism*, a prolonged and painful erection that lasts more than several hours, is the main dysfunction of the male resolution phase. Although not a "dysfunction" properly speaking, the longer and more gradual resolution phase of women (see Figure 13-1) may become a source of distress if a postorgasmic male partner simply rolls over and goes to sleep. Interpersonal tension produced by this inattentiveness often leads to sexual withdrawal.

The elaboration of the presenting sexual problem has three goals: (1) a detailed description of the behavior, (2) determination of its onset relative to the illness, surgery, or medication regimen, and (3) information about any prior episodes of this problem in the life of the patient. It is for the last two goals that a complete psychosexual and psychosocial history is obtained.

The Psychiatric Interview

The preferred sequence for the interview is first to meet with the patient and sexual partner together for an initial exploration of the sexual problem or concern, next to meet separately with the patient and the partner, and finally to discuss issues of treatment with both.

During the initial meeting the psychiatrist establishes rapport with the couple and seeks to answer the following questions: Who initiated seeking professional help for the sexual problem? What are the investments each has in sexual life together? Who leads the description of the problem? How is responsibility for it apportioned? What level of communication exists between them? How have they responded *as a couple* to any limitations the medical illness may presently or in the future impose?

The individual interview with the identified patient includes a complete psychosexual and psychosocial history as well as a mental status examination to document the presence of signs and symptoms of a coexisting psychiatric disorder. The history also provides a developmental framework within which it is helpful to understand the patient's reaction to both the medical illness and the sexual dysfunction (Fagan, Meyer, & Schmidt, 1986). This would include an assessment of object relations and defensive style. Of particular importance is, of course, the sexual history per se. Table 13-1 outlines one possible format for taking a complete sexual history.

The individual interview with the partner follows the same format as that of the identified patient: psychosexual and psychosocial histories (with sexual data stressed) as well as mental status examination. Although some adjustments are made, dictated by clinical sensitivity, for example, decrease of emphasis on first-rank schizophrenic symptomatology, it is better to err on the side of overinclusiveness in the interview with the partner. The partner, even of a medically ill patient, may be implicated in the etiology of the dysfunction and most certainly will be called upon to collaborate in its remedy. Even if the treatment is a change in medications, the partner must be willing to participate in a renewed sexual life.

The final phase of the interview sequence is a conjoint session in which the treatment recommendations are made to the couple. Although the recommendations may seem relatively straightforward to the psychiatrist (e.g., change medications; have NPT studies performed), they are often complex to the patients. One must be prepared to spend time responding to anxious questions, especially from more obsessive patients. Time and patience expended at this point yield greater compliance with treatment recommendations, especially when they involve marital or sexual therapy.

When a medically ill patient with a sexual dysfunction does not have a sexual partner, there must be gentle probing to investigate why the patient is alone. Issues of shame, isolation, institutionalization, and fear of spreading disease may socially isolate patients. Evaluation of their social situation is necessary.

Further Diagnostic Procedures

The psychiatrist must either perform a sufficiently complete physical examination (see Table 13-2) or verify that one has been done by another physician. Likewise, the psychiatrist should make sure that an adequate laboratory data base has been established to permit a comprehensive diagnosis

Table 13-1

Data Covered for Sexual History

Childhood
   First sex play with peers
   Family sleeping arrangements
   Sex play with siblings
   Sexual abuse, incest, or molestation
   Parental attitudes toward sex
   Sources of sexual knowledge

Pubertal
   Menarche or first ejaculation: subjective reaction
   Secondary sex characteristics: subjective reaction
   Body image
   Masturbation fantasies and frequency
   Homoerotic fantasies and behavior
   Dating experiences (physical intimacies)
   Intercourse
      Age at first occurrence
      Reaction to first intercourse

Young adult
   Lengthy or live-in relationships
   Pattern of sexual activities with others
   Paraphilic behaviors
   Previous marriages
      Courtship
      Parental attitudes toward spouse
      Sexual activity (dysfunction?)
      Reasons for termination of marriage
   Veneral disease

Adult
   Present primary sexual relationship
      Development of relationship
      Significant nonsexual problems (e.g., money, alcohol, in-laws)
      Infertility; contraceptive practices
      Children (problems?)
   Sexual behaviors
      Extramarital affairs
      Intercourse frequency during relationship
      Variety of sexual behaviors (e.g., oral-genital, masturbation)
      Previous dysfunction (in either partner)
      Elaboration of onset and history of present problem (without partner present)
      Perception of partner's reaction to problem
      Homosexual activity
      Possible exposure to AIDS

Table 13-2.
Components of Physical examination of Sexually Dysfunctional Patients

Organ Systen	Physical Examinations
Endocrine system	hair distribution
	gynecomastia
	testes
	thyroid gland
Vascular system	peripheral pulses
Gastrointestinal	hepatomegaly, or atrophic liver with peripheral neuropathy due to alcoholism
Genitourinary	Prostate (in male)
system	Pelvic examination (in female)
Nervous system	
Sacral innervation	
S1–S2	mobility of small muscles of the foot
S2–S4	internal, external anal sphincter tone
	bulbocavernosus reflex (in male)
S2–S5	perianal sensation
Peripheral sensation	
Deep tendon	
reflexes	
Long tract signs	

Source: Wise TN & Schmidt CW (1985). Diagnostic approaches to sexuality in the medically ill. In RC Hall & TP Beresford (Eds), *Handbook of psychiatric diagnostic procedures* (Vol 2). New York: Spectrum.

that integrates psychologic, social, or biomedical factors.

Medical History

The medical history of the patient should center on the symptomatology or history of endocrine, vascular or neurologic diseases that may impair sexual functioning as well as the medications that have been used to treat those diseases or symptoms. A detailed alcohol and drug history must also be taken.

A family history of chronic diseases should be obtained. Medical conditions that commonly affect sexual response in both sexes are outlined in Table 13-3; Tables 13-4 and 13-5 further describe the effects of organic factors on each sex. Drugs that

commonly affect sexual function are listed in Table 13-6. Alcohol and drug abuse, beta-adrenergic blockers, centrally acting antihypertensives, and antiandrogens are among the best established exogenous causes of sexual dysfunction.

Endocrine Studies

Endocrine studies of medical patients should include measurement of fasting blood sugar and assays of follicle-stimulating hormone (FSH), luteinizing hormone (LH), testosterone, and prolactin, as well as a general survey, such as the SMA-12 or SMA-18, for liver and renal disease. For menustruating women, the interpretation of LH and FSH values depends on the time in the cycle when the blood sample is ob-

Table 13-3

Medical Conditions that May Affect Sexual Responses in Both Sexes

Medical Condition	Sexual Disorder
Cardiovascular	
Angina pectoris	Inhibited desire
Vascular disease: Large vessel (Leriche syndrome)	Inhibited excitement (pelvic vascular insufficiency)
Small vessel (pelvic vascular insufficiency)	Inhibited excitement
Neurological	
Alcoholic neuropathy	Inhibited excitement, inhibited orgasm
Multiple sclerosis	Decreased desire, inhibited excitement, inhibited orgasm
Cord lesions:	
Lower motor	Inhibited reflex excitement (psychogenic excitement and reflex ejaculation may be preserved)
Upper motor	Inhibited psychogenic excitement (reflex excitement and ejaculation may be preserved)
Temporal lobe lesions	Decreased or increased desire
Endocrinological	
Diabetes mellitus	Inhibited excitement; retrograde ejaculation (men) Inhibited orgasm (women)
Other (thyroid deficiency states, Addison's disease, Cushing's disease, hypopituitarism, hyperprolactinemia)	Decreased desire, variable effect on excitement
Other	
Any chronic systemic disease	Decreased desire, inhibited excitement
Chronic pain	Decreased desire
Degenerative arthritis and disk disease of lumbosacral spine	Inhibited desire, inhibited excitement
Radical pelvic surgery	Inhibited excitement, inhibited orgasm

Source: Schmidt CW (in press). Sexual disorders. In A Harvey, A Owens, VA McKusick (Eds), *Principles and practices of medicine.* New York: Appleton-Century-Croft.

tained. Formal endocrine consultation may be helpful in planning the hormonal evaluation.

Vascular Studies

Standard vascular studies are the Doppler studies of penile blood flow and a measurement of the penile-brachial index (PBI, the ratio of penile systolic pressure to brachial systolic pressure. Gerwertz and Zarins (1985) suggest that a vascular etiology for erectile impotence is possible when the PBI is less than 0.75. In the presence of normal values, further invasive procedures, such as a pelvic angiography, should be deferred unless abnormal results are ob-

Table 13-4.
Medical Conditions that May Cause Sexual Dysfunction in Women

Medical Condition	Sexual Disorder
Dyspareunia (painful intercourse)	Inhibited desire, inhibited
Agenesis of the vagina	excitement, inhibited orgasm,
Clitoral phymosis	and vaginismus may occur
Imperforate hymen, rigid hymen, tender hymenal tags	with any of the organic
Infections of the external genitalia:	factors listed at the left.
Herpes genitalis, labial cysts, furnucles, Bartholin cyst	
infections	
Infections of the vagina:	
Herpes genitalis	
Candida albicans	
Trichomonas	
Injuries due to birth trauma:	
Episiotomy scars, tears, uterine prolapse	
Irritations of the vagina:	
Chemical dermatitis (douches)	
Atrophic vaginitis	
Intercourse with insufficient lubrication	
Surgical complications:	
Ovarian approximation to vagina	
Posthysterectomy scarring	
Shortened vagina	
Miscellaneous pelvic problems	
Cystitis, urethritis, urethral prolapse	
Endometriosis, ectopic pregnancy, pelvic inflammatory	
disease, ovarian cysts and tumors, pelvic tumors	
Intrauterine device complications	
Reproductive endocrine problems	
Ovarian failure	
Hysterectomy without estrogen replacement	
Polycystic ovary disease	

Source: Schmidt CW (in press). Sexual disorders. In A Harvey, A Owens, VA McKusick (Eds), *Principles and practices of medicine.* New York: Appleton-Century-Croft.

tained from nocturnal penile tumescence studies.

Neurologic Assessment

Neurologic assessment includes a review of motor, sensory, and autonomic nervous system. As shown in Table 13-1, the lumbosacral spinal pathways merit spe-

cial attention as essential to sexual functioning. Cystometrogram or urinary flow studies can grossly define autonomic function in this area. Recent advances in determining the location of autonomic nerves from the pelvic plexus to the corpora cavernosa (Lepor, Gregerman, Crosby, et al., 1985) have made possible a nerve-spar-

Table 13-5.

Medical Conditions that May Affect Sexual Responses in Men

Organic Factor	Sexual Disorder
Dyspareunia (genital pain during intercourse)	Inhibited desire, inhibited
Disturbed penile anatomy (chordee, Peyronie's disease, traumatic fracture, traumatic amputation)	excitement, and inhibited orgasm may occur with any
Penile skin infections	of the organic factors listed at
Prostatic infections	the left.
Testicular disease (orchitis, epididymitis, tumor, trauma)	
Urethral infections (gonorrhea, nonspecific urethral infections)	
Hypogonadal androgen-deficient states (Klinefelter's syndrome, testicular agenesis, Kallman's syndrome, testicular tumors, orchitis, hyperprolactinemia, castration, primary testicular failure, pituitary hypogonadism)	Inhibited desire, inhibited excitement, inhibited orgasm
Mechanical problems (inguinal hernia, hydrocele)	Inhibited excitement
Surgical procedures:	
Abdominoperineal bowel resection	Inhibited excitement
Lumbar sympathectomy	Inhibited orgasm
Radical perineal prostatectomy	Inhibited excitement
Retroperitoneal lymphaedenectomy	Retrograde ejaculation

Source: Schmidt CW (in press). Sexual disorders. In A Harvey, A Owens, VA McKusick (Eds), *Principles and practices of medicine*. New York: Appleton-Century-Croft.

ing technique for retropubic prostatectomies. (Walsh, Lepor, & Eggleston, 1983) Such patients should therefore not be considered a priori surgically impotent. Neurologic patients with bladder and spasticity problems are more likely to have sexual dysfunction (Valleroy & Kraft, 1984).

Nocturnal Penile Tumescence Studies

Nocturnal penile tumescence (NPT) studies (Karacan, 1982) are helpful in ruling out predominantly organic etiology in medical patients. Presented with an identified pathologic condition, the physician may be inclined to attribute the erectile dysfunction to the medical illness or postsurgical status. With the two exceptions of hyperprolactinemia and vascular steal syndrome, a nor-

mal NPT can be interpreted to indicate adequate neurologic and vascular competency for coital erections. NPT studies also incidentally provide polysomnographic data which may assist in the diagnosis and treatment of a sleep apnea or major depression (as suggested by decreased REM latency and increased REM density). In addition to data on the frequency, duration, and rigidity of tumescence episodes, NPT studies can establish the relationship between penile blood flow and bulbocavernosus and ischiocavernosus muscle activity (Karacan, Aslan, & Hirshkowitz, 1983). This is especially important in the assessment of neurologically impaired men.

Interpretation of NPT studies is complex. Concerns about technical difficulties and basic assumptions of NPT have been raised that may impinge upon reliability and

Table 13-6.

Some Drugs That May Affect Sexual Response

Drug	Sexual Disorder
Antihypertensives and cardiovascular	
Acetazolamide	decreased desire
Atenolol	inhibited excitement
Bethanidine	inhibited excitement
Chlorthalidone	decreased desire
Clofibrate	decreased desire
Clonidine	inhibited excitement
Digoxin	decreased desire
Disopyramide	inhibited excitement
Guanethidine	inhibited excitement, no ejaculation
Hydralazine	inhibited excitement
Methyldopa	decreased desire, inhibited excitement, inability to ejaculate
Phenoxybenzamine	No ejaculation
Pentolinium	inhibited excitement, inability to ejaculate
Prazosin	inhibited excitement
Propranolol	decreased desire, inhibited excitement
Reserpine	decreased desire, inhibited excitement, decreased or no ejaculation, breast enlargement
Spironolactone	decreased desire, inhibited excitement
Thiazide diuretics	inhibited excitement
Timolol	decreased desire, inhibited excitement, no ejaculation
Drugs often abused	
Alcohol	decreased desire, inhibited excitement
Heroin	inhibited excitement
Methadone	decreased desire, inhibited excitement
Sedative-hypnotics	Inhibited excitement
Psychoactive drugs	
Antidepressants	
Amitriptyline	changes in libido, inhibited excitement, inability to ejaculate
Cyclobenzaprine	changes in libido
Doxepin	changes in libido, inhibited excitement
Imipramine	changes in libido, inhibited excitement, inability to ejaculate
Phenelzine	inhibited excitement
Trazodone	spontaneous erections or priapism in men; increased libido in women
Anxiolytic agents	
Benzodiazepines	changes in libido

317

Table 13-6 *(continued)*

Drug	Sexual Disorder
Antipsychotic agents	
Fluphenazine	changes in libido, inhibited excitement, inability to ejaculate
Haloperidol	changes in libido, inhibited excitement, inability to ejaculate
Lithium	inhibited excitement
Mesoridazine	changes in libido, inhibited excitement, inability to ejaculate
Prochlorperazine	changes in libido, inhibited excitement, inability to ejaculate
Thioridazine	changes in libido, inhibited excitement, inability to ejaculate
Trifluoperazine	changes in libido, inhibited excitement, inability to ejaculate
Gastrointestinal drugs	
Chlordiazepoxide	decreased desire
Cimetidine	decreased desire, inhibited excitement
Dicyclomine hydrochloride	inhibited excitement
methantheline bromide	inhibited excitement
propantheline bromide	inhibited excitement
Hormonal drugs	
Estrogens	decreased desire in men
Hydroxyprogesterone caproate	inhibited excitement
Methandrostenolone	decreased desire
Norethandrolone	decreased desire, inhibited excitement
Norethindrone	decreased desire, inhibited excitement
Progesterone	decreased desire, inhibited excitement
Others	
Aminocaproic acid	no ejaculation
Fenfluramine	decreased desire, inhibited excitement
Homatropine methylbromide	inhibited excitement
Metronidazole	decreased desire
Naproxen	inhibited excitement, no ejaculation
Phenytoin	decreased sexual activity

Source: DxRx, 1, 2 (1985); Wise TN (1984, May). How drugs can help or hinder sexual function. *Drug Therapy,* pp 137–149. See also Drugs that cause sexual dysfunction (1983). *Medical Letter on Drugs and Therapeutics, 25,* 73–76, for a more complete list with references.

validity. Segraves, Schoenberg, and Segraves (1985) cite previous studies in which, although NPT studies showed only partial sleep tumescence, the subjects later reported full erections with masturbation and intercourse. Segraves, Schoenberg, et al. (1985) describe one insulin-dependent diabetic with documented peripheral neuropathy who had a virtually flat nocturnal tumescence record. Subsequently he was able to have intercourse in an extra-marital situation. As Segraves, Schoenberg, et al. (1985) note, "These cases are a potent reminder that we have minimal information concerning the general physiological activation responsible for nocturnal erections and have no evidence that this arousal is equivalent in intensity to environmental stimuli" (p 177). Recently depression has been clearly shown to depress NPT response and appear "organic." The depression commonly found in medically ill patients may thus confound NPT data (Thase, Reynolds, Glanz, et al., 1987).

If NPT studies are abnormal and there are no additional signs or symptoms of organic etiology or of major depression, further vascular and neurologic studies are indicated. Presuming that Doppler blood flow and penile-brachial index have been obtained in the physical examination or as part of the NPT procedure, further vascular studies include arteriography of the aortic bifurcation, the internal iliac, and the internal pudendal arteries. When venous drainage problems are suspected, as when the glans penis does not engorge, a corporeal cavernosogram should be obtained (DePalma, 1984). Further neurologic studies include cystometrography and the testing of pudendal nerve conduction velocity (sacral latency testing).

More recently a home monitor for continuous measurement of NPT and penile rigidity has been developed (Bradley, Timm, Gallagher, et al., 1985; Kaneko & Bradley, 1986). Although the assumption of this device—that radial stiffness is related to axial rigidity—awaits further validation, the unit may provide reliable and valid NPT studies to those patients who did not previously have access to sleep laboratories because of geographic or financial restrictions.

Other home devices, such as the "stamp test" or tension gauges to assess nocturnal tumescence, are frequently used. There is little consensus about their reliability and validity. The working hypothesis is that circumferential tumescence equates with tip-to-base rigidity. This may not be the case, especially in some medical conditions. In diabetic men, for example, an engorged but still flaccid penis might break the devices and be considered a positive stamp test yet be inadequate for coital penetration.

Intracavernosal Injection

Recently intracavernosal injection of vasodilators such as phenoxybenzamine (alpha-adrenergic blocker) (Brindley, 1983) and papaverine hydrocloride with phentolamine mesylate (Zorgniotti & LeFleur, 1985) have been employed both diagnostically and therapeutically for presumed vascular and neurogenic impotence. At the present stage of development of pharmacologic erection challenge, caution should be used in interpreting negative (no erection) results. In one study, 50 percent of those with normal NPT did not have any response to intracavernosal papaverine injection (Buvat, Buvat-Herbaut, Dehaene, et al., 1986).

The extent of effort, time, and financial resources put into diagnostic studies of erectile and other sexual dysfunctions should be limited by treatment options. What the physician and patient will do with the knowledge gained is a question that should be asked prior to each diagnostic procedure. Advances in erection therapy (pharmacologic treatment) that permit temporary artificial erections may reduce the number of studies ordered.

Psychologic Assessment

Psychologic self-report instruments that assess either psychosocial distress or sexual functioning (Derogatis & Melisaratos, 1979) provide a valuable component in the full assessment of the medical patient with a sexual disorder. In some instances a patient will admit to a sexual behavior in a self-report format that concern for social desirability prevents in a face-to-face interview (DeLeo & Magni, 1983). Conte (1983) has written an excellent review and evaluation of self-report measurements of sexual functioning.

Multiple attempts to divide the etiologies of erectile dysfunction into strictly organic and psychogenic categories have not proven replicable. This failure may reflect a fault in the theoretical dichotomy of etiologies. Organic and psychologic factors in sexual functioning are not dichotomous but orthogonal factors. Each contributes to the sexual response—even in those patients whose sexual dysfunction appears directly caused by a medical condition.

Of particular utility with medical patients is the Psychological Adjustment to Illness Scale (PAIS). The PAIS (Derogatis, 1986) can be administered in a 20–30-minute semistructured interview or given in a self-report (PAIS-SR) format. It contains 7 subscales (including a sexual relationship scale), which measure different domains of psychosocial adjustment following illness. The PAIS provides normative values for the following clinical groups: lung cancer patients, renal dialysis patients, acute burn patients, and essential hypertensives.

TREATMENT ISSUES

General Issues

The initial treatment issue for the sexual problem of a medical patient is to ensure that the pathologic processes of the illness are ameliorated as much as possible. The second issue is to convey to the patient that the goal of sexual therapy (regardless of the mode of intervention) is to maximize whatever sexual abilities remain that can be developed within the patient's esthetic and ethical parameters. With illness taking control from some areas of the patient's life, he or she should experience sexual therapy as a means of regaining initiative in a relationship and securing pleasure for self and partner.

The premorbid baseline of the patient's sexual function should be noted. It is patently more difficult to recover and improve a premorbid low baseline than assist a patient back to a relatively sound baseline that may have existed before the illness.

If one suspects that the sexual dysfunction is pharmacologically caused (Table 13-6), then a drug holiday, if possible, may be employed as a diagnostic-therapeutic measure. When a drug is implicated, efforts should be made to achieve the same effects with a different drug or the same drug at a lower dosage. The sexual inhibiting effects of some drugs, such as antihypertensives, can cause patients to unilaterally discontinue the regimen and thereby put themselves at serious medical risk. Concern about the effects of drugs on sexual functioning, therefore, is not "merely" a concern about patient's sexual lives. If the etiology of the sexual disorder is alcohol or substance abuse, treatment should be aimed at controlling the abuse.

Illness, injury, and surgery, especially that involving breasts and genitalia, may have severe effects on body image and upon the patient's self-concept as spouse or lover (Stoudemire, Techman, & Graham, 1985). Sexual desire often is decreased even though the capacity for sexual functioning may remain intact. For the premorbidly psychologically healthy, a brief schedule of individual therapy (5 or 6 sessions) followed by conjoint therapy (3 or 4 sessions) usually is sufficient to assist the patient and partner through the adjustment crisis. Those with characterological or severe neurotic traits require more extensive psychotherapy when faced with these traumata. Another group for whom problems of body image exist are the head-injured. Problems of body image and sexual identity in the head-injured have been treated successfully with cognitive restructuring, social skills training, assertiveness training, and behavioral assignments. (Valentich & Gripton, 1986). Disturbances of body image relating to sexual dysfunction are also discussed by Riether and Stoudemire in Chapter 19.

Medical-Surgical Treatments

Disorders of Desire

Inhibited sexual desire due to illness-related fatigue and malaise should be acknowledged. In chronic debilitating illnesses such as multiple sclerosis, a realistic candor about the inadequacy of waiting for spontaneous sex is in the patient's interest. The clinician may encourage the patient and spouse to plan for sex by conserving energy and allotting time for sexual rendezvous.

Estrogen replacement therapy in women who have undergone hysterectomy and oophorectomy does not appear to improve libido and sexual function (Dennerstein, Wood, & Burrows, 1977; Utian, 1975), but topical or systemic estrogen reduces the occurrence of dyspareunia due to lack of lubrication and vaginal atrophy in posthysterectomy and postmenopausal women. Systemic estrogen replacement therapy may have a positive effect on a woman's mood and sense of well-being and secondarily, therefore, on her baseline of interest in and desire for sexual activity.

A man with abnormally low plasma testosterone levels not due to pituitary or hypothalamic disease may be administered testosterone cypionate (200 mg intramuscu-

larly every other week). This is a treatment for *decreased desire* in the presence of abnormally low testosterone levels. Testosterone replacement is *not* a treatment for erectile dysfunction.

Patients with pituitary disease may require postsurgical replacement therapy. To restore fertility in cases of pituitary destruction Jones (1985) describes a regimen of 1500–2000 IU of human chorionic gonadotropin intramuscularly twice weekly until normal plasma testosterone levels are restored. Then one ampule of human menopausal gonadotropin is given every other day for at least six months.

Bromocriptine (1.25 mg daily up to 2.5 mg twice daily) may be helpful in restoring both libido and erectile function for patients with hyperprolactinemia and low plasma testosterone levels (Carter, Tyson, Tolis, et al., 1978). Patients with high prolactin levels and demonstrable tumors will require both surgical resection and bromocriptine treatment (Prescott, Kendall-Taylor, Hall, et al., 1982).

The use of centrally acting agents to increase sexual desire and performance is yet inconclusive, though it appears that most interest has been generated in the aphrodisiac effects of serotonin antagonists and dopamine agonists (Segraves, Madsen, Carter, et al., 1985). Yohimbine, an α_2-adrenergic blocker (2 mg orally 3 times daily), has been reported to moderately improve sexual desire and arousal in some patients (Condra, Morales, Surridge, et al., 1986).

Disorders of Excitement

Little is known about the response to treatment in women with disease processes that impair sexual excitement. As in men, side effects of drugs can be minimized by decrease, substitution, or discontinuance of the drug. Dyspareunia due to vulvovaginal conditions and atrophic vaginitis can usually be eliminated. A nonpetroleum vaginal lubricant rather than jellies, which may provide a nidus for infection, should be prescribed for those women whose diseases have been implicated in inhibited sexual excitement. If recurrent urinary tract infection is associated with the disease, as in diabetes and multiple sclerosis, cunnilingus should be avoided as a possible contributing factor.

The recent development of pharmacologically induced erections by intracavernosal autoinjections of vasodilating drugs (Zorgniotti & LeFleur, 1985) has direct application in a treatment program for organically impaired men as well as for those men who do not benefit from sex therapy. Although some vascular compromise may be compatible with a good response to vasodilator injection, a certain (yet to be quantified) minimum level of vascular competency is required. A PBI-pulsation ratio less than 0.5, coupled with a maximum penile rigidity less than 350 grams, successfully discriminated those who responded unsuccessfully to papaverine in one report (Brendler, Allen, Engel, et al., 1986).

Pharmacologic erection treatment has the most promise for men with neurogenic impotence due to multiple sclerosis, pelvic nerve dysfunction, spinal cord injury, transverse myelitis, and diabetes mellitus. Goldstein, Payton, Saenez de Tejada, et al. (1985) reported on the pharmacologic erection treatment of 22 men with neurologic impotence over a 15-month period. Using test doses of 0.42–0.83 mg or phentolamine mesylate and 12.5–25.0 mg of papaverine hydrochloride in a total volume of 0.5–1.0 ml, erections were maintained for a period of 45 minutes to 6 hours and ejaculation was achieved by most. Priapism from the initial dosage was managed with corporal epinephrine (10 μg) irrigation. Goldstein et al. (1985) reported no systemic complications or major local penile problems despite multiple injections. Others (Brendler et al., 1986) have reported a high sensitivity of neurologic patients to the papaverine and

have reduced the dosage according to the response of the patient.

The surgical implantation of a penile prosthesis enables a man to have penetration and, to the extent possible prior to surgery, ejaculation and orgasm (Coleman, Listiak, Braatz, et al., 1985). Subsequent to surgery the man will not be able to have an erection without the prosthesis. Patients with manual dexterity limitations (or at risk for them because of disease such as multiple sclerosis) should be advised against a prosthesis requiring fine digital movements for inflation or deflation.

Reports of patient satisfaction with penile prostheses have been consistently high, although most studies have serious methodologic weaknesses (Collins & Kinder, 1984). One exception to this was a preoperative and postoperative study done by Berg and colleagues (1984) to identify predictors of successful adjustment following implantation of a penile prosthesis. Favorable predictors were (1) patient ambivalence about the operation, (2) a mature relationship between patient and partner, (3) some sexual activity before *and* after the onset of impotence, and (4) good mental health. Indicators of unfavorable prognosis were (1) a psychogenic component to the erectile dysfunction and (2) unrealistic expectations of what the prosthesis would accomplish for sexual and relational satisfaction.

When consulting to urologists concerning both penile implantations and pharmacologic erection treatment, psychiatrists should urge the involvement of spouses in the preoperative discussion of implantation and should assess carefully the quality of expectations for the treatment held by the patient and his wife.

There have been recent favorable reports of a pump cylinder that produces a vacuum around a flaccid penis. The resulting engorgement (erection) is preserved and utilized in coitus by a constriction band slipped onto the base of the penis after the erection is achieved. Further information can be obtained from Nu-Potent, Inc., Box 1478, 1246 Jones Street, Augusta, GA 30903.

Disorders of Orgasm

Apart from managing local vaginal conditions and discontinuing possible causal drugs, there are no organic therapies for anorgasmia in women secondary to a disease process. In those women with identified neuronal damage, including diabetic neuropathy, the goal of therapy should therefore be to assist the patient (and spouse) to adjust to the permanent limitations caused by the disease.

In men, lack of ejaculatory reflex should be distinguished from retrograde ejaculation, and the condition should be explained to the patient. If retrograde ejaculation is anticipated as a result of impending surgery (e.g., retroperitoneal lymphadenoctomy), adequate fertility counseling and sperm bank information should be given to the patient. Imipramine (25–50 mg/day) has been used to restore anterograde ejaculation in these patients (Nijman, Jager, Boer, et al., 1982).

Premature ejaculation is treated behaviorally with sensate focus techniques (Masters & Johnson, 1970), which may at times be complemented by anxiolytic medication. In men, primary or longstanding anorgasmia (without an identified organic cause) requires intensive psychotherapy to effect improvement.

Disorders of Resolution

Priapism, unless treated within four hours, may lead to penile ischemia, fibrosis, and permanent impotence. It is treated with an injection of epinephrine directly into the penis. Trazodone may cause priapism as a side effect during the treatment of depression. Because of the risk of permanent erectile impairment, this side effect must be regarded as a medical emergency. Male patients being treated with trazodone should be informed of this potential side effect, and advised to seek immediate treatment if it occurs. Two patients on trazodone reported 30–60-minute erections with no subjective sexual arousal (Sacks, Miller, Gunn, et al., 1985). They were switched to nortriptyline without further episodes of abnormal erections.

Psychologic Treatments

Offering psychologic treatment to medical patients with sexual dysfunction does not imply that there is a clear choice between medical-surgical interventions and those of a psychologic nature. Treatment is determined by etiology. For the medical patient (as for the healthy), sexual dysfunction is a biopsychosocial disorder. Treatment of the sexual dysfunction will be concerned with the patient's physical condition, the patient's psychologic state, and the social and relational adjustment the patient is making to the illness.

A useful model for treatment of the sexual problems of the medical patient is the PLISSIT model developed by Annon and Robinson (1978). The physician gives permission (P) to the patient to discuss his or her sexual concerns and apprehensions by initiating the discussion with an appropriate and solicitous question. In response to the questions that the patient and spouse may have about the effects of the illness or surgery upon sexual functioning, the clinician provides limited information (LI). Limited information is sufficient factual information to enable informed choice without overloading the patient with accurate but excessive detail. As rapport is established between physician and patient, specific suggestions (SS) are given by the clinician regarding maximizing sexual relations given the limitations imposed by the medical condition. In some cases, the patient must be referred to someone who can provide (IT) intensive therapy in an individual or couple modality. Each of these interventions can be demonstrated using cardiovascular disease as an example:

Permission

Without the clinician's inquiry into their sexual concerns and problems, most patients will remain silent about them. DeLeo and Magni (1983) reported that only 10 percent of patients on antihypertensive medication spontaneously reported impotence. Systematic questioning increased the incidence to 26 percent. When the patients were given a questionnaire to complete in privacy, 47 percent admitted impotence.

Spouses also need to be given the opportunity to air their concerns about the patient's illness and sexuality. This is especially the case for partners of patients who have had a myocardial infarction (MI) or coronary artery bypass surgery (Papadopoulos et al., 1986).

Limited Information

MI patients and their spouses have less anxiety and less fear of "coital death" when a health professional makes concerted efforts to address their sexuality as part of the rehabilitation program. Hellerstein and Friedman (1970) have described the cardiovascular demands of sexual intercourse. During coitus, blood pressure generally rises to approximately 160 mm Hg systolic with a concurrent heart rate of 150 beats a minute. This has been compared to a brisk walk around a city block or climbing two flights of stairs. Exercise testing establishing sufficient aerobic exercise balance can thus be used to establish the probable cardiac safety of resuming intercourse. Prior to discharge from hospital, such patients and their spouses should be given some concrete means of appreciating the cardiovascular demands of intercourse. Resumption of full sexual activity can occur 8–12 weeks following an acute infarct. In the interim, couples should continue to engage in caressing and other expressions of sexual tenderness to which they have been accustomed.

For the first few months of recovery, apprehension and reluctance are typical feelings about sexual activity. Beyond 6 months, male MI patients have been reported to have no significant difference in incidence in sexual dysfunction when matched with controls for age, hypertension, diabetes, and smoking habits (Dhabuwala, Kumar, & Pierce, 1986). Men who were sexually active before their MI who persist in avoiding sexual activity beyond six months after MI should thus be considered to have sexual dysfunction. They should be educated as to the limited risk that coitus entails for them. Problems persisting after education will require psychotherapy or sexual therapy.

Specific Suggestions

When intercourse is attempted by a post-MI patient, the couple may find that a side-by-side or female-superior position places less isometric tension and cardiovascular demand on the male patient and is thus preferable for them. Prophylactic nitroglycerin can be suggested to patients who experience mild angina during coital activity.

In addition to cardiovascular patients, those with chronic illnesses or conditions, such as multiple sclerosis or ostomy, can be encouraged to participate in one of the numerous patient self-help organizations. Such organizations regularly feature speakers or workshops on sexual problems commonly experienced by persons with the illness particular to the groups. In addition to these specific medical illness groups, there is a national organization with local chapters that offers support and information to couples about erectile dysfunction. Impotence Anonymous (IA, 119 South Ruth Street, Maryville, TN 37801-5746) is oriented toward surgical implants and may be particularly helpful for patients who are considering a penile prosthesis.

Intensive Therapy

The information, suggestions, and reassurance that can be obtained in two or three medical office visits may suffice for many medical patients to remedy the sexual dysfunction. For others, the psychologic component of the sexual problem may require a referral to someone who can provide a specialized mode of treatment. Formal psychiatric consultation should be obtained at this point. Psychiatrists and other sexual therapists with specific, detailed knowledge of the patient's medical problems will obtain the best results.

The initial psychiatric differential diagnosis is whether the sexual dysfunction is a psychosexual dysfunction or is secondary to another DSM-III-R Axis I disorder, such as major mood disorder, which must be treated first. If there is no other Axis I disorder that requires prior treatment and the etiology of the sexual dysfunction is presumed intrapsychic, then individual psychotherapy is indicated. This may subsequently be supplemented by group therapy.

If interpersonal factors are implicated in the etiology of the sexual dysfunction, a conjoint modality is indicated. If marital or relational issues predominate, these must be attended to first, by employing the techniques of family therapy. If sexual dysfunction is fairly discrete, then more behavioral therapy (e.g., sensate focus) may suffice. In practice, conjoint therapy initiated because of a sexual problem almost always involves both marital and specifically sexual therapy.

ACKNOWLEDGMENTS

The authors wish to thank Thomas N. Wise, M.D., for his helpful comments and suggestions concerning this chapter.

REFERENCES

Abel GG, Becker JV, Cunningham-Rather J, et al. (1982). Differential diagnosis of impotence in diabetics: The validity of sexual symptomatology. *Neurology and Urodynamics*, *1*, 57–69.

Alzate H (1985) Vaginal eroticism and female orgasm: A current appraisal. *Journal of Sex and Marital Therapy*, *11*, 271–284.

Annon JS & Robinson CH (1978). The use of vicarious learning in the treatment of sexual concerns. In J LoPiccolo & L LoPiccolo (Eds), *Handbook of sex therapy*. New York: Plenum.

Barrett M (1982). *Sexuality and multiple sclerosis*. New York: National Multiple Sclerosis Society.

Bradley WE, Timm GW, Gallagher JM, et al. (1985). New method for continuous measurement of nocturnal penile tumescence and rigidity. *Urology*, *26*, 4–9.

Brendler CB, Allen RP, Engel RM, et al. (1986). NPT predicts response to pharmacological erection. Paper read at the Mid-Atlantic American Urological Association annual meeting, Bermuda.

Brindley GS (1983). Cavernosal alpha-blockade: A new technique for investigating and treating erectile impotence. *British Journal of Psychiatry*, *143*, 332–337.

Buvat J, Buvat-Herbaut M, Dehaene JL, et al. (1986). Intracavernous injection of papaverine a reliable screening test for vascular impotence? *Journal of Urology*, *135*, 476–478.

Carter JN, Tyson JE, Tolis G, et al. (1978). Prolactin-secreting tumors and hypogonadism in 22 men. *New England Journal of Medicine*, *299*, 847–852.

Coleman E, Listiak A, Braatz G, et al. (1985). Effects of penile implant surgery on ejaculation and orgasm. *Journal of Sex and Marital Therapy*, *11*, 199–205.

Collins GF & Kinder BN (1984). Adjustment following surgical implantation of a penile prosthesis: A critical overview. *Journal of Sex and Marital Therapy*, *10*, 255–271.

Condra M, Morales A, Surridge DH, et al. (1986). The unreliability of nocturnal penile tumescence recording as an outcome of measuremnt in the treatment of organic impotence. *Journal of Urology, 135*, 280–282.

Conte HR (1983). Development and use of self-report techniques for assessing sexual functioning: A review and critique. *Archives of Sexual Behavior, 12*, 555–576.

DeLeo D & Magni G (1983). Sexual side effects of antidepressant drugs. *Psychosomatics, 140*, 1076–1082.

Dennerstein L, Wood C, & Burrows GD (1977). Sexual response following hysterectomy and oophorectomy. *Obstetrics and Gynecology, 49*, 92–96.

DePalma RG (1984, October). Vascular assessment of sexual dysfunction. Paper read at Society for Sex Therapy and Research annual meeting, New York.

Derogatis LR (1986). The Psychosocial Adjustment to Illness Scale (PAIS). *Journal of Psychosomatic Research, 30*, 77–91.

Derogatis LR, Fagan PJ, Schmidt CW, et al. (1986). Psychological subtypes of anorgasmia: A marker variable approach. *Journal of Sex and Marital Therapy, 12*, 197–210.

Derogatis LR & Melisaratos N (1979). The DSFI: A multidimensional measure of sexual functioning. *Journal of Sex and Marital Therapy, 5*, 244–280.

Dhabuwala CB, Kumar A, & Pierce JM (1986). Myocardial infarction and its influence on male sexual functioning. *Archives of Sexual Behavior, 15*, 499–504.

Fagan PJ, Meyer JK, & Schmidt CW, Jr (1986). Sexual dysfunction in an adult developmental perspective. *Journal of Sex and Marital Therapy, 12*, 1–12.

Gerwertz BL & Zarins CK (1985). Vasculogenic impotence. In RT Segraves and HW Schoenberg (Eds), *Diagnosis and treatment of erectile disturbances* (pp 105–114). New York: Plenum.

Goldstein I, Payton T, Saenez de Tejada I, et al. (1985). Neurologic impotence: An advance in treatment. Paper read at the annual meeting of the Society for Sex Research and Therapy, Minneapolis.

Hellerstein HK & Friedman EH (1970). Sexual activity and the postcoronary patient. *Archives of Internal Medicine, 125*, 987–999.

Heslinga K, Schellen AM, & Verkuyl A (1974) *Not made of stone: The sexual problems of handicapped people.* Springfield, IL: Charles C Thomas.

Jensen SB (1985). Sexual relationships in couples with a diabetic partner. *Journal of Sex and Marital Therapy, 11*, 259–270.

Jones TM (1985). Hormonal factors in erectile dysfunction. In RT Segraves and HW Schoenberg

(Eds), *Diagnosis and treatment of erectile disturbances* (pp 115–158). New York: Plenum.

Kaneko S & Bradley WE (1986). Evaluation of erectile dysfunction with continuous monitoring of penile regidity. *The Journal of Urology, 136*, 1026–1029.

Kaplan HS (1979). *Disorders of sexual desire.* New York: Brunner/Mazel.

Kaplan HS (1981). *The new sex therapy.* New York: Brunner/Mazel.

Karacan I (1982). Nocturnal penile tumescence as a biological marker in assessing erectile dysfunction. *Psychosomatics, 23*, 349–360.

Karacan I, Aslan C, & Hirshkowitz M (1983). Erectile mechanisms in man. *Science, 220*, 1080–1082.

Kolodny RC, Masters WH, & Johnson VE (1979). *Textbook of sexual medicine.* Boston: Little, Brown and Co.

Lepor H, Gregerman M, Crosby R, et al. (1985). Precise localization of the autonomic nerves from the pelvic plexus to the corpora cavernosa: A detailed anatomical study of the adult male pelvis. *The Journal of Urology, 4*, 207–212.

Masters WH & Johnson VE (1966). *Human sexual response.* Boston: Little, Brown and Co.

Masters WH & Johnson VE (1970). *Human sexual inadequacy.* Boston: Little, Brown and Co.

Meyer JK, Schmidt CW, & Wise, TN (Eds) (1983). *Clinical management of sexual disorders* (2nd Ed). Baltimore: Williams & Wilkens.

Nijman JM, Jager S, Boer PW, et al. (1982). The treatment of ejaculation disorders after retroperitoneal lymph node dissection. *Cancer, 50*, 2967–2971.

Papadopoulos C, Shelly SI, Piccolo M, et al. (1986). Sexual activity after coronary bypass surgery. *Chest, 90*, 681–685.

Prescott RW, Kendall–Taylor P, Hall, K, et al. (1982). Hyperporlactinaemia in men: Response to bromocriptine therapy. *Lancet, 1*, 245–249.

Sacks M, Miller F, Gunn J, et al. (1985). Unusual erectile activity as a side effect of trazodone. *Hospital and Community Psychiatry, 36*, 298.

Schreiner-Engel P, Schiavi RC, Vietorisz D, et al. (1985). Diabetes and female sexuality: A comparative study of women in relationships. *Journal of Sex and Marital Therapy, 11*, 165–175.

Schwartz MF, Bauman J, & Kolodny RC (1981). Prolactin level in men presenting with sexual dysfunction. Paper read at annual meeting of Society for Sex Therapy and Research, New York.

Segraves RT (1982). Male sexual dysfunction. Paper read at annual meeting of Society for Sex Therapy and Research, Charleston, SC.

Segraves RT, Madsen R, Carter CS, et al. (1985). Erectile dysfunction associated with pharmacological agents. In RT Segraves and HW

Schoenberg (Eds), *Diagnosis and treatment of erectile disturbances* (pp 23–63). New York: Plenum.

Segraves RT, Schoenberg HW, & Ivanoff J (1983). Serum testosterone and prolactin levels in erectile dysfunction. *Journal of Sex and Marital Therapy*, 9, 19–26.

Segraves RT, Schoenberg HW, & Segraves KA (1985). Evaluation of the etiology of erectile failure. In RT Segraves & HW Schoenberg (Eds), *Diagnosis and treatment of erectile disturbances* (pp 165–196). New York: Plenum.

Stoudemire A, Techman T, & Graham SD (1985). Sexual assessment of the urologic oncology patient. *Psychosomatics*, 26, 405–410.

Thase ME, Reynolds CF, Glanz LM, et al. (1987). Nocturnal penile tumescence in depressed men. *American Journal of Psychiatry*, 144, 89–96.

Utian WH (1975). Effect of hysterectomy, oophorectomy and estrogen therapy on libido. *International Journal of Obstetrics and Gynaecology*, 13, 97–100.

Valentich M & Gripton J (1986). Facilitating the sexual integration of the head-injured person in the community. *Sexuality and Disability*, 7, 28–42.

Valleroy ML & Kraft GH (1984). Sexual dysfunction in multiple sclerosis. *Archives of Physical and Medical Rehabilitation*, 65, 125–128.

Walsh PC, Lepor H, & Eggleston JC (1983). Radical prostatectomy with preservation of sexual function: Anatomical and pathological considerations. *Prostate*, 4, 473–485.

Wise TN (1985). Sexual dysfunctions following diseases of the reproductive organs. *Advanced Psychosomatic Medicine*, 12, 136–139.

Wise TN & Schmidt CW (1985). Diagnostic approaches to sexuality in the medically ill. In RC Hall & TP Beresford (Eds), *Handbook of psychiatric diagnostic procedures* (Vol 2). New York: Spectrum.

Zorgniotti AW & LeFleur RS (1985). Auto-injection of the corpus cavernosum with a vasoactive drug combination for vasculogenic impotence. *The Journal of Urology*, 133, 39–41.

Gene G. Abel
Joanne-L. Rouleau
Barry J. Coyne

14
Behavioral Medicine Strategies in Medical Patients

BEHAVIORAL THERAPY AND BEHAVIORAL MEDICINE

This chapter will present basic principles of behavior therapy and illustrate how selected behavioral strategies may be applied to the treatment of medical patients. Since a comprehensive treatment of behavioral therapy in the medical population is beyond the scope of this chapter, the discussion is limited to the most common disorders that psychiatrists are likely to encounter in the medical setting in which behaviorally oriented techniques are useful as part of the overall treatment plan. The disorders selected for discussion are eating disorders, Type A personality traits, hyperventilation, "drop attacks," and "shy bladder" syndrome (psychogenic urinary retention). Behavioral techniques in the management of chronic pain are discussed in Chapter 17, by Houpt, behavioral techniques for cardiovascular risk factor reduction are discussed by Abrams, Raciti, Guise, et al. in Chapter 15, and sexual

dysfunction is discussed in Chapter 13, by Fagan and Schmidt.

Definitions

The definition of behavior therapy currently endorsed by the Association for the Advancement of Behavior Therapy and approved by the American Psychiatric Association refers to a general approach rather than specialized techniques or a unified theoretical frame (Franks & Wilson, 1973). Behavior therapy is distinguished from other approaches to treating human behavior problems by using principles based upon research and experimental social psychology, which are systematically applied to patients and simultaneously evaluated. The field of behavioral medicine is in part an application of behavioral therapy theory and principles to the management of disorders within the medical population. For example, Pomerleau and Brady (1979) defined behavioral medicine as "the clinical use of techniques derived from the experimental analysis of behavior—behavior

PRINCIPLES OF MEDICAL PSYCHIATRY
ISBN 0-8089-1883-4

Copyright © 1987 by Grune & Stratton, Inc.
All rights reserved.

therapy and behavior modification—for the evaluation, prevention, or treatment of physical disease or physiological dysfunction" and "the conduct of research contributing to the functional strategies and understanding of behavior associated with medical disorders in health care." In general, however, strictly defining behavioral medicine as the application of behavioral therapy to the medical population is probably too strict. Behavioral medicine is more broadly defined as "the field concerned with the development of behavioral science knowledge and techniques relevant to the understanding of physical health and illness and the application of this knowledge and techniques to prevention, diagnosis and rehabilitation" (Schwartz & Weiss, 1978).

This chapter will focus primarily on specific behavioral therapy techniques as a guide for clinical psychiatrists in choosing which type of medical patients and conditions may be responsive to a behavioral approach. (In many circumstances, however, behavioral techniques can and should be integrated with individual psychodynamic therapy, family therapy, or pharmacologic strategies.) For further reading and more detailed accounts of behavioral techniques, readers are referred to comprehensive texts on behavioral medicine and behavioral therapy, found in the reference list.

The Behavior Therapy Approach: Basic Treatment Approach

According to Kazdin (1978), the behavior therapy approach to treatment can be summarized in seven rules. *First*, therapist and patient must agree upon the specific, objective goals of treatment. *Second*, selected strategies for treatment and assessment must match the treatment goal. *Third*, treatment strategies must work *directly* to reach criterion or target behaviors required by the specific treatment goals.

Fourth, the therapist must accept the patient's problems and goals in the patient's own terms instead of inferring some underlying disposition or thoughts that directly influence the patient's behavior. *Fifth*, current conditions rather than historical determinants should shape the course of treatment. *Sixth*, specifying treatment in objective terms will facilitate replication. Finally, the therapist should rely upon basic research in behavioral psychology as the primary source for specific therapeutic techniques.

BASIC TECHNIQUES AND APPLICATION TO MEDICAL SETTINGS

Illness behavior, if more strongly reinforced than wellness behavior, may persist long after its organic cause has disappeared. Behavioral approaches have been used successfully with patients suffering from a variety of conditions for which organic causes could not be found, as well as with patients having difficulty coping with a persistent medical illness or physical disability. The following nine behavior therapy methods have potential applications with medical patients.

Systematic Desensitization

Developed by Joseph Wolpe (1958, 1969), systematic desensitization (a form of counterconditioning) means substituting an emotional response that is appropriate or adaptive to a given situation for one that is inappropriate or maladaptive. Counterconditioning describes any procedure using learning principles to train the patient to substitute one type of response for another. In desensitization, relaxation is specifically substituted for anxiety.

Modeling

Following the work of Bandura (1969, 1971), modeling procedures have been applied extensively in behavior therapy. In its basic form, modeling is quite simple. The patient is exposed to one or more other individuals, actually present (live) or filmed (symbolic), who demonstrate appropriate behaviors to be learned by the patient. Exposure to models should include exposure to the stimuli and situations that surround the model's behavior so that not only the target behavior, but also its appropriateness to relevant stimuli can be demonstrated. Ideally, the adoption of specific modeled behaviors should also provoke changes in the affects and attitudes that accompany the behavior. Many modeling techniques involve the immediate participation of the patient, who will perform the modeled behavior after its demonstration by the model. Verbal reinforcement often follows the patient's performance.

Contingency Management

In behavior therapy, reinforcement always increases the frequency of a behavior. By definition, there are two types of reinforcers, positive and negative. A *positive reinforcer* is any stimulus event whose contingent application will increase the likelihood of the behavior preceding it, while a *negative reinforcer* is any event whose contingent withdrawal increases the rate of the behavior preceding it (Skinner, 1969). Care must be taken that the reinforcer is available only following the display of appropriate behavior; usually, it is the close pairing in time between any action and its consequences that establishes the link between a behavior and its contingent reinforcement. In behavior therapy, a systematic strategy of presenting and withdrawing contingent rewards and punishments is called contingency management.

Prior to establishing a contingency management program, assessment procedures must determine the frequency of the target behavior during a baseline period in order to confirm a diagnosis. Once treatment begins, the frequency of the target behavior will indicate the relative effectiveness of the behavior modification program. Finally, frequencies should be recorded for some time following termination of treatment to verify the continuing beneficial effect of treatment.

In all behavioral techniques, it is essential for the therapist to identify the particular antecedent stimuli, situations, and conditions that consistently elicit the patient's inappropriate behavior as well as those conditions that consistently follow the inappropriate behavior and act as maintenance factors or reinforcers. Prior to the initiation of treatment in a contingency management program, the relative power of each reinforcer in the patient's environment should also be determined. There are different types of reinforcers, such as material reinforcers (candy, tokens, money), social reinforcers (smiles, praise, physical contact), or activity reinforcers (phone calls, walking privileges). An observant therapist or nursing staff will quickly discover those conditions for each patient that make for effective contingent reinforcement (McFarlane, Bellissimo, & Upton, 1982). The incentive value and power of particular reinforcers is different for each patient; so contingency management strategies must be individualized.

Once powerful reinforcers are identified, the therapist must establish when contingent reinforcement will be delivered. Immediate reinforcement seems best; usually, the longer the time between the completion of a behavior and the delivery of a reinforcer, the less effect the reinforcer will have (Ware & Terrell, 1961). When the patient is expected to acquire an entire sequence of desired behaviors, the therapist can set a policy that reinforcement should be administered following each component of the sequence as well as at its end. As therapy progresses, delaying reinforcement until the entire sequence is completed can also be highly effective. Some controversy exists whether the patient should be consciously aware of reinforcement contingencies in order for learning to occur (Spielberger and DeNike, 1966). When a reinforcer follows a long sequence of behaviors, however, or when reinforcement is delayed following the completion of a behavior, its effectiveness can be increased by clearly spelling out the contingency.

Adherence to medical treatment regimens in particular can be viewed as a function of specific situational factors (Shelton & Levy, 1981). The more the therapist can directly influence the patient's environment, the more effective contingency management will be.

Contingency Management Program in Treatment of Anorexia Nervosa

Evaluation. Behavioral analysis of a 57-year-old anorectic woman suggested that the antecedent of the patient's weight loss was a lack of social interactions following her family's move to a new state and her husband's continual absence on business trips. The patient's weight loss was rewarded by the extensive attention she received from her family and medical staff while in the cachectic state (Miller, 1983). The patient's history of noncompliance with traditional psychotherapy, coupled with her marked hostility and anger when interviewed, suggested that any discussion of "why" she failed to eat would be unproductive (Goldfarb, Dykens, & Gerrard, 1985; Halmi, 1974). This was confirmed by her gastroenterologist, who reported that over the two years she had been in his care, the patient persistently evaded coping with her needed weight gain.

Behavioral intervention. Because the patient's refusal to eat and resulting weak-

ness had placed her in an environment where hospital staff could observe her specific behavior, contingency management was selected as the major treatment intervention. This operant conditioning treatment (1) identifies an excessive behavior that needs to decrease in frequency or a deficit behavior that needs to increase in frequency (in this case, weight gain); (2) develops an objective measure of the target behavior (the patient's weight as measured by the nurse-recorded analytic scale each morning, with the patient wearing the same minimal hospital garment after voiding); and (3) sets the behavioral criterion (0.25-pound weight gain from the patient's previous highest weight) needed to be reinforced by something the patient considers a reward (Bhanji & Thompson, 1974). *Most positive reinforcers are generally identified by their high frequency in the patient's natural environment or, in this case, by their high frequency in the hospital environment.* The therapist and staff observed the patient frequently talking on the telephone, watching television, smoking about 30 cigarettes a day, and enjoying talks with other patients on her hospital floor. The following treatment strategy was promptly implemented.

1. Protocol for Medical Staff
   (a) Discontinue patient's television, phone, and visiting privileges, and limit her cigarette intake to 15 a day.
   (b) Confine patient to her room.
   (c) Weigh patient each morning at 6:00 A.M., after voiding and in hospital gown.
2. Contingency Rules
   (a) If patient gains 0.25 pound above previous highest weight, she enters step 1 of reinforcement program (see below).
   (b) If patient sustains 3 consecutive days of Step 1, she enters Step 2.

(c) If patient sustains 3 consecutive days of Step 2, she enters Step 3.
3. Reinforcement Program
   Step 1.   Access to TV and 30 cigarettes per day.
   Step 2.   Step 1 plus use of the telephone.
   Step 3.   Steps 1 and 2 plus visiting privileges and freedom to leave her room.

Following implementation of this contingency management program, the patient (and eventually her husband) gave impassioned pleas for exceptions to the contingency program or attempted to justify its termination so that she would not be upset. These maneuvers by the patient and her family were met consistently with the unimpassioned response "This is the method we feel will be most effective in allowing you to leave the hospital as rapidly as possible." As was expected, the busy hospital staff, with constantly changing shifts, initially needed repeated clarification and reassurance about the criteria for the various steps of reinforcement.

A major advantage of the program, given the hospital setting, was its simplicity. *Critical to such a program is the proper identification of positive reinforcers that the patient so highly values that she will change her behavior to obtain them* (Pomerleau & Brady, 1979). In this case, positive reinforcers were identified simply by observing the patient for 30 minutes in the hospital environment and talking with her about what she enjoyed within that setting. After an initial 7–10 days of attempting to disrupt the contingency program, the patient learned that the staff were steadfast in their resolve to carry out the program and were consistent in rewarding her for weight gain. She began steadily gaining weight and within 4 weeks was discharged after gaining 20 pounds.

In all contingency management programs, various artifacts can creep into the treatment that make it less than perfect. In this case, the patient began her treatment while receiving IVs and hyperalimentation, factors that produced either sudden weight loss or weight gain unrelated to the patient's eating behavior. No attempt was made to rectify the system for these contaminants since such adjustments would be exhausting to the therapist, the staff, and probably the patient herself. More extensively detailed discussions of the behavioral treatment of anorexia nervosa may be found in Bruch (1973) and Mizes (1985).

Behavior Therapy and Relaxation Procedures

Proper evaluation of a treatment's effectiveness requires using measures that both reflect the severity of the problem and would be responsive to effective treatment. Behavioral approaches always strive to assess three separate components of the patient's functioning: (1) the patient's self-report regarding symptoms, (2) psychophysiologic measures that are concomitant with the patient's medical symptoms, and (3) direct observations of overt motor behavior associated with the problem (Keefe, 1979).

One of the most common tools in behavior therapy is relaxation training. Progressive relaxation (Jacobson, 1938) is a method in which the patient is taught to systematically tense and then relax all the parts of the body while concentrating on the sensations produced by relaxation and learning to progressively produce deeper relaxation. Autogenic training (Schultz & Luthe, 1969) consists of concentrated imagery of warmth and heaviness. Transcendental meditation involves deep breathing and repetition of a single word (mantra).

Biofeedback has been used separately or in combination (biofeedback-assisted relaxation) with one of the other relaxation techniques to help the patient to learn muscular relaxation by providing immediate information, or feedback, from instruments that measure the electrical activity of muscles. Often, the patient's knowledge that he or she is succeeding serves as a reward to facilitate further success. As the following case history illustrates, biofeedback may also have more subtle effects, such as helping patients to select successful coping strategies and to increase their sense of self-control.

Muscle Relaxation and Biofeedback in Treatment of Type A Behavior

Evaluation. A 57-year-old male was referred to cardiology because of persistent chest pain and depressive features following myocardial infarction and coronary artery bypass. Clinical observation of the patient's behavior revealed the characteristics of the Type A personality pattern. He exuded dominance and control over others, maintained an authoritarian attitude regarding nearly all issues, and displayed rapid speech with frequently hostile, angry comments. He reported that he worked 7 days a week and that a typical day off began Friday night at 7:00 P.M., when he would leave work, go home, take his boat to the lake, fish all night long, and then go back to work Saturday morning feeling that he had enjoyed a day's relaxation and should now get back to work.

When his authoritarian, controlling personality style was not well accepted by others, he experienced marked anxiety, which was exacerbated by more frequent intrusions of chest pain into his daily life. With each onset of pain, his attitude was to ignore it and continue working, which inevitably led to persistent chest pain that would plague him through the night.

Behavioral intervention. To evaluate the frequency of his symptoms and to identify his attitudes and emotions toward them, a self-report form was developed. This "homework" allowed an ongoing daily appraisal by the patient (Shelton & Levy, 1981) of the various components of his anxiety, chest pain, and Type A behavior. In addition to treatment with antidepressants for his depression, the patient was taught progressive muscle relaxation. This nonpharmacologic intervention assisted the patient in controlling anxiety and also taught him how to become more aware of the early situational antecedents that provoked his anxiety, such as not getting his way or being unable to control situations. To further assist in the patient's control of anxiety, he also underwent muscle biofeedback assessment and treatment.

Biofeedback involves recording one or more of the patient's physiologic responses and displaying that information to the patient to see if he can alter his physiologic responding once he correlates his emotional feelings with his physiologic responses (Burish, 1981). Biofeedback can be used as both an assessment tool and a treatment strategy. With this patient, biofeedback was first used to evaluate whether specific situations related to his Type A personality pattern would provoke an elevated electromyographic (EMG) response and subsequent chest pain. In this case, to objectively evaluate physiologic provocative responses from the patient, the therapist presented him with brief, two-minute audiotaped scenes that specifically aggravated him as an individual with Type A personality, such as hearing the boss lavishly praising a younger competitor, being criticized for not working hard enough and being continually interrupted when trying to talk (Abel & Blanchard, 1976; Abel, Blanchard, Barlow, et al., 1975). For many patients, elevated EMG provides an objective assessment of anxiety. In this case, elevation of EMG occurred as he recalled being angry with people, or recalled becoming anxious by attempting to be perfect in various work situations.

The medical patient is frequently reluctant to conceptualize emotional factors as contributing to his physical symptoms and often finds it exceedingly difficult to trust the opinion of a psychiatrist or psychologist, possibly because of widely prevalent negative attitudes toward such professionals in our culture. Psychophysiologic assessment, by contrast, provides a means of cutting through this distrust by presenting the patient with powerful "concrete" evidence that demonstrates a connection between emotional factors and the body's physiologic reactivity.

This particular patient initially was skeptical that his anger and anxiety could affect his body's physiologic responding. During one particular session early in his biofeedback training, however, he had marked difficulty controlling his EMG tensions within his normal range. Puzzled by the elevated EMG, the biofeedback technician questioned the patient about his thoughts. The patient reported that he had been thinking angrily about another hospitalized patient with whom he had exchanged hostile words the day before. The patient was instructed to ignore those thoughts for the moment and to proceed with biofeedback by attempting to relax. After the session, he was shown the EMG printout, which demonstrated the elevated tension associated with his anger and the dramatic drop in EMG elevation that accompanied diverting his attention from anger to relaxation. Here was objective evidence that made it impossible for the patient to ignore the relationship between anger and his body's physiologic responding (EMG). At that moment he dedicated himself to learning how to control his anger and anxiety and to using both muscle relaxation and biofeedback procedures to assist in his therapy.

Effective treatment in a therapy session alone, however, is of limited value. Gains within treatment sessions must extend or generalize to the patient's natural environment so that the patient is able to control his physiologic responses without mechanical assistance (Young & Blanchard, 1980). As this patient's training continued, the physiologic recordings demonstrated a significant reduction in the patient's overall EMG activity when receiving biofeedback, which generalized to when he was sitting quietly without biofeedback. In addition, he reported that when awakened by angina attacks during the night, he successfully applied the techniques he had learned during biofeedback training to control his anxiety, which eventually resulted in the elimination of his chest pain episodes.

The patient was not "cured" by biofeedback alone. Antidepressants, assertiveness training, progressive muscle relaxation exercises, awareness of the antecedents of chest pain and anxiety, family therapy, education to alter the Type A personality pattern (Friedman & Rosenman, 1974), and biofeedback were all components of a total treatment program directed at his primary symptomatology. In this case, however, biofeedback motivated the patient for treatment by providing the objective evidence that cut through his reluctance to see how emotional factors contributed to his physical illness.

Procedures to Increase Effectiveness of a Behavioral Treatment Approach

Assuming that the behavior therapist has adopted an effective treatment approach, what sort of evidence should he use to convince the patient that Behavior X is responsible for Problem Y? In some cases, in order to enhance the potential impact of a treatment procedure as well as to maximize the patient's compliance, a demonstration of the relation between the patient's behavior and symptom can be highly effective.

An effective means of assessing a patient's problem is direct observation of the patient's motor behavior during symptom development. The closer the therapist can come to actually witnessing the development of symptomatology, the better the patient's and the therapist's understanding of what strategies may help treat the patient's symptom complex. In some cases, symptoms can be provoked involuntarily, as in the following example of a patient with hyperventilation syndrome.

Behavioral Diagnostic Technique (Provocative Test) in Treatment of Hyperventilation

Evaluation. A 38-year-old woman with limited intellectual functioning gave a two-year history of "spells." The symptoms she described appeared to be panic attacks with hyperventilation (Lum, 1975, 1981). To evaluate and treat this patient's symptoms, the therapist told the patient that she would undergo a breathing test, but he did not inform her that the test was likely to provoke her symptoms. Her lack of awareness was necessary in order to block any demand characteristic of the test and, more importantly, to allow the patient to better realize that any symptoms that were provoked were identical to those she had been having during her "spells." Following medical clearance, she was first taught to breathe at a rate (15 excursions a minute) indicated by the therapist, who raised and lowered his hand to signal when the patient should inhale and then exhale. The patient was verbally reinforced for following the therapist's instructions to breathe, and when she was questioned about how she felt, no symptoms were reported. Her breathing was then rapidly accelerated to 30 breaths a minute, a rate that was to be maintained until the patient became symptomatic (or for 5 minutes without symptoms). In this patient's case, within $1\frac{1}{2}$ minutes she developed marked flushing of her face and numbness of her hands, and within $2\frac{1}{2}$ minutes she developed the tightness of

her fingers and toes typically occurring with her hyperventilation. Two minutes into the provocative test, she also became less attentive to the examiner and began reporting her typical chest pain, along with tachycardia, marked shortness of breath, and sensations of passing out. The patient was asked to describe each of these symptoms and to report if she had ever had these before and under what conditions. In each case she reported the symptoms as identical to those that developed during her spells. By $3\frac{1}{2}$ minutes into the provocative test, she asked to stop because she feared her symptoms would get out of control.

Treatment. The therapist then reduced her pace of breathing to 15 breaths a minute and instructed her to place her right hand over her chest and her left hand over her abdomen and to breathe, not with chest excursion, but with abdominal excursion (diaphragmatic breathing). The patient was also instructed to breath through her nose or purse her lips in order to cut down on the exchange of air, and thereby decrease carbon dioxide expulsion from her lungs. As the patient's breathing was paced at the new lower rate, there was a dramatic reduction of her symptoms described above. The patient was then asked why her symptoms had decreased. She reported that it must have something to do with her breathing, since rapid breathing had brought on the symptoms she usually had with her "spells" and slower breathing eliminated those symptoms. At this point, the therapist reiterated the patient's insights about the relationship between her symptoms and her way of breathing.

Subsequent treatment included training the patient in appropriate abdominal breathing while lying supine, sitting, standing, and, most importantly, walking and exerting herself. The importance of the latter element is that many patients with hyperventilation syndrome precipitate their symptoms during the course of their work, when exertion leads to tachycardia, which triggers the anxiety–hyperventilation cycle (Moreyra, McGough, Hosler, et al., 1982).

Shaping Procedures

Many patients suffer a common problem of not being able to assert themselves. In the medical patient, such lack of assertiveness may take the form of being unable to perform specific medical care skills. Diabetic patients' inability to check their own blood glucose, obese patients' inability to increase their physical activities to promote weight loss, the inability of the man with erectile dysfunction to touch his partner sexually without focusing on his erection response—all are examples in which the patient may need to acquire skills in order to deal with a specific medical problem. Physicians, however, may be so far removed from the realities of their patients' lack of skills that they find it difficult to understand why the patients do not just go ahead and do what the physicians request. This attitude generally emanates from a physician's inability to appreciate the patient's limitations when asked to emit those skills necessary for compliance with the physician's regimen. Often the physician fails to appreciate that seemingly simple assignments actually involve complex skills that must be learned one small step at a time through a procedure called "shaping."

This technique is also called *successive approximation* or *response differentiation* (Bandura, 1969). If a behavior is not emitted by an individual, it cannot be reinforced. Shaping is used, therefore, to induce the performance of new behaviors by the initial reinforcement of behaviors that are already present in the individual's response repertoire and that have some continuity with the desired behavior. In the following case we will see how the acquisition of sequential behaviors was increased by social reinforcement and shaping procedures.

Verbal Reinforcement and Shaping Treatment for Noncompliance with Physical Rehabilitation in a Patient with "Drop Attacks"

Evaluation. A 62-year-old widow was referred by neurology for treatment of possible depression. She had been an energetic, self-sufficient, responsible woman, working 5 days a week and enjoying a full social life until 2 years prior to her referral, when she developed "drop attacks," episodes in which without warning she would suddenly lose control of her skeletal muscles and collapse. Falling without muscle tone, she was unable to prepare for the impact of the fall, and in 2 years she had suffered numerous lacerations, a skull fracture, various fractured ribs, and a fractured vertebra. Extensive neurologic workups and attempts at drug intervention had not reduced the frequency of these attacks. Her neurologist was puzzled because throughout her most recent 4-week hospitalization, when asked to ambulate again using a walker, the patient refused.

When interviewed, the patient was attentive and engaging and could easily identify the etiology of her noncompliance. Her last 2 years had been filled with drop attack episodes. Falling to the ground, even if she sustained no fractures in the fall, was terrifying. Since she had not risked ambulating in more than a month, the patient anticipated that she would inevitably become an invalid and have to be cared for by others. These thoughts led her to be depressed.

Behavioral intervention. Following institution of antidepressant medication, a behavioral analysis was conducted to assess the patient's fears and her skills at ambulation. In spite of staff on either side to assist her in moving from bedside to her walker, the patient became suprisingly anxious and fearful. Although merely standing at her walker was anxiety-provoking for the patient, it soon became apparent that her most terrifying fear was the prospect of having to get up from the floor. When lowered to the floor by staff (as if she had suffered a drop attack), in proximity to a chair for climbing support, the patient immediately became so frightened and confused that she gave up any attempt to raise herself. Because the patient, when lying in bed, responded to the attention and concern she received from the hospital staff, an operant or instrumental approach was chosen to increase her use of the walker and to train her to stand up from the floor. While on the neurology service, she had received attention from staff regardless of whether she was attempting to ambulate, attempting to stand up from the floor, or simply lying in bed. *On the behavioral medicine unit, attention from the staff was made contingent upon her practicing walker ambulation and getting up from the floor, with minimal attention given to her while simply lying in bed.*

The patient received social reinforcement in the form of praise and encouragement from staff during each training session when she practiced her needed skills. Each complex skill, however, was divided into small, separate components. Behaviors that are problematic for a patient need to be divided into small, manageable steps so that reinforcement can be given frequently for even minor attempts at mastering each component of a complex behavior (such as using a walker or rising from the floor). Training the patient to stand up included training her to wait on the floor until she was no longer frightened before mentally organizing the steps of getting up, to identify the furniture that would be supportive for rising, to turn furniture into position while still lying on the floor, to move her legs under her body so that her limbs could work in unison to "climb up" the furniture, to pause halfway to rest so that she had adequate energy to complete the full climb, to climb up the furniture until standing erect, to rest while standing before attempting to ambulate, and so on. She received separate training sessions on each compo-

nent of this complex task, and after several days of training, the patient regained her ability to walk.

Dividing a complex skill into manageable components presents the opportunity for frequent reinforcement and allows the patient to gain confidence without having to complete an entire complex task. This successive-approximation, or shaping, strategy has frequent application in skills training of the medical patient. Once a skill is acquired, successful performance of a complex task improves mood and self-esteem.

Flooding or Response Prevention

Some medical patients do not have problems of behavioral deficits that require the training of new behaviors, but instead perform dysfunctional behaviors that need to decrease in frequency. Ideally, it is best if appropriate behavior can be strengthened in a patient's repertoire, since sometimes this weakens or eliminates the excessive dysfunctional behavior. At times, however, this is not possible and more invasive, generally aversive procedures must be taught to the patient.

A variety of behavioral techniques have been developed to eliminate or reduce the frequency of problem behaviors (Rimm & Masters, 1974). Of the seven basic extinction procedures (extinction by contingency management procedures, negative practice, stimulus satiation, implosive therapy, graduated extinction, covert extinction, and flooding), the following sections will illustrate several of these approaches.

The therapeutic technique of *flooding* has its roots in laboratory experiments on the establishment and extinction of avoidance responses (Soloman, 1964). The two terms of flooding and response prevention both stand for the same general technique of exposing an individual to anxiety-provoking stimuli while preventing the occurrence of avoidance behaviors. In practice, patients are exposed to the actual feared stimuli in vivo without chance of escape while they experience high levels of anxiety.

Exposure Extinction

Exposure extinction is an additional technique designed to eliminate fear and avoidance behavior by the exposure of the individual to the fear-evoking stimuli. Although similar to desensitization and flooding, significant differences exist. Exposure extinction differs from desensitization in that no competing response replaces the response of anxiety. In desensitization, Wolpe (1958, 1969) proposed that relaxation provides a competing response to anxiety arousal. Exposure extinction also differs from flooding in that no specific care is taken to prevent avoidance responses at high anxiety.

A variety of phobic symptoms can be treated by exposing patients to their fears under conditions from which they cannot escape. The result of such an exposure technique is prompt reduction of anxiety to the feared environment or situation. Fear development and avoidance behaviors are best explained from a behavioral perspective by what is called the *two-factor theory of fear and learning*. In the first step, classical conditioning, anxiety is associated with a specific situation or behavior. Over time and as a result of generalization, this anxiety becomes associated not only with that specific environment, but with environments similar to the original anxiety-provoking situation. The second component of fear learning involves operant conditioning and avoidant responses. In an attempt to avoid the anxiety associated with the feared situation, the individual escapes from or avoids the situation. Escaping from the feared situation is momentarily associated with anxiety reduction. Because anxiety reduction is a strong reinforcer, further avoidance of the feared situation is maintained by the constant reinforcement that follows avoidance of or escape from the feared situation. The fear–avoidance pattern becomes chronic.

Anxiety Reduction through Exposure to the Feared Situation and Extinction of Avoidance Behavior in Treatment of the "Shy Bladder" Syndrome

Evaluation. A 33-year-old man was referred from urology because of a "shy bladder." All his life he recalled being highly anxious when urinating in public rest rooms. Throughout grade school and high school, this fear led him to reduce his fluid intake prior to going to school in order to avoid urinating there. His fears about urinating in public facilities continued after graduation and eventually extended to his work site: in the 12 years prior to referral, he had never urinated in any of the rest rooms of the office building in which he worked. With an advanced position in his company, he sought treatment because of a recently initiated drug awareness program in which employees were asked to submit urine samples for drug screening. He had never been able to provide physicians with a urine sample on demand.

Behavioral intervention. After initiating a behavioral analysis of the patient's phobia through interview and self-report forms (Kazdin, 1974), the therapist walked with the patient into various rest rooms to identify the precise characteristics and surroundings that provoked the patient's anxiety. To provide further quantification of his fear response, the patient was asked to rate his anxiety before, during, and after entrance into each rest room. As is traditionally the case with such individuals, rest rooms with frequent use, open stalls, and especially stalls with no dividers between the urinals were most provocative of the patient's anxiety and inability to urinate

(Abel & Blendinger, 1985; Anderson, 1977). The patient was next asked to "water-load" by drinking 16 ounces of soda $1\frac{1}{2}$ hours prior to each future therapy session. With high urges to urinate, he was then accompanied by the therapist to an anxiety-provoking public rest room where he was asked to imagine his usual thought about entering such a feared situation. He was told to enter the rest room and approach the urinal, unzip his pants, and carry out all of the physical and cognitive steps of urination except actually voiding. This procedure was repeated at several public rest rooms with those characteristics that especially provoked his fears.

After 4–5 days of entering rest rooms in proximity to the therapist's office, the patient was then asked to carry out the same procedure at work and in social surroundings to bring about generalization of the treatment. To the patient's surprise, his fears began to decrease drastically, and as the therapist expected, on a number of such occasions the patient was unable to comply with instructions not to void, since his fear under such circumstances was reduced and, as a result of his water loading, his urges to urinate were high. He subsequently voided on a number of such occasions, which gave him considerable encouragement and further reduced his fear (Wolpe, 1958).

As a result of the treatment, the patient's life changed markedly. In the past the patient had avoided work and social situations that might necessitate his urinating in another's presence. He began socializing, attending parties and mixing more with work colleagues, as his social limitation was now markedly reduced.

For the final step of his treatment, the patient had to overcome his greatest fear: urinating on demand for laboratory testing. During the course of the treatment program, the therapist took the patient to a hospital laboratory and had him void in the very rest room used for collecting urine samples. With his urinary urges high and anxiety lowered, the patient was overjoyed by his ability to void under this formerly anxiety-provoking situation. His follow-up treatments required him to maintain his gains by frequent exposure to previously fearful situations, new rest rooms.

In vivo exposure with subsequent extinction of avoidance behavior is an exceedingly powerful treatment with wide applicability to a variety of fears.

Covert Sensitization

Covert sensitization involves having the patient imagine performing a problem behavior and then imagine a punitive or aversive consequence of performing that problem behavior. These two cognitions should be matched in the patient's imagination for as long as the problem behavior continues to occur (Cautela, 1970). In the next clinical case, covert sensitization was used to extinguish bulimic behavior by asking the patient to cognitively pair the antecedents of binge behavior with its possible negative consequences.

Covert Sensitization in Treatment of Bulimia

Evaluation. A 29-year-old woman was referred by her internist for treatment of bulimia. Her life was organized around binge-purge episodes. Working a different shift than her husband, she would leave work after an afternoon of planning her binge menu. A quick trip to the grocery store would procure half-gallons of ice cream, dozens of cookies and doughnuts, pastries, potato chips, and any food that suited her fancy. Locking her apartment door, she would attack the food and relish its consumption, knowing that she could eat anything she wanted, since vomiting was to follow. Futile attempts to conceal her binge-vomit episodes and pleas by her family and herself to give up her bulimia eventually overwhelmed the patient.

Behavioral intervention. Behavioral analysis revealed that the majority of the patient's bulimic episodes occurred in the late afternoon, evening, or early morning— periods when her husband was not at home and her 3- and 4-year-old daughters were with sitters or asleep. The patient's binge-purge episodes did not occur on the spur of the moment, however, but began hours earlier as she ruminated about binge-purging and planned her menu (Fairburn, 1982).

One method of decreasing high-frequency behaviors is to associate them with negative events or consequences (Abel, Becker, Cunningham-Rathner, et al., 1984). Covert sensitization (Janda & Rimm, 1972) is a behavioral method in which patients are taught, first, to imagine the thoughts, images, and feelings antecedent to their dysfunctional behavior; second, to imagine very negative (usually social) consequences that could result from their behavior; and third, to repeat that cycle over a 15-minute session so that the antecedents begin to prompt cognitions of the negative, aversive consequences. In this manner the early antecedents are extinguished and the subsequent dysfunctional behavior does not follow.

In this case there were a number of negative social consequences that might result from bulimia. For example, her two children were becoming aware of her binge-purge episodes. The patient feared that they might acquire an interest in binge-vomiting, simply modeling after her. She also feared that her husband might leave her on realizing that she had not ceased her binge-purge behavior as promised.

To ensure compliance with the treatment, the patient was asked to verbalize and tape-record her 15-minute covert sensitization scenes (Abel et al., 1984), during which the adverse consequences of her behavior were described in grim detail.

After listening to the audiotapes, the therapist critiqued them and then taught the patient, first, how to make the aversive scenes even more aversive and, second, how to promote frequent pairings or associations between the antecedents of the binge-purge behavior and the possible social consequences that were most fearful to her. Such feedback by the therapist was not only instructional; it also provided the patient with attention and social reinforcement (DiMatteo & DiNicola, 1982). Once the patient had acquired the skills to develop such scenes within the therapy setting, she practiced developing covert sensitization tapes while at home. Finally, she was asked to use this symptom reduction technique in her natural environment whenever she had urges to ruminate about binge-purging. Following several weeks of covert sensitization, the patient's binges ceased.

SPECIFIC CHARACTERISTICS OF PATIENTS WHO BENEFIT FROM BEHAVIOR THERAPY

The characteristics of some patients' symptoms make them more amenable to behavior therapy. The factors listed below should help guide the clinician in making the decision whether to pursue a behavioral approach.

Observable Behavior

For a behavior therapy program to be implemented, the patient, the clinician, or others in the patient's environment must be able to know when contingent intervention should be implemented. For example, if nursing personnel were to institute a treatment contingent on a patient's increased anxiety, a behavioral program would be difficult to follow if the nurses could not observe outward signs of the patient's internally felt anxiety. If the emotional episodes of the patient were marked by hand wringing, pacing, or tachycardia, these signs would provide observable behavior to carry out a contingency program.

Fluctuation of the Symptom

If observers are to respond to a behavior, it should have specific antecedents that influence whether the symptom occurs more frequently or with greater intensity. The therapist has to evaluate whether fluctuations of the symptom suggest the presence of specific antecedents that worsen the patient's condition. For example, if a patient seeks treatment because of hypertension but shows no fluctuation of the symptom, behavioral treatment will be more difficult. If the patient's blood pressure fluctuates, however, then it increases the likelihood that behavioral analysis will identify antecedents that aggravate the symptom.

A Social Environment That Can Observe Behavior and Respond to It Consistently

Treatment interventions necessitate a response from the social environment in which the behavioral excess or deficit occurs. In some situations, patients themselves can respond following the occurrence of symptomatic behaviors, but this generally requires attentive patients who are anxious to reduce their symptoms. When patients are less motivated to reduce their symptoms or are incapable of organizing their thoughts and actions following the occurrence of the symptom, other people in the patient's environment must be available to implement treatment interventions. This responsive environment does not mean that the treatment personnel must be highly trained in behavioral therapy. It does, however, require that they be observant of the patient's symptoms and able to respond with consistency.

A Frequent Occurrence of the Symptom

If the patient is to learn a new response or if different consequences are to be taught to the patient following the occurrence of the symptom, such learning requires repetition if the new response is to be acquired. Repetition of the consequences of the behavior necessitates a fairly high frequency of the symptom. If a diabetic's hypoglycemic episodes occurred once every four months, a behavioral treatment would probably be ineffective, since implementation of the treatment would occur so infrequently. On the other hand, if the patient's blood glucoses could be monitored with frequent blood glucose checks, and treatment implemented not only after clinical episodes of hypoglycemia but after hypoglycemic episodes identified solely by blood chemistries, this would increase the frequency of implementing the treatment.

Adequate Time for Treatment Intervention

Learning requires repetition. Behavioral treatment interventions, therefore, require an adequate passage of time so that patients can repetitively see the consequences of their behavior. When clinical realities, however, require immediate intervention, behavioral interventions may be contraindicated. Acutely suicidal patients threatening to end their lives necessitate psychiatric hospitalization to protect them. Such suicidal patients can be treated with behavioral approaches for the cognitive distortions that increase their suicidal ideation, but such treatment takes time. Clinical necessity of protecting a patient's life would warrant a prompt protective hospi-

Table 14-1

Objective Behavioral Approaches to Diagnosis, Treatment, and Patient Compliance

	Objective Criteria for Diagnosis	Treatment Approach	Objective Criteria for Compliance with Treatment Approach
Anorexia nervosa	Weight lost, observation of eating behavior	Contingency management	Weight recording by therapist
Bulimia nervosa	Patient's tape recording of bulimic episode	Covert sensitization	Listening to audiotaped treatment sessions
Type A behavior	Psychophysiologic assessment of electromyography	Progressive muscle relaxation, EMG biofeedback	Psychophysiologic assessment of electromyography
Hyperventilation	Hyperventilation provocative test	Controlled breathing	Direct observation of patient's breathing by therapist
Shy bladder	Inability to void in public rest rooms	Extinction of avoidance behavior and exposure	Direct observation of voiding training
Drop attacks	Direct observation of motor skills performance	Muscle relaxation and ambulation skills training	Observation of ability to ambulate, use of pedometer

343

talization rather than a less immediate cognitive treatment intervention.

SUMMARY

Rather than attempt to define various psychiatric syndromes in need of treatment, behavioral approaches recognize the variability of symptoms over time and environments and therefore attempt to break down all problematic behavior into behavioral excesses and behavioral deficits. In this chapter, behavior therapy strategies have been presented for assessment, treatment, and compliance evaluations in six typical cases. The strategies used are summarized in Table 14-1. No brief discussion of behavior therapy can allude to all possible treatment interventions, since designing effective strategies is limited only by the therapist's imagination (Miller, 1983).

FURTHER INFORMATION

Readers interested in obtaining information about the most recent developments in behavioral medicine are advised to write two organizations that actively promote advances in this field.

1. Ms. Jude Woodward, The Society of Behavioral Medicine, Box 8530, University Station, Knoxville, TN 37996. The society publishes both *Annals of Behavioral Medicine* and *Behavioral Medicine Abstracts*.

2. Dr. Andrew Bawm, The Academy of Behavioral Medicine, Department of Medical Psychology, Uniformed Services University of the Health Sciences, Bethesda, MD 20814. The academy publishes, through Academic Press, *Perspectives on Behavioral Medicine*, a yearly volume of the annual proceedings of the academy.

REFERENCES

Abel GG, Becker JV, Cunningham-Rathner J, et al. (1984). *Treatment manual: The treatment of child molesters*. Monograph available from the authors, Emory Clinic, Department of Psychiatry, Atlanta, Georgia, 30322.

Abel GG & Blanchard EB (1976). The measurement and generation of sexual arousal in male sexual deviates. In M Hersen, R Eisler, & PM Miller (Eds), *Progress in behavior modification* (Vol 2, pp 99–136). New York: Academic Press.

Abel GG, Blanchard EB, Barlow DH, et al. (1975). Identifying specific erotic cues in sexual deviation by audio-taped description. *Journal of Applied Behavior Analysis, 8*, 247–260.

Abel GG & Blendinger D (1985). Behavioral urology. In JO Cavenar (Ed), *Psychiatry* (Vol 2, Section 98, pp 1–11). Philadelphia: JB Lippincott.

Anderson LT (1977). Desensitization *in vivo* for men unable to urinate in a public facility. *Journal of Behaviour Therapy and Experimental Psychiatry, 8*, 105–106.

Bandura A (1969). *Principles of behavior modification*. New York: Holt.

Bandura A (1971). Psychotherapy based on modeling principles. In AE Bergin & SL Garfield (Eds),

Handbook of psychotherapy and behavior change. New York: Wiley.

Bhanji S & Thompson J (1974). Operant conditioning in the treatment of anorexia nervosa: A review and retrospective study of 11 cases. *British Journal of Psychiatry, 124*, 166–172.

Bruch H (1973). *Eating disorders, obesity and anorexia*. New York: Basic Books.

Burish TG (1981). EMG biofeedback in the treatment of stress-related disorders. In CK Prokop & LA Bradley (Eds), *Medical psychology: Contributions to behavioral medicine* (pp 395–421). New York: Academic Press.

Cautela JR (1970). The use of covert sensitization in the treatment of alcoholism. *Psychotherapy: Theory, Research, and Practice, 7*, 86–90.

DiMatteo MR & DiNicola DD (1982). *Achieving patient compliance: The psychology of the medical practitioner's role*. New York: Pergamon Press.

Fairburn CG (1982). Binge eating and its management. *British Journal of Psychiatry, 141*, 631–633.

Franks CM & Wilson GT (1973). *Annual review of behavior therapy: Theory and practice*. New York: Brunner/Mazel.

Friedman M & Rosenman RH (1974). *Type A behavior and your heart.* New York: Knopf.

Goldfarb LA, Dykens EM, & Gerrard M (1985). The Goldfarb Fear of Fat Scale. *Journal of Personality Assessment, 49*(3), 329–332.

Halmi KA (1974). Anorexia nervosa: Demographic and clinical features in 94 cases. *Psychosomatic Medicine, 36,* 18–25.

Jacobson E (1938). *Progressive relaxation.* Chicago: University of Chicago Press.

Janda LW & Rimm DC (1972). Covert sensitization in the treatment of obesity. *Journal of Abnormal Psychology, 80,* 37–42.

Johnson-Sabine EC, Wood KH, & Wakeling A (1984). Mood changes in bulimia nervosa. *British Journal of Psychiatry, 145,* 512–516.

Kazdin AE (1974). Self-monitoring and behavior change. In MJ Mahoney & CE Thoresen (Eds), *Self-control: Power to the person* (pp 218–246). Monterey, CA: Brooks/Cole.

Kazdin AE (1978). Behavior therapy: Evolution and expansion. *Counseling Psychologist, 3,* 34–37.

Keefe FJ (1979). Assessment strategies in behavioral medicine. In JR McNamara (Ed), *Behavioral approaches to medicine: Application and analysis* (pp 101–129). New York: Plenum Press.

Lum LC (1975). Hyperventilation, the tip of the iceberg. *Journal of Psychosomatic Research, 19,* 375.

Lum LC (1981). Hyperventilation and anxiety state. *Journal of the Royal Society of Medicine, 74,* 1–4.

McFarlane AH, Bellissimo A, & Upton E (1982). Atypical anorexia nervosa: Treatment and management on a behavioral medicine unit. *Psychiatric Journal of the University of Ottawa, 7*(3), 158–162.

Miller NE (1983). Behavioral medicine: Symbiosis between laboratory and clinic. *Annual Review of Psychology, 34,* 1–31.

Mizes JS (1985). Bulimia: A review of its symptomatology and treatment. *Advances in Behaviour Research and Therapy, 7,* 91–142.

Moreyra AE, McGough WE, Hosler M, et al. (1982). Clinical improvement of patients with chest pain and normal coronary arteries after coronary arteriography: The possible role of hyperventilation syndrome. *International Journal of Cardiology, 2,* 306–308.

Pomerleau OF & Brady JP (Eds) (1979). *Behavioral medicine: Theory and practice.* Baltimore: Williams & Wilkins.

Rimm DC & Masters SC (1974). *Behavior therapy: Techniques and empirical findings.* New York: Academic Press.

Schultz JH & Luthe W (1969). *Autogenic therapy.* New York: Grune & Stratton.

Schwartz GE & Weiss SM (1978). Yale conference on behavioral medicine: A proposed definition and statement of goals. *Journal of Behavioral Medicine, 1,* 3–12.

Shelton JL & Levy RL (Eds) (1981). *Behavioral assignments and treatment compliance: A handbook of clinical strategies.* Champaign, IL: Research Press.

Skinner BF (1969). *Contingencies of reinforcement: A theoretical analysis.* New York: Appleton.

Solomon RL (1964). Punishment. *American Psychologist, 19,* 239–253.

Spielberger CD & DeNike LD (1966). Descriptive behaviorism versus cognitive theory in verbal operant conditioning. *Psychological Review, 73,* 306–326.

Ware R & Terrell G (1961). Effects of delayed reinforcement on associative and incentive factors. *Child Development, 32,* 789–793.

Wolpe J (1958). *Psychotherapy by reciprocal inhibition.* Stanford, CA: Stanford University Press.

Wolpe J (1969). *The practice of behavior therapy.* Oxford: Pergamon.

Young LD & Blanchard EB (1980). Medical applications of biofeedback training—a selective review. In S. Rachman (Ed), *Contributions to medical psychology* (Vol 2, pp 215–254). New York: Pergamon Press.

David B. Abrams, Michael A. Raciti
Laurie Ruggiero, Barrie J. Guise
Michael J. Follick

15
Cardiovascular Risk Factor Reduction in the Medical Setting

Although more than half of all chronic diseases can be prevented through changes in life-style, cardiovascular disease, notably coronary heart disease (CHD) and stroke, constitutes the primary preventable cause of death and disability. In the United States, more than a quarter of a million heart attacks occur annually and account for over $40 billion in health care costs. Although CHD has a complex and multifactorial etiology (Stamler, 1979), it is generally accepted that both fixed and modifiable risk factors lead to the development of atherosclerosis, which causes narrowing of the arteries and often results in heart attack or stroke (Matarazzo, 1984).

The development of CHD begins in childhood, lasts decades, and is a slow, silent process. Few warning signs precede the acute and often fatal first event. For these and other reasons, intervention prior to the clinical manifestation of CHD (primary prevention through life-style modification) is generally regarded as the only effective method of controlling the problem (Breslow, 1978, 1979). Despite a strong awareness among most medical professionals of the importance of life-style modification, the diagnosis, treatment (or referral), and continued follow-up of patients with potentially modifiable risk factors is not yet a routine part of medical practice. Both acute medical events and primary care settings, however, provide opportunities to diagnose and begin a life-style intervention.

Life-style modification is a process of change that should be viewed within a chronic disease and prevention framework rather than an acute care model. The technology of life-style change involves the ongoing application of behavioral principles, a caring relationship, and effective health education and communication skills rather than isolated brief verbal prescriptions, drugs, or surgical techniques. Specific biobehavioral technologies now exist for effective life-style modification (Brownell, 1986; Davidson & Davidson,

PRINCIPLES OF MEDICAL PSYCHIATRY
ISBN 0-8089-1883-4

1980; Lichtenstein, 1982). Ideally, improving one's health is a never-ending process that takes place throughout the life span.

The appropriate targets for life-style change should be just as aggressively pursued as any other psychiatric or medical signs and symptoms. Generally, the more difficult patients require the specialized techniques of health care professionals who are trained in behavioral medicine. Less difficult patients can be successfully helped with encouragement and support from the medical practitioner or the office staff and with self-help materials. Risk factor screening should be implemented to increase the likelihood that patients who are at risk for CHD will have their behavioral risk factors identified as early as possible so that effective life-style modification procedures can be implemented.

This chapter will present a step-care approach to the behavioral modification of selected life-style habits. Life-style factors for CHD will be briefly identified, and structured approaches to behavioral intervention described. The challenge of matching patient characteristics to treatment alternatives will be explored, using smoking and obesity as examples. Some common problems in adherence and compliance will also be addressed.

LIFE-STYLE FACTORS IN CHD

Space does not permit a comprehensive review of the evidence linking life-style to mediating mechanisms and disease endpoints. A consistent body of epidemiologic and laboratory research has demonstrated, however, that the following factors are associated with increased risk of developing CHD: sex (male), family history, diabetes, cigarette smoking, elevated serum lipoprotein levels, high blood pressure, overweight, sedentary life-style, and particular patterns of stress-related behavior (Matarazzo, Weiss, Herd, et al., 1984). It has

reasonably been presumed that the following factors can reduce the risk of CHD: reduction in serum cholesterol, control of total calories to attain an ideal body weight, cessation of cigarette smoking, and management of blood pressure within normal limits. Regular exercise has general positive effects. Possibly important is the reduction or modification of specific aspects (e.g., repressed anger) of the Type A coronary prone behavior pattern in vulnerable individuals (Friedman, Ulmer, Brown, et al., 1986)

The risk factors present in any one individual can be synergistic with respect to CHD risk. Life-style risk factors can also complicate existing medical conditions that are highly associated with cardiac disease, as in the case of obesity and type II adult-onset diabetes (Abrams, Steinberg, Follick, et al., 1986). Kannel and Gordon (1979) suggest that "because it reversibly promotes atherogenic traits like hypertension, diabetes, and hyperlipidemia, reduction of overweight is probably the most important measure aside from the avoidance of cigarettes that is available for the control of cardiovascular disease" (p 265).

In a step-care approach to assessment and treatment, it is important to emphasize the need to intervene with individuals at moderate risk as well as those at severe risk for CHD, in order to make an effective public health impact on reducing the prevalence of chronic disease associated with CHD (Abrams, Elder, Carlton, et al., 1986). Individuals who are 20 percent or more overweight, have serum cholesterol over 180 mg/dl, or have mild hypertension (in the range of 90 mm Hg diastolic or 140 mm Hg systolic) and the recently diagnosed type II diabetic, are in many ways ideal candidates for life-style change interventions (Matarazzo et al., 1984). A focus on diet, nutrition, and exercise can go a long way toward prevention of CHD risk through the mediating mechanisms of weight reduction, control of hypertension, and an increased high density lipoprotein cholesterol to total cholesterol ratio (Simopoulos, 1986; Simopoulos & Van Itallie, 1984). Unfortunately, the reality of medical practice is that those in the low to moderate risk categories are more likely to be left to their own devices than those in the high-risk populations and those individuals who already have manifest signs of CHD, such as angina pectoris or myocardial infarction.

Behavior modification principles have been applied to both the post-MI patient and others for stress management, smoking cessation, weight control, exercise, borderline hypertension control, and dietary modification to reduce cholesterol. The remainder of this chapter, however, will describe the general behavioral approach to treatment within a behavioral medicine model and will then focus on cigarette smoking, obesity, and noncompliance as examples of a step-care approach to diagnosis and management to prevent the onset of CHD.

THE BEHAVIORAL MEDICINE MODEL

The establishment of behavioral medicine clinics for primary prevention and life-style modification is of relatively recent origin. Once patients have been identified as having a modifiable risk factor, clinic staff coordinate both the multidisciplinary evaluation and appropriate treatment of the patient. Behavioral medicine clinics can function effectively for inpatients in general medical settings (e.g., as part of a psychiatry consultation service), for outpatients, and as a "wellness center" for prevention in the community. Psychologists, psychiatrists, and other health professionals (e.g., cardiologists, nutritionists, exercise physiologists, nurse-educators) collaborate in a multidisciplinary team approach to diagnosis and management. Such clinics are playing an increasingly important role in the delivery of primary preven-

tion services and in solving related behavioral problems, such as issues of patient noncompliance with medical regimens and psychosocial adjustment to medical conditions.

In general terms, a variety of biologic, psychologic, and sociocultural variables are assessed, and these patient characteristics are used to determine the severity of risk, the difficulty of changing the life-style problem, and the most appropriate treatment modality. Chronic maladaptive life-style habits can sometimes reflect more severe psychopathology, as in patients with addictions or eating disorders. A small minority of the cases can thus require more formal psychologic or psychiatric intervention. In most cases, however, severe psychopathology is absent, and a reasonable approach to treatment can be formulated that involves individual or group behavior modification protocols usually lasting from 4 weeks to 1 year. Programs emphasize at least two distinct phases: (a) skills acquisition and acute treatment and (b) maintenance or relapse prevention (Brownell, 1982; Lichtenstein, 1982).

The general principles of behavior modification have evolved to the point where they could ideally be available for routine clinical service in the medical setting (Follick, Gottlieb, & Fowler, 1986). Martin and Prue (1984), however, point to at least four major stumbling blocks to the success of behavioral medicine clinics: First, in the disease model of service delivery and acute care, the absence of signs and symptoms of disease leads to an underemphasis on health, wellness, and prevention. Second, hospital staff tend to think of solutions to problems in terms of medications, procedures, and use of medical equipment. Furthermore, physicians may feel that it is time-consuming, intrusive, and uncomfortable to talk to patients about personal habits. Physicians have not been trained sufficiently in behavioral counseling skills and education techniques that would enhance success and increase referrals (Wechsler, Levine, Idelson, et al., 1983). Consequently, referrals are not made except in extreme cases. Third, programs for life-style change are quite variable, and some minimal interventions and commercial programs are of questionable value. Professionals are reluctant to recommend change when they do not have confidence in the procedures. Finally, it is possible that behavioral medicine programs are underutilized because of their association with a traditional role of psychology and psychiatry—the treatment of mental illness—rather than the new technology of life-style modification. Concerted efforts are required on the part of all health professionals to overcome these barriers to the diagnosis and treatment of life-style problems (Martin & Prue, 1984).

OBESITY

Estimates of the prevalence of obesity in the American population range from at least 15 percent to as high as 50 percent, depending upon the criteria being used (Bray, 1976; Van Itallie, 1979). There is increasing evidence that obesity (20 percent or more over ideal weight) is a precursor of CHD development (Hubert, 1986). Furthermore, health care providers are now recognizing that obesity can play an important role in other diseases, such as hypercholesterolemia, essential hypertension, and diabetes. The management of obesity is also considered a significant tool in the reduction of cardiac risk factors (Simopoulos, 1986). Obesity does not yield easily to treatment. Although there is increasing evidence of a genetic influence on obesity (e.g., Foch and McClearn, 1980), there are also strong psychologic reasons for its high prevalence and resistance to change (Brownell, 1982, 1986). The most promising treatments now available are based on a comprehensive biopsychosocial approach

to weight management (Brownell, 1982; Abrams, 1984).

Patient Assessment

In deciding when to intervene and at what level, there are several dimensions of patient characteristics used to assess severity: biological, psychological, and social factors are considered (1) medical risk status and specific metabolic disorders; (2) psychologic factors related to motivation, abnormal eating patterns, and poor exercise habits; and (3) social factors, including potential support from the family, friends, and the work environment.

Stunkard (1984) proposes three categories of obesity: (a) mild (0–30 percent over ideal weight); (b) moderate (30–100 percent); and (c) severe (100 percent or greater). Increased medical risk from obesity alone begins in the moderate range and encompasses the severe category. In conjunction with other risk factors, however (e.g., smoking, hypertension, diabetes, family history of heart disease, and hypercholesterolemia), it has been suggested that even mild obesity should be treated (Brownell, 1986).

Biobehavioral factors must also be evaluated to help determine which program might be best for a particular patient. A review of the patient's weight history, eating habits, and previous attempts to lose weight (with a focus on what went wrong) can be helpful. Patients may report eating in response to psychologic events (such as stress, depression, or social anxiety). They may reveal fatigue, dizziness, or cravings for protein, carbohydrates, or sugar, which could reflect biochemical imbalances (e.g., hypoglycemia). They may have an underlying compulsive eating disorder such as binge eating, or bulimia.

Interpersonal and sociocultural factors should also be evaluated. The educational level, economic situation, and living environment of the patient may make it more difficult for the patient to change life-style.

Social support (or lack of it) can also play a crucial role. Sometimes spouses, parents, or family are unaware of their power to support and sustain change; alternatively, they can unwittingly sabotage treatment efforts because of their own life-style habits or values. The assessment of the patient's environment often suggests a need to involve other members of the family in lifestyle change efforts. Significant others' involvement can promote the long-term maintenance of change (Brownell, 1982).

Patients should be prepared for treatment by ensuring appropriate attitudes, goals, and expectations. One major barrier to successful weight loss is unrealistic expectations about speed and ease of weight loss. Patients should be discouraged from seeking rapid weight loss, or fad diets. One drawback of all fad diets is that patients eventually feel deprived and must stop the diet. This is when they typically return to their prior eating habits. The greater the involvement of biopsychosocial factors in a patient's obesity, the stronger the need for combined forms of therapy including several specialists.

The basic philosophy of behavior modification is that in order to lose weight and keep it off, a person must gradually learn new eating behaviors and exercise habits that can be maintained for a lifetime. There are no "magic cures" that will produce lasting weight loss. Weight loss demands persistent effort and realistic expectations. Education and ongoing support over many months may be necessary for success, and there is always the danger of losing motivation, especially if expectations were too high and goals have not been achieved.

Patient–Treatment Matching: A Step-Care Model

Brownell (1986) has proposed a step-care approach to weight loss, which is perhaps the most rational and cost-effective way to proceed. The challenge to the phy-

sician is to determine which type of treatment is most appropriate for a particular patient. As cost, risk, and invasiveness increase with each step, it should be recommended to patients that they begin at the lowest step not yet given a fair test. The most costly and risky procedures should be reserved for those patients who have not responded to previous programs.

In general, mild to moderately obese individuals should be encouraged to seek treatment in low-cost self-help or commercial programs. Those who have already failed in such treatments and those who are moderately to severely obese should consider more intensive interventions. Finally, severely overweight patients and those who have failed with a variety of conventional treatments might be appropriate candidates for the more aggressive combinations of behavior modification with pharmacotherapy, medical diets, or the use of gastroplasty surgery.

Treatment Options

Minimal Interventions: Self-Help and Commercial Programs

Although self-help manuals and books to help people lose weight abound, almost no systematic evaluation of the effectiveness of these materials has been undertaken. Often the qualifications and experience of the group leader will determine the effectiveness of the program. Self-help protocols based on behavioral principles are currently being developed and tested (Black & Trelfall, 1986). The few reports that have examined the effectiveness of self-help programs suggest that they are most appropriate for mildly overweight individuals who are highly motivated and have good social supports. Furthermore, their content varies from scientifically validated methods to dangerous diets. Such programs must be reviewed on an individual basis before they can be endorsed.

The most widely recognized commercial weight reduction group is Weight Watchers. It is based on standard behavioral modification techniques (Stuart & Davis, 1972). It can be very helpful to individuals for both weight loss and maintenance because Weight Watchers utilizes goal setting, self-reporting with public weigh-in, and social pressure and support from other participants. Weight Watchers is widely available and relatively inexpensive. The public nature of the treatment, however, and the social pressure to lose weight do not appeal to some patients. There are several similar support groups available to patients, such as TOPS (Take Off Pounds Sensibly). Overeaters Anonymous is essentially modeled after Alcoholics Anonymous and is usually reserved for those with more serious compulsive eating problems. It can provide needed support to individuals in a confidential atmosphere but is not a substitute for individual psychotherapy. Other commercial programs may be rather expensive and are best for individuals who are mildly overweight or those individuals who need ongoing support to maintain their weight loss.

The little research information that exists on commercial programs suggests that modest weight losses can be expected but that high attrition rates are also common. Generally highly motivated, self-selected individuals use these services. Those that have tried and failed to lose weight on several occasions by any of these methods should be strongly encouraged to seek more intensive levels of care. Recent evidence suggests that repeated unsuccessful efforts to lose weight can be medically dangerous and make each future attempt more difficult (Brownell, 1986).

Moderate Interventions:
Behavior Modification Programs.

Perhaps the most widely researched and evaluated of all weight loss programs is the professionally led behavior modification approach (Brownell, 1982, 1986). Generally, it is based on the energy-balance model of caloric restriction and increases in caloric expenditure through exercise (Brownell, 1982, 1986). Specialized diets are not typically employed, but general caloric restriction, while selecting from the four main food groups, is recommended. Nutritional counseling can easily be employed as well, especially when there is a need for a special diet (e.g., with patients who have hypertension or diabetes).

The model is implemented using the principles of behavior modification based on the assumption that people's eating patterns are learned over time (Brownell, 1982). Consequently, participants are first taught to observe and record their maladaptive eating patterns (amounts and types of food, time of day, moods, etc.) and are then provided with the specific training modules necessary to modify these unhealthy eating and exercise habits. Common behavioral components typically employed include self-monitoring (of food intake), goal setting and self-reinforcement, and various stimulus control procedures (e.g., restrictions on access to food, on timing of meals, on location of meals, and on portion size). Patients typically are taught to slow down their eating, to use alternative skills in managing moods (e.g., relaxation training), to use social support (assertiveness), to apply problem-solving skills, and to change their ways of thinking about food (cognitive restructuring). For more details about clinical techniques, see Abrams (1984).

Research indicates that moderate weight loss of 10–20 pounds can reliably be achieved through behavioral treatment methods (Brownell, 1982, 1986; Jeffery, 1987). The rate of weight loss is ideally between 0.5 and 2 pounds per week so that changes can be made gradually and in a medically safe manner. Furthermore, recent evidence suggests that behavioral weight loss programs have a beneficial impact on serum lipoprotein levels (Follick, Abrams, Smith, et al., 1984) even when only moderate losses are achieved (9–12 pounds). These benefits have been found to be sustained to 6 months after treatment.

Maintenance of weight loss continues to be a problem, as long-term recidivism (more than one year) has been estimated to be as high as 75 percent regain of initial weight (Jeffery, 1987). Several behavioral programs, however, have reported good maintenance of weight loss. The inclusion of the patient's spouse (or significant other) offers much promise for improving maintenance over time (Brownell, Heckerman, Westlake, et al., 1978). Integrating programs into the natural environment, for example, at the work place or in the school system, is also showing promise (Abrams & Follick, 1983; Brownell & Kaye, 1982). Other methods that have been tested for improving maintenance include use of booster sessions (Kingsley & Wilson, 1977), relapse prevention (Perri, Shapiro, Ludwig, et al., 1984), and cognitive-behavioral packages (Perri, MacAdoo, Spevak, et al., 1984).

When exercise is combined with calorie restriction, it becomes an effective strategy for weight loss and maintenance. Exercise will (1) increase energy expenditure, (2) counteract ill effects of obesity, (3) suppress appetite, (4) increase basal metabolism, and (5) minimize loss of lean tissue. Exercise in obese persons can have a positive influence on plasma insulin, lipids, blood pressure, and coronary efficiency, and it has psychologic benefits as well, such as counteracting fatigue or depression (Björntorp, 1978; Bray, 1976; Epstein & Wing, 1980; Folkins & Sime, 1981). Many experts now consider exercise to be one of the best strategies for the maintenance of weight loss and the improvement of health status (Donahoe, Lin, Kirschenbaum, et al., 1984).

Maximal Interventions: Combination of Behavioral and Medical or Surgical Interventions

Over the years, numerous medically supervised diets and surgical interventions for the management of obesity have been developed. Typically, these programs are reserved for those individuals with severe obesity that poses a definite and sometimes imminent risk to their health. Consequently, these programs tend to be aggressive and to carry with them a significant degree of risk in the form of side effects and complications. Very low-calorie diets (VLCD) are perhaps the most prevalent and hold promise as a treatment for moderate to severe obesity (Bistrain, 1978; Howard & Bray, 1981; Wadden & Stunkard, 1986; Wadden, Stunkard, & Brownell, 1983). They are far safer when limited to periods of three months. Although such programs can produce a relatively large weight loss in a short period of time (e.g., 20 kg in 12 weeks), they are plagued by just as rapid relapse. Behavioral modification programs are now being combined with VLCD's to increase adherence and compliance and to help ensure the maintenance of weight loss (Brownell, 1986; Wadden & Stunkard, 1986).

Recidivism also frequently follows vertically banded gastroplasty surgery, which is the most common surgical intervention employed for the morbidly obese (over 100 percent overweight) and which has a reported 50–60 percent long-term rate of success (Kral & Kissileff, 1987). Many surgeons are now also noting the problem of "late weight gain," which represents a lack of maintenance of weight loss. Patients undergoing these procedures may thus lose as much as 120 pounds over 12–18 months, only to gain back much of the lost weight over the next 2 years. Although the patients retain a reduced stomach size, some alter their eating patterns over time so that they end up consuming a continuous stream of low-volume, high-calorie foods. They thus defeat the procedure through undesired adjustments in their eating behaviors. This, once again, emphasizes the importance of using behavior modification techniques together with medical treatment in a comprehensive biopsychosocial approach.

SMOKING CESSATION

Cigarette smoking is thought to be the single most important of the known modifiable risk factors for CHD in the United States. A smoker's risk of death from CHD is 70–300 percent greater than a nonsmoker's. Heavy smokers and female smokers who use oral contraceptives are at particular risk. Unless there are major changes in the smoking habits of Americans, 24 million people (or 10 percent of all persons now living) will die prematurely of CHD due to smoking. Fortunately, smokers who quit have significantly lower mortality rates from CHD than persons who continue to smoke (United States Department of Health and Human Services, 1982).

Recent discoveries about the biobehavioral basis for smoking are helping to identify a more comprehensive biopsychosocial approach to diagnosis and treatment. Nicotine is an "ideal drug" for modulating moods and alleviating fatigue and stress (Abrams, Monti, Elder, et al., 1987). It stimulates the release of beta-endorphin and vasopressin, which reduce pain, increase stress tolerance, and improve memory, concentration, and speed of information processing (Pomerleau & Pomerleau, 1984). Not surprisingly, some smokers become psychologically dependent on the stress-dampening and reinforcing effects of smoking. For others, smoking can be used to mask boredom, fatigue, or social anxiety or to modulate anger or frustration.

Many smokers who quit report making anywhere from two to seven *unsuccessful* attempts before they finally succeed (Lichtenstein, 1982). Any attempt at quitting should be looked at as a learning experience rather than as a failure resulting in guilt, avoidance, and hesitation about trying again. Physicians should be on guard against becoming frustrated, feeling helpless, and giving up on patients. Helping patients quit smoking should also be approached in stepwise fashion, if necessary,

over several years. Although physicians do not have to provide all the time-consuming treatment, they are in a unique position to play a critical role in motivating the smoker to quit and in persisting with support until success is achieved (Wells, Ware, & Lewis, 1984). There are data to indicate that physician advice alone may be the single most cost-effective method of motivating patients to attempt to stop smoking (Sachs, 1984). Some studies (e.g., Burt, Illingworth, Shaw, et al., 1974) suggest that if every physician in the United States took a few moments to tell a patient of the specific and devastating health risks of smoking, several million smokers would quit who otherwise would continue to smoke. Further, Coletti and Supnick (1980) demonstrated that brief telephone contacts 3 and 6 months after a smoking cessation program greatly improved maintenance. This underscores the power of physician attention and advice in motivating smokers to consider quitting and in exploring various available treatment options.

Patient Assessment

It is important to assess patient characteristics before deciding on the appropriate level of intervention. Four major characteristics need to be evaluated. These are (1) readiness or motivation to change, (2) degree of biologic addiction, (3) degree of psychologic dependence, (4) history of attempts to quit, and (5) degree of positive social support and negative support (e.g., another smoker in the household).

If the patient is not strongly motivated to change, then motivating him or her becomes the first priority before deciding on treatment options. Counseling, education, and "assertive interactions" with the patient, coupled with follow-up visits to show that the physician is "really serious," can have a strong impact on moving the unmotivated smoker toward being ready to take action (Wells, Ware, & Lewis, 1984).

Behavioral techniques and role playing of counseling skills are now being used to train physicians to be more effective at persuading patients to consider change.

Assuming an individual is ready for action, the rule of thumb is that smokers should receive a more intensive (maximal) treatment program if they (1) are biologically addicted (smoke more than 25 cigarettes per day, usually smoke within 30 minutes of awakening during the morning, and report smoking even during a cold or other minor respiratory illness), (2) are psychologically dependent (smoke as part of their "image," for stress management, or to help cope with social interactions), and (3) have tried to quit on their own and failed. Smokers who report severe withdrawal symptoms may be candidates for nicotine chewing gum as an adjunct to comprehensive behavioral treatment. By contrast, first-time quitters and those individuals who are less biologically addicted and less psychosocially dependent are candidates for minimal levels of treatment, such as self-help or other brief interventions (Abrams & Wilson, 1986).

A review of the patient's previous attempts to quit can be revealing (Best, 1976). They may show, for example, that the patient was unable to quit although able to cut down (suggesting biologic addiction) or that the patient quit for a period but slipped back into smoking when stressed, angry, or depressed (suggesting psychologic dependence). If the patient relapsed in a social situation, then social anxiety or lack of assertiveness may be a problem that needs correcting before the next quit attempt.

By exploring the patient's status and history on biopsychosocial dimensions, one can decide how to move the patient in a stepwise fashion through three possible levels of treatment: (1) minimal interventions (self-help, commercial programs, hypnosis), (2) intermediate interventions (behavior modification), and (3) maximal interventions (behavior modification plus pharmacologic treatments).

Treatment Options

Minimal Interventions

In order to compare programs, it is useful to know that the spontaneous quit rate of the general population is 1–3 percent per year. Data on the effectiveness of self-help programs are sparse. The American Lung Association program (Freedom from Smoking in 20 days) and a companion maintenance manual (*A Lifetime of Freedom from Smoking*) achieved a 20 percent initial quit rate, with 18 percent not smoking at 12-month follow-up (Davis, Faust, & Ordentlich, 1984). Another study evaluated materials provided by the American Cancer Society ("I Quit Kit") and two behavioral self-help books. The "I Quit Kit" tended to do slightly better. Overall abstinence was 7 percent at 6 months (Glasgow, Shafer, & O'Neill, 1981). It is likely that these rates underestimate the usefulness of self-help interventions. Although these cessation rates may seem disappointing, even small increases above the spontaneous rate of 3 percent per year can have enormous public health benefits.

Several studies suggest the potential power of brief intervention in physicians' offices. In one study of 28 general practitioners, patients received one of four treatments: (a) no intervention, (b) questionnaire only, (c) physician advice to quit, and (d) advice to quit plus informational leaflet and follow-up interview. Only the fourth condition resulted in significantly lower smoking rates at 1-year follow-up (5.1 percent abstinent versus 0.3–3.3 percent in the other three groups) (Russell, Wilson, & Taylor, 1979). The finding that physician advice is improved when follow-ups and support are provided is consistent with behavioral principles.

In general, hypnosis, acupuncture,

brief commercial interventions, and brief mass-media interventions are difficult to evaluate because of the absence of objective data. Several studies suggest, however, that exposure to these types of interventions can be effective for some patients, at least in the short run. One drawback of brief forms of treatment is that they may not provide follow-up or teach maintenance skills to prevent relapse after quitting. It is also important to note that the quality of these programs can be quite variable. The better programs report a success rate between 10 percent and 25 percent at 6-month follow-up. Generally, it is the lighter, less dependent smokers who are highly motivated to quit and who have excellent social support for quitting that are the preferred candidates for brief or minimal interventions.

Intermediate Interventions

If minimal interventions have been attempted without success or if the individual is more biologically or psychologically dependent on cigarettes, then treatment programs of 4–8 weeks' duration should be considered. These programs teach skills for quitting, managing acute withdrawal, and maintenance or preventing relapse (Abrams & Wilson, 1986; Lichtenstein, 1982).

Behavioral approaches to quitting include nicotine fading, stimulus control, and aversive techniques. Nicotine fading involves switching to a lower-nicotine brand of cigarettes and reducing the number of cigarettes smoked per day on a systematic basis over a period of 3–5 weeks (Foxx & Brown, 1979). Gradual reduction of nicotine is designed to minimize withdrawal symptoms. Stimulus control involves rearranging the environment and self to make smoking more and more difficult (removing all ashtrays, smoking only in one room of the house, buying packs instead of cartons).

Although aversive strategies are unlikely to be widely accepted by consumers, they have yielded some of the most successful outcomes. Aversive strategies may be justified when benefits outweight the risks and less aversive methods have already been tried unsuccessfully. Smoking rapidly until tolerance is reached (feelings of nausea and dizziness) is the most common aversive procedure. Since rapid smoking increases heart rate, carboxyhemoglobin, and other blood gases, there have been questions raised about its safety in patients with signs of cardiovascular disease. Close medical supervision is necessary in such cases (Sachs, Hall, Pechacek, et al., 1979).

Behavioral strategies for assisting with acute withdrawal symptoms include relaxation and deep breathing techniques, use of coping images, and teaching patients how to formulate positive self-statements and counteract negative thoughts (cognitive restructuring). (For more details on these and other behavioral methods, see Abrams & Wilson, 1986, or Lichtenstein, 1982).

Most current programs include a variety of techniques rather than one strategy. Reviews of the behavioral literature indicate that at one-year follow-up the average participant in the typical behavioral program has a 20–40 percent chance of being abstinent. The more successful programs report abstinence as high as 35–50 percent (Lichtenstein, 1982). Furthermore, a large percentage of nonabstinent participants report smoking fewer cigarettes or cigarettes lower in tar and nicotine content, although abstinence is the preferred goal of smoking cessation programs. Those who reduce should still keep trying to stop at some future time, to obtain maximum health benefits and to avoid the ever-present danger of "backsliding" to their original smoking rate if they continue to smoke. There is no "safe" cigarette (Abrams & Wilson, 1986).

Maximal Interventions

Programs that add nicotine chewing gum or other pharmacologic procedures (e.g., clonidine) to behavior modification should be considered for the chronic and more difficult-to-treat heavy smoker who has tried to quit repeatedly without success (Fagerstrom, 1978, 1982). Given the evidence that nicotine dependence is an important factor for some smokers, it would seem logical that a pharmacologic agent might help to alleviate withdrawal symptoms and facilitate cessation (Hughes & Miller, 1984). Once cessation has been achieved and maintained, gradual withdrawal from the agent can then be dealt with separately. It is important to note that trials to date have used nicotine gum in combination with formal behavioral programs. These trials have reported 30–60 percent success rates at 6-month to 1-year follow-up. Use of gum alone, without a formal behavioral treatment program that addresses psychosocial factors, is not recommended and may severely reduce efficacy (Abrams & Wilson, 1986), because simply using a pharmacologic agent to reduce withdrawal is considered an incomplete treatment of a complex habit.

Maintenance Strategies

Behavioral techniques for maintenance and prevention of relapse are of recent origin and hold much promise, since 60 percent of those who quit smoking will relapse within the first 3 months of quitting (Marlatt and Gordon, 1985). Techniques for relapse prevention should include a detailed analysis of *high-risk situations.* These are people, places, or emotional states that the smoker feels are most likely to precipitate a return to smoking. Individuals are taught how to cope with these situations, using rehearsal and other techniques to resist temptation. If they should have a slip back into smoking (one or two cigarettes), they are provided with techniques to prevent the slip from becoming a full-blown relapse. Additional support and follow-up are usually provided during the critical 3–6 months after quitting, when

people are most vulnerable to relapse (e.g., telephone hot lines).

In summary, even a small amount of physician time can make a large impact on helping patients to become motivated for quitting smoking and then to take action, quit, and resist relapse. A step-care plan can be adopted with every smoker in the office practice and in the hospital. More time and effort is placed on high-risk individuals and those who are willing to contemplate change. Those who are not yet ready to quit are still targeted for systematic counseling, education, and follow-up. Effective behavioral methods are available in training physicians to communicate quitting messages more effectively. Beyond physician advice (which can be very effective), there are self-help and comprehensive programs that can be used. Clinics specializing in behavioral medicine are available in some areas, with specially trained health psychologists to deal with more recalcitrant patients. Widespread efforts by physicians to help patients quit smoking can make a substantial impact on chronic disease and disability in the United States over the next decades.

ADHERENCE TO TREATMENT: MANAGING COMPLIANCE AND NONCOMPLIANCE

Compliance has been defined as "the extent to which the patients' behavior (in terms of taking medications, following diets, or executing other life-style changes) coincides with the clinical prescription" (Sackett & Haynes, 1976, p 1). At one time or another, many patients have been advised by their physicians to quit smoking or lose weight. One major obstacle to pharmacologic and behavioral strategies for risk-factor modification is noncompliance. Although the technology to modify CHD risk factors exists, all of our knowledge is useless if individuals do not make the recommended life-style changes or follow the prescribed medical regimen.

Research has indicated that, in general, 50 percent of patients are noncompliant with long-term pharmacologic or behavioral regimens. Specifically, 30–80 percent (depending on regimen) are noncompliant with medication protocols, while over 50 percent fail to comply with life-style modification programs after 6 months (Haynes, Taylor, & Sackett, 1979). It has been reported that 20–50 percent of patients fail to keep appointments with health professionals, with the best results corresponding to appointments scheduled by the patients themselves (Dunbar & Agras, 1980). The importance of the physician's role in preventing, identifying, and remediating noncompliance is obvious.

Patient Assessment

Clinical practice has identified a number of patient characteristics believed to be associated with compliance. These include such factors as demographic information, personality characteristics or psychopathology, intellectual functioning, physical capacities, financial and psychosocial resources, cultural norms, and health beliefs. Although patient characteristics are useful for treatment planning on a case-by-case basis, research has suggested that they are poor predictors of compliance with medical recommendations (Haynes, 1976). As one might suspect, if the factors associated with compliance fail to predict compliance, it is difficult for physicians to assess whether or not their patients will follow advice. Indeed, research suggests that patients are better predictors of their own health care behavior than are health professionals (Dunbar & Stunkard, 1979; Gordis, 1976). Clinicians might do well, therefore, to ask their patients directly to predict their expected compliance and to identify potential compliance problems. In order to improve patient compliance with treatment recom-

mendations, we recommend a two-level intervention: minimal intervention (patient–provider interaction, patient education) and maximal intervention (behavioral techniques).

Intervention Strategies

Minimal Interventions

Perhaps the most salient factor in enhancing compliance is the patient–provider relationship (Baekeland & Lundwall, 1975). Studies have identified several stylistic components that promote compliance. These include displaying a warm and empathic manner, allowing the patient collaborative input in treatment planning, giving individualized instruction, and interacting with the patient on a conversational level (Korsch & Negrete, 1972). A number of points about patient education may also be beneficial in enhancing compliance. These include providing simple and clear instructions, being careful not to overload the patient with information, providing multiple modes (written materials, verbal instructions) of presenting educational material, providing well-organized instruction, and evaluating the patients recall of the medical recommendations provided. The potential benefits of attending to these interpersonal factors is greatly enhanced by continuity of care, such as specific follow-up on a regular basis (both by telephone and in person). Research indicates that although patient education is important to enhance understanding of medical recommendations, it is often not sufficient to ensure full compliance with recommendations (Haynes, 1976).

Even if the patient–provider relationship is satisfactory and the patient demonstrates a good understanding of the recommendations, the specifics of the treatment regimen will influence the patient's ability to follow through. A number of features of a health care regimen can influence compliance. Among these are (1) the complexity of the regimen, (2) the duration of time over which the regimen continues, (3) the likely side effects of the regimen, and (4) the extent to which compliance is economically feasible for the patient. In general, the more complex, long-lasting, unpleasant, and expensive the regimen, the less likely it is that the patient will follow it (Blackwell, 1973; Haynes, 1976).

Several recommendations address these features and thereby increase the likelihood that patients will comply with treatment recommendations. First, a treatment regimen should be designed so that the complexity is minimized (e.g., as few medications on as simple an administration schedule as possible) (Dunbar & Agras, 1980). If a regimen must be complex and requires several behaviors on the part of the patient, it may be prescribed in such a way as to change one behavior at a time. This sort of approach has intuitive appeal and has demonstrated efficacy in the learning of other behaviors (Bandura, 1969, 1977). Also of importance is the expected duration of the regimen. Frequent patient–provider contacts for the purpose of follow-up and feedback throughout the course of a long-term regimen are believed to improve maintenance of adherence (Masur, 1981).

The potential benefits versus risks of a given treatment may play an important role in the likelihood that recommendations are carried out. The expectations of patients regarding treatment efficacy and risks, such as severity and duration of side effects, are often overlooked. The extent to which the patient is prepared to experience a particular side effect also appears to influence compliance (Dunbar & Agras, 1980). Finally, consideration of every possible detail of the regimen is of no value if the behaviors necessary to comply place a prohibitive financial burden on the patient. The cost of medications and of life-style prescriptions should be taken into account.

Maximal Interventions

Oftentimes, despite a good physician–patient relationship and the physician's best efforts to educate the patient and to tailor the treatment regimen to individual needs, the patient still does not follow through with the recommended treatment. It is at this point that physicians should consider consultation with a behavioral psychologist or psychiatrist. Behavioral professionals approach refractory compliance problems with techniques including cueing and prompting, self-monitoring, reinforcement and shaping, and contingency contracting. It is important for physicians to address directly the issue of compliance at follow-up sessions. Patients may not report side effects or other difficulties with their medication regimen unless specifically asked.

Cueing is based simply on the principle that the patient may respond to programmed stimuli or reminders in the environment to prompt the completion of the various regimen components. A number of studies have reported success in improving compliance when environmental cues are used (e.g., Baekland & Lundwall, 1975). The prompts used ranged from strategically placed stickers to medication calendars to electronically programed medication dispensers (Dunbar & Agras, 1980). Simpler cueing strategies (e.g., telephone or postcard reminders) have also proven useful (Larsen, Olsen, Cole, et al., 1979).

Self-monitoring has long been utilized for both assessment and treatment purposes. This method requires that patients keep records of their own behaviors specific to the treatment regimen. Although the utility of this technique has not been widely studied, it has received some empirical support (Dunbar, 1977). The success of the technique may be attributed to the focus of patients' attention on their own behavior, as well as the additional attention necessarily provided by the health care professional in this process (Masur, 1981).

Response reinforcement and shaping are mainstays of behavioral techniques to increase the occurrence of desired behaviors. An arrangement may be set up by which the patient may receive a predetermined reward for each behavior that, first partially and then increasingly, approaches fulfillment of the prescribed treatment regimen. A contract refers to the formalization of the process, in which specific rules and consequences are developed and agreed upon by the patient and are administered according to the patient's regimen-related behavior. This technique has been demonstrated to improve adherence to a complex post–myocardial infarction medical regimen (Dapcich-Miura & Hovell, 1979).

Although more systematic research is certainly needed in order to better design successful behavioral interventions for noncompliance, early studies indicate that the two levels discussed are relatively low-cost, low-risk ways to improve patient compliance with treatment regimens. Behavior modification programs for life-style change employ similar methods, and pro-grams may simultaneously address life-style change and compliance with specific medical prescriptions. Such strategies can be used for other problems of noncompliance with medical recommendations.

In summary, this chapter provides brief examples of the potential fruitful collaboration of biomedical and behavioral science in the health care delivery system. An increasing emphasis is placed on primary prevention. Implementation of prevention protocols takes place in public health, community, primary care, and traditional medical settings. There is increasing evidence that a comprehensive biopsychosocial approach can achieve results that are superior to those of unidimensional specialty services, regardless of whether they are medical or psychologic. This is all the more true when dealing with complex behavioral-biologic interactions, as in the case of CHD, with its multifactorial etiology. The multidisciplinary team approach, using technologies from behavioral and biomedical sciences, provides a promising potential solution to the chronic disease problem, for which medical procedures are often palliative at best.

REFERENCES

Abrams DB (1984). Current status and clinical developments in the behavioral treatment of obesity. In CM Franks (Ed), *New directions in behavior therapy*. New York: Haworth Press.

Abrams DB, Elder JP, Carlton RA, et al. (1986). Social learning principles for organizational health promotion: An integrated approach. In MF Cataldo & TJ Coates (Eds), *Health and industry: A behavioral medicine perspective*. New York: John Wiley & Sons.

Abrams DB & Follick MJ (1983). Behavioral weight loss intervention at the worksite: Feasibility of maintenance. *Journal of Consulting and Clinical Psychology, 51*, 226–233.

Abrams DB, Monti P, Elder J, et al. (1987). Psychosocial stress and coping in smokers who relapse or quit. *Health Psychology, 6*, 289–303.

Abrams DB, Steinberg J, Follick MJ, et al. (1986). Obesity and type II diabetes: Behavioral medicine's contribution. *Behavioral Medicine Abstracts, 7*, 1–4.

Abrams DB & Wilson GT (1986). Habit disorders: Alcohol and tobacco dependence. In AJ Frances & RE Hales (Eds), *American Psychiatric Association Annual Review* (Vol 5). Washington, DC: American Psychiatric Press.

Baekeland F & Lundwall L (1975). Dropping out of treatment: A critical review. *Psychological Bulletin, 82*, 738–783.

Bandura A (1969). *Principles of behavior modification*. New York: Holt, Rinehart & Winston.

Bandura A (1977). Self-efficacy: Toward a unifying theory of behavioral change. *Psychological Review, 84*, 191–215.

Best JA (1976). Tailoring smoking withdrawal procedures to personality and motivational differences. *Journal of Consulting and Clinical Psychology, 4,* 1–8.

Bistrain BR (1978). Clinical use of protein-sparing modified fast. *Journal of the American Medical Association, 21,* 2299–2302.

Björntorp P (1978). Exercise and obesity. *Psychiatric Clinics of North America, 1,* 691–696.

Black DR & Trelfall WE (1986). A stepped approach to weight control: A minimal intervention and a bibliotherapy problem-solving program. *Behavior Therapy, 17,* 144–157.

Blackwell B (1973). Patient compliance. *New England Journal of Medicine, 289,* 249–253.

Bray GA (1976). *The obese patient.* Philadelphia: WB Saunders.

Breslow L (1978). Risk factor interventions for health maintenance. *Science, 200,* 908–912.

Breslow L (1979). A positive strategy for the nation's health. *Journal of the American Medical Association, 242,* 2093–2095.

Brownell KD (1982). Obesity: Understanding and treating a serious, prevalent, and refractory disorder. *Journal of Consulting and Clinical Psychology, 50,* 820–840.

Brownell KD (1986). Public health approaches to obesity and its management. *Annual Review of Public Health, 7,* 521–533.

Brownell KD, Heckerman CL, Westlake RJ, et al. (1978). The effect of couples training and partner cooperativeness in the behavioral treatment of obesity. *Behavior Therapy, 16,* 323–333.

Brownell KD & Kaye FS (1982). A school-based behavior modification, nutrition education, and physical activity program for obese children. *American Journal of Clinical Nutrition, 35,* 277–283.

Burt A, Illingworth D, Shaw TDR, et al. (1974). Stopping smoking after myocardial infarction. *Lancet 1,* 304–306.

Colletti G & Supnick JA (1980). Continued therapist contact as a maintenance strategy for smoking reduction. *Journal of Consulting and Clinical Psychology, 48,* 665–667.

Dapcich-Miura ED & Hovell MD (1979). Contingency management of adherence to a complex medical regimen in an elderly heart patient. *Behavior Therapy, 10,* 193–201.

Davidson PO & Davidson SM (1980). *Behavioral medicine: Changing health lifestyles.* New York: Brunner/Mazel.

Davis AL, Faust R, & Ordentlich M (1984). Self-help smoking cessation programs: A comparative study with 12-month follow-up by the American Lung Association. *American Journal of Public Health, 74,* 1212–1217.

Donahoe CP, Lin DH, Kirschenbaum DS, et al. (1984). Metabolic consequences of dieting and exercise in the treatment of obesity. *Journal of Consulting and Clinical Psychology, 52,* 827–836.

Dunbar JM (1977). Adherence to medication regimen: An intervention study with poor adherers. Unpublished doctoral dissertation, Stanford University, Palo Alto, CA.

Dunbar JM & Agras WS (1980). Compliance with medical instructions. In J Ferguson, C Taylor (Eds), *The comprehensive handbook of behavioral medicine* (Vol 3). Prentice-Hall, NJ: Spectrum Publications.

Dunbar JM & Stunkard AJ (1979). Adherence to diet and drug regimen. In R Levy, B Rifkind, B Dennis, et al (Eds), *Nutrition, lipids, and coronary heart disease.* New York: Raven Press.

Epstein LH & Wing RR (1980). Aerobic exercise and weight. *Addictive Behaviors, 5,* 371–388.

Fagerstrom KO (1978). Measuring degree of physical dependence to tobacco smoking with reference to individualization of treatment. *Addictive Behaviors, 3,* 235–241.

Fagerstrom KO (1982). A comparison of psychological and pharmacological treatment in smoking cessation. *Journal of Behavioral Medicine 5,* 343–351.

Foch TT & McClearn GE (1980). Genetics, body-weight and obesity. In AJ Stunkard (Ed), *Obesity* (pp 48–71). Philadelphia: WB Saunders.

Folkins CH & Sime WE (1981). Physical fitness training and mental health. *American Psychologist, 36,* 373–389.

Follick MJ, Abrams DB, Smith TW, et al. (1984). Behavioral intervention for weight loss: Acute versus long-term effects on HDL & LDL cholesterol level. *Archives of Internal Medicine, 44,* 1571–1574.

Follick MJ, Gottlieb B, & Fowler J (1986). Behavior therapy and coronary heart disease: Lifestyle modification. In HJ Sobel (Ed), *Behavior therapy in terminal care: A humanistic approach.* New York: Harper & Row.

Foxx RM & Brown RA (1979). Nicotine fading and self-monitoring for cigarette abstinence as controlled smoking. *Jounal of Applied Behavior Analysis, 12,* 111–125.

Friedman M, Ulmer D, Brown B, et al. (1986). Alteration of type A behavior and its effect on cardiac recurrences in post myocardial infarction patients: Summary results of the recurrent coronary prevention project. *American Heart Journal, 112,* 653–665.

Glasgow RE, Schafer L, & O'Neill HK (1981). Self-help and amount of therapist contact in smoking cessation programs. *Journal of Consulting and Clinical Psychology, 49,* 659–667.

Gordis I (1976). Methodologic issues in the measurement of patient compliance. In DI Sackett & RB Haynes (Eds), *Compliance with therapeutic regimens* (pp 51–66). Baltimore: Johns Hopkins University Press.

Haynes RB (1976). Introduction. In RB Haynes, DW Taylor, & DL Sackett (Eds), *Compliance in health care*. Baltimore: Johns Hopkins University Press.

Haynes RB, Taylor DW, & Sackett DI (Eds) (1979). *Compliance in health care*. Baltimore: Johns Hopkins University Press.

Howard AN & Bray GA (Eds) (1981). Proceedings of a symposium on evaluation of very-low-calorie diets. *International Journal of Obesity*, 5, 193–352.

Hubert HB (1986). The importance of obesity in the development of coronary risk factors and disease: The epidemiologic evidence. *Annual Review of Public Health*, 7, 493–502.

Hughes JR & Miller SA (1984). Nicotine gum to help stop smoking. *Journal of the American Medical Association*, 20, 2855–2858.

Jeffery RW (1987). Behavioral treatment of obesity. *Annals of Behavioral Medicine*, 9 (1), 20–24.

Kannel W & Gordon T (1979). Physiological and medical concomitants of obesity: The Framingham study. In GA Bray (Ed), *Obesity in America* (NIH Publication No. 79-359). Bethesda, MD: National Institutes of Health.

Kingsley RG & Wilson GT (1977). Behavior therapy for obesity: A comparative investigation of long-term efficacy. *Journal of Consulting and Clinical Psychology*, 45, 288–298.

Korsch BM & Negrete VF (1972). Doctor-patient communication. *Scientific American*, 227, 66–74.

Kral JG & Kissileff HR (1987). Surgical approaches to the treatment of obesity. *Annals of Behavioral Medicine*, 9(1), 15–19.

Larsen EB, Olsen E, Cole W, et al. (1979). The relationship of health beliefs and a postcard reminder for influenza vaccination. *Journal of Family Practice*, 8, 1207–1211.

Lichtenstein E (1982). The smoking problem: A behavioral perspective. *Journal of Consulting and Clinical Psychology*, 50, 804–819.

Marlatt GA & Gordon JR (1985). *Relapse prevention*. New York: Guilford Press.

Martin JE & Prue DM (1984). Health marketing in a hospital setting. In LW Frederiksen, LJ Solomon, & KA Brehony (Eds), *Marketing health behavior*. New York: Plenum.

Masur FT (1981). Adherence to health care regimens. In CK Prokop & LA Bradley (Eds), *Medical psychology: Contributions to behavioral medicine*. New York: Academic Press.

Matarazzo JD (1984). Behavioral health: A 1990 challenge for the health services professions. In JD Matarazzo, SM Weiss, JA Herd, et al. (Eds), *Behavioral health: A handbook of health enhancement and disease prevention*. New York: John Wiley & Sons.

Matarazzo JD, Weiss SM, Herd JA, et al. (Eds) (1984). *Beahvioral Health: A handbook of health enhancement and disease prevention*. New York: John Wiley & Sons.

Perri MG, MacAdoo WG, Spevak PA, et al. (1984). Effects of multicomponent maintenance program on long-term weight loss. *Journal of Consulting and Clinical Psychology*, 53, 480–481.

Perri MG, Shapiro RM, Ludwig CT, et al. (1984). Maintenance strategies for the treatment of obesity: An evaluation of relapse prevention training and post-treatment contact by mail and telephone. *Journal of Consulting and Clinical Psychology*, 53, 404–413.

Pomerleau OF & Pomerleau CS (1984). Neuroregulators and the reinforcement of smoking: Towards a bio-behavioral explanation. *Neuroscience and Biobehavioral Reviews*, 8, 503–513.

Russell MH, Wilson C, & Taylor C (1979). Effect of general practitioners advice against smoking. *British Medical Journal*, 2, 231–235.

Sachs DPL (1984). Office strategies to help your patients stop smoking. *Journal of Respiratory Disease*, 5, 35–40.

Sachs DPL, Hall RG, Pechacek TF, et al. (1979). Clarification of risk-benefit issues in rapid smoking. *Journal of Consulting and Clinical Psychology*, 47, 1053–1060.

Sackett DL & Haynes RB (1976). *Compliance with therapeutic regimens*. Baltimore: Johns Hopkins University Press.

Simopoulos AP (1986). Obesity and body weight standards. *Annual Review of Public Health*, 7, 481–492.

Simopoulos AP & Van Itallie TB (1984). Body weight, health and longevity. *Annals of Internal Medicine*, 100, 285–289.

Stamler J (1979). Dietary and serum lipids in the multifactorial etiology of atherosclerosis. *Archives of Surgery*, 113, 21–25.

Stuart RB & Davis B (1972). *Slim chance in a fat world*. Champaign, IL: Research Press.

Stunkard AJ (1984). The current status of treatment of obesity in adults. In AJ Stunkard & E Stellar (Eds), *Eating and its disorders*. New York: Raven Press.

United States Department of Health and Human Services (1983). The health consequences of smoking: Cardiovascular disease: A Report of the Surgeon General. Bethesda, MD: Public Health Service Office on Smoking and Health.

Van Itallie TB (1979). Obesity: Adverse effects on health and longevity. *American Journal of Clinical Nutrition, 32,* 2723–2733.

Wadden TA & Stunkard AJ (1986). Controlled trial of very low calorie diet, behavior therapy, and their combination in the treatment of obesity. *Journal of Consulting and Clinical Psychology, 54,* 482–488.

Wadden TA, Stunkard AJ, & Brownell KD (1983).
Very low calorie diets: Their efficacy, safety, and future. *Annals of Internal Medicine, 99,* 675–684.

Wechsler H, Levine S, Idelson RK, et al. (1983). The physician's role in health promotion: A survey of primary-care practitioners. *New England Journal of Medicine, 308,* 97–100.

Wells KB, Ware JE & Lewis CE (1984). Physicians' practices in counseling patients about health habits. *Medical Care, 22,* 240–246.

Richard J. Goldberg
Michael S. Sokol
Leah Oseas Cullen

16
Acute Pain Management

The psychiatrist in the medical-surgical setting encounters a variety of issues involving
difficulties with the management of acute
pain. These issues include recognition and
alleviation of psychosocial stresses and depression; advocacy of proper medical diagnoses and management; systems problems
that result from lack of coordination among
providers; the need for the provision of
adjunctive nonpharmacologic approaches
to pain, such as hypnosis and relaxation;
and the education of resident and nursing
staff regarding the proper use of analgesics.
This chapter addresses the most common
problems that involve analgesic pharmacology, providing the basic information
needed for their solutions. The majority of
these problems involve recognizing inadequate prescribing practices of narcotics and
managing the complications associated with
their use.

DOSE AND FREQUENCY

The most common cause of inadequate
acute pain management is the underuse of
narcotic analgesics. In fact, many doctors
prescribe *less than half* the effective analgesic dose for their patients with pain
(Marks & Sachar, 1973; Sriwatanakul,
Weis, Alloza, et al., 1983). In addition to
doses that are inadequate, narcotics are
often prescribed at time intervals that extend beyond the effective half-life of the
drug. The use of suboptimal doses and
excessive time between dose intervals may
result from physician orders, nursing administration, or patient bias. Some patients
may attempt to endure pain and earn the
respect of the nurses and doctors as a
"good" patient. It is not unusual to find
patients on every-4–6-hour schedule of
meperidine, when this drug usually requires
administration every 3-to-4 hours. When
patients start to complain of severe pain at
3.5 hours after their last dose, they are
often thought of as "addicted" or excessively preoccupied with medication. In
fact, such patients may only be expressing
the fact that their pain has reemerged because their dose time has gone beyond the
effective duration of the narcotic. Table
16-1 lists usual dose ranges for commonly

PRINCIPLES OF MEDICAL PSYCHIATRY
ISBN 0-8089-1883-4

Table 16-1
Usual Dose Ranges of Commonly Prescribed Narcotics*

Agent	Usual Dose Range (milligrams)	Comment
Codeine	30–60 PO q.4–6 hr.	Usually combined with an NSAID
Oxycodone	5–10 PO q.4–6 hr.	Comes as tablets with 5 mg oxycodone plus aspirin or acetaminophen†
Pentazocine	25–50 PO q.4–6 hr.	Mixed agonist-antagonist; may cause psychotic symptoms†
Butorphanol	1–4 IM q.3 hr.	Mixed agonist-antagonist; less respiratory depression
Meperidine	50–100 SC or IM q.2–3 hr.	Rapid onset of action; has a psychotoxic metabolite
	50–100 PO q.3–4 hr.	
Morphine	2–8 SC or IM q.4 hr.	Sedating; may lower blood pressure
	5–30 PO q.4 hr.	
Hydromorphone	1–2 SC or IM q.3 hr.	
	2–4 IV q.3 hr.	
	2–8 PO q.4 hr.	
Methadone	5–20 PO q.6–8 hr.	Long half-life; lower dose in renal failure

Note:

* Commonly used dose ranges are *not* equianalgesic (see Table 16–4). Higher or lower doses may be appropriate for particular patients, depending upon severity of pain, duration of treatment, tolerance, body weight, pharmacokinetics, drug interactions, and use of adjuncts.
† Mixed agonist-antagonists must not be given together with other narcotics.

Table 16-2
Analgesic duration (with
Oral Dosing)

Analgesic	Duration of Action
Morphine	4–7 hours
Meperidine	3–5 hours
Methadone	4–6 hours
Hydromorphone	4–6 hours
Pentazocine	4–7 hours
Codeine	4–7 hours
Propoxyphene	4–7 hours
Oxycodone	4–6 hours

prescribed analgesics, and Table 16-2 lists the average duration of action.

The consultant dealing with a pain patient who continues to complain despite "usually adequate treatment" should first look at the dose and frequency of analgesic actually delivered. Ask patients what level of relief they get within the first hour after their dose. If relief in that time is inadequate, the dose is too low. If pain relief is complete but reemerges before the next dose, then the duration between doses is too long. *It is indispensable to look directly at the actual drug administration record, not at orders or progress notes, to confirm what has actually been given to the patient and on what schedule.* Narcotics should be given on a schedule corresponding to their analgesic half-life (Table 16-2). Regarding dose, there is no rule that 75 mg of meperidine, for example, is the right dose for everyone. Some patients require 75 mg, others 150 mg, for the same effect.

One concern about giving high narcotic doses is respiratory depression, especially if the patient is also on benzodiazepines. Respiratory depression can be treated by naloxone, the drug of choice for reversal of respiratory depression secondary to narcotics. Rapid reversal however, can precipitate acute withdrawal, with psychotomimetic symptoms and exacerbation of pain. It is, therefore, suggested that a dilute solution of naloxone (0.4 mg in 10 ml of saline) be given slowly, titrated against the patient's respiratory rate until just enough of the solution has been given to reverse the respiratory depression (Foley, 1985a). Patients should be closely followed after this with frequent respiratory rate checks, as naloxone has a short half-life, and patients may have to be redosed if taking longer-acting agents (methadone or levorphanol) (Foley, 1985a).

Fixed versus As-Needed Dose Schedules

When a diagnosis of acute pain has been made, physicians need to consider whether analgesics should be prescribed on an as-needed (PRN) or a fixed schedule. Severe, continuous pain is better treated on a fixed schedule for the following reasons (Goldberg & Tull, 1983):

1. A schedule based on the half-life of the narcotic prevents reemergence of pain before the next dose.
2. The dose required to treat reemergence pain resulting from an as-needed schedule is often larger than would be required to prevent it using a fixed schedule (Reuler, Girard, & Nardone, 1980; Shimm, Logue, Maltbie, et al., 1979).
3. Patients on an as-needed schedule are in a dependent position, which requires them to ask for medication in a way that may be interpreted as excessive preoccupation with medication, or experienced by the patient as humiliating.
4. Elderly patients and those who are cognitively impaired and in pain may lose track of time or have difficulty calling the nursing staff to ask for medication.

Exceptions to the usual fixed-dosage schedule are patients with impaired hepatic metabolism (extensive liver disease or elderly patients older than 80 years), in whom the drug's half-life may be prolonged, and patients with night pain only (Twycross & Lack, 1984, chap 9).

Narcotic analgesics should be given during the night for patients whose sleep is being interrupted by pain or who awaken in the morning with excessive reemergence pain. Lack of sleep creates a vicious cycle of increased pain, which causes more lack of sleep (Moldofsky, Scarisbrick, England, et al., 1975). Conversely, if a patient is sleeping well and is not awakening with increased perception of pain and its consequent anxiety, then there is no need to schedule analgesic doses during the patient's sleep time.

Some clinicians will double the nighttime narcotic dose to maintain analgesic control without unnecessary awakening of patients. For the elderly or frail patient, the bedtime dose may be increased by only 50 percent (Twycross & Lack, 1984, Chap 9). With the newer "slow-release" morphine preparations (Roxanol SR, Roxane Laboratories, Columbus, OH; MS Contin, Purdue Frederick, Norwalk, CT), the every-8–12-hour dosing also allows for continuous analgesia without nighttime interruption. It is also important to ascertain whether the pain problem is the result of some intermittent procedure such as debridement, dressing changes, or physical therapy. In such instances, the most important intervention would be to provide a narcotic dose prior to the intervention.

An alternative narcotic scheduling method is known as "reverse PRN." This involves offering the medication to the patient on a scheduled basis, allowing the patient to accept or refuse the dose. This reverse PRN method ensures that the medication is made available but also helps the patient maintain some autonomy over titrating the dose (Goldberg & Tull 1983; Sriwatanakul et al., 1983).

A major concern among physicians and nurses is the fear of creating an addicted patient. This fear is largely unwarranted. For example, in a large review of 11,882 nonaddicted Medicare inpatients who received narcotics, in only four cases was iatrogenic narcotic addiction documented (Porter & Jick, 1980). Fear of addiction and lack of knowledge of pharmacokinetic profiles extend also to nursing staff, who frequently choose lower doses when dose range choices are ordered (Sriwatanakul et al., 1983).

THE EFFECTIVE USE OF NARCOTICS

The effective use of analgesics is based upon an assessment of whether the pain is acute or chronic, a definition of the specific pain syndrome, and an understanding of the clinical pharmacology of the drug prescribed (Foley, 1982). In patients with severe, acute pain, morphine represents the standard narcotic against which all others are compared. Unlike the mixed agonist-antagonist analgesics, morphine has no ceiling effect. In addition, it is neither more nor less likely to cause physical dependence than any other equianalgesic narcotic. Analgesic narcotics that are more potent, with shorter half-lives, such as hydromorphone, are much more difficult to titrate. Narcotics with longer half lives, such as methadone, tend to accumulate in tissues and precipitate more central nervous system (CNS) and respiratory side effects (Gourlay, Cherry & Cousins, 1986).

Butorphanol is an alternative narcotic agonist-antagonist analgesic. Its duration of action is comparable to morphine and provides analgesia comparable to morphine with 2 mg of butorphanol equivalent to 10 mg morphine intramuscularly (IM) or intravenously (IV) (Heel, Brogden, Speight, et al., 1978). It does not come in an oral form. It has a lower incidence of psychotomimetic side effects than pentazocine. Unlike other narcotics, butorphanol does not produce a dose-related increase in respiratory depression (Nagashima, Karamanian, Malovany, et al., 1976; Popio, Jackson, Ross, et al., 1978), though it can be reversed with naloxone, just as with the other narcotics. It has minimal effects on blood pressure, though its use may be limited following myocardial infarction because of effects on increasing pulmonary artery pressure and end diastolic pressure. To avoid precipitation of acute withdrawal, it cannot be given to patients already on narcotics. Other narcotics can be begun after about 4 hours following the last butorphanol dose. This drug is also thought to induce less tolerance of analgesic effects than other narcotics (Vandam, 1980).

Sustained-release morphine has recently become available in the form of 30 mg controlled-release tablets. This medication is recommended to be given every 12 hours or every 8 hours, respectively. The use of a sustained-release preparation may not be the regimen of choice in acute, severe pain, but in the patient whose acute pain has been stabilized on oral morphine or other oral narcotics and whose pain is judged to remain severe and continuous for some time, time-released morphine may be a viable option. The obvious advantage of such a medication is the convenience in dosing time for both patient and staff. Moreover, the slow release mechanism may result in fewer peak and trough fluctuations and, therefore, may cause fewer side effects, such as nausea and vomiting (Walsh, 1984). Finally, due to the fact that the tablets are slow release and the morphine sulfate is contained in a matrix, the controlled-release morphine is less likely to become an illicit street drug and may be more palatable and socially acceptable to the patient than the current morphine sulfate aqueous solution or morphine sulfate USP tablets. As suggested earlier, this form of administration probably is less useful for the patient just being started on oral morphine sulfate therapy. Titrating the dose to the pain may result in toxic side effects until a total oral milligram dose is established with shorter-acting morphine sulfate. The nature of the acute pain may require more frequent dosing or higher doses and tighter control because of pain breakthrough.

Oral versus Parenteral Use

Oral analgesic administration offers simplicity and economy, avoids the discomforts and potential complications of repeated injections, makes the patient less dependent on others for his care, and may even obviate the need for hospitalization in some cases (Beaver, 1980). There are, however, two specific instances when the use of parenteral narcotics is warranted. The first instance is in the case of acute, severe pain requiring immediate relief, as in the trauma, burn, heart attack, or postoperative patient. The second instance is in the case of the patient with severe pain in which oral medications fail to provide adequate relief, when tolerance has developed, or when the patient is no longer able to swallow (Moertel, 1980).

When one has determined the necessity of using parenteral narcotics for the control of pain, several variables should be considered. Parenterally administered narcotics have a rapid onset of action with a shorter duration of effect compared with orally administered narcotics. Peak concentrations may vary three- to fivefold between patients, and the time required to reach peak concentration varies as well. Moreover, for a given patient, differences in meperidine concentration as small as 0.05 μg/ml can represent the difference between no relief and complete analgesia (White, 1985). One study has documented that meperidine concentrations, when given IM every 3–4 hours, will equal or exceed the minimal analgesic concentration for only 35 percent of the dosing period because of the highly variable absorption

Table 16-3
Intravenous Morphine Drip

I.   Discontinue previous narcotics and sedatives.

II.   Obtain baseline vital signs and level of alertness.

III.   Loading dose: 2–5 mg IV every 15 minutes until pain is relieved.

IV.   Maintenance dose: Total loading dose/hour; check vital signs every 15 minutes for first hour, then every hour for the next 6 hours, then every 6 hours for the next 24 hours, then every shift.

Calculation of Morphine Infusion Rates to Be Given in D_5W (May Also Be Given in D_5NS)

Morphine (mg)	Amount of Solution (ml)	Rate (ml/h or microdrop/h)
250	1,000	Hourly morphine $\times$ 4
500	1,000	Hourly morphine $\times$ 2

V.   Dosage should not be increased by more than one-third of previous hourly dosage. If one increases hourly dosage rate, then vitals must be rechecked every 15 minutes for 1 hour and every hour for next 6 hours.

VI.   As the mixing of such solutions requires time and care by hospital pharmacy, one must give adequate advance notice to the hospital pharmacy for IV morphine solution preparation.

VII.   Upper range of infusion is generally 300 mg/hour, although most persons are controlled on much lower doses (and some infusion rates may be higher in tolerant individuals).

Source: Citron ML (1984, December). How would you treat severe cancer pain refractory to oral analgesics? *Drug Therapy*, pp 11, 15, 19.

and the narrow therapeutic window (Austin, Stapleton & Mather, 1980).

Intravenous Narcotics

The IV route is best reserved for the following situations (Portnoy, 1986):

1. Acute trauma, burn, or heart attack patients
2. Severely cachectic patients in whom IM routes are not tolerated
3. Patients with severe bleeding diatheses, or low platelet counts, for whom IM injections or suppositories are contraindicated.
4. Cases in which IM routes are not desirable (as with pediatric patients) and the oral route is not possible.

Unfortunately, the IV bolus route causes a duration of analgesia that is quite short-lived because of rapid drug uptake by tissue and rapid elimination. As a result of this diminished duration of action, larger and more frequent doses are needed for breakthrough pain, thus precipitating a higher incidence of respiratory depression, sedation, nausea, and vomiting. Finally, the demand for repeated IV narcotic boluses may become a time-consuming function for nursing personnel.

As a result of these disadvantages of IV bolus narcotic administration, analgesic researchers have devised several models of continuous opioid infusion. Intravenous drip may be rate-controlled by medical and nursing staff or in some cases by the patients themselves. According to Graves,

Table 16-4
Conversion of Narcotics
to Oral Morphine
Equivalents and Relative
Potencies

To convert oral dose of any narcotic to an equivalent oral dose of morphine, multiply by:

0.15 for propoxyphene
0.2 for meperidine
1/3 for codeine
1/3 for pentazocine
2 for oxycodone
3 for methadone
8 for dilaudid

To convert I.M. dose of any narcotic to an equivalent oral dose of morphine, multiply by:

1.5 for pentazocine
6 for methadone
40 for hydromorphone
3 for morphine
0.8 for meperidine
5 for butorphanol

Divide by 3 to get equivalent dose of I.M. morphine.

Foster, Batenhorst, et al. (1983), minimal sedation and fewer side effects can be achieved with patient-controlled analgesia. Moreover, the potential for overdose can be minimized if small bolus doses (1–2 mg/hour of morphine) are used, with a mandatory dosing-free interval between successive doses (White, 1985). Table 16-3 presents a method for initiating a morphine IV drip. For a complete review of the guidelines used in the management of continuous opioid infusions, refer to White (1985) and Portnoy (1986). For the most part, it is preferable to maintain patients on oral analgesics for as long as possible, because administration by the IV (or intrathecal) routes has been associated with rapid development of tolerance (Foley, 1985b).

Conversions among Different Narcotics

There are several situations where improper narcotic conversion leads to psychiatric consultation. Typically, these conversions involve a change from the parenteral to the oral route, encountered frequently in postoperative situations. When a patient is changed precipitously from parenteral meperidine to oral acetominophen and codeine, the acute decrease in narcotic dose can be dramatic, leading to iatrogenic withdrawal, a dramatic increase in pain complaints, and an agitated patient. In the case of a switch from the parenteral to the oral route, one must recognize that increases in total mg per dose are necessary to maintain the same level of analgesia. Differences in oral-to-parenteral analgesic efficacy are due to limited gastrointestinal absorption and a first-pass hepatic metabolism. Original data by Houde, Wallenstein, and Beaver (1965) indicated a 6:1 oral/parenteral ratio for morphine, but the results of this single-dose study do not hold for regular administration and show that sixfold increased oral doses will cause oversedation and respiratory depression. For patients on regular schedules of morphine, the oral/parenteral ratio can be considered 3:1. In the case of meperidine, the oral/parenteral ratio is 4:1.

When calculating conversion from a parenteral to an oral narcotic, or to sort out the total narcotic dose in situations where many different analgesics have been used, it is helpful to convert all analgesics to a standard reference (Goldberg, Mor, Wiemann, et al., 1986). This conversion among narcotics is easily facilitated by converting all drugs to oral morphine equivalents (Table 16-4). From a methodologic viewpoint, the information for this table comes primarily from pain relief studies in cancer patients, whose acute pain needs and analgesia metabolism may be different from those of the noncancer patient. In addition, the time–effect curves for studying various doses of analgesia generally result from single-dose experiments. Single-dose studies neglect the kinetic changes that take place following repeated dosing, especially in narcotics with long half-lives, such as methadone. Finally, the conversion table presented does not acknowledge the probable differences in pain relief associated with age, sex, race, or quality of pain (Kaiko, Wallenstein, Rogers, et al., 1982).

The Development of Tolerance

Another variable that accounts for pain relief problems is the development of tolerance. The tolerant patient is the one who notices a shortened duration of analgesic effect and an eventual decrease in pain relief. The rate of development of tolerance varies; however, "since tolerance to most of the adverse dose-limiting effects of narcotics, including respiratory and general CNS depressant effects, develops concomitantly with tolerance to analgesic effect, even substantial tolerance can usually be surmounted and adequate analgesia restored by increasing the narcotic dose" (Beaver, 1980). Tolerance needs to be differentiated, however, from loss of pain control due to new or advancing disease. Cross-tolerance is incomplete with most narcotics. Switching parenteral narcotics, therefore, may be helpful. Because cross-tolerance is incomplete, Foley (1985b) recommends calculating the dosage of the new drug via morphine equivalents equal to the new preparation and reducing the dose by one-half to start. The dosage of the new narcotic may then be titrated upward, based on the patient's response. When a patient is not responding to one narcotic, however, the problem is usually inadequate dose or duration rather than tolerance. Yet, any patient who is exposed to continuous doses of narcotics may develop tolerance, often in as soon as 5–7 days. It is often

necessary, therefore, to increase the dose in order to obtain the same pain relief. Unfortunately, staff often get anxious about continuing narcotics for very long and attempt to decrease the dose just at the time when the patient has developed tolerance and an *increase* actually is called for. The consultant needs to explain this phenomenon and should anticipate some resistance to the recommendation to increase narcotics for a "problem" patient just at the time when the staff expected a solution that included tapering narcotics. If tolerance has developed in a patient, a greater-than-expected oral dose may be required when switching from parenteral. Alternatively, cross-tolerance may not be complete in some patients, which may account for an overly sedated or "narcotic toxic" patient following a switch in medications.

Prevention of Narcotic-Induced Constipation

Constipation is a problem that faces all patients on narcotic analgesics. This effect appears to be dose-dependent. When narcotics bind to opiate receptors in the gut (Foley, 1982), the result is increased tone with markedly diminished propulsive contractions in both the small and large intestines. The resulting delay in the passage of the intestinal contents causes considerable dessication of the feces, which in turn retards their advance through the colon. Moreover, greatly enhanced anal sphincter tone, combined with inattention to the normal sensory stimuli for the defecation reflex due to narcotic-induced CNS effects, further contribute to narcotic-induced constipation (Jaffe & Martin, 1980). The constipating effect of narcotic analgesics is not due entirely to local effects of intestinal action. Naloxone injected into the cerebral ventricles acts to abolish the constipating effects of morphine injected in small quantities into the cerebral ventricles of rats (Parolaro, Sala & Gori, 1977).

Constipation can be uncomfortable and disturbing to patients and may result in the need for manual disimpaction. Severe cramping pain can also result, or narcotics may lead to a functional ileus. Therefore, severe constipation should be avoided and treated preventively. There is one circumstance in which narcotic-induced changes in colonic motility may be life threatening. Patients with chronic ulcerative colitis, when treated with opioids during acute attacks, may develop a life-threatening toxic dilation of the colon, termed *toxic megacolon* (Garrett, Sauer, & Moertel, 1967).

Stimulant cathartics, by virtue of their direct and local effects on longitudinal peristalsis, are useful in treating narcotic-induced constipation. All anthraquinone derivatives, which are stimulant cathartics, are effective in preventing constipation, but senna compounds (e.g., Perdiem granules, Rorer, Fort Washington, PA, or Senokot tablets, Purdue Frederick, Norwalk, CT) are better accepted than cascara or aloe. Some clinicians have proposed that there is a fixed dose relation: one-half of Senokot (concentrated senna) tablet reverses the constipating effect of 4 mg IM morphine or its equivalent (Maguire, Yon, & Miller, 1981).

The most practical and useful regimen to prevent and treat narcotic-induced constipation is the following, described by Twycross and Lack (1984).*

1. Ask about patient's usual bowel habits and use of laxatives.
2. Do a rectal examination to check for fecal impaction.
3. Be aware that fluid stool, especially

*Adapted from Twycross RG & Lack SA (1984). Therapeutics in terminal cancer, London: Pitman Publishing pp 56–63.

with incontinence, may mean high fecal impaction.

4. Record bowel motions each day in the appropriate log.
5. Encourage fluids (i.e., water, prune juice) and foods that have a laxative effect if bowels do not move spontaneously.
6. For patients on morphine or alternative strong narcotic, prescribe:
   a. Casanthranol 30 mg with docusate 100 mg. (Peri-Colace, Mead Johnson, Evansville, IN), 1 capsule 1 to 4 times a day. Dose to be adjusted by nurse according to result.
   b. If casanthranol with docusate causes abdominal cramps, change to docusate alone (available as a generic) 100 mg. alone 1 to 4 times daily.
   c. If casanthranol with docusate (2 capsules q.i.d.) is ineffective, give milk of magnesia and cascara suspension (25 ml milk of magnesia; 5 ml cascara aromatic fluid extract) 30 ml q.h.s. in addition.
7. If no movement by next morning, manually assess location of stool in rectum. If good contact with rectal mucosa seems possible, use bisacodyl (Dulcolax, Boehringer Ingelheim Ltd., Ridgefield, CT) 10 mg suppository.
8. If a suppository is not feasible or ineffective, administer an oil retention enema and/or Fleets enema followed by soap-suds enema (SSE) if no result.
9. Manually disimpact if necessary.
10. Whenever possible, strong patient preferences for bowel care should be honored and a requisite physician order sought.

The compositions of available laxatives are listed in Table 16-5. This regimen may be

Table 16-5
Composition of Laxatives

Laxative	Composition
Peri-Colace	
Capsule	casanthranol 30 mg
	docusate 100 mg
Solution (per 5 ml)	casanthranol 10 mg
	docusate 20 mg
Colace (docusate sodium)	
Capsule	docusate 100 mg
Solution (per 5 ml)	docusate 50 mg
Dialose (docusate potassium)	docusate 100 mg
Capsule	
Senokot	
Tablet	sennoside B 7.5 mg
Dulcolax	
Tablet	bisacodyl 5 mg
Suppository	bisacodyl 10 mg
Milk of magnesia	
Suspension (per 5 ml)	magnesium hydroxide 350 mg
Concentrate (per 5 ml)	magnesium hydroxide 1050 mg
Magnesium citrate	
Solution (per 10 oz)	magnesium citrate 17.45 g
Cascara sagrada and milk of magnesia	
Suspension (per 5 ml)	magnesium hydroxide 350 mg in cascara sagrade
Metamucil	
Powder packets	psyllium mucilloid 5 g/10 g, dextrose 5 g/10 g

followed on a chronic basis as long as narcotics are needed for analgesia.

IS PAIN REAL?:
USE OF PLACEBOS IN THE
MEDICAL SETTING

Placebo, which is Latin for "I shall please," is a term that evokes great emotion in both health care givers and recipients. A placebo is an inert substance, given in any form and without inherent pharmacologic property, that, by virtue of the environment in which it is taken, the psychologic state of the recipient, and the specific neurophysiologic processes of the recipient, may have a desired effect on a given disorder. Unfortunately, there remains significant misunderstanding within the medical community regarding placebos and their purpose (Goldberg et al., 1979). As pointed out by Goodwin in a study of 60 house officers and 39 nurses, the majority of physicians and nurses greatly underestimate the percentage of patients who experience pain relief when given a placebo. Placebos are typically given to disliked patients suspected of exaggerating their pain, failing to respond to usual medical regimens, or both. Placebo use is often rationalized by the staff as a means of avoiding "dangerous" or "possibly addicting" treatment. Positive responses to placebo are often misinterpreted by physicians as evidence that pain has no physiologic basis. Several studies have shown that overdemanding and complaining patients are, if anything, less likely to respond to placebo than patients well liked by the hospital staff (Goodwin, Goodwin, & Vogel, 1979).

Thirty to 40 percent of patients are placebo responders. In addition, not only does pain respond to placebo, but in the studies comparing 10 mg IM morphine to placebo, nausea and anxiety respond as well (Beecker, 1955). In an enlightening study comparing pain relief in postoperative oral surgery in 51 subject, placebo analgesia was felt to be effective by activating endogenous endorphins, therefore supporting a "true" physiologic rather than psychologic basis for placebo analgesia (Levine, Gordon & Fields, 1978). Not only are placebos recognized for their analgesic properties, but, like morphine, they become less effective at the same dose, creating a tolerance effect.

When placebo use is encountered or contemplated, the physician should ask, "What is happening in this treatment system?" Typical answers include the following: inadequate narcotic medication is being used; the personality style of the patient has prompted the staff to become unduly suspicious; the patient and staff are caught in ongoing interpersonal conflict (Goldberg & Tull, 1983). In conclusion, there seems to be no significant role for placebos except in research protocols.

ALLERGY AND BEHAVIORAL SIDE EFFECTS OR NARCOTICS

Psychiatric consultation may be requested when the patient develops some behavioral disturbance and the issue is raised whether this represents a reaction to narcotics.

Allergic and Idiosyncratic Reactions

Idiosyncratic reactions, such as nausea, vomiting, and dizziness, to morphine and related opioids are often described by patients as an "allergy" to narcotics. Actually, true allergic phenomena to narcotics are uncommon and are usually manifested by urticaria, skin rashes, and dermatitis. More severe anaphylactoid reactions are extremely rare. In a review of the medical literature from entries in *Index Medicus* from 1966 to 1982, there were no documented cases of anaphylaxis following oral or intramuscular administration of specific narcotics (Levy & Rockoff, 1982). True anaphylaxis has been described for both IV codeine and IV meperidine (Levy & Rockoff, 1982; Shanahan, Marshall, & Garrett, 1983). It is felt that those persons who are known to have the "aspirin-intolerance syndrome" have a higher likelihood of having more severe allergic reactions to morphine, morphine derivatives, and codeine (Samter & Beers, 1968).

The mechanism by which opiates cause allergic reactions is via histamine release. Comparatively, codeine appears to have a more potent histamine releasing action than morphine in equianalgesic doses (Shanahan et al., 1983). Both in vitro and in vivo studies have shown that increased doses of morphine cause increased histamine release from human skin that is not antagonized by naloxone. This implies that the mechanism of histamine release is not via specific receptors and that naloxone is unlikely to be of value in blocking an allergic phenomenon (McLelland, 1986). Recognizing that allergic reactions to morphine are due to histamine release, potent H_1 antihistamines such as diphenhydramine or doxepin are effective inhibitors of the common allergic responses (Sullivan, 1982). More recently, oral ketotifen, a histamine release inhibitor used commonly outside the United States, has been demonstrated to suppress the wheal and flare reactions of intradermal codeine (Wang, Wang, & Chang, 1985).

When severe pain requires narcotics in a narcotic-allergic patient, there are several options available. Obviously, a non-narcotic analgesic should be considered, recognizing the hematologic and gastric risks associated with high-dose aspirin and nonsteroidal agents. Another option when narcotics cannot be used is the parenteral phenothiazine analgesic methotrimeprazine (Rogers, 1981). This drug appears to have some analgesic effect (possibly by raising the pain threshold), but published reports are equivocal and do not show the analgesic effect to be independent of the sedative or tranquilizing effects. This drug is described further in the following section.

No research data could be found describing the degree of cross-reactivity of allergic responses within the family of opioid narcotics. If one obviously needs to use a narcotic analgesic, an allergic response to morphine does not necessarily imply an allergy to a chemically related congener, such as codeine. As there are other families of narcotic analgesics, an alternative would be to use a member of the phenylpiperidine family, such as meperidine, or a member of the agonist-antagonist family, such as pentazocine.

Specific Psychotoxicities of Narcotics

All narcotics have some psychotoxic potential, with more specific problems associated with meperidine, pentazocine, nalbuphine, and butorphanol tartrate. Narcotics produce analgesia, drowsiness, changes in mood, and mental clouding, though analgesia should occur without loss of consciousness. As the dose is increased, the subjective effects, including pain relief, become more pronounced. Moreover, in individuals, the euphoric effects become greater. For a given degree of analgesia, the mental clouding produced by therapeutic doses of morphine is considerably less pronounced and of a different character than that produced by alcohol or barbiturates. Morphine and its related analgesics rarely produce the garrulous, jocular, and emotionally labile behavior seen with alcohol or barbiturate intoxication. Finally, extremely high doses of morphine (and the majority of related congeners) produce convulsions at dose levels in excess of those required for analgesia (Jaffe & Martin, 1980).

Meperidine is a phenylpiperidine analgesic that produces a pattern of CNS effects similar to morphine, with some differences. The corneal reflex in systemic meperidine analgesia tends to be obtunded or abolished, and some patients develop dysphoria. More specifically, the accumulation of normeperidine, the N-demethylated metabolite, especially in patients with renal failure or cancer, may cause CNS excitation with seizures, myoclonus, or toxic psychosis. These CNS excitatory signs generally occur with meperidine doses greater than 1200 mg/day. The CNS toxicity of meperidine is much more likely to occur via the intravenous route, however, and may occur at doses as low as 350 mg/day (Szeto, Inturrisi, Houde, et al., 1977).

Life-threatening reactions may follow the administration of meperidine to patients being treated with monoamine oxidase inhibitors. These reactions consist of hypertension, excitation, delirium, hyperpyrexia, convulsions, respiratory depression, and death (Jaffe & Martin, 1980).

Pentazocine is a mixed opiate agonist-antagonist. Because of its antagonist characteristics, pentazocine should never be prescribed for anyone already on opiates because it will precipitate a sudden withdrawal syndrome. Moreover, at doses greater than 60 mg given parenterally, anxiety, nightmares, dissociative sensations, dysphoria, and hallucinations have been reported, especially in the elderly (Houde, 1979). Because of such phenomena, especially in the elderly, pentazocine is best avoided in the hospitalized patient (Kane & Pokorny, 1975; Taylor, Galloway, Petrie, et al., 1978). Nalbuphine and butorphanol tartrate are other opiate agonist-antagonists. They also should never be prescribed to persons known or suspected of being on opiates. Nalbuphine is known to precipitate an abstinence syndrome in individuals dependent on 60 mg or more of morphine a day. At doses greater than or equal to 70 mg parenterally, it has been reported to cause racing thoughts, depressed mood, and hallucinations (Houde, 1979).

WAYS TO AUGMENT NARCOTIC ANALGESIA

Although potentiators of narcotic analgesics have been used for over 20 years, relatively few controlled studies of their effectiveness have been done. In most causes, analgesic adjuvants are best reserved for situations where it is important for the patient to have a lower narcotic dose or to counteract sedation.

Hydroxyzine

Hydroxyzine is an antihistamine often used as a coanalgesic. The mechanism of analgesic effects of antihistamines is unknown and remains speculative. They may act as analgesics through interaction with an unknown histaminergic system (i.e., H_3 receptors), through an interaction with biogenic amines or the sympathetic nervous system, or through an interaction with one or more chemical mediators, such as substance P, bradykinins, or opioids (Rumore & Schlichting, 1986). Although it is common clinical practice to prescribe hydroxyzine in 25 mg IM doses in combination with IM narcotics, this practice appears to be based mostly on anecdotal support. Some clinical studies have compared hydroxyzine and morphine to morphine alone, or hydroxyzine and meperidine to meperidine alone, using a dose of 100 mg of hydroxyzine. These studies support an additive analgesic effect for hydroxyzine at that dose (Hupert, Yacoub, & Turgeon, 1980; Stambaugh, 1979). The analgesic effect of 100 mg of hydroxyzine has been demonstrated to be equivalent to about 8 mg of IM morphine (Belville, Dorey, Capparell, et al., 1979). Finally, when using hydroxyzine with a narcotic analgesic, the dose should be given on the same schedule as the narcotic. The primary side effect is sedation.

Stimulants

Stimulants represent another class of analgesic adjuvants most useful in patients with coexisting sedation, loss of alertness, or depressive symptoms. In a large double-blind study involving 450 patients, Forrest, Brown, Brown, et al. (1977) demonstrated the augmentation of morphine analgesia with either 5 mg or 10 mg of oral dextroamphetamine. At these doses, the analgesia was judged to be respectively 1.5 and 2 times the analgesia of the given morphine dose alone. Moreover, dextroamphetamine offset the sedating effects of the morphine without significantly changing vital signs (Forrest et al., 1977). Amphetamine coprescribing is not common practice because of several concerns. Tolerance of its alerting effects has been recognized to occur within weeks, leading to the necessity of higher doses, and at doses greater than 40 mg, paranoia and hallucinations have been known to occur (Ellinwood, 1969). Finally, amphetamines may suppress sleep and appetite. In order to avoid the carry-over of alerting effects into the evening, dextroamphetamine or methylphenidate, should be prescribed, starting with 5 mg orally in the morning and at noontime, increasing the dose slowly if necessary. Frail, elderly patients with coexisting heart disease can begin with 2.5 mg morning and noon.

Some of the concerns about the side effects of stimulants may be exaggerated. A retrospective review of 66 medical and surgical patients treated with dextroamphetamine or methylphenidate for depression demonstrated minimal side effects. Of those patients who did develop possibly drug-related side effects, the effects were mild, were reversible with drug discontinuation, and showed no correlation with the dosage prescribed or the age of the patient. These side effects included maculopapular rash, nausea, sinus tachycardia, and confusion in two patients with concurrent dementia (Woods, Tesar, Murray, et al., 1986). The use of psychostimulants is also discussed in Chapter 4 by Stoudemire and Fogel.

Cocaine

Cocaine is the most powerful euphoriant known and has been touted as an analgesic augmenter for years. In fact, Coca-Cola originally contained cocaine and was marketed as both a stimulant and an analgesic. Unfortunately, despite its intermittent use in Brompton's solution, no study has demonstrated any general analgesic properties of cocaine. Cocaine may, however, induce mood elevation that may be interpreted as pain relief (Warfield, 1985).

Steroids

Steroids are important analgesic adjuncts for acute pain syndromes associated with metastatic bone disease, epidural cord compression, headache due to increased intracranial pressure and tumor infiltration of brachial and lumbar plexuses, or other peripheral nerve involvement. Steroids are felt to provide analgesia via their peripheral anti-inflammatory effects, as well as central effects on neurotransmitters (Foley, 1985a). For patients with epidural cord compression, 100 mg of dexamethasone IV given with radiation may provide significant pain relief in up to 85 percent of patients (Foley, 1985a) After initial treatment, this dose may be tapered and maintained at 16 mg of dexamethasone while radiation is completed. For nerve infiltration, dosages of 4–16 mg of dexamethasone during radiation therapy may significantly reduce pain. In addition, steroids may have additional benefits of increased appetite, weight gain, and improvement of mood. Care, however, must be taken with the coadministration of nonsteroidal anti-inflammatory drugs because of the increased risk of gastrointestinal (GI) side effects (ulcers and GI bleeding).

Brompton's Mixture

Perhaps the most widely publicized "analgesic cocktail" is the "Brompton cocktail." This combination was first advocated in 1896 by Snow to treat pain associated with advanced cancer and was reintroduced in the 20th century at the Brompton Chest Hospital in Great Britain. Brompton's original formula consisted of an elixir containing morphine or heroin combined with cocaine in a vehicle of syrup, alcohol, and chloroform water. This elixir is often combined with a phenothiazine, providing agents that control pain and counteract side effects at multiple levels within the nervous system. Some people have felt that heroin may provide superior analgesia to morphine in the cocktail, but this advantage has never been documented (Kaiko, Rogers, Wallenstein, et al., 1981). Moreover, there appears to be no advantage of the Brompton cocktail over a simple aqueous morphine solution for treating intractable pain in patients with advanced malignant disease (Melzack, Mount, & Gordon, 1979; Schad, 1980). Finally, Twycross and Lack (1984) state, "It is more nauseating (due to the syrup content) and may cause a burning sensation in the throat (due to the alcohol)." They conclude, "The traditional mixture of morphine sulphate and cocaine in a vehicle of syrup, alcohol, and chloroform water offers no advantages over a simple solution of morphine sulphate in chloroform or tap water."

Neuroleptics

Neuroleptics represents another class of narcotic potentiators. Despite their widespread use, over 20 years ago Moore and Dundee (1961) drew attention to the fact that phenothiazines do not have significant analgesic properties In fact, no well-controlled study exists to document the coanalgesic effects of phenothiazine in pain patients. The primary use of phenothiazines in terminal cancer patients remains antiemetic or anxiolytic in conjunction with morphine (Goldberg & Cullen, 1986).

A unique member of the phenothiazine group is methotrimeprazine (Levoprome, Lederle, Wayne, NJ). It has been reported to have two-thirds the analgesic potency equivalent of morphine in single-dose studies using 15 mg (Foley, 1985a). It may be especially useful in patients with pain and nausea, with narcotic tolerance, constipation, respiratory depression, or narcotic allergy. Moreover, its mechanism of action appears to be outside the realm of direct opiate-receptor analgesia (Foley, 1985a). Treatment should begin with a test dose of 5 mg IM to see if significant orthostatic

hypotension or sedation results. If not, doses of 10 mg to 20 mg IM every 6 hours may be used (Foley, 1985a). This drug is available for IM use only.

Fluphenazine, at doses of 1 mg every 6–8 hours in combination with amitriptyline, has been reported to be useful in the treatment of certain neuropathic conditions, such as diabetic neuropathy and postherpetic neuralgia (Davis, Lewis, Gerich, et al., 1977; Taub, 1973). Again, no controlled studies have documented this effect.

The basis of the use of haloperidol as a coanalgesic largely rests on anecdotal reports. In one controlled study using 34 patients, haloperidol was compared to placebo as a postoperative analgesic in doses of 5 and 10 mg. The results of this study demonstrated no difference in postoperative analgesia, although good sedation and antiemesis were obtained (Judkins & Karmer, 1982). In a retrospective review of 424 cancer patients receiving morphine alone or morphine and haloperidol in doses up to 30 mg, reduction in the need for morphine was seen at both low and high doses of haloperidol (Hanks, Thomas, Trueman, et al., 1983). Although haloperidol has been reported to be useful as a coanalgesic in doses of 0.5–1.0 mg two or three times a day (Foley, 1985a), its use seems most appropriate for the management of agitated delirium in the patient requiring pain management.

Antidepressants

Antidepressants are also used as analgesic adjuvants. The analgesic effects of antidepressants are possibly mediated centrally by enhancement of transmission in serotonin pathways (Basbaum & Fields, 1978; Carasso, Yehuda, & Streifler, 1979; Watson & Evans, 1985). Moreover, the inability of naloxone to influence their analgesic actions in a rat nociceptive assay supports a nonopiate system mechanism

(Spiegel, Kolb & Pasternak, 1983). Despite the first report, by Paoli, Darcourt, and Corsa in 1960, describing the use of imipramine for chronic pain, studies in humans demonstrating enhancement of morphine analgesia have been lacking. Naturally, depression itself may lead to an exaggerated perception of pain, and chronic pain may, conversely, lead to depressive symptoms. The demonstration of independent analgesic effects is thus difficult. Amitriptyline and imipramine, however, in doses of 50 mg–100 mg, have been shown in various uncontrolled studies to be effective in the treatment of postherpetic neuralgia, headaches, and diabetic neuropathy. In one double-blind study, desipramine, but not amitriptyline, was shown to augment morphine analgesia (Levine, Gordon, Smith, et al., 1986). The analgesic effects of antidepressants have been reviewed recently (France, Houpt, & Ellinwood, 1984). In patients for whom there are no contraindications, amitriptyline or imipramine may be used as an analgesic potentiator at a starting dose of 25–50 mg, increasing every 4–7 days by 25 mg, provided anticholinergic and sedative side effects are tolerated. Although there are no clinical studies using trazodone, it may also be a useful coanalgesic in light of its strong serotonergic effects and low anticholinergic profile. Doxepin is primarily active via serotonin mechanisms and tends to have less anticholinergic side effects than amitriptyline.

Other Agents

Two new drugs may find a use as narcotic alternatives or coanalgesics in the future. One uncontrolled study describes the successful use of clonazepam to treat neuralgic pain with allodynia (Bouckoms & Litman, 1985). Finally, an experimental cholecystokinin antagonist, proglumide, has been studied in 80 human subjects in doses of 50–100 μg IV and found to significantly potentiate the analgesic effects of

small doses of morphine (Price, von der Gruen, Miller, et al., 1985). Further work along these lines may elucidate new mechanisms for controlling pain. The use of adjuvant analgesics in the management of chronic pain is further discussed by Houpt in Chapter 17 of this book.

Nonnarcotic Analgesics

The adjunctive use of nonnarcotic analgesics should not be overlooked, even in situations of severe acute pain, though the nonnarcotic analgesics are generally used for mild to moderate pain. They possess similar characteristics that distinguish them from narcotic analgesics, and their actions are not dependent on centrally acting opioid receptors.

Nonsteroidal anti-inflammatory drugs (NSAID), of which aspirin of the salicylate family is the best known, control pain via the inhibition of prostaglandin synthetase function, thus preventing the formation of prostaglandin $E_2(PGE_2)$. This compound is known to sensitize certain tissues to the pain-producing effects of substances such as bradykinin (Inturrisi, 1985). Most painful conditions are associated with some inflammation, which is remediated by these drugs. Although originally marketed as possessing antiarthritic properties, these drugs have a role in treating a variety of painful conditions, including postoperative pain, dysmenorrhea, headaches, and metastatic bone pain. Moreover, in contrast to narcotic analgesics, nonsteroidal anti-inflammatory agents do not cause dependence or physical tolerance. These agents may however, cause upper gastrointestinal bleeding, diminished platelet function, and salt and water retention.

Nonsteroidal anti-inflammatory drugs include the following drug families with the following representative members: salicylates (aspirin), paraaminophenol (acetaminophen), pyroles (indomethocin and sulindac), propionic acids (ibuprofen and naproxen), and oxicams (piroxicam). Of all these drugs, acetominophen is the least effective anti-inflammatory with the pyroles, propionic acids and oxicams differing from aspirin primarily with respect to their higher analgesic potential and better patient tolerance (Inturrisi, 1985).

The nonaspirin NSAIDs differ primarily in their pharmacokinetics and duration of analgesic action, with their side effects and toxicities being essentially the same (Amadiio, 1984). These drugs may cause central nervous system side effects, including nervousness, anxiety, insomnia, drowsiness, and visual disturbance (Krips & Barger, 1980; Sotsky & Tossell, 1984; Steele & Morton, 1986; Thornton, 1980). The most severe CNS side effects are associated with indomethacin. These side effects include several frontal headaches, vertigo, mental confusion, severe depression, psychosis, and hallucinations. (Flower, Moncada, & Vane, 1980). The psychotomimetic effect of indomethacin may be related to its serotoninlike chemical configuration (Kantor, 1982).

Although there is a body of literature describing increased analgesic efficacy when combined NSAIDs with narcotic analgesics in cancer-related pain (Ferrer-Brechner & Ganz, 1984; Weingart, Sorkness, & Earhart 1985), there are no significant data describing increased analgesic efficacy when combining NSAIDs and antidepressants. Such combinations, however, may be useful in patients with moderate pain and depressive symptomatology. If pain is due to a significant component of inflammation or due to bony metastases, pain relief may be more likely. By avoiding marcotics if possible for such pain, one avoids the side effects, such as drowsiness and constipation, as well as the possibility of physical dependence and tolerance.

NARCOTIC WITHDRAWAL

If narcotics are taken on a regular basis, physical dependence will develop. Physical dependence generally occurs in patients taking oral narcotics for more than 3-4 weeks and, along with tolerance, is a characteristic feature of the opioids. Physical dependence on opioids is best defined as a condition that is associated with withdrawal symptoms after an abrupt discontinuation or significant decrease in dosage. The emergence or withdrawal symptoms occurs more rapidly and more intensely with the use of drugs with shorter half-lives. Withdrawal symptoms are best described as a noradrenergic hyperactivity state and include abdominal pain, diarrhea, muscle aching, yawning, rhinorrhea, and lacrimation.

Narcotic withdrawal (or abstinence) symptoms may create an acute management problem and occur on a predictable and observable basis. They usually appear in order of severity. The consultant is often faced with a decision about "covering" the habit of an alleged addict admitted to the hospital. Many addicts will exaggerate their habit in order to obtain a free high in the hospital. The naive clinician who conscientiously converts what the addict claims to a maintenance dose may inadvertently overdose the patient, since the actual amount may be much less than the patient claims, either because of lying or because the actual amount of narcotic in a "bag" of heroin is less than advertised. It is prudent, therefore, to watch for objective signs of withdrawal before initiating zealous coverage. Objective withdrawal symptoms can be rated using a checklist such as that in Table 16-6. Significant objective symptoms, but not subjective anxiety or drug craving alone, warrant attention with increased narcotic coverage.

There are several options available for discontinuing narcotics in patients who

Table 16-6
Narcotic Checklist

| Name: |
| Date and time: |

Blood pressure
Temperature
Respirations
Pulse Rate

Opiate Craving
Anxiety
Yawning
Perspiration
Lacrimation
Rhinorrhea
Interrupted Sleep
Mydriasis
Goose Flesh
Tremors
Hot/Cold Flashes
Aching Bones/Muscles
Anorexia
Restlessness
Nausea/Vomiting
Diarrhea
Spontaneous Orgasm

Dose & Comments

have become physically dependent on them. One possibility is slow weaning from the specific narcotic to minimize the development of withdrawal symptoms. Bedtime doses should be decreased last in order to minimize sleep disruption. For morphine, a 10–25 percent decrease each day is reasonable. The main drawbacks are the necessity to tolerate some withdrawal symptoms and the extension of drug use over time, especially when the process is initiated on the day the patient is otherwise medically ready to leave the hospital.

Another option is a methadone withdrawal. Methadone was first synthesized by German chemists and used clinically by the late 1940s. The pharmacologic actions of single doses of methadone are qualitatively identical to those of morphine. The outstanding properties of methadone are its effective analgesic activity, its efficacy by the oral route, its extended duration of action in suppressing withdrawal symptoms in physically dependent individuals, and its tendency to show persistent effects with repeated administration (Jaffe & Martin, 1980). A narcotic dependent patient may be put on an equivalent dose of oral methadone (see Table 16-4). Because of an approximately 15-hour half-life after a single dosage and a 22-hour half-life after chronic administration (Inturrisi & Verebey, 1972; Verebey, Volavka, Mules, et al., 1975), the withdrawal symptoms associated with methadone are less intense but more prolonged. The withdrawal process frequently takes up to 30 days, and many drug-dependent individuals require months before they feel free of abstinence symptoms.

Use of Clonidine in Narcotic Withdrawal

The attractiveness of using clonidine is that opiates can be rapidly withdrawn. Clonidine is an alpha-2-adrenergic agonist that substantially diminishes withdrawal symptomatology by replacing opiate-mediated inhibition with alpha-2-adrenergic-mediated inhibition of brain noradrenergic activity, primarily in the locus ceruleus (Gold, Pottash, Sweeney, et al., 1980). Clonidine has no affinity for opiate receptors and thus supports a parallel function that opiate receptors and noradrenergic receptors have in the brain. The disadvantages of using clonidine are the development of sedation and orthostatic hypotension, a slight risk of inducing hallucinations (which stop on drug discontinuation), and some increase in the more subjective signs of withdrawal, including insomnia, restlessness, anorexia, muscle aching, and craving sensations

Table 16-7
Sample Inpatient Clonidine Withdrawal Regimens for 70-Kilogram Man

I.

Day 1:   0.4 mg p.o. test dose in morning, with a repeat 0.4 mg p.o. at bedtime if no
            significant side effects from clonidine

Day 2–10:   0.5 mg every morning (8 A.M.)
            0.2 mg every afternoon (4 P.M.)
            0.5 g every evening (11 P.M.)

Day 11–14: Reduce dose on a daily basis by 50 percent of the previous day's dose until stopping
            on day 14.

II. For moderate to severe opioid dependence
Day 1:   0.3 mg po q3h while awake
Day 2:   0.2 mg po q6h while awake
Day 3:   0.2 mg po q8h while awake
Day 4:   0.1 mg po q12h
Day 5:   Discontinue medication

III. For habit of less than 7 bags of heroin/day
Day 1:   0.2 mg po q3h while awake
Day 2:   0.2 mg po q6h while awake
Day 3:   0.2 mg po q8h while awake
Day 4:   0.1 mg po q12h
Day 5:   Discontinue medication

Source: Clonidine (Catapres) in detoxification (1985). In AJ Gelenberg (Ed), *Biological therapies in psychiatry* (vol 8, pp 13, 16). Littleton, MA: PSG Publishing Co., Inc.
    Hypotension, sedation, and dry mouth are the major side effects.

(Brown, Salmon, & Rendell, 1980; Jasinski, Johnson, & Kocher, 1985). Additionally, it is possible that the concurrent use of tricyclic antidepressants may antagonize clonidine's opiate withdrawal blocking effects via the same mechanism by which they are known to antagonize clonidine's antihypertensive action—direct inhibition of one or more centrally located regulators of sympathetic outflow (Gold, Redmond, & Kleber, 1978; Haggerty & Slatkoff, 1981).

The technique for a clonidine detoxification (see Table 16-7) involves stopping all opiates and beginning clonidine at an every-4–6 hours dosage of 6 μg/kg/24 hours (doses of clonidine are rounded to the nearest tenth of a milligram). This dosage may be gradually increased to 17 μg/kg/24 hours (and the schedule may be spread up to

every 8 hours) over the next week, depending on the individual's objective and subjective signs of opiate withdrawal. If the signs of opiate withdrawal appear gone within a week, the clonidine must be tapered over 3–4 days to prevent the mild hyperadrenergic state caused by abrupt clonidine discontinuation. During the first 24–48 hours of clonidine therapy, close attention must be paid to the patient's blood pressure in order to recognize clinically significant hypotension. The day-by-day withdrawal procedure is well described in more detail in the literature (Charney & Kleber, 1980; Gelenberg, 1985; Traub, 1985).

There are currently two new opiate withdrawal regimens being described in the literature. The first is the combining of clonidine and naltrexone at the onset of the withdrawal regimen (Charney, Heninger and Weber 1986). This regimen is generally too complex for most general hospital settings, especially in patients with concurrent medical illness. In any case, elective narcotic withdrawal should not be undertaken in patients who are acutely ill, since it adds an additional physiologic stress and may complicate the interpretation of signs and symptoms of other disorders.

Another new regimen for opiate withdrawal, currently undergoing clinical trials, is the use of a clonidine analogue, lofexidine. Lofexidine is an investigational analogue of clonidine and is being administered on an experimental basis in dosages of 0.4–2 mg/day in divided doses every 2–6 hours. According to one open trial using 30 opiate-dependent outpatient volunteers, 21 successfully completed the detoxification, with only 2 of the 9 noncompleters attributing their treatment failure to unacceptable withdrawal discomfort. Lofexidine showed significant antiwithdrawal efficacy but no dizziness, profound sedation, or lowering of blood pressure, even at doses as high as 20 mg/day. Lofexidine might, therefore, prove to be a safer and more clinically useful treatment than clonidine (Washton, Resnick, & Geyer, 1983). Finally, although clonidine is widely accepted as a treatment for opiate withdrawal, clonidine is not currently recognized by the Food and Drug Administration as a pharmacotherapeutic agent for opiate withdrawal.

TREATMENT OF ACUTE PAIN IN NARCOTIC ADDICTS

The need to treat acute pain in a methadone maintenance patient or in an illicit narcotic addict generally raises pharmacologic and systems problems. It is not common for such patients to be overtreated or undertreated because of a lack of understanding of addiction management.

Treating pain in patients receiving methadone or naltrexone for drug addiction requires knowledge of the pharmacology of these drugs. Methadone is a synthetic opiate agonist that has strong analgesic properties but produces much less euphoria and sedation than morphine. It is used, therefore, in the detoxification and maintenance treatment of addicts as a substitute for other narcotics to suppress the opiate-agonist abstinence syndrome. Naltrexone is a pure opiate antagonist that attenuates or produces a complete but reversible block of the pharmacologic effects of narcotics, including euphoria and analgesia. It may precipitate mild to severe withdrawal in individuals physically dependent on opiates. It is thought that naltrexone displaces opiates from their CNS receptors in a competitive fashion. It is thus used in formerly addicted patients to block the euphoric effects of narcotics, thereby eliminating the reinforcement for continued use.

In patients on methadone maintenance, it is useful to keep the management of addiction separate from the management of pain. The methadone can be continued for opiate maintenance therapy and a different narcotic chosen to treat the pain. When methadone maintenance is established, the pain can be treated as if the patient were not an addict, except that a 50 percent greater than normal analgesic dose must be used for each dose of analgesic (because of tolerance). Generally, the physician or staff are reluctant to be seen as supporting the patient's "habit"; therefore, addicted patients are often given too little analgesia, whereas the pharmacology of the addition actually necessitates a greater analgesic dosage (Goldberg, 1980). Once the underlying cause of pain is resolved, a reduction of 20 percent daily in the methadone dose may be attempted during hospitalization if one wishes to withdraw methadone maintenance. Ideally, the patient can be discharged to a methadone program.

For patients on naltrexone, the use of narcotic analgesics may be ineffective. Unfortunately, no literature has been found to describe the specifics of treatment of severe pain in patients on naltrexone. It is possible to overcome naltrexone blockade of opiate receptors by using large doses of narcotics.

The alternatives that are available are obviously limited. Obviously, if one can use a nonnarcotic analgesic, such as aspirin or NSAID, with a sedating coanalgesic, such as 100 mg IM hydroxyzine, adequate analgesia may be possible. Another possibility may be to use methotrimeprazine (Levoprome) in doses up to 20 mg IM every 6 hours, as discussed elsewhere in this chapter.

REFERENCES

Amadio P, Jr (1984). Peripherally acting analgesics. In Appropriate management of pain in primary care practice [symposium]. *American Journal of Medicine, 77,* 38–53.

Austin KL, Stapleton JV, & Mather LE (1980). Multiple intramuscular injections—a major source of variability in analgesic response to meperidine. *Pain, 8,* 47–62.

Basbaum AI & Fields HL (1978). Endogenous pain control mechanisms: Review and hypothesis. *Annals of Neurology, 4,* 451–462.

Beaver, WT (1980). Management of cancer pain with parenteral medication. *Journal of the American Medical Association, 244,* 2653–2657.

Beecker, HK (1955). The powerful placebo. *Journal of the American Medical Association, 159,* 1602–1606.

Belville, JW, Dorey F, Capparell D, et al. (1979). Analgesic effects of hydroxyzine compared to morphine in man. *Journal of Clinical Pharmacology, 19,* 290–296.

Bouckoms AJ & Litman RE (1985). Clonazepam in the treatment of neuralgic pain syndrome. *Psychosomatics, 26,* 933–936.

Brown MJ, Salmon D, & Rendell M (1980). Clonidine hallucinations. *Annals of Internal Medicine, 93,* 456–457.

Carasso RL, Yehuda S, & Streifler M (1979). Clomipramine and amitriptyline in the treatment of severe pain. *International Journal of Neuroscience, 9,* 191–194.

Charney DS, Heninger GR, & Kleber HD (1986). The combined use of clonidine and naltrexone as a rapid, safe, and effective treatment of abrupt withdrawal from methadone. *American Journal of Psychiatry, 143,* 831–837.

Charney DS & Kleber HD (1980). Iatrogenic opiate addiction: successful detoxification with clonidine. *American Journal of Psychiatry, 137,* 989–990.

Davis JL, Lewis SB, Gerich JE, et al. (1977). Peripheral diabetic neuropathy treated with amitriptyline and fluphenazine. *Journal of the American Medical Association, 238,* 2291–2292.

Ellinwood EH, Jr (1969) Amphetamine psychosis: A multidimensional process. *Seminars in Psychiatry, 1,* 208–266.

Ferrer-Brechner T & Ganz P (1984). Combination therapy with ibuprofen and methadone for chronic cancer pain. In Ibuprofen [symposium]. *American Journal of Medicine, 77,* 78–83.

Flower RJ, Moncada S, & Vane JR (1980). Analgesic-antipyretics and anti-inflammatory agents: Drugs employed in the treatment of gout. In AG Gilamn, LS Goodman, & A Gilman (Eds), *The pharmacological basis of therapeutics* (pp 682–728). New York: MacMillan.

Foley KM (1982). The practical use of narcotic analgesics. *Medical Clinics of North America, 66,* 1091–1104.

Foley, KM (1985a). Non-narcotic and narcotic analgesics: Applications. In KM Foley (ed), New York: Memorial Sloan Kettering Cancer Center. [syllabus of postgraduate course] (pp 135–148). *Management of cancer pain*

Foley KM (1985b). The treatment of cancer pain. *The New England Journal of Medicine, 313,* 84–95.

Forrest WH, Jr, Brown BW, Jr, Brown CR, et al. (1977). Dextroamphetamine with morphine for the treatment of postoperative pain. *New England Journal of Medicine, 296,* 712–715.

France RD, Houpt JL, & Ellinwood EH (1984). Therapeutic effects of antidepressants in chronic pain. *General Hospital Psychiatry, 6,* 55–63.

Garrett JM, Sauer WG, & Moertel CG (1967). Colonic motility in ulcerative colitis after opiate administration. *Gastroenterology, 53,* 93–100.

Gelenberg AJ (Ed) (1985). Clonidine (Catapres) in detoxification: Caveats and issues. *Biological Therapies in Psychiatry, 8,* 15–16.

Gold MS, Pottash AC, Sweeney DR, et al. (1980). Opiate withdrawal using clonidine. *Journal of the American Medical Association, 243*, 343–346.

Gold MS, Redmond DE, Jr, & Kleber HD (1978). Clonidine blocks acute opiate withdrawal symptoms. *Lancet, 2*, 599–602.

Goldberg RJ (1980). *Strategies in psychiatry for the primary physician.* Darien, CT: Patient Care Publications.

Goldberg RJ & Cullen LO (1986). Use of psychotropics in cancer patients [No. 8 in a series]. *Psychosomatics, 27*, 687–700.

Goldberg RJ, Leigh H, Quinlan D (1979). The current status of placebo in hospital practice. *General Hospital Psychiatry, 1*, 196–201.

Goldberg RJ, Mor V, Wiemann M, et al. (1986). Analgesic use in terminal cancer patients: Report from the National Hospice Study. *Journal of Chronic Diseases, 39*, 37–45.

Goldberg RJ & Tull RK (1983). *The psychosocial dimensions of cancer.* New York: Free Press.

Goodwin, JS, Goodwin JM, & Vogel AV (1979). Knowledge and use of placebos by house officers and nurses. *Annals of Internal Medicine, 91*, 106–110.

Gourlay GK, Cherry DA, & Cousins MJ (1986). A comparative study of the efficacy and pharmacokinetics of oral methadone and morphine in the treatment of severe pain in patients with cancer. *Pain 25*, 297–312.

Graves DA, Foster TS, Batenhorst RL, et al. (1983). Patient-controlled analgesia. *Annals of Internal Medicine, 99*, 360–366.

Haggerty JL & Slatkoff S (1981). Clonidine therapy and meperidine withdrawal. *American Journal of Psychiatry, 138*, 698.

Hanks GW, Thomas PJ, Trueman T, et al. (1983). The myth of haloperidol potentiation. *Lancet, 2*, 523–524.

Heel RC, Brogden RN, Speight TM, et al. (1978). Butorphanol: A review of its pharmacological properties and therapeutic efficacy. *Drugs 16*, 473–505.

Houde RW (1979). Analgesic effectiveness of the narcotic agonist-antagonists. *British Journal of Clinical Pharmacology, 7*, 2975–3085.

Houde RW, Wallenstein SL, & Beaver WT (1965). Clinical measurements of pain. In G de Stevens (Ed), *Analgetics.* New York: Academic Press.

Hupert C, Yacoub M, & Turgeon LR (1980). Effect of hydroxyzine on morphine analgesia for the treatment of postoperative pain. *Anaesthesia and Analgesia, 59*, 690–696.

Inturrisi CE (1982). Narcotic drugs. *Medical Clinics of North America, 66*, 1061–1071.

Inturrisi CE (1985). Non-narcotic and narcotic analgesics. In KM Foley (Ed). *Management of cancer pain* (pp 135–148). New York: Memorial Sloan Kettering Cancer Center.

Inturrisi CE & Verebey K (1972). Disposition of methadone in man after a single oral dose. *Clinical Pharmacology and Therapeutics, 13*, 923–930.

Jaffe JH & Martin WR (1980). Opioid analgesics and antagonists. In AB Gilman LS Goodman & A Gilman (Eds), *The pharmacological basis of therapeutics.* New York: MacMillan.

Jasinski DR, Johnson RE & Kocher TR (1985). Clonidine in morphine withdrawal. *Archives of General Psychiatry, 42*, 1063–1066.

Judkins KC & Karmer M (1982). Haloperidol as an adjunct in the management of postoperative pain. *Anaesthesia, 37*, 1118–1120.

Kaiko RF, Rogers AG, Wallenstein SL, et al. (1981). Analgesic and mood effects of heroin and morphine in cancer patients with postoperative pain. *New England Journal of Medicine, 304*, 1501–1504.

Kaiko RF, Wallenstein SL, Rogers AG, et al. (1982). Narcotics in the elderly. *Medical Clinics of North America 66*, 1079–1089.

Kane FJ & Pokorny A (1975). Mental and emotional disturbance with pentazocine (Talwin) use. *Southern Medical Journal, 68*, 808–811.

Kantor TG (1982). Control of pain by nonsteroidal anti-inflammatory drugs. *Medical Clinics of North America 66*, 1053–1059.

Kruis R & Barger R (1980). Paranoid psychosis with sulindac [Letter to the editor]. *Journal of the American Medical Association, 243*, 1420.

Lee R & Spencer PSJ (1977). Antidepressants and pain. *Journal of Internal Medical Research, 5*(Suppl 1), 146–156.

Levine JD, Gordon NC, & Fields HL (1978). the mechanism of placebo analgesia. *Lancet, 2*, 654–657.

Levine JD, Gordon NC, Smith R, et al. (1986). Desipramine enhances opiate postoperative analgesia. *Pain, 27*, 45–49.

Levy JH & Rockoff MA (1982). Anaphylaxis to meperidine. *Anaesthesia and Analgesia, 61*, 301–303.

Maguire LC, Yon JL, & Miller E (1981). Prevention of narcotic-induced constipation [letter]. *New England Journal of Medicine, 305*, 1651.

Marks RM & Sachar EJ (1973). Undertreatment of medical inpatients with narcotic analgesics. *Annals of Internal Medicine, 78*, 173–181.

Martin WR, Jasinski DR, Haertzen CA, et al. (1973). Methadone—a re-evaluation. *Archives of General Psychiatry, 28*, 286–295.

McLelland J (1986). The mechanism of morphine-induced urticaria. *Archives of Dermatology, 122*, 138–139.

Melzack R, Mount BM, & Gordon JM (1979). The

Brompton mixture versus morphine solution given orally: Effects of pain. *Canadian Medical Association Journal*, *115*, 435–438.

Moertel CG (1980). Treatment of cancer pain with orally administered medications. *Journal of the American Medical Association*, *244*, 2448–2450.

Moldofsky H, Scarisbrick P, England R, et al. (1975). Musculoskeletal symptoms of non-REM sleep disturbance in patients with "fibrositis syndrome" and healthy subjects. *Psychosomatic Medicine*, *38*, 341–351.

Moore J & Dundee JW (1961). Alterations in response to somatic pain associated with anaesthesia: 7. The effects of nine phenothiazine derivatives. *British Journal of Anaesthesia*, *33*, 422–431.

Nagashima H, Karamanian A, Malovany R, et al. (1976). Respiratory and circulatory effects of intravenous butorphanol and morphine. *Clinical Pharmacology and Therapeutics*, *19*, 738–745.

Paoli F, Darcourt G, & Corsa P (1960). Note preliminaire sur l'action de l'imipramine dans les états douloureux. *Revue Neurologique*, *102*, 503–504.

Parolaro D, Sala M, Gori E (1977). Effect of intracerebroventricular administration of morphine upon intestinal motility in rats and its antagonism with naloxone. *European Journal of Pharmacology*, *46*, 329–338.

Popio KA, Jackson DH, Ross AM, et al. (1978). Hemodynamic and respiratory effects of morphine and butorphanol. *Clinical Pharmacology and Therapeutics*, *23*, 281–287.

Porter J & Jick H (1980). Addiction rare in patients treated with narcotics. *New England Journal of Medicine*, *302*, 123.

Portnoy RK (1986). Continuous infusion of opioid drugs in the treatment of cancer pain: Guidelines for use. *Journal of Pain and Symptom Management*, *1*, 223–228.

Price DD, von der Gruen A, Miller J, et al. (1985). Potentiation of systemic morphine analgesia in humans by proglumide, a cholecystokinin antagonist. *Anaesthesia and Analgesia*, *64*, 801–806.

Reuler JB, Girard DE, & Nardone DA (1980). The chronic pain syndrome: Misconceptions and management. *Annals of Internal Medicine*, *93*, 588–596.

Rogers A (1981). Twenty-one problems in pain control and way to solve them. *Your Patient and Cancer*, September 65–75.

Rumore MM & Schlichting DA (1986). Clinical efficacy of antihistaminics as analgesics. *Pain*, *25*, 7–22.

Samter M & Beers RF (1968). Intolerance to aspirin: Clinical studies and consideration of its pathogenesis. *Annals of Internal Medicine*, *68*, 975–983.

Schad R (1980). Brompton's mixture for chronic pain. *Southern Medical Journal*, *73*, 1420–1421.

Shanahan, EC, Marshall AG, & Garrett CPO (1983). Adverse reactions to intravenous codeine phosphate in children. *Anaesthesia*, *38*, 40–43.

Shimm DS, Logue GL, Maltbie AA, et al. (1979). Medical management of chronic cancer pain. *Journal of the American Medical Association*, *241*, 2408–2412.

Snow H (1986). Opium and cocaine in the treatment of cancerous disease. *British Medical Journal*, *11*, 718.

Sotsky SM & Tossell JW (1984). Tolmetin induction of mania. *Psychosomatics*, *25*, 626–628.

Spiegel K, Kolb R, & Pasternak GW (1983). Analgesic activity of tricyclic antidepressants. *Annals of Neurology*, *13*, 462–465.

Sriwatanakul K, Weis OF, Alloza JL, et al. (1983). Analysis of narcotic analgesic usage in the treatment of postoperative pain. *Journal of the American Medical Association*, *250*, 926–929.

Stambaugh JE (1979). Pharmacologic and pharmacokinetic consideration in analgesic regimens. *Hospital Practice*, *14*, 35–39.

Steele TE & Morton WA, Jr (1986). Salicylate-induced delirium. *Psychosomatics*, *27*, 455–456.

Sullivan TJ (1982). Pharmacologic modulation of the whealing response to histamine in human skin: Identification of doxepin as a potent in vivo inhibitor. *Journal of Allergy and Clinical Immunology*, *69*, 260–264.

Szeto HH, Inturrisi CE, Houde R, et al. (1977). Accumulation of normeperidine, an active metabolite of meperidine, in patients with renal failure or cancer. *Annals of Internal Medicine*, *86*, 738–741.

Taub A (1973). Relief of postherpetic neuralgia with psychotropic drugs. *Journal of Neurosurgery*, *39*, 235–239.

Taylor M, Galloway DB, Petrie JC, et al. (1978). Psychotomimetic effects of pentazocine and dihydrocodeine tartrate. *British Medical Journal*, *2*, 1198.

Thornton TL (1980). Delirium associated with sulindac [Letter to the editor]. *Journal of the American Medical Association*, *243*, 1630–1631.

Traub SL (1985). Clonidine for opiate withdrawal. *Hospital Formulary*, *1*, 77–80.

Twycross RG & Lack SA (1984). *Therapeutics in terminal cancer*. London: Pitman Publishing.

Twycross RG & Lack SA (1986). *Oral morphine in advanced cancer*. Beaconsfield, Bucks, England: Beaconsfield Publishers.

Vandam LD (1980). Butorphanol. *New England Journal of Medicine*, *302*, 381–384.

Verebey K, Volavka J, Mule S, et al. (1975). Methadone in man: Pharmacokinetic and excretion studies in acute and chronic treatment. *Clinical Pharmacology and Therapeutics*, *18*, 180–190.

Walsh TD (1984). Oral morphine in chronic cancer pain. *Pain 18*, 1–11.

Wang SSM, Wang SR, & Chang BN (1985). Suppressive effects of oral ketotifin on skin responses to histamine, codeine, and allergen skin tests. *Annals of Allergy*, *55*, 57–61.

Warfield CA (1985). Psychotropic agents for pain control: Clinical guidelines. *Hospital Practice*, *20*, 141–143.

Washton AM, Resnick RB, & Geyer G (1983). Opiate withdrawal using lofexidine, a clonidine analogue with fewer side effects. *Journal of Clinical Psychiatry*, *44*, 335–337.

Watson CPN & Evans RJ (1985). A comparative trial of amitriptyline and zimelidine in post-herpetic neuralgia. *Pain*, *23*, 387–394.

Weingart WA, Sorkness CA, & Earhart RH (1985). Analgesia with oral narcotics and added ibuprofen in cancer patients. *Clinical Pharmacy*, *4*, 53–58.

White PF (1985). Patient controlled analgesia: A new approach to the management of postoperative pain. *Seminars in Anaesthesia*, *4*, 255–266.

Woods SW, Tesar GE, Murray GB, et al. (1986). Psychostimulant treatment of depressive disorders secondary to medical illness. *Journal of Clinical Psychiatry*, *47*, 12–15.

Jeffrey L. Houpt

17
Chronic Pain Management

Chronic pain is defined as pain of at least six months' duration that interferes with an individual's functioning. In contrast to acute pain, total relief cannot be anticipated, there is no adaptive function for the pain, there are no autonomic signs, and treatment is based on a richer interplay of biologic and psychosocial factors. Adaptation to pain or minimizing pain with corresponding greater functioning become treatment goals.

ASSESSMENT

Assessment of the chronic pain patient includes evaluation of the specific way in which psychologic factors play a role in pain. Psychologic factors interact with chronic pain in at least three ways: (1) through psychophysiologic mechanisms, (2) through operant mechanisms, and (3) through overt psychiatric comorbidity (France & Keefe, 1986).

Psychophysiologic Mechanisms

Tension headaches, migraine headaches, temporomandibular joint pain, peptic ulcer pain, and irritable bowel pain all are thought to be significantly related to psychologic factors through psychophysiologic mechanisms. Stress via neural mechanisms initiates physiologic events responsible for the pain. Patients often are unaware of the stressful event and are, in fact, said to be *alexithymic* (Postone, 1986), that is, unable to describe feelings and fantasies in words. Consequently, eliciting important emotional information requires a special adaptation of the psychiatric interview.

Three methods of assessment are recommended to enhance the data gathered from patients with alexithymia. First, it is useful to follow the routine format for a medical history in a rigid fashion. This involves sequentially reviewing the history of present illness, past history, family history, social history, and mental status examination. The psychiatrist is encouraged not to pursue affective leads as might otherwise be done. The interviewer should insist on *specific dates* in every segment of the medical history. One can often make important connections relatively easily between stressful events and the exacerbation of symptomatology simply by juxtaposing

PRINCIPLES OF MEDICAL PSYCHIATRY
ISBN 0-8089-1883-4

dates from the social history with the history of the present illness. This technique allows the needed information to be elicited; the connections are out of the patient's awareness. The connections between stressful events, affect, and pain symptoms should not be pointed out to the patient at the first interview.

Second, the patient is encouraged to keep a diary of events. This diary not only provides a baseline for the treatment program, but may also illuminate the relationship of life events to symptomatology. The patient is asked to record a pain rating each hour, based on a scale in which 0 = none and 10 = worst pain. The patient is further encouraged to keep notes on activities at each entry. Some clinicans provide the patient with a visual analogue scale (VAS) (Huskisson, 1974). This scale consists of a 10-cm line anchored at the left with "no pain at all" and at the right by "unbearable pain." Patients are asked to mark where their pain falls on the scale.

Finally, the diary is reviewed with the patient at each visit. Whether or not the diary is filled out is a major indicator of motivation. Fluctuations in scores from the VAS provide clues to noxious environmental events. The patient is questioned about activities at times of high recordings. No variation or fluctuation in pain ratings suggests that psychologic issues are highly relevant to the pain reports.

The diary also has treatment implications. Comparisons of one week or month with another provide positive feedback to patients, who, too often, are not aware of improvement. Setbacks can be softened by remembering past improvements and by an optimistic attitude that "we should be able to recapture previous ground."

Finally, the family should be carefully interviewed in order to ascertain their assessment of the patient's problem. They are often quite readily able to pinpoint the nature of the difficulty if simply asked, "What, in your opinion, makes these symptoms worse?" or "Do you have any idea what causes the symptoms?" Family members may often pinpoint a stressful event exacerbating pain, when patient interviews and diaries do not, simply because the patient believes that the symptoms could not be related to anything so mundane.

Operant Mechanisms

Some patients' pain complaints and pain behavior are exacerbated by socioenvironmental factors. For them, a chronic pain life-style is positively reinforced by certain life-style factors. For others, socioenvironmental factors lead to stoic denial, thus affecting pain behavior and complaints in the exact opposite direction. In either instance, the experience and activity of the pain patient is significantly altered by operant mechanisms. The importance of operant factors is often independent of the degree of physiologic basis for the pain. Diagnosing "psychogenic" pain based on evidence of operant mechanisms alone is thus too simplistic.

Operant mechanisms can perpetuate pain behavior. Mechanic (1972) has pointed out that our society removes sick people from normal social obligations, such as work or familial responsibility, and absolves them from blame for their condition (i.e., the "sick role"). Once a family has made the determination that the member is sick, a series of rewarding responses is thus set in motion that, by themselves, can cause pain behavior to be perpetuated beyond the normal course of the actual painful experience. After a period of time a psychologic homeostasis is effected within the family, in which pain and illness behavior become the norm. Other family members make adjustments that may in turn be rewarding to them; for example, a spouse now has an excuse not to take on an unwanted responsibility as well. Such a sequence leads to a rigid family culture that resists change.

The consequences to the family can best be investigated during the social history unless it comes up more naturally earlier. The patient can easily be asked, "How has this affected your relationship with your spouse? children? parents? in-laws?" and so on. "How are they adjusting to this?" If an appropriate lead-in is presented, one might say, "It must be difficult for them as well." Additional questions include "How is life different for the family from the way it was before?" "How has this affected your spouse? your interest in sex? sexual performance?" and so on.

Assessing operant factors in chronic pain syndromes requires meticulous attention to the patient's everyday activities. The patient is asked to describe how each day is spent, and the interviewer uses questions to determine the activity of all persons in the social field. The diary described earlier is often useful as a stimulus for probing the patient's daily activities. For example, if the patient reports a routine of getting up at six-thirty, having a cup of coffee, and then going back to bed at ten o'clock in the morning and sleeping until two in the afternoon, the interviewer wants to know who is present at six-thirty, who is present at ten, and what interaction takes place.

The interviewer also wants to assess the impact of the chronic pain syndrome on the patient's life. This involves questions about the economic and legal implications of the illness, as well as the within-family consequences of the illness. Questions concerning compensation are best handled matter-of-factly in the context of the present illness. After the person has explained the injury and the nature of the symptoms, it is logical to inquire whether or not the patient is receiving any compensation for these, whether any further litigation is planned, what the patient has been told about the proposed outcome of his injury, and, given that information, what the patient's plans are.

Psychiatric Comorbidity in Chronic Pain Patients

The development of a psychiatric disorder significantly alters the course of chronic pain. Diagnosis of a concurrent psychiatric disorder alters treatment in that attention must be directed to the psychiatric disorder per se. Psychiatric assessment of chronic pain patients requires evaluation for depression, anxiety, somatization disorder, schizophrenia, somatoform pain disorder, and substance abuse.

Major Depression versus Depressive Symptoms

The concurrence of chronic pain and depression has been repeatedly observed in a variety of conditions (Cabot, 1911; Sternbach, 1973; Timmermans & Sternbach, 1976). From the point of view of treatment, distinguishing between major depression and depressive *symptoms* without full syndromal major depression is critical.

Major depression, as defined by DSM-III-R criteria, requires prominent and persistent dysphoria or anhedonia and the presence of vegetative signs. Psychiatrists frequently are concerned with the utility of DSM-III-R criteria in the face of a physical illness. There is both clinical and research evidence, however, that the traditional criteria, which include vegetative signs, are in fact useful (France, Krishnan, Houpt, et al., 1984). A patient with chronic pain who meets DSM-III-R criteria for major depression should receive pharmacologic antidepressant treatment regardless of the possible influence of chronic pain on vegetative symptoms. (See Chapter 2, by Cohen-Cole and Harpe, on the "inclusive" approach to diagnosis.) Further, patients with endogenous symptoms, such as anhedonia, diurnal variation, actual weight loss, and early morning awakening, should receive drug treatment even if they do not meet full diagnostic criteria for a major mood disorder. It is impossible to predict based on signs and symptoms *alone* which patients with depressive features enmeshed with their chronic pain syndrome will have a positive response to antidepressant treatment. Empirical trials of antidepressant medication may permit a pharmacologic "dissection" of patients who have a strong affective component to their condition that serves to exacerbate pain. A family history of depression is also a useful marker and, when positive, should lead the clinician to consider a clinically significant depression.

Differentiation of patients with major depression from those with depressive symptoms is thus accomplished primarily by descriptive criteria, which have varying degrees of sensitivity in the chronic pain population. Neuroendocrine tests, such as the dexamethasone suppression test or the TRH stimulation test, may provide confirmation, but they allow at most the same degree of specificity and sensitivity that they do in depressive syndromes without pain. Distinguishing *syndromal major depression* from *depressive symptoms* associated with chronic pain is important because many patients with mild depressive symptoms will benefit from antidepressants at relatively lower doses, whereas patients with major depression will usually require higher doses. The use of antidepressants will be considered in more detail later in this chapter.

Anxiety

Symptoms of anxiety are commonplace in chronic pain syndromes. Motor tension, vigilance, scanning, and apprehension are common, whereas autonomic hyperactivity is not usually present. Agoraphobia and panic disorder, however, are not common. When they do occur in chronic pain patients, they should be vigorously treated. Pharmacologic treatment and biofeedback-assisted relaxation are often useful. Pharmacologic approaches are also considered later in this chapter.

Somatization Disorder

It is important for clinicians to identify those patients who chronically experience and complain of somatic symptoms as a way to maintain self-esteem and establish relationships. Typically, these people have a history of somatic complaints extending from childhood and involving symptoms other than pain, such as dizziness, blurred vision, and so on. In such instances, the physician needs to recognize the role the symptom plays in maintaining psychologic homeostasis and must direct treatment to the issues of self-esteem and the need for a supportive relationship. Support, encouragement for functioning, conservative pharmacotherapy, and regularly scheduled appointments that are not contingent on new or worsening symptoms are thus indicated. (See Chapter 8, by Smith and Ford, on somatoform disorders.)

Schizophrenia

The psychiatrist should keep in mind that schizophrenics are often unable to describe their pain syndrome accurately. For example, a patient was transferred to an acute psychiatric unit for a neuroleptic-induced catatonia, and after treatment for the catatonia, she would not put weight on her right leg. It finally dawned on the staff that not stepping on her foot might be a way for her to splint from pain. She was found, in fact, to have a large fecal impaction, and its removal allowed her to resume walking.

Schizophrenic patients occasionally may offer pain complaints, such as headache or back pain, when they are in fact suffering from exacerbations of psychosis. The pain in this case remits with antipsychotic treatment. A history of recurrent, stereotypic pain complaints in association with schizophrenic relapses supports this diagnosis.

Somatoform Pain Disorder

This disorder requires the highest level of interviewing skill on the part of the psychiatrist because it requires the ability to elicit information sufficient to formulate the case psychodynamically. Phenomenologically, the only feature present is the disparity between objective findings and pain complaints; the clinician has to elicit the supporting data so that an inferential connection can be made between the timing of an event and the onset of the symptom. Such an assessment requires an understanding of the individual's life history, including how the patient manages feelings. One clue is the concurrence of the origin of pain and an event of psychodynamic importance. Although the patient may deny the importance of the event, the patient's life narrative will allow the psychiatrist to determine its meaning. One example is the woman who becomes symptomatic at the time her late adolescent daughter is achieving independence and leaving home. One such patient, the oldest in her family, was forced to give up her adolescence to care for her siblings. She consequently married early, assuming more responsibility rather than less, and became symptomatic when her youngest daughter was about to leave home.

Substance Abuse

In chronic pain syndromes, the abuse of alcohol as well as other sedative hypnotics is often a significant factor. An accurate history often requires additional information from family members. Treatment requires withdrawal from the sedative hypnotic. Patients with significant alcohol and sedative-hypnotic abuse problems will require specific treatment for those conditions before any adequate effort can be made to control their pain.

Disability Syndromes and
Malingering

Some patients are thought to seek financial gain from injuries and pain complaints. Those aware of their deceit are termed malingerers. Eliciting information about financial reward is required in all evaluations; however, the use of the elic-

ited material is problematic. Obviously, the presence of financial reward is not, by itself, sufficient evidence for determining malingering. Nevertheless, three caveats serve in treating patients receiving financial reward for pain complaints. First, seek to have the financial issues settled prior to treatment. Second, if it is not possible to settle the financial issues, determine the goal of treatment: is it to enable the patient to return to work, or just to live more comfortably without returning to work? If the latter pertains, begin treatment. Third, if treatment is intended to return the patient to work, set incremental goals, and continue treatment only if they are being met. If they are not being met, discontinue treatment and await closure of the financial issues.

TREATMENT

Initiating Treatment

Treatment begins with the initial assessment. It may involve directing the patient to maintain a diary of all activities and medications in order to gain more information, it may involve referral for additional consultations, or it may involve a specific intervention if the issues are clear enough from the first assessment.

Treatment options involve either inpatient or outpatient treatment and may involve a number of disciplines. In chronic pain, consultation from an anesthesiologist, neurologist, or neurosurgeon is often indicated. The use of behavioral paradigms, including biofeedback training, often involves psychologists. In certain forms of pain, such as chronic low back pain, physical therapy also takes on an important role, as do the services of a nutritionist for those who are overweight.

The decision whether to treat someone as an inpatient or as an outpatient involves judgment based on several factors. Narcotic dependence often requires an inpatient program, although some patients dependent only on oral narcotics can begin with an outpatient trial of detoxification. If unsuccessful, inpatient treatment is again considered. The decision also depends to a large degree on the nature of the pain syndrome. Chronic low back pain often can be helped by an inpatient stay because of the intensity of the intervention allowed. Comprehensive inpatient programs allow psychologists, physical therapists, nutritionists, and multiple medical specialists to create an intensity of treatment that cannot be accomplished on an outpatient basis. Inpatients with chronic low back pain can learn techniques during hospitalization that can then be transferred to a successful outpatient program. Patients with chronic headaches, on the other hand, are infrequently hospitalized unless there is a question of narcotic dependence involved.

The decision whether or not to admit to an inpatient unit is ultimately one of cost–benefit ratio. What is best for an individual depends on the nature of the ailment, the ability of the family or living environment to assist, results of past efforts at outpatient care, and the treatment resources available. All of these issues may require discussion with third-party payors, whose reluctance to pay for inpatient care may dissipate when they are reminded of the costs associated with prior unsuccessful treatment.

Course of Treatment

Whether on an inpatient or outpatient basis, the following treatment sequence generally ensues: pharmacologic and behavioral management early on, family assessment and intervention, and, in selected cases, an individual growth-oriented psychotherapy. The treatment process can be likened to peeling the layers of an onion. The patient must first be stabilized pharmacologically, then assisted to behave in ways that produce the least amount of pain. Of-

ten, treatment requires family instruction and intervention so that improvement can be sustained in the home environment. And, finally, for some patients, a more growth-oriented psychotherapy is the final step in total rehabilitation. Not all patients are required to go through all stages. A patient with trigeminal neuralgia may respond to carbamazepine treatment alone, whereas a patient with chronic low back pain may require all stages of treatment.

Pharmacologic Principles

There are three categories of drugs useful to the psychiatrist in the management of chronic pain patients: (1) nonnarcotic analgesics, (2) narcotic analgesics, (3) psychotropic medications, and (4) anticonvulsants.

Table 17-1 lists the most commonly prescribed nonnarcotic analgesics, including the nonsteroidal anti-inflammatory drugs (NSAIDs). As a group, these drugs are effective general analgesics with some specific anti-inflammatory properties. They are used for mild or moderate pain and are free of addictive potential. Table 17-1 also lists the usual doses and some common side effects.

Narcotics, which are used for moderate to severe pain are discussed in detail in Chapter 16 by Goldberg, Sokol, and Cullen. Tables 16-1 and 16-2 list the commonly prescribed narcotic agents. These drugs are potent analgesics and have addictive potential. Conversion from one narcotic to another is accomplished by use of dose equivalencies presented in Table 16-4.

Pain should be treated promptly (Posner, 1982). If drug doses are placed so far apart that pain is allowed to recur, analgesia become less effective. There is both experimental and clinical evidence to suggest that too little analgesia eventually leads to excessive amounts of analgesics in order to effect pain relief. Too little or too infrequent analgesia often leads to psychi-

Table 17-1
Commonly Prescribed Nonnarcotic Analgesics

Drug	Usual Oral Dose (mg)	Comment
Aspirin	600 q3–4h	Gastric distress, GI bleeding
Acetaminophen	650 q3–4h	Useful with aspirin allergy, bleeding diathesis; overdose can cause severe hepatic toxicity; no significant anti-inflammatory effect
Ibuprofen	400 q4–6h; do not exceed 3200/d	Does affect bleeding time but probably less than aspirin; anti-inflammatory response similar to aspirin; gastric distress less than aspirin; useful in arthritides
Indomethacin	25 q8h; do not exceed 150–200/d	As analgesic, probably not superior to aspirin; useful in arthritides; can cause corneal deposits and retinal disturbance; may aggravate depression
Naproxen	250 q6–8h; do not exceed 1250/d	Similar to ibuprofen; may cause less GI upset
Sulindac	150 q12h; do not exceed 400/d	Similar to ibuprofen and naproxen; needs to be taken only two times a day
Piroxicam	20 qd	Long half-life, requires single daily dose

Note: Patients vary in their pharmacokinetic and pharmacodynamic responses to aspirin and the NSAIDs. Dosages should be individualized. In the case of aspirin, salicylate levels may aid in determining optimal dosage.

atric consultation because of the patient's distress, which can be expressed maladaptively.

Combinations of narcotics and non-narcotics are effective. Combinations of narcotics and nonsteroidal anti-inflammatory drugs (NSAIDs) often have greater effect than either group alone (Posner, 1982). Likewise, combinations of analgesics and antidepressants (both cyclic and MAOI) can have synergistic effects on pain control. For moderate chronic pain, the combination of a low-dose tricyclic with an NSAID often suffices. For more severe pain, antidepressants appear to potentiate narcotics and prolong duration of subjective relief. Bedtime antidepressants, in particular, diminish nocturnal awakenings with pain. Combinations of analgesics with neuroleptics and with stimulants have also

been advocated; these are not satisfactory for long-term use because of the risk of tardive dyskinesia (TD) in the first case and of tolerance or dependence in the second.

Narcotics have a potential for abuse, but narcotic dependence is unusual if pain is later relieved (Posner, 1982). Stated alternatively, narcotics are used in the relief of acute pain but are not usually indicated in chronic pain. One clear exception is those chronic pain conditions which are preterminal, such as cancer pain. In these instances, pain relief is a goal in its own right.

Unfortunately, one cannot always avoid the use of narcotics in chronic pain patients. For those patients who take codeine or oxycodone episodically, there is little problem. If, however, a patient requires regular dosing of codeine or oxycodone as an outpatient, one should attempt periodic withdrawal and drug-free "holidays" for these patients. Escalating doses of codeine or oxycodone are an indication for inpatient withdrawal or at least a second opinion to see if alternative treatments might be possible. A consistent pattern of intramuscular injections of meperidine (Demerol) or similar drugs often requires inpatient withdrawal and treatment.

In the case of chronic pain, intramuscular injections should not be used. Pain must be relieved with oral medications. The rationale is to unlink the stimulus of injection from the effect of powerful analgesics: pain relief and euphoria. Withdrawal from narcotics should be carried out after pain has been relieved. Treatment should allow for the relief of pain using whatever amount of oral opiate is necessary, and only afterward should withdrawal take place. This withdrawal can be carried out easily with a "pain cocktail." To mix a pain cocktail, all narcotics are converted to an equivalent dose of methadone, which is then dissolved in Robitussin liquid to make 30 cc. The methadone dose is decreased by 5 mg or 10 percent (whichever is larger) each day, while keeping the amount of liquid medication constant at 30 cc (Fordyce, Fowler, Lehman, et al., 1973). An example of how this is accomplished follows:

Forty y/o wm, otherwise in good health, is admitted for chronic low back pain. The first full day in the hospital he requires 2 oxycodone tablets q3–4 h (for total of 12 tablets) for pain relief.

12 oxycodone = 5 mg oxycodone × 12 tablets = 60 mg/d

60 mg oxycodone/d = 40 mg methadone/d (see dose equivalencies, Table 16-3)

Therefore orders are written as follows:

Day 1: 10 mg (1 cc) methadone delivered in 29 cc Robitussin (A. H. Robins) (total 30 cc) PO at 7 A.M., 1 P.M., 6 P.M., and h.s.

Day 2: 10 mg (1 cc) methadone in 29 cc Robitussin (total 30 cc) PO at 7 A.M., 6 P.M., and h.s. 5 mg (0.5 cc) methadone in 29.5 cc Robitussin (total 30 cc) PO at 1 P.M.

Day 3: 10 mg (1 cc) methadone in 29 cc Robitussin (total 30 cc) PO at 7 A.M. and h.s. 5 mg (0.5 cc) methadone in 29.5 cc Robitussin (total 30 cc) PO at 1 P.M. and 6 P.M.

The orders continue in this manner. If patient is not showing signs of increased pain, then one would increase the rate of withdrawal by decreasing by 10 mg methadone/d.

The patient is informed that the medication is going to be reduced but is not told the amount. Patients need to be assured that although there may be times of difficulty as their medicines are readjusted, under no circumstances will they be allowed to suffer needlessly.

The third group of drugs useful to the psychiatrist in treating chronic pain problems are those drugs with psychotropic properties. Although little is known of their mode of action, they are often very useful. Prudent clinical practice makes use of these drugs, but also requires honest appraisal and discontinuance if not successful. As can be seen from Table 17-2, amitriptyline, carbamazepine, lithium, and MAO inhibitors are all useful in specific conditions.

In addition, anxiolytics and antidepressants are also useful as an adjunctive treatment for secondary symptoms of anxiety or clinical depression.

Anticonvulsants, particularly phenytoin and carbamazepine, can be useful in three distinct types of pain syndromes. First, they may help pain due to neuralgia. Applications in trigeminal neuralgia and glossopharyngeal neuralgia are well documented, but anecdotal accounts indicate that these drugs may also help posttraumatic or postsurgical pain of peripheral nerve origin. A careful neurologic examination or neurologic consultation is needed to estab-

Table 17-2

Specific Conditions for Which Psychotropics Are Useful (Partial List)

Condition	Psychotropic*
Chronic low back pain	Amitriptyline or doxepin 25–50 mg/d (more if patient is depressed)
Cluster headaches	Methysergide 2mg tid or qid, with 3–8-wk drug-free periods each 3 mo Lithium 900–1500 mg/d × 4 wk Amitriptyline or doxepin 50–200 mg/d
Glossopharyngeal neuralgia	Carbamazepine
Migraine headaches	NSAID Aspirin 300 mg, with codeine 30-60 mg; limit to 2–3/wk Ergotamine tartrate 2–4 tabs immediately, with total of up to 8 tabs per attack Amitriptyline or doxepin or doxepin 50–100 mg (build up slowly; give more if patient is depressed) Propranolol Methysergide
Myofascial pain syndrome	Local anesthetics Phenelzine 15 mg PO qid
Other neuralgias	Carbamazepine Phenytoin
Postherpetic neuralgia	Amitriptyline or doxepin 75–300 mg/d with fluphenazine 1–3 mgm/d
Reflex sympathetic dystrophies	Peripheral nerve or sympathetic block with local aethetic Amitriptyline or doxepin
Tabes dorsalis	Carbamazepine
Trigeminal neuralgia (tic douloureux)	Carbamazepine

* Where anticonvulsants are suggested, adjust dose to usual therapeutic range for epilepsy, unless a lower dose relieves symptoms.

lish the likelihood of a neuralgic component to chronic pain; coincident parathesias or local alterations in sensation are diagnostic clues. When sedation or muscle relaxation is sought in addition to anticonvulsant effects, clonazepam may be considered. Second, anticonvulsants may be useful adjuncts to pain management in individuals with proxysmal EEG abnormalities and episodic exacerbations of pain, whether or not a diagnosis of epilepsy is warranted by the history. Third, they may help patients with true lancinating or "electric" pains.

Use of Adjuvant Psychotropics

Psychotropic medications are prescribed to control symptoms of anxiety and depression. As already described, the most common symptoms of anxiety are motor restlessness and tension, and they can be effectively treated with hydroxyzine, 25 milligrams orally three times a day. Hydroxyzine is not habituating, and its anti-histaminic effects provide negative feedback limiting the total amount desired. This becomes important, since chronic pain syndromes are by definition of long duration, thus making benzodiazepines undesirable because of their tendency to produce physical dependence. Because hydroxyzine potentiates narcotics, nonnarcotic analgesics, and barbiturates, patients must be observed for excessive drowsiness or incoordination. The potentiation of the analgesia, however, supports its use in pain patients. Buspirone, a new nonsedating anxiolytic, would appear to be another rational choice, but not data are yet available to document its efficacy in the chronic pain population.

France, Houpt, and Ellinwood (1984) have reviewed the literature on the use of antidepressants in chronic pain syndromes. As their review suggests, most evidence is anecdotal, though there are a handful of controlled studies suggesting the efficacy of antidepressants in various chronic pain syndromes. Clinical lore and a modest amount of research suggest the importance of serotonergic pathways in inhibiting pain. Tricylic antidepressants such as amitriptyline or doxepin thus tend to be used commonly in chronic pain syndromes without major depression. Lower doses, such as 50–75 milligrams per day, have often proved effective. In addition, clinicans have noted that the effect often occurs within 2 or 3 days rather than requiring a 2-to-4-week period before proving effective.

Higher doses (for example, 150–300 milligrams of amitriptyline or its equivalent of other antidepressants per day) typically are required to treat major depression. Patients suffering a major depressive disorder also differ from the former group of patients in that their pain symptoms improve in a 2-to-4-week period of time, as the depression improves. Consequently, adequate evaluation of patients for major depressive disorder is absolutely essential to the proper pharmacologic treatment of pain patients.

Chlorpromazine and other neuroleptics, such as haloperidol, potentiate narcotics, and thus are sometimes used in acute pain or severe preterminal cancer pain. These drugs, however, have little use in other chronic pain syndromes (except postherpetic neuralgia) because of the potential for tardive dyskinesia.

Behavioral Approaches

Keefe and Bradley (1984) have divided behavioral approaches to chronic pain into self-management techniques and operant techniques. Self-management techniques include biofeedback, cognitive approaches, and multimodal approaches. Operant techniques, on the other hand, include paradigms in which the desired behavior is rewarded and undesired behavior is ignored.

Biofeedback is a technique whereby the patient is taught to control muscle activity. Surface electrodes are placed over target muscles, and feedback about electromyographic (EMG) activities is provided by means of audio or visual display. Most commonly, electrodes are placed on the frontalis muscles over the forehead, and the patient is taught to relax in conjunction with EMG training. An impressive literature establishes its usefulness in muscle contraction headaches (Budzynski, 1978), and there are also reports suggesting its usefulness in migraine headaches (Blanchard & Andrasik, 1982), chronic low back pain, and phantom limb pain (Keefe & Bradley, 1984).

Cognitive behavioral approaches include a variety of techniques. Routinely, patients are taught to imagine pleasant events, to focus on distracting elements in the environment, or to concentrate on other sensations as a way to combat their pain. These approaches are individualized for the patient according to those events in the patient's life that promote distraction. These approaches are often combined with assertiveness training and other cognitive behavioral intervention that might be appropriate for a given individual's maladaptive thoughts and behavior.

For both biofeedback and cognitive behavioral therapies, the patient is encouraged to practice daily. Depending on the clinical condition, the patient may practice on a fixed schedule (one, two, or three times a day) or in response to a pain episode. These exercises are discussed with the patient, with timing and number determined from data in the daily diary. The overall effort is to place patients in control of their behavior, and thus their advice is sought in this process. Patients must continue to be seen on a regular basis to monitor and reinforce the use of these behavioral techniques.

Operant conditioning is based on the notion that behavior is controlled by its consequences. As a result, the likelihood of a behavior's continuing is increased when positive reinforcements become contingent on the behavior. Pain behavior (e.g., complaints of pain, grimacing) thus increases when there is positive reinforcement for it. Fordyce et al. (1973) have established the value of operant conditioning in some chronic low back pain patients. In a program in which nursing staff withheld positive reinforcement for pain behaviors (e.g., complaints of pain) but provided attention for well behaviors (e.g., increased activity), and in which pain medications were given on a fixed schedule rather than "as needed," chronic low back pain patients showed significant improvement. They used a "pain cocktail" to withdraw patients from narcotics, as described earlier in this chapter.

The decision whether to use operant approaches or one of the other behavioral strategies depends on the patient and the problem involved (Keefe & Bradley, 1984). Generally, operant approaches are used when there are no (or minimal) physical findings and when there is a high level of pain behavior. Self-management techniques are used when there is more evidence of tissue damage, shorter duration of symptoms, or less evidence that positive environmental reinforcement will be effective.

Cognitive behavioral strategies have the advantage of placing patients in control of their behavior and thus have the potential for increasing self-esteem. Operant conditioning procedures, inasmuch as they ignore pain complaints, face some difficulty in that they confuse patients and referral sources, for whom pain was the reason for which referral was made. It thus requires much cooperation from the patient, family, and referral source.

Engaging the family as an ally in an operant strategy requires gaining their confidence and then clearly outlining the program in a joint meeting of family and patient. One immediately tries to sidestep the issue of blame and guilt. For example, "I want to outline a program that has worked for other pain patients. You must stop making meals for this patient, and you must not pay attention to the [pain behavior]. The patient does have pain—no one is to blame—but our job now is to get beyond it." Assignments are given and, if not followed, are reexplained. Continued noncompliance requires further analysis of the noncompliant behavior and usually formal family therapy.

Behavior therapy should be viewed both as a specific treatment in the management of chronic pain disorders and as an organizing precept around which extensive rehabilitative programs are developed. In the simplest terms, the patient needs to be placed in a structured environment that assists the patient to cope better throughout all 24 hours of the day. Knowledge of behavior therapy principles are of much importance in this respect. Behavioral programs initiated on an inpatient basis must have outpatient follow-up to prevent extinguishing of newly learned coping techniques learned as inpatients.

Somatic Approaches

Surgical procedures include nerve blocks, nerve stimulators, rhizotomy, cordotomy, and pituitary ablation. The use of rhizotomy, cordotomy, or pituitary ablation requires a discrete pathophysiologic syndrome for which the definitive surgical procedure is indicated. Such a determination requires neurologic and neurosurgical consultation.

Minimally invasive somatic approaches to chronic pain include nerve blocks and nerve stimulators. Nerve blocks are based on the premise that the injection of anesthetics into an appropriate neurostructure can cause a reversible interruption of nerve conduction. The duration of blockade can be determined by choice of local anesthetic. Procaine is short acting, lidocaine is intermediate acting, and bupivacaine long acting. Local pharmacologic effects can be increased by the concomitant use of a vasoconstrictor such as epinephrine. Further, in some low back pain patients, further enhancement can be accomplished by the epidural injection of steroids as well.

Nerve blocks can be categorized by the neurostructure injected. They consist of spinal (subarachnoid), epidural, paravertebral, somatic nerve, sympathetic ganglion, peripheral nerve, and local infiltration blocks. Most commonly used are epidural, sympathetic, and local infiltration blocks (Urban, 1984).

Nerve blocks have both diagnostic and therapeutic importance. From a diagnostic point of view, consistent results from a series of blocks can help to identify a specific pathologic diagnosis. In this respect, nerve blocks may provide the data for a surgical or ablative procedure.

Repeated nerve blocks are valuable in chronic pain if they effectively interrupt motor and sympathetic reflexes in addition to blocking nociceptive impulses. Clinically, their effect may often last longer than would be anticipated pharmacologically. They may cure or ameliorate causalgia or myofascial pain syndromes.

Permanent blocks using such vehicles as alcohol, phenol, heat, or cold are not commonly used because of their poor long-term effects (Urban, 1984). They are occasionally used to treat cancer pain. Psychiatrists who work within a multidisciplinary pain team may fill the role of advising against unsuccessful continued nerve blocks.

Nerve stimulators are increasingly used in chronic pain syndromes. It has long been acknowledged that increasing afferent impulses with counterirritation properties has been useful to modulate pain. Not until recently, however, has technology been available to capitalize on this finding.

The simplest method involves the use of transcutaneous electrical nerve stimulators (TENS). In this procedure, electrodes are attached to the skin and then attached by wire to a suitable generator. Percutaneous stimulators are used less frequently, since they involve implanting electrodes into a neurostructure, as, for example, in the epidural space. The success with percutaneous stimulation in the epidural space in chronic low back pain has encouraged a more widespread use of transcutaneous stimulators. Nerve stimulators are applied on a trial-and-error basis, and patients must experiment with different electrode placements, waveforms, and stimulus intensities before concluding that the stimulation is not helpful. TENS probably is more helpful in pain of musculoskeletal or nerve root origin than in pain of visceral or CNS origin.

CONCLUSION

Treatment of the patient with chronic pain requires adherence to sound pharmacologic and behavioral principles. Maximal recovery from chronic pain often requires family intervention and, in some cases, individual psychotherapy. Psychiatric disorders, when present, require their own treatment. In addition, adjuvant psychotropics are frequently useful in chronic pain.

Chronic pain syndromes are best treated in a multidisciplinary setting. Anesthesiology, neurosurgery, psychiatry, psychology, and nursing all have important roles to play. In addition to providing patients access to these various specialties, multidisciplinary settings allow the professionals to become more efficient by virtue of interacting daily. The psychiatrist fills an important role as the primary psychopharmacologist and psychodiagnostician and formulator of an integrated biopsychosocial treatment plan.

REFERENCES

Blanchard EB & Andrasik F (1982). Psychological assessment and treatment of headache: Recent development and emerging issues. *Journal of Consulting and Clinical Psychology, 50*, 859–879.

Budzynski T (1978). Biofeedback in the treatment of muscle contractions (tension) headache. *Biofeedback and Self Regulation, 3*, 409–435.

Cabot RC (1911). *Differential diagnosis*. Philadelphia: WB Saunders.

Fordyce WE, Fowler US, Lehman JR, et al. (1973). Operant conditioning in the treatment of chronic pain. *Archives of Physical Medicine and Rehabilitation, 54*, 399–408.

France RD, Houpt JL, & Ellinwood EH (1984). Therapeutic effects of antidepressants in chronic pain. *General Hospital Psychiatry, 6*, 55–64.

France RD & Keefe FJ (1986). Chronic pain. In JO Cavenar (Ed), *Psychiatry* (Vol 2, Ch 104). Philadelphia: Lippincott.

France RD, Krishnan KRR, Houpt JL, et al. (1984). Differentiation of depression from chronic pain with the dexamethasone suppression test and DSM-III. *American Journal of Psychiatry, 141*, 1577–1579.

Huskisson EC (1974). Measurement of pain. *Lancet, 2*, 1127–1131.

Keefe FJ & Bradley LA (1984). Behavioral and psychological approaches to the assessment and treatment of chronic pain. *General Hospital Psychiatry, 6*, 49–54.

Mechanic D (1972). Social psychological factors affecting the presentation of bodily complaints. *New England Journal of Medicine, 286*, 1132–1139.

Posner JB (1982). Pain. In JB Wyngaarden & LH Smith Jr (Eds), *Cecil textbook of medicine* (Vol 2, p. 416). Philadelphia: WB Saunders.

Postone N (1986). Alexithymia in chronic pain patients. *General Hospital Psychiatry, 8*, 163–167.

Sternbach RA (1973). Psychological aspects of pain and the selection of patients, *Clinical Neurosurgery, 21*, 323–333.

Timmermans G & Sternbach RA (1976). Human chronic pain and personality: A canonical correlation analysis. *Advances in Pain Research and Therapy, 1*, 307–310.

Urban BJ (1984). Treatment of chronic pain with nerve blocks and stimulation. *General Hospital Psychiatry, 6*, 43–48.

Michael G. Goldstein

18
Intensive Care Unit Syndromes

Medical patients with life-threatening ill-nesses and surgical patients recovering from cardiac, neurosurgical, or other major surgical procedures are likely to experience emotional distress and develop distur-bances of thinking and behavior. The high-tech setting of intensive care, with its noise, bright lighting, lack of privacy, and imper-sonality may itself exacerbate the psychiat-ric intensive care syndromes to be de-scribed in this chapter. The intensive care unit (ICU) staff, too, are stressed by high responsibility, the fast pace, and the often grave nature of their patients' conditions.

The first section of this chapter will describe psychiatric aspects of patient man-agement, focusing on the cardiac care unit. This section will describe typical psychiat-ric syndromes in the medical intensive care setting. Next, the psychiatric aspects of the management of patients undergoing cardiac surgery will be discussed as an example of typical problems in the care of critically ill or surgical patients. Subsequent sections describe the general assessment and man-agement of delirium, brief reactive psycho-sis, and post-traumatic stress disorders in

the intensive care setting, the management of patients receiving mechanical ventila-tion, and the evaluation and management of ICU staff issues.

THE CARDIAC CARE UNIT

It has been estimated that 1,500,000 people will have a myocardial infarction (MI) each year in the United States, and 1,000,000 will survive the acute event (American Heart Association, 1985). A number of authors have described psycho-logic and psychiatric reactions after a myo-cardial infarction (Blumenthal, 1982; Feuerstein, Labbé, & Kuczmierczyk, 1986; Follick, Gottlieb, & Fowler, 1981; Gentry & Williams, 1979; Hackett & Rosenbaum, 1984; Krantz, 1980; Razin, 1985; MJ Stern, 1984; TA Stern, 1985). The Cardiac Care Unit (CCU) is the setting for many of these reactions. These reactions and possible therapeutic interventions will be discussed in this chapter. The other phases of care of these patients will be discussed in the chap-ter on cardiology (see Chapter 22).

Anxiety

Anxiety is ubiquitous during the first 24 hours and is most intense just after admission. Many factors contribute to the experience of anxiety, including fears of death or disability, misconceptions about the meaning of a myocardial infarction and its course, misunderstanding of information provided by staff, misinterpretation of the displays and alarms from the cardiac monitors in their rooms, and restriction on ability to perform usual activities, which may be associated with feelings of helplessness and loss of control (Cassem & Hackett, 1971; Krantz, 1980; TA Stern, 1985). Patients are also concerned about the life problems that they were confronting prior to admission and the effects that the illness and hospitalization might have on their ability to handle these problems (Cay, Vetter, Philip, et al., 1972; Thomas, Sappington, Gross, et al., 1983). Patients who witness a cardiac arrest may be especially likely to develop anxiety (TA Stern, 1985).

Anxiety usually diminishes as patients feel more secure with the knowledge that they are being closely monitored. Simply surviving the first hours reduces panic. Denial, which is hazardous during the prehospital phase of unstable angina or a myocardial infarct, may actually protect the patient during the CCU phase as it serves to reduce anxiety and associated cardiovascular stimulation. Transfer from the CCU to a general medical floor or an intermediate care unit is often accompanied by a marked increase in anxiety, attributed by many to the loss of constant supervision and intensive monitoring (Klein, Liner, Zipes, et al., 1968; Philip, Cay, Vetter, et al., 1979).

Biological factors may also influence the experience of anxiety in the CCU. Patients who are treated with sympathomimetic drugs, such as theophylline or terbutaline, for concomitant pulmonary disease or with isoproterenol for cardiac rhythm disturbances, may develop anxiety as an adverse reaction to these drugs. Anxiety may also be a manifestation of a drug withdrawal reaction to alcohol, sedatives, opiates, or antidepressants. The onset of withdrawal symptoms will depend on the half-life of the particular drug. (See Chapter 10 on alcohol and drug abuse.)

The management of anxiety in the CCU includes both pharmacologic and nonpharmacologic approaches. Nonpharmacologic approaches include providing accurate medical information, explaining the role and meaning of the monitoring equipment, providing emotional support and reassurance, and reinforcing the appropriate use of denial (see the following subsection) (Cohen-Cole, 1985; Cohen-Cole & Bird, 1986a; Mumford, Schlessinger, & Glass, et al., 1982; Thomas, Sappington, & Gross, et al., 1983) Teaching patients relaxation techniques that they may use as needed may also be an effective strategy to reduce anxiety and enhance self-control and self-efficacy, though no standardized, controlled study has assessed this in the CCU or ICU. Patients receiving brief cognitively oriented psychotherapy in the CCU had fewer manifestations of depression and anxiety as well as shorter hospital stays, fewer medical complications, and less functional disability at follow-up, when compared with no-treatment controls (Gruen, 1975). Cromwell, Butterfield, Brayfield, et al. (1977) found that patients receiving information about their illness had a shorter CCU stay, but only if this was coupled either with an opportunity for participation in their care or with diversion. This suggested that if patients are given information about their condition, they should also be given something to do about it.

Several authors recommend that anxiolytic medications be used routinely in the CCU (Cassem & Hackett, 1971; TA Stern, 1985), but there are no controlled studies assessing their efficacy in this setting. Though anxiolytics are usually well tolerated in the CCU setting, they may produce excessive sedation, impair cognition, and exacerbate delirium. Further discussion of the use of anxiolytics can be found in the chapter on psychopharmacology (see Chapter 4). Treatment of withdrawal states and other psychiatric conditions that produce anxiety should also be undertaken, and this is discussed in Chapters 4, 6, and 10.

Denial

Denial, broadly defined as suppression of part or all of the meaning of an event to diminish painful affect, is common in patients admitted to the CCU after a myocardial infarction. Denial, however, can be an effective mechanism to reduce anxiety and fear (Doehrman, 1977; Krantz, 1980). Denial independently predicts rapid medical stabilization of unstable angina (Levenson, Kay, Monteferrante, et al., 1984) and may protect the patient from death during the immediate postinfarction period (Hackett, Cassem, & Wishnie, 1968). Recent studies, however, have not confirmed an effect of denial on overall mortality from myocardial infarction (Levenson et al., 1984).

Denial during the acute phase of recovery from a myocardial infarction usually should not be confronted or challenged. Denial may, however, lead to impatience and intolerance for restrictions on activity, resistance to medical therapy and recommended procedures, and occasionally a desire to sign out of the CCU against medical advice. Struggles between patient and staff over these issues may lead to psychiatric consultation. A combination of education and brief medical psychotherapy will usually lead to adequate adherence to the treatment plan (Cohen-Cole, 1985; Cohen-Cole & Bird, 1986a; Cohen-Cole & Bird, 1986b). If these efforts are ineffective, a family meeting is often useful, as family members may be able to convince the patient that compliance with treatment is important.

Some patients will respond to a request to comply "for their family's sake." Chapter 11 discusses such intervention in its section on personal leverage.

Depression

Depressed mood typically becomes more prominent after the third hospital day, when denial begins to diminish and patients become more aware of the implications of their illness (Cassem & Hackett, 1971). For most patients dysphoria is self-limited and does not require pharmacologic intervention. Minor depressive reactions usually respond to medical psychotherapy or to initiation of formal rehabilitation efforts (Razin, 1985; TA Stern, 1985). Some patients, however, will go on to develop a major depressive episode.

Others have reviewed the assessment and treatment of depression in the medical setting (Klerman, 1981) (See Chapter 2). Some general guidelines for the management of depression in the intensive care setting follow. Before initiating pharmacologic treatment for depression, it is important to consider whether any medications or concurrent medical conditions may be contributing to depressive symptoms. Beta blockers may contribute to the development of depressive symptoms, especially if lipophilic drugs, such as propranolol, are used (Paykel, Fleminger, & Watson, 1982; Petrie, Maffucci, & Woosley, 1982). Less lipophilic beta blockers, such as atenolol or nadolol, or calcium channel blockers are less likely to produce depressive symptoms and should be substituted for the lipophilic beta blockers. If symptoms have persisted for more than 2 weeks, and if there is no evidence of an organic cause for depression, major depressive episodes should be treated. The type, dose, and timing of psychopharmacologic treatment or ECT, if needed, will depend on the physiological status of the patient (Goldstein & Guttmacher, in press; Levenson & Friedel, 1985; Stern, 1985).

Delirium

Delirium may occur in CCU patients, especially the elderly or those with preexisting organic brain disease (Cassem & Hackett, 1971; Neshkes & Jarvik, 1982). The general assessment and management of delirium is described in Chapter 6, by Slaby and Cullen. Factors particularly likely to contribute to the development of delirium in the CCU setting will be discussed here.

Lidocaine is frequently used in the CCU as treatment for or prophylaxis against ventricular arrhythmias in proven or suspected myocardial infarction. Systemic side effects have been reported to occur in 7–50 percent of patients receiving lidocaine in this setting, and central nervous system (CNS) side effects account for a significant portion of these (Rademaker, Kellen, Tam, et al., 1986). A well-controlled study found the incidence of confusion in CCU patients receiving lidocaine to be 11 percent, though patients under 75 and those with severe heart failure were excluded from study. More than half of the occurrences of confusion were severe enough to warrant alteration of therapy. Symptoms were much more common in the first 12 hours of administration than in the subsequent 36 hours. Though there was no clear relationship between the development of toxicity and lidocaine levels in this study, lidocaine-induced delirium definitely is dose related within individuals. Thus, reduction in lidocaine dose may be helpful if delirium occurs (Rademaker, et al., 1986). Tocainide and mexiletine, two recently released oral cogeners of lidocaine, are also especially likely to precipitate delirium.

Delirium may also result from medical complications of acute cardiac illness, such as hypoxia, hypotension, congestive heart failure, and embolic stroke. Therefore, a complete neurologic reexamination is indicated when delirium develops suddenly in a post-MI patient. Withdrawal from alcohol, sedatives, and hypnotics may cause delirium as well, and the cause may be missed, as complete alcohol and drug histories are frequently omitted when acutely ill cardiac patients are hospitalized.

While a search for an underlying pathologic process that would explain the delirium is under way, treatment of agitation is essential. The approach to the agitated critically ill patient is described later in this chapter. Haloperidol is the neuroleptic agent of choice for delirious agitation in patients with cardiac disease, unless the patient has a condition that would be exacerbated by its use (Sos & Cassem, 1980; Tesar & Stern, 1986).

Special mention should be made of the neurologic and psychiatric sequelae of cardiac arrest, which often are unrecognized (Reich, Regestein, Murawski, et al., 1983). Though some studies have found little evidence of neurologic sequelae after cardiac arrest (Bedell, Delbanco, Cook, et al., 1983; Longstreth, Inui, Cobb, et al., 1983), careful assessments of cognitive and psychologic status have shown that these patients may develop subtle signs of persistent cognitive impairment or changes in mood and behavior. Symptoms and signs include fatigue, distractibility, inability to learn new skills, impaired recall, apathy, irritability, petulance, emotional disinhibition, and disturbances of impulse control, insight, empathy, judgment, and social perceptiveness. (Reich et al., 1983; Volpe, Holtzman, & Hirst, 1986). Because of the relative preservation of recognition memory, the absence of motor findings, and the prominent psychologic and behavioral features, patients with subtle organic sequelae from cardiac arrest may have their symptoms attributed to depression or the effects of medication (Reich et al. 1983; Volpe et al., 1986). Careful cognitive assessment of these patients is warranted to improve diagnosis and subsequent management (see Chapter 3).

CARDIAC SURGERY

Cardiac surgery has become a common procedure in the United States. Approximately 190,000 patients underwent coronary artery bypass grafting (CABG) in 1983, and tens of thousands more undergo other cardiac operations (American Heart Association, 1985). The experience of these patients in the intensive care setting will be described in the following section.

Delirium and Other Neuropsychiatric Sequelae of Cardiac Surgery

The incidence of delirium after cardiac surgery is much higher than after general surgery (Goldman & Kimball, 1985). The reported incidence of delirium after cardiac surgery ranges from 12 percent to 70 percent (Breuer, Furlam, Hanson, et al., 1983; Dubin, Field, & Gastfriend, 1979; Goldman & Kimball, 1985). Several factors may influence the risk of delirium after cardiac surgery, the most important of which are the nature of the procedure, the presence of preexisting central nervous system dysfunction, a history of a previous MI, the age of the patient, the length of time on cardiopulmonary bypass, the degree of intraoperative hypotension, the duration of surgery, and the severity of the patient's condition in the recovery room (Dubin et al., 1979; Goldman & Kimball, 1985; Kornfeld, Heller, & Frank, 1978). Delirium is twice as frequent after open-heart surgery (e.g., valve replacement) as it is after closed-heart surgery (e.g., CABG) (Dubin et al., 1979; Goldman & Kimball, 1985; Rabiner, Willner, & Fishman, 1975). Transient neurologic complications occur in a majority of patients after cardiac surgery (Shaw, Bates, Cartlidge, et al., 1985), but persistent disability related to impairment in neurologic function occurs in less than 5

percent (Shaw, Bates, Cartlidge, et al., 1986).

Recent studies using neuropsychologic tests have uncovered significant abnormalities in cognitive function shortly after cardiac surgery in 30–75 percent of patients (Raymond, Conklin, Schaeffer, et al., 1984; Savageau, Stanton, Jenkins, et al., 1982a; Smith, Treasure, Newman, et al., 1986; Sotaniemi, 1983). Correlates of significantly reduced test performance include age greater than 67 years, elevated left ventricular pressure, enlarged heart, and the use of propranolol and chlordiazepoxide. Perioperative correlates include total time of operation greater than 7 hours, duration of cardiopulmonary bypass pump time, blood loss, hypotension, difficult intubation, and insertion of an intra-aortic balloon pump. Postoperative factors included electrolyte abnormalities, longer stays in the ICU, bizarre behavior or disorientation, and depression scores (Savageau et al., 1982a). Available evidence suggests, however, that these neuropsychologic abnormalities are transient in the majority of patients, with fewer than 5 percent exhibiting persistent deficits months after surgery (Raymond et al., 1984; Savageau, Stanton, Jenkins, et al., 1982b; Smith et al., 1986). One follow-up study has shown that some individuals actually show improvement in cognitive function from preoperative levels after cardiac surgery (Willner & Rabiner, 1979). Controlled studies confirm that cardiac surgery produces more neurologic and neuropsychologic abnormalities immediately after surgery than general, thoracic, or major vascular surgery, but group differences disappear after several weeks (Raymond et al., 1984; Smith et al., 1986).

Several mechanisms have been proposed to explain the increased incidence of neuropsychiatric sequelae after cardiac surgery. These include embolization of atheroma secondary to the altered flow of cardiopulmonary bypass; microbubbles from cardiopulmonary bypass; air embolism; inadequate cerebral perfusion associated with low-flow, prolonged cardiopulmonary bypass and with extracranial and intracranial arterial occlusive disease; disruption of sleep-wake cycles; effects of anesthetics or other pharmacologic agents used intraoperatively or postoperatively; sensory deprivation; and preoperative psychologic state (Bojar, Najafi, DeLaria, et al., 1983; Goldman & Kimball, 1985; Henriksen, 1984; Larson, 1984; Milano & Kornfeld, 1984; Shaw et al., 1986; Slogoff, Girgis, & Keats, 1982). The development of psychopathology or persistent cognitive dysfunction after cardiac surgery is a predictor of mortality in the 5 years after surgery (Willner & Rabiner, 1979).

The incidence of delirium after cardiac surgery has decreased over the last decade (Goldman & Kimball, 1985; Milano & Kornfeld, 1984). Factors contributing to this decline include improved surgical technique, which has limited total operation and cardiopulmonary bypass time; modification in intensive care settings, which have decreased noise and sensory monotony; recognition of premorbid factors that increase risk of complications; and preoperative preparation of the patient (Goldman & Kimball, 1985; Lazarus & Hagens, 1968; Milano & Kornfeld, 1984).

ASSESSMENT OF DELIRIUM

Several points regarding the assessment of delirium in the intensive care setting need to be emphasized. *Withdrawal states are sometimes overlooked in the intensive care setting*, for several reasons (Tesar & Stern, 1986). Obtaining a history of substance abuse may be difficult with a critically ill or unconscious patient. The autonomic signs that accompany withdrawal may be masked by the patient's acute illness. Finally, though toxic screens may establish drug or alcohol use, there are no laboratory results that confirm the diagnosis of drug withdrawal. Patients in the ICU are likely to have impairments of several organ systems, any one of which might produce delirium.

Hypoxia and hypotension, common sequelae in the critically ill, may produce transient or permanent brain injury. The psychiatrist should personally review vital sign records and blood gas reports to evaluate this possibility.

Factors that would not produce an organic brain syndrome independently may interact additively or synergistically to produce delirium. In particular, the CNS side effects of pharmacologic agents may be additive or synergistic. Many of the drugs frequently used in the intensive care unit can induce delirium or other organic mental disorders. These drugs are listed in Table 18-1.

MANAGEMENT OF DELIRIUM

As in any setting, the first step in managing delirium is to attempt to ameliorate or reverse the medical conditions contributing to the alteration in mental state. Abnormal behavior is simultaneously addressed, with pharmacologic and nonpharmacologic interventions.

Nonpharmacologic Interventions

Nonpharmacologic interventions that are particularly useful in the intensive care setting are listed in Table 18-2. They are directed at enhancing patients' cognitive function; enhancing communication among patient, family, and staff; preventing self-harm or harm to staff; minimizing environmental stresses; maximizing patients' comfort; and providing support and reassurance.

Explanation and education by staff about illness, procedures, and technical

Table 18-1

Pharmocologic Agents Commonly Contributing to Organic Brain Syndromes
in the Intensive Care Setting

Class of Agent	Agent
Anesthetics	All (especially fentanyl)
Anticholinergics	Atropine
Anticonvulsants	Barbiturates
	Carbamazepine
	Phenytoin
Antihistamines	
Nonselective	Diphenhydramine
	Promethazine
H$_2$ blockers	Cimetidine
	Ranitidine
Cardiac agents	
Antiarrhythmics	Lidocaine
	Mexiletine
	Procainamide
	Quinidine
Beta blockers	Metoprolol
	Propranolol
Cardiac glycosides	
	Digitalis
Corticosteroids	All (also ACTH)
Narcotics	All (especially Meperidine)
Sedative-hypnotics	
Barbiturates	All
Benzodiazepines	All

equipment may help reduce patients' confusion. Communication with patients in an intensive care setting may be hampered by endotracheal intubation or a neurologic condition that impairs language function. Writing notes to staff and family should be encouraged. If the patient is unable to write, the patient may be able to point to letters or words on a chart that has been specially designed for this purpose. If this is not possible, a system of tapping or blinking may permit useful communication. Technical communication aids have recently been developed that permit vocalization despite intubation (Venus, 1980; Walsh & Rho, 1985). Once extubated, a patient with a tracheostomy may speak with the assistance of a fenestrated tracheostomy tube. Family visitation, in general, should be encouraged.

Both sensory deprivation and sensory overload, in the form of excessive noise, may lead to behavioral alterations and potentiation of delirium in the ICU (Hansell, 1984). Excessive noise levels, which have been documented to exist in intensive care units, may lead to sleep deprivation, irritability, and impaired cognitive performance (Bentley, Murphy, & Dudley, 1977; Hansell, 1984). Sleep deprivation and dis-

Table 18-2

Nonpharmacologic Management of Organic Brain Syndromes in the Intensive
Care Setting

Goal of Intervention	Methods
Enhance cognitive function	Reorient frequently Clock, calendar, radio, television in room Provide explanations, education
Enhance communication between patient, family and staff	Encourage writing if unable to speak; use letter board, hand or blink signals if unable to speak or write Encourage family visitation
Prevent self-harm or harm to staff	Use mittens and restrain, using least restraints necessary
Minimize environmental stresses	Provide sensory stimulation, but limit noise from alarms, equipment Maintain semblance of day–night cycle (i.e., dim lights at night) Transfer to general medical floor as soon as feasible Preoperative orientation and visit, when possible
Maximize patients' comfort	Control pain adequately Mobilize (i.e., bed to chair) Permit rest, limit unnecessary awakenings
Provide support and reassurance	Empathy, opportunity to ventilate, support, reassurance

turbance of the normal sleep pattern (suppression of stages 3 and 4 and REM sleep) are ubiquitous in the intensive care and coronary care setting (Aurell & Elmquist, 1985). Though noise, pain, and medications play a major role in contributing to sleep problems in the intensive care unit, some authors suggest that the sleep pattern abnormality is due to the effects of anesthesia or the systemic effects of surgery or illness on the brain's sleep-wake regulating mechanism (Aurell & Elmquist, 1985). To diminish sleep disruption, it is useful to limit noise and maintain some semblance of a day–night cycle (i.e., dim lights at night).

It is especially difficult in the ICU to distinguish between agitation associated with pain and agitation due to delirium.

Pain is often undertreated in the hospital setting (Marks & Sachar, 1973). Though narcotic analgesics may contribute to the development or persistence of delirium, analgesia should not be withheld when pain is known to be present or likely. Critically ill patients who have cancer and bone metastases, severe burns, or recent major surgery will need narcotics if they are conscious. It is best to continue to treat such patients with a moderate dose of a narcotic on a regular fixed schedule to avoid peaks and valleys of blood levels due to intermittent, as-needed (PRN) dosing. Meperidine should not be used in repeated doses intravenously because of the cumulative central nervous system toxicity of a major metabolite, normeperidine (Foley, 1985). Further discussion of acute pain management can be found in Chapter 16, by Goldberg, Sokol, and Cullen.

Pharmacologic Treatment

Controlled studies to test the effectiveness of pharmacologic agents in treating delirium in the ICU have not been done. The recommendations that follow are based upon a review of the clinical literature (Cassem, 1984; Sebastian, 1985; Tesar & Stern, 1986; Wells, 1985). The use of neuroleptics, benzodiazepines, and a group of alternative agents will be discussed below.

Neuroleptics

Neuroleptics remain the drugs of choice in the management of the agitated intensive care patient with delirium, with few exceptions (Cassem, 1984; Cummings, 1985; Eisendrath & Link, 1983; Tesar & Stern, 1986). Although benzodiazepines are a reasonable alternative to neuroleptics in many medical settings, neuroleptics are preferable to benzodiazepines, barbiturates, opiates, and other sedatives in the intensive care setting for several reasons. Neuroleptics do not produce significant respiratory depression, and they are less likely than benzodiazepines, barbiturates, and opiates to further impair cognitive function. Though low potency phenothiazines have minor cardiovascular effects, haloperidol has been shown to have a very safe cardiovascular profile (Donlon, Hopkin, Schaffer, et al., 1979; Dudley, Rowlett, & Loebel, 1979; Settle & Ayd, 1983; Sos & Cassem, 1980; Tesar, Murray, & Cassem, 1985; Tesar & Stern, 1986). The use of haloperidol in agitated ICU patients is discussed in detail later. Though they are safe in most ICU situations, neuroleptics should be avoided or used very cautiously in patients with acute central nervous system injuries because of the increased risk of respiratory paralysis in these patients (Hershey & Hales, 1984). Alternative agents should

also be considered for patients who have evidence of preexisting neurologic disorders such as Parkinson's disease or seizures, and those patients who have developed severe toxicity from neuroleptics in the past.

In the intensive care unit setting, the ideal neuroleptic would have minimum cardiovascular, hepatic, or respiratory toxicity and would be available in parenteral forms. Intravenous (IV) neuroleptics would be most advantageous for two reasons. They would permit more rapid relief of signs and symptoms and, second, would produce more reliable blood levels in critically ill patients, who may have poor adsorption from intramuscular injections because of poor muscle perfusion. Haloperidol is the neuroleptic of choice in the intensive care setting because of its minimal effects on cardiac function, blood pressure, and respiratory function and its low incidence of hepatic or renal toxicity (Donlon et al., 1979; Settle & Ayd, 1983; Shulman, 1984). Administration of IV haloperidol has also been found to be safe in the intensive care unit setting (Dudley et al., 1979; Tesar & Stern, 1986; Tesar et al., 1985; Thompson & Thompson, 1983). Although IV use of haloperidol has not yet been approved by the Food and Drug Administration, this does not preclude its use when indications for IV use are documented. The intravenous line must be flushed with saline before haloperidol is administered if heparin is being used, since haloperidol may precipitate with heparin.

Low-potency phenothiazines are inferior to haloperidol in the intensive care setting for several reasons. They have effects on cardiac conduction, anticholinergic effects, which can contribute to delirium, and alpha-adrenergic receptor blocking effects, which can produce hypotension and drug interactions with antihypertensive medications (Richelson, 1984). Molindone, a nonphenothiazine neuroleptic with low anticholinergic effects and a safe cardiovascular profile, is not available in parenteral form, limiting its usefulness in treating delirium in the intensive care setting (Paper, 1985; Richelson, 1985).

The use of IV haloperidol in the ICU. Tesar and Stern (1986) have described a protocol for the use of IV haloperidol in the intensive care setting that is based on the experience of the psychiatric consultation service at Massachusetts General Hospital. Table 18-3 depicts a modified version of their protocol.

The initial dose of IV haloperidol is determined by several factors, including the severity of agitation, the risks of agitation to the patient, the patient's age, and the patient's previous response to haloperidol, if known. For mild agitation that is not presenting an immediate danger to the patient, a dose between 0.5 and 2.0 mg is chosen, based on the patient's age and history of previous response. In general, elderly patients should be strarted on a low dose because of the possibility of increased sensitivity to the drug's effects (Salzman, 1984). For moderate or severe agitation or agitation that is presenting an immediate danger to the patient (e.g., an evolving myocardial infarction, the presence of an intra-aortic balloon pump), higher initial doses are usually needed, from 2.0 to 10 mg. Some authors advocate the use of even higher initial doses (Tesar & Stern, 1986), but initial doses greater than 10 mg have not been found to be any more effective (Adams, 1984).

After the response to the initial dose has been observed, subsequent doses of haloperidol are based on the level of sedation or calm achieved. Because the peak effect of IV haloperidol occurs rapidly, *doses can be repeated as often as every 20–30 minutes.* If there is no change in the level of agitation 20–30 minutes after the first dose, the dose is doubled. If some calming is noted, the previous dose is repeated. Once adequate calming has been obtained, the interval between doses is increased. Frequent adjustments usually are needed over the first 24–48 hours. Once the patient has been stable for 24 hours, haloperidol should be continued on a regular

Table 18-3

Treatment Guidelines for the Use of Intravenous Haloperidol in the Intensive Care Setting

Starting Dose	
Degree of Agitation	Dose
Mild	0.5–2.0 mg
Moderate–severe	2.0–10 mg

Titration and maintenance
1. Allow 20–30 minute before the next dose.
2. If agitation is *unchanged*, administer double dose every 20–30 minutes until patient begins to calm.
3. If patient is calming down, repeat the last dose at next dosing interval.
4. Adjust dose and interval to patient's clinical course. Gradually increase the interval between doses until the interval is 8 hours, then begin to decrease dose.
5. Once stable for 24 hours, give doses on a regular schedule and supplement with PRN doses.
6. Once stable for 36–48 hours, begin attempts to taper dose.
7. When agitation is very severe, very high boluses (up to 40 mg) may be required (see text).

Source: Modified from GE Tesar & TA Stern (1986). Evaluation and treatment of agitation in the intensive care unit. *Journal of Intensive Care Medicine, 1,* 137–148.

schedule. A useful formula to estimate the daily haloperidol requirement after rapid sedation is to provide half of what was required over the first 24 hours, in two or three divided doses (Eisendrath & Link, 1983). For example, if 40 mg of haloperidol was necessary to control agitation during the first 24 hours, a total of 20 mg is ordered for the next 24 hours in divided doses (e.g., 10 mg every 12 hours).

Until recently, it was felt that there was little advantage in using more than a 10 mg bolus of IV haloperidol at a time or more than 100 mg a day (Tesar et al., 1985). In two recently reported series of critically ill patients, however, very high doses of haloperidol were used to treat agitation without adverse cardiovascular or neurologic effects. Tesar et al. (1985) described the treatment of 4 patients who developed agitation while being treated with intra-aortic balloon counterpulsation for severe unstable angina. Single doses as high as 75 mg and 24-hour totals of as much as 530 mg were used. One patient recieved almost 1500 mg of haloperidol over 5 days without apparent neurologic or cardiovascular complications, though a brief period of hypotension and bradycardia was noted after the addition of propranolol to the regimen. Adams (1984) describes the use of a combination of high-dose haloperidol (10 mg/h) and lorazepam (10 mg/h), an intermediate-acting benzodiazepine, for the treatment of delirium in critically ill cancer patients. Many patients received 240 mg/day of each medication for as long as 15 consecutive days. Again, no significant toxicity was attributed to the haloperidol or the lorazepam, though several of the patients died from complications of their illness. Lorazepam may be problematic, however, because of its tendency to produce amnesia. Surprisingly, there were no reports of significant extrapyramidal toxicity, despite the very high doses of haloperidol (Tesar et al., 1985).

There are, as yet, no controlled studies that compare low- and high-dose neuroleptic regimens in delirious patients. Caution is warranted when considering the use of high-dose neuroleptics to treat delirium in intensive care patients, until more clinical data regarding the effectiveness and safety of this practice are available. Reports of hypotension during concurrent haloperidol and propranolol use suggests cautious use of haloperidol in patients receiving beta blockers (Alexander, McCarty, & Griffen, 1984; Tesar et al., 1985).

Benzodiazepines

Benzodiazepines are alternatives to neuroleptics for managing agitation associated with delirium in the intensive care setting. Some authors actually prefer benzodiazepines to haloperidol in this setting, because benzodiazepines are less likely to exacerbate seizures or produce acute dystonic reactions, akathisia, and other extrapyramidal syndromes (Sebastian, 1985; Wells, 1985). (See also Chapter 4 of this volume, by Stoudemire and Fogel.) They are the agents of choice in treating alcohol or benzodiazepine withdrawal and are also preferred in the presence of status epilepticus, neuroleptic malignant syndrome, and severe Parkinson's disease. They may worsen the cognitive dysfunction of delirium, however, particularly when underlying dementia is present or high doses are used (Salzman, 1984). This is especially true of agents with long half-lives, such as diazepam and chlordiazepoxide, which tend to accumulate, particularly in the elderly (Salzman, 1984). Their respiratory depressant effects increase the risks of respiratory failure and may make weaning from a ventilator more difficult.

Lorazepam is the benzodiazepine of choice for treating agitation in the intensive care setting. Advantages include a relatively short half-life (10–12 hours), no active metabolites, and elimination that is not significantly affected by age or liver disease

(Salzman, 1984). Lorazepam is also available in parenteral form and is the only benzodiazepine that has reliable intramuscular absorption. The initial dose is 0.5–2 mg. Doses can be repeated every hour intramuscularly and every 30 minutes intravenously, and the dose can be increased to 5 mg, if necessary.

Midazolam is a new parenteral benzodiazepine that is being promoted for intravenous sedation for short diagnostic or endoscopic procedures, for sedation before general anesthesia, and as an adjunct to anesthesia regimens (Medical Letter, 1986). Because of its rapidity of action, short half-life (elimination half-life of 1–4 hours), and decreased local irritation, it may become the benzodiazepine of choice for the treatment of delirium in the ICU. Clinical experience with midazolam in the ICU, however, remains limited thus far. Like other benzodiazepines, it may also produce respiratory depression and hypotension. Its half-life is prolonged in the elderly and those with hepatic disease (Byatt, Lewis, Dawling, et al., 1984; Medical Letter, 1986). Benzodiazepine antagonists may eventually prove useful for promoting rapid recovery after infusion of benzodiazepines in the ICU. The experimental drug Ro 15-1788 has been shown to antagonize the effects of benzodiazepines, with few side effects ("Sedation in," 1984).

Other pharmacologic approaches have also been used to treat agitated patients with delirium in the intensive care setting. When patients have not responded to other approaches and agitation is interfering with necessary treatments, such as medical ventilation or intra-aortic balloon counterpulsation, it may be necessary to resort to the use of anesthetic agents or paralytic agents, such as pancuronium bromide, metocurine, or D-tubocurarine (Rie & Wilson, 1983; Tesar & Stern, 1986). In these circumstances, collaboration with an anesthesiologist is advised.

BRIEF REACTIVE PSYCHOSIS AND POSTTRAUMATIC STRESS DISORDERS IN THE ICU

Virtually all patients in the intensive care setting are experiencing the psychologic and physical stresses of having a life-threatening serious illness. The stress of having a life-threatening illness is then compounded by the environmental stresses of the intensive care setting. Weakness, fatigue, impairment of cognitive function, restrictions on mobility, and barriers to communication are ubiquitous in the ICU. Serious burns and multiple traumata are especially difficult to cope with because they are often accompanied by severe pain, disfigurement, loss of body parts; multiple surgeries and procedures, and a prolonged hospital and intensive care stay (Avni, 1980; Mendelsohn, 1983). (See chapter 19, on surgery and trauma, by Riether and Stoudemire.)

Brief Reactive Psychosis

Patients experiencing the combination of the acute stress of a life-threatening illness and the environmental stressors of the intensive care environment may develop symptoms or signs of psychosis. In the absence of delirium or another organic mental disorder, the diagnosis of brief reactive psychosis (American Psychiatric Association, 1987) may be made. Some have used the term "ICU syndrome" or "ICU psychosis" when describing the reactions of some patients to the stress of the intensive care environment. This term is misleading, however, (Cassem, 1984; Tesar & Stern, 1986) because psychosis occurring in the intensive care setting almost always is a manifestation of an organic mental disorder. *Environmental and psychologic stressors and organic factors interact to produce both organic mental disorders and stress response disorders.*

Posttraumatic Stress Disorder and Other Stress Response Syndromes

Patients in the ICU may also develop severe stress response syndromes. Horowitz provides a thorough description of stress syndromes and a guide to their treatment in his book *Stress Response Syndromes* (Horowitz, 1986). The diagnostic criteria for posttraumatic stress disorder (PTSD), published by the American Psychiatric Association in DSM-III-R, are based largely on his work (APA, 1987). The criteria for PTSD are listed in Table 18-4.

The diagnosis of posttraumatic stress disorder is made when intrusive thoughts and feelings, maladaptive denial, and associated signs and symptoms are present, Table 18-4. When the full syndrome is not present, a diagnosis of an adjustment disorder may be appropriate, though the DSM-III-R criteria are not easily applied in the medical setting (APA, 1987). Psychological factors affecting physical condition is an alternative diagnosis.

Horowitz (1986) has described a num-

Table 18-4

Diagnostic Criteria, Posttraumatic Stress Disorder

A. The person has experienced an event that is outside the range of usual human experience and that would be markedly distressing to almost anyone.

B. The traumatic event is persistently reexperienced in at least one of the following ways:
1. recurrent and intrusive distressing recollections of the event;
2. recurrent distressing dreams of the event;
3. sudden acting or feeling as if the traumatic event were recurring;
4. intense psychological distress at exposure to events that symbolize or resemble an aspect of the traumatic event, including anniversaries of the trauma.

C. Persistent avoidance of stimuli associated with the trauma or numbing of general responsiveness, as indicated by at least three of the following:
1. efforts to avoid thoughts or feelings associated with the trauma;
2. effects to avoid activities or situations that arouse recollections of the trauma;
3. inability to recall an important aspect of the trauma;
4. markedly diminished interest in significant activities;
5. feeling of detachment or estrangement from others;
6. restricted range of affect;
7. sense of a foreshortened future.

D. Persistent symptoms of increased arousal include the following:
1. difficulty falling or staying asleep;
2. irritability or outbursts of anger;
3. difficulty concentrating;
4. hypervigilance;
5. exaggerated startle response;
6. physiologic reactivity on exposure to events that symbolize or resemble an aspect of the traumatic event.

E. Duration of the disturbance (symptoms in B, C, and D) of at least one month

ber of psychotherapeutic, behavioral, and pharmacologic interventions to treat a patient who is having intrusive symptoms. These include reducing external demands and stimulus levels, promoting rest, permitting temporary idealization and dependency, providing information and education, helping the patient to differentiate fantasy from reality, suppressing strong negative emotion with anxiolytics or sedatives, and using desensitization procedures and relaxation. Denial states are usually not challenged in the intensive care setting unless they interfere with effective care (e.g., wanting to sign out of the hospital against advice) or decision making (e.g., to have necessary surgery).

PSYCHOLOGIC CARE OF PATIENTS REQUIRING MECHANICAL VENTILATION AND DIFFICULTY IN WEANING

Patients requiring mechanical ventilation because of respiratory failure or other respiratory disorders often experience emotional distress (Cassem, 1984; Gale & O'Shanick, 1985; Mendel & Khan, 1980). Dependence on the machine, loss of control, communication difficulty, fears of death and disability, sensory alteration, and sleep deprivation are some of the psychologic stressors faced by these patients (Cassem, 1984; Gale & O'Shanick, 1985). Many of these patients experience considerable anxiety as they are weaned from the ventilator (Bowden, 1983; Cassem, 1984; Gale & O'Shanick, 1985; Mendel & Khan, 1980; Tesar & Stern, 1986). At times, this may lead to much difficulty in weaning, as hyperventilation and panic may lead to early fatigue and inadequate gas exchange. Anxiety may be exacerbated when patients are not properly informed about the weaning process, when weaning begins before the patient is physically or mentally ready to be weaned, or

when trials on a T-tube or a low rate of intermittent mandatory ventilation (IMV) are ordered so that they terminate only when the patient tires. This latter method of weaning leads to the repeated experience of breathlessness and anxiety, which may become associated with the weaning *process*, producing a classically conditioned learned response. Subsequent T-tube or low-rate IMV trials may trigger conditioned anxiety, which leads to early fatigue and more anxiety and breathlessness in a vicious circle. The experience of "failure" with this method may also frustrate and demoralize a patient if the weaning process is prolonged.

Criteria to assess whether a patient is physically ready to be successfully weaned are readily available and will not be discussed in detail here (Francis, 1983; Gale and O'Shanick, 1985; Petty, 1984; Rie & Wilson, 1983). The patient must be alert and well rested. Delirium or other organic mental disorders are likely to make weaning difficult if respiratory function is close to the minimum requirements for weaning. Associated agitation should thus be well controlled before attempts are made to begin the weaning process. Gale and O'Shanick (1985) discuss psychologic parameters to determine weaning readiness and include absence of delirium, understanding by the patient of the weaning process, and a positive and hopeful attitude in the patient regarding weaning.

Patients should be informed well in advance of the procedures to be followed during the weaning process. They should be assured that they will be watched closely and that adjustments will be made if they have any difficulty. To avoid the development of conditioned anxiety and the repeated experience of failure, trials on a T-tube or low-rate IMV should be ordered so that they terminate after a predetermined period of time. The first trial should be no longer than 30 minutes (Francis, 1983; Petty, 1984). During each trial, especially the first, pulmonary function is monitored and patients are observed closely for signs of fatigue and distress. If the patient tolerates the first trial well, the duration of subsequent trials is gradually lengthened until extubation seems likely to succeed. Patients are given an opportunity to rest for at least an hour between trials, and weaning should be suspended during the late evenings and overnight. Encouragement is helpful, and patients should be praised for their efforts and success. If they express discouragement or impatience with the weaning process, it is very important to provide them with concrete feedback about their progress. Sedatives should be avoided, as they may contribute to fatigue and depress respiratory function. Anxiety and fears frequently can be managed with medical psychotherapy and by reassurance from ICU staff (Gale & O'Shanick, 1985; Mendel & Kahn, 1980). Relaxation training also may help. Severe anxiety and agitation should be treated with low-dose haloperidol.

STAFF ISSUES

The staff working in intensive care settings are exposed to multiple stresses. These include the high volume and rapid pace of the work, the high level of clinical responsibility, the severity and high mortality of patients' illnesses, understaffing, and environmental stresses, such as noise and overcrowding (Caldwell & Weiner, 1981; Stehle, 1981). Nursing staff have few opportunities to rest or escape from the intensive care unit for relief. In modern intensive care units, nurses are called upon to attend to multiple and diverse tasks, which include attending to patient comfort, assessing clinical status, administering medications, intravenous solutions, and blood products, providing enteral and parenteral nutrition, attending to multiple lines and tubes, and monitoring multiple physiologic parameters. They must become familiar with an ever-expanding array of technologic aids that have been developed to care for critically ill patients. Strong feelings about patients and grief over the death of patients are a constant stress for these nurses. Dealing with prolonged care of poor-prognosis patients and having to help families deal with their grief are especially stressful, especially for pediatric intensive care nurses (Caldwell & Weiner, 1981; Woolston, 1984). Intrastaff conflict in the face of great responsibility for clinical care is also a significant stressor (Caldwell & Weiner, 1981; Bailey et al., 1980).

Despite impressions that ICU nurses are highly stressed, studies comparing stress among intensive care nurses with stress among nurses working in other settings have yielded inconsistent results (Cronin-Stubbs & Rooks, 1985; Eisendrath, Link, & Matthay, 1985; Gentry, Foster, & Froehling, 1972). Recent studies have not found differences in levels of stress between intensive care nurses and medical-surgical nurses (Cronin-Stubbs & Rooks, 1985; Eisendrath et al., 1985).

The level of stress experienced by physcians in the intensive care setting has not been well studied. One systematic study of house-staff stress in the intensive care setting found that ICU rotations were not rated more stressful than other clinical rotations (Eisendrath et al., 1985). Of note, the ranking of stresses by house officers in this study was fairly consistent with the results of similar studies of intensive care nurses. Prolonged care of poor-prognosis patients was ranked as most stressful. Dealing with death, feeling insecure about clinical responsibility, and communication problems with staff were also rated as rather stressful (Eisendrath et al., 1985).

Studies that have surveyed strategies for coping with the stress of working in intensive care units have also focused on the experience of nurses. Nurse support groups are described as helpful, though controlled studies of their effectiveness are lacking (Caldwell & Weiner, 1981; Weiner & Caldwell, 1981; Weiner & Caldwell, 1983–1984). Support groups seem to work best if they are initiated in response to a felt need, if the group is highly structured and does not allow early discharge of intense negative feelings, and if the group's problems are primarily interpersonal rather than environmental or administrative (Weiner, Caldwell, & Tyson, 1983). Thus, open-ended, unstructured "gripe groups" are not helpful and may actually increase dissatisfaction.

Comprehensive stress management programs for ICU nurses have been developed, which appear to be quite effective (Bailey, Walker, & Madsen, 1980). These behaviorally oriented programs utilize structured training modules that focus on the development of specific skills. Modules address patient care issues, interpersonal and communication issues, personal stress reduction, and administrative issues. A

workshop format is utilized, led by skilled trainers on off-duty time. Written materials are distributed, and skills are demonstrated and practiced during sessions. Evaluation of the stress program is an important component, as it allows participants and trainers to get feedback about the impact of the program (Bailey et al., 1980).

Interventions to decrease the stress of ICU physicians have not been studied. However, the study assessing stress among house officers rotating through the ICU found that humor, opportunities to communicate with other staff, the opportunity to recover from sleep deprivation and regular activities outside the ICU helped house staff to cope with the stresses of the rotation (Eisendrath et al., 1985). The psychiatric consultant can also play a valuable role by providing house staff and attending physicians with covert emotional support while performing consultations on patients in the intensive care setting.

REFERENCES

Adams F (1984). Neuropsychiatric evaluation and treatment of delirium in the critically ill cancer patient. *Cancer Bulletin, 36*, 156–160.

Alexander HE, McCarty K, & Griffen MB (1984). Hypotension and cardiopulmonary arrest associated with concurrent haloperidol and propranolol. *Journal of the American Medical Association, 252*, 87–88.

American Heart Association (1985). *1986 heart facts*. Dallas: American Heart Association.

American Psychiatric Association (1987). *Diagnostic and statistical manual of mental disorders* (3rd ed, revised). Washington, DC.

Aurell J & Elmquist D (1985). Sleep in the surgical intensive care unit: Continuous polygraphic recording of sleep in nine patients receiving postoperative care. *British Medical Journal, 290*, 1029–1032.

Avni J (1980). The severe burns. *Advances in Psychosomatic Medicine, 10*, 57–77.

Bailey JT, Walker D, & Madsen N (1980). The design of a stress management program for Stanford intensive care nurses. *Journal of Nursing Education, 19*, 26–29.

Bentley S, Murphy F, & Dudley H (1977). Perceived noise in surgical wards and an intensive care area: An objective analysis. British Medical Journal, 2, 1503–1506.

Bedell SE, Delbanco TL, Cook EF, et al. (1983). Survival after cardiopulmonary resuscitation in the hospital. *New England Journal of Medicine, 309*, 569–576.

Blumenthal JA (1982). Assessment of patients with coronary heart disease. In FJ Keefe & JA Blumenthal (Eds), *Assessment strategies in behavioral medicine* (pp 37–97). Orlando: Grune and Stratton.

Bojar RM, Najafi H, DeLaria GA, et al. (1983). Neurological complications of coronary revascularization. *Annals of Thoracic Surgery, 36*, 427–432.

Bowden P (1983). Psychiatric aspects of intensive care. In J Tinker & M Rapin (Eds), *Care of the critically ill patient* (pp 787–797). Berlin: Springer-Verlag.

Breuer AC, Furlan AJ, Hanson MR, et al. (1983). Central nervous system complications of coronary artery bypass graft surgery: Prospective analysis of 421 patients. *Stroke, 14,* 682–687.

Byatt CM, Lewis LD, Dawling S, et al. (1984). Accumulation of midazolam after repeated dosage in patients receiving mechanical ventilation in an intensive care unit. *British Medical Journal, 289,* 799–800.

Caldwell T & Weiner MF (1981). Stresses and coping in ICU nursing: 1. A review. *General Hospital Psychiatry, 3,* 119–127.

Cassem NH (1982). Cardiovascular effects of antidepressants. *Journal of Clinical Psychiatry, 43* (no. 11, sec 2), 22–28.

Cassem NH (1984). Critical care psychiatry. In WC Shoemaker, WL Thompson, & PR Holbrook (Eds), *Textbook of critical care* (pp 981–989). Philadelphia: WB Saunders.

Cassem NH & Hackett TP (1971). Psychiatric consultation in a cardiac care unit. *Annals of Internal Medicine, 75,* 9–14.

Cay EL, Vetter N, Philip AE, et al. (1972). Psychological status during recovery from an acute heart attack. *Journal of Psychosomatic Research, 16,* 425–435.

Cohen-Cole SA (1985). Interviewing the cardiac patient: I. A practical guide for assessing quality of life. *Quality of Life in Cardiovascular Care, 2,* 7–12.

Cohen-Cole SA & Bird J (1986a). Interviewing the cardiac patient: II. A practical guide for helping patients cope with their emotions. *Quality of Life in Cardiovascular Care, 2,* 53–65.

Cohen-Cole SA & Bird J (1986b). Interviewing the cardiac patient: III. A practical guide to educate and motivate patients to cooperate with treatment. *Quality of Life in Cardiovascular Care, 2,* 101–112.

Cromwell RL, Butterfield EC, Brayfield FM, et al. (1977). *Acute myocardial infarction: Reaction and recovery.* St. Louis: CC Mosby.

Cronin-Stubbs D & Rooks CA (1985). The stress, social support, and burnout of critical care nurses: The results of research. *Heart and Lung, 14,* 31–39.

Cummings JL (1985). Acute confusional states. In *Clinical Neuropsychiatry* (pp 68–74). Orlando: Grune and Stratton.

Doehrman SR (1977). Psycho-social aspects of recovery from coronary heart disease: A review. *Social Science and Medicine, 11,* 199–218.

Donlon PT, Hopkin J, Schaffer CB, et al. (1979). Cardiovascular safety of rapid treatment with intramuscular haloperidol. *American Journal of Psychiatry, 136,* 233–234.

Dubin WR, Field HL, & Gastfriend DR (1979). Postcardiotomy delirium: A critical review. *Journal of Thoracic and Cardiovascular Surgery, 77,* 586–594.

Dudley DL, Rowlett DB, & Loebel PJ (1979). Emergency use of intravenous haloperidol. *General Hospital Psychiatry, 1,* 240–246.

Eisendrath SJ & Link N (1983). Mental changes in the ICU, detection and management. *Drug Therapy, 13,* 18–26.

Eisendrath SJ, Link N, & Matthay M (1985). Intensive care unit: How stressful for physicians. *Critical Care Medicine, 14,* 95–98.

Feuerstein M, Labbé EE, & Kuczmierczyk AR (1986). Coronary heart disease. In M. Feuerstein, EE Labbé, & AR Kuczmierczyk (Eds), *Health psychology, a psychobiological perspective* (pp 317–380). New York: Plenum Press.

Foley KM (1985). Medical progress: The treatment of cancer pain. *New England Journal of Medicine, 313,* 84–95.

Follick MJ, Gottlieb BS, & Fowler JL (1981). Behavior therapy and coronary heart disease: Lifestyle modification. In HJ Sobel (Ed), *Behavior therapy in terminal care: A humanistic approach* (pp 253–298). New York: Harper and Row.

Francis PB (1983). Acute respiratory failure in obstructive lung disease. *Medical Clinics of North America, 67,* 657–668.

Gale J & O'Shanick GJ (1985). Psychiatric aspects of respirator treatment and pulmonary intensive care. *Advances in Psychosomatic Medicine, 14,* 93–108.

Gentry WD, Foster SB, & Froehling S (1972). Psychological response to situational stress in intensive and non-intensive care settings. *Heart and Lung, 1,* 793.

Gentry WD & Williams RB (Eds) (1979). *Psychologic aspects of myocardial infarction and coronary care.* St. Louis: CV Mosby.

Goldman LS & Kimball CP (1985). Cardiac surgery: enhancing postoperative outcomes. In AM Razin (Ed), *Helping cardiac patients: Behavioral and psychotherapeutic approaches* (pp 113–156). San Francisco: Jossey-Bass.

Goldstein MG & Guttmacher LB (in press). Treatment of the cardiac impaired depressed patient. *Psychiatric Medicine.*

Gruen W (1975). Effects of brief psychotherapy during the hospitalization period on the recovery process in heart attacks. *Journal of Clinical and Consulting Psychology, 43,* 232–233.

Hackett TP, Cassem NH, & Wishnie HA (1968). The cardiac care unit: An appraisal of its psychologic hazards. *New England Journal of Medicine, 279,* 1365–1370.

Hackett TP & Rosenbaum JF (1984). Emotion, psychiatric disorders, and the heart. In E Braunwald

(Ed), *Heart disease: A textbook of cardiovascular medicine* (pp 1826–1844). Philadelphia: WB Saunders.

Hansell HN (1984). The behavioral effects of noise in man: The patient with "intensive care unit psychosis." *Heart and Lung*, *13*, 59–65.

Henriksen L (1984). Evidence suggestive of diffuse brain damage following cardiac operations. *Lancet*, *1*, 816–820.

Hershey SC & Hales RE (1984). Psychopharmacologic approach to the medically ill patient. *Psychiatric Clinics of North America*, *7*, 803–816.

Horowitz MJ (1986). *Stress response syndromes* (2nd ed). Northvale, NJ: Jason Aronson.

Klein RF, Liner VA, Zipes DP, et al. (1968). Transfer from a cardiac care unit. *Archives of Internal Medicine*, *122*, 104–108.

Klerman GL (1981). Depression in the medically ill. *Psychiatric Clinics of North America*, *4*, 301–317.

Kornfeld DS, Heller SS, & Frank KA (1978). Delirium after coronary bypass surgery. *Journal of Thoracic and Cardiovascular Surgery*, *76*, 93–96.

Krantz DS (1980). Cognitive process and recovery from heart attack: A review and theoretical analysis. *Journal of Human Stress*, *6*, 27–38.

Larson PB (1984). Coronary heart disease: Etiology, diagnosis and surgical treatment. In JB Pimm & JR Feist (Eds), *Psychological risks of coronary bypass surgery* (pp 9–20). New York: Plenum Press.

Lazarus HJ & Hagens JH (1968). Prevention of psychosis following open-heart surgery. *American Journal of Psychiatry*, *124*, 1190–1195.

Levenson JL & Friedel RO (1985). Major depression in patients with cardiac disease: Diagnosis and somatic treatment. *Psychosomatics*, *26*, 91–102.

Levenson JL, Kay R, Monteferrante J, et al. (1984). Denial predicts favorable outcome in unstable angina pectoris. *Psychosomatic Medicine*, *46*, 25–32.

Levy AB, Davis J, & Bidder TG (1984). Successful treatment of endogenous depression with alprazolam in a patient with recent cardiac disease: Case report. *Journal of Clinical Psychiatry*, *45*, 480–481.

Longstreth WT, Inui TS, Cobb LA, et al. (1983). Neurologic recovery after out-of-hospital cardiac arrest. *Annals of Internal Medicine*, *98*, 588–592.

Marks RM & Sachar EJ (1973). Undertreatment of medical inpatients with narcotic analgesics. *Annals of Internal Medicine*, *78*, 173–181.

The Medical Letter on Drugs and Therapeutics. (1986) Midazolam 28, 73–76.

Mendel JG & Khan FA (1980). Psychological aspects of weaning from mechanical ventilation. *Psychosomatics*, *21*, 465–471.

Mendelsohn IE (1983). Liaison psychiatry and the burn center. Psychosomatics, *24*, 235–243.

Milano MR & Kornfeld DS (1984). Psychiatry and surgery. In L Grinspoon (Ed), Psychiatry update: The American Psychiatric Association annual review (Vol 3, pp 256–277). Washington, DC: American Psychiatric Press.

Mumford E, Schlessinger HJ, & Glass GV (1982). The effects of psychological intervention on recovery from surgery and heart attacks: An analysis of the literature. *American Journal of Public Health*, *72*, 141–152.

Neshkes RE & Jarvik LF (1982). Clinical psychiatry and cardiovascular disease in the aged. *Psychiatric Clinics of North America*, *5*, 171–179.

Paykel ES, Fleminger R, & Watson JP (1982). Psychiatric side effects of antihypertensive drugs other than reserpine. *Journal of Clinical Psychopharmacology*, *2*, 14–39.

Paper M (1985) Clinical experience with molindone hydrochloride in geriatric patients. *Journal of Clinical Psychiatry*, *46* (8, Sec 2), 26–29.

Petrie WM, Maffucci RJ, & Woosley RL (1982). Propranolol and depression. *American Journal of Psychiatry*, *139*, 92–94.

Petty TL (1984). Acute respiratory failure in chronic obstructive pulmonary disease. In WC Shoemaker, WL Thompson, & PR Holbrook (Eds), *Textbook of critical care* (pp 264–272). Philadelphia: WB Saunders.

Philip AE, Cay EL, Vetter NJ, et al. (1979). Short-term fluctuations in anxiety in patients with myocardial infarction. *Journal of Psychosomatic Research*, *23*, 277–280.

Rabiner CJ, Willner AE, & Fishman J (1975). Psychiatric complications following coronary bypass surgery. *Journal of Nervous and Mental Disorders*, *160*, 342–348.

Rademaker AW, Kellen J, Tam YK, et al. (1986). Character of adverse effects of prophylactic lidocaine in the coronary care unit. *Clinical Pharmacology and Therapeutics*, *40*, 71–80.

Raymond M, Conklin C, Schaeffer J, et al. (1984). Coping with transient intellectual dysfunction after coronary bypass surgery. *Heart and Lung*, *13*, 531–539.

Razin AM (1985). Coronary artery disease: Reducing risk of illness and aiding recovery. In AM Razin (Ed), *Helping cardiac patients: Behavioral and psychotherapeutic approaches* (pp 157–193). San Francisco: Jossey-Bass.

Reich P, Regestein QR, Murawski BJ, et al. (1983). Unrecognized organic mental disorders in survivors of cardiac arrest. *American Journal of Psychiatry*, *140*, 1194–1197.

Richelson E (1984). Neuroleptic affinities for human brain receptors and their use in predicting adverse effects. *Journal of Clinical Psychiatry*, *45*, 331–336.

Rie MA & Wilson RS (1983). Acute respiratory failure. In J Tinker & M Rapin (Eds), *Care of the critically ill patient* (pp 311–340). Berlin: Springer-Verlag.

Salzman C (1984). *Clinical geriatric psychopharmacology*. New York: McGraw-Hill.

Savageau JA, Stanton BA, Jenkins CD, et al. (1982a). Neuropsychological dysfunction following elective cardiac operation: 1. Early assessment. *Journal of Thoracic and Cardiovascular Surgery*, *84*, 585–594.

Savageau JA, Stanton BA, Jenkins CD, et al. (1982b). Neuropsychological dysfunction following elective cardiac operation: 2. A six-month reassessment. *Journal of Thoracic and Cardiovascular Surgery*, *84*, 595–600.

Sebastian P (1985). Delirium. In JM Rippe, RS Irwin, JS Alpert, & JE Dalen (Eds), *Intensive care medicine* (pp 1079–1083). Boston/Toronto: Little, Brown.

Sedation in the intensive-care unit [Editorial] (1984). *Lancet*, *1*, 1388–1389.

Settle EC & Ayd FJ (1983). Haloperidol: A quarter century of experience. *Journal of Clinical Psychiatry*, *44*, 440–448.

Shaw PJ, Bates D, Cartlidge NEF, et al. (1985). Early neurological complications of coronary bypass surgery. *British Medical Journal*, *291*, 1384–1387.

Shaw PJ, Bates D, Cartlidge NEF, et al. (1986). Neurological complications of coronary artery bypass graft surgery: Six month follow-up study. *British Medical Journal*, *293*, 165–167.

Shulman R (1984). Haloperidol therapy for agitated cardiac patients. *International Drug Therapy Newsletter*, *19*, 8.

Slogoff S, Girgis KZ, & Keats AS (1982). Etiologic factors in neuropsychiatric complications associated with cardiopulmonary bypass. *Anesthesia and Analgesia*, *61*, 903–911.

Smith PLC, Treasure T, Newman SP, et al. (1986). Cerebral consequences of cardiopulmonary bypass. *Lancet*, *1*, 823–825.

Sos J & Cassem NH (1980). Managing postoperative agitation. *Drug Therapy*, *10*, 103–106.

Sotaniemi K (1983). Cerebral outcome after extracorporeal circulation: Comparison between prospective and retrospective evaluation. *Archives of Neurology*, *40*, 75–77.

Stehle JL (1981). Critical care nursing stress: The findings revisited. *Nursing Research*, *30*, 182–186.

Stern MJ (1984). Psychosocial rehabilitation following myocardial infarction and coronary artery bypass surgery. In NK Wenger & HK Hellerstein (Eds), *Rehabilitation of the coronary patient* (pp 453–471). New York: John Wiley & Sons.

Stern TA (1985). The management of depression and anxiety following myocardial infarction. *Mt. Sinai Journal of Medicine*, *52*, 623–633.

Tesar GE, Murray GB, & Cassem NH (1985). Use of high-dose intravenous haloperidol in the treatment of agitated cardiac patients. *Journal of Clinical Psychopharmacology*, *5*, 344–347.

Tesar GE & Stern TA (1986). Evaluation and treatment of agitation in the intensive care unit. *Journal of Intensive Care Medicine*, *1*, 137–148.

Thomas SA, Sappington E, Gross HS, et al. (1983). Denial in coronary care patients—an objective reassessment. *Heart and Lung*, *12*, 74–80.

Thompson TL & Thompson WL (1983). Treating postoperative delirium. *Drug Therapy*, *13*, 30–40.

Venus B (1980). Five year experience with Kistner tracheostomy tube. *Critical Care Medicine*, *8*, 106–109.

Volpe BT, Holtzman JD, & Hirst W (1986). Further characterization of patients with amnesia after cardiac arrest: Preserved recognition memory. *Neurology*, *36*, 408–411.

Walsh JJ & Rho DS (1985). A speaking endotracheal tube. *Anesthesiology*, *63*, 703–705.

Weiner MF & Caldwell TA (1981). Stresses and coping in ICU nursing: #2. Nurse support groups on intensive care units. *General Hospital Psychiatry*, *3*, 129–134.

Weiner MF & Caldwell T (1983–1984). The process and impact of an ICU nurse support group. *International Psychiatry in Medicine*, *13*, 47–55.

Weiner MF, Caldwell T, & Tyson J (1983). Stresses and coping in ICU nursing: Why support groups fail. *General Hospital Psychiatry*, *5*, 179–83.

Wells CE (1985). Organic syndromes: Delirium. In HI Kaplan & BJ Sadock (Eds), *Comprehensive textbook of psychiatry* (4th ed, pp 838–851). Williams & Wilkins.

Willner AE & Rabiner CJ (1979). Psychopathology and cognitive dysfunction five years after open-heart surgery. *Comprehensive Psychiatry*, *20*, 409–418.

Woolston JL (1984). Psychiatric aspects of a pediatric intensive care unit. *Yale Journal of Biological Medicine*, *57*, 97–110.

Anne Marie Riether
Alan Stoudemire

19
Surgery and Trauma

In this chapter the basic issues of the surgical patient will be explored with regard to loss and changes in body image. Cosmetic surgery and reconstructive surgery will be examined. Special considerations for the spinal-cord-injured patient, the burned patient, and the heart transplant patient will be discussed as well. Surgery specific to females will be reviewed, as well as the sexual concerns of spinal-cord-injured and ostomy patients. The head-injured patient will be presented, with special attention to accompanying delirium and behavioral and affective changes. Also discussed will be mutilating cancer surgery and the special issues of patients undergoing amputation.

PSYCHOLOGICAL REACTIONS
TO SURGERY

Patients undergoing surgery are presented with challenges to their body integrity and may experience a change in body image. The two major fears of surgical patients, which appear to be the basis for their anxiety anger or depression, are the

threat of death and the fear of bodily injury and the loss of body parts (Surman, 1978). This physical assault upon the body may be accompanied by pain and feelings of powerlessness and uncertainty. Patients may also have fears regarding their diagnosis and the extent of disease, as well as their prognosis for recovery.

Surgery is a narcissistic injury to the body, which often occurs while patients are separated from their usual support systems, such as family, friends, and employment. This may cause patients to regress and become more dependent on others to care for them. This regression may be partially adaptive, to facilitate patients entrusting their care to "strangers." Regression during illness is usually transient and becomes pathologic only when dependent behaviors become fixed or manipulative, or lead to problems with noncompliance, depression, or psychosis (see Chapter 1, by Green).

The unconscious (and sometimes conscious) conflicts that arise when a patient is operated upon may be very similar to "normal" childhood fears. There may be fear of falling asleep (dying), fear of being alone

PRINCIPLES OF MEDICAL PSYCHIATRY
ISBN 0-8089-1883-4

(abandonment), fear of the dark (death), fear of surgery (mutilation anxiety), fear of parental rejection (nonapproval from the surgeon), fear of not being able to care for oneself (dependency), fear of humiliation (if control of sphincter tone is lost), and fear of strangers.

In an attempt to specifically determine the preoperative fears of patients, Ryan (1975) studied 50 patients about to undergo various surgical procedures. The possibility of having cancer was the predominant fear among the patients he studied. He also found that women expressed their fears more openly than men, and that none of the patients had previously mentioned their fears to their surgeon or anesthesiologist unless they were specifically asked.

The Value of Preoperative Teaching and Preparation

There have been numerous studies showing the value of preoperative teaching and preparation in decreasing postoperative requests for analgesics and promoting shorter hospital stays (Egbert, Battit, Turndorf, et al., 1963; Egbert, Battit, Welch, et al., 1964). Others have reported decreased postoperative delirium in groups of patients receiving preoperative preparation by a psychiatrist (Layne & Yudofsky, 1971; Lazarus & Hagens, 1968). Wallace (1984), in studying patients about to undergo a minor gynecologic procedure, found that patients who received routine care plus a maximally informative preparation booklet had lower stress responses on measures of preoperative fear and anxiety, heart rate, and blood pressure. They reported less pain after surgery, and their behavioral recovery, as measured by time to begin eating, drinking, and becoming ambulatory was quicker than that of a control group that received minimal or no preoperative preparation. At 1- and 6-week follow-up, the prepared group showed less

self-reported anger, anxiety, depression, and fatigue, and had increased vigor. A number of other studies have shown that psychologic preparation for elective surgery reduces hospital stays (Johnson, 1966), and reduces physical complications such as postoperative vomiting (Dumas, 1963).

In addition to these cognitive approaches for preoperative preparation, specific behavioral methods are also useful. Instruction in self-care behaviors such as preoperative relaxation exercises, deep breathing techniques, coughing, and leg exercises may be particularly helpful (Johnson, 1984).

Sometimes when a physician attempts to prepare a patient for surgery the patient may not hear what is being said. In a study of cardiac patients undergoing open-heart surgery, all the patients "forgot" large portions of the preoperative discussion, which had been tape-recorded. Four to 6 months postoperatively some patients denied hearing certain details regarding the procedure or the surgical risk (Robinson & Merav, 1976). These patients may have used denial or repression to deal with their illness and fears of surgery, or perhaps they were so transiently overwhelmed by the multiple stresses of hospitalization that they were not able to fully integrate the new information.

Since surgery involves stresses that threaten a patient's autonomy and independence, some degree of worry and fear may serve an adaptive function. Patients who worry prior to an operation may actually strengthen the coping skills they will use in dealing with the surgical experience. This might be similar to the "working through" stage of a grief process, in which the end result is the acceptance of the loss and a reduction in the anxiety and fear. Also, this fear or worry might help the patient to practice visualizing different outcomes of the surgery and postoperative course and thereby to gain a sense of mastery and control of the potential outcome.

Patients may have fantasies about their operation, which they will never share unless asked. One way to get this information is to ask patients to draw a picture of what they think the procedure is. In doing this, misinformation can be corrected, and a clearer understanding of proposed surgery can be promoted.

Patients may not understand the proposed surgery because of ignorance about basic anatomy or physiology. For example, a study of 81 patients that attempted to assess lay knowledge of bodily functions showed that only 23 percent had a vague understanding of basic anatomy. Some common misconceptions were that the stomach was the same as the abdominal cavity and that *duodenum* was the name of an ulcer and not part of the gastrointestinal tract. Six percent confused the rectum and anus with the vagina and uterus (Pearson & Dudley, 1982). A preoperative visit to discuss the proposed procedure, the expected outcome and possible complications will help to clarify the patient's goals and explore the patient's motivation for the surgery and will be helpful in assessing the patient's psychologic health and coping skills.

POSTOPERATIVE DELIRIUM

Postoperative delirium is not rare, nor is it limited to specific surgical procedures or a specific type of patient. One study found 10–15 percent incidence of general surgical patients age 65 and older to be delirious after their operations (Millar, 1981), and another found a 78 percent delirium in a random sample of 200 general surgical patients (Titchner, Zwerling, & Gottschalk, 1956). Operations known to have a particularly high incidence of postoperative delirium include ophthalmologic procedures and cardiac surgery.

Postoperative delirium may not appear until the third or fourth postoperative day and may be related to the cumulative effect of medications, metabolic disorders, decreased sensory input, and decreased sleep. Usually delirium comes on abruptly and is short-lived. Periods lasting longer than a week should alert the physician to search for additional specific causes prolonging the delirium.

In assessing the etiology of postoperative delirium, an accurate record of all the patient's medicines with their total daily doses should be recorded, and special attention should be paid to narcotic analgesics, cardiac drugs, and any medications with anticholinergic activity. This should be based on nurses' records rather than the doctor's order sheet, as errors in transcription or administration are occasionally made. The usual spectrum of toxic, metabolic, and infectious causes should be considered, as well as embolic phenomena in patients at risk. The assessment and management of delirium is further discussed in Chapter 6, by Slaby and Cullen and in Chapter 18, by Goldstein.

THE BURN PATIENT

The severely burned patient is likely to exhibit a spectrum of emotions, from fear and anxiety to anger and depression (West & Shuck, 1978). Sometimes, however, immediately after the burn, patients may appear to have a dissociated calm, in contrast to the emotional reactions of their family and friends (Imbus & Zawacki, 1977). Later, there may be emotional lability or periods of delirium, psychosis, or pathologic regression and passivity. In one study two-thirds of severely burned adults exhibited psychiatric complications of such severity as to be deemed life-threatening (Steiner & Clark, 1977).

Unlike patients with chronic illnesses, burn patients frequently have been well all of their lives and suddenly find themselves in the hospital with a blackened body, in excruciating pain, lying nude before strangers who are telling them that they need to debride their already raw skin. Burn patients have suffered a narcissistic injury and must grieve this loss of body image. Pathologic regression may result when the grief process is arrested (Steiner & Clark, 1977). When this occurs, the patient may refuse to sign the consent form for proposed skin grafts. Furthermore, burn patients are often totally dependent on others for their most basic bodily needs, such as fluid intake, nutrition, pain control, and prevention of sepsis. For patients with conflicts over this dependency, noncompliance with treatment may serve as an effective, although maladaptive, route to a sense of autonomy and control.

Many times burn patients are on a respirator as well, and may not be able to verbalize their fears. A note pad by the bedside, or written flash cards with frequent responses that patients can point to, may be helpful. For those patients who can talk, opportunities for catharsis should be provided. Emotional venting may also be useful for the patient's family and for burn unit staff.

Burn patients may become delirious or develop a characteristic "burn psychosis" (West & Shuch, 1978) that may be a harbinger of sepsis or electrolyte imbalance or may represent an encephalopathy directly related to the burn (Andreasen, Hartford, Knott, et al., 1974). "Burn psychosis" can be treated symptomatically with a low dose of neuroleptic while other causes of delirium are sought and corrected. Chlorpromazine has been reported to be especially useful because of its sedative, antipruritic, antiemetic, and narcotic-analgesic-potentiating effects in this group of patients (Harper, 1978).

The pain of severe burns is freqently treated with a combination of narcotics and anxiolytics. The ample use of medications is of critical importance in breaking the anxiety–pain cycle, and benzodiazepines may be useful as a premedication prior to debridement. The reader is referred to Chapters 16 and 17 for more specific recommendations on pain management. Ketamine, which is frequently used to reduce the pain of debridement, may cause terrifying nightmares in some patients (Surman, 1978).

Burn patients may become depressed over repeated grafting, being immobilized, and the reality of scarring, possible contractures, and loss of function. Patients with facial or genital burns often voice suicidal ideation. Medical psychotherapy and, in some cases, antidepressants should be offered.

Patients beginning physical therapy and rehabilitation after their burns have begun to heal may experience difficulty in dealing with their decreased function or in looking into the mirror for the first time. After having been considered normal on the burn unit, the patient may experience stares or intrusive questions after leaving the unit. Some patients then experience a "social death" (Ravenscroft, 1982), in which they withdraw from activities involving others and lead a schizoid existence.

Patients may become very self-conscious about scarring to their faces and may request reconstructive procedures. Most facial scars, however, should be treated conservatively, utilizing elastic pressure masks for 1 or 2 years. Attempts to reconstruct earlier than 2 years following the burn are often unsuccessful, since the tissue remains hyperactive for at least 1 year after injury (Curreri, 1979). Psychotherapy may help patients tolerate the long wait for reconstruction.

Children in the Burn Unit

Children who are burned often have difficulty understanding painful procedures and may feel that they have been bad and are being punished by physical pain and separation from their families (West & Shuck, 1978). When a child is burned, there is often grief or anger in the parents over the circumstances in which the child was burned. They may become overprotective of the child or be emotionally unable to visit the child because of their own grief. Therapy for the family may mitigate these problems.

Depending on the age of the child when burned, it may be therapeutic to attempt to give the child some sense of mastery or control over the experience. Allowing children to help in removing their bandages or having them apply bandages to a doll may ease dressing changes. Some children tolerate debridement better if they bring a toy into the tub with them. Other games such as burn-bath play, in which the child is allowed to sit in the tub without being debrided, may help ease the child's fears of the tub (Ravenscroft, 1982).

Studying the burned child helps us to understand the development of body image in adults. Deutsch (1955) postulated that the sensory organs of touch, pain, sight, and position facilitate the formation of early body images and concepts. Stoddard (1982) studied the burned child at different ages of development with special attention to the developing body image. He drew inferences about the emerging development of self, based on work with burned infants, school-aged children, and teenagers. He found that children under 2 years of age depend on their mother for a stable sense of body image. He felt that separation from mother after bodily trauma is experienced as bodily hurt and that disfigurement at this stage of life is incorporated into the child's sense of body image and is linked to separation from mother. Also, any disfigurement at this early age leads to increased fears that they are like the unlovable monsters of their fantasy life (Stoddard, 1982). Often, children at this age know the parts of their body that hurt, and they think of these parts as bad. These "bad" parts grow with

them into adulthood, and some authors believe that they may have cognitive distortions as a result (Stoddard, 1982).

The school-aged child is aware of a change in body image after the burn and grieves the loss. These children can frequently act out the trauma in their play as they talk through situations with their dolls. Children's drawing at this age can also reflect changes in body image. Guilt and fears of punishment are frequent and may be related to incompletely resolved oedipal conflicts.

The teenage years are a period of change and a time when body image is very important to a "sense of self." It is a time of intense narcissistic investment in body image. If the burns involve organs with sexual meanings, such as the face, genitals, breasts, or hands, "there will be fears of sexual inadequacy, bodily annihilation, or castration" (Stoddard, 1982). Teenage burn victims will frequently have dreams of being "normal" again and might have unconscious guilt "that their burn was a punishment for their emerging sexual or aggressive feelings" (Stoddard, 1982).

As with adults, if attention to disruption in body image is not worked through, the child might not develop a reintegrated body image. This might lead to body image conflicts, social isolation, or sexual conflicts.

CARDIAC TRANSPLANTATION

Receiving a new heart involves an internal change of body image and, in a sense, an integration of two persons that "match": one terminally ill, the other one dead. This foreign body surgically implanted into the donor represents the death of one person and the possibility of life for another. This may lead the recipient to experience "survival guilt." This guilt, occurs when an individual survives because of the death of someone else, which, in the language of the unconscious, means that the other person had to be killed (Blancher, 1978; Castelnuovo-Tedesco, 1973).

A heart transplant recipient incorporates an object that formerly kept another person alive. In one reported case, a patient became severely regressed after surgery when he learned that he had a woman's heart. In his very primitive, regressed state, he worried that he had "stolen what did not or should not belong to him, namely, his mother's heart" (Castelnuovo-Tedesco, 1970). Later, as part of a postoperative state, he heard his mother calling to him that she was coming back to retrieve what belonged to her; and by this process she could absorb and incorporate him just as he had done earlier when he acquired her heart" (Castelnuovo-Tedesco, 1970).

Unconscious fears of mutilation may lead to preoperative anxiety in these patients, for patients realize at some level that their beating hearts will be taken out of the body and that their only chance for survival involves replacing the heart with a dead person's heart. There may be fears of annihilation (Castelnuovo-Tedesco, 1973), and the patient may exhibit pathologic regression that might interfere with the incorporation of the donor heart into the internal body image. Very little is known about one's sense of internal body image; some patients, on hearing they have received a heart from the opposite sex, worry about their sexual identity postoperatively (Kraft, 1971).

The most common coping mechanism in the heart transplant patient is denial (Mai, 1986). Frequently, the recipient will deny any feelings or emotions connected with the transplant. This denial may be a way of dealing with the unconscious ambivalent feelings that some patients have regarding their transplant. Although these patients may often have dreams involving theft or wrongful acts, they are frequently not aware of any anxiety or guilt in receiving someone else's heart. Other patients

reduce the heart into "just a pump" or "just a muscle" and talk about it as a "worn-out part" that is being replaced by a "new" one. The difference, however, is that it is not a "spare part," but one that represents the life-and-death struggle, possible freedom from pain, and prolongation of life. In studying renal transplant patients, Kemph (1966) found that although the recipients may deny any feelings toward the donors, their responses on the Thematic Apperception Test (TAT) were preoccupied with theft, robbing, and punishment. This seems to suggest that these conflicts and affects associated with the transplant have become unconscious through repression and may be undetected if projective testing is not done. The dreams of transplant patients may offer another approach to their unconscious conflicts.

Preoperative screening of patients for a heart transplant includes assessing the psychologic implications of the decision. The patient and the family should be interviewed prior to being placed on a transplant list, and the entire transplant team, including surgeon, cardiologist, psychiatrist, social worker, and clinical nurse specialist, should feel comfortable in the selection of a particular patient. Patients with unrealistic expectations, previous histories of noncompliance, self-destructive behaviors, or histories of psychosis or severe character pathology are relatively poor candidates for a heart transplant. Patients with a history of alcoholism or other drug addictions might be required to receive treatment for chemical dependency and have a minimum of 6 months of continuous sobriety before undergoing surgery, if such a delay would not be life-threatening. These patients might also be required to take disulfiram or have random drug screens as part of their preoperative assessment and care.

Because denial is so prominent in patients with chronic illness, they may deny the extent of their myocardial disease and so have a difficult time postoperatively adjusting to any limitations or complications of the surgery (since they were never "that ill" in the first place). The fantasies of the patient regarding a transplant need to be explored because some patients who have undergone severe postoperative depressions had almost magical preoperative expectations of their surgery (Kraft, 1971). To facilitate adjustment, prediction of the psychologic impact that the transplant will have on the recipient and his family should be attempted. A patient who has been totally dependent on a spouse for emotional, financial, and physical support may have difficulty, or even be overwhelmed, at the prospect of being independent and self-sufficient. Discussing the fears and expectations of the other family members is also important because often the family system has developed a homeostatic balance that will be upset as one of its members changes roles. Finally, not to discuss the possible death of the patient (either with or without surgery) is in a true sense participating in a "conspiracy of silence" and may contribute to a feeling that the physician does not really understand the gravity of the situation (Kemph, 1967, 1971).

Patients with extended family support, who are able to discuss the possibility of death openly, and who want to prolong life to do specific things appear to have fewer psychologic difficulties following the transplant (Christopherson & Lunde, 1971). After surgery, they seem more able to achieve their preoperative goals and integrate their new self-image as a transplant survivor. These patients are more compliant with treatment and appear to assume increasing responsibility for their recovery while adjusting to a less dependent role in their family. Conversely, those persons who view surgery as a mutilating assault upon their bodies or who are severely depressed or actively suicidal appear to be high risks for psychiatric morbidity (Christopherson & Lunde, 1971).

Christopherson (1976) emphasized a series of stages seen in the majority of transplant cases that might aptly be seen as rites of passage. First there is fear and anger when transplantation of a heart is discussed with the patient. The patient may deny being that sick of may feel angry at the disease. Next there may be a period of waiting after the patient is placed on a list. During this time, the patient may adjust to the idea and begin to idealize the surgeon. On hearing of another cardiac transplant patient's death, the patient might reduce any conflict by believing that their match will be "perfect" with no chance of rejection. Personality traits may become more pronounced: obsessive patients may gather statistics on the operation, whereas paranoid patients may become suspicious when another patient on the transplant list is matched with a donor and they are not. Dependent patients may become more demanding toward their families, and borderline patients may act out more and attempt to split the transplant team, creating chaos if the underlying dynamics are not appreciated. After working through these stages, there may be relief and readiness to proceed when the donor is found. In the immediate postoperative period, there is often a period of euphoria that may be due to high steroid doses (Christopherson, 1976). During this time, the patient should be observed closely and given needed support. In the event of a threatened rejection or complication, there may be severe depression, sadness, and fear of abandonment.

Much has been written about postoperative delirium and anxiety in heart patients (Dublin, Field, & Gastfriend, 1979; Kornfeld, Heller, Frank, et al., 1978; Nadelson & Notman, 1976; Sadler, 1981). Cardiac surgery is associated with a high incidence of psychiatric postoperative complications, from acute brain syndromes to major mood disorders and psychosis. These "psychiatric conditions" may, however, be the first sign of a neurologic or infectious complication. In a retrospective study of 83 patients with cardiac transplants, 54 percent had at least one neurologic complication, 16 percent had more than one, and 20 percent died from their neurologic complications (Hotson & Pedley, 1976). Because of the high dosages of steroids used in these patients, they are at risk for viral and fungal infections such as candidiasis and aspergillosis, with metastatic abscesses and meningeal involvement. Many patients with early infections have only mild signs of cognitive impairment and may have normal EEGs. If these mental status changes are blamed on metabolic encephalopathy or "ICU psychosis," the infection may be found only on postmortem examination. Steroids themselves may lead to a reversible, acute psychosis, including hallucinations, paranoid delusions, or depression. Other steroid-induced psychopathology includes hypomanic behavior, euphoria, panic attacks, dissociative experiences, and episodes of depersonalization (Kraft, 1971).

Family members may look upon the transplant recipient with fear and awe. After so many years of cardiac disability, they may fear the patient will "drop dead," and therefore they could be overprotective. They may have difficulty adjusting to the new independent role of their parent or spouse and may attempt to take charge or control of his or her activities. Home visits or passes from the hospital during the recovery period may help the family adjust. They also will aid in the early identification of family problems requiring more formal family intervention.

SPINAL CORD INJURY

Individuals with a traumatic spinal cord injury are faced with a possible loss of their mobility, sensation, sexual functioning, and control over even their most basic bodily functions. After being stabilized medically, patients often worry about the

ways their disability will affect their job and career choice, as well as their family and social relationships. Changes occur in an individual's body image, but there is no new "picture" to assimilate. Instead, the patient looks the same but has lost control over movement and can no longer feel sensation in some parts of the body.

In the past, all spinal-cord-injured patients were thought to go through a period of deep depression or mourning, and patients who seemed to accept their disability were thought to be denying the extent of their injury and simply not dealing with it (Hughs, 1980). Possibly because of increasing knowledge of the psychologic and medical needs of these patients, it appears that the "universal" major depression of these patients may have been overstimated and that if it does occur within the first few months of recovery, it is not as severe or prolonged as expected (Green, Pratt, & Grigsby, 1984). Although few long-term studies of these patients are reported in the literature, there are increasingly more reports of spinal-cord-injured patients adjusting to their injury within the first year (Cook, 1979; Richards JS, 1986). In a study of the self-concept of 71 paraplegics and quadraplegics at least 4 years after the date of injury, Green and colleagues (1984) found that although scales measuring physical appearance and sexual functions were more negative than noninjured norms, all other areas of self-concept, including social functioning and ethical and moral sense of self, were more positive than a control group of noninjured persons. The variable most strongly correlated with a positive self-concept was the patient's perception of independence and mobility, regardless of the severity of injury. Individuals who believed that they were as physically independent as possible had more positive self-concepts than those who perceived themselves as less independent than they were capable of being.

Understanding the injured patient's

fears and difficulties in recovery is essential. As with any sudden physical injury, there may be a period of shock and anxiety over the present and fears for the future. In an attempt to summarize the factors that determine feelings of well-being and satisfaction with life, Decker and Schultz (1985) interviewed 100 middle-aged and elderly spinal-cord-injured persons. The most frequent fear was lack of adequate income, followed by fear of deteriorating health and forced dependency on others. The majority of people indicated they were not depressed, and individuals reporting an increased sense of well-being were the younger individuals with more education who were working and requiring little assistance with daily activities.

Until recently, rehabilitation programs frequently addressed the medical, vocational, and psychologic needs of these patients but overlooked the diagnosis, management, and rehabilitation of sexual functioning. Too often, if the patient did not bring up sexual concerns, they did not get addressed. Since performance in sexual intercourse is often confused with one's sexuality, neglecting the sexual issues of a patient may inadvertently give the message that the physician is relating to the patient as an asexual human being.

To talk about these intimate issues, the psychiatrist must be comfortable talking about sex and must be knowledgeable about sexual physiology and the implications of spinal cord injury in sexual functioning. A thorough history of the patient's preinjury sexual practices, with specific questions about overall satisfaction, heterosexual or homosexual preferences, masturbation, frequency of sexual activity, history of sexual dysfunction, sexual fantasies, and any strong moral or religious beliefs as they relate to sexual practices, should be recorded (King, Klein, & Remenyi, 1985). Although the patient may have many questions regarding the ability to have coitus, to ejaculate, or to become pregnant and have children, the psychiatrist should guard against making premature predictions.

Immediately after injury, there is a period of spinal shock, which may last up to 6 weeks (Boller & Frank, 1982). Usually this means that all spinal cord reflex action below the injury is suppressed. In the male this includes reflex penile erection and the bulbocavernosus and scrotal reflexes. In both sexes, the rectal sphincter reflexes are abolished or severely depressed (Boller & Frank, 1982).

After this initial period of spinal shock, the important considerations for an individual's sexual functioning will be determined by the level of the injury and whether it is a complete or an incomplete cord injury. Regardless of the prognosis based on the spinal cord level, it is always advisable to encourage the patient to experiment with sexual touching activities to see what feels pleasurable.

Because erections are found even in patients with spinal cord lesions at the sacral spinal cord level, it is postulated that *both* the parasympathetic and the sympathetic nervous system are involved. In the noninjured patient both of these systems would act together to produce erections. In the patient with an injury at the sacral cord level, direct physical stimulation of the genitals may produce a *reflexogenic erection*, mediated by the parasympathetic nervous system. Another type of erection appears to be produced by mental stimuli and is not dependent on physical stimulation. This type, *psychogenic erection*, appears to be mediated by the sympathetic nervous system (Boller & Frank, 1982).

Knowledge of these two types of erections helps to account for the fact that many men with relatively high spinal cord injuries can experience reflexogenic erections by direct physical stimulation of their genitals. Although this erection is often brief (and generally is without ejaculation), coitus is sometimes possible (Boller & Frank, 1982).

Table 19-1
Effects of Spinal Cord Injury on Sexual Functioning

Injury Level	Effect	Comments
Spinal shock	Rectal sphincter contraction profoundly depressed or abolished	Suppression of reflex activity at all spinal cord levels below the lesion 1–6 weeks after injury
	Males Profoundly depressed or abolished: 1. Reflex penile erection 2. Bulbo cavernosus reflex 3. Scrotal reflexes	Spinal shock caused by contusion usually followed by spontaneous improvement; hemorrhage usually produces permanent disability; laceration produces permanent impairment
Cauda equina	Autonomic bladder Loss of external urethral sphincter tone Loss of anal sphincter tone Anal reflex absent	Lesions of nerve root at L2 and lower. Injuries to cauda equina and conus medullaris similar; most often result from space-occupying lesions
	Males 1. Usually loss of erection 2. Ejaculation occasionally occurs	Effects on sexual behavior most severe of spinal cord injuries and least reversible
	Females 1. Vaginal sensation often absent 2. Vaginal secretion present as part of genital reflex 3. Injuries above sacral segments do not interfere with fertility 4. Increased frequency of urinary tract infections	
Lumbar	May have sexual activity	Sexual activity probably mediated by sympathetic nervous system via preganglionic fibers at the lower thoracic and upper lumbar level
	Males 1. Psychogenic erection may occur 2. Ejaculation with orgasm occasionally occurs	
	Females See cauda equina	

Thoracic and cervical	Males	Erections, when present, usually short-lived
	1. Psychogenic erection rare	
	2. Spontaneous erection common	
	3. Reflex-stimulated erection common	
	4. Coitus sometimes possible	
	5. Orgasm and seminal emission rare	
	6. Sperm count low, with few motile sperm	
	Females	
	See cauda equina	

Source: Boller F & Frank E (1982) *Sexual dysfunction in neurologic disorders: Diagnosis, management, and rehabilitation* (pp 41–44). New York: Raven Press.

Conversely, patients with lesions of the cauda equina may have lost the ability to have an erection although sometimes ejaculation may occur. Finally, some men with lesions of the lumbar cord may be able to obtain psychogenic erections and, in some cases, ejaculation (Boller & Frank, 1982). Very few spinal-cord-injured men, however, are able to retain their reproductive capacity, even when they are able to ejaculate, because the semen usually is not normal. Sperm counts in these patients are generally low, and motility is decreased (Boller & Frank, 1982). It is theorized that chronic urinary tract infections from indwelling Foleys or inability to control scrotal temperature may lead to this decrease in fertility (King et al., 1985).

In spinal-cord-injured women there is frequently no sensation during intercourse, and vaginal secretions are variable (Boller & Frank, 1982; King et al., 1985). Although orgasm is absent, some authors claim that with sexual touching of areas innervated by spinal cord segments above the lesion (such as the breast), there may be "transfer of erotic zones from one region of the body (the vagina) to another (the breasts)" (Kolodny, 1979). Also, some patients claim that with erotic touching and sexually stimulating thoughts a mental, or "phantom," orgasm may occur (King, et al., 1985; Kolodny, 1979).

Unlike males with spinal cord injuries above the sacral level, a woman usually maintains her fertility. In fact, in a review of 187 pregnancies in female paraplegics, Goller and Paeslack (1972) found no increase in the number of spontaneous first-trimester abortions. If a patient does not wish to become pregnant, however, she should be aware of the increased risk of thrombophlebitis with oral contraceptives in spinal-cord-injured patients and the increased risk of irritation or penetration of the uterus with an intrauterine device because of decreased sensation in the pelvis. (Kolodny, 1979).

Table 19-1 summarizes the effects of spinal cord injury on sexual functioning.

Specific Recommendations for Spinal-Cord-Injured Patients

Because so many patients fear accidental bowel or urine spillage, the patient may wish to have sexual activity after bowel evacuation and bladder emptying. This can usually be accomplished fairly easily, since most spinal-cord-injured patients are on a daily schedule. A man with an indwelling Foley can fold the tubing over the penis, running it along the shaft, and then apply a condom over the penis and the catheter (King et. al., 1985). A woman with an indwelling Foley can empty the bag before sexual activity and then tape the catheter to her leg.

Depending on the patient's previous sexual activities and experiences, the patient may engage in a variety of sensual touching and sexual activities. Patient and partner may engage in mutual masturbation, massage with and without oils, oral-genital stimulation, anal stimulation, and experimentation with vibrators. It is important for the psychiatrist to be sensitive to the concerns and wishes of the couple and to be available for empathic listening and specific suggestions. For the male who is unable to achieve an erection, a technique called "stuffing," whereby the woman takes the flaccid penis in her hand and places it in the vagina, may be helpful (Masters & Johnson, 1970). If the woman contracts her vaginal muscles, sometimes a reflexogenic erection may occur.

Some spinal-cord-injured patients may prefer having a surgically implanted penile prosthesis. Follow-up studies on this operative alternative have reported patient satisfaction in the 89–95 percent range (Gerstenberger, Osborne, & Furlow, 1979; Malloy & Voneschenbach, 1977). Although most penile implants have been in diabetic males, Golji (1979) studied 20 spinal-cord-injured males at 3 and 27 months after surgery. All the patients studied reported increased sexual satisfaction, and 18 out of 20 wished they had had the implant earlier.

Regardless of the extent of the spinal cord injury, when patients' sexual concerns and issues are addressed in an unhurried atmosphere, the physician is helping the patients to recover another aspect of their lives—sexual functioning. Each patient should be evaluated by a psychiatrist, and follow-up sexual therapy should be available either from the psychiatrist or from a trained sexual therapist of an allied mental health discipline.

CANCER SURGERY

In the past, a diagnosis of cancer brought to mind incurableness, loss of function, disfigurement, pain, dependence, and death. Though the prognosis for many forms of cancer is no longer so bleak, patient fears are the same as in the past. Two questions come to mind: "Am I going to die?" and "Will I be in pain?" Sometimes there is the pressure of time when dealing with a malignancy, so these questions may go unanswered. The consulting surgeon, whom, frequently, the patient has just met, gives the result of the biopsy, followed by such words as "We need to operate to give you the best chance for a cure." The patient, although intellectually comprehending these words, may be left with the profound psychologic impact that these words leave: *cancer . . . operation . . . chance for cure.* The avalanche of feelings and emotions is often covered up by words that need to be translated and addressed. The patient may intially refuse to believe the diagnosis or insist that the biopsy is wrong. This denial may then be replaced by anger, and the anger may be projected onto the physician, the family, or God. The patient may feel that the cancer is a punishment for past transgressions (especially if the cancer involves the sexual organs) and may feel guilty. Finally, the patient may become anxious and fearful of metastatic spread, while attempting to retain hope for a surgical "cure."

An individual's ability to integrate the diagnosis and treatment options can often be predicted from the patient's style of coping with previous life stresses, as well as from assessment of the psychologic and social resources currently available. The physician should employ the patient's emotional support system as much as possible when honestly discussing treatment options. Possible side effects, disfigurement, and possible complications, including death, need to be explained and discussed.

There should be ample time for the patient to ask questions and clarify points of confusion. Often, the patient might not "hear" what is being said, and questions will be repeated, but the most important message to communicate to the patient is concern, understanding, and openness to questions.

Whatever cancer is being treated, the patient needs to know the treatment options and the recommendations of the treatment team (often the family doctor and a surgical specialist). In the case of metastatic spread, the patient should not be stripped of hope and should always feel there is a treatment plan (even if the plan is to make the patient comfortable and treat the pain). Emphasis should always be on what *can* be done rather than what will *not* work. Possible disfigurement and, if realistic, possible reconstructive procedures should be discussed. Sexual concerns should be addressed, especially with the gynecologic or urologic patients and with those individuals for whom a mastectomy or colostomy is a possibility. Table 19-2 is a summary of the impact of urologic treatment on sexual functioning.

The supportive psychiatric care of these patients is discussed in Chapter 23.

In the following sections, specific issues concerning amputation of the extremities, breast and gynecologic cancer, genitourinary surgery, and colostomies will be addressed in detail.

Gynecologic Cancer

Gynecologic cancer surgery may have profound psychologic impact on a woman. It may bring up issues of earlier losses as well as fears about future physical attractiveness and sexual functioning. For some women, self-esteem and identity are strongly linked to their physical appearance.

A woman's breasts may be symbolic of early childhood nurturance, femininity, attractiveness, and sexuality (Nadelson &

Notman, 1979). Diseases of the breast may therefore have emotional or psychologic effects that go beyond the confines of the diseased tissue. For a woman undergoing a lumpectomy for a breast nodule that appears to be relatively encapsulated, there may be a fear of microscopic spread and the uncertainty of a cure. In the case of a recurrence, there may be intense guilt and anger for not having had a more invasive procedure, such as a mastectomy, to begin with. For the woman who has undergone a mastectomy, there may be issues of loss coupled with worries about the carcinoma that has invaded her body. There may be further pharmacologic interventions and insults, leading to the loss of hair and nausea and vomiting. Steroids may lead to weight gain as well as changes in mood. The patient may become euphoric or even psychotic on high doses, and severely depressed while they are being lowered. Further loss of the feminine appearance may be secondary to androgen therapy, which may lead to hirsutism.

A hysterectomy usually leaves minimal external scarring, but the psychologic impact is well-documented in the literature. A woman may feel that her femininity has been taken from her, especially if she desires more children. There may be unconscious guilt for possibly causing the cancer by some past romantic affair, sexual transgression, or promiscuity. Some authors have reported an increased incidence of depression in women following this type of surgery (Polivz, 1974; Richards, 1973). It appears that the women most susceptible to posthysterectomy depression are those who have little marital support, who are under 40 years of age, and who wanted more children (Nadelson & Notman, 1979).

Unfortunately, few reports have made attempts to describe the premorbid psychologic makeup of women who have had a hysterectomy for nonmalignant uterine pathology. It is possible, therefore, that what we are reporting as a "posthysterectomy

Table 19-2

Impact of Urologic Treatment on Sexual Functioning

Procedure or Surgery	Possible Complication and Therapeutic Considerations
Transurethral resection for benign prostatic hypertrophy (TURP)	Retrograde ejaculation Loss of erectile capacity rare if it was normal preoperatively
Radical (total) prostatectomy for cancer	May result in complete absence of emission, ejaculation, and erection Erectile dysfunction decreased if pelvic nerve plexus innervating corpus cavernosa is spared
Radiation therapy for prostate cancer	May cause erectile impotence Higher rate of dysfunction with external beam than with radiation implants Complications related to arterial vascular occlusion
Orchiectomy, estrogen therapy, or both for advanced prostatic carcinoma	80% will loss potency Libido suppressed both by effects of castration on testosterone and by estrogen treatment
Cystectomy and radiation for bladder cancer	Ideal loop diversion above the field of radiotherapy to create a permanent stoma is the treatment of choice
Cystectomy for bladder cancer in women	May damage innervation in perineum May have loss of lubrication and orgasm due to loss of sensation Possible reduction in size of vaginal vault Possible scarring, contributing to painful intercourse
Cystectomy for bladder cancer in men	Loss of semen Ejaculation response may remain intact Only a few men will retain erectile potency
Partial penile amputation for tumors of glans, foreskin, coronal sulcus, and distal shaft	Length of penis reduced At times may have sufficient residual tissue for successful vaginal penetration May experience orgasm and ejaculation through stimulation of prostate, testes, and perineal and scrotal regions, with ejaculation occurring through a penile urethrostomy
Total penectomy with perineal urethrostomy for cancer of the penis	More damaging psychologically Adequacy for vaginal penetration and masturbation varies with length of remaining phallus

Chemotherapy or radiotherapy for testicular tumors	Infertility may result because of decreased sperm concentrations
	Sperm banking and fertility counseling important
Retroperitoneal lymphadenectomy for testicular cancer	Majority of men will have dysfunctional ejaculations due to sympathetic nerve damage
	Erection, libido, and orgasmic sensation unchanged
	90% of patients have retrograde ejaculation
	Anterograde ejaculation may be restored by treatment with imipramine 25–50 mg/day
	L-sympathomimetic on receptors in the bladder neck and proximal urethra
Ileal conduit surgery or urinary diversion	Males may feel demasculinized
	Women may perceive the operation as a bodily violation
	May feel less attractive sexually

Source: Stoudemire A, Techman T, & Graham SD, (1985). Sexual assessment of the urologic oncology patient. *Psychosomatics*, 26, 405–410.

syndrome" may have been present before surgery and may have actually aggravated or intensified the gynecologic symptoms. In a prospective study of 49 women receiving hysterectomies for disorders other than cancer, Martin, Roberts, and Clayton (1980) found that 53 percent of the women had a history of psychiatric illness, and 27 percent fulfilled the DSM-III criteria for somatization disorder (Briquet's syndrome). Cohen, Robins, Purtell, et al., (1953) also reported that gynecologic operations were seven times more frequent in "hysterics" than in control subjects.

In light of these findings, a patient who presents with dramatic or vague symptoms or a predominantly positive review of systems, for which little objective evidence can be found, a psychiatric consultation should be obtained prior to surgery. Finally, in treating a woman after a hysterectomy has been performed, knowledge of whether bilateral oophorectomy was done is important. In oophorectomized patients, hormone replacement can lead to significant improvement in feelings of well-being. Even when estrogen is being replaced, some women will do better psychologically on more or less estrogen, or with cyclic progestin therapy added. Bilateral oophorectomy, however, does not imply complete estrogen deficiency, since fragments of ovarian tissue as well as the adrenal glands, continue to produce estrogen (Martin, et al., 1980).

For the woman who has undergone extensive pelvic exenteration surgery, the physical assault may be extensive, including the removal of the rectum, distal colon, bladder, iliac vessels, uterus, tubes, and ovaries in addition to the entire pelvic floor (Silberfarb, 1984). Vaginal reconstructive surgery should be discussed in appropriate patients and may lessen the feelings of mutilation and help the patient reconstruct her body image. Frank, open discussions of sexual concerns and issues should be begun by the treating physician or by a psychiatric consultant. The patient may feel that her first priority is to worry about the cancer and that sexual issues are a personal matter not to be discussed with the surgeon. Scanty information may lead to misconceptions in the patient as well as her partner.

The patient may avoid sex because of dyspareunia from decreased lubrication after radiation, while fears of "catching" the radiation or cancer or anxiety about hurting his partner may lead to impotence in the male.

OSTOMY SURGERY

Patients undergoing surgery in which an ostomy is planned will not only experience a change in body image, but will also have to struggle with a variety of complex emotions and feelings regarding the ostomy. Unlike aesthetic surgery, no one "wants" an ostomy, and there may be concerns about sexual attractiveness and social acceptability, as well as a fear of a recurrence of the disease for which the surgery was performed (Watson, 1985). Often patients have only a vague understanding, prior to surgery, of how an ostomy functions, and they may appear more concerned with the technical aspects of surgery, anesthesia, and the surgical "cure." In the immediate postoperative period, the patient may focus mainly on incisional pain, advancement of diet, and regaining strength. Sometimes it is not until patients are being taught how to care for their stoma that they begin to deal with the loss of the diseased body part and a changed body image. Postoperatively, patients may be not only dealing with a break in their body integrity, but also attempting to incorporate into their body image a new surgically made opening in the anterior abdominal wall. The patient must also grieve the loss of control over one of the most basic of human bodily functions: elimination. Because the stoma has no sphincter mechanism, the colostomy patient may worry about passing flatus, having an odor, or leaking. The patient may feel overwhelmed by learning new ostomy management skills and dealing with this previously hidden internal organ. Some patients who refer to the stoma as "it" or the "bag" may be reacting to the ostomy in a detached way, as if it belonged to the surgeons who created it (Gloeckner, 1984).

This difficulty in redefining one's body image can have a profound impact on the patient's acceptance of responsibility for the care of the ostomy. An enterostomal therapist may provide invaluable assistance in helping the patient deal with these technical and emotional issues. In addition, self-help groups affiliated with the Ileostomy Association, the Urinary Conduit Association, and the International Ostomy Association are found in many communities. Members of these groups share firsthand experiences, providing emotional and psychologic support for the new ostomy patient. In addition, they may provide hints regarding irrigation techniques, dietary practices to prevent constipation, diarrhea, or excessive flatus, and overall stomal care.

Issues of altered body image, worries about sexual attractiveness, and fear of odor or leakage are similar for patients with ileal conduits, colostomies, and ileostomies. In a retrospective study of 40 ostomy patients, the most negative statements regarding body image were made in the first year after surgery (Dlin & Perlman, 1971), followed by perceived improvement in attractiveness in the following years (Gloeckner, 1984). Those with an ileostomy had the highest self-rating scores on sexual attractiveness. Patients who were not symptomatic preoperatively and who had the most complications and problems with their ostomy after surgery had the lowest postoperative attractiveness scores (Gloeckner, 1984).

Although the impact of mutilating surgery may be very traumatic for the emotionally unprepared patient, it appears that most patients who are given emotional support and psychiatric intervention when needed can resume full and well-adjusted lives. In a long-term follow-up of 344 ileostomy patients at the Mayo Clinic, 84 percent felt that the management of their ileostomy was not a major problem, and 92 percent were satisfied with their way of living. Most patients felt they were not restricted by their ostomy (82 percent), and 95.6 percent returned to their previous employment. Sexual habits did not change in 87.2 percent, and one-third of the married women became pregnant and had normal vaginal deliveries (Roy, Sauer, Beahrs, et al., 1970).

Showing patients the ostomy appliance they will most likely be wearing after surgery may raise some important questions preoperatively, including sexual concerns. In a survey that assessed the psychosexual response to ileostomies and colostomies among 500 ostomy association members, it was found that there was little or no discussion with patients before or after surgery about sexual issues (Dlin, Perlman, and Ringold, 1969).

Discussion of sexual issues is best handled by a psychiatrist who is familiar with the sexual problems encountered by ostomy patients. To postpone these discussions until the patient is ready to go home, or to wait until the patient brings up specific questions, may lead to misconceptions and undue anxiety in the patient and spouse. A complete psychosocial history should be taken from these patients; this may be the best introduction to detailed discussion of sexual functioning after surgery. Whenever possible, the patient's sexual partner should be included in discussions of sexual function, to alleviate miscommunication and fears about "breaking the news." Information should be given regarding possible problems with impotence, ejaculation, changes in libido, dyspareunia, fertility, and childbearing. In a study of 40 patients with a permanent ostomy, 30 percent stated that their partner reacted with a "fear of hurting me," which could have been alleviated by including the sexual partner in the preoperative and postoperative discussions (Gloeckner & Starling, 1982)

Although coital practice and frequency among married ileostomates do not differ from the general population (Grüner, 1983; Grüner, Naas, Fretheim, et al., 1977), some patients may have psychologic problems related to their stoma, especially in the first year after surgery. They may experience depression or anxiety and may worry about sexual attractiveness. It is during this critical time that psychotherapy can help patients return to their previous level of sexual functioning (Dlin & Perlman, 1971).

A survey conducted by the Ileostomy Association of Great Britain and Ireland found that only 40 percent of the patients with sexual problems after ileostomies felt comfortable discussing these issues with their primary physician (Burnham, Lennard-Jones, & Brooke, 1977). Other studies report that, frequently, patients have little or no preoperative discussion of possible sexual problems and little or no sexual guidance (Jones, Breckman, & Hendry, 1980). Dlin and Perlman (1971), in their interview of 146 ostomy patients over the age of 50, found that only 11 percent had received any sexual counseling before or after surgery.

Patients about to undergo extensive dissection for carcinoma will be dealing with the emotional crisis of having cancer as well as worries and fears about postoperative dysfunction. Patients are often reluctant to bring up issues of possible sexual dysfunction because of modesty, embarrassment, or the feeling that the doctor is interested in discussing "more important things." The reported incidence of sexual difficulties following abdominal-perineal resection for cancer ranges from 53–100 percent, with an average of 75 percent (Bernstein, 1972). Although there have been few studies on the sexual dysfunction of women after pelvic exenteration, dyspareunia sometimes occurs, possibly as a result of the perineal scarring. There may also be decreased lubrication because of pain or psychologic factors in women after abdominal-perineal resection (CH Young, 1982). For the woman with dyspareunia, the female-superior position might be more comfortable, and decreased lubrication can be alleviated by saliva or a vaginal lubricant (Young, 1982). For women who are concerned about conception and pregnancy after surgery, the majority of previously fertile women can conceive and give birth to healthy babies following ostomy surgery (Burnham et al., 1977). Although Daly (1968) felt that fertility might be reduced in women with ileostomies, he found that primary closure of pelvic peritoneum might decrease this incidence. Women who do not wish to become pregnant should be informed that birth control pills have, at times, been found unabsorbed in the ostomy appliance because of increased intestinal motility and that the failure to be absorbed negates their contraceptive effectiveness (CH Young, 1982).

For the male with partial postoperative impotence, a change in position while having sex might help. "Sometimes with the woman sitting 'astride' it is possible for both partners to introduce the penis into the vagina" (CH Young, 1982). Also, a penile or penoscrotal ring can be helpful by decreasing venous return, permitting erection and penetration. For total impotence in the male, a penile prosthesis may be considered (Carson, 1983; Collins & Kinder, 1984; Merrill, 1983; Schlamowitz, Beutler, Scott et al., 1983). For the male homosexual couple, although they may continue with manual and oral sexual activity, the ostomy should not be used for intercourse because of the risk of disrupting it (CH Young, 1982).

HEAD INJURY

A head injury may produce structural damage that is seen on a CT scan at the site of the trauma, or there may be evidence of trauma on the opposite side, as in a contre-coup injury. In these severe head injuries postoperative psychologic disability correlates well with other measures, such as the presence of coma or the duration of posttraumatic amnesia. Sometimes, however, there may be extensive damage that is not visualized anatomically but that is reflected in the behavior of the head-injured patient. This may be due to shearing and stretching of nerve fibers or secondary to microscopic damage to the white-matter tracts (Kwentus, Hart, Peck, et al., 1985; Ommaya & Gennarelli, 1974; Oppenheimer, 1968).

By contrast, in mild head injuries, the important determinants are personality and the presence or absence of significant neuropsychologic impairment. In the mildly head-injured patient, a combination of personality assessment and neuropsychologic testing is helpful in assessing individual patients.

As with all other conditions, it is important to be aware of the premorbid functioning of the individual, including a history of previous psychiatric problems, drug or alcohol use, and previous coping skills under stress. Other factors to consider in evaluating an individual patient are the age of the patient at the time of the injury, the etiology of the trauma, and evidence of damage to other internal organs (Kwentus et al., 1985; Newcombe, 1982). Lishman (1973), in his review of the psychiatric sequelae of head-injured patients, noted that impaired eye movements and pupillary reactions, endocrine abnormalities, increased intracranial pressure over 20 mm Hg, abnormal evoked potentials, and EEG slowing were associated with a worse outcome.

Although it may be difficult to quantify the severity of the head injury for an individual patient and to make predictive statements about the patient's future functioning, periods of unconsciousness longer than 6 hours frequently have psychiatric and intellectual consequences, and periods longer than 3 weeks have been associated with severe cognitive and psychiatric impairment (Kwentus et al., 1985).

Several authors have found that the most useful clinical measure of the severity of head trauma as it relates to cognitive and long-term memory impairment and psychiatric complications is the period of posttraumatic amnesia (PTA) (Kwentus et al., 1985; Newcombe, 1982). Furthermore, persistent anterograde amnesia and impaired new learning are predictive of long-term neurologic sequelae and permanent disability (Warren, Goethe, & Peck, 1984).

A patient with a severe head injury may be unconscious for a brief period or may take several weeks to "wake up." As patients become more aware of their surroundings, they may become delirious. Fluctuations in mental state are commonly seen during delirium and should be explained to the family, who may be confused or frightened by the patient's behavior. Withdrawal states need to be ruled out in any head-injured delirious patient, as many people with head injuries have been abusing alcohol and drugs at the time of their accident. Toxic screens and alcohol levels drawn at the time of initial presentation assist in identifying patients at risk.

Sometimes there may be a Korsakoff syndrome, in which the patient attempts to compensate for memory impairment by filling in the gaps with fabrications (Stam, 1967). This process, often referred to in the literature as confabulation, is usually time-limited, even if memory defects persist.

As with other patients with delirium, head-injured patients may have an altered sleep-wake cycle, periods of confusion that are worse in the evenings, agitation, or combativeness or emotional withdrawal. As discussed elsewhere, a low-dose neuroleptic may be useful. Recently, there has been evidence to suggest that propranolol can be a useful alternative for delirious agitation. The reader is referred to Chapter 4 for a more detailed discussion of this topic. In some cases, this delirium may not resolve and may evolve into a posttraumatic dementia (Kwentus et al., 1985). Multiple mild head injuries may sometimes produce aggregate effects. An example of this is the dementia that may occur in professional boxers, who can show cortical atrophy and intellectual deficit even if they have never been knocked out.

Damage to specific areas of the brain may lead to distinctive cognitive deficits or to organic mood disorders or behavioral syndromes. Damage to the dominant hemisphere may lead to language difficulties, including aphasia, dysnomia, or dyslexia and dyspraxia, and damage to the left temporal lobe may lead to problems with verbal memory (Kwentus et al., 1985). Damage to any of these areas may lead to subtle changes in attention, concentration, and memory.

Although it may at times be difficult to assess the mood states in head-injury patients because of emotional lability or neuropsychologic deficits, it is important to realize that even a minor head injury may influence the patient's emotional state on an organic basis (Levin & Grossman, 1978). Frontal damage and temporal damage are most often correlated with affective disorders; Robinson and Szetela (1981), in their review of stroke patients with left-sided damage, claimed that an individual's depressive symptoms could be correlated to the proximity of the damage to the frontal poles. They hypothesized that there may be damage to the norepinephrine fibers in this area and that the brain may become relatively depleted of norepinephrine.

Personality changes are associated with frontal lobe damage. Depending on the extent and location of the damage, the patient may become apathetic, indifferent, or pseudodepressed or may become euphoric and appear manic, with a pseudosociopathic type of disinhibition (Jarvie, 1954). The patient who appears depressed may benefit from a trial of antidepressants

(Tyler, McNelly, & Dick, 1980). If manic symptoms appear as part of an organic manic state, lithium may be used (Williams & Goldstein, 1979; LD Young, Taylor, & Holmstrom, 1977). Brain-injured patients, however, may be more sensitive to lithium neurotoxicity, and levels shoud be maintained at the lower end of the therapeutic range. In the case of a major depressive disorder unresponsive to antidepressant therapy, electroconvulsive therapy is not contraindicated and should be considered (Ruedrich, Chu, & Moore, 1983). Sometimes the location of the neurologic lesion plays a very important role in the way an affective disorder is seen clinically. Patients with right-sided lesions may talk about feeling sad but may go untreated because aprosodia makes their affect appear shallow or bland. On the other hand, patients with left-sided lesions may look severely depressed but be unable to discuss it because they cannot verbally express their distress due to aphasia (Kwentus, Hart, Peck, et al., 1985).

Temporal lobe injuries are frequently associated with personality changes and may be accompanied by temporal lobe seizures, sometimes in conjunction with violent outbursts. Patients should be advised to avoid alcohol and sedative drugs that may disinhibit aggressive behavior. In patients with complex partial seizures, a "temporal lobe personality" may develop, often characterized by hyposexuality, hypergraphia, circumstantiality, and talkativeness (Kwentus, et al., 1985).

Although much of the previous discussion has been in reference to severe head injuries, sometimes minor injuries lead to what is commonly known as the postconcussion syndrome. The main features are complaints of headaches, dizziness, difficulty concentrating, and poor memory (Kwentus et al., 1985). Further, it appears that these symptoms are not correlated with the duration of posttraumatic amnesia or the severity of the head injury (Kay,

Derr, & Lassman, 1971). The causes of these symptoms are varied and may relate to microscopic lesions in the brain or to extracranial injury, such as cervical whiplash. Anxiety, depression, or nervousness may develop for psychodynamic, as well as organic, reasons. Physical treatment may include a cervical collar, muscle relaxants, or nonnarcotic analgesics. Medical psychotherapy is indicated for more severe or permanent psychologic symptoms. The possibility of secondary gain from continued morbidity should always be considered, and patients should be asked about pending litigation.

Even in patients with apparently trivial head injury, neuropsychologic screening is advisable when there are persistent disabilities. A minority of patients with apparently mild injuries will show significant cognitive deficits relevant to their psychologic symptoms and disability. Similarly, an EEG should be obtained in severe or persistent cases of apparent postconcussion syndrome, particularly if there are paroxysmal symptoms, such as dizzy spells or lapses of memory. Although neuropsychologic testing and EEG often contribute useful diagnostic information in this situation, CT scanning is not indicated unless there are significant unexpected abnormalities on EEG, neuropsychologic testing, or neurologic examination (see Chapter 3 for further details on neurodiagnostic procedures).

Neuroleptics should be avoided in patients with a history of head trauma because of these patients' enhanced sensitivity to CNS side effects and because drugs that have catecholamine receptor blocking effects may impair recovery from head trauma (O'Shanick & Parmelee, in press). Benzodiazepines may have disinhibitory effects on behavior in these patients and impair neuropsychological performance. If psychotropics are needed for behavioral and affective instability in head trauma patients, carbamazepine should be considered a first line drug of choice. Lithium carbonate should also be considered in this clinical context. Nocturnal and intermittent agitation may be handled with doses of trazodone, 200 mg as needed (O'Shanick & Parmelee, in press).

ELECTIVE COSMETIC SURGERY

Cosmetic surgery differs from traumatic or general surgery in that most of the time the patients are not medically ill and are not undergoing a procedure to relieve pain or prolong life. It is a surgery to purposely alter body image; therefore it can be expected to have impact on an individual's self-concept and identity.

The concept of body image has been studied since its introduction by Schilder (1950). Although cosmetic surgery may produce an abrupt change in the outward appearance of a person, there is not always a corresponding change in body image. The concept of body image is a concept of psychologic variables, which include cognitive understanding, sensory input, and comparisons made by the individual between self and others. A person's body image is shaped by the emotional responses he or she receives from peers (Belfer, Harrison & Murray, 1979; Murray, Mulliken, Kaban, et al., 1979; Schilder, 1950). These reactions cannot be underestimated, since research has shown that attractive individuals are more likely to be seen as intelligent, friendly, successful, sensitive, interested, and outgoing (Arndt, Travis LeFebvre et al., 1986; Dion, Berscheid, & Walster, 1972).

There may be temporary alterations in body image, such as pregnancy, acne, or broken bones, but, generally, these changes are not incorporated into the "psychological picture of oneself" (Henker, 1979).

Murray and colleagues (1979), in their review of the literature, reasoned that a patient must work through several stages before the mental concept of body image undergoes change. Initially, there is the decision to have an operation, followed by the surgical experience. Next, there is the immediate postoperative period, which is followed by the reintegration phase, in which the patient adjusts to or incorporates a new body image. When the individual has a congenital or traumatic deformity, he postulated, early correction may be important in the prevention of distortion of body image, isolation from peers, and psychologic difficulties (Murray et al., 1979).

Some patients, however, may have a distorted sense of their body size. Individuals who have been obese most of their lives may still see themselves as fat even after losing large amounts of weight (Glucksman & Hirsch, 1969). Sometimes this distorted body image may have delusional proportions and cause the patient to greatly exaggerate a minimal defect. In DSM-III-R (American Psychiatric Association, 1987) this disorder is designated as body dysmorphic disorder and is characterized by the belief that the body is grossly deformed. At times there may indeed be a cosmetic deformity; however, the defect is greatly exaggerated. Since as many as 2 percent of cosmetic surgical consultations may be secondary to this disorder, a psychiatrist should carefully assess a patient who is requesting surgery for a minimal defect (Andreasen & Bardach, 1977; Connolly & Gipson, 1978; Stoudemire, in press). Patients requesting surgery because of body image distortions first need psychiatric therapy to address their underlying psychodynamic issues. The role of the psychiatrist is to sort out the relative contributions of reality and fantasy in producing the patient's dissatisfaction. When the realistic issues are large, surgery is unequivocally indicated, and the psychiatrist needs to help the patient with realistic expectations of the proposed change and incorporation of this change after the operation. When the realistic component is small, the psychiatrist's job is to address the underlying dynamics leading to the conflict and, if possible, talk the patient and surgeon out of the procedure.

Sometimes even psychologically healthy individuals have body image distortions secondary to pain in a particular body part. Because the individual is so obsessionally focused on that part, it may occupy a larger part of the patient's mental body schema. Although some patients may discuss the details of their deformity quite openly, they may have a hidden emotional agenda, which becomes clear only after the surgery. The body part being operated on may have a special meaning for the patient or may have an unconscious significance that may result in psychologic conflicts postoperatively.

The results of treatment for cosmetic surgery patients will generally affect their relationships with others, eliciting varying responses with psychologic meaning for the patient. Although most authors report few long-term psychiatric complications in appropriately screened cosmetic surgical patients (Reich, 1969), there may be a period of reactive anxiety and depression in the immediate postoperative period (Thomson, Knorr, & Edgerton, 1978). In a study of 599 patients, Reich (1969) reported reactive depression and anxiety in 31 percent of patients. These reactions, however, may be a reflection of preoperative difficulties. In a prospective psychologic study of 50 female face-lift patients, Goin, Burgoyne, Goin, et al. (1980) found that there was a high frequency of postoperative depressive reactions in patients who showed depressive features on preoperative psychologic testing. They placed greater emphasis on the premorbid function and characterological styles of the patients than on the symbolic meaning of the operation.

Guidelines for patient selection are found in many textbooks of plastic surgery, but it is generally accepted that those patients judged to be poor candidates on

psychologic grounds are those who are excessively fearful, who have unrealistic or magical expectations, who have minimal deformities, who are male, or who have histories of psychosis, recent loss, or current depression (Groin et al., 1980). The patient with a history of many elective surgical procedures is also a high-risk patient, who may have a somatization disorder or a personality disorder. Patients with overly dependent, masochistic, or narcissistic personality traits may request surgery as a derivative of their personality disorder and, under the "crisis" of surgery, may become regressed, self-destructive, or dissatisfied, depending on their life-long characterological style. When the sugeon is unsure about the patient's ability to handle surgery or the patient's expectations are unclear, psychiatric consultation should be obtained.

Although alteration of any part of the body may have psychologic impact, structures such as the face, breast, and genitalia are more affect-laden. The face is the organ most often used for identification and is intimately tied with recognition. Our profiles, facial movements, and characteristic features are the ways other people see us. Similarly, we recognize emotions in others by "reading" their faces.

The face also has the sensory structures that enable us to see, touch, smell, hear, and taste. Blepharoplasties, rhinoplasties, chin implants, otoplasties, and rhytidectomies (facelifts) are common surgical procedures that may alter these sensory organs. The most prominent feature on one's face is the nose, and rhinoplasty is the most commonly requested operation.

The link between self esteem and body image was assessed by Gillies (1984) when she asked patients to identify the part of their body they felt was their "self core," or the seat of their identity. Most responded that it was behind the bridge of their nose or in their midchest. Surgery in this area may therefore be influencing not only how the patients look but also how they feel about themselves.

The body part that is being altered by surgery may symbolize an unconscious conflict for the individual. Some psycho-analytic authors feel that because the nose contains erectile tissue similar to the genitals, feelings of sexual inadequacy may be displaced from the genitals to the nose (Schaeffer, 1920). Other authors suggest that a male patient who is dissatisfied with his nose may be defending against a feeling that his profile is effeminate, or an unconscious fear that he is homosexual (Hill & Silver, 1950).

In the light of these varying issues and potential psychologic conflicts, Meerloo (1956) wrote that plastic surgery "intervenes in a complicated psychological battle." Furthermore, he suggested that the patient who seeks surgery for a minimal disfigurement may actually be hoping that the physician will refuse to operate, thereby giving validation that the disfigurement is minimal.

Changing the way one looks is making an evaluation on the body—an assessment that some parts are "good" and others are "bad" and need change. Updegraff and Menninger (1934) felt that persons with sexual conflicts or low self-image may displace these conflicts onto a body part they view as defective. Other authors propose that some individuals may believe their deformity is a punishment for wrongdoings (Meerloo, 1956).

Specific surgeries of the breast and genitalia are reviewed in other sections of this chapter, but the surgeon needs to be mindful of the symbolic meanings of these structures in the patient's mind. The patient's fantasies and expectations regarding surgery should always be assessed, and the inividual hoping that the surgeon's knife may mend a broken marriage or improve business success should be considered at high risk for postoperative psychologic problems. On the other hand, for the pa-

tient with a marked deformity, plastic surgery may "reconstruct" the body image and improve the self-image.

AMPUTATIONS

The psychiatric implications of a surgical amputation are different for various groups of patients. For the elderly patient with vascular disease and nonhealing ulcers, it may be a welcome relief from pain, for the individual with cancer, the amputation may be a sacrifice in exchange for the hope of a surgical cure. An amputation might be a sudden life-saving measure to prevent sepsis in the case of gangrene or the end result of a failed revascularization procedure in a trauma patient.

As with other types of surgery, the patient undergoing an amputation should be evaluated for preexisting psychiatric difficulty, and ego strengths should be assessed. As much as possible, the meaning of the amputation with regard to the patient's self-concept and body image should be determined. An amputation of a lower extremity of a dancer will produce more grief than the amputation of a nonfunctional extremity in a paraplegic. Similarly, a traumatic amputation will more greatly affect an active child than a retired sedentary individual. Irrespective of age, however, there will be issues of incorporating a new body image, and regardless of the precipitating causes leading to the amputation, the patient will be dealing with the loss and with grief for the amputated limb.

Patients may be fearful about their future and the impact this surgery may have on their family and friends. They may wonder where the body part was sent after the amputation and may unconsciously fear that other body organs may be disposed of in a similar fashion. To regard an amputation strictly as a surgical procedure with low mortality is to deny the tremendous impact of this disfiguring surgery. There is often sadness and mourning in the immediate postoperative period, and patients may talk about their loss as if they had lost a family member (Ruby, 1978).

Socially, there may be changes in the patient's relationships with peers. Children may be taunted as "Peg Leg" or "Hopalong" or "Captain Hook," and adults may get curious stares or be whispered about. Young adults may worry about the effect an amputation may have on their careers or ability for promotions and may be concerned about changes in sexual functioning, attractiveness, and desirability.

Initially, patients may have difficulty looking at or touching the stump and may need psychiatric intervention to help them adjust to their changed body image.

In older patients whose amputation was due to vascular insufficiency, there may be relief from painful ischemic disease, but some authors have found these patients to be particularly at risk for depression and to be preoccupied with issues of death and dying (Caplan & Hackett, 1963). Pathologic reactions that may signal the need for additional therapy include no reaction at all to the loss, a state of euphoria or unfounded optimism, prolonged depression or anxiety, severe overreaction to the loss, aggressive or asocial behavior, and masochism.

A significant prevalence of major depressive reactions was found by Kashani, Frank, Kashani et al. (1983) in a prospective study of 65 amputees. The most common cause for the amputations in their series was vascular disease, and 34 percent of the patients were found to be depressed on clinical interview, according to DSM-III criteria for major depression. There were also higher frequencies of depression among the female amputees (50 percent), while only 30 percent of the males had depressive symptoms. It appears that geriatric amputees are likely to have significant psychiatric morbidity. Vegetative symptoms or "depressive equivalents" should be treated with antidepressant drugs and medical psychotherapy.

REFERENCES

American Psychiatric Association (1980). *Diagnostic and Statistical manual of mental disorders* (3rd ed., p 104). Washington, DC.

American Psychiatric Association (1986). *Diagnostic and statistical manual of mental disorders* (3rd ed, rev). Washington, DC.

Andreasen NC & Bardach J (1977). Dysmorphophobia: Symptom or disease? *American Journal of Psychiatry, 134*, 673–676.

Andreasen NJC, Hartford CE, Knott JR, et al. (1974). Cerebral deficiencies after burn encephalopathies. *New England Journal of Medicine, 290*, 1487–1488.

Arndt EM, Travis F, Lefebvre A, et al. (1986). Beauty and the eye of the beholder: Social consequences and personal adjustment for facial patients. *British Journal of Plastic Surgery, 39*, 81–84.

Belfer ML, Harrison AM, & Murray JE (1979). Body image and the process of reconstructive surgery. *American Journal of Diseases of Children, 133*, 532–535.

Bernstein WC (1972). Sexual dysfunction following radical surgery for cancer of rectum and signoid colon. *Medical Aspects of Human Sexuality, 6*, 156–163. Blancher RS (1978). Paradoxical depression after heart surgery: A form of survival syndrome. *Psychoanalytic Quarterly, 47*, 267–284.

Boller F & Frank E (1982). *Sexual dysfunction in neurologic disorders: diagnosis, management, and rehabilitation* (pp 14–20, 41–44). New York: Raven Press,

Burnham WR, Lennard-Jones JE, & Brooke BN (1977). Sexual problems among married ileostomists: Survey conducted by the Ileostomy Association of Great Britain and Ireland. *Gut, 18*, 673–677.

Caplan LM & Hackett TP (1963). Emotional effects of lower limb amputation in the aged. *New England Journal of Medicine, 269*, 1166–1171.

Carson CCM (1983). Inflatable penile prosthesis: Experience with 100 patients. *Southern Medical Journal, 76*, 1139–1141.

Castelnuovo-Tedesco P (1970). Psychoanalytic considerations in a case of cardiac transplantation. In A Silvano (Ed), *The world biennial of psychiatry and psychotherapy* (Vol 1, pp 336–352). New York: Basic Books.

Castelnuovo-Tedesco P (1973). Organ transplant, body image, psychosis. *Psychoanalytic Quarterly, 42*, 349–363.

Christopherson L (1976). Cardiac transplantation. Need for patient counseling. *Nursing Mirror, 143*, 34–36.

Christopherson LK & Lunde DT (1971). Selection of cardiac transplant recipients and their subsequent psychological adjustment. *Seminars in Psychiatry, 3*, 36–45.

Cohen ME, Robins E, Purtell JJ, et al. (1953). Excessive surgery in hysteria. *Journal of the American Medical Association, 151*, 977–986.

Collins GF & Kinder BN (1984). Adjustment following surgical implantation of a penile prosthesis: A critical overview. *Journal of Sex and Marital Therapy, 10*, 255–271.

Connolly FH & Gipson M (1978). Dysmorphophobia—a long term study. *British Journal of Psychiatry, 132*, 568–570.

Cook D (1979). Psychological adjustment to spinal cord injury: Incidence of denial, depression and anxiety. *Rehabilitation Psychology, 26*, 97–104.

Curreri PW (1979). Burns. In SI Schwartz, GT Shires, FC Spencer, et al. (Eds), *Principles of surgery* (3rd ed, Vol 1, pp 298–299). New York: McGraw-Hill.

Daly DW (1968). The outcome of surgery for ulcerative colitis. *Annals of the Royal College of Surgeons, 42*, 38–57.

Decker SD & Schultz R (1985). Correlates of life satisfaction and depression in middle-aged and elderly spinal cord-injured persons. *American Journal of Occupational Therapy, 39*, 740–745.

Deutsch F, Murphy WF (1955). The application of psychoanalytic concepts in psychosomatic disease. In *The Clinical Interview, Volume 1: Diagnosis* (pp 138–142). New York: International Universities Press.

Dion KK, Berscheid E, & Walster E (1972). What is beautiful is good. *Journal of Personality and Social Psychology, 24*, 285–290.

Dlin BM, Perlman A, & Ringold E (1969). Psychosexual response to ileostomy and colostomy. *American Journal of Psychiatry, 126*, 374–381.

Dlin BM & Perlman A (1971). Emotional response to ileostomy and colostomy in patients over the age of 50. *Geriatrics, 26*, 112–118.

Dublin WR, Field HL, & Gastfriend DR (1979). Postcardiotomy delirium: A critical review. *Journal of Thoracic Cardiovascular Surgery, 77*, 586–594.

Dumas RG (1963). Psychological preparation for surgery. *American Journal of Nursing, 8*, 52–55.

Egbert LD, Battit GE, Turndorf H, et al. (1963). Value of preoperative visit by anesthetist: Study of doctor–patient rapport. *Journal of the American Psychiatric Association, 185*, 553–555.

Egbert LD, Battit GE, Welch CE, et al. (1964). Reduction of postoperative pain by encouragement and instruction of patients: A study of doctor patient rapport. *New England Journal of Medicine, 270*, 825–827.

Gerstenberger DL, Osborne D, & Furlow WL (1979). Inflatable penile prosthesis: Follow-up study of patient–partner satisfaction. *Urology, 14*, 583–587.

Gillies DA (1984). Body image changes following illness and injury. *Journal of Enterostomy Therapy, 11*, 186–189.

Gloeckner MR (1984). Perceptions of sexual attractiveness following ostomy surgery. *Research in Nursing Health, 7*, 87–92.

Gloeckner MR & Starling JR (1982). Providing sexual information to ostomy patients. *Diseases of the Colon and Rectum, 25*, 575–579.

Glucksman M & Hirsch J (1969). The response of obese patients to weight reduction: The perception of body size. *Psychosomatic Medicine, 31*, 1–7.

Golji H (1979). Experience with penile prosthesis in spinal cord injury patients. *Journal of Urology, 121*, 288–289.

Goller H & Paeslack V (1972). Pregnancy damage and birth complications in the children of paraplegic women. *Paraplegia, 10*, 213–217.

Green B, Pratt CC, & Grigsby TE (1984). Self-concept among persons with long-term spinal cord injury. *Archives of Physical and Medicine Rehabilitation, 65*, 751–754.

Goin MK, Burgoyne RW, Goin JM, et al. (1980). A prospective psychological study of 50 female face-lift patients. *Plastic and Reconstructive Surgery, 65*, 436–442.

Grüner OP, (1983). Sexual problems after rectal surgery and operated colitis. *Praxis, 72*(28), 948–952.

Grüner OP, Naas R, Fretheim B, et al. (1977). Marital status and sexual adjustment after colectomy: Results in 178 patients operated on for ulcerative colitis. *Scandinavian Journal of Gastroenterology, 12*, 193–197.

Harper G (1978). The burn unit. In TP Hackett & NH Cassen (Eds), *Massachusetts General Hospital handbook of general hospital psychiatry* (pp 405–414). St. Louis: CV Mosby.

Henker FO (1979). Body-image conflict following trauma and surgery. *Psychosomatics, 20*, 812–820.

Hill G & Silver AG (1950). Psychodynamic and aesthetic motivation for plastic surgery. *Psychosomatic Medicine*, *12*, 345–355.

Hotson JR & Pedley TA (1976). The neurological complications of cardiac transplantation. *Brain*, *99*, 673–694.

Hughes F (1980). Reaction to loss, coping with disability and death. *Rehabilitation Counseling Bulletin*, *23*, 251–256.

Imbus SH & Zawacki BE (1977). Autonomy for burned patients when survival is unprecedented. *New England Journal of Medicine*, *297*(6), 308–311.

Jarvie HF (1954). Frontal lobe wounds causing disinhibition. *Journal of Neurology, Neurosurgery and Psychiatry*, *17*, 14–32.

Johnson JE (1966). The influence of purposeful nurse patient interaction on the patient's post-operative course. *American Nurses Association Monographs*, *2*, 16–22.

Johnson JE (1984). Coping with elective surgery. *Annual Review of Nursing Research*, *2*, 107–132.

Jones MA, Breckman B, & Hendry WF (1980). Life with an ileal conduit: Results of questionnaire survey of patients and urological surgeons. *British Journal of Urology*, *52*, 21–25.

Kashani JH, Frank RG, Kashani SR, et al. (1983). Depression among amputees. *Journal of Clinical Psychiatry*, *44*, 256–258.

Kay DWK, Derr TA, & Lassman LP (1971). Brain trauma and the postconcussion syndrome. *Lancet*, *11*, 1052–1055.

Kemph JP (1966). Renal failure, artificial kidney and kidney transplant. *American Journal of Psychiatry*, *122*, 1270–1274.

Kemph JP (1967). Psychotherapy with patients receiving kidney transplant. *American Journal of Psychiatry*, *124*, 77–83.

Kemph JP (1971). Psychotherapy with donors and recipients of kidney transplants. *Seminars in Psychiatry*, *3*, 145–158.

King NJ, Klein RM, & Remenyi AG (1985). Sexual counselling with spinal cord injured patients. *Australian Family Physician*, *14*, 47–50.

Kolodny RC (1979). Sex and the handicapped. In RC Kolodny, WH Masters, & VE Johnson (Eds), *Textbook of sexual medicine* (pp 353–380). Boston: Little, Brown.

Kornfeld DS, Heller SS, Frank KA, et al. (1978). Delirium after coronary artery bypass. *Journal of Thoracic and Cardiovascular Surgery*, *76*(1), 93–96.

Kraft IA (1971). Psychiatric complications of cardiac transplantation. *Seminars in Psychiatry*, *3*, 58–69.

Kwentus JA, Hart RP, Peck ET, et al. (1985). Psychiatric complications of closed head trauma. *Psychosomatics*, *26*, 8–17.

Layne OL & Yudofsky SC (1971). Postoperative psychosis in cardiotomy patients: The role of organic and psychiatric factors. *New England Journal of Medicine*, *284*, 518–520.

Lazarus HR & Hagens JH (1968). Prevention of psychosis following open heart surgery. *American Journal of Psychiatry*, *124*, 1190–1195.

Levin H & Grossman R (1978). Behavioral sequelae of closed head injury. *Archives of Neurology*, *35*, 720–727.

Lishman WA (1973). The Psychiatric sequelae of head injury: A review. *Psychological Medicine*, *3*, 304–318.

Mai FM (1986). Graft and donor denial in heart transplant recipients. *American Journal of Psychiatry*, *143*, 1159–1161.

Malloy TR & Voneschenbach AC (1977). Surgical treatment of erectile impotence with inflatable penile prosthesis. *Journal of Urology*, *118*, 49–51.

Martin RL, Roberts WV, & Clayton PJ (1980). Psychiatric status after hysterectomy: A one-year prospective follow up. *Journal of the American Medical Association*, *244*, 350–353.

Masters WH & Johnson VE (1970). *Human sexual inadequacy* (pp 93–315). Boston: Little, Brown.

Meerloo J (1956). The fate of one's face. *Psychiatric Quarterly*, *30*, 31–43.

Merrill DC (1983). Clinical experience with Scott inflatable penile prosthesis in 150 patients. *Urology*, *4*, 371–375.

Millar HR (1981). Psychiatric morbidity in elderly surgical patients. *British Journal of Psychiatry*, *138*, 17–20.

Murray JE, Mulliken JB, Kaban LB, et al. (1979). Twenty year experience in maxillocraniofacial surgery: An evaluation of early surgery on growth, function and body image. *Annals of Surgery*, *190*, 320–330.

Nadelson CC & Notman MT (1979). Disease and illnesses specific to women. In G Usdin & JM Lewis (Eds), *Psychiatry in general medical practice* (pp 475–497). New York: McGraw-Hill.

Nadelson T (1976). The psychiatrist in the surgical intensive care unit. *Archives of Surgery* III, 113–117.

Newcombe F (1982). The psychological consequences of closed head injury: assessment and rehabilitation. *Injury: the British Journal of Accident Surgery*, *14*, 111–136.

Ommaya AK & Gennarelli TA (1974). Cerebral concussion and traumatic unconsciousness: Correlations of experimental and clinical observations on blunt head injuries. *Brain*, *97*, 633–654.

Oppenheimer DR (1968). Microscopic lesions in the brain following head injury. *Journal of Neurology, Neurosurgery and Psychiatry*, *31*, 299–306.

O'Shanick GJ & Parmelee D (in press). Psychopharmacologic agents in the treatment of brain injury in AL Christensen & DW Ellis (Eds). *Neuropsychological Treatment of Head Injury*.

Pearson J & Dudley H (1982). Bodily perceptions in surgical patients. *British Medical Journal, 284*, 1545–1546.

Polivz J (1974). Psychological reactions to hysterectomy: A critical review. *American Journal of Obstetrics and Gynecology, 118*, 417–426.

Ravenscroft K (1982). The burn unit. *Psychiatric Clinics of North America, , 419–432*.

Reich J (1969). The surgery of appearance: Psychological and related aspects. *Medical Journal of Australia, 2*, 5–13.

Richards JS (1986). Psychological adjustment to spinal cord injury during first postdischarge year. *Archives of Physical and Medical Rehabilitation, 67*, 362–365.

Richards DH (1973). Depression after hysterectomy. *Lancet, 2*, 430–433.

Robinson G & Merav A (1976). Informed consent recall by patients tested postoperatively. *Annals of Thoracic Surgery, 22*, 209–212.

Robinson RG & Szetela B (1981). Mood change following left hemisphere brain injury. *Annals of Neurology, 9*, 447–453.

Roy P, Sauer W, Beahrs OH, & Farrow GM (1970). Experience with ileostomies: Evaluation of long term rehabilitation in 497 patients. *American Journal of Surgery, 119*, 77–86.

Ruby LK (1978). Acute traumatic amputation of an extremity. *Orthopedic Clinics of North America, 9*, 679–692.

Ruedrich SL, Chu CC, & Moore SL (1983). ECT for major depression in a patient with acute brain trauma. *American Journal of Psychiatry, 140*, 928–929.

Ryan DW (1975). A questionnaire survey of preoperative fears. *British Journal of Clinical Practice, 29*, 3–6.

Schaeffer JP (1920). *The nose and olfactory organ* (pp 271–272, 300–301). Philadelphia: Blakeston.

Sadler PD (1981). Incidence, degree, and duration of postcardiotomy delirium. *Heart Lung* 10, 1084–1092.

Schilder P (1950). *The image and appearance of the human body* (pp 11–16, 238–304). New York: International Press.

Schlamowitz KE, Beutler LE, Scott FB, et al. (1983). Reactions to the implantation of an inflatable penile prosthesis among psychogenetically and organically impotent men. *Journal of Urology, 129*, 295–298.

Silberfarb PM (1984). Psychosexual impact of gynecologic cancer. *Medical Aspects of Human Sexuality, 18*, 212–223.

Stam FC (1967). Traumatic and posttraumatic psychosyndromes. *Psychiatria, Neurologia, and Neurochirurgia, 70*, 175–186.

Steiner H & Clark WR (1977). Psychiatric complications of burned adults: A classification. *Journal of Trauma, 17*, 134–143.

Stoddard FJ (1982). Body image development in the burned child. *Journal of the American Academy of Child psychiatry, 21*, 502–507.

Stoudemire A (in press). Somatoform disorders, factitious disorders, and malingering. In J Talbott, RE Hales, & S Yudofsky (Eds), *Textbook of psychiatry*. Washington, DC: American Psychiatric Press.

Stoudemire A, Techman T, & Graham SD (1985). Sexual assessment of the urologic oncology patient. *Psychosomatics, 26*(5), 405–410.

Surman O (1978). The surgical patient. In TP Hackett & NH Cassem (Eds), *Massachusetts General Hospital handbook of general hospital psychiatry* (pp 65–92). St. Louis: CV Mosby.

Thomson JA, Knorr NJ, & Edgerton MT Jr (1978). Cosmetic surgery: The psychiatric perspective. *Psychosomatics, 19*, 7–15.

Titchner JL, Zwerling I, Gottschalk L, et al. (1956). Psychosis in surgical patients. *Surgical Gynecology and Obstetrics, 102*, 59–65.

Tyler S, McNelly H, & Dick L (1980). Treatment of posttraumatic headache with amitriptyline. *Headache, 20*, 213–216.

Updegraff HL & Menninger KA (1934). Some psychoanalytic aspects of plastic surgery. *American Journal of Surgery, 25*, 554–558.

Wallace LM (1984). Psychological preparation as a method of reducing the stress of surgery. *Journal of Human Stress, 10*, 62–77.

Warren JB, Goethe KE, & Peck EA (1984). Neuropsychological abnormalities associated with severe head injury. *Journal of Neurosurgical Nursing, 16*, 30–35.

Watson PG (1985). Meeting the needs of patients undergoing ostomy surgery. *Journal of Enterostomy Therapy, 12*, 121–124.

West DA & Shuck JM (1978). Emotional problems of the severely burned patient. *Surgical Clinics of North America, 58*, 1189–1204.

Williams K & Goldstein G (1979). Cognitive and affective responses to lithium in patients with organic brain syndrome. *American Journal of Psychiatry, 136*, 800–803.

Young CH (1982). Sexual implications of stoma surgery (Part 1). *Clinics in Gastroenterology, 2*, 383–395.

Young LD, Taylor I, & Holmstrom V (1977). Lithium treatment of patients with affective illness associated with organic brain symptoms. *American Journal of Psychiatry, 134*, 1405–1407.

George Molnar
Giovanni A. Fava

20
Intercurrent Medical Illness in the Schizophrenic Patient

The responsibility for managing physically ill schizophrenic patients has become an increasingly frequent challenge for psychiatrists in general hospitals. Among the factors that have led to this increasing frequency are the expended role of general hospitals in the mental health system, the development of medical-psychiatric units, and deinstitutionalization. Equally important, contemporary psychiatrists have become increasingly involved in the medical diagnosis and treatment of their patients.

Despite the existence of community mental health centers and state hospitals, the general hospital has become the focal point for delivery of mental health care in the United States (Greenhill, 1979). As a consequence of the deinstitutionalization movement, general hospitals serve large numbers of former state hospital patients, as well as first-time patients who in the past would have been admitted to state institutions. Over one-third of admissions to psychiatric units in public general hospitals

suffer from schizophrenia (Bachrach, 1979).

The delivery of medical care to patients with chronic schizophrenia is relatively underdeveloped despite the high rate of medical illness (much of it neglected), found in this population. Schizophrenic patients within the general medical and general hospital settings require integrated medical and psychiatric care. Newly developing medical-psychiatric units appear especially well suited to serve this function.

PHYSICAL ILLNESS AND SCHIZOPHRENIA

With higher mortality and morbidity than the general population, schizophrenic patients form a vulnerable group. There is general agreement that, overall, the relative risk of death in schizophrenia is twice that in the community population (Baldwin, 1979). Though "unnatural deaths," particularly those from suicide, have been found to be the leading cause of the excess mortality in cohorts of schizophrenic patients compared with age-matched controls, schizophrenic patients also have a mortality from medical causes that is two to four times greater than a comparison group (Allebeck and Wistedt, 1986; Tsuang, Woolson, & Fleming, 1980).

Chronic mental patients are also more likely than the population at large to be in poor physical health (Karasu, Waltzman, Lindenmayer, et al., 1980). Estimates of the prevalence of physical illness among such patients range from 33 to 60 percent; even more striking, in approximately 50 percent of psychiatric patients who were found to have a medical illness after undergoing a thorough medical screening, the existence of the condition was unknown both to the patient and to the referring physician (Hall, Gardner, Stickney, et al., 1980; Koranyi, 1979).

Koranyi (1979) defined the relationship between medical illness and psychiatric symptoms as *causative* when the medical illness is considered responsible for the psychiatric symptoms, as *aggravating* when the medical illness augments but does not cause a psychiatric disorder, and as *coexisting* when the medical and psychiatric conditions are relatively independent. Our discussion, will primarily deal with coexisting and aggravating medical illnesses.

The reciprocal influences between medical illness and psychosis are complex. In patients with schizophrenia, anecdotal accounts describe the remission of psychosis following an intercurrent medical illness. Mayer-Gross, Slater, and Roth (1969) noted the reduction of psychiatric symptoms during acute febrile illness in schizophrenic patients. On the other hand, schizophrenic symptoms may begin following medical illness or trauma. The phenomenon of remission of schizophrenia when medical illness supervenes merits further investigation (Lipper and Werman, 1977).

Epidemiologic studies have addressed the question of the relative prevalence of various medical diseases in schizophrenic patients compared with the general population or control groups (Ananth & Englesmann, 1984; Baldwin, 1979; Tsuang, Perkins, & Simpson, 1983). Tsuang et al. (1983) reported an increased incidence of gastrointestinal cancer and of cardiovascular and infectious diseases and a decreased incidence of rheumatoid arthritis in schizophrenia. Studies of immunologic and psychophysiologic dysfunctions in schizophrenia have been conducted in attempts to shed light on the biologic and psychophysiologic mechanisms predisposing schizophrenic patients to illness Neuchterlein, 1984; McGuffin, Farmer, & Rajah, 1978). These studies are of considerable theoretical interest but are not conclusive.

Detecting Physical Illness in Schizophrenic Patients

The detection of previously unknown medical illness in schizophrenic patients requires a high index of suspicion and systematic medical screening. The basic and most important screen is a careful medical history and physical examination.

Hoffman and Koran (1984) identified disease-related, patient-related, and physician-related causes as contributing to the failure to diagnose physical illness in mental patients. In known schizophrenic patients, an important cause of misdiagnosis is the tendency to attribute all mental symptoms to the schizophrenia although similar symptoms may be induced by physical illness. Because of this assumption, underlying medical conditions such as endocrine diseases, metabolic disorders, brain tumors, and toxic and viral encephalopathies may be missed. Symptoms due to medical illness are commonly labeled delusional (Varsamis & Adamson, 1976). To avoid this error, potential medical causes should be considered when a new mental or physical symptom appears or existing symptoms prove refractory to the usual treatment.

When patients are agitated and otherwise uncooperative or have very poor hygiene, it can be very difficult to perform a thorough medical evaluation. Incomplete portions of the medical evaluation should be completed within a specifically designated time, and mechanisms to check that evaluations are complete should be incorporated in the routines of clinics and inpatient units. Because of their suspiciousness and threatening behavior, paranoid patients also present difficulties in the evaluation and management of their medical problems. Reiteration of information on the medical treatment is sometimes useful. Of course, not all hostile, suspicious, or angry patients are paranoid; a psychiatric interview to clarify the source of the patient's negative affects may need to precede a formal medical history and examination.

Screening for Medical Problems

Schizophrenic patients who present for psychiatric admission often have no evident medical problem or have one of lower priority than the immediate behavioral issue. Nevertheless, subjection of all patients to a medical screening protocol greatly increases the yield of diagnosed and treatable conditions. A written policy specifying the medical screening protocol is useful for staff orientation, quality assurance and other administrative purposes. On the authors' service, the admission routine includes a medical history, a physical examination, and laboratory tests including a complete blood count, a blood chemistry panel (Na, K, Cl, CO_2, blood urea nitrogen (BUN), serum creatinine, blood sugar, and total protein), a serum glutamic oxaloacetic transaminase (SGOT) test, and a urinalysis. After admission, vital signs are monitored regularly. Rather than including a larger number of routine tests, thereby incurring greater expense and risking more false positives, additional diagnostic tests are ordered as clinically indicated. Frequently ordered supplementary tests are serum calcium, thyroid function (T3, T4, TSH), and an expanded liver function battery. (These supplementary tests are routinely done on the editors' units, where the rates of concurrent medical illness are extremely high. Local epidemiology and referral patterns should be considered when developing a screening battery.) An electrocardiogram (EKG) is ordered in individuals over 40; when tuberculosis or other pulmonary disease is suspected, a chest X ray is done. In particular, chest X rays are ordered in malnourished, indigent patients at epidemologic risk for tuberculosis. When organic brain dysfunction is suspected, as it should be in all first episodes of schizophreniform psychosis, an electroencephalogram (EEG) is ordered, provided the patient can cooperate: this examination is useful in differentiating acute "functional" psychosis from delirium. Since many schizophrenic patients are also substance abusers, blood or urine toxicology screens are often done. If blood levels of the patient's medications are available and are known to be clinically meaningful, they should be obtained. When risk factors are identified, AIDS testing and hepatitis B testing should be done, not only for the patient's benefit but also to protect staff by instituting appropriate infectious precautions in case of positive result. As indicated by the medical history and physical findings, diagnostic tests for syphilis, gonorrhea, and the newer venereal diseases should be ordered.

Since schizophrenic patients often take poor diets and suffer from malnutrition, a nutritional assessment is important. The appearance of the skin, hair, nails, and mouth, as well as reference to height–weight tables, helps to furnish an indication of the nutritional status. A complete blood count (CBC) with differential, iron, B_{12}, etc., and folate levels will help diagnose nutritional anemias. A low lym-

phocyte count (below 1500) and a low serum albumin level are useful laboratory
indices of protein–calorie malnutrition.

PSYCHOPHARMACOLOGY

Despite progress in psychosocial and
rehabilitative approaches, antipsychotics
are still the mainstay of treatment of schizophrenia (Donaldson, Gelenberg, &
Baldessarini, 1985). No antipsychotic drug
is generally more effective than any other in
the treatment of schizophrenia (Baldessarini, 1985). When a physical illness is
present, however, side effects and
pharmacokinetic properties provide a rationale for using one antipsychotic rather than
another (Baldessarini, 1985; Norman, Sloman, & Burrows, 1985; Shader, Weinberger, & Greenblatt, 1978). Low-potency
phenothiazine antipsychotics have relatively more cardiovascular side effects than
high-potency agents (Norman et al., 1985).
Among the antipsychotics, haloperidol and
molindone are relatively devoid of cardiovascular side effects and are among the
least likely to induce orthostatic hypotension.

The anticholinergic effects of antipsychotics should be considered in patients
with cardiovascular, gastrointestinal,
genitourinary, and ocular diseases in which
such effects may be harmful. The anticholinergic effects of antipsychotics must also
be considered when these agents are used
in conjunction with antiparkinson drugs
and antispasmodics that also have anticholinergic actions. With respect to anticholinergic action, thioridazine and chlorpromazine are most potent, loxapine is
intermediate, and trifluoperazine, fluphenazine, perphenazine, haloperidol, thiothixene, and molindone have relatively
weak cholinergic-blocking effects (Baldessarini, 1985). Since susceptibility to the
central anticholinergic syndrome (anxiety,
delirium, agitation, hallucinations, hyper-

pyrexia, myoclonus, convulsions, and stupor) increases with age (van der Kolk,
Shader, & Greenblatt, 1978), the correct
selection of an antipsychotic agent is especially important in older patients, who are
more susceptible to anticholinergic effects.
For these patients, high-potency agents
generally should be used, unless a quite low
dose of a low-potency agent is sufficient to
control the patient's psychosis. Anti-
parkinson agents such as benzotropine
mesylate and trihexyphenidyl are also
strongly anticholinergic. To avoid unwanted anticholinergic actions, amantadine
or diphenhydramine may be used to prevent or treat neuroleptic-induced parkinsonism.

Neuroleptics may be used cautiously
in patients with existing liver disease (Maxwell, Carrella, Parkes, et al., 1972; Read,
Laidlaw, & McCarthy, 1969). Rarely, however, a phenothiazine is responsible for
inducing cholestatic jaundice. In such case
the responsible agent should be discontinued and replaced by an antipsychotic of a
different chemical class. Since the liver
retains considerable reserve capacity to
metabolize antipsychotics, the presence of
impaired liver function does not automatically disqualify use of antipsychotics. The
effects of antipsychotics on seizure threshold are also of clinical relevance. Low-
potency aliphatic phenothiazines (particularly chlorpromazine) are more likely to
decrease the seizure threshold, whereas
high-potency antipsychotics (particularly
fluphenazine, molindone, and thiothixene)
are less likely to induce seizures (Itil, 1978).

Baldessarini (1985) reviewed a series
of interactive drug effects involving
antipsychotics. The metabolism of antipsychotics can be enhanced by such drugs
as barbiturates (phenobarbital) and anticonvulsants (carbamazepine, phenytoin),
which induce microsomal drug-meta-
bolizing enzymes. In such cases, a compensatory increase in neuroleptic dosage may
be necessary to obtain the desired antipsy-

chotic action. Antipsychotics inhibit the actions of direct dopaminergic agonists and thus interfere with the antiparkinsonian action of L-dopa. In patients requiring both L-dopa and an antipsychotic, slow manipulation of drug dosages is needed, with careful observation of neurologic and psychiatric status. For a more complete discussion of the use of neuroleptics and other psychoactive drugs, the reader is referred to Chapter 4 by Stoudemire and Fogel.

Tardive Dyskinesia and Neuroleptic Malignant Syndrome

As the number of patients on neuroleptics and the duration of exposure to these drugs increase, tardive dyskinesia (TD) and neuroleptic malignant syndrome (NMS) are being seen more frequently in clinical practice. Though symptom complexes similar to these two syndromes are known to occur independently of neuroleptic treatment and in subjects not affected by schizophrenia, TD and NMS are of primary interest to psychiatry as the most prominent side effects of the use of neuroleptics to treat schizophrenia. Because of their serious medical and liability implications, it is critical for physicians working with the mentally ill to be informed about the risk factors associated with the onset of TD and NMS and about the preventon, detection, and treatment of these syndromes.

Tardive Dyskinesia

The lifetime prevalence and annual incidence of TD in schizophrenic patients on long-term neuroleptic maintenance have been estimated as 23 percent and 2.9 percent, respectively (Chouinard, Annable, Mercier, et al., 1986). According to controlled studies, the risk factors most consistently associated with increased prevalence of TD are advancing age and, to a lesser extent, female sex (Kane and Smith, 1982). Additional risk factors, including duration

of neuroleptic treatment, cumulative neuroleptic dose, organic central nervous system (CNS) disease, and use of high-potency antipsychotics, are less consistently associated with TD. Initially believed to be irreversible, TD has since been shown to be partially or totally reversible in some patients over a period of several weeks to several years. Unlike drug-induced parkinsonism, TD appears after protracted rather than initial neuroleptic treatment, does not respond to anticholinergics, and is unmasked or exacerbated by discontinuing the neuroleptic.

Medical complications of TD include dysarthria, edentulousness, gait disturbance and abnormal posture, respiratory distress, and dysphagia (Yassa and Jones, 1985). Swallowing and respiratory difficulties related to TD may have serious medical consequences. In case of dysphagia, nutritional management includes a feeding program prepared in consultation with a professional dietician, based on the type and degree of swallowing impairment (Weiden and Harrigan, 1986).

To prevent, minimize, or delay the onset of TD, patients should be exposed to the lowest effective neuroleptic dose for the shortest time possible. The continued need for neuroleptic treatment must be continually reevaluated and documented at least every six months. Intermittent medication schedules are being studied (Herz, Szymanski, & Simon, 1982); they may be effective in patients who are followed very closely and who do not relapse immediately after discontinuation of neuroleptics. All neuroleptics can induce TD; patients on maintenance neuroleptics should therefore be monitored carefully for abnormal movements. Use of the Abnormal Involuntary Movement Scale (AIMS) at regular intervals offers a simple standard method for determining the presence and severity of TD symptoms (Guy, 1976). Patients on maintenance neuroleptics should be informed about the risks and benefits of such medication, with specific and documented mention of TD. Informed consent should be repeated and documented every 6 months. (Munetz & Roth, 1985; Shader et al., 1978). When maintenance neuroleptic treatment is prescribed, it is advisable to obtain the patient's signature on a consent form in addition to documenting the rationale for the treatment and the discussion with the patient and family members in the medical record.

Neuroleptic Malignant Syndrome

Related to Stauder's, or lethal, catatonia and to malignant hyperthermia, NMS is probably not a unitary syndrome (Levinson & Simpson, 1986). It has been defined in terms of a spectrum of neuroleptic-related neurotoxicity, with varying combinations of extrapyramidal, cortical, and autonomic dysfunction (Fogel & Goldberg, 1985). With a mortailty rate of 15–30 percent, NMS is the most lethal adverse effect of neuroleptics (Sternberg, 1986). The symptoms and treatment of NMS are discussed in Chapter 4. Though NMS was considered rare, recent studies report higher NMS prevalence rates: Pope, Keck, and McElroy (1986) reported a 1.4 percent prevalence for diagnosed cases; if milder NMS variants are included, the prevalence rate among neuroleptic-treated patients may reach 10 percent (Addonizio, Susman, & Roth, 1986). Most cases are related to high-potency antipsychotics, but NMS has been reported with all commonly used antipsychotics, whether used alone or in combination with antidepressants or lithium. Predisposing conditions such as medical illness, dehydration, fever, exhaustion, or malnutrition place patients at higher risk for NMS (Sternberg, 1986). To reduce the risk, such aggravating conditions should be identified and treated vigorously (Harpe & Stoudemire, 1987).

NMS may recur upon reexposure to neuroleptics (Shalev, Hermesh, Aizenberg, et al., 1985). Since the need to treat schizo-phrenic patients with antipsychotics is often unavoidable, a cautious approach to reexposure to the same or, preferably, a different neuroleptic is recommended. Reexposure is based on frequent monitoring, low initial doses, and gradual upward titration after informed consent has been obtained (Guze & Baxter, 1985). Prophylactic antiparkinson medication, especially amantadine may reduce the risk of recurrence.

TREATMENT OF PREGNANT SCHIZOPHRENIC PATIENTS

Pregnant schizophrenic patients referred to general hospitals for inpatient care tend to be grossly disorganized, to be admitted on an involuntary status, and to have scant family, social, and community supports (Muqtadir, Hamann, & Molnar, 1986; Spielvogel & Wile, 1986). Treatment plans for such patients should be coordinated with the respective departments for obstetric and antenatal care and should include management of the delivery. The presence in the delivery room of a psychiatry staff member familiar with the patient improves the patient's cooperation during labor and facilitates the task of delivery room staff. Since infants born of schizophrenic mothers have a higher perinatal death rate than those born of normal mothers (Rieder, Rosenthal, Wender, et al., 1975), all pregnancies in schizophrenic women should be considered high-risk. Nevertheless, in a series of 18 deliveries in which the mothers had been treated on a medical-psychiatric unit, healthy infants were delivered in all instances (Muqtadir et al., 1986). The sample is small, but the finding suggests that comprehensive care in a protected environment may diminish perinatal risk.

Though conclusive evidence of teratogenic effects linked to antipsychotics has not been established, case reports of congenital malformations associated with the use of this drug class during the first trimester of pregnancy produce much concern about their use in pregnant patients. Use of antipsychotics and other drugs in pregnant schizophrenic women requires a strong and well-documented rationale, since medication prescribed for the mother may reach the fetus through the placenta and the neonate through breast milk. Usually, however, the risk to the mother and the fetus from uncontrolled psychosis is greater than the risk from judicious use of antipsychotics. Use of antipsychotics during lactation is discussed in Chapter 29.

Electroconvulsive treatment (ECT) of psychosis in pregnant patients is a viable alternative to medication (Nurnberg & Prudie, 1984). When conducted with proper technique and the patient adequately relaxed and oxygenated during the procedure, ECT can be safely conducted in any stage of pregnancy (see Chapter 5).

Pregnant schizophrenic women often cannot provide reliable information on their state, have difficulty cooperating with prenatal examinations and obstetric procedures during labor and delivery, and often disregard the signs of impending labor. Therefore, during pregnancy, schizophrenic patients should receive close obstetric and medical monitoring, including weekly or biweekly physical examination. Their attitudes about the pregnancy and custody of the baby frequently reflect ambivalence and may be distorted by their impaired reality testing. Involvement of responsible family members if available and appropriate social agencies such as children's protective services are usually necessary to plan for aftercare for mother and newborn. Family planning also emerges as an important and difficult topic with this group of patients, who in many cases go on to have serial pregnancies.

THE SCHIZOPHRENIC PATIENT AND SURGERY

Under optimal circumstances, the surgeon prepares the patient for surgery, explains the procedure, and discusses what may be anticipated in terms of postoperative pain, discomfort, and body-image alteration (Baudry & Wiener, 1975). Very often circumstances are not optimal in this regard. When a sufficiently knowledgeable and experienced psychiatrist prepares the patient for surgery, the postoperative course is much less stormy.

The use of anesthetic procedures and agents in schizophrenic patients undergoing surgery also raises important practical issues. Spinal anesthesia should be avoided in behaviorally unstable patients because they may be agitated or otherwise unable to cooperate. When low-potency phenothiazine antipsychotics are used in combination with halothane, enflurane, and isoflurane, there is considerable risk of a profound hypotensive reaction (Janowsky, Risch, & Janowsky, 1981). The potent alpha-adrenergic blocking action of these drugs causes patients to become functionally hypovolemic. Patients scheduled for elective surgery for which halogenated anesthetics are planned, should thus be switched to appropriate doses of high-potency neuroleptics. In emergency situations, however anesthesiologists are almost always able to manage the hypotension that may occur with the halogenated anesthetics in patients on phenothiazine antipsychotics.

Patients with schizophrenia may develop exacerbations of psychosis during the postoperative period, perhaps precipitated by stress, pain, or mild delirium. Some exacerbations, however, result from *failure* of the surgeon to reorder antipsychotic medication when postoperative orders are written. The psychiatrist should always confirm that antipsychotics have been reordered. If the patient will be prohibited from taking anything by mouth for several days following surgery, parentenal antipsychotics should be given.

MEDICAL-PSYCHIATRIC UNITS

Recently, special wards for patients with concomitant psychiatric and medical illnesses have been established in some general hospitals. Much as general hospital psychiatric services were in the 1950s, however, these medical-psychiatric units are still in an early phase of development. Though they have generated considerable interest, no single model prevails. At present, there are almost as many variants as there are medical-psychiatric units, each differing from the other with respect to the auspices under which it operates, its mission, the patient popualtion, and admission criteria (Fogel & Stoudemire, 1986; Fogel, Stoudemire, & Houpt, 1985; Goodman, 1985; Koran & Barnes, 1982; Markoff, Yano, Hsu, et al., 1981; Molnar, Fava, & Zielezny, 1985; Stoudemire & Fogel, 1986; Stoudemire, Kahn, & Brown, 1985; Young & Harsch, 1986). (See also Chapters 32 and 33.)

The recognition that standard medical and psychiatric inpatient services are inadequate to treat patients with concomitant medical and psychiatric illness provided the stimulus for the development of these units. Quite apart from attitudinal factors, which often militate against managing problems identified with the other specialty, the staff of medical-surgical units lack the expertise necessary to manage agitated or suicidal patients, and staff of standard psychiatric units often find it difficult to treat patients requiring more than a minimal level of medical and medical nursing care.

Medical-psychiatric units appear to offer effective treatment to schizophrenic patients requiring medical-surgical care short

of intensive care. They can be used to treat acute medical and psychiatric conditions definitively, to stabilize chronic conditions, and to offer patients and their families education about the medical illnesses and their treatments (Fava, Wise, Molnar, et al., 1985).

AMBULATORY CARE

Reflecting the historic separation of medical and psychiatric services (Goldman, 1982), ambulatory care for schizophrenic patients continues for the most part to be conducted in outpatient departments or community clinics without systematic ongoing links with medical care. The desirability of such links is made evident by findings such as those of Koranyi's (1979) large study of psychiatric clinic patients, according to which almost half suffered from one or more physical illnesses. Of these, almost half were undiagnosed by the referring physician. These findings point out the necessity on the one hand, for medical orientation on the part of the psychiatrist and, on the other, for aftercare medical-psychiatric clinics (Fava et al., 1985; Garai & Goldsmith, 1979).

HEALTH ATTITUDES AND PATIENT EDUCATION

Though it is controversial whether psychiatric patients are less compliant than other medical patients when they have a physical illness (Blackwell, 1982), neglected care of physical illness is commonly observed in psychiatric settings (Talbott & Linn, 1978). Harmful personal habits, such as excessive smoking and drinking, are quite common among schizophrenic patients, as among other high-cost users of hospital care (Zook & Moore, 1980). A high incidence of bronchogenic carcinoma has been noted in schizophrenic patients who are heavy smokers (Masterson & O'Shea, 1984). Drug abuse is also frequent in schizophrenia, complicating diagnosis and treatment.

As do other medical patients (Giloth, 1985) chronic mental patients need education to make informed decisions about their health, to manage their illnesses, and to implement care in the home. Patient education services can contribute substantially to the efficiency of hospital and ambulatory care. Group formats are particularly effective for achieving these purposes. Medically ill schizophrenic patients and their families should be instructed about the psychotropic and other medications prescribed, the need to adhere to treatment schedules, and ways to maintain a healthy diet and other favorable health habits.

CONSENT FOR MEDICAL TREATMENT

When physically ill schizophrenic patients are psychotic or otherwise present severely impaired judgment, questions arise as to their competence to provide consent for medical or surgical treatment. Civil commitment laws permit the involuntary hospitalization of patients only for the evaluation and treatment of psychiatric disorders and definitely do not imply permission for nonemergency medical or surgical treatment over the patient's objection or in case of the patient's incompetence to provide informed consent for such treatment (Fogel, Mills, & Landen, 1986). Except for treatment administered under the emergency doctrine in case of danger to life or limb, consent for major medical or surgical treatment must be obtained from the patient if the patient is competent. An involuntary admission status does not imply lack of competence to make decisions about medical care; this requires a separate evaluation. In most jurisdictions, except in an emergency, it is necessary to have recourse to the courts to administer even psychopharmacologic treatment over an involuntary patient's objection. Because of the liability potential inherent in such situations, the usual guidelines for careful documentation of the need and rationale of the proposed medical treatment and its potential benefits and risks should be followed. A second opinion is advisable in doubtful or controversial cases. When a patient is found mentally incompetent to consent to medical treatment, court proceedings become necessary to establish a temporary guardianship.

REFERENCES

Addonizio G, Susman VL, & Roth SD: (1986). Symptoms of neuroleptic malignant syndrome in 82 consecutive inpatients. *American Journal of Psychiatry, 143,* 1587–1590.

Allebeck P & Wistedt B (1986). Mortality in schizophrenia: A ten-year follow-up based on the Stockholm County Inpatient Register. *Archives of General Psychiatry, 43,* 650–653.

Ananth J & Engelsmann F (1984). Relationship between schizophrenia and psychosomatic illness: A review. *Neuropsychobiology* 12, 138–141.

Bachrach LL (1979). General hospitals taking greater role in providing services for chronic patients. *Hospital and Community Psychiatry, 30,* 488.

Baldessarini RJ (1985). Drugs and the treatment of psychiatric disorders. In AG Gilman, LS Goodman, TW Rall & F Murad (Eds), The pharmacological basis of therapeutics (pp 387–445). New York: MacMillan.

Baldwin JA (1979). Schizophrenia and physical disease. *Psychological Medicine, 9,* 611–618.

Baudry FD & Wiener A (1975). The surgical patient. In JJ Strain & S Grossman (Eds), *Psychological care of the medically ill* (pp 123–137). New York: Appleton-Century-Crofts.

Blackwell B (1982). Treatment compliance. In Greist

JH, JW Jefferson, & RL Spitzer (Eds), *Treatment of mental disorders*. Oxford: Oxford University Press.

Chouinard G, Annable L, Mercier P, et al. (1986). A five-year follow-up study of tardive dyskinesia. *Psychopharmacology Bulletin, 22*, 259–263.

Dawson ME & Nuechterlein KH (1984). Psychophysological dysfunctions in the development course of schizophrenic disorders. *Schizophrenia Bulletin, 10*, 204–232.

Donaldson SR, Gelenberg AJ, & Baldessarini RJ (1985). The pharmacologic treatment of schizophrenia: A progress report. *Schizophrenia Bulletin, 9*, 506–527.

Fava GA, Wise TN, Molnar G, et al. (1985). The medical-psychiatric unti: A novel psychosomatic approach. *Psychotherapy and Psychosomatics, 43*, 194–201.

Fogel BS & Goldberg RJ (1985). Neuroleptic malignant syndrome [Letter to the editor]. *New England Journal of Medicine, 313*, 1292.

Fogel BS, Mills MJ, & Landen JE: (1986). Legal aspects of the treatment of delirium. *Hospital and Community Psychiatry, 37*, 154–158.

Fogel BS & Stoudemire A (1986). Organization and development of combined medical—psychiatric units (Part 2). *Psychosomatics, 27*, 417–428.

Fogel BS, Stoudemire A, & Houpt JL (1985). Contrasting models for combined medical and psychiatric inpatient treatment. *American Journal of Psychiatry, 142*, 1085–1089.

Garai T, & Goldsmith W (1979). Medical teamwork in a psychiatric clinic. *Hospital and Community Psychiatry, 30*, 848–849.

Giloth B (1985, October). Incentives for planned patient education. *Quality Review Bulletin*, pp 295–301.

Goldman HH (1982). Integrating health and mental health services. *American Journal of Psychiatry, 139*, 616–620.

Goodman B (1985). Combined psychiatric-medical inpatient units: The Mount Sinai model. *Psychosomatics, 26*, 179–189.

Greenhill MH (1979). Psychiatric units in general hospitals. *Hospital and Community Psychiatry, 30*, 169–182.

Guy W (1976). *ECDEU assessment manual for psychopharmacology* (pp 534–537). Washington, DC: U.S. Government Printing Office.

Guze BH & Baxter LR, Jr (1985). Current concepts: Neuroleptic malignant syndrome. *New England Journal of Medicine, 313*, 163–166.

Hall RC, Gardner ER, Stickney SK, et al. (1980). Physical illness manifesting as psychiatric disease. *Archives of General Psychiatry, 37*, 989–995.

Harpe C & Stoudemire A (1987). Aetiology and treat-

ment of the neuroleptic malignant syndrome. *Medical Toxicology, 2*, 166–176.

Herz MI, Szymanski HV, & Simon JC (1982). Intermittent medication for stable schizophrenic outpatients: An alternativeto maintenance medication. *American Journal of Psychiatry, 139*, 918–922.

Hoffman RS, & Koran LM (1984). Detecting physical illness in patients with mental disorders. *Psychosomatics, 25*, 654–660.

Itil TM (1978). Effects of psychotropic drugs in qualitatively and quantitatively analyzed EEG. In WG Clark & J. DelGiudice (Eds), *Principles of psychopharmacology* (pp 261–277). New York: Academic Press.

Janowsky EC, Risch C, & Janowsky DS (1981). Effects of anesthesia on patients taking psychotropic drugs. *Journal of Clinical Psychopharmacology, 1*, 14–20.

Kane JM, & Smith JM (1982). Tardive dyskinesia: Prevalence and risk factors, 1959 to 1979. *Archives of General Psychiatry, 39*, 473–481.

Karasu TB, Waltzman SA, Lindenmayer JP, et al. (1980). The medical care of patients with psychiatric illness. *Hospital and Community Psychiatry, 31*, 463–472.

Koran LM, & Barnes LE (1982). The Stanford comprehensive medicine unit: Integrating medical and psychiatric care. In J Kuldan (Ed), *New directions for mental health services: Treatment for psychosomatic problems* (Monograph No. 15) San Francisco; Jossey-Bass.

Koranyi EK (1979). Morbidity and rate of undiagnosed physical illness in a psychiatric clinic population. *Archives of General Psychiatry, 36*, 414–419.

Levinson DF, & Simpson GM (1986). Neuroleptic-induced extrapyramidal symptoms with fever—heterogeneity of the neuroleptic malignant syndrome. *Archives of General Psychiatry, 43*, 839–848.

Lipper S, & Werman DS (1977). Schizophrenia and intercurrent physical illness: A critical review of the literature. *Comprehensive Psychiatry, 18*, 11–22.

Markoff RA, Yano BS, Hsu J, et al. (1981). The mixed medical-psychiatric unit: An alternative approach to inpatient psychiatric care. *Hospital and Community Psychiatry, 32*, 561–564.

Masterson E,& O'Shea B (1984). Smoking and malignancy in schizophrenia. *British Journal of Psychiatry, 145*, 429–432.

Maxwell JD, Carrella M, Parkes JD, et al. (1972). Plasma disappearance and cerebral effects of chlorpromazine in cirrhosis. *Clinical Science, 43*, 143–151.

Mayer—Gross W, Slater E, & Roth M (1969). *Clinical*

psychiatry (pp 259–260). London: Baillier, Tindell and Cassel.

McGuffin P, Farmer AE,& Rajah SM(1978). Histocompatibility antigens and schizophrenia. *British Journal of Psychiatry, 132,* 149–151.

Molnar G, Fava GA, & Zielezny M (1985). Medical-psychiatric unit patients compared with patients in two other services. *Psychosomatics, 26,* 203–209.

Munetz MR, & Roth LH (1985). Informing patients about tardive dyskinesia. *Archives of General Psychiatry, 42,* 866–871.

Muqtadir S, Hamann MW,& Molnar G (1986). Management of psychotic pregnant patients in a medical-psychiatric unit. *Psychosomatics, 27,* 31–33.

Norman TR, Sloman GJ,& Burrows GD (1985). Adverse effects, cardiotoxicity and drug interactions of antipsychotic drugs. In GD Burrows, TR Norman, & B Davies (Eds), *Antipsychotics* (pp 253–267). Amsterdam: Elsevier.

Nurnberg HG, & Prudie J (1984). Guidelines for treatment of psychosis during pregnancy. *Hospital and Community Psychiatry, 35,* 67–71.

Pope HG, Keck PE, & McElroy SL (1986). Frequency and presentation of neuroleptic malignant syndrome in a large psychiatric hospital. *American Journal of Psychiatry, 143,* 1227–1233.

Read AE, Laidlaw J, & McCarthy CF (1969). Effects of chlorpromazine in patients with hepatic disease. *British Medical Journal, 3,* 497–499.

Rieder RO, Rosenthal D, Wender P, et al. (1975). The offspring of schizophrenics. Fetal and neonatal deaths. *Archives of General Psychiatry, 32,* 200–211.

Shader RI, Weinberger DR, & Greenblatt DJ (1978). Pharmacological approaches to the medically ill patient. In TB Karasu & RI Steinmuller (Eds), *Psychotherapeutics in medicine.* (pp 117–155). Orlando: Grune & Stratton.

Shalev A, Hermesh H, Aizenberg D, et al. (1985). Neuroleptic malignant syndrome [Letter to the editor]. *New England Journal of Medicine, 313,* 1292.

Spielvogel A, & Wile J (1986). Treatment of the psychotic pregnant patient. *Psychosomatics, 27,* 487–492.

Sternberg DS (1986). Neuroleptic maligant syndrome: The pendulum swings. *American Journal of Psychiatry, 143,* 1273–1275.

Stoudemire A, & Fogel BS (1986). Organization and development of combined medical-psychiatric units (Part 1). *Psychosomatics, 27,* 341–345.

Stoudemire A, Kahn M, Brown JT, et al. (1985). Masked depression in a combined medical-psychiatric unit. *Psychosomatics, 26,* 221–230.

Talbott R, & Linn L (1978). Reactions of schizophrenics to life-threatening disease. *Psychiatric Quarterly, 40,* 218–227.

Tsuang MT, Perkins K, & Simpson JC (1983). Physical diseases in schizophrenia and affective disorder. *Journal of Clinical Psychiatry, 44,* 42–46.

Tsuang MT, Woolson RF,& Fleming JA (1980). Premature deaths in schizophrenia and affective disorders. *Archives of General Psychiatry, 37,* 979–983.

van der Kolk B, Shader RI, & Greenblatt DJ (1978). Autonomic side effects of psychotropic drugs. In MA Lipton, A DiMascio, & KF Killan (Eds), *Psychopharmacology: A generation of progress* (pp 1009–1020). New York: Raven Press.

Varsamis J & Adamson JD (1976). Somatic symptoms in schizophrenia. *Canadian Psychiatric Association Journal, 21,* 1–6.

Weiden P, & Harrigan M (1986). A clinical guide for diagnosing and managing patients with drug-induced dysphagia. *Hospital and Community Psychiatry, 37,* 396–398.

Yassa R, & Jones BJ (1985). Complications of tardive dyskinesia: A review. *Psychosomatics, 26,* 305–313.

Young LD, & Harsch HH (1986). Inpatient unit for combined physical and psychiatric disorders. *Psychosomatics, 27,* 53–60.

Zook CJ, & Moore FD(1980). High-cost users of medical care *New England Journal of Medicine, 302,* 996–1002.

Mark J. Mills
Marcia L. Daniels

21
Medical-Legal Issues

The hospital-based psychiatrist is frequently asked by colleague physicians to provide expertise on medical-legal problems; the psychiatrist should thus possess sufficient knowledge of both pertinent psychiatric and legal issues as they apply to that setting. The role of the hospital-based psychiatrist is to provide a thorough consultation, appropriate clinical assessment, and when requested, treatment. It is up to the courts and the legislatures to provide the appropriate judicial rulings and laws. In this chapter, common and important medicolegal issues that require psychiatric expertise will be described, and guidelines for the hospital-based psychiatrist will be provided.

COMPETENCE

Strictly speaking, the determination of competence is a legal issue (Applebaum & Roth, 1981; Mills 1985; Roth, Appelbaum, Sailee, et al., 1982; Roth, Meisel, & Lidz, 1977). As a general rule, under the law, all individuals are presumed competent until proven otherwise. As a practical matter, however, psychiatrists are often asked if a patient is competent. Consider the following case:

A 50-year-old male with diabetes and depression is hospitalized with a fever and a foot ulcer. He has previously lived on his own and managed his affairs without difficulty. He is started on appropriate medical treatment, but his fever persists and his ulcer worsens. At times, the staff notes that he appears confused. Psychiatric consultation is requested to determine why the patient is confused and to learn if the patient is competent to consent to continuing treatment. The psychiatrist determines that the patient is fully oriented and cognitively intact, although his responses to questions are slow, his mood is depressed, and his affect is blunted. Under the law, the patient is presumed competent, and the mental status exam, as well as the rest of the psychiatric consultation, fails to reveal any information that would warrant a court assessment of the patient's competency. The medical team continues to assess and treat the patient, and the psychiatrist agrees to continue to evaluate the patient with regard to his bouts of confusion and the abnormal mood and affect findings. No metabolic abnormalities or bodily fluid abnormalities are found, but the patient's fever and ulcer persist. Repeat mental status exams, however, reveal that the patient has developed a delirium. A local surgical procedure is urgently required because of the worsening of the foot infection. Once again the psychiatrist is asked if the patient is competent to consent to continuing diagnostic and treatment procedures.

The role of the psychiatrist is to provide the medical team with information as to the patient's mental status and, in the process, to assess several facets of competency. Further, the informed hospital-based psychiatrist will be sufficiently knowledgeable about legal requirements that he will be able to advise the treatment teams when consultation with the hospital's general counsel or risk manager is advisable. Still, however, the psychiatrist does not determine if the patient is competent; if necessary, that is a role of the courts.

Several facets of competency should be routinely assessed (Roth, et al., 1977). First, does the patient possess a clear choice in regard to any diagnostic and treatment procedure? Second, is the choice reasonable? Third, is the choice rational? Fourth, does the patient possess the ability to reason? Fifth, is the patient able to understand the relevant information needed to make a choice? In other words, is the patient able to choose, understand, reason, and appreciate the pertinent issues.

In the case described, the psychiatrist reported that the patient was confused and disoriented to place and time and did not appear to understand the significance of his medical condition nor to understand the rationale for particular treatments. He was not able to make a clear decision regarding his treatment preferences and needs. The responsibility of the psychiatrist at this point would typically be to assist the medical team in initiating access to the hospital general counsel or to the judicial process.

The plan would be to formally assess the patient's competence with respect to the specific clinical issue, as it was the belief of the psychiatrist (and the rest of the medical team) that the patient was not competent. Note, however, that *only the court makes this legal determination of competence.* If the court finds the patient incompetent, then a guardian may be appointed to make decisions for the patient.

In the interim, the team should generally not proceed with additional new treatments (unless it is an emergency), as it is unclear that the patient is competent to consent to such additional care. Unfortunately, in most jurisdictions, competency proceedings may take weeks to complete. In the case described above, treatment is urgently indicated, although not on an emergency basis. Depending on the jurisdiction in which the patient is receiving treatment, several options are open to the medical team. For example, in some states, hot lines are available on a 24-hour basis that provide for a judge to authorize urgently needed treatment. In other states, spousal consent is recognized under specifically delineated conditions. In states where rapid judicial access is unavailable, other mechanisms may be found to facilitate treatment authorization. If the situation described above were emergent, then authorization for treatment would not be necessary, as the circumstances (the immediately life-threatening nature of the patient's condition) would imply that a reasonable person would consent to treatment. In such emergent circumstances, consent is implied (Fogel, Mills, & Landen, 1986; Mills, Winslade, Lyon, et al., 1984).

In some clinical situations, however, the situation is pressing, but does not reach the "immediately life-threatening" threshold implicit in the word *emergent.* When the patient's condition requires urgent treatment, when there is no rapid access to the judical process, and when there is no guardian or conservator already in place, then a substitute decision maker should be found. Such decision makers might include a close relative of the patient, the hospital's chief of staff, the chief of one of the major clinical services, a senior colleague, or the medical center's risk manager or general counsel. The authorization of one of these people does not substitute for a competency hearing. Such authorization, known as *vicarious consent*, is appropriate only when the need for diagnostic and treatment procedures is urgent and access to the courts cannot be obtained in a sufficiently timely fashion. The courts understand, however, that a patient's condition may be sufficiently grave to require urgent treatment, well before a hearing can be convened, and yet not be so grave as to fit the "immediately life-threatening" definition of an emergency.

In the case described, several points merit review. First, it is the responsibility of the psychiatrist to know the appropriate tests for competency. It is the function of the psychiatrist to conduct a thorough evaluation of the patient, including a biopsychosocial assessment as well as serial mental status examinations, and to provide feedback to the treating team as to the findings. Relevant psychodynamic factors should be included in the report. The reliability and accuracy of information provided to the patient and obtained from the patient should also be noted. In the case described, family and other sources of information about the patient were not available. To the extent possible, the psychiatrist should try to obtain pertinent information about the patient from several sources. It should further be noted that psychiatric illness, per se, is not grounds for clinicians to presume, nor for courts to find, a patient incompetent. Competency in regard to medical issues may be situational and thus requires continued assessment as the patient's medical condition evolves.

The essence of competence is that a particular patient at a particular time has the capacity to make a meaningful choice about a particular clinical alternative. Common sense and legal precedents suggest that for patients to exercise such a choice, they must have knowledge of the preferred therapeutic intervention, including its benefits and risks, as well as knowledge of alternative treatments (if any) and the likely consequences of no treatment. Further, the law requires that the patient be able to utilize or weigh this information. The law generally does not require, however, that a patient weigh such information "fully." Thus, patients who have some obvious, but circumscribed, cognitive or emotional deficit may well be able to be competent and to provide consent. For example, patients with schizophrenia, depression, or mild dementia may be competent for a particular medical choice, or (although less revelant to physicians) for making a nonmedical choice, such as writing a will or voting (Appelbaum & Roth, 1981; Fogel et al., 1986; Mills, 1985; Mills et al., 1984; Roth, et al., 1982; Roth, et al., 1977).

CONSENT ISSUES

Over the past thirty years, the modern doctrine of informed consent has emerged. In the 1950s, the court held that in order for patients to give consent, they had to receive "full disclosure" regarding the risks of the preferred procedures (Salgo, 1957). In subsequent legal determinations, the courts redefined the duty of the physician to disclose to the patient what a "reasonable medical practitioner" would disclose (*Natanson v Kline*, 1960). The most recent and most universally applied standard provided by the courts has been to define the duty of the physician to disclose to a patient what a "reasonable patient" would want disclosed (Mills, Hsu, & Berger, 1980). Implicit in the "reasonable patient" doctrine is that patients will want more information when the procedures consented to are more complex and when the hazards are greater. Also implicit in this standard is that what is reasonable for one patient may not be reasonable for another; that is, this standard explicitly recognizes the variability of the patient's "subjectivity" (Mills, 1985; Mills et al. 1980; *Natanson v Kline*, 1960; *Salgo v Leland Stanford, Jr, University Board of Trustees*, 1957).

Consider the following case:

A 20-year-old female is admitted for evaluation of an abdominal mass. She is belligerent and refuses to consent to routine noninvasive diagnostic procedures, after initially agreeing to undergo diagnostic evaluation. A psychiatric consultation is requested to evaluate the patient's belligerence and her refusal to consent to the diagnostic procedures. The psychiatrist determines that the patient has a personality disorder but that she is neither psychotic nor disoriented. Her family members provide corroborating information that she is often combative and ambivalent. The psychiatrist reports his findings to the medical team and, with the patient's consent, provides a brief psychotherapeutic intervention to lessen the patient's distress. The patient decides to stay in the hospital and at a subsequent time consents to the evaluation of her abdominal mass.

There are three components of informed consent that should be assessed routinely (*Kaimowitz v Michigan Department of Mental Health*, 1973). First, is the patient competent to provide consent? That is, does the patient have the intelligence and the ability to judge the information presented? Second, has the patient been given sufficient knowledge about the proposed procedures? Specifically, what are the benefits to the patient, to others with a similar condition, and to society? What is the risk of harm if the procedure is done or if it is delayed? What other risks exist? Third, has the consent been obtained in a voluntary manner? Specifically, for informed consent to be obtained, a patient must not be coerced into a consent, nor

may a patient be given improper inducements to consent.

In the case described, the psychiatrist determined that the three components of consent had been addressed and that there were no grounds to assume that the patient was incapable of giving informed consent. There are situations, however, when the psychiatric assessment reveals that the patient is not capable of providing informed consent. When such situations arise, several options are available to the treating team, depending on the urgency of the situation. Consider the following case:

A 65-year-old male with Alzheimer's disease is admitted for treatment of pneumonia. A psychiatric consultation is requested to determine if the patient can consent to treatment. The patient is disoriented and at times unaware that he has an acute medical problem. Information from the family reveals that he is not able to care for himself and that family members provide his routine daily care, food, and shelter. The patient does not have a court-appointed guardian to make decisions on his behalf. The psychiatrist determines that the patient has a significant dementing condition and does not appear to be competent to give informed consent. Nor does he understand the risks and benefits of proposed procedures. The responsibility of the psychiatrist is to report these findings to the treating team and to help facilitate access to the appropriate court proceedings.

Implied Consent

As already noted, proceedings to determine competency and to appoint a guardian may take weeks to complete. In the interim, several options should be considered. First, if the medical condition is such that emergency treatment is needed, the doctrine of *implied consent* may be invoked and treatment initiated (Fogel, Mills & Landen, 1986). Specifically, this allows the treating physician to evaluate and treat the emergent condition and to do so even against the apparent will of the patient.

When the evaluation and treatment of the medical condition are *not* emergent, then the physician has at least four alternatives. A second opinion can be obtained concerning the nature of the medical condition, the need for proposed procedures, and the alternatives that may be available. The hospital's legal counsel can be consulted. Such consultation does not substitute for court authorization, but it can be useful in order to obtain an independent assessment from someone who is at a distance from the treating team. Further, seeking such consultation may allay the fears that family members may have regarding treatment choices, as such consultations often provide clarification and amplification regarding proposed treatments. Another alternative is to involve the family in the evaluation and treatment process. This is most useful when there is time for consultation, when several procedures are equally effective, and when family members are genuinely interested in the patient's welfare. If there is any question as to the family's interest, if family members disagree, if treatment issues are complex or risky, or if there are only distant family members available, then this alternative should be used only adjunctively. That is, it is almost always useful to consult the patient's family, but their opinion is not necessarily that of the patient, or that which the patient would have desired but for the present incompetence (Mills, 1985).

Court Proceedings

The most appropriate alternative is to seek court authorization for patients who cannot give informed consent. In such a situation, a court can appoint a guardian to make decisions for the patient. The wishes of the family, as well as information from the treating team and from consultants, can be considered. Since a court proceeding allows the relevant clinical information to be considered and because the court may deliberate both about what is best for a patient and about what the particular patient might want, such a process is appropriate if the medical condition allows a time delay before treatment needs to be initiated.

In this regard, it is important to note that the court may evaluate a proposed treatment from at least two perspectives, or it may mix the two: what is "best for the patient"—a so-called objective standard—and what "the patient would have wanted but for the present incapacity"—a so-called subjective standard. Various jurisdictions and clinical contexts tend to sway the court to employ one standard or the other. It is also important to note that the process of coming into court with counsel can be time-consuming for the patient, family, and clinicians, as well as expensive and possibly demeaning for the patient. Most clinicians thus avoid seeking court intervention. Studies suggest that clinicians fail to seek court attention even when patients are seriously impaired cognitively. Sometimes this may be because the clinician believes the risks of the proposed treatment are few and the benefits great. Oftentimes, however, it is either because the clinician has failed to appreciate the severity of the patient's mental condition or because the clinician is reluctant to spare time dealing with the largely unfamiliar legal system (Mills, 1985).

Consent for Neuroleptics

Finally, but still relating to matters of consent, it is useful to recall that the courts have recently required extra care when obtaining consent for the use of neuroleptics (*Clites v Iowa*, 1980; Gelenberg, 1982; Wettstein, 1983). In at least three separate rulings involving substantial judgments or settlements, the courts have attributed the development of tardive dyskinesia to the administration of neuroleptics and have held, in effect, that the patients might have chosen not to receive such medication had they been more completely informed of its risks. Although it is still too early to know if such cases will become common, extra care is warranted when obtaining consent for antipsychotics. In general, psychiatrists should carefully and periodically (every 6 months or so) note in the medical record the indications for the use of neuroleptics, explicitly discuss how the patient has been informed of the risks and benefits, and particularly note the patient's acceptance (or refusal) of the medication. In addition, it should be documented that the medications are still needed if extended treatment is considered and that the drugs are being used at the lowest possible effective dose. As in other cases in which patients' illnesses may render them incompetent, the psychiatrist will want to consider consulting the hospital general counsel in order to obtain a guardianship if the patient's acceptance or refusal of medications appears to be for irrational reasons. It is also useful to obtain an Abnormal Involuntary Movement Scale (AIMS) assessment every 6 months on patients being treated with antipsychotics and, most important, to consult an expert colleague on diagnosis and treatment alternatives should the patient begin to develop signs of tardive dyskinesia (Gutheil, 1980; Mills, 1985).

CIVIL COMMITMENT

In most jurisdictions, the psychiatrists are empowered under specific conditions to restrain patients against their will for purposes of brief evaluation and (in most jurisdictions) treatment (Lonsdorf, 1983; Mills, 1986). If a psychiatrist restrains a patient who later is found not to be committable, the psychiatrist is not held liable, so long as the conditions for initiating commitment

were considered and malice was absent. Although the history of commitment law initially favored institutionalization of almost anyone deemed in need of treatment, subsequent legal rulings have tended to strike a balance between the need for treatment and the individual's right to freedom. In fact, a number of psychiatrist commentators believe that the pendulum has swung too far and that too often concern for patients' rights overwhelms concern for patient's welfare. There has also been a reduction in the procedural differences between civil and criminal commitment proceedings, so those civilly committed have many of the same rights (for example, the right to counsel) that the criminally committed have had.

Consider the following case:

A 40-year-old male is hospitalized in order to undergo chemotherapy for metastatic cancer. He is noted by the staff to be despondent. A psychiatric consultation is rquested to evaluate his affect and mood. Evaluation reveals that the individual has a major mood disorder and is actively suicidal. The patient subsequently requests that all medical treatments be discontinued. He is fully oriented, and his cognitive processes are intact. The patient refuses any psychiatric treatment for his depression and continues to verbalize suicide plans. The psychiatrist should provide feedback to the medical team regarding the patient's condition and assist in initiating commitment proceedings.

The general intent of commitment laws is to allow evaluation and treatment of patients who lack the ability to care for themselves as a result of a mental disorder. In the case just mentioned, commitment of the individual would permit clinical interventions, including evaluation and (in most jurisdictions) treatment of the patient's mental disorder. Psychiatric intervention may occur in the setting in which the patient is or may occur in a specialized mental health facility. Commitment of the hospitalized patient might thus necessitate transfer of the patient to another facility. Commitment of a patient, however, does not automatically allow treatment of the patient's underlying medical disorder (his carcinoma). Commitment in the case described would thus not allow the treating team to initiate chemotherapeutic procedures for metastatic disease.

Since such patients are not so infrequently encountered, it is useful to have considered an approach to them. When a patient has a functional psychiatric illness, commitment and treatment allow time and psychiatric treatment to be effective. In many instances, as the patient's psychiatric illness remits, the patient will again be able to make more appropriate decisions about medical treatment. If the psychosis does not diminish or if the patient's therapeutic choices are persistently irrational, the clinician will generally want to consult the medical center's legal counsel and to plan on using the legal system to find a conservator or guardian for the patient.

PATIENTS' RIGHTS TO TREATMENT AND REFUSAL OF TREATMENT

Although there has been relatively little case law on the right to treatment, the legal doctrine has had a major impact. Conversely, there have been a plethora of legal rulings in regard to the right to refuse treatment, but at least until recently, the impact of these rulings has been relatively minor (Mills, 1982, 1985). In 1971, a federal court ruled that an individual had a constitutionally derived right to treatment (Wyatts, 1970s). Subsequent rulings have generally reaffirmed and narrowed this right (Mills, 1982; *O'Connor v Donaldson*, 1975; *Romeo v Youngberg*, 1980; *Youngberg v Romeo*, 1982). The impact of the right-to-treatment rulings, especially through the consent decree process, has been to mandate that jurisdictions provide minimal treatment for individuals in such need. The hospital-based psychiatrist needs to be cognizant of this right because some of the programs created in response to this right have become politically volatile and economically unstable. Practically, this often means that certain publicly funded treatment centers are unfortunately crowded or underfunded.

The courts have approached the right to *refuse* treatment in a different manner. A number of rulings have been made that generally support a constitutionally derived liberty interest to refuse treatment (*AE and RR v Mitchell*, 1980; Mills, 1985; Mills, Yesavage, & Gutheil, 1983; *Mills v Rogers*, 1982; *Lessard v Schmidt*, 1972; *Rennie v Klein*, 1979; *Rogers v Okin*, 1979), but the courts have also attempted to balance the patient's right to refuse care against the need to provide patients with access to care. Some jurisdictions have created elaborate mechanisms, including mental health advocates and quasi-judicial proceedings, to protect both patients' rights and patients' needs. Recently, however, state, as opposed to federal, courts have begun to consider the right-to-refuse-treatment issue (*Goedecke v Colorado*, 1979; *In re KKB*, 1980). Because their perspective is different, they look first to the state (not federal) constitution and laws, and an increasing number have found that state laws prohibit the treatment of legally committed patients. Because, from the clinical perspective, treatment is the ostensible purpose of commitment, such rulings, although not yet widespread, are viewed by most psychiatrists as countertherapeutic.

The appropriate role of the hospital-based psychiatrist is to be aware of the pertinent rulings in his jurisdiction in regard to patients' rights, and to model behavior for the medical team consistent with the current applicable law.

CONFIDENTIALITY

Patients have a longstanding common-law right to confidentiality (Jonsen, Siegler, & Winslade, 1982). The psychiatrist's general obligation in regard to confidentiality is often confused with privilege, the statutory right that patients generally have to keep their communications with their physician private, unless they specifically waive this right. It is thus prudent to obtain a patient's consent regarding release of any communication. Exceptions to this right vary across jurisdictions, but a general guideline is that confidentiality must give way where public peril begins (Mills, 1985; *Tarasoff v Regents of the University of California*, 1976). Furthermore, clinical information should be disclosed when such information is relevant, let alone essential, to the completion of an emergency assessment. Information should also be disclosed when patients are referred for treatment. The extent of information released without a patient's consent should be limited to that which absolutely must be revealed in order for appropriate evaluation and treatment to be initiated.

Consider the following case:

A 70-year-old female presents for evaluation of memory loss. Extensive evaluation reveals that the patient most likely has multi-infarct dementia. There are no findings to suggest that the patient is incompetent. The patient requests that family members not be informed of her condition. The patient's spouse subsequently calls the treating physician and demands to know about his wife's condition and prognosis.

The physician should explain that the patient has requested that no information be released but that the physician will discuss the spouse's request with the patient. The physician should also counsel the spouse to discuss the matter directly with the patient. The physician may, and generally should, elect to explore with the patient the reasons for the decision and to assess the appropriateness of that decision. In the case described, the physician met privately with the patient. She decided to grant permission for the physician to talk with her spouse. At this point, the role of the physician is to discuss with the patient the reasons for her change of mind. Once assured that the patient wants the physician to speak to her spouse, the physician is free to do so. In sum, disclosure should be keyed to the patient's wishes and needs. Since patients are often ambivalent, it is best to proceed gradually, unless an emergency situation exists.

An aspect of confidentiality of growing importance is that arising from *Tarasoff*-like cases (1976). *Tarasoff* was a California case that established the *duty to protect,* often incorrectly called the "duty to warn." The essence of that duty, one that is recognized in a growing minority of states, is that psychotherapists (and this probably includes hospital-based psychiatrists) must be unusually sensitive to clinical material that suggests a patient is planning to harm another and perhaps another's property. Psychiatrists generally may discharge this duty by ensuring that the patient is not released from the hospital until perceived as no longer dangerous or until ordered released by the court. Additionally, some jurisdictions specifically allow that warning the intended victims or notifying the police will provide immunity from suit even if the threatened harm occurs (Mills, 1985).

LEAVING AGAINST MEDICAL ADVICE

Leaving treatment against medical advice is the absolute right of the competent patient (McCartney, 1985; Mills, 1985). Patients who want to leave against medical advice often do so because they believe they have been mismanaged, misinformed, or misunderstood. Most often the desire to leave the hospital under these circumstances is the result of a number of interactions between the patient and at least some of the providers. Consider the following case:

A 30-year-old male, admitted for treatment of inflammatory bowel disease urgently desires to leave the hospital. He has previously been subdued but cooperative with the treating team. On the morning of the threatened discharge, he tells the staff that he is fed up, does not want to talk with anyone, and has called his family to come and take him home. A psychiatric consultation is requested. The psychiatrist talks briefly with the patient and also reviews the hospital course. On mental status examination, the patient is found to be cognitively intact but angry. Although the patient is receiving steroids, there are not sufficient findings to suggest that the patient is incompetent to consent or refuse to consent to his care. The patient refuses to talk further with the psychiatrist and refuses to sign a paper acknowledging his decision to leave against medical advice.

The function of the psychiatrist in this situation is to provide an evaluation of the patients mental status and to try to determine what has happened to promote the patient's decision to leave against medical advice. Often psychiatrists will partially ally themselves with the patients and in the process will discover why the patients believe they have been treated improperly. Empathic and objective discussions with the patient may help to clear up misunderstandings and allow for the patient to continue to receive care, if that is indicated. An additional strategy that may be helpful is to offer the patient a cooling-off period. For example, in the case described, the patient could be offered an overnight pass to allow him time to reconsider his decision. If the patient chooses to leave the hospital, the psychiatrist may still be helpful to the treatment team in assisting them to understand and to accept the patient's decision.

In the case described, the patient was competent and elected to exercise his right to leave the hospital. In many situations, the patient will provide information about why he makes a particular decision, but in this case that information was not forthcoming. Still, as long as patients are competent, they have the right to leave the hospital, and they do not have to sign any release to do so. Signed releases are for the convenience of the institution and its staff; when a patient leaves without a release, the treating team should carefully chart the patient's requests and the attempted interventions. The psychiatrist should also meet with the treating team in an effort to discover what may have prompted the leaving. The patient may have distorted the situation or may have needed to control the environment as a way of containing the dependency and helplessness that can occur in hospital settings. Some additional reasons that may promote patient departures include staff conflict that gets displaced onto the patient, staff miscommunications with the patient, and staff diffusion of care. Finally, one has to always consider that the patient may have a specific psychiatric disorder, such as psychosis, dementia, or a personality disorder, that has been previously undetected (McCartney, 1985).

FAMILIES AND THE LAW

Patient's families often have an important role in the course and care of the hospitalized patient. It is thus important that the medical team appreciate the individual cultural, religious, ethnic, and socioeconomic aspects of both the patient and the family. Family members who are treated abruptly or who are resented because of the demands they place on the medical team are more likely to be litigious. It is important for the medical team to understand that family members may act in seemingly inappropriate ways because of the difficulties they have in coping with a patient's illness. When possible, it is prudent to talk with a family about the concerns they have regarding the patient. Evaluation of potential roles that family members can take in providing care for the patient should also be considered. With the patient's permission, providing education to the family about the patient's condition and then setting appropriate limits regarding family behavior in the hospital can be beneficial in providing better care. Just as with patients, maintaining a supportive and empathic stance with family members should be a primary aim. As with patients, when family members feel abandoned or misunderstood, they are more apt to be litigious.

SPECIAL TOPICS

A variety of special topics need discussion albeit in a pithier fashion than such topics as competence and consent.

Guardians and Conservators

One source of confusion for many physicians is the differences between guardianship and conservatorship and between the probate code and the civil commitment code (Morris, 1980; Steinbrook & Lo, 1984). Because the laws of the fifty states vary so widely, there is no uniform distinction between a guardian and a conservator. Still, in many jurisdictions, conservators are those "guardians" who are appointed to look after a patient with psychiatric problems. (A source of additional confusion is that the law has not followed the recent developments in neurobiology that largely blur the historically useful distinctions between functional and organic illness.) More important, however, is the distinction between the probate code and the mental health code. The probate code is the old portion of the law designed to deal with conveying property in an orderly fash-

ion upon the death of an individual. For centuries, those laws have recognized that a person might become so ill that another, acting under the authority of the state, would need to make decisions, particularly about the use of assets for that person. Traditionally, probate code guardians have had the power to consent to a patient's medical treatment. In contrast, mental health code guardians are the product of the civil commitment reforms of the sixties and seventies. In most juridictions, they do not have the power to consent to treatment for conditions other than those defined as psychiatric.

Temporary Guardians and Durable Power of Attorney

Because guardians and conservators, regardless of the source of their statutory authority, have considerable power, their appointment has been protected by elaborate due process requirements, generally in the form of judicial hearings. These hearings are sufficiently time-consuming that the process, as discussed above, is often too slow to respond to evolving medical needs. Some jurisdictions allow for the appointment of a temporary guardian, whose powers are quite limited in duration and who, therefore, can be appointed with less protracted judicial scrutiny.

Similarly, the time-consuming nature of court processes has served to inspire other legal mechanisms to deal with a patient's incapacity. One of the newest and potentially most useful mechanisms is the *durable power of attorney. Durable* power of attorney, *endures* past the time when a patient becomes incompetent, in contrast to an *ordinary* power of attorney expires when a patient becomes incompetent. Furthermore, the individual who holds power of attorney may not make medical decisions for the patient unless this power is specifically included in the legal documents establishing the power of attorney. In those jurisdictions (still relatively few) in which durable power of attorney is recognized, it allows a still-competent person to anticipate future incompetence and to conditionally delegate the authortiy to another to make decisions, including medical ones, in the event of the person's incompetence. As such, the durable power of attorney usually obviates the need for costly and complicated guardianship arrangements.

The Living Will and "Do Not Resuscitate" Orders

Related to the durable power of attorney is the living will. In such a document, the testator (maker of the will) outlines certain requests regarding treatment or care in the future. Because such wills are not as personal as durable powers of attorney, they appear less apt to circumvent traditional guardianship laws and are thus recognized in more jurisdictions. The problem with such wills is that they may not very effectively guarantee the testator's requests (Stephens, 1986).

"Do not resuscitate" (DNR) orders are increasingly familiar in virtually all medical centers and may be one of the requests embodied in a living will. Such orders are widely accepted in this country as long as medical center policy has been assiduously followed and state laws have not been violated. Because most states have not regulated DNR orders, medical centers are the de facto policy makers in this regard. Given the fact that physicians' biases are strongly toward maintaining life, it is not surprising that most medical centers severely restrict the use of such orders by requiring collegial (often medical state board) review and by specifying the relatively few conditions (brain death, terminal illness, and intractable pain are common) in which such orders will be countenanced (Deciding, 1983).

SUMMARY

As with nearly every aspect of medicine, when a clinician is unfamiliar with a particular issue, a consultation is prudent. The hospital-based psychiatrist has an important function as a consultant who can understand and provide knowledge about pertinent medicolegal issues in the hospital setting. Analogously, the legally informed psychiatrist also periodically seeks the advice and assistance of hospital counsel as novel issues arise. Psychiatrists can serve as advocates for patients as well as for the hospital and society. By doing so, they set the tone for both optimal patient care and a reduction in medical-legal problems.

REFERENCES

AE and RR v Mitchell, No C8–466 (D Utah 1980)

Appelbaum PD & Roth LH (1981). Clinical issues in the assessment of competency. *American Journal of Psychiatry, 138,* 1462–1467.

Clites v Iowa, Law No. 46274 (Iowa Dist Ct, Pottawatamie County August 7, 1980).

Deciding to Forego Life-Sustaining Treatment: Ethical, Medical, and Legal Issues in Treatment Decisions (1983). Washington, DC: President's Commission for the Study of Ethical Problems in Medicine and Biomedical and Behavioral Research.

Fogel BS, Mills MJ, & Landen JE (1986). Legal aspects of the treatment of delirium. *Hospital and Community Psychiatry, 37,* 154–158.

Gelenberg AJ (1982). $375,000 for tardive dyskinesia. *Biological Therapeutic Psychiatry, 3,* 41–42.

Goedecke v. Colorado, 603 P2d 123 (Colo S Ct 1979).

Gutheil TG (1980). Paranoia and progress notes. A guide to forensically informed psychiatric record-keeping. *Hospital and Community Psychiatry, 31,* 479–482.

Jonsen A, Siegler M, & Winslade WJ (1982). *Clinical Ethics.* New York: Macmillan.

Kaimowitz v Michigan Department of Mental Health, Div No 73-19434-AW (Cir Ct, Wayne County, Mich 1973). Abstracted in 13 Criminal L Rep 2452. Reprinted in AD Brooks (1974), *Law Psychiatry and the Mental Health System* (New York: Little, Brown) and in 1 Mental Disability L Rep 147.

In re KKB, No 51, 467 (Okla S Ct Jan 15, 1980).

Lessard v Schmidt, 349 F Supp 1078 (ED Wisc 1972), remanded.

Lonsdorf RG (1983). The involuntary commitment of adults: An examination of recent legal trends. *Psychiatric Clinics of North America, 6,* 651–660.

McCartney JR (1985). Management of refusal of medical treatment. *International Journal of Psychiatry in Medicine, 15,* 31–36.

Mills, MJ (1982). The right to treatment; Little law but much impact. In L Grinspoon (Ed), *Psychiatry.* Washington DC: American Psychiatric Association Press.

Mills MJ (1985). Legal issues in psychiatric treatment. *Psychiatric Medicine, 2,* 245–261.

Mills MJ (1986). Civil commitment of the mentally ill: An overview. *Annals, American Association of Political and Social Sciences, 484,* 28–41.

Mills MJ, Hsu L, & Berger PA (1980). Informed consent: Psychotic patients and research. *Bulletin of the American Academy of Psychiatry and Law, 8,* 119–132.

Mills MJ, Winslade WJ, Lyon MA, et al. (1984). Clinicolegal aspects of treatment of demented patients. *Psychiatric Annals, 14,* 209–211.

Mills MJ, Yesavage JA, & Gutheil JG (1983). Continuing case-law development in the right to refuse treatment. *American Journal of Psychiatry, 140,* 715–719, 1983.

Mills v Rogers, 102 S Ct 2442 (1982).

Morris GH (1980). The use of guardianships to achieve—or to avoid—the least restrictive alternative. *International Journal of Law and Psychiatry, 3,* 97–115.

Natanson v Kline, 186 Kan 393, 350 P2d 1093 (1960).

O'Connor v Donaldson, 422 US 563 (1975).

Rennie v Klein, 476 F Supp 1294 (D NJ 1979).

Rogers v Okin, 478 F Supp 1342 (DC Mass 1979).

Romeo v Youngberg, 644 F2d 147 (3d Cir 1980).

Roth LH, Appelbaum PS, Sailee R, et al. (1982). The dilemma of denial in the assessment of competency to refuse treatment. *American Journal of Psychiatry, 139,* 910–913.

Roth LH, Meisel A, & Lidz CW (1977). Tests of competency to consent to treatment. *American Journal of Psychiatry, 134,* 249–284.

Salgo v Leland Stanford, Jr, University Board of Trustees, 317 p2d 170 (1957).

Steinbrook R & Lo B (1984). Decision making for incompetent patients by designated proxy. *New England Journal of Medicine, 310,* 1598–160l.

Stephens RL (1986). "Do not resuscitate" orders: Ensuring the patient's participation. *Journal of the American Medical Association, 255,* 240–24l.

Tarasoff v Regents of the University of California, 118 Cal Rptr 129 (1974); 131 Cal Rptr 14 (1976).

Wettstein RM (1983). Tardive dyskinesia and malpractice. *Behavioral Science Law, 1,* 85–107.

Wyatt v Aderholt, CA No 72-2634 (5th Cir Aug 15, 1972); Wyatt v Aderholt, 503 F2d 1305 (5th Cir 1974). Wyatt v Hardin, CA No 3195-N (MD Ala Feb 7, 1975); Wyatt v Ireland, CA No 3195-N (Md Ala Oct 25, 1979); Wyatt v Stickney, 325 F Supp 781 (MD Ala 1971a); Wyatt v Stickney, 334 F Supp 1341 (MD Ala 1971b); Wyatt v Stickney, 334 F Supp 373 (MD Ala 1972a); Wyatt v Stickney, 334 F Supp 387 (MD Ala 1972b).

Youngberg v Romeo, 457 US 307 (1982).

PART II

Specific Disease Categories

James L. Levenson

22
Cardiovascular Disease

EPIDEMIOLOGY OF CARDIOVASCULAR DISEASE

Almost 20 percent of the U.S. population has cardiovascular disease and one-fourth of them suffer limitation of activity (Kannel & Thom, 1985). One out of every three men, and one in ten women, will develop significant cardiovascular disease before age 60 (Gordon & Kannel, 1971). Hypertension has a prevalence of 60 million, which is 26 percent of the total population and 36 percent of the adult population (National Heart, Lung, and Blood Institute, 1982). Coronary heart disease affects 6 million, with American males having a one-in-five chance of developing the disease before age 60 (Kannel & Thom, 1985). There are 800,000 new heart attacks and 450,000 recurrences each year (National Heart, Lung, and Blood Institute, 1982).

Despite advances in treatment and risk-factor reduction, cardiovascular disease remains the leading cause of death in the United States, accounting for half of all deaths. One-third of deaths in persons over age 35 are due to coronary heart disease

(Kannel & Thom, 1985). Cardiovascular disease accounts for the highest amount of total health care expenditures, short-stay hospital days, and worker disability allowances, accounting for one-third of all Social Security disability benefits (National Heart, Lung, and Blood Institute, 1982; U.S. Department of Health and Human Services, 1983).

The treatment of cardiovascular disorders has been increasingly aggressive in recent years. Cardiac catheterization, coronary artery bypass grafting, percutaneous coronary angioplasty, and permanent pacemakers have become routine procedures, and cardiac transplantation is no longer regarded as experimental. From 1960 to 1980, the percentage of hypertensives receiving medication increased from 36 to 56 percent (Kannel & Thom, 1985). Cardiopulmonary resuscitation has been widely taught in the community at large.

By chance alone, the high prevalence of both cardiovascular and psychiatric disorders would produce frequent concurrence. In addition, patients with significant cardiovascular disease appear to be at increased risk for developing psychopathology, particularly depression (Levenson & Friedel, 1985; Vazquez-Barquero, Acero, Ochoteco, et al., 1985). Anxiety and depression are frequent after myocardial infarction (MI) (Cassem & Hackett, 1977; Hackett, Cassem, & Wishnie, 1968; Lloyd & Cawly, 1978; Stern, Pascale, & Ackerman, 1977), and anxiety, depression, and delirium commonly follow cardiac surgery (Dubin, Field, & Gastfriend, 1979; Freyhan, Gianelli, O'Connell, et al., 1979) (see also Chapter 18, by Goldstein). Despite the extensive literature describing psychiatric symptoms in the cardiac patient, the specific incidence of psychiatric disorders remains unclear. Rather than use criterion-based diagnoses, most studies have focused on psychologic symptoms, which may be due to transient reactions, drug side effects, major psychiatric disorders, or cardiac disease itself. Studies utilizing symptom-oriented instruments document significant psychopathology in 20–45 percent of patients with cardiac disease (Lloyd & Cawly, 1978; Vazquez-Barquero, et al., 1985). Clinically, depression appears the most common psychiatric disorder encountered in patients with heart disease or hypertension, with delirium, substance abuse, and somatoform disorders also common.

PSYCHOLOGIC ASPECTS

The close interrelationship between human emotion and the heart has long been recognized. Most intense affects, including rage, anxiety, elation, and sexual excitement, produce changes in cardiac function, particularly increased heart rate. Many cultures regard the heart as the seat of the emotions, the organ of love, the abode of conscience, and the center of strength. We speak of people as brokenhearted, heartless, hearty, or having a heavy heart.

Emotional Consequences of Cardiac Illness

The onset of symptomatic cardiac disease is a potent provocation for anxiety (in this section, anxiety and depression are used to denote affects, rather than diagnoses). Angina, arrhythmias, and acute heart failure produce anxiety related to fears of heart attack, disability, and sudden death. Psychodynamically, the individual's anxiety may contain varying degrees of fears of annihilation, passivity and impotence, object loss, and guilt. The experience of anxiety is often somatically magnified by the acute autonomic and physiologic concomitants of acute cardiac disease (cold sweats, nausea, lightheadedness, shortness of breath, chest tightness, etc.). One who has lost friends or family with cardiac disease, particularly when a sudden unexpected death has been witnessed, may already have anticipatory anxiety before ever experiencing the first cardiac symptom.

Angina and arrhythmias share many symptoms with panic attacks and, like panic, may lead to increasing anticipatory anxiety and phobic avoidance of the seeming precipitants of acute attacks. Fortunately, medical treatment is usually effective in preventing or aborting acute cardiac symptoms, and the acute anxiety most often recedes rather than generalizing. Even pharmacologically or surgically ineffective treatments may relieve angina and the attendant anxiety, through potent placebo effects (Benson & McCallie, 1979). When anxiety does persist, the patient may become a "cardiac cripple," too frightened to risk an active life.

Chronic cardiac illness evokes depression through narcissistic injury, object loss, and guilt. Narcissistic injury occurs through the loss (or threat of loss) of functions, including limitations on occupational, recreational, and sexual activities. Death is the ultimate catastrophe for the self, but the losses associated with premature death carry different meanings depending on the person's particular emotional investments. A patient may feel robbed of seeing children grow up, providing for dependents, finishing a lifework, or reaching a hard-earned retirement. The physician measures the progress of the disease by how few steps the patient can take and how many pillows are needed to sleep, tangible reminders to patients of their limitations. Sexual dysfunction is common in men and women with cardiac disease (Abramov, 1976; McLane, Krop, & Mehta, 1980; Mehta & Krop, 1979). Each of these real and feared losses adds another blow to the individual's narcissism and produces feelings of depression.

Each attack or hospitalization evokes a vivid sense of mortality and the threat of separation from loved ones. When cardiac disease is familial, the symptoms evoke grief-laden memories of the deaths of parents or other close family members. The patient's cardiac symptoms may thus serve for identification with the lost objects. This identification underlies the common fantasy in patients with familial heart disease that they will die of a heart attack at the same age as a parent did. Elderly patients with heart disease experience a similar echo of object loss and grief in their cardiac symptoms as they witness one by one the deaths of their peers, many of which are due to cardiovascular disease.

Patients may blame themselves for failing to stop smoking, lose weight, exercise, or comply with medical treatment, or simply to "having a weak heart." More unconsciously, a patient may experience guilt stemming from previous object losses caused by heart disease. If the patient had unconsciously wished for the death of a cardiac sufferer, then heart disease may be felt as retribution for this forbidden wish. Depression may occur in a patient who does well medically after a heart attack or cardiac surgery, deriving from "survivor guilt" (Blacher, 1978). (See also Chapter 19

by Riether and Stoudemire.) People with survivor guilt feel guilty that they have lived when loved ones previously did not, sometimes because they were able to receive medical or surgical treatment not available to the lost objects.

As cardiac disease may lead to depression, depression in turn may be expressed in cardiac symptoms. Affect is commonly somatized into chest pain, both in those with significant heart disease and in those without (Bass, Wade, & Gardner, 1983). Chest pain is a frequent "depressive-equivalent" in children as well as adults (Kashani, Lababidi, & Jones, 1982). Acute grief often includes a sensation of chest tightness, and later memory of the loss (conscious or unconscious) may appear as the somatic symptom (Miller, 1978)—the depressed are often brokenhearted.

Rather than denying their fears and losses, some patients are overwhelmed by them. They may become fearful of activity, especially work and sex (a fear sometimes called "cardiac neurosis"). Since any strong emotion tends to cause an increase in heart rate, they may become emotionally constricted in attempting to avoid "stressing the heart." They internalize the approach of the coronary care unit, where they felt safer and cared for, and so respond to each new pain or chest sensation as occasion for "rule-out-MI"procedures. Feeling doomed, they may nihilistically give up on trying to modify risk factors: "Why stop smoking if I'm about to be executed?"

For those who are not immobilized by extreme denial or crippling pessimism, the psychologic tasks of changing life-style and modifying risk factors still remain difficult. Smoking, overeating, and compulsive working are all often fueled by anxiety or depression and are especially hard to give up when the new stress of cardiac disease has been added. Bad habits create a maladaptive, hard-to-change behavioral homeostasis. Cessation of smoking may exacerbate overeating. Attempting to exercise while still overweight and smoking can be self-defeating, as can trying to lose weight without exercising.

Physicians' Countertransference

The psychiatrist evaluating a cardiac patient with psychologic symptoms should consider the possibility of relevant countertransference reactions in the internist or cardiologist responsible for the patient's primary care. These reactions may relate in a circular fashion to the patient's difficulties. Physicians old enough to be at risk for coronary disease will tend to identify with some of their cardiac patients. While this could potentially enhance their ability to empathize with patients, it may instead lead them to distance themselves. If patients are very frightened by their heart disease, physicians may withdraw to avoid their own resonant anxiety. If patients are strong deniers, physicians unconsciously worried about their own mortality may collude in the denial, distancing themselves not only from the patients but from the disease as well.

Younger physicians are more likely to err in the other direction. Enthusiastically launching an attack on risk factors, they may become almost messianic in their approach to the patient. Concerned over some patients' denial of illness, they may try to directly overcome their defenses. Benevolently, even feeling morally obligated to do so, the physician may attempt to "reason with" (i.e., scare) the patient by reciting a litany of disastrous consequences if the patient will not stop smoking, lose weight, and so on. This usually increases the patient's anxiety, in turn increasing the need to deny illness. Frustrated, the physician may then become angry, feeling and communicating (sometimes nonverbally) to the patient that the disease is self-induced, the result of an indulgent, undisciplined,

self-destructive lifestyle. Even a subtle and unconscious tendency to blame the patients for their illness may affect the patients adversely, as many patients are already feeling guilty, hopeless and depressed over the same issue.

BIOLOGICAL ASPECTS

Heart failure causes symptoms that may be misinterpreted as representing a primary psychiatric disorder. Mild to moderate heart failure produces insomnia (orthopnea and paroxysmal nocturnal dyspnea), anorexia, fatigue, weakness, and constipation, symptoms that may be mistakenly attributed to depression. In more severe heart failure, subtle or overt encephalopathy may occur, including confusion, cognitive dysfunction, drowsiness, apprehension, poor judgment, and even psychosis. These symptoms are the consequence of ischemia—decreased perfusion of the brain and other organs—which includes hypoxia, decreased delivery of nutrients (particularly glucose), and increased accumulation of waste products (leading to acidosis). Hepatic congestion in heart failure may impair the ability to metabolize and excrete many drugs, sometimes leading to further encephalopathy. With left heart failure, pulmonary congestion further exacerbates hypoxia.

Heart failure may be acute or chronic. In chronic, end-stage heart failure, the ensuing *cardiac cachexia* may be very difficult to distinguish from severe depression, with its extreme weakness and lethargy, anorexia and weight loss, social withdrawal, and loss of the will to live. These symptoms may reflect not only brain ischemia, but poor perfusion of kidneys, liver, and other organs, leading to multiple organ dysfunction. The diagnostic distinction between cardiac cachexia and depression is an important one, for antidepressants will not relieve symptoms due to low cardiac output, and they add the risk of even further hypotension. The presence of cardiac cachexia is suggested on physical examination by palpating extremities that are cool, pale, or cyanotic, with weak or absent pulses, reflecting poor perfusion. Objective estimation of cardiac index and ejection fraction (e.g., by arteriography or radionuclide ventriculography scan) may also help in deciding whether a patient's symptoms are "proportionate" to the cardiac disease. Cachexia cannot be explained solely on a cardiac basis if the ejection fraction is 40 percent but might well be with an ejection fraction of 10–20 percent. (This is a general guideline; an exact cutoff cannot be given because the interpretation of the ejection fraction depends on heart size.) A cardiac index greater than 2 l/M^2 is inconsistent with cardiac cachexia. (See also Chapter 2, by Cohen-Cole and Harpe.)

Besides heart failure, neuropsychologic deficits may result from cardiac surgery (Sotaniemi, Juolasmaa, & Hokkanen, 1981), congenital heart disease (Newberger, Silbert, Buckley, et al., 1984), cardiac arrest (Bass, 1985), and endocarditis (Bademosi, Falase, Jaiyesimi, et al., 1976). Older patients with coronary artery disease often also have other vascular disease, especially cerebrovascular disease, and even minor reductions in blood pressure may sometimes result in cognitive dysfunction.

A variety of acute cardiovascular events, including arrhythmias, coronary ischemia (angina), acute valve dysfunction, and systemic and pulmonary embolism, may lead to acute sympathetic discharge, with a surge in circulating catecholamines, which may be experienced by the patient as anxiety or even panic. Particularly in the elderly and in patients with known heart disease, the abrupt onset of acute anxiety should lead the physician to consider the possibility of an acute cardiac event, rather than just to suppress the anxiety with an antianxiety drug.

PRACTICAL DIAGNOSIS AND MANAGEMENT

Differential Diagnosis

Cardiac disease, as already noted, may mimic psychiatric disorders. Congestive heart failure frequently includes symptoms that may be mistaken for major depression, particularly in the elderly, though, of course, depression commonly occurs in patients who also have cardiac disease. The presence of a "true" depression is suggested by pronounced feelings of guilt or worthlessness, suicidal ideation, anhedonia, and functional disability and affective disturbance that are out of proportion to the degree of heart failure (see Chapter 2). Such laboratory tests as the dexamethasone suppression test, the thyrotropin-releasing hormone stimulation test, and sleep studies are of limited help in determining whether a cardiac patient has an autonomous depression, because these tests have not been specifically validated in medically ill patients (most studies of these tests actually exclude the medically ill) (Levenson & Friedel, 1985). False positives may result from serious physical illness or medications.

Reversible cognitive impairment associated with low cardiac output must also be distinguished from dementia in the patient with heart failure. The elderly are especially at risk for being considered primarily demented. The simplest method for determining whether the individual is temporarily encephalopathic rather than demented is to perform serial mental status examinations as the degree of heart failure varies. If improvement in cardiac output corrects cognitive deficits, the patient is not likely to have a primary dementia. Although an electroencephalogram (EEG) would be likely to show diffuse, nonfocal slowing in a reversible, low-output encephalopathy, this finding is not specific and does not rule out dementia. If the cognitive diagnosis remains in doubt, formal neuropsychologic assessment should be obtained (see Chapter 3, by Fogel and Faust). Physicians should also keep in mind that many cardiac drugs may worsen cognitive impairment either directly or by further contributing to systemic hypotension.

Panic attacks and cardiac arrhythmias share many of the same symptoms (shortness of breath, palpitations, lightheadedness, and autonomic arousal) and may be confused with each other. Psychologic stressors can play an important role in the precipitation of either, including life-threatening ventricular arrhythmias (Lown, DeSilva, Reich, et al., 1980). Most often, it is panic disorder that is misdiagnosed as an arrhythmia, usually as paroxysmal atrial tachycardia (PAT). Both panic disorder and PAT occur mostly in a young, otherwise healthy, predominantly female population. Diagnostic confusion may be compounded by treatment, since some drugs for PAT, such as beta blockers, may at least partially ameliorate panic symptoms. A careful history will usually lead to a correct diagnosis. Syncope, with actual loss of consciousness, is unusual in panic disorder but common with serious arrhythmias. Attacks of arrhythmia tend to be less stereotypical compared to panic. Panic attacks last typically 5–10 minutes, whereas arrhythmias vary from seconds to days. The development of agoraphobia points to a diagnosis of panic disorder. When in doubt, ambulatory electrocardiographic (Holter) monitoring can be used to document the presence or absence of arrhythmias. Hyperventilation may be used to try to provoke typical symptoms during the period of monitoring. A hyperventilation test without some form of monitoring is inconclusive, since both panic attacks and arrhythmias may sometimes be induced by hyperventilation. The relationship between panic attacks and mitral valve prolapse is discussed in Chapter 7.

Insomnia is a frequent symptom in both psychiatric and cardiac illness, and may mislead both diagnosis and treatment. The cardiac patient's sleep difficulties usually have some specifiable characteristics. Heart failure produces *orthopnea*, that is, shortness of breath and inability to sleep in the recumbent position. The patient characteristically uses several pillows in order to sleep. With more severe failure, paroxysmal nocturnal dyspnea develops, with severe shortness of breath and wheezing, not always relieved immediately on sitting up. Nocturnal angina awakens the patient with typical chest pain with or without associated features such as left arm numbness. If the clinician fails to discern the cardiac cause of insomnia and treats the patient with hypnotics, at best there will be little or no benefit, and the correct intervention will be missed. At worst, the hypnotic will further compromise an already impaired respiratory drive or exacerbate sleep apnea.

Somatoform disorders (hypochondriasis, somatization disorder, conversion, somatoform pain disorder, and Munchausen's syndrome) and cardiac disease are sometimes mistaken for each other but also frequently coexist. A somatizing patient may learn all too well how easy it is, by complaining of the right symptoms to a physician, to precipitate the "rule-out-MI" cascade, with a guaranteed stay in the CCU. Although the physical examination and EKG can "rule in" cardiac disease, they do not exclude it acutely. This may also lead to errors in the other direction, with cardiac symptoms misdiagnosed as psychogenic. For example, patients with variant angina or coronary vasospasm may have "clear coronaries" on arteriography, and electrocardiographic changes are usually manifest only during an attack. Early cardiomyopathy may be difficult to discern on physical examination, and the patient's weakness may be misattributed to depression or hypochondriasis.

Psychiatrists are often asked to see

individuals with "atypical" chest pain, to aid in correct diagnosis. The cardiologist will often turn to exercise testing. In addition to the standard exercise electrocardiogram (EKG) treadmill test, newer tests are useful that combine radionuclide imaging with exercise stress (Froelicher, 1983; Patterson, Liberman, Morris, et al., 1986). Thallium imaging is utilized to assess myocardial perfusion during exercise. The gated blood pool scan (radionuclide ventriculography) employs technetium to measure changes in left ventricular ejection fraction and wall motion during exercise. Except for the intravenous injection of radionuclide, both of these tests are noninvasive.

How accurate are exercise tests in determining whether an individual has coronary artery disease (CAD)? Their sensitivity and specificity vary with the specific criteria utilized, the degree of effort made by the exercising patient, and the prevalence of CAD in the population studies. All tests have some false positives and some false negatives. Tomographic thallium imaging (most reliable) and gated blood pool scanning (reliability 85–90 percent) are both more reliable than the EKG treadmill test in determining whether CAD is present (Patterson et al., 1986). For a symptomatic patient who is at low risk for CAD (e.g., a young woman with nonanginal or atypical chest pain and few or no risk factors), a radionuclide study would be very helpful in ruling out CAD. In contrast, for a patient with a high probability of disease (e.g., a 45-year-old man with a history typical of angina pectoris), noninvasive exercise tests are not useful for diagnosis because the high likelihood of having CAD is little affected by test results.

Special Considerations in Psychotherapy

Psychologic interventions with cardiac patients are made by nonpsychiatric physicians as well as by mental health professionals, aimed at anxiety, depression, denial, compliance, and modifiable risk factors. To intervene effectively, the clinician must look beyond the symptom to its function and meaning for the particular patient. For patients overwhelmed by anxiety or depression, the first therapeutic task may be to strengthen the patient's defenses, whereas for those with excessive denial, a reduction in defenses may be desirable (see Chapter 1, by Green, on medical psychotherapy).

Anxiety may derive from a multitude of different fears. If physicians wrongly presume they know why patients are anxious, without asking, then the patients are likely to feel misunderstood. For one patient the fear of sudden death may be most frightening, but another may be preoccupied with fears of limitations on sexual activity, and the two should not be approached in the same way. Reassurance given facilely, without investigating the patient's fears, can undermine the physician–patient relationship, as patients may regard it as empty reassurance offered by a physician not really interested in what they are actually feeling. Appropriate psychotherapeutic interventions can be matched to specific fears. Unrealistic fears can be reduced by cognitive interventions, for example, telling the patient that it is not true that after a heart attack, one must give up sexual activity. Medical psychotherapy is indicated if fears persist despite reasonable efforts at education and reassurance.

Effective therapeutic intervention in depression requires an understanding of its roots for the individual cardiac patient, just as in anxiety. For some, therapy is aimed at improving damaged self-esteem and self-denigrating pessimism after an MI. For others, unresolved grief over previous losses, sometimes with survivor guilt, must be worked through. The narcissistic injury of the MI may result in a hostile, irritable depression suggesting narcissistic character pathology.

Denial is common in patients with cardiac disease, varying in its timing, strength, and adaptive value. "Silent" or "atypical" myocardial infarctions and sudden deaths may occur when denial prevents the individual from acknowledging his symptoms and promptly seeking medical care. The length of delay between the onset of symptoms of an MI and hospitalization is a powerful predictor of morbidity and mortality (Doehrman, 1977). The patient's spouse or others close by may be able to overcome the patient's denial and convince the patient to seek care. Unfortunately, physicians seldom have an opportunity to affect such denial, except through education of the general public.

Denial during hospitalization has adaptive value, perhaps even reducing morbidity and mortality (Levenson, Kay, Monteferrante, et al., 1984; Levine, Warrenburg, Kerns, et al., 1987). Patients with such denial minimize their symptoms, displace them to less threatening organ systems (angina becomes dyspepsia), and pay little heed to cardiac monitors and alarms. *If not excessive*, such denial reduces anxiety but does not prevent the patient from accepting and cooperating with medical treatment. For some, this defensive reaction is firm and requires from physicians only that they not interfere with it. For others, the denial is fragile, and the physician must judge whether the defense should be supported and strengthened, or whether the patients would do better giving up the denial to be able to share their fears with someone directly. When denial is extreme, patients may refuse vital treatment or threaten to leave against medical advice. Here the physician must try to help reduce denial, but not through a direct assault on the patient's defenses. Since such desperate denial of reality usually reflects intense underlying anxiety, trying to scare the patient into cooperating will intensify the denial. A better strategy is to avoid directly challenging the patient's claims while simultaneously reinforcing the staff's concern for the patient and maximizing the patient's sense of control, as discussed in Chapter 11 in the section called "Giving a Sense of Control."

Denial after hospital discharge may also be helpful or harmful. Too little denial with unstable adaptive defenses may leave the patient flooded with fears of disability and death, and result in a "cardiacneurosis." Excessive denial may result in a counterphobic rush back to full-time work, disregard for the cardiac rehabilitation plan, ignoring of modifiable risk factors, and a cavalier attitude toward cardiac drugs. The physician's task is to try to help patients find a middle course between adaptive denial and expression of grief-related affect, which includes realistic assessment of their life sitaution and hope for rehabilitation.

Denial is one of several factors that may interfere with treatment adherence and risk-factor reduction. Depression, anxiety, habituation and addiction, character style, family dynamics, unrecognized size effects, and sociocultural factors all may impede a change in lifestyle. Simply cajoling patients to change without regard to the source of resistance often results in guilt, demoralization, and alienation from the physican. Smoking, for example, is an addictive disorder and should be treated as such, not just as an indication of self-destructiveness or weak willpower.

Psychosocial interventions may also be aimed at psychosocial risk factors for coronary disease. Social isolation and life stresses are associated with increased mortality in coronary disease (Ruberman, Weinblatt, Goldberg, et al., 1984), and their reduction may improve outcome (Frasure-Smith & Prince, 1985). Although psychotherapeutic (especially behavioral) treatments have shown promise in reducing psychosocial risk factors, the small number of studies, with their methodologic limitations, have not provided conclusive evidence of their effectiveness (Blanchard & Miller, 1977; Razin, 1984, 1985a, 1985b). More recent long-term studies have shown positive benefits of altering Type A behavior in preventing recurrences in post-MI patients (Freidman, Thoresen, Gill, 1986).

A variety of nonpharmocologic treatments involving behavior change, safe but underutilized, may help reduce hypertension (Kaplan, 1985), particularly biofeedback (Engel, Glasgow, & Gaardner, 1983; Patel, Marmot, & Terry, 1981). Behavioral treatment alone, however, would be inappropriate for moderate to severe hypertension. Among mild hypertensives, it is not yet clear who might be the best candidates for behavior therapy or how long beneficial effects will last. Behavior therapies for hypertension are ineffective for patients who are unmotivated to continue practicing the techniques on their own; they should receive drug treatment. On the other hand, some individuals with mild hypertension who do not wish to take antihypertensive medication because of side effects or because they put a high value on a drug-free approach may opt for a trial of behavioral treatment. Although the practicality and long-term benefits of relaxation techniques and biofeedback in controlling even mild hypertension are questionable, occasional patients seem to do well with them.

Cardiac rehabilitation, an essential part of overall treatment, involves early ambulation during hospitalization, outpatient prescriptive exercise training, and education of patient and family (Wenger & Hellerstein, 1984), often including sexual counseling (McLane et al., 1980). Although exercise training is often said to reduce mild anxiety and depression in cardiac patients (Cassem & Hackett, 1977; Wenger & Hellerstein, 1984), major psychopathology may prevent patients from benefiting from traditional rehabilitation programs (Cay, 1982). For the psychiatrically ill cardiac patient, optimal treatment combines specific psychiatric treatment with a cardiac rehabilitation program designed for the individual. For major psychopathology, psychiatric intervention should precede entry into rehabilitation, to reduce symptoms that would interfere with participation. For difficult personality disorders, it is usually best to individualize rehabilitation, with realistic tailoring of goals. A schizoid or paranoid patient, for example, may have serious difficulty in participating in group meetings.

Drug Treatment

Antidepressants

Among the antidepressants, the tricyclics have been available the longest and are therefore the best known. The well-established cardiac effects of tricyclics include changes in conductivity (quinidinelike effects), increases in heart rate, and orthostatic hypotension (Glassman & Bigger, 1981). Antidepressants do not have clinically significant effects on stable congestive heart failure (Veith, Raskind, Caldwell, et al., 1982). Many studies of the effects of tricyclic antidepressants on the electrocardiogram have shown statistical, but generally clinically insignificant, increases in the PR, QRS, and QT intervals, but most were not done in patients with cardiac disease. Studies of antidepressant treatment in patients with chronic heart disease generally have not found clinically significant increases in the PR, QRS, or QT intervals (Hayes, Gerner, Fairbanks, et al., 1983; Veith et al., 1982). Increases in heart rate were similarly found to occur less frequently than expected.

Orthostatic hypotension is the most common serious cardiovascular effect of tricyclic antidepressants encountered in cardiac patients, especially in the elderly. Depressed cardiac patients are much more likely than other patients with depression to have hypotension as a side effect, often related to their concurrent use of cardiac or antihypertensive drugs or to impaired left ventricular function (Glassman, Walsh, Roose, et al., 1982). In the elderly, orthostatic hypotension may contribute to vascular insufficiency, which in turn can lead to syncope and falls. The patient may become bedridden, or a fall may cause a hip fracture. These risks can be reduced by addressing other causes of hypotension in the elderly cardiac patient, such as overtreatment with diuretics, nitrates, or antihypertensives, and giving specific attention to adequate hydration. In some hypertensive patients, the hypotensive effects of tricyclics may actually prove beneficial (Zachariah & Rosenbaum, 1982).

Before starting a patient on an antidepressant, congestive heart failure should be corrected, and potassium, digitalis, and quinidine levels should be within normal limits. Patients with serious conduction delays are at risk for complete heart block if treated with antidepressants (with the possible exception of trazodone), though it does not inevitably occur (Roose, Glassman, Giardina, et al., 1987; Vieweg, Yazel, & Ballenger, 1984). If such treatment appears strongly indicated, implantation of a pacemaker will reduce the risk of antidepressant-induced heart block (Alexopoulos & Shamoian, 1982; Levenson & Friedel, 1985). If cardiac function is stable, antidepressant treatment can often be initiated on an outpatient basis with careful monitoring of blood pressure and periodic monitoring of the EKG until therapeutic blood levels are achieved. With new, changing, or unstable cardiac disease, the patient should be monitored in the hospital during the introduction of antidepressants. A low starting dose (generally 10–25 mg at bedtime) should be used. For most medically stable patients, the dose can be raised by 25 mg every few days until a therapeutic dose is reached or limiting side effects are encountered. With serious unstable cardiac disease, such as a new myocardial infarction, it is advisable to delay the introduction of antidepressants. How long to delay after myocardial infarction depends on how stable cardiac function is. After an uncomplicated MI with rapid recovery, antidepressants can usually be started safely after approximately 4 weeks. Complications such as threatened extension of the infarct, hypotension, uncontrolled arrhythmias, severe heart failure, and major new conduction disturbances would be contraindications to beginning tricyclics. The use of cyclic antidepressants in the post-MI period is discussed in detail in Chapter 4, by Stoudemire and Fogel.

There is little evidence to support the widespread beliefs that one or another antidepressant is much safer in the cardiac patient (Luchins, 1983). The nature of the cardiac disease and the character of the depression should influence the particular choice of antidepressant. For example, for a patient who has premature ventricular beats and depression-related insomnia, imipramine would be a good choice because of its antiarrhythmic (Connolly, Mitchell, Swerdlow, et al., 1984; Giardina, Bigger, Glassman, et al., 1979) and mildly sedating properties, although this drug has a high degree of associated orthostatic hypotension. Trazodone would be useful for patients when the anticholinergic or quinidinelike effects of other antidepressants are unwanted, but it may contribute to increased ventricular irritability in some patients at risk (Janowsky, Curtis, Zisook, et al., 1983; Lippman, Bedford, Manshadi, et al., 1983). Newer antidepressants tend to be marketed as "safer" in cardiac patients, but there is generally a lack of data to back up such claims. Side-effect profiles of the cyclic antidepressants in respect to use in medically compromised cardiac patients are discussed in detail in Chapter 4.

Lithium

At therapeutic and toxic levels lithium may cause changes in the EKG and occasionally may cause arrhythmias. Lithium has been used cautiously but safely in patients with severe cardiac disease by beginning with a low dose, increasing slowly, and watching for side effects (Levenson, Mishra, Bauernfeind, et al., 1986). Because of age-related decline in the renal glomerular filtration rate, elderly patients generally require about two-thirds the maintenance dose of lithium for younger patients. If cardiac disease further decreases renal perfusion, the maintenance dose is even lower. Conservative use of lithium in the elderly cardiac patient is also warranted by the frequent concurrence of low-salt diets, diuretics, and changing fluid and electrolyte status, all of which may profoundly affect lithium levels.

Monoamine Oxidase Inhibitors

There is much less clinical experience or study of the use of monoamine oxidase (MAO) inhibitors to treat depression in the presence of cardiac disease, particularly in the elderly. MAO inhibitors include a wide variety of different drugs, each with a different side-effect profile. All, however, can cause significant resting and orthostatic hypotension (Goldman, Alexander, & Lunchins, 1986), raising the same concerns discussed with regard to the cyclic antidepressants. In some hypertensive patients, this may be a beneficial rather than an adverse effect. MAOIs appear to have little effect on heart rate or cardiac conduction (Goldman et al., 1986). An additional consideration is that the patient must be willing and able to follow the dietary and drug restrictions imposed by the use of an MAO inhibitor.

Antipsychotics

Although antipsychotics may occasionally affect cardiac conduction or rhythm, hypotension is the major adverse cardiovascular effect. This occurs much *less* frequently with higher-potency, less anticholinergic drugs (e.g., haloperidol), which can be used safely even with severe acute cardiac disease or soon after cardiac

surgery (Risch, Groom, & Janowsky, 1982). Pimozide appears to have greater effects on prolonging the QT interval than other neuroleptics.

Benzodiazepines

Given orally, benzodiazepines are essentially free of cardiovascular side effects, and numerous studies have documented their safety even in the immediate post-MI period (Risch et al., 1982). Except for lorazepam and midazolam, benzodiazepines should not be given intramuscularly, because they are erratically absorbed, particularly if cardiac output is diminished. Intravenous administration, if too rapid, may acutely cause hypotension.

Stimulants

Stimulants such as dexedrine and methylphenidate have been advocated by some for the short-term treatment of depression in the seriously medically ill (Woods, Tesar, Murray et al., 1986). Because careful longitudinal studies have not supported their antidepressant properties, and because of the potential for drug dependence, their use remains controversial. Since hypertension or the presence of arrhythmias appears to constitute a contraindication, many clinicans have been especially reluctant to try stimulants in elderly patients with cardiac disease. Their safe use has been described, however, in patients with arrhythmias, congestive heart failure, coronary artery disease, or hypertension (Woods et al., 1986). Stimulants seem to be most appropriate when one cannot afford to wait for a response to tricyclics. Most patients who respond favorably do so within 24–48 hours. Stimulant treatment may be especially helpful when depressive immobilization impedes medical recovery. The use of psychostimulants is also discussed in Chapter 4 by Stoudemire and Fogel.

Disulfiram

Disulfiram itself has no significant cardiovascular side effects. The concurrent ingestion of even small amounts of *alcohol*, however, may produce heart failure, shock, arrhythmias, MI, respiratory depression, and sudden death. It would be prudent to reserve disulfiram for only those alcoholic cardiac patients who are highly reliable.

Other Drugs

Carbamazepine, a tricyclic compound, may exacerbate congestive heart failure or coronary artery disease and may produce hypotension or hypertension, arrhythmias, and atrioventricular block. Precautions identical to those taken with cyclic antidepressants should therefore be taken with this drug. Beta blockers like propranolol should not be used as antianxiety agents in patients with congestive heart failure, because they may exacerbate it.

Electroconvulsive Therapy

Electroconvulsive therapy (ECT) may be safer than antidepressants for some patients with cardiac disease. ECT produces short-lived but frequent increases in heart rate and blood pressure as well as changes in conduction and arrhythmias. The risks associated with ECT are greater in elderly cardiac patients than in younger, healthier patients (Burke, Rutherford, Zorumski, et al., 1985). ECT can be used safely in patients with significant cardiac disease, (Dec, Stern, & Welch, 1985), but the answer to the question which is safer, ECT or antidepressants, is variable and depends on the cardiac and general medical status of the patient (Dec et al., 1985; Levenson & Friedel, 1985). ECT appears to involve a brief but precipitous period of risk, compared with antidepressants, which can be introduced gradually but with a sustained period of risk. The choice of treatment in an individual patient should be made through

close collaboration between psychiatrist and cardiologist (see also Chapter 5, by Weiner and Coffey).

Psychiatric Side Effects of Cardiovascular Drugs

Psychiatric side effects are common with cardiovascular drugs (Table 22-1). Among the antiarrhythmic agents, lidocaine is the most common cause of central nervous system (CNS) excitement and psychosis. It is well known that digitalis toxicity may include the visual illusion of yellow halos around lights, but it can also produce anorexia, depression, and delirium. The visual symptoms may sometimes be present but not be volunteered by the patient unless specifically asked by the physician. It is often unappreciated that mental symptoms may be the earliest symptoms of digitalis intoxication and may serve as an early warning of potentially life-threatening toxicity. Psychiatric symptoms may occur even at physiologically "normal" drug levels (Eisendrath & Sweeney, 1987).

Depressive symptoms have commonly been seen in many patients receiving antihypertensive drugs, especially reserpine, beta blockers, and methyldopa (Avorn, Everitt, & Weiss, 1986; DeMuth & Ackerman, 1983; Goodwin & Bunney, 1971). (Clonidine may have a heavily sedating effect that can mimic a depressive profile.) Most commonly, such "depressions" are characterized by vegetative symptoms (insomnia, weakness, poor concentration, lethargy, decreased libido), with psychologic symptoms (self-deprecation, hopelessness, guilt, suicidal ideation) less frequent. Beta blockers that enter the CNS less readily (e.g., atenolol, nadolol) may cause less depression and less of other psychiatric side effects than other beta blockers (e.g., propranolol, metoprolol). Among antihypertensive agents, captopril has been shown to have smaller psychiatric side effects (including sexual dysfunction)

Table 22-1
Psychiatric Side effects of Cardiac Drugs

Drugs	Psychosis	Anxiety or Agitation	Depression	Cognitive Deficits or Confusion	Insomnia	Lightheadedness or Dizziness
Antiarrhythmics						
Lidocaine	X	X		•		X
Tocainide	X	X	rare	X		X
Flecainide		X				X
Phenytoin	•	•		X	•	•
Mexiletine	X	X			X	X
Quinidine		X		X		
Procainamide	•	•	•			
Disopyramide	rare	•	rare			X
Amiodarone			•	•		X
Bretylium	•	•		•		X
Verapamil			•			•
Digitalis	•	•	•	•	•	
Antihypertensives						
Methyldopa	•		X	X	X	X
Beta-blockers	•		X	•	X	
Reserpine	X	•	X		•	•
Clonidine	•	•	X	•	X	•
Hydralazine	•	•	•	•		•
Prazosin	•	•	X			X
Guanethidine			•			X
Minoxidil						
Captopril	rare?	•	rare?	•	•	
Enalapril		•			•	X
Sodium Nitroprusside		•				•
Diuretics*		•	X	X		X
Antianginal						
Diltiazem, nifedipine	X	•		•	•	
Nitrates						
Inotroprics						
Amrinone						
Dopamine						
L-dopa	X	X	X	X	X	X

X = occasional, • = uncommon, rare = isolated case report
* Via electrolyte or fluid imbalance.

than methyldopa or propranolol (Croog, Levine, Testa, et al., 1986).

When diuretics cause hypokalemia or hypovolemia, a similar organic affective disorder may occur. Diuretic-induced hypokalemia is frequently overlooked, especially in the elderly. Anorexia, lethargy, weakness, constipation, and depressive affect are common. Less often, irritability, anxiety or delirium occur. When the motor weakness associated with (unrecognized) hypokalemia is severe, sometimes extending to paralysis, a misdiagnosis of conversion disorder may be made (Lishman, 1978).

With antihypertensives or diuretics, some patients thus thought to be "reactively depressed" over their cardiovascular disease are actually suffering iatrogenic symptoms. Other cardiac drugs (including calcium channel blockers, captopril, tocainide, and flecainide) may also produce anorexia and weight loss due to drug-induced abnormalities of taste and smell (Levenson, 1985).

Drug Interactions

The most common adverse effect of combining psychotropic and cardiac drugs is hypotension, since many in each class can themselves produce hypotension (antidepressants, antipsychotics, MAO inhibitors; antihypertensives, diuretics, antiarrhythmics, vasodilators). Since cyclic antidepressants, and to a lesser extent antipsychotics, may prolong the PR, QRS, and QT intervals, clinicians should be aware of their synergistic effects on conduction time with other antiarrhythmics (e.g., quinidine, procainamide, flecainide, and amiodarone) to avoid producing atrioventricular block or a long-QT syndrome. If a psychotropic is being initiated in a cardiac patient who is already on one of these antiarrhythmics, it would be prudent to initiate treatment in the hospital. Antidepressants and some phenothiazines block the antihypertensive effects of guanethidine and bethanidine by blocking the uptake of the latter drugs into neurons. Methyldopa has precipitated symptoms of lithium toxicity in patients receiving both drugs, even at nontoxic lithium levels. Methyldopa may also cause haloperidol toxicity on a previously well-tolerated dose. In general,

methyldopa should be avoided in patients with psychiatric complications.

Thiazide diuretics and salt-restricted diets may both raise lithium levels into the toxic range, but neither constitutes an absolute contraindication to lithium treatment, as lithium dosing can be adjusted downward. Nonthiazide diuretics (e.g., furosemide) have less pronounced effects on lithium levels. During an acute diuresis, such as that produced in congestive heart failure when cardiac drugs rapidly improve cardiac output and renal perfusion, adjustment of lithium dosage can be very difficult because of rapid and unpredictable changes in sodium and fluid balance. In such a case, a neuroleptic is safer than lithium until the period of acute diuresis is over. In patients who chronically receive diuretics, lithium treatment can be safely continued, as long as the dose is adjusted for any further change in diuretics, salt intake, or cardiac output (see Chapter 4 for further treatment of this topic).

It is well known that the administration of sympathomimetic agents to patients on MAO inhibitors may cause a hypertensive crisis. The combination of MAO inhibitors with beta blockers, methyldopa, or reserpine has also been warned against, but few data are available. Phenothiazines and beta blockers together may produce mutual enhanced drug effects through mutual inhibition of their hepatic metabolism. Barbiturates will tend to decrease the effects of digoxin and quinidine via the induction of hepatic enzymes. Verapamil may induce carbamazepine toxicity by inhibiting liver enzymes (MacPhee, Thompson, McInnes, et al., 1986). Trazodone may increase blood levels of digoxin or phenytoin.

SPECIAL TOPICS

Pacemakers

Permanent pacemakers involve the implantation of a foreign body within the heart, and produce different stresses than other types of cardiac surgery (Phibbs & Marriott, 1985). In other types of cardiac surgery, the patient can feel "cured," but a pacemaker is a constant reminder of illness and possible sudden death. Anxiety is common early after implantation. Depression may appear after hospital discharge, especially in patients with strong needs to be independent and in control (Blacher & Basch, 1970).

Mitral Valve Prolapse and Panic Disorder

Mitral valve prolapse (MVP) and panic disorder share many symptoms, including tachycardia, palpitations, lightheadedness, atypical chest pain, dyspnea, and fatigue. Patients with either may appear highly anxious. Some, but not all, studies have found a significantly increased incidence of MVP in panic disorder, with a range of 0–50 percent (Dager, Comess, & Dunner, 1986; Liberthson, Sheehan, King, et al., 1986). The divergence in findings appears due in large part to differing criteria for MVP.

The relationship between MVP and panic disorder remains controversial and poorly understood. It is not clear whether one predisposes toward the other or they share a common underlying etiologic factor. In a patient with panic disorder with mild mitral valve prolapse seen on echocardiogram and no history of heart disease, antibiotic prophylaxis for dental and other procedures is not necessary. More significant MVP may indicate antibiotic prophylaxis; a cardiologist should be consulted in doubtful cases.

REFERENCES

Abramov LA (1976). Sexual life and sexual frigidity among women developing acute myocardial infarction. *Psychosomatic Medicine*, *38*, 418–425.

Alexopoulos GS & Shamoian CA (1982). Tricyclic antidepressants and cardiac patients with pacemakers. *American Journal of Psychiatry*, *139*, 519–520.

Avorn J, Everitt DE, & Weiss S (1986). Increased antidepressant use in patients prescribed B-blockers. *Journal of the American Medical Association*, *255*, 357–360.

Bademosi O, Falase AO, Jaiyesimi F, et al. (1979). Neuropsychiatric manifestations of infective endocarditis: A study of 95 patients at Ibadan, Nigeria. *Journal of Neurology, Neurosurgery and Psychiatry*, *39*, 325–329.

Bass C, Wade C, & Gardner WN (1983). Unexplained breathlessness and psychiatric morbidity in patients with normal and abnormal coronary arteries. *Lancet*, *1*, 605–608.

Bass E (1985). Cardiopulmonary arrest: Pathophysiology and neurological complications. *Annals of Internal Medicine*, *103*, 902–927.

Benson H & McCallie DP (1979). Angina pectoris and the placebo effect. *New England Journal of Medicine*, *300*, 1424–29.

Blacher RS (1978). Paradoxical depression after heart surgery: A form of survivor syndrome. *Psychoanalysis Quarterly*, *47*, 267–283.

Blacher RS & Basch SH (1970). Psychological aspects of pacemaker implantation. *Archives of General Psychiatry*, *22*, 319–23.

Blanchard EB & Miller ST (1977). Psychological treatment of cardiovascular disease. *Archives of General Psychiatry*, *34*, 1402–1413.

Burke WJ, Rutherford JL, Zorumski CF, et al. (1985). Electroconvulsive therapy in the elderly. *Comprehensive Psychiatry*, *26*, 480–486.

Cassem NH & Hackett TP (1977). Psychological aspects of myocardial infarction. *Medical Clinics of North America*, *61*, 711–721.

Cay EL (1982). Psychological aspects of cardiac rehabilitation: Unsolved problems. *Advances in Cardiology*, *31*, 237–241.

Connolly SJ, Mitchell LB, Swerdlow CD, et al. (1984). Clinical efficacy and electrophysiology of imipramine for ventricular tachycardia. *American Journal of Cardiology*, *53*, 516–521.

Croog SH, Levine S, Testa MA, et al. (1986). The effects of antihypertensive therapy on the quality of life. *New England Journal of Medicine*, *314*, 1657–64.

Dager SR, Comess KA & Dunner DL (1986). Differentiation of anxious patients by two-dimensional echocardiographic evaluation of the mitral valve. *American Journal of Psychiatry, 143*, 533–535.

Dec GW Jr, Stern TA, & Welch C (1985). The effects of electroconvulsive therapy on serial electrocardiograms and serum cardiac enzyme values. A prospective study of depressed hospitalized inpatients. *Journal of the American Medical Association, 253*, 2525–2529.

DeMuth GW & Ackerman SH (1983). Alphamethyldopa and depression: A clinical study and review of the literature. *American Journal of Psychiatry, 140*, 534–538.

Doehrman SR (1977). Psychosocial aspects of recovery from coronary heart disease: A review. *Social Science and Medicine, 11*, 199–218.

Dubin WR, Field HL, & Gastfriend DR (1979). Postcardiotomy delirium: A critical review. *Journal of Thoracic and Cardiovascular Surgery, 77*, 586–594.

Eisendrath SJ & Sweeney MA (1987). Toxic neuropsychiatric effects of digoxin at therapeutic serum concentrations. *American Journal of Psychiatry, 144*, 506–507.

Engel BT, Glasgow MS, & Gaardner KR (1983). Behavioral treatment of blood pressure: 3. Follow-up results and treatment recommendations. *Psychosomatic Medicine, 45*, 23–29.

Frasure-Smith N & Prince R (1985). The ischemic heart disease life stress monitoring program: Impact on mortality. *Psychosomatic Medicines, 47*, 431–445.

Freidman M, Thoresen CE & Gill JJ (1986). Alteration of Type A behavior and its effect in cardiac recurrences in post myocardial infarction patients: Summary results of the recurrent coronary prevention project. *American Heart Journal, 112*(4), 653–665.

Freyhan FA, Gianelli S, Jr, O'Connell RA, et al. (1979). Psychiatric complications following open heart surgery. *Comprehensive Psychiatry, 12*, 181–195.

Froelicher VF (1983). *Exercise testing and training*. Chicago: Year Book Medical Publishers.

Giardina EG, Bigger JT, Jr, Glassman AH, et al. (1979). The electrocardiogram and antiarrhythmic effects of imipramine hydrochloride at therapeutic plasma concentrations. *Circulation, 60*, 1045–1052.

Glassman AH & Bigger JT (1981). Cardiovascular effects of therapeutic doses of tricyclic antidepressants: A review. *Archives of General Psychiatry, 38*, 815–820.

Glassman AH, Walsh BJ, Roose SP, et al. (1982). Factors related to orthostatic hypotension associated with tricyclic antidepressants. *Journal of Clinical Psychiatry, 43*(2),35–38.

Goldman LS, Alexander RC, & Luchins DJ (1986).

Monoamine oxidase inhibitors and tricyclic antidepressants: Comparison of their cardiovascular effects. *Journal of Clinical Psychiatry, 47*, 225–229.

Goodwin FK & Bunney WE (1971). Depressions following reserpine: A re-evaluation. *Seminars in Psychiatry, 3*, 435–448.

Gordon T & Kannel WB (1971). Premature mortality from coronary heart disease: The Framingham study. *Journal of the American Medical Association, 215*, 1617–1625.

Hackett TP, Cassem NH, & Wishnie HA (1968). The coronary-care unit: An appraisal of its psychological hazards. *New England Journal of Medicine, 279*, 1365–1370.

Hayes RL, Gerner RH, Fairbanks L, et al. (1983). ECG findings in geriatric depressives given trazodone, placebo, or imipramine. *Journal of Clinical Psychiatry, 44*, 180–183.

Janowsky D, Curtis G, Zisook S, et al. (1983). Ventricular arrhythmias possibly aggravated by trazodone. *American Journal of Psychiatry, 140*, 796–797.

Kannel WB & Thom TJ (1985). Incidence, prevalence, and mortality of cardiovascular diseases, in JW Hurst, RB Logue, CE Rackley, et al. (Eds), *The heart, arteries, and veins* (6th ed, pp 557–565). New York: McGraw-Hill.

Kaplan NM (1985). Non-drug treatment of hypertension. *Annals of Internal Medicine,102*, 359–373.

Kashani JH, Lababidi Z, & Jones RS (1982). Depression in children and adolescents with cardiovascular symptomatology: The significance of chest pain. *Journal of the American Academy of Child Psychiatry, 21*, 187–189.

Levenson, JL (1985). Dysosmia and dysgeusia presenting as depression. *General Hospital Psychiatry, 7*, 171–173.

Levenson JL & Friedel RO (1985). Treating major depression in cardiac patients. *Psychosomatics, 26*, 91–102.

Levenson JL, Kay R, Monteferrante J, et al. (1984). Denial predicts favorable outcome in unstable angina pectoris. *Psychosomatic Medicine, 46*, 25–32.

Levenson JL, Mishra A, Bauernfeind RA, et al. (1986). Lithium treatment of mania in a patient with recurrent ventricular tachycardia. *Psychosomatics, 27*, 594–596.

Levine J, Warrenburg S, Kerns R, et al. (1987). The role of denial in recovery from coronary heart disease. *Psychosomatic Medicine, 49*, 109–117.

Liberthson R, Sheehan DV, King ME, et al. (1986). The prevalence of mitral valve prolapse in patients with panic disorders. *American Journal of Psychiatry, 143*, 511–515.

Lippman S, Bedford P, Manshadi M, et al. (1983).

Trazodone cardiotoxicity. *American Journal of Psychiatry*, *140*, 1383.

Lishman WA (1978). *Organic psychiatry: The psychological consequences of cerebral disorder* (pp 659–660). Oxford: Blackwell Scientific Publications.

Lloyd GG & Cawly RH (1978). Psychiatric morbidity in men one week after first acute myocardial infarction. *British Medical Journal*, *2*, 1453–1454.

Lown B, DeSilva RA, Reich P, et al. (1980). Psychophysiologic factors in sudden cardiac death. *American Journal of Psychiatry*, *137*, 1325–1335.

Luchins DJ (1983). Review of clinical and animal studies comparing the cardiovascular effects of doxepin and other tricyclic antidepressants. *American Journal of Psychiatry*, *140*, 1006–1009.

MacPhee GJA, Thompson GG, McInnes GT, et al. (1986). Verapamil potentiates carbamazepine toxicity: A clinically important inhibitory interaction. *Lancet*, *1*, 700–703.

McLane M, Krop H, & Mehta J (1980). Psychosexual adjustment and counseling after myocardial infarction. *Annals of Internal Medicine*, *92*, 514–19.

Mehta J & Krop H (1979). The effect of myocardial infarction on sexual functioning. *Sexual Disability*, *2*, 115–121.

Miller SP (1978). Amenorrhea and anniversary reaction in a woman presenting with chest pain. *American Journal of Psychiatry*, *135*, 120–121.

National Heart, Lung, and Blood Institute (1982, October). *Tenth report of the director, National Heart, Lung, and Blood Institute: Vol 2. Heart and vascular disease*. Bethesda, MD: National Institute of Health et al (1984).

Newberger JW, Silbert AR, Buckley LP, et al. (1984). Congnitive function and age at repair of transposition of the great arteries in children. *New England Journal of Medicine*, *310*, 1495–99.

Patel C, Marmot MC, & Terry DJ (1981). Controlled trial of biofeedback-aided behavioral methods in reducing mild hypertension. *British Medical Journal (Clinical Research)*, 282, 2005–2008.

Patterson RE, Liberman HA, Morris DC, et al. (1986). Noninvasive assessment of coronary artery disease. In AR Leff (Ed). *Cardiopulmonary exercise testing* (pp 139–181). Orlando: Grune & Stratton.

Phibbs B & Marriott HJL (1985). Complication of permanent tranvenous pacing. *New England Journal of Medicine*, *312*, 1428–1432.

Razin AM (1984). Psychotherapeutic intervention in angina: 1. A critical review. *General Hospital Psychiatry*, *6*, 250–257.

Razin AM (1985a). Coronary disease: Reducing risk of illness and aiding recovery. In AM Razin (Ed), *Helping cardiac patients* (pp 157–197). San Francisco: Jossey-Bass.

Razin AM (1985b). Psychotherapeutic intervention in angina: 2. Implications for research and practice. *General Hospital Psychiatry*, *7*, 9–14.

Risch SC, Groom GP, & Janowsky DS (1982). The effects of psychotropic drugs on the cardiovascular system. *Journal of Clinical Psychiatry*, *43*, 16–31.

Roose SP, Glassman AH, Giardina EGV, et al. (1987). Tricyclic antidepressants in depressed patients with cardiac conduction disease. *Archives of General Psychiatry*, *44*, 273–275.

Ruberman W, Weinblatt E, Goldberg JD, et al. (1984). Psychological influences on mortality after myocardial infarction. *New England Journal of Medicine*, *311*, 552–559.

Sotaniemi KA, Juolasmaa A, & Hokkanen ET (1981). Neuropsychologic outcome after open-heart surgery. *Archives of Neurology*, *38*, 2–8.

Stern MJ, Pascale L, & Ackerman A (1977). Life-adjustment post-myocardial infarction. *Archives of Internal Medicine*, *137*, 1680–1685.

U.S. Department of Health and Human Services, Social Security Administration (1983, November). *Characteristics of Social Security disability beneficiaries* (SSA Publication No 13-11947). Washington, DC: U.S. Government Printing Office.

Vazquez-Barquero JL, Acero JAP, Ochoteco A, et al. (1985). Mental illness and ischemic heart disease: Analysis of psychiatric morbidity. *General Hospital Psychiarty*, *7*, 15–20.

Veith RC, Raskind M, Caldwell J, et al. (1982). Cardiovascular effects of the tricyclic antidepressants in depressed patients with chronic heart disease. *New England Journal of Medicine*, *306*, 954–959.

Vieweg WVR, Yazel JJ, & Ballenger JC (1984). Tricyclic antidepressant use in a patient with bundle branch blocks and ventricular ectopy. *Journal of Clinical Psychiatry*, *45*, 353–355.

Wenger NK & Hellerstein HK (1984). *Rehabilitation of the coronary patient* (2nd ed). New York: John Wiley & Sons.

Woods SW, Tesar GE, Murray GB, et al. (1986). Psychostimulant treatment of depressive disorders secondary to medical illness. *Journal of Clinical Psychiatry*, *47*, 12–15.

Zachariah PK & Rosenbaum AH (1982). Stabilization of high blood pressure with tricyclic antidepressants and lithium combinations in hypertensive patients. *Mayo Clinic Proceedings*, *57*, 625–628.

Lynna M. Lesko
Mary Jane Massie
Jimmie C. Holland

23
Oncology

In 1986, approximately 930,000 people were diagnosed with cancer. Of the 43 million Americans now living, 30 percent will develop some form of malignancy, and three out of four families will be affected. Four out of ten patients who get cancer in 1987 will be surviving the illness 5 years after diagnosis. Several cancers that had a very poor prognosis twenty years ago, such as acute lymphocytic leukemia in children, Hodgkin's disease, Ewing's and osteogenic sarcoma, Wilm's tumor, and testicular cancer, are being cured today.

Cancer has remained, however, a disease equated with hopelessness, pain, fear, and death. Its diagnosis and treatment often produce psychologic stresses due to the actual symptoms of the disease, as well as to the patient's and family's perceptions of the disease and its stigma. The universal patient fears have been termed the *six D's* (Holland, Rowland, Lebovits, et al., 1979): *death*; *dependency* on family, spouse, and physician; *disfigurement* and change in body appearance and self-image, sometimes resulting in loss of or changes in sexual functioning; *disability* interfering

with achievement of age-appropriate tasks in work, school, or leisure roles; *disruption* of interpersonal relationships; and, finally *discomfort* or pain in later stages of illness. Currently, cancer treatment includes multimodal treatment regimens (surgery, chemotherapy, radiation), drugs used in high doses or administered by various routes (intrathecal, intracarotid, or intrahepatic), and innovative procedures such as bone marrow transplantation, all adding to a larger number of cancer survivors. Consequently, as the study of survivorship in cancer patients is begun, a seventh issue can be added—*disengagement* from the cancer diagnosis, treatment, and hospital and the patient role and reentry into a near-normal life-style.

The patient's ability to manage these stresses depends on medical, psychologic, and social issues. These include (1) the disease itself (i.e., site, symptoms, clinical course, type of treatment required), (2) prior level of adjustment, especially to medical illness, (3) the threat that cancer poses in attaining age-appropriate developmental tasks and goals (i.e., adolescence,

PRINCIPLES OF MEDICAL PSYCHIATRY
ISBN 0-8089-1883-4

495

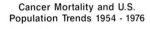

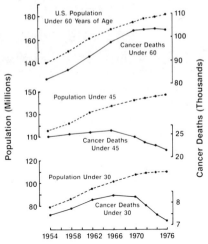

Source of Data: U.S. Public Health Service Statistics

Fig. 23-1. Cancer mortality and U.S. population trends 1954–1976. (Source: U.S. Public Health Statistics.

career, family), (4) cultural and religious attitudes, (5) the presence of emotionally supportive persons in the patient's environment, (6) the patient's potential for physical and psychologic rehabilitation, and (7) the patient's own personality and coping style (Holland, 1982a).

Why are physicians beginning to focus on the psychologic concerns of patients with cancer? Figure 23-1 summarizes data from the National Cancer Institute on cancer mortality trends in the United States from 1954 through 1976. Cancer deaths in persons under the age of 30 years have dropped sharply since 1966, largely because of dramatic improvements in survival from certain cancers. Patients under 45 years have had a clear but less impressive decline in cancer mortality. Those under 60 show a plateau in mortality, which began in 1968. Optimism about improved survival has increased, especially concerning pediatric and elderly patients. Treatments are now more rigorous, involving multimodal approaches and multidrug regimens. Proce-

dures such as bone marrow transplantation, once experimental, are becoming standard treatments employed earlier in the course of a patient's disease.

More rigorous treatment, however, requires a higher level of patient participation and responsibility. In keeping with the patient's increased responsibility is a more frank disclosure of prognosis, diagnosis, and treatment options by physicians. Patients and families appear more interested in treatment issues and quality of life both during and after treatment than in the past. Patients no longer accept global statements such as "You should be grateful just to be alive." Since patients survive longer, there are more delayed effects of treatment. Consequently, professional attention has turned from death and dying issues to the emotional, physical, and behavioral consequences of rigorous treatment regimens. Quality of life and delayed treatment effects have become important clinical and research issues.

In this chapter are reviewed the normal responses to cancer, the most frequently encountered psychiatric disorders, psychotherapeutic, pharmacologic, and behavioral management of these disorders, and several special topics, such as central nervous system side effects of cancer treatment, nausea and vomiting, anorexia, drug interactions, and terminal illness.

PSYCHIATRIC DISORDERS IN CANCER PATIENTS

Prevalence of Psychiatric Disorders

There have been many myths about the psychologic state of cancer patients. Assumptions have varied from "*All* patients are depressed and need psychiatric intervention" to "Patients manage well and few need help." Prevalence studies counter these attitudes. The Psychosocial Collabo-

SPECTRUM OF PSYCHIATRIC DISORDERS IN CANCER
(Derived from PSYCOG Prevalence Data)

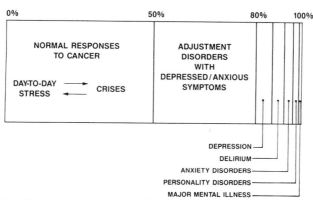

Fig. 23-2. Spectrum of psychiatric disorders in cancer (Derived from PSYCOG Prevalence Data).

rative Oncology Group (PSYCOG) reported a study of 215 randomly selected hospitalized and ambulatory patients at three major cancer centers (Derogatis, Morrow, Fetting, et al., 1983). Using DSM-III diagnostic criteria, 47 percent of patients met criteria for a psychiatric disorder, and 53 percent did not. Of the 47 percent who had a recognizable psychiatric disorder, 68 percent had an adjustment disorder with depressed, anxious, or mixed mood, 13 percent had major depression, 8 percent had an organic mental disorder, 7 percent had a personality disorder, and 4 percent had an anxiety disorder. The spectrum of depressive disorders, encompassing adjustment disorder with depressed mood and major depression, accounted for the majority of diagnoses. Nearly 90 percent of the psychiatric disorders observed were either reactions to or manifestations of disease or treatment. Only 11 percent represented prior psychiatric problems, such as personality and anxiety disorders (Fig. 23-2). Patients with cancer are thus largely psychologically healthy individuals who have emotional distress related to illness

Bukberg, Penman, and Holland (1984) examined the prevalence of depression in hospitalized cancer patients, using modified DSM-III criteria that eliminated physical symptoms. These authors found that 24 percent were severely depressed, 18 percent were moderately depressed, and 14 percent had depressive symptoms of "sadness." The remaining 44 percent showed no symptoms of depression, despite their cancer. The factor *most* significantly related to severe depression was physical function. Seventy-seven percent of those who were most depressed were also the most physically impaired, although distinguishing vegetative signs of depression from physical symptoms is difficult in greater levels of illness, making interpretation of findings difficult. These findings are similar to a study by Plumb and Holland (1977), who found that 23 percent of cancer patients were significantly depressed. Two studies of patients on general medical floors (Moffic & Paykel, 1975; Schwab, Bialow, Brown, et al., 1967) found a similar prevalence of depression, supporting the belief that patients with malignancies are no more or less depressed than patients with equally physically debilitating illness. In summary, approximately 25 percent of all cancer patients, irrespective of their hospital and physical status, may be experiencing significant depression. Diagnosis of depression in physically ill patients is also discussed in Chapter 2, by Cohen-Cole and Harpe.

Cancer-related Suicide

In the United States, suicide is the ninth leading cause of death (12.5 deaths for every 100,000 people) (Resnik, 1980), but accurate data are difficult to obtain about suicide in patients with cancer. There is a general consensus among care givers in the cancer setting that relatively few patients actually commit suicide. Three studies, in Finland (Louhivouri & Hakama, 1979), Connecticut (Fox, Stanek, Boldy, et al., 1982), and Sweden (Bolund, 1985), indicate that although few cancer patients commit suicide, they may be at a somewhat greater risk than the general population. Death certificates often do not indicate suicide in patients with advanced illness, however, and the actual rate may be underreported.

Factors associated with an increased risk of suicide in cancer patients include an advanced stage of disease, a poor prognosis, mild delirium with poor impulse control, poorly controlled pain, depression, preexisting psychiatric or personality disorders (prior alcohol abuse or suicide attempts), physical and emotional exhaustion, and social isolation. Patients with risk factors should be monitored more closely as being at higher risk. Most of the patients who have suicidal ideation do not carry out attempts, and the thought of suicide provides a sense of ultimate control: "If it gets too bad, I can always commit suicide" (Holland, 1982a). Suicidal risk is slightly increased in patients with head and neck cancer. Since tumors in the mouth and pharynx are associated with alcohol and tobacco abuse, often with preexisting personality disorder, these patients may be at greater risk for that reason. Breitbart (in press) found that patients with acquired immune deficiency syndrome (AIDS) con-

stituted a large proportion of patients seen in consultation for evaluation of suicidal risk.

Clinical evaluation and management principles, in the presence of advanced cancer or AIDS, must take into account the patient's short expected survival. Although the psychiatrist must assess the patient for major depression or other predisposing conditions and treat them, suicidal risk must be evaluated in light of short expected survival and the desirability of keeping the patient at home with family or significant others. At times, the psychiatrist must simply recognize the risk of rational suicide and discuss it with the family and the oncologist, rather than recommend psychiatric hospitalization. Evaluation and management of suicidal patients in the medical setting are discussed by Davidson in Chapter 9.

DIAGNOSIS AND MANAGEMENT

The most frequent disorders in cancer patients are anxiety, depression, delirium, nausea and vomiting, anorexia, and pain. Each is discussed in the following subsections in relation to their diagnosis and management.

Anxiety

Anxiety in the oncologic setting is either *acute*, related to disease symptoms or treatment, or *chronic*, which antedates the cancer and is exacerbated by the illness. Acute anxiety occurs at several points: (1) while awaiting the diagnosis of cancer, (2) while awaiting procedures and tests (bone marrow aspiration, wound debridement, lumbar puncture), (3) prior to major treatment (surgery, chemotherapy, radiation), (4) while awaiting test results, (5) with change of treatment, (6) after learning of relapse, and (7) on the anniversary of illness-related events. Pain, hypoxia, endocrine abnormalities, drug withdrawal, and medications may also produce symptoms of anxiety.

The chronic anxiety states that may cause problems during cancer include generalized anxiety disorders, simple phobias (e.g., claustrophobia during radiologic or diagnostic scanning), fear of needles, and panic states provoked by stressful events. All may require use of anxiolytic drugs, supplemented in many cases by behavioral techniques (relaxation or distraction) or psychotherapy. Hypnosis (self-hypnosis) may be useful in good hypnotic subjects.

Acute and chronic anxiety states in cancer usually are treated with benzodiazepines. Antipsychotic medications, however, in low doses (e.g., thioridazine 10 mg TID) can be used with severe anxiety when a therapeutic dose of a benzodiazepine is not effective. Antihistamines can be used for patients who have serious respiratory impairment and for those in whom physicians have other reasons to be concerned about suppression of central respiratory mechanisms by the benzodiazepines. Anxiety accompanied by hyperventilation frequently occurs in lung cancer patients who are short of breath. Concerns about compromising respiratory function should not preclude a trial of an anxiolytic, since the patient's shortness of breath may be markedly improved when the secondary anxiety is improved. Low-dose neuroleptics are the preferable alternative in patients with CO_2 retention. Beta blockers (e.g., propranolol) and tricyclic antidepressants (e.g., imipramine) may ameliorate both panic and phobic symptoms in patients for whom they are not medically contraindicated (see Chapter 4, by Stoudemire and Fogel, on psychopharmacology in the medically ill). Buspirone may also be considered, but this drug has so far not been used extensively in medical settings.

In patients with hepatic disease related to cancer or its treatment, the benzodiazepines of choice are the short-acting compounds that are metabolized primarily by conjugation and are excreted by the kidney (e.g. oxazepam and lorazepam). In control of anxiety before chemotherapy or painful procedures, the short-acting benzodiazepine, lorazepam, is useful because it produces anterograde amnesia after both oral and intravenous administration (Healey, Pickens, Meisch, et al., 1983). It can be given intravenously as part of the antiemetic regimen with some chemotherapeutic agents that produce severe emesis (e.g., cisplatin). Lorazepam is also rapidly absorbed via the sublingual route. Lorazepam does *not* decrease the number or frequency of emetic events; however, patients remember little of their vomiting episodes (Laszlo, Clark, Hanson, et al., 1985). Lorazepam reduces the motor restlessness caused by metoclopramide, commonly given to reduce emesis. Intravenous anesthetics such as fentanyl or ketamine have been used effectively in children undergoing bone marrow aspiration or biopsy. They have an anesthetic and tranquilizing effect within minutes of intravenous administration. Ketamine, however, can produce dreamlike states with visual hallucinations, which are distressing to most adults.

Anxiety during terminal illness may be due to poorly controlled pain or hypoxia. It responds to intravenous morphine sulphate and a benzodiazepine or neuroleptic as needed. Recommended starting doses of morphine sulphate are highly variable (0.5–100 mg/h); maximum doses vary widely (4–480 mg/h) (see Portnoy, Moulin, Roger, et al., 1986). Benzodiazepines should usually be avoided in terminally ill patients with delirium because of their tendency to enhance confusion; low-dose neuroleptics are preferred. (See Chapter 16, by Goldberg, Sokol, and Cullen, on acute pain management.)

Depression

Depression in cancer patients results from (1) stress related to the cancer diagnosis and treatment, (2) medications (steroids, interferon, or other chemotherapeutic agents), (3) a biologically determined depression (endogenous depression), which is not related to a precipitating event, or (4) recurrence of a bipolar mood disorder. The first two are the most common, but it can be very difficult to determine with certainty whether a depression appearing in cancer is related to a preexisting mood disorder. Whereas the diagnosis of depression in physically healthy patients depends depends heavily on the somatic symptoms of anorexia, fatigue, and weight loss, these indicators are of little value in the assessment of a cancer patient, since they are common to both cancer and depression. Diagnosis must rest upon psychologic, not somatic, symptoms: anhedonia, dysphoric mood, feelings of helplessness or hopelessness, loss of self-esteem, worthlessness, suicide, or guilt. Psychotic depression is rare in the cancer patient, except when associated with steroids. Cancer patients who are at higher risk for depression are those with poor physical state, inadequately controlled pain, advanced stages of illness, and preexisting mood disorders. (See Chapter 1, by Cohen-Cole & Harpe.)

In addition to medical psychotherapy, the antidepressant agents that are used in the oncology setting are (1) tricyclic antidepressants, (2) second-generation antidepressants, (3) lithium carbonate, (4) monoamine oxidase inhibitors (MAOIs), and (5) sympathomimetic stimulants. The tricyclic antidepressants are used most commonly. For reasons that are unclear, many patients with neoplasms and depression respond to doses far below those effective in physically healthy depressed patients. The starting dose is therefore low, beginning with 10–25 mg at bedtime, increased by 25 mg every 2–3 days until a beneficial effect is seen. Usually this is achieved by 125 mg/day. Elderly patients and those prone to constipation (e.g., patients on opiate analgesics) will usually benefit from concurrent use of 100–300 mg/day of docusate. Patients are maintained on the tricyclic for 4–6 months after their symptoms have improved; then the dose is tapered gradually and discontinued. Patients should be followed carefully for signs of relapse, and patients prone to recurrent depression should be maintained on antidepressants indefinitely.

The choice of the tricyclic depends upon the nature of the depressive symptoms, concurrent medical problems, the side effects of the medication, and the route of access. As do other medically ill patients, the depressed patient who is agitated or has insomnia will benefit from a tricyclic with sedating effects (amitriptyline, doxepin). Patients with psychomotor retardation will benefit from compounds with less sedating effects, such as nortriptyline or desipramine. The patient who has stomatitis secondary to radiotherapy or chemotherapy, or urinary retention or slow intestinal motility, should be given a tricyclic with low anticholinergic potency, such as nortriptyline or desipramine. Patients who are unable to take medication in pill form, because of oral, pharyngeal, or esophageal surgery, restricted oral intake or severe esophagitis, may be able to take an elixir (nortriptyline, doxepin) or an intramuscular form (amitriptyline, imipramine). Because of the discomfort caused by the volume of the injected vehicle, 50 mg is usually the maximum dosage that can be delivered per IM injection.

Although intravenous use of tricyclic antidepressants has not been approved in the United States, several studies from Europe indicate their efficacy and safety via this route. Because cancer patients have a number of reasons to have altered pharmacokinetics, tricyclic blood levels should be obtained in patients who fail to respond to usual dosages or who show unusually severe side effects at low doses.

Patients who have been receiving lithium carbonate prior to their cancer diagnosis may be maintained on it. Close monitoring is especially important during pre- and postoperative periods, when fluid intake is low; during chemotherapy, when hydration is mandatory; and when patients are receiving a nephrotoxic drug such as cisplatin. The use of lithium to stimulate granulocyte production in neutropenic patients or to prevent leukopenia during chemotherapy has been attempted. The stimulation effects, however, appear to be minimal and transient; mood changes have not been noted in these patients. Corticosteroids, prednisone, and dexamethasone, commonly used in cancer treatments, can cause a range of psychiatric disorders including, mania and depression. There are several reports in the literature regarding the potential usefulness of lithium carbonate for prevention of steroid-induced mood changes (Goggans, Wishberg, & Koran, 1983). We have not found lithium helpful in preventing steroid-related affective symptoms and prefer to use neuroleptics should psychotic symptoms appear.

If a cancer patient has responded to a monamine oxidase inhibitor (MAOI) prior to medical illness, its continued use is appropriate. Most psychiatrists in the oncology setting, however, are reluctant to prescribe an MAOI in patients who often already have dietary restrictions or nutritional deficiencies. If MAOIs are used, meperidine should not be prescribed for pain, because of the possibility of a fatal hypertensive crisis. Furthermore, dosages of other narcotics may have to be reduced because MAOI's may potentiate their effects and may retard their metabolism.

The psychostimulants dextroamphetamine and methylphenidate are sometimes used with cancer patients who are depressed. Used in the terminal phase of illness, amphetamines often improve appetite, promote an increased sense of well-being, and counter the sedative effects of opiates. The starting dose if 2.5 mg of dextroamphetamine given twice daily (in the morning and early afternoon); dosages are increased each day until the desired effect is obtained, or until side effects such as tachycardia or insomnia limit further increases. (See also Chapter 4 by Stoudemire and Fogel).

Electroconvulsive therapy (ECT) can be used for depressed cancer patients in whom treatment with antidepressants poses unacceptable side effects or for patients with psychotic or dangerously suicidal features.

Delirium

Delirium is common in cancer, due both to the *direct* involvement of the central nervous system (CNS) by tumor and to the *indirect* effects on the CNS of toxic-metabolic consequences of the disease or its treatment. The prevalence of delirium in cancer patients has ranged from about 5 percent to 25 percent in various studies (Table 23-1). These differences are based on variations in populations sampled. Some studies report prevalence rates based on screening all hospital admissions (Derogatis, Morrow, Fetting, et al., 1983; Folstein, Fetting, Lobo, et al., 1984) sequentially for diagnosable psychiatric disorders, whereas others report the frequency of organic mental disorders among patients referred for a suspected psychiatric problem (Hinton, 1972; Levine, Silberfarb, & Lipowski, 1978; Massie & Holland, 1984). Older age, preexisting dementia, and levels of physical disability are confounding factors that prohibit interpretation of data to arrive at a uniform

Table 23-1

Prevalence of Delirium in Hospitalized Cancer Patients

Author	Number of Patients	State or Type of Disease	Organic Mental Syndrome (OMS) (%)	Comments
Hospitalized patients (referred for psychiatric consultation)				
Massie et al. (1983)	334	All Stages	25	
Levine et al. (1978)	100	All stages	40	All OMS "chronic" and "acute" DSM-II
Shevits et al. (1976)	1000	Cancer and noncancer (gen. hosp.)	16	All OMS "chronic" and "acute" DSM-II
Massie et al. (1987)	546	All stages	20	
Hinton (1972)	50	Terminal illness	10	
Massie et al. (1983)	13	Terminal illness	85	
Hospitalized patients (not only those referred for psychiatric consultation				
Davies (1973)	46	Advanced cancer	27	Patients screened for OMS & depression
Folstein (1984)	83	Consecutive admissions	26	
Derogatis et al. (1983)	215		8	Included deliria, dementia with depression, organic mood syndrome, atypical organic brain syndrome, organic personality disorder
Posner (1979)		CNS complication of cancer	15	
Hospitalized patients on general medical and surgical services (cancer and noncancer patients)				
Adams (1984)		Gen. surgical patients ≥ 65 yrs.	10–15	
Lipowski (1983)		Gen. medical patients "elderly"	16	

502

prevalence rate. At Memorial Sloan-Kettering Hospital, 15 percent of 546 inpatients seen by a psychiatric consultation service met diagnostic criteria for delirium (Massie & Holland, 1984).

As in other medical settings, early symptoms of delirium are often unrecognized or misdiagnosed by medical or nursing staff as depression. Yet, early recognition of delirium is important, since the underlying etiology may be a treatable complication of cancer. When faced with an abrupt behavioral change in a cancer patient, the physician must investigate a number of potential causes of delirium. Those causes can be classified as follows:

1. Direct effects
   a. Primary tumor
   b. Metastatic lesions
2. Indirect effects
   a. Infections (CNS and non-CNS)
   b. Vascular complications
   c. Metabolic problems
      Organ failure
      Electrolyte imbalances
   d. Treatment effects
      Chemotherapeutic agents
      Steroids
      Radiation
      Medications: analgesics,
      anticholinergic drugs,
      antibiotics
   e. Nutrition
      Malnutrition of chronic illness
   f. Remote effects
      Paraneoplastic syndromes
      Tumors that secrete
      psychoactive substances

Particularly frequent metabolic problems include hyponatremia, hypercalcemia, malnutrition, and liver failure. Thyroid or adrenal status may be altered. Patients with hematologic malignancies and AIDS are at especially high risk for opportunistic infection. Other cancers, such as those of the lung and the breast, frequently metastasize to the brain. The design of the "delirium workup" is tailored to the patient's specific cancer.

Chemotherapeutic agents may produce delirium; this effect is dealt with in detail later in this chapter.

As they are for other medically ill patients, neuroleptics are the mainstay in the management of delirious agitation. Patients who are debilitated require a low starting dose. Haloperidol is the most commonly prescribed antipsychotic drug in this setting because of its low incidence of cardiovascular and anticholinergic effects and because of the availability of several forms of administration (elixir, pill, parenteral). Though not FDA-approved for intravenous (IV) administration, it is often administered that way in cancer centers when patients are thrombocytopenic and unable to take medications intramuscularly (IM), when stomatitis or extensive oropharyngeal surgery makes them unable to take any drug orally (PO), and when rapid sedation is mandatory, as with severely agitated patients with thrombocytopenia. The use of IV haloperidol is discussed by Goldstein in Chapter 18.

NAUSEA AND VOMITING

Nausea and vomiting are frequent and distressing complications of some cancers, and are also common side effects of chemotherapy and radiation. If untreated, vomiting leads to dehydration, disturbances in serum electrolytes, malnutrition, metabolic imbalance, aspiration pneumonia, and occasionally esophageal tears. Sometimes oncologists are forced to give less than an optimal dose of a chemotherapeutic regimen because of nausea or vomiting. If nausea or vomiting is severe and untreated, some patients will abandon traditional chemotherapeutic treatment (because of an intolerable quality of life) and seek out unproven remedies (which are a potential risk for shortened survival). Considerable effort has gone into finding safe and effective antiemetics to ensure patients' ability to tolerate curative treatment regimens.

The etiology of nausea and vomiting in the oncologic patient encompasses (1) physiologic and metabolic, (2) treatment-related, and (3) psychologic causes. The following are common causes:

1. Physiologic and Metabolic
   a. Bowel obstruction
   b. Uremia
   c. Hepatic dysfunction
   d. CNS disorders (tumor, metastases, increased intracranial pressure)
   e. Fluid and electrolyte imbalance
   f. High fever
   g. Endocrine abnormalities
2. Treatment-related
   a. Chemotherapeutic agents
   b. Radiation
   c. Analgesics
   d. Antibiotics
3. Psychologic (psychophysiologic)
   a. Anticipatory nausea and vomiting
   b. Anxiety
   c. Anorexia nervosa, bulimia

Metabolic and physiologic causes of vomiting are easily identified, but may be difficult to treat. They include bowel obstruction due to tumor, metastases, or mechanical or drug-related ileus, fluid and electrolyte imbalance, metabolic abnormalities of ketoacidosis and uremia or hepatic dysfunction, hypercalcemia, high fever, endocrine dysfunction (i.e., adrenocortical insufficiency), and central nervous system dysfunction (primary brain tumor, metastatic disease, increased intracranial pressure). Since early satiety is a feature of advanced abdominal cancer, large meals can contribute to anorexia and nausea. Frequent small and visually appealing meals may reduce nausea and result in greater caloric intake. Causes of vomiting unrelated to cancer diagnosis should never be overlooked: gastritis, ulcer, pancreatitis, renal or biliary colic, and myocardial infarction.

Treatment-related nausea or vomiting is one of the most common problems faced by the cancer patient. Radiation, chemotherapy agents, narcotic drugs, and some IV antibiotics all may produce nausea. Figure 23-3 lists chemotherapy agents commonly used in cancer patients and their potential for producing emesis (Gralla, 1983). Their route of administration and the individual variation among patients and treatment cycles affect the incidence and severity of emesis. Chemotherapeutic agents also vary in their mechanism of emetic action. For example, cisplatin, a highly emetic chemotherapeutic agent, acts primarily on the gastrointestinal tract, producing vomiting by stimulation of the vagus nerve. In contrast, 5-fluorouracil causes vomiting by directly stimulating the chemoreceptor trigger zone (CTZ).

Behavioral and psychologic causes of nausea and vomiting are also common. Nausea and vomiting in anticipation of chemotherapy or radiation follows a classical behavioral conditioning paradigm (see the following subsection, on anorexia, and a later subsection on behavioral interventions.). Present treatment approaches use antiemetics and anxiolytics combined with relaxation or other behavioral techniques. Nausea and vomiting may result from a number of other psychologic and behavioral causes. Anxiety related to unfamiliar treatments (e.g., radiation equipment or IV infusions and new procedures) can be extreme enough to produce nausea. It is well managed by anxiolytics such as alprazolam, lorazepam, or diazepam. Finally, there is the rare patient who develops cancer in the context of a preexisting eating disorder in which one of the symptoms is vomiting (anorexia nervosa or bulimia).

There are several classes of pharmacologic agents with proven efficacy in the management of chemotherapy-related nausea and vomiting: phenothiazines, butyrophenones, cannabinoids, or combinations of steroids, antihistamines, anxiolytics, and phenothiazines. The following drugs can be used as antiemetics:

1. Dopamine antagonists
   Chlorpromazine
   Prochlorperazine
   Metoclopramide
   Haloperidol
2. Adjuvants
   a. Anticholinergics and antihistaminics
      Hydroxyzine pamoate
      Scopolamine
      Diphenhydramine
   b. Adrenergic stimulants
      Dextroamphetamine
   c. Cannabinoids
      Delta-9-tetrahydrocannabinol (THC)
   d. Benzodiazepines
      Lorazepam
   e. Steroids
      Dexamethasone
      Methylprednisolone

Each requires a specific dosage and schedule to be effective. In addition, patients vary in their responses, so no one drug or dose can be assumed to be the best for all patients. The choice of antiemetic agent depends on (1) the emetogenic potential of the chemotherapy agent and its route of action, (2) the etiology of the symptoms, (3) the route of administration and the side effects of the antiemetic drug, and (4) concurrent medical problems.

Phenothiazines produce their antiemetic effects by partial inhibition of the CTZ via their antidopaminergic properties. They are effective for patients receiving nitrosoureas and methotrexate, but they are usually ineffective when used *alone* in patients receiving the most highly emetogenic chemotherapeutic agent, cisplatin. Since antiemetic effects of this class of neuroleptics require a dosage similar to that used in antipsychotic treatment, extrapyramidal side effects of acute dystonias, akathisia, muscle rigidity, or akinesia are common. They are less common with the low-potency phenothiazines. Prochlorperazine and chlorpromazine can be administered parenterally, rectally, and orally (tablet or elixir).

Metoclopramide, a procainamide derivative and CNS dopamine antagonist with peripheral gastrointestinal cholinergic effects, was used for years in diabetic patients to increase the tone of the lower esophageal sphincter, promote gastric emptying and increase the motility of the upper gastrointestinal tract. It was found more recently to be highly effective in controlling chemotherapy-related emesis when given in higher doses (Gralla, Itri, Pisko, et al., 1981). Given at 2 mg/kg IV one-half hour prior to chemotherapy, and repeated every 2 hours for 2–5 doses, it is more effective for emesis resulting from cisplatin than is chlorpromazine (3.0 mg/kg) or haloperidol (1.0 mg/kg) (Gralla, Itri, Pisko, et al., 1981). As with other dopamine antagonists, side effects of long-term use of metoclopramide include tardive dyskinesia.

Butyrophenones, especially haloperidol, are potent inhibitors of the CTZ. Haloperidol at 1–3 mg IV or PO Q 3–6 H. has shown significant antiemetic activity. Its effect against the highly emetogenic drugs, such as doxorubicin and cisplatin, however, has not been substantiated in controlled studies.

Cannabinoids, such as delta-9-tetrahydrocannabinol (THC) and synthetic cannabinols have proved to have antiemetic efficacy for several chemotherapeutic agents (e.g., high-dose methotrexate) when compared with placebo. It is felt that the cannabinoids act centrally to raise the nausea and vomiting threshold of the emetic center. The average oral THC dose is 5–10 mg/M^2 (7.5–15 mg), given 2 hours before chemotherapy and repeated every 3–4 hours for 24–48 hours. Side effects are considerable for many patients, especially the elderly, who complain of dysphoria and confusion. Some authors feel that smoking marijuana is more effective than oral tablets

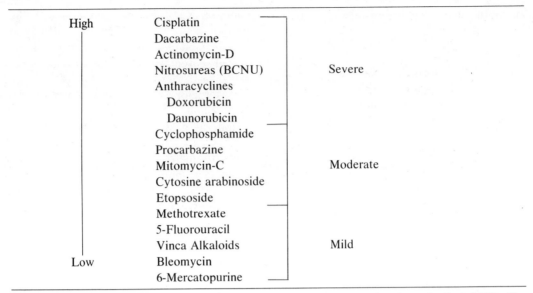

Fig. 23-3. Chemotherapy agents causing nausea and vomiting. Modified from Gralla J (1985). The control of nausea and vomiting in GJ Bosel (Ed) *Current concepts in Medical Oncology* (pp 47–54), New York: Gold Publishers.

because of incomplete intestinal absorption of the pill.

Antihistamines (diphenhydramine or hydroxyzine) commonly used in labyrinthine-induced vomiting, or motion sickness, have a minor role in the management of oncologic patients with treatment-induced emesis. As sole agents they are inferior to the more commonly used dopamine antagonists.

Other antiemetic agents, such as steroids and anxiolytics, have been effective adjunctive antiemetics when used in combinations. Dexamethasone (3–20 mg PO or IV) and methylprednisolone (200–500 mg IV) have some antiemetic activity. Parenteral lorazepam given prior to or concurrently with the infusion of chemotherapy may reduce vomiting and produces a mild amnesia for vomiting episodes, thus appearing promising as a way to inhibit the development of anticipatory nausea and vomiting. The most effective regimens for emesis control currently combine several agents: metoclopramide, steroids, and lora-

zepam (Gralla, 1983). These medications are given only a few hours before chemotherapy, and they are continued by IV infusion during treatment and up to 24–36 hours after completion of the chemotherapy infusion. Most combined antiemetic regimens are designed for use with highly emetogenic chemotherapy protocols (Strum, McDermed, Steng, et al., 1984).

ANOREXIA

Anorexia is one of the most common symptoms of cancer. Anorexia and related weight loss may be caused by the disease, by its treatment, or by psychologic disorders. Medical causes are related to tumor, bowel obstruction, fever, reduced food intake, metabolic abnormalities (hepatic and renal dysfunction), and ectopic hormone production by tumors. Loss of appetite develops because of surgery, radiation, and chemotherapy. Head and neck surgery may change facial architecture and limit food intake. Gastrectomy, pancreatectomy, and bowel resection may produce malabsorption and anorexia. Radiation produces acute side effects of glossitis, stomatitis, esophagitis, and altered sense of taste, all making it difficult to eat. Many of the chemotherapeutic agents, besides causing ulcerations of the gastrointestinal tract, produce nausea, vomiting, and anorexia. Antibiotics, antifungal agents, and pain medications produce anorexia. Cancer treatment alters the taste of food, the pleasure of eating, and the normal anatomic and metabolic processes.

Psychiatric syndromes and behavioral dynamics are often overlooked as the cause of appetite loss. Sometimes anorexia occurs in the context of depression or anxiety in the cancer patient. In such cases it may be difficult to determine cause and effect. Anorexia, in rare instances, can emerge as a symptom of a previous psychiatric illness. Adolescents and young adults with eating disorders, such as anorexia nervosa and bulimia, bring to the cancer setting a complex set of preexisting psychologic and behavioral dynamics.

Learned food aversions also may play an important role in cancer-related anorexia. "Learned food aversions are acquired aversions to specific foods or tastes which develop as a result of the association of those foods with unpleasant internal responses (nausea and vomiting)" (Bernstein, 1986). This behavioral phenomenon is similar to classical conditioning paradigms, in which animals learn to associate a conditioned stimulus (taste) with an unconditioned stimulus (symptoms of the illness). Bernstein and colleagues have examined learned food aversions in pediatric cancer patients receiving chemotherapy, constituting the first demonstration of such a phenomenon in humans. Children were randomly assigned to a control group or an experimental group. Those in the experimental group were offered a novel flavor of ice cream shortly before their scheduled chemotherapy treatment. All children were tested for food aversion at 1–4 weeks. Those exposed to the novel food were three times as likely to have developed a food aversion.

Management of anorexia can involve educational, behavioral, and pharmacologic approaches. Consultation from a nutritionist provides very valuable ideas for patients—for example, small frequent meals with high caloric content, appetizing recipes, visually appealing presentations, and avoidance of strongly flavored foods. Often a nutritional consultant is mandatory when a patient has undergone head and neck surgery and requires special pureed foods or prosthetic devices. Quite often, simple behavioral techniques are overlooked by the disinterested patient or distraught family member. The ambience of the mealtime can be very important in encouraging eating. Having a family member share a meal, serving a favorite wine or beer, or using special table settings can add social aspects that individuals associate with a pleasant meal. Operant conditioning, in which rewards such as family visits or watching TV or movies are contingent on weight gain or caloric intake have been successful in patients with anorexia nervosa, but there has been no effort to apply these behavioral methods to patients with cancer.

Anorexia may also result from anxiety or worry about poor intake, anticipatory anxiety, or nausea before a meal. Fear, anxiety, worry, and anorexia may become coupled to one another. In these situations, behavioral techniques such as relaxation and self-hypnosis can lower anxiety and the anticipatory phenomena around eating.

Several pharmacologic agents are useful in promoting gain: antihistamines, steroids, cannabinoids (THC), tricyclic antidepressants, and low doses of amphetamines. Pharmacologic management is more often used in terminally ill patients, however, whereas educational or behavioral techniques are used earlier in the course of illness and during active treatment.

Patients with significant malnutrition who remain anorectic despite pharmacologic and environmental manipulations require formal nutritional support, such as gastrostomy feedings or total parenteral nutrition (TPN). Untreated malnutrition can produce or exacerbate both mood disorders and delirium.

PAIN

In the PSYCOG study (Derogatis et al., 1983), each of the 215 patients rated the severity of their pain. Of patients who received a psychiatric diagnosis, 39 percent indicated the severity of their pain as greater than 50 mm on a 100-mm visual analog scale. The psychiatric diagnosis of those patients was predominantly adjustment disorder with depressed or mixed mood (69 percent) or major depression (15 percent). In contrast, only 19 percent of patients who did *not* receive a psychiatric diagnosis had significant pain. This finding of increased frequency of psychiatric disturbance in patients with pain has been reported by others. Ahles, Blanchard, and Ruckdeschel (1983) compared cancer patients with and without pain and found that patients with pain obtained higher scores on measures of depression, anxiety, hostility, and somatization. Sternbach (1974) noted that anxiety symptoms often accompany acute pain, whereas depression is found in patients with chronic pain. Psychologic symptoms of anxiety or depression may be either a consequence of or a contributor to pain, and treating both usually has the effect of reducing pain (Peteet, Tay, Cohen, et al., 1986).

The data just cited confirm clinical observations that psychiatric symptoms (e.g., anxiety, depression) of patients who are in pain must *initially* be considered as a *consequence* of uncontrolled pain. Acute anxiety, depression, despair (when the patient believes the pain means disease progression), irritability, agitation, uncooperativeness, anger, and change in sleep patterns are common emotional and behavioral symptoms of pain. Psychiatrists should first assist in the management of pain and then reassess the patient's mental state *after* pain is adequately controlled to determine whether the patient's symptoms are psychiatric in nature. In summary, the cancer patient with pain has an enhanced risk of developing psychiatric disorders commonly seen in cancer. Clearly, depression, anxiety, and mixed symptoms of depression and anxiety are the most common problems.

Pharmacologic therapy remains the mainstay of treatment of acute and chronic pain. The analgesic medications most commonly used are divided into these major categories (Moulin & Foley, 1984): (1) aspirin, acetaminophen, and nonsteroidal anti-inflammatory drugs, which peripherally produce analgesia via inhibition of the enzyme prostaglandin synthetase; (2) narcotic agonists and antagonists, which act centrally and peripherally by binding to opiate receptors and activating endogenous pain suppression; and (3) adjuvant drugs (antidepressants, antipsychotics) that act centrally to control pain by poorly understood mechanisms (Foley, 1984).

Foley (1986) advocates an extensive assessment of the pain in a patient prior to attempting to treat it. Pain can be considered in 5 categories: (1) acute cancer-related pain secondary to disease or treatment (surgery, chemotherapy, radiation), (2) chronic pain related to tumor progression or treatment, (3) cancer-related pain and preexisting chronic pain, (4) cancer-related pain with history of drug addiction, and (5) pain in terminally ill patients.

Excellent guidelines for pharmacologic management of pain are available (Foley, 1984, 1986). These principles include (1) treating the psychologic as well as the physical symptoms of the pain, (2) using a specific drug for specific pain (aspirin or nonsteroidal anti-inflammatory drugs are used for mild to moderate pain, and oral or parenteral narcotics for moderate to severe pain), (3) learning the pharmacology of the specific pain medication—analgesic dose for each route of administration, peak time and duration of analgesia, pharmacokinetics, and toxic side effects (e.g., sedation, respiratory depression, nausea, vomiting, constipation), (4) administering analgesics regularly, (5) being flexible in changing medications but allowing each analgesic an adequate trial, (6) watching for development of analgesic tolerance, physical dependence, and withdrawal, (7) not using placebos, (8) considering use of combinations of drugs to enhance analgesia (e.g., narcotic analgesic with nonnarcotic analgesic, dextroamphetamine, hydroxyzine, or amitriptyline, Walsh, 1986), and (9) adequately managing pain in terminal illness by morphine infusions when possible (Portnoy et al., 1986). (See also Chapters 16 and 17, on pain management.)

NEUROPSYCHIATRIC AND PSYCHOLOGIC SIDE EFFECTS OF CHEMOTHERAPEUTIC AGENTS

Many chemotherapeutic agents do not cross the blood–brain barrier to any significant degree, and therefore produce few direct side effects on the central nervous system. Delirium is associated, however, with the use of methotrexate (especially with intrathecal or high-dose intravenous administration), 5-fluorouracil, the vinca alkaloids (vincristine, vinblastin), bleomycin, carmustine (BCNU), cisplatin, L-asparaginase, procarbazine, Ara-C, and prednisone (Young & Posner, 1980). Cerebellar ataxia occurs infrequently from Ara-C, 5-fluorouracil, BCNU, and procarbazine. The vinca alkaloids, chemotherapeutic agents

derived from the periwinkle plant, used extensively in the treatment of leukemia and lymphoma, produce a peripheral neuropathy that can be severe and extremely painful for years after treatment is discontinued.

Corticosteroids are used in cancer treatment for several purposes: (1) to reduce cerebral edema associated with metastatic or primary brain tumor, (2) as a chemotherapeutic agent for leukemia and lymphoma, (3) combined with radiation therapy to the spine when there are signs of cord compression, and (4) increasingly, as an adjunct antiemetic agent in combination with metoclopramide, haloperidol, diphenhydramine, or lorazepam for chemotherapy protocols that utilize highly emetogenic drugs.

The initial psychologic response to steroids, euphoria and irritability, occurs independent of the dose. Some effects are beneficial, providing a sense of well-being, increased appetite, and weight gain. Many effects, however, are uncomfortable: insomnia, restlessness, hyperactivity, muscle weakness, fatigue, and depression. Severe effects are usually seen with higher doses but can occur at small doses. Cessation of steroids can produce depression. Exaggerated responses to steroids—for example, profound mood disturbance, such as mania, or severe depression or delirium—are less common. These drug-induced changes may be accompanied by hallucinations, paranoia, and delusions and are clinically indistinguishable from primary affective illness. These responses may appear when the dose is abruptly increased, tapered, or discontinued. Patients who require steroids as part of their chemotherapy, or who develop a spinal cord compression that demands emergency treatment, are given steroids even if they have a history of affective lability. Patient's moods should be carefully monitored, and psychopharmacologic treatment should be prescribed when necessary. If steroid reactions occur during a rapid taper, the steroid dose should be increased and then lowered more gradually.

Interferon

The newest chemotherapy agents include biologic response modifiers: alpha, beta, and gamma interferon, interleukins, tumor necrosis factor (cachectin), and B cell growth factor (BCGF). To date, interferon has been used in clinical studies in patients with hairy cell leukemia, chronic myelocytic leukemia, Kaposi's sarcoma, and renal cell carcinoma. Intramuscular administration of interferon in dose ranges of 2–50 million units per day produces flu-like symptoms of lethargy, anorexia, nausea, or depression, somnolence, confusion and paresthesia (Rohatiner, Prior, Burton, et al., 1983; Smedley, Katrak, Sikora, et al., 1983). These symptoms appear to be dose dependent and disappear upon discontinuation of the drug. Symptoms of fatigue, malaise, and depression are sometimes severe enough to compromise patient compliance. The psychologic side effects of the other new agents have been less carefully documented and studied. Interleukin-2/Lak, however, has significant neurotoxicity and may cause delirium with violent agitation (Denicoff, Rubinow, Pappa, et al., 1987).

OTHER MEDICATIONS CAUSING CNS SIDE EFFECTS

Amphotericin B is used regularly for the treatment of fungal infections in immunologically compromised cancer patients. Because it is poorly absorbed via the gastrointestinal tract, it is administered intravenously. It can cause anaphylaxis, fever, rigors, anorexia, and impaired renal function. Various neurologic side effects, including delirium, have been reported with intrathecal administration. Patients treated with the methyl ester of amphotericin B

may be particularly susceptible to CNS effects (Ellis, Sobel, & Nielsen, 1982). Ellis et al. (1982) reported 14 patients who developed progressive severe neurologic dysfunction including dementia, akinesia, mutism, hyperreflexia, tremor, and white-matter degeneration. Symptoms were dose dependent and were most severe with doses greater than 9.0 grams. Often, it is difficult to distinguish CNS effects of antifungal medication from those of fever, CNS infection, or metabolic abnormalities.

Acyclovir is a relatively new antiviral drug that has proved efficacious for the prophylaxis and treatment of herpes simplex and varicella zoster virus. It is used widely in patients who are immunologically compromised by AIDS, bone marrow transplantation, or leukemia. The use of parenteral acylovir (750–3000 mg/M^2/day) has been associated with minimal drug toxicity. Wade and Meyers (1983) reported reversible neurotoxicity in 6 of 143 bone marrow transplant recipients studied. Symptoms, which developed in a median of 8 days after the initiation of treatment, included lethargy ($N = 5$), agitation ($N = 5$), tremor ($N = 5$), disorientation ($N = 1$), and transient hemiparesthesias ($N = 1$). The authors noted that these patients may have been predisposed to neurologic side effects by previous intrathecal methotrexate therapy, total body irradiation, preexisting CNS leukemia, herpes virus infections, or the concurrent use of interferon. Improvement in all patients with discontinuation of acylovir, however, suggested that the transient CNS toxicity was secondary to the antiviral agent rather than to other causative agents.

NEUROPSYCHIATRIC SIDE EFFECTS OF RADIATION TREATMENT

Whole-brain radiation, combined with intrathecal methotrexate, enhances the development of encephalopathy. Rowland,

Glidewell, Sibley, et al. (1984) retrospectively studied children with acute lymphocytic leukemia who were treated with intrathecal methotrexate and cranial radiation as prophylaxis against CNS recurrence. They found that children who received both radiation and intrathecal methotrexate had a mean IQ 10 points lower than that of children who received only intrathecal methotrexate. Soft neurologic signs and abnormalities in growth hormone were also evident. Radiation causes a transient syndrome in children, known as the radiation somnolence syndrome. This occurs several weeks after radiation and is caused by demyelination. The doses of radiation required to treat brain tumors at times produce cognitive impairment and occasionally lead to progressive dementia.

Radiation necrosis of the brain may result from therapeutic antineoplastic irradiation of the central nervous system (McMahon & Vahora, 1986). Radiation effects on the brain may be divided into three basic groups, based on time of appearance of clinical symptoms. Acute reactions may occur during radiation treatment because of brain edema, are usually transient, and may be treated symptomatically with steroids. Early delayed reactions, due to demyelination, appear from several weeks to months later and are also relatively transient. Late delayed reactions are reactions (months to years later) due to brain necrosis and determined by (1) total radiation dose, (2) fractionated dose of radiation (amount given per day), (3) time frame in which the radiation was given, (4) presence of concurrent intracranial disease, (5) concurrent chemotherapy, and (6) variations in sensitivity of the brain due to tumor effects. Computerized tomography (CT) scanning findings may include diffuse low-density, isodense, or high-density lesions, ventriculomegaly, cortical atrophy, white-matter attenuations, and intracranial hemorrhage. Clinically, radiation necrosis of the brain may present not only with symptoms of an organic mental disorder but also with personality changes and depression. The depressive component of the syndrome has been reported to respond to antidepressant treatment despite the presence of underlying brain damage (McMahon & Vahora, 1986).

SPECIAL CONSIDERATIONS IN PSYCHOTHERAPEUTIC AND PHARMACOLOGIC TREATMENT

The therapeutic approaches used in cancer are a combination of psychotherapeutic, pharmacologic, and behavioral techniques. Psychopharmacologic management is effective for anxiety syndromes, depression, delirium, schizophrenia, bipolar disorder, pain syndromes, nausea, vomiting, and insomnia. Behavioral interventions, including relaxation, biofeedback, systematic desensitization, hypnosis, and guided imagery, are helpful for pain and anxiety during procedures, nausea and vomiting, and cancer-related eating disorders. Psychotherapeutic approaches include professionally led groups, individual therapy, and self-help individual treatment (patient to patient volunteers) and self-help groups (Make Today Count, Cansurmount, Candlelighters).

Psychotherapeutic Interventions with Cancer Patient

Medical Psychotherapy

Medical psychotherapy with cancer patients includes utilizing educational techniques, answering questions, correcting facts, and giving reassurance. Interpretation and explanation of psychologic dynamics often leads to exploration of more effective coping mechanisms. The medical psychiatrist often explains laboratory results, treatment options, and predicted side effects of treatment, provides information about hospital procedures and community support services, helps patients and families learn to negotiate the medical system, and defines normal symptoms of psychologic stress.

Such treatment begins by focusing on current issues; however, exploration of reactions to cancer often includes exploration of situations unrelated to illness. Some patients with cancer may become interested in more exploratory or analytically oriented psychotherapy. The young cancer patient frequently chooses to continue psychotherapy to explore life issues of growing up, separating from family, starting career, family, and marriage, while under active cancer treatment or during survivorship.

In addition, the therapist must be knowledgeable of the medical aspects of the patient's disease, its prognosis, treatment, and common side effects. The therapist must be flexible in approach; the focus of treatment shifts as illness changes. The therapist often becomes the patient's advocate in the medical system, with family members, or with employers. Patient cancellations or no-shows are quickly followed up by phone rather than left to interpretation, since physical status can change quickly. Sometimes psychotherapy is continued by telephone for those patients too ill to come to the office regularly.

Group Psychotherapy

Group psychotherapy may be advantageous for the cancer patient, allowing the patient to receive support from others (patients or nonpatients) who have experienced and have conquered similar problems of medical illness. The cancer patient in a group setting can easily learn that there are a range of normal reactions to illness and a range of healthy adaptive coping styles and strategies, which others have employed to make adjustment to illness easier. Group participation helps decrease the sense of isolation and alienation, as the

cancer patient and his family can see that they are not alone in adjusting to illness. Groups for cancer patients and families are often formed for patients with the same disease (e.g., Hodgkin's disease, breast cancer, or leukemia) or for patients at the same stage of different diseases or separately for family members. Initially, therapists had some concern about having the dying patient in a group with patients who were fairly recently diagnosed or whose long-term prognosis was good. Spiegel, Bloom, and Yalom (1981) have reported on their success in leading groups for patients with breast cancer at all stages of disease, ranging from recently diagnosed patients to the terminally ill. These types of groups, when directed by skilled leaders, can be highly rewarding for many patients. The principles of group therapy for the non–medically ill person apply for group therapy with cancer patients.

Self-Help and Mutual Support Programs

Self-help and mutual support programs are alternative support for patients and families. Life crises, such as bereavement, separation, divorce, drug addiction, or life-threatening illness, often provide the impetus for individuals to seek emotional support from others experiencing the same trauma. Historically, in cancer, self-help and mutual support programs started after World War II, when the American Cancer Society began a visitors program offering practical help for patients at home. The International Laryngectomy Association was founded in 1942, and Reach to Recovery was officially sponsored by the American Cancer Society in 1952 to meet the needs of women undergoing mastectomies. As colostomies became a common procedure during gastrointestinal cancer, ostomy clubs were started.

Most self-help support networks for cancer patients work closely with professional medical services, thereby offering social support as an adjunct to medical care. Self-help groups include those run by parents of pediatric cancer patients (Candlelighters), cancer patient visitor's programs (Reach to Recovery, International Laryngectomy Society, ostomy clubs), and others (Make Today Count, Cansurmount, Compassionate Friends). At the Memorial Sloan-Kettering Cancer Center, the Patient to Patient Volunteer Program has been implemented; it is a program in which volunteers visit every newly admitted cancer patient. Volunteers see patients who have the same cancer diagnosis as they once had, or one similar to it. Such volunteers help decrease the sense of alienation and isolation of patients because of their unique knowledge and sensitivity, which comes with having had the same experience. Veteran patient volunteers facilitate coping in the newly diagnosed patient by (1) being a source of credible information based on their own past patient experiences, (2) demonstrating constructive ways of managing and living despite illness, (3) providing the motivation for rehabilitation and enhancement of self-worth, (4) encouraging patients to participate in their own treatment, and (5) serving as a "surrogate patient," with whom spouses and family members can ask questions and express feelings. The veteran patient also provides education to the public and professionals about the needs of cancer patients (Mastrovito, Moynihan, in press).

Sexual Counseling and Rehabilitation

Gynecologic cancers make up at least 17 percent of all malignancies of women and include (in decreasing order of incidence) cancers of the uterus, the ovary, the cervix, the vulva, the vagina, and the fallopian tube. Treatment is usually surgical, followed by radiation or chemotherapy or both. Many gynecologic cancers have a good prognosis. Increasingly, there is recognition of the need for psychosexual rehabilitation after gynecologic cancer treatment, for patients irrespective of age. A psychiatrist trained as a sex therapist brings special expertise to surgical teams caring for women undergoing radical gynecologic procedures and men undergoing prostate surgery. All health professionals, however, can learn how to identify and refer a patient whose concerns about sexuality and possible sexual dysfunction require additional professional help (Auchincloss, 1984).

Auchincloss (1984) suggests it is the job of the oncologic professional to initiate the subject of sexuality with all patients. Patients are often embarrassed or may even assume that after cancer one's sex life should no longer exist. Married patients may have had precancer sexual problems, which are compounded by cancer treatment. Single patients face dating and potential marriage (partner) issues. Elderly patients and patients who have undergone extensive gynecologic reconstructive surgery or those who are sterile secondary to radiation are likely to be ignored by staff. Evaluation includes obtaining a sexual history, including that of the partner, noting preexisting sexual problems, and addressing the patient's current treatment-specific questions and fears. The therapist must be informed about side effects or sequelae of surgery, radiation, or chemotherapy in order to supply information and practical suggestions. Patients with persistent concerns about body image, sexual desire, and sexual function should be referred to professionals who are trained in sexual rehabilitation. Treatment techniques include supportive psychotherapy, behavioral techniques such as relaxation, and gradual reeducation in sexual functioning. Sexual aspects of cancer surgery are also discussed in Chapter 19, on surgery and trauma, and also in Chapter 13, on sexual dysfunction in the medically ill.

Behavioral Interventions

Behavioral techniques include passive relaxation with visual imagery, progressive muscle relaxation, electromyographic (EMG) feedback, systematic desensitization, and cognitive distraction (Burish & Lyles, 1981; Morrow & Morrell, 1982; Redd, Andresen, & Minagawa, 1982). These methods are useful as adjuvant treatments, combined with pharmacologic agents for pain and during chemotherapy infusions, and as a primary intervention for children undergoing painful procedures such as bone marrow biopsies or venipuncture.

Research efforts have been directed toward the usefulness of passive relaxation and cognitive distraction during chemotherapy infusions and for anticipatory nausea and vomiting (ANV), which may occur before hospital visits. ANV before chemotherapy or radiation follows a classical behavioral conditioning paradigm and is a far more common symptom than has been previously recognized (Pratt, Lazar, Penman, et al., 1984). ANV can occur hours or even days before chemotherapy administration and often occurs in patients who receive *repeated* cycles of a chemotherapy regimen or *highly* emetogenic drugs, in those who experience *severe* posttreatment nausea and vomiting, and in those who have *high* levels of anxiety or alterations of taste and smell associated with the chemotherapy infusion. Studies at Memorial Sloan-Kettering Cancer Center involving long-term survivors of Hodgkin's disease reveal that symptoms of nausea and vomiting can be elicited as long as 10 years after treatment had been completed (Cella, Pratt, & Holland, 1986). Present treatment approaches for this phenomenon include use of combinations of behavioral methods with anti-emetic and antianxiety agents (Stoudemire, Cotanch, & Laszlo, 1984).

Elderly Patients

The psychologic and social impact of cancer in the elderly is significant, since the elderly cancer patient must bear two stigmas in our society: having cancer and being old. One common myth about cancer in the elderly is that it is a uniformly fatal disease. Data suggest that cancer is now a far more treatable disease in older individuals than it was in the past (Fig. 23-1).

Cancer treatment in the elderly is complicated by (1) concurrent chronic diseases such as hypertension, heart disease, and diabetes; (2) greater toxicity of chemotherapeutic agents excreted by the kidneys (e.g., cisplatin, methotrexate); (3) physical debilitation, which prevents vigorous rehabilitation after surgery or during convalescent care; (4) cognitive slowing, which makes education and rehabilitation difficult; and (5) lack of family involvement, sometimes due to geography. Early diagnosis and treatment of cancers in the elderly produce best prognosis, but unfortunately, older individuals more often neglect early symptoms (e.g., pain, blood in stool, coughing of blood, weakness, and fatigue) of cancer than do younger individuals. Procrastination in care and treatment also results from fear of the financial burden of treatment, less education, or pessimism and fatalistic attitudes. Lack of awareness of community health care services and absence of an existing relationship with a physician also contribute to delay in the elderly.

Terminal Illness and Hospice Care

In the care of the terminally ill patient, the art and the science of medicine and psychiatry are blended. Often the art is strongly influenced by the care giver's own personality and by the history that family and patient bring with them and their psychosocial values and issues (Holland, 1982b). Conflicts that arise regarding decisions about care may lead to requests for psychiatric consultation and intervention.

Terminally ill patients are those who have not responded to known curative measures, and treatment is aimed at providing maximal comfort during their limited life span. Physicians, patients, and family attitudes variably define the life span remaining for a terminal patient as a few hours to a few months. As more effective resuscitative and life support measures have become available in critical care medicine, *terminal illness* has become more difficult to define. Potential death and recovery exist simultaneously, especially in critical care and dialysis units in cancer hospitals. When the label "dying" is assigned a patient, attitudes and behaviors of staff and family and friends often assume a different character. These attitudes may tend to isolate or alienate the patient from those whom the patient most needs at a crucial time. We often forget that the person who is dying has not changed, only the life expectancy has changed; emotional needs only intensify.

To Tell or Not to Tell

Should patients know of their critical state, what should they be told, and how and when? There is a trend toward greater candor in discussions of medical facts with both the patient and the family. Novack, Plumer, Smith, et al. (1979) conducted a study in Rochester, New York, in 1979 and reported that 97 percent of physicians favored telling cancer patients their diagnosis, in contrast to 90 percent who did not tell in 1961. Most patients prefer to know about their illness. Those who need to deny the truth will continue to do so.

The "conspiracy of silence" still remains in much of Europe and the East.

Recent articles in the lay press have again emphasized the patient's right to be told the truth. The necessity of each physician's knowing each patient and that patient's capacity to "hear the truth" cannot be overemphasized. Most patients, even children, want to be told the seriousness of their illness, but they also want to hear the ways in which family and professionals will help. By discussing with patients and families the availability of such supportive measures as pain control and alternative forms of nutrition, by offering flexibility in providing care outside the hospital, and by having an understanding of the patient's perceptions of their stages of illness, physicians communicate their pledge to provide continued care for dying patients. Currently, there is a trend in the United States to allow terminally ill children to die at home; this requires a compassionate and sophisticated team approach to caring for the patient's medical symptoms and the psychologic needs of the patient's family and friends.

Perceptions of Terminal Illness

A patient's *perception* of terminal illness depends on several issues: medical or physical factors in the course of illness (pain, relapse) and patient-related concerns (cultural attitudes about death, coping mechanisms, developmental life stage). The patient's or family's first perception of a "sense" of terminal disease results from an increase in the severity of medical problems, delirium, development of pain, organ failure, a rapid course irrespective of adequate medical management, or the level of care given by the health care team. A patient's and family's *acceptance* of terminal illness depends on many cultural and religious factors.

The psychologic stages of denial, depression, anger, bargaining, acceptance, and resolution, as defined by Kubler-Ross

(1969), do not occur in any patterned progression. In a study of 90 patients with advanced cancer, Plumb and Holland (1977) were unable to relate nearness to death to level of depressive symptoms, acceptance, or decathexis. More typically, patients show daily changes in optimism and pessimism, related to medical events. Intellectual problem solving and information gathering are mechanisms to provide control over unknown prognosis, side effects, drugs, and general feelings of hopelessness. Patients who "cope well" during terminal illness have the ability to blend problem solving methods with the right amount of denial and hope.

The stage of the life cycle in which fatal illness occurs has a strong impact on how death will be perceived, since both attitudes and views toward death change with age. (Holland et al., 1979). The young adult, like the adolescent, recognizes the finality of death. Death is apt to be viewed as the adversary that must be fought, and anger, hostility, and bitterness may be strong in terminal stages. The mature adult, often at the peak of intellectual output and work, often has established social and family roles. Here, death strikes at the time of feeling one has "made it" in terms of work, family, and children. The older adult, sensing diminishing responsibilities and thinking toward the "rewards of older age" feels that death must be faced, but "not yet." There are also an increased sense of vulnerability to disease and an altered sense of "time left" instead of "time since birth." Since old age is normally a time for taking stock and increased introspection, death is approached more realistically and can be an openly accepted outcome. The elderly adult usually has a realistic view of life expectancy and may be more concerned about the stages of terminal illness and the manner of dying than about death itself. Of great concern are thoughts of not being a burden, particularly to one's children. The frequency of losses of significant others—

especially spouse, friends, and siblings—may contribute to a pervasive sadness, and sometimes the meaning of living is substantially reduced. Life review in a few supportive sessions may permit the patient to put memories in order and rework past events—functions that become more urgent as terminal illness ensues (Viederman, 1982).

Care of the terminally ill has traditionally been delegated to and accepted as a responsibility by various religious groups. Calvary Hospital in New York, started by Dominican nuns in the late 1800s, is a specialized facility for care of terminally ill patients, primarily those with cancer. Twenty years ago, the issues of dying patients were made publicly visible by Cicely Saunders, who founded St. Christopher's Hospice in London, England. This was the beginning of the hospice movement, which has since spread to the United States. Unfortunately, the decision whether a terminally ill patient is cared for at home or in a hospice setting can be made hastily, with only a few family members present and without involving the patient. The decision can be governed by financial restraints or job requirements of supporting family or by the lack of such family. Ideally, mental health professionals can be consulted at this stage to best fit the needs of the patients, family needs, and doctor and community resources. Irrespective of whether a terminally ill patient is cared for at home or in the hospice setting, psychiatric consultation can be beneficial in the care of patients who are terminally ill and their families. Issues that should be addressed by such consultants in the care of such patients are

1. What is the extent of the patient's and family's understanding of terminal illness, their coping mechanisms, and their cultural or religious mind set?
2. Is there a preexisting psychiatric syndrome (of patient or family member), a

problem with pain control, drug abuse, or delirium, which makes management of such a patient complex for the physician?

3. Has the pattern of family function been one that suggests ability to maintain cohesion and retain adequate social support during this period and previous periods of stressful illness and death?

4. Are there internal or external family resources to indicate that the family's self-image can be maintained throughout the illness and during bereavement?

5. Do the patient and the family have an open communication with professional staff and their primary physicians so that a sense of trust in care and decision making can be sustained throughout the illness?

6. Do they have the physical and psychologic stamina, the financial support, and the educational ability to juggle work schedules and changes in work and family responsibilities and to interpret changes in medication and physical care, besides assuming day-to-day responsibilities?

Other Pharmacologic Considerations

Movement Disorders Secondary to Antiemetic Agents

All the antiemetics that are from the neuroleptic class of drugs may produce movement disorders, classically described in the psychiatric literature from their dopamine antagonist characteristics. As mentioned before, chlorpromazine, haloperidol, and metoclopramide are all antiemetics with dopamine antagonist properties, thereby potentially producing dystonic reactions, akathisias, and tardive dyskinesia.

Dystonic reactions and akathisia have been reported as common side effects with such agents; however, there have been few reports of long-term side effects, such as tardive dyskinesia. These short-term effects have responded to anticholinergic medications. Of note, metoclopramide is capable of producing tardive dyskinesia not only after prolonged *long-term oral* use (Lazzara, Stoudemire, Manning, et al., 1986 Wilholm, Mortimer, Boethius, et al., 1984), but also after short-term, high-dose parenteral use (Breitbart, 1986).

Hematologic Side Effects of Psychotropic Drugs

The incidence of hematologic problems associated with psychotropic drugs is very small (e.g., the incidence of agranulocytosis varies from 1:10,000 to 1:3,000) (Balon & Berchou, 1986). The exact rates are unknown among medically ill patients, and it is presumed that cancer does not contribute to a patient's susceptibility to these side effects. Danielson, Douglas, Herzog, et al. (1984) reported on drug-induced blood disorders (pancytopenia, hemolytic anemia, thrombocytopenia, and granulocytopenia) at a health maintenance organization in the northwestern U.S. from 1972 through 1981. During this 10-year period of surveillance of 200,000 members, only 26 persons were hospitalized for hematologic side effects secondary to medications. The rate of side effects was 1 for every 100,000 persons for each year. Most cases reported were thrombocytopenia caused by sulfa and quinidine. Only 1 of the 26 cases of hematologic side effects was related to a psychotropic drug (amitriptyline).

According to Balon and Berchou (1986), the most frequently reported hematologic side effects of psychotropic medications are agranulocytosis, leukopenia, eosinophilia, thrombocytopenia, purpura, and anemia; less frequently reported side effects are thrombocytosis, leukocytosis, altered platelet function, and immunologic alterations. White middle-aged women may be at greater risk for development of agranulocytosis than are others. Hematologic toxicity usually develops after several weeks of drug therapy and involves various mechanisms: bone marrow suppression, direct toxicity to bone marrow elements, liver function impairment, immune-related destruction, or direct peripheral blood toxicity. The most frequently reported hematologic side effects are associated with neuroleptics and antidepressants. Agranulocytosis with neuroleptics is rare (1:4,000 to 1:10,000) and occurs more often with low-potency drugs. Anemia and agranulocytosis is secondary to antidepressants are more rare than those caused by the neuroleptics. In summary, hematologic side effects of psychiatric drugs are very rare and usually disappear after discontin-

uation of the medication, without adverse sequelae. Psychotropics are often prescribed for life-threatening periods of delirium or depression and should not be withheld because of concern for rare hematologic side effects.

AKNOWLEDGMENTS

The authors wish to acknowledge and show appreciation of other Memorial Sloan-Kettering Cancer Center colleagues whose works and clinical experiences are mentioned in this chapter: Sarah Auchincloss, M.D., William Breitbart, M.D., David Cella, Ph.D., Stewart Fleishman, M.D., Rene Mastrovito, M.D., William Redd, Ph.D., Julia Rowland, Ph.D.

REFERENCES

Adams F (1984). Neuropsychiatric evaluation and treatment of delirium in the critically ill cancer patient. *The Cancer Bulletin of the University of Texas, MD Anderson Hospital and Tumor Institute, 36*, 156–160.

Ahles TA, Blanchard EB, & Ruckdeschel JC (1983). Multidimensional nature of cancer-related pain. *Pain, 17*, 227–288.

Auchincloss S (1984). Gynecological cancer: Psychological and sexual sequelae and management. In MJ Massie & LM Lesko (Eds), *Current Concepts in psycho-oncology* (pp 25–26). New York: Gold Publishers.

Balon R & Berchou R (1986). Hematologic side effects of psychotropic drugs. *Psychosomatics, 27*, 119–127.

Bernstein I (1986). Etiology of anorexia in cancer. *Cancer, 58*, 1881–1886.

Bolund C (1985). Suicide and cancer: 1. Demographic and social characteristics of cancer patients who committed suicide in Sweden 1973–1976. *Journal of Psychosocial Oncology, 3*, 17–30.

Breitbart W (1986). Tardive dyskinesia associated with high dose intravenous metoclopramide. *New England Journal of Medicine, 315*, 518.

Breitbart W (in press). Suicide in patients with cancer. In JC Holland & JH Rowland (Eds), *Handbook of

psychiatric oncology*. New York: Oxford University Press.

Bukberg JB, Penman DT, & Holland JC (1984). Depression in hospitalized cancer patients. *Psychosomatic Medicine, 46*, 199–212.

Burish TG & Lyles JN (1981). Effectiveness of relaxation training in reducing adverse reactions to cancer chemotherapy. *Journal of Behavioral Medicine, 4*, 65–78.

Cella D, Pratt A, & Holland JC (1986). Persistent anticipatory nausea, vomiting and anxiety in cured Hodgkins Disease patients after completion of chemotherapy. *American Journal of Psychiatry, 143*, 641–643.

Danielson DA, Douglas SW, Herzog P, et al. (1984). Drug induced blood disorders. *Journal of the American Medical Association, 252*, 3257–3260.

Davies RK, Quinlan DM, McKegney FD, et al. (1973). Organic factors and psychological adjustment in advanced cancer patients. *Psychosomatic Medicine, 35*, 464–471.

Denicoff KD, Rubinow DR, Pappa M, et al. (1987). Neuropsychiatric toxicity of interleukin-2/Lak. CME Syllabus and Proceedings Summary, Abstract No. 31A. Presented at the 140th Annual Meeting of the American Psychiatric Association, Chicago, IL.

Derogatis LR, Morrow GR, Fetting J, et al. (1983). The prevalence of psychiatric disorders among cancer patients. *Journal of the American Medical Association, 249,* 751–757.

Ellis, WG, Sobel RA, & Nielsen SL (1982). Leukoencephalopathy in patients treated with amphotericin B methyl ester. *Journal of Infectious Disease, 136,* 125–137.

Foley K (1984). Pharmacologic management of pain. In MJ Massie & LM Lesko (Eds), *Current concepts in psycho-oncology.* (pp 29–32) New York: Gold Publishers.

Foley K (1986). Non-narcotic and narcotic analgesics: Applications in K Foley (Ed), *Management of cancer pain* (pp 135–152). New York: Gold Publishers.

Folstein MF, Fetting JH, Lobo A, et al. (1984). Cognitive assessment of cancer patients. *Cancer, 53,* 2250–2257.

Fox BH, Stanek EJ, Boldy SC, et al. (1982). Suicide rates among cancer patients in Connecticut. *Chronic Disease, 35,* 85–100.

Goggans FC, Wishberg LJ & Koran LM (1983). Lithium prophylaxis of prednisone psychosis: A case report. *Journal of Clinical Psychiatry, 44,* 111–112.

Gralla RJ (1983). Metoclopramide as an antiemetic agent. In RJ Gralla (Ed), *Supportive care of the cancer patient*: New York: Biomedical Information.

Gralla RJ (1985). The control of nausea and vomiting in patients in GR Bosel (Ed), *Current concepts in medical oncology* (pp 47–54), New York: Gold Publishers.

Gralla RJ, Itri LM, Pisko SE, et al. (1981). Antiemetic efficacy of high dose metoclopramide: Randomized trials with placebo and procholorperazine in patients with chemotherapy, induced nausea and vomiting. *New England Journal of Medicine, 305,* 905–909.

Healey M, Pickens R, Meisch R, et al. (1983). Effects of clorazepate, diazepam, lorazepam and placebo on human memory. *Journal of Clinical Psychiatry, 44,* 4436–439.

Hinton J (1972). Psychiatric consultation in fatal illness. *Proceedings of the Royal Society of Medicine, 65,* 29–32.

Holland, JC (1982a). Psychological aspects of cancer. In JF Holland & E Frei (Eds), *Cancer medicine.* Philadelphia: Lea & Febiger.

Holland JC (1982b). Psychological issues in the care of the terminally ill. In: F Flach (Ed), *Directions in psychiatry.* New York: Hatherleigh.

Holland JC, Rowland J, Lebovits A, et al. (1979). Reactions to cancer treatment: Assessment of emotional response to adjunct radiotherapy. *Psychiatric Clinics of North America, 2,* 347–358.

Kubler-Ross E (1969). *On death and dying.* New York: Macmillan.

Laszlo J, Clark RA, Hanson DC, et al. (1985). Lorazepam in cancer patients treated with cisplatin: A drug having antiemetic, amnesic and anxiolytic effects. *Journal of Clinical Oncology, 3,* 864–869.

Lazzara RR, Stoudemire A, Manning D, et al. (1986). Metoclopramide induced tardive dyskinesia: A case report. *General Hospital Psychiatry, 8,* 107–109.

Levine PM, Silberfarb PM, & Lipowski ZJ (1978). Mental disorders in cancer patients: A study of 100 psychiatric referrals. *Cancer, 42,* 1385–1391.

Lipowski ZJ (1983). Transient cognitive disorders (delirium, acute confusional states) in the elderly. *The American Journal of Psychiatry, 140,* 1426–1436.

Louhivouri KA & Hakama M (1979). Risk of suicide among cancer patients. *American Journal of Epidemiology, 109,* 59–65.

Massie MJ & Holland JC (1984). Current concepts in psychiatric oncology. In L Greenspan (Ed), *Psychiatric update III.* Washington, DC: American Psychiatric Press.

Massie, MJ, Holland JC (in press). Consultation and liaison issues in cancer care.

Massie, MJ, Holland J, & Glass E (1983). Delirium in terminally ill cancer patients. *The American Journal of Psychiatry, 140,* 1048–1050.

Mastrovito R & Moynihan R (in press). Self help and mutual support programs in cancer. In JC Holland & JH Rowland (Eds), *Handbook of psychiatric oncology.* New York: Oxford University Press.

McMahon T & Vahora S (1986). Radiation damage to the brain: Neuropsychiatric aspects. *General Hospital Psychiatry, 8,* 437–441.

Moffic H & Paykel ES (1975). Depression in medical inpatients. *British Journal of Psychiatry, 126,* 346–353.

Morrow GR & Morrell BS (1982). Behavioral treatment for the anticipatory nausea and vomiting induced by cancer chemotherapy. *New England Journal of Medicine, 306* 1476–1480.

Moulin D & Foley K (1984). Management of pain in patients with cancer. *Psychiatric Annals, 14,* 815–822.

Novack DH, Plumer R, Smith RL, et al. (1979). Changes in physicians' attitudes toward telling the cancer patient. *Journal of the American Medical Association, 241*(9), 897–900.

Peteet J, Tay V, Cohen G, et al. (1986). Pain characteristics and treatment in an outpatient cancer population. *Cancer, 57,* 1259–1265.

Plumb MM & Holland JC (1977). Comparative studies of psychological function in patients with advanced cancer: 1. Self reported depression symptoms. *Psychosomatic Medicine, 39*, 264–276.

Portnoy RK, Moulin DF, Roger A, et al. (1986). Intravenous infusion of opioids in cancer pain: Clinical review and guidelines for use. *Cancer Treatment Reports, 70*, 575–581.

Posner JB (1979). Delirium and exogenous metabolic brain disease in PB Beeson, W McDermott, & JB Wyngaarden (Eds), *Cecil textbook of medicine* (pp 644–651). Philadelphia: WB Saunders.

Pratt, A, Lazar R, Penman D, et al. (1984). Psychological parameters of chemotherapy-induced conditioned nausea and vomiting: A review. *Cancer Nursing, 1*, 483–490.

Redd, WH, Andresen GV, & Minagawa Y (1982). Hypnotic control of anticipatory emesis in patients receiving cancer chemotherapy. *Journal of Consulting and Clinical Psychology, 50*, 14–19.

Resnik HLP (1980). Suicide. In I Kaplan, A Freedman, & BJ Saddoch (Eds), *Comprehensive textbook of Psychiatry* (Vol 3). Baltimore: Williams & Wilkins.

Rohatiner AZS, Prior PF, Burton AC, et al. (1983). Central nervous system toxicity of interferon. *British Journal of Cancer, 47*, 419–442.

Rowland JH, Glidewell OJ, Sibley RF, et al. (1984). Effects of different forms of central nervous system prophylaxis and neuropsychologic function in childhood leukemia. *Journal of Clinical Oncology, 2*, 1327–1335.

Schwab JJ, Bialow M, Brown J, et al. (1967). Diagnosing depression in medical inpatients. *Annals of Internal Medicine, 67*, 695–707.

Shevitz SA, Silberfarb PM, & Lipowski ZJ (1976). Psychiatric Consultants in a general hospital: A report of 1000 referrals. *Diseases of the Nervous System, 37*, 295–300.

Smedley H, Katrak M, Sikora K, et al. (1983). Neurological effects of recombinant human interferon. *British Medical Journal, 286*, 262–264.

Spiegel D, Bloom J, & Yalom I (1981). Group support for patients with metastatic cancer. *Archives of General Psychiatry, 45*, 333–339.

Sternbach RA (1974). *Pain patients: Traits and treatment.* New York: Academic Press.

Stoudemire A, Cotanch P, & Laszlo J (1984). Recent advances in the pharmacologic and behavioral management of chemotherapy induced emesis. *Archives of Internal Medicine, 144*, 1029–1033.

Strum SF, McDermed JE, Steng BR, et al. (1984). Combination metoclopramide and dexamethasone: An effective antiemetic regimen in outpatients receiving cisplatin chemotherapy. *Journal of Clinical Oncology, 2*, 1057–1063.

Viederman M (1982). Psychotherapeutic management of depression in the medically ill. In JC Holland (Ed), *Current concepts in psychology* (pp 29–39). New York: Gold Publishers.

Wade, JC & Meyers JD (1983). Neurological symptoms associated with parenteral acyclovir treatment after marrow transplantation. *Annals of Internal Medicine, 98*, 921–925.

Walsh TD (1986). Controlled study of imipramine and morphine in chronic pain due to advanced cancer. *Proceedings of the American Society of Clinical Oncology, 5*, Abstract No. 929, p 237.

Wilholm B-E, Mortimer O, Boethius G, et al. (1984). Tardive dyskinesia associated with metoclopramide. *British Medical Journal, 288*, 545–547.

Young, DF & Posner JB (1980). Nervous system toxicity of the chemotherapeutic agents. In PJ Viken & GW Bruyn (Eds), *Handbook of clinical neurology: Vol 39. Neurological manifestations of systemic diseases, part II.* New York: Elsevier Biomedical Press.

M. Eileen McNamara

24
Neurology

The interface of neurology and psychiatry has received much scholarly attention in the last two decades, with the growth of behavioral neurology and neuropsychology, and with advances in basic neurosciences that permit a rational exploration of pathophysiology. This chapter will discuss the four most commonly occurring neurologic disorders for which psychiatric complications are highly prevalent: stroke, multiple sclerosis, Parkinson's disease, and epilepsy.

ETIOLOGY OF STROKE

Cerebral infarction has many etiologies. Most commonly, carotid atherosclerotic plaques ulcerate, dislodging "white emboli" that travel distally and lodge in cerebral blood vessels, causing occlusion and ischemia. Alternatively, atheromata may cause stenosis and occlusion of carotid arteries with hemodynamic compromise of cerebral blood flow. As the incidence of atherosclerotic vascular disease increases with age, so does the incidence of stroke

(Barnett, 1980; Beal, Williams, Richardson, et al., 1981; Bogousslavsky & Regli, 1986).

Cardiac disease is also a significant cause of cerebral embolism, often resulting in large and functionally devastating strokes. Atrial fibrillation with hemostasis and development of clot within a dilated left atrium accounts for approximately half of cardiogenic emboli, with other etiologies including rheumatic valvular disease, cardiomyopathy, endocarditis, and acute myocardial infarction. With the advent of computed brain tomography (CT scan), the old clinical maxim that cardiac emboli produce hemorrhagic stroke whereas carotid disease produces bland stroke has been disproven (Cerebral Embolism Task Force 1986; Komrad, Coffey, Coffey, et al., 1984).

Another common cause of stroke, with paricular prevalence in the elderly, is hyaline degeneration of the small midline perforating arteries of the brain, which results in lacunar infarctions. These small infarcts most commonly occur in the periventricular white matter of the frontal lobe and the head of the caudate nucleus. Because of the anatomic locations, which

PRINCIPLES OF MEDICAL PSYCHIATRY
ISBN 0-8089-1883-4

interrupt frontal neuronal pathways, lacunar infarcts most often result in frontal lobe symptoms of emotional lability, gait apraxia, abulia, incontinence, and so on. At times, small infarcts are so numerous that diffuse softening of the white matter occurs, known as Binswanger's disease. Hypertension is the most common underlying cause of lacunar infarction, with alternate etiologies including high blood viscosity, vasculitis, and amyloid angiopathy .(Caplan, 1980; Cosgrove, LeBlanc, Meagher-Villemure, et al., 1985; Ishii, Nishihara, & Imamuia, 1986; Kinkel, Jacobs, Polachini, et al., 1985; Pullicino, Nelson, Kendall, et al., 1980).

Stroke is not only a disease of the elderly. Three percent of all strokes occur in young adults, and the incidence is probably increasing due to the prevalence of cocaine abuse. Migraine, alcohol, mitral valve prolapse, trauma, autoimmune disease, and the use of oral contraceptives have been identified as other contributing factors (Adams, Butler, Biller, et al., 1986; Dorfman, Marshall, & Enzmann, 1979; Hillbom & Kaste, 1981; AC Jackson, Boughner, & Barnett, 1984; Schoenberg, Whisnant, Taylor, et al., 1970).

PSYCHIATRIC PRESENTATIONS OF STROKE

The abrupt onset of hemiparesis in middle cerebral artery infarction is dramatic and immediately obvious, but the presentation of cerebrovascular ischemia can be far more subtle. Posterior cerebral artery infarctions may produce no motor symptoms, and a left posterior infarct may have as its sole overt manifestation the acute onset of a fluent aphasia. Patients suffering such infarcts, whose speech is confused and nonsensical, are occasionally misdiagnosed as psychotic and admitted to psychiatric units. Since examination of the patient's visual fields usually reveals a right

homonymous hemianopsia, it is lamentable that clinicians often omit this simple test (Benson, 1973; Geschwind, 1971).

Right hemisphere infarctions may also be mistaken for psychiatric illness. Delirium, delusions, and bizarre behavior may be the presentation of right-sided stroke, particularly if there is preexisting cortical atrophy (Hier, Mondlock, & Caplan, 1983; Levine & Grek, 1984). Right temporal strokes occasionally cause secondary hypomania.

Rostral basilar artery infarction may also result in disturbances of behavior and vision with a paucity of motor symptoms. With high brain stem infarction, patients may have vivid visual and auditory hallucinations with intact reality testing. The patients may also be disoriented and may reply bizarrely to questions (Caplan, 1980; Cascino & Adams, 1986). Bilateral paramedian thalamic infarction from occlusion of a Y-shaped branch of the posterior circulation, the thalamosubthalamic perforating artery, may produce profound subcortical dementia from very small lesions (Guberman & Stuss, 1983).

The prompt diagnosis of stroke has more than nosologic significance. Regardless of etiology, whether carotid, cardiac, lacunar, aneurysmal, or due to systemic disease, strokes often recur. Further neurologic damage may be prevented by timely medical intervention. Moreover, evidence is accumulating that part of the neuronal injury that occurs in stroke may not take place immediately but may occur over several hours to days and may be reversible if treated rapidly. For example, cerebral edema develops usually between 2 and 5 days after a large stroke, and it may be so severe as to cause brain herniation and death. Treatment of this edema can be lifesaving (Raichle, 1983; Ropper & Shafran, 1984).

Because it is impractical to refer all patients with behavioral abnormalities to a neurologist, psychiatrists should be familiar with methods to confirm or exclude a diagnosis of stroke. A screening neurologic examination with visual fields and auscultation for carotid bruits should be performed on every patient. It is an error to believe that CT scan will exclude the possibility of cerebrovascular infarctions, as often new strokes will not be visible for several days. Moreover, lacunar strokes are often below the resolution of CT scans, although nuclear magnetic resonance imaging scans may be more helpful in this regard. An electroencephalogram (EEG) may show focal slowing before changes are demonstrated on radiographic studies, but lacunar infarcts usually do not produce any EEG changes. A high index of suspicion is warranted when patients are elderly, hypertensive, or diabetic, are substance abusers, or have a history of cardiac disease.

Poststroke Depression

The most prevalent and most studied of poststroke psychiatric syndromes is depression. Folstein, Maiberger, and Mc-Hugh (1977) examined 20 consecutive stroke patients admitted to a rehabilitation hospital, and found a 45 percent prevalence of depression indicated by the Present State Examination and Hamilton Rating Scale. Orthopedic patients with a similar degree of physical disability had only a 10 percent prevalence of depression. Finklestein, Benowitz, Baldessarini, et al. (1982) in a similar investigation found a 48 percent prevalence of depression.

In an effort to better define the clinical characteristics of poststroke depression, Robinson and associates evaluated patients hospitalized for stroke and followed them longitudinally, defining depression by DSM-III criteria. At the time of initial examination, 26 percent of 103 patients met criteria for major depression, and a further 20 percent met criteria for dysthymia. At 6-month follow-up, the prevalence of major depression had increased to 34 percent, and

another 26 percent of patients had dysthymia. Only 40 percent of all patients remained nondepressed. A 12-month study of participants in a stroke clinic for ambulatory patients suggests that major depression that develops after a stroke has a natural course of about 8 months (Robinson & Price, 1982; Robinson, Lipsey, & Price, 1985).

Although depressed mood in stroke patients has often been attributed to a reactive response to physical disability, available data do not support this conclusion. Degree of depression has not correlated with degree of disability. Patients with physical disability from other causes have not demonstrated such a high incidence of depression.

Etiology of Poststroke Depression

The etiology of depression after cerebrovascular accident is unknown, although several hypotheses present themselves. The abrupt onset of a stroke, often without premonitory warnings such as transient ischemic attacks, coupled with the devastating and obvious impairments produced by stroke, with widespread effects on functioning, can be a traumatic and frightening experience for patients and families. Whereas other illnesses, such as myocardial infarction, may threaten life, brain injury threatens the sense of self. Patients will often say that they would rather die than "become a vegetable," and the threat of another stroke, despite therapy, is always a possibility.

Some authors have noted an increase in depression associated with specific locations of stroke, and they postulate a neuroanatomic etiology of mood disorder in stroke. Robinson reported that the highest frequency of depression was seen with left anterior brain infarctions and that the closer the left hemisphere lesion was to the frontal pole, the more severe the depression. When infarcts occurred in the right hemisphere, depressive symptoms correlated with proximity to the occipital pole (Robinson, Kubos, Starr, et al., 1984). This study, however, excluded patients with severe comprehension deficits, presumably patients with left posterior infarctions. Also, patients with right anterior, frontal-parietal infarctions may appear apathetic and euphoric, so their depressions may be difficult to detect with standard, unmodified interviews and rating scales. It is therefore unclear if there is truly an anatomic left-right or anterior-posterior gradient for depression, or whether the observed association is an artifact of patient selection and diagnostic procedure.

Animal models, however, suggest that there is a true asymmetry in the brain in response to stroke that may underlie the development of depression. In rats with experimentally induced right middle cerebral artery ischemic lesions, there was widespread subsequent depletion of norepinephrine and dopamine, both in injured and uninjured cortex, both ipsilateral and contralateral to the lesion site (Robinson, 1979). Norepinephrine was decreased within twelve hours by 75 percent, with similar depletions in the locus ceruleus, where the noradrenergic cell bodies are located. A similar widespread depletion of dopamine, to below 50 percent of control levels, also occurred in the substantia nigra and ventral tegmental area. Interestingly, identical lesions made in the left middle cerebral artery did not produce significant changes in norepinephrine and dopamine. Further, this hemispheric asymmetry in response to stroke was observed only in male rats (Lipsey, Spencer, Rabins, et al., 1986). Female rats had depletions with both right- and left-sided lesions.

Recently, studies have examined poststroke patients by using radiolabeled ligands to examine receptor binding by positron emission tomography (PET scans). Preliminary investigations suggest that poststroke patients have decreased serotonin receptor binding with left hemi-sphere infarcts, with the opposite finding—increased serotonin binding—in right hemisphere infarcts. Such an asymmetry might also underlie the observed increase in depression following left hemisphere stroke (Riesenberg, 1986).

Other Poststroke Psychopathology

Other psychiatric disturbances have also been reported to follow stroke, but these are less well studied. Mania has been reported with right hemisphere lesions, but the discrimination between true mania and its mimic, frontal lobe disinhibition, has been problematic. In other reports it is unclear whether the excitable behavior observed is due to a central lesion per se or is more related to secondary epileptogenesis (Cummings & Mendez, 1984; Jampala & Abrams, 1983; Krauthammer & Klerman, 1978).

Paranoia has also been observed as a consequence of stroke, particularly in patients with left posterior lesions and fluent aphasia. These patients are unable to comprehend language, and as Benson notes, "in the most severe cases the patient literally does not understand that he does not understand." Patients may believe that others are plotting against them and, unaware that the problem lies within themselves, become delusional and agitated. Similar phenomena have been observed in deafness and may underlie some instances of late onset schizophreniform psychoses (Benson, 1973; BL Miller, Benson, Cummings, et al., 1986).

Psychiatric diagnosis in the stroke patient may be made difficult by the presence of neurologic impairments that complicate the presentation. Infarcts of the left hemisphere, producing aphasia, may render patients incapable of communicating their moods verbally. Lesions of the right hemisphere, which appears to be dominant for communication of mood by gestures, facial expression, and prosody, may cause a dissociation between subjective feelings of mood and overt expressions of affect. Flat, monotonous, and uninflected speech may mask the presence of a mood disorder. Similarly, bland denial of illness, anosognosia, produced by right parietal infarctions, may also obscure the presence of depression (Ross, 1981; Ross & Rush, 1981). Multiple lacunar infarcts often produce organic emotional lability or abulia, which can confound diagnosis (Ishii et al., 1986).

Disturbances of sleep and appetite and other "vegetative" symptoms, usually helpful in the diagnosis of depression, may also be misleading in the poststroke patient. These functions may be affected by neurologic lesions themselves, by medications, and by environment. Disinterest in self-care, poor motivation, withdrawal, negativism, irritability, anhedonia, anxiety, and sluggishness appear to be more consistent indications of depression in the poststroke patient. Interviews with the family and the caretakers of the patients may also provide valuable information about mood and behavior that the patient is unable to give (Finklestein et al., 1982; Lipsey et al., 1986; Reding, Orto, Willensky, et al., 1985; Reding, Orto, Winter, et al., 1986; Ross & Rush, 1981).

Treatment of Poststroke Depression

The treatment of poststroke depression is similar to that of other depressive disorders, but with some special considerations.

The leading cause of death in poststroke patients is cardiac disease. Vascular disease that occurs in the carotids also occurs in the coronary arteries, and myocardial infarction, angina, congestive heart failure, and conduction abnormalities are common associated diagnoses. The stroke patient should have a cardiologic evaluation, and psychotropic drug therapy should take cardiac risk factors into account (Heyman, Wilkinson, Hurwitz, et al., 1984; Rokey, Rolak, Harati, et al., 1984).

Hypertension is another common associated finding in stroke. Either hypertension *or* hypotension may be hazardous to the patient with coronary and cerebrovascular disease. Moreover, stroke patients may be more sensitive to the hypotensive side effects of psychiatric medications than other patients.

Seizures develop in more than 10 percent of stroke patients. Since tricyclics and neuroleptics affect seizure threshold, an EEG should be obtained before institution of these drugs. Patients with frankly paroxysmal EEGs or a history of seizures should be covered with anticonvulsants before tricyclics or neuroleptics are instituted. Of course, short-term neuroleptics may occasionally be necessary to control agitation before an EEG can be obtained, and low dosages of high potency neuroleptics are preferable in this situation.

Stroke patients are frequently on multiple medications at the time of evaluation. Propranolol, captopril, clonidine, and methyldopa, used in the treatment of hypertension, may produce depression and other psychiatric symptoms. Digitalis, tocainide, calcium channel blockers, and other cardiac medications are also associated with significant psychotropic effects (Cocito, Favale, & Reni, 1982; DeMuth & Ackerman, 1983; Erman & Guggeheim, 1981; Kopin, 1979; Schaut & Schnoll, 1983; SH Snyder & Reynolds, 1985; Vincent, 1985; Zubenko & Nixon, 1984).

Medications may interact to affect protein binding and clearance rates. Oral anticoagulants (e.g., warfarin) may interact with a number of psychiatric medications, with subsequent changes in coagulation times. Prothrombin times therefore should be checked more frequently in patients on anticoagulants when psychiatric medication is being initiated or changed. Propranolol may elevate levels of chlorpromazine and other neuroleptics. Because many drug–drug interactions remain to be explored, relevant serum drug levels should be measured whenever new medications are introduced or dosages are changed (Wood & Feely, 1983).

Depression can be successfully treated in poststroke patients. Lipsey, Robinson, Pearlson, et al. (1984) administered nortriptyline to poststroke patients, beginning at 20 mg at bedtime and increasing slowly over 4 weeks to 100 mg and/or until therapeutic blood levels were achieved. Patients who were able to tolerate the medication evidenced a significant decrease in depression as measured by the Hamilton and the Zung Depression Rating Scales. Seven of 17 patients were unable to complete treatment because of side effects, chiefly delirium. Trazodone also has been reported to be efficacious in poststroke depression. Reding and colleagues (1986) employed 50 mg, increased every 3 days to a maximum of 200 mg, but only a small minority of patients were able to tolerate this dose. A significant proportion of patients developed side effects, chiefly oversedation. Successfully treated patients had a better functional outcome from rehabilitation. Depression rating scales were not performed.

The ideal timing for initiation of antidepressant therapy poststroke is unknown. It is advisable to wait 3–4 weeks after the acute stroke, as most associated cardiovascular complications will have declared themselves within this time, and patients with intense but brief reactive depressions may have begun to show some spontaneous recovery.

Electroconvulsive therapy (ECT) has also been given to patients with poststroke depression, but the safety of this procedure for patients with cerebrovascular disorders is not fully established, as long-term follow-up studies have not been reported. Murray, Shea, & Conn (1986) retrospectively reported the successful use of ECT in 14 patients, but there was a lengthy average time between stroke and ECT, up to 12 years. Given the reduced life expectancy for most poststroke patients, one must question whether these patients who survived so long were representative of typical stroke patients. Only one patient was reported to have suffered a complication of ECT, cardiac arrhythmia, but the criteria for patient exclusion were not documented. The incidence of cardiac disease, carotid stenosis, vascular malformations, and other lesions commonly associated with cerebral infarction were not reported. Given that ECT is commonly associated with transient marked elevations in blood pressure, as well as transient cardiac arrhythmia, the presence of such lesions may be a significant risk factor.

In conclusion, although clinical considerations warrant the empirical drug treatment of poststroke depression, more rational treatment will await further clarification of pathophysiology and further controlled studies of treatment outcome.

MULTIPLE SCLEROSIS

Young adults are the chief victims of multiple sclerosis (MS). Epidemiologic studies suggest that the disease is probably acquired in childhood, and that there follows a clinically quiescent period of several years before the onset of symptoms. Onset of clinical multiple sclerosis is unusual before the age of 10 and in senescence. The risk of acquiring MS is highly correlated with the geographic location of the patient's childhood. Patients who lived in New Orleans until the age of 15 have a 1-in-10,000 risk of developing MS, whereas the risk for patients who were raised in Canada is nearly 13 times higher. To a certain extent the risk of MS is a function of distance from the equator. Patients who in adulthood migrate from a high-risk area to a low-risk area retain an increased risk for MS, supporting the hypothesis of an infectious etiology with a long latency period. Detailed epidemiologic investigations of discrete epidemics of MS in the Faroe Islands (associated with the influx of the British Army) and in Newfoundland (linked with outbreaks of canine distemper) also provide indirect but supportive evidence of an an infectious etiology (Kurtzke & Hyllested, 1986; Pryse-Phillips, 1986).

Other lines of evidence suggest an autoimmune factor in MS. Cerebrospinal fluid (CSF) studies of patients frequently indicate elevated gamma globulin, composed of heterogeneous molecules of polyclonal origin. Subsets of gamma globulin with restricted heterogeneity, oligoclonal bands, are found in more than 90 percent of patients with MS. The presence of such bands, however, is only modestly related to the activity of the disease and is not specific to MS. The bands are found in many active neurologic diseases, including acute stroke, infection, and neuropathies, where their presence is thought to represent an immune response to neurologic injury (Chu, Sever, & Madden, 1983; Farrell, Kaufmann, Gilbert, et al., 1985; Link & Laurenzi, 1979; JR Miller, Burke, & Bever, 1983). Further, when gamma interferon was administered intravenously (IV) to 19 MS patients, 6 (32 percent) experienced an acute flare of their disease, suggesting a partial role of immunologic function in pathogenesis. Conversely, immunosuppression with adrenocorticotropin (ACTH) or cyclophosphamide has been somewhat effective in arresting acute exacerbations of the illness (Hauser, Dawson & Lehrich, 1983; Raymond, 1986). Waksman, Director of Research for the National Multiple Sclerosis Society (quoted in "In Pursuit of Quarry," 1986), has said, "Many of us think that [we're] dealing with an autoimmune disease started by a viral infection, but where the virus doesn't have to persist [once the infection is underway]."

The characteristic lesions of MS are plaques of scattered, circumscribed demyelination in the central nervous system (CNS). Such plaques occur predominantly in white matter, with a predilection for periventricular areas, optic nerves, and spinal cord. They may occur anywhere in the CNS, however, including cranial and spinal nerve roots. Microscopically, there is destruction of myelin sheaths and, to a lesser extent, of neuronal fibers. Lymphocytes, macrophages, immunoglobins, and complement are found in active disease. Later, acute inflammation may be replaced by reactive gliosis. Signs and symptoms are chiefly due to interference with neuronal conduction by the demyelinating plaques.

The great variations in locations, numbers, and recurrences of plaques among individual patients account for the very broad spectrum of the clinical presentation. Multiple sclerosis has justifiably been proposed to replace syphilis as "The Great Imitator." Initial symptoms may include motor or sensory impairment, visual loss, diplopia, ataxia, incontinence, vertigo, and changes in mental status. Later, as the disease progresses, initial symptoms may be partially or completely resolved, only to be replaced or joined by a panoply of new symptoms as fresh plaques occur elsewhere in the CNS.

Multiple sclerosis may be more common than previously realized. Postmortem studies and newer diagnostic techniques indicate that the characteristic demyelinating plaques of MS are found more frequently than expected from clinical history (Gabarski, Gabrielsen, Gilman, et al., 1985). Recent studies are also calling into question the basic course of the disease, once regarded as a relapsing and remitting illness (Gebarski et al., 1985; Poser, 1985). Poser (1985), in fact, suggests that the "clinical manifestations of MS are the externally observable parts of an underlying, essentially *continuous* process."

To improve diagnosis, numerous criteria for the classification of MS have been proposed. One of the most widely accepted divides patients into *clinically definite*, *probable*, and *possible* categories (Rose, Ellison, Myers, et al., 1976), which reflect persistent difficulties in confidently diagnosing MS. The criteria for these classifications are as follows:

1. Clinically definite multiple sclerosis
   a. i. Relapsing and remitting course with at least two bouts separated by no less than 1 month, or
      ii. Slow or stepwise progressive course extending over at least 6 months
   b. Documented neurological signs attributable to more than one site of predominantly white-matter central nervous system pathology
   c. Onset of symptoms usually between ages 10 and 50
   d. No better neurologic explanation
2. Probable multiple sclerosis
   a. i. History of relapsing and remitting symptoms but without documentation of signs and presenting with only one neurologic sign commonly associated with multiple sclerosis, or
      ii. A documented single bout of symptoms with signs of multifocal white-matter disease with good recovery, and followed by variable symptoms and signs
   b. No better neurologic explanation
3. Possible multiple sclerosis
   a. i. History of relapsing and remitting symptoms without documentation of signs, or
      ii. Objective neurologic signs insufficient to establish more than one site of central nervous system white-matter pathology
   b. No better neurologic explanation

Neurodiagnostic techniques may assist in accurate differential diagnosis, not only to discriminate multiple sclerosis from other neurologic illness, but also to confirm the presence of disease. This is particularly important in patients whose symptoms are vague and fleeting. Not infrequently, such patients are initially thought to be hysterical.

As discussed earlier, oligoclonal bands are found in the CSF of over 90 percent of patients. Such oligoclonal bands "may represent an immune response to neurological injury that is prominent in disorders with a particularly intense or continuous antigenic stimulus" and are rarely found in patients without definable neurologic illness (Grimaldi, Roos, Nalefski, et al., 1985; JR Miller et al., 1983).

When there is active destruction of brain tissue, whether from MS or from other illness, elevations of myelin basic protein (MBP) will be found in the CSF. An important component of myelin, MBP is liberated into CSF during breakdown of white matter in about one-half of the acute exacerbations of MS. Presumably, the percentage of positive results in active disease is limited by the distance of pathologic areas from CSF. The presence of MBP provides strong evidence in support of neurologic disease and against the diagnosis of hysteria (Cohen, Brooks, Herndon, et al., 1980; Jacque, DeLassalle, Rancurel, et al., 1982).

Evoked potentials are another useful procedure in the diagnosis of neurologic illness, subclinical and overt, as they may reveal the presence of unsuspected lesions. Conduction delays in visual, auditory, or somatosensory evoked potentials indicate dysfunction along their respective pathways. Abnormalities persist during clinical remissions. When correctly performed and interpreted, evoked potentials may be a sensitive indicator of illness in a wide variety of disorders, including MS (Chiappa,

1980). (See Chapter 3, by Fogel and Faust, on neurodiagnostic procedures.)

Neuroradiologic studies also contribute to the diagnosis of cerebral MS. On nonenhanced CT scans, hypodensities in the white matter corresponding to established MS plaques may be visualized. The addition of contrast to imaging will sometimes demonstrate transient enhancing lesions corresponding to destruction of the blood–brain barrier in periods of acute exacerbations. Scanning with "double-dose" contrast after a 1-hour delay may maximize the detection of lesions with this technique (Barrett, Drayer, & Shin, 1985; Ebers, Vinuela, Feasby, et al., 1984; Sears, McCammon, Bigelow, et al., 1982). The occurrence of adverse reactions to high-dose contrast is a drawback of this technique.

More sensitive and safer than CT scans for the detection of MS plaques is nuclear magnetic resonance imaging (MRI). The better resolution of MRI scans, without using contrast agents, and their ability to detect lesions in brain stem and spinal cord usually obscured by artifacts on CT scans make this procedure a clearly superior technique (Bogousslavsky, Fox, Cavey, et al., 1986; Kirshner, Tsai, Runge, et al., 1985). (See Chapter 3.)

Bursts of enthusiasm for new technologies should not obscure the maxim that laboratory investigations are never a replacement for clinical acumen. None of the above tests are specific for MS. Several disorders may imitate MS. A full discussion of these illnesses is beyond the scope of this chapter, and readers interested in the extensive differential diagnosis of MS are referred to standard neurologic texts and the following references: Abramowitz and Kasdon (1982); Britt, Connor, and Enzmann (1981); Elkin, Leon, Grenell, et al. (1985); Moore and Cupps (1983); Reik, Smith, Khan, et al. (1985); Rundell and Wise (1985); Snider, Simpson, Nielsen, et al. (1983).

Psychiatric Presentation

The neuropsychiatric symptoms of MS are as wide and varied as the motor and sensory symptoms. Euphoria has been regarded as the classic mental symptom of MS since its description by Cottrell and Wilson in 1926. "Euphoria" may be the presentation of parietal lobe anosognosia or of frontal lobe disinhibition, but detailed neuropsychiatric definitions are lacking. The presence of euphoria has been found to correlate with intellectual deterioration (Surridge, 1969).

Dementia, varying in severity from mild to profound, develops as numerous association tracts are disrupted by plaques. It has long been recognized as one of the most distressing developments of MS. Apphasia, impulsivity, perseveration, and memory impairment may all be found early or late in the disease (Jambor, 1969; Young, Saunders, & Ponsford, 1976).

In more recent years, attention has turned to the high incidence of depression in MS. Although early reports were anecdotal, more current investigations have examined larger series of patients, with control populations. Kahana, Leibowitz, and Alter (1971) reported the results of a national survey of MS patients in Israel. They found, in addition to the expected findings of euphoria and dementia, a significant incidence of depression and a suicide rate for MS patients that was 14 times higher than the general population.

Whitlock and Siskind (1980) examined 30 patients with MS and compared them with 30 patients with other chronic neurologic diseases, matched for age, sex, and degree of disability. Using the Beck Depression Inventory and an interview procedure, they found that the incidence of depression in MS patients was significantly higher than in controls, both during their illness and before it. Eight of the MS patients, but none of their controls, suffered from depression prior to the onset of neurologic symptoms. Correcting for age and the expected incidence of depression in the general population, the incidence was still significantly higher. About half the MS patients suffered from an "endogenous" depression since the onset of illness, in contrast to only 17 percent of neurologic controls. The authors concluded that "serious affective illness can be a presenting or complicating features of MS."

In a detailed epidemiologic study, Schiffer and Babigian (1984) found a prevalence rate of 20 percent for psychiatric disturbances in multiple sclerosis; depression accounted for more than half of the diagnoses. By contrast, amyotrophic lateral sclerosis (ALS), which is much more grim and an inexorably fatal disease, showed much less associated depression. This suggests that the high rate of depression in MS may be disease-specific.

Schiffer, Caine, and Bamford (1983) further defined the prevalence and presentation of depression in MS by interviewing patients using not only the Beck inventory but also the Schedule for Affective Disorders and Schizophrenia (SADS). Other important refinements of this study were that the patients received neuropsychologic testing to quantify cognitive impairment. Nine patients with predominantly cerebral involvement and 7 patients with predominantly spinal cord involvement (defined both clinically and radiologically) were matched with 15 normal controls by age, sex, and education. The 9 patients in the cerebral MS group had 11 depressive episodes. Two of the patients with predominantly spinal MS had 1 episode of depression each. The incidence of depression in the control subjects was zero. Neither neurologic disability, duration, and pattern of illness nor cognitive impairment differentiated the two MS groups. This study further strengthens the contention that depression seen with MS may be a direct result of cerebral involvement.

Dalos, Rabins, Brooks, et al. (1983)

further clarified this issue by studying 64 MS patients prospectively with monthly ratings for 1 year. The prevalence of emotional disturbance was 90 percent in progressive illness, 39 percent in stable patients, and 12 percent in controls, who were spinal-cord injured.

Mania and bipolar disorder have also been linked to MS, but the literature on this subject is smaller and less detailed. In one of the most interesting reports, psychiatric diagnoses were assigned using an interview utilizing the Schedule for Affective Disorders and Schizophrenia (SADS) and Research Diagnostic Criteria (RDC). The result was that a twofold increase in bipolar disorder was found in MS patients compared with population controls (Schiffer, Wineman, & Weitkamp, 1986).

Therapy

Although more scientific investigation is needed to delineate the incidence and clinical features of psychiatric disturbance in MS, several features of the illness suggest plausible hypotheses both for etiology and for treatment. At a psychologic level, MS is a fearsome illness. It strikes young adults at a crucial time in their psychosocial development. Further, the prognosis for an MS patient is uncertain, so planning for the future is difficult. The uncertainty of when one will have the next symptom, or become blind, demented, or crippled, can be terrifying. The symptoms of MS—gait problems, incontinence, blindness, and so on—can be demoralizing to patients and their families and increase their feelings of helplessness.

Physical and occupational therapy may improve mood as well as maximize body functioning. The National Multiple Sclerosis Society, with its many local branches, affords patients and their families support and education as well.

The medications employed to treat multiple sclerosis may themselves be the cause of psychiatric problems and should be periodically reassessed. Steroids are often used for flares of MS and have long been notorious for causing depression, mania, and psychosis (Glaser, 1953). Baclofen, which is used in the treatment of spasticity, may cause agitation and psychosis with hallucinations, particularly upon withdrawal (Arnold, Rudd, & Kirshner, 1980; Kirubakaran, Mayfield, & Rengachary, 1984). At least in one case, baclofen was observed to suppress muscle rigidity in an MS patient who developed all other components of the neuroleptic malignant syndrome (Rodgers and Stoudemire, in press), thus covertly delaying the diagnosis. In MS patients on neuroleptics and baclofen, fever, autonomic immobility, and delirium may represent NMS even if rigidity is absent. The creatinine phosphokinase (CPK) level is the most helpful diagnostic test.

Neuropsychologic testing is often of value in helping to clarify how much neurologic factors are coloring the patient's presentation. Easy tearfulness can be a sign of depression or of pseudobulbar palsy. Missed appointments and inattention to medications may be due to denial, or can be early signs of dementia. Objective neuropsychologic data may aid families, who otherwise might misattribute symptoms or experience rejection where none is intended, and aid patients who might receive unwarranted criticism or otherwise suffer from the misinterpretation of their behavior.

When the patient is depressed, antidepressant medication may be used, although there is surprisingly little literature on this subject. MS patients may be sensitive to low doses of medication and require less than standard dosages. Tricyclics may cause exacerbation of tremor; this can sometimes be treated effectively with beta blockers or benzodiazepines. They can also exacerbate ataxia. Patients with cerebral involvement may be exquisitely sensitive to anticholinergic effects of tricyclics, with the development of sedation and confusion. The bladder difficulties of patients may improve or worsen with tricyclics, depending on their specific urodynamics. Tricyclics should be started at low dosage and increased slowly, and the patient should be re-examined after dosage increases. Amitriptyline can be helpful for the emotional incontinence of pseudobulbar palsy, even when the patient is not depressed. Schiffer, Hernedon, and Rudick (1985) found that a dosage of 50–75 mg a day often helped to relieve this symptom.

Trazodone, which has been reported to be helpful in elderly patients with dementia and behavior disturbance (DM Simpson & Foster, 1986), may be helpful in MS, although this has not been specifically addressed in the literature. Excessive sedation and ataxia have been found to be limiting factors in its use with MS patients.

Carbamazepine is frequently used to treat some of the paroxysmal symptoms of MS, such as trigeminal neuralgia; a mood-stabilizing effect has been observed when this done. Lithium tends to produce ataxia, tremor, and confusion in MS patients and is often poorly tolerated. The polyuria that frequently results from lithium use may aggravate problems with incontinence. For MS patients with bipolar symptoms, carbamazepine might thus be preferable to lithium. If lithium is used, a relatively low blood level is advisable, and amiloride might be used if polyuria aggravates incontinence.

MS patients also appear to be particularly sensitive to extrapyramidal side effects of neuroleptics, so relatively low doses should be used, and prophylactic antiparkinson medication should be strongly considered, particularly with high-potency neuroleptics. Amentadine would be the first choice, as it lacks anticholinergic effects and may reduce fatigue in MS patients.

Given the uncertain nature of MS, perhaps the most useful thing the clinician can do is to provide stable and consistent support, advice, and advocacy for the patient. Families may also benefit from an opportunity to work through the stress, anxiety, and guilt that may be engendered. Divorce, loss of employment, poverty, and social isolation also cripple patients with MS and add to the patient's despair. Knowing that there is an informed and caring person who will not abandon them may make their losses more bearable.

PARKINSON'S DISEASE

"A more melancholy object I never beheld. The patient, naturally a handsome, middle-sized, sanguine man, of cheerful disposition, and an active mind, appeared much emaciated, stooping, and dejected." (James Parkinson, 1817.)

There has been an intense reemergence of interest in Parkinson's disease in recent years because of the discovery of the toxic effects of MPTP (N-methyl-4-phenyl-1,2,3,6-tetrahydropyridine). Beginning in the late 1970s, sporadic outbreaks of severe Parkinson's syndrome were noted in young drug abusers in California, Maryland, and Vancouver, British Columbia. Among these was a 23-year-old college student who in 1977 developed severe bradykinesia, rigidity, and mutism and was initially thought to have catatonic schizophrenia until a response to L-dopa revealed the surprising diagnosis of Parkinson's syndrome. The patient was referred to the National Institute of Mental Health (NIMH), where the patient's psychiatrist, G. Davis, in a skilled piece of detective work, obtained a history that the patient had been synthesizing illicit drugs. Investigating this clue, Dr. Davis visited the patient's home and collected the glassware used for the production of synthetic meperidine. Contaminating the glassware were found several pyridines, including MPTP. Eventually, MPTP was shown

by Langston and others to be the culprit of the patient's illness, causing degeneration of the substantia nigra in humans and producing Parkinson's syndrome (Ballard, Tetrud, & Langston, 1985; Langston, Ballard, Tetrua, et al., 1983). Prior research on Parkinson's had always been hampered by a lack of animal models for the disease. Now with the availability of MPTP, there has been a marked increase in research in the field (SH Snyder & D'Amato, 1986).

Parkinson's disease has been a puzzle to medical science since its description in 1817 by James Parkinson, who reported a clinical syndrome he termed *paralysis agitans*. The apparent contradiction inherent in the title, paralysis with agitation, conveys the sense of the seemingly paradoxical symptoms of the illness. On the one hand, victims of the illness have profoundly slowed voluntary movement, with akinesia, rigidity, and abulia, coupled with a masked face and unblinking stare. On the other hand, the patients may have tremor at rest and with movement, explosive pseudobulbar weeping and laughing, pressured pallilalic speech, festination, and akathisia, all suggesting an agitated state. Oliver Sacks, in his philosophically profound and emotionally compelling book *Awakenings* (1973), writes, "The Parkinsonian has indeed lost, and quite fundamentally, his inner sense of scale and pace. Hence the incontinent accelerations and retardations, the magnifications and minifications, to which he is prone." As Dr. Sacks indicates, it is both simplistic and incorrect to view Parkinson's disease as purely a disorder of movement, as the observed muscular activity and the mental state of the patient are inextricably linked. Though this point is often overlooked by physicians, it is well known to patients. Physical slowing is reflected in slowing of thought processes, and bursts of intense emotion are coupled with increased psychomotor activity. This is of course true for many other states: the abulia of depression, the restless movements of mania, the nervous fidgeting of worry, the increase in tardive dyskinesia with stress.

Janice Stevens (1973) has discussed the striking anatomic and functional similarities of two of the brain's major dopaminergic systems, the nigrostriatal and the mesolimbic. This anatomic homology may underlie some of the linkages of motor activity and emotion that are seen Parkinson's disease, but the details are unknown.

Classically, Parkinson's disease has been regarded as idiopathic degeneration of dopaminergic neurons in the substantia nigra of the midbrain, resulting in loss of "motor impulse" to the corpus striatum. Actually, there is evidence of widespread catecholamine dysfunction. Degeneration and loss of dopamine are also seen in the ventral tegmental area, which projects to the cingulate, entorhinal, and frontal cortex and to the nucleus accumbens, olfactory tubercle, and central amygdaloid nucleus (Javoy-Agid & Agid, 1980; SH Snyder & D'Amato, 1986). Further, there is evidence of degeneration of the locus ceruleus, which has extensive noradrenergic projections (Riederer, Birkmayer, Seemann, et al., 1977). Additionally, Parkinson's patients have evidence of serotonergic alteration, with decreased binding sites for serotonin in the basal ganglia and some regions of cerebral cortex (Raisman, Cash, & Agidmy, 1986), and the cerebrospinal fluid shows evidence of decreased serotonin turnover (Mayeux, Stern, Cote, et al., 1984). With such evidence of involvement of several neurotransmitters known to be important in behavior, the association of Parkinson's disease with neuropsychiatric disorders is not surprising.

Clinically, Parkinson's disease usually occurs in mid to late life and gradually progresses over 10 or 20 years. Males and females are affected equally, with a prevalence of about 1 percent of the population over 50 and 2 percent of the population over

70. Initial symptoms may include resting tremor of one hand, usually progressing to generalized symptoms of tremor, bradykinesia, and rigidity. Seborrhea is frequent. Later, gait impairment, retropulsion, dysphagia, dysautonomia, and secondary orthopedic changes may occur. There is, however, considerable variability in the rates of progression of various symptoms. For all ages of onset, however, mortality is increased above controls, often from sepsis, malnutrition, or pulmonary embolus (Duvoisin, 1986; Rajput, 1984).

Dementia has consistently been reported to be a concomitant of Parkinson's disease, with estimates of prevalence varying but correlated with the length of illness. Sweet, McDowell, Feigenson, et al. (1976) found dementia in one-third of 100 patients followed for 6 years, with deficits increasing over time. Mortimer, Pirozzolo, Hansch, et al. (1982) studied 60 patients with idiopathic Parkinson's disease who were receiving dopaminergic medications and found that they had marked cognitive problems with memory, abstract reasoning, and concept formation, consistent with a subcortical dementia. Other authors have noted an association between Parkinson's and Alzheimer's diseases, diagnosed both clinically and pathologically (Boller, Mizutani, Roessmann, et al., 1980), although this has been disputed (Ball, 1984; Mann & Yates, 1983; Perry, Tomlinson, Candy, et al., 1983).

The dementia of Parkinson's disease may have diverse etiologies, and its classification and pathogenesis are the subject of intense investigation. Depletion of neurons and formation of Lewy bodies in the nucleus basalis of Meynert occur in idiopathic Parkinson's disease (Nakano & Hirona, 1984), and cell death is most severe in demented patients (Whitehouse, Hedreen, White, et al., 1983). According to Nakano and Hirona (1984), in the majority of cases, neuronal loss is not associated with other pathologic changes of Alzheimer's disease, such as senile plaques or neurofibrillatory tangles, but Hakim and Mathieson (1979) have reported a nearly universal occurrence of such changes. Chui, Mortimer, Slager, et al. (1986) have reported that the clinical distinctions between the so-called cortical and subcortical dementias of Parkinson's may be more apparent than real and that both presentations correlate with neuronal loss in subcortical nuclei. Hornykiewicz and Kish (1984) report that demented Parkinson patients, irrespective of the presence or absence of Alzheimer's neuropathology, have a disturbance of central cholinergic function. Whether this cholinergic deficiency is necessary or sufficient to result in dementia is unclear.

Regardless of etiology, the development of dementia in the later stages of Parkinson's represents a difficult problem for the patient and the physician. The dementia is inexorable and does not respond to antiparkinson medication. Rather, such patients may develop delirium, agitation, and psychosis on small doses of the drugs required to ameliorate motor symptoms, presenting a therapeutic impasse. In assessing dementia in Parkinson's, the clinician should first consider whether the patient indeed has true Parkinson's disease or instead has any of a variety of illnesses that produce extrapyramidal signs accompanied by dementia. Chief among these would be progressive supranuclear palsy (PSP), also known as Steele-Richardson syndrome, which presents with bradykinesia, retropulsion, and rigidity and may be accompanied by a fulminant dementia (Jackson, Jankovic, & Ford, 1983). Early loss of vertical eye movements and absence of tremor help to differentiate this illness. PSP responds poorly to dopaminergic medication but may respond partially to methysergide (Rafal & Grimm, 1981) or amitriptyline (Kvale, 1982).

Another mimic of Parkinson's disease is multi-infarct dementia, particularly with lacunar infarcts of the basal ganglia. Such patients also have stopped posture, shuffling gait, rigidity, and dementia (Ishii et al., 1986; Tolosa & Santa-Maria, 1984). Patients usually, but not always, have a history of hypertension (Fisher, 1982). The classic stepwise deterioration in function is a history that is often difficult to obtain in clinical practice. CT head scan may be useful in detecting small midline lacunae but may be normal. The magnetic resonance scan (MRI) is a superior test, detecting up to eight times the number of lacunae visualized on CT (DeWitt, Buonanno, Kistler, et al., 1984). Therapy for multi-infarct dementia is directed toward prevention of further lacunar infarcts (JR Miller et al., 1983). Postsynaptic dopamine agonists, such as bromocriptine, may be helpful in improving bradykinesia, and drug treatment of associated depression may improve mood and function.

Several other illnesses may also mimic Parkinson's disease, including olivopontocerebral degeneration, carbon monoxide intoxication (Klawans, 1982), and tumors (Leenders, Findley, & Cleeves, 1986). Extrapyramidal syndromes may also be induced by neuroleptics, which include not only antipsychotics, but also antiemetic agents such as metoclopramide (Patel, Seth, & Meador, 1986).

Depression in Parkinson's Disease

Depression is highly prevalent in Parkinson's disease and may be linked to the occurrence of dementia. Although estimates of the prevalence of depression have varied with the instruments employed for assessment (Harvey, 1986; Robins, 1976), there is consensus that depression is far more common in Parkinson's disease patients than in the general population. Recently Mayeux and colleagues examined 49 consecutive patients with Parkinson's disease and found that 20 percent met DSM-III criteria for major depression and 10 percent met criteria for dysthymia. Depression was correlated with low CSF 5-HIAA, suggesting a reduction in central serotonin. The patients exhibited sleep disturbance, fatigue, psychomotor retardation, loss of self-esteem, and guilt. Treatment with a serotonin precursor (L-5-HTP) resulted in improvement of depressive symptoms and a return of CSF 5-HIAA levels to normal (Mayeux, Stern, Sano, et al., 1986; Mayeux, Stern, Williams, et al., 1986).

Atypical depression has also been found to be associated with Parkinson's disease. Defining atypical depression by the prominence of panic and anxiety associated with depressed mood, Rubin, Kurlan, Schiffer, et al. (1986) found an incidence of 7.6 percent, which is significantly higher than the general population prevalence.

In 55 Parkinson's patients were evaluated for depression with the Beck Depression Inventory and were simultaneously assessed for dementia with a modified Folstein Mini-Mental State Examination (Mayeux, Stern, Rosen, et al., 1981). Forty-seven percent of the patients were found to be significantly depressed, and degree of depression correlated with the degree of cognitive impairment. Mayeux et al. (1981) postulated two types of intellectual impairment in Parkinson's: Alzheimer's disease in 30 percent and, in another 50 percent, a dementia manifested as a mood disorder accompanied by impaired cognitive skills and inattention, but not a global dementia. Huber, Shuttleworth, and Paulson (1986) also found a nearly universal occurrence of depression and impairments of recent memory in Parkinson's disease patients, with a subset of 35 percent showing more profound intellectual decline.

There are also suggestions that depression may exacerbate Parkinson's disease. Rats depleted of dopamine may appear and behave normally until stressed, at which time parkinsonian signs emerge. Neurologic impairments were related both to the extent of dopamine depletion and to the intensity of stress in an additive fashion, a "biopsychosocial" rat model (AM Snyder, Stricker, & Zigmond, 1985). Clinicians may note an analogous phenomenon in patients who appear to have increased symptoms when stressed or depressed.

That depression may precipitate Parkinson's disease is also suggested by a recent study that examined 34 patients with recent onset of Parkinson's disease who were not yet receiving dopaminergic drugs. Patients were evaluated by the Columbia University Parkinson Scale and the Northwestern Disability Scale to quantify their degree of Parkinson's. Patients were also assessed for depression past and current, using DSM-III criteria and the Beck Depression Inventory, and were assessed for cognitive impairment with a modified Mini-Mental State Examination. Of the 34 patients, 11 had a history of depression. For 10 of these 11, depression preceded the onset of symptoms of Parkinson's by 1 or more (sometimes many) years. For 4 of these patients, the first parkinsonian symptoms appeared shortly after the onset of a moderately severe depression. Also, depressed patients tended to be younger than other newly diagnosed Parkinson's patients, and the authors suggested that "aminergic dysfunction . . . may make the patient with latent Parkinson's disease, already having loss of nigral cells, develop Parkinsonism earlier" (Santamaria, Tolosa, & Valles, 1986).

Psychosis

Psychosis is a frequent concomitant of late Parkinson's but is not well characterized in the literature. A common presentation is of "lilliputian" visual hallucinations with impaired reality testing in a clear sensorium. The patient will report little people under the furniture, at the window, and so on. The hallucinations are usually entertaining, but occasionally paranoid delusions and agitation may accompany the presentation. The symptoms are usually related to dopamine agonist treatment but at times are seen with anticholinergics alone.

Depressive psychosis may also be seen, with mood-congruent auditory hallucinations and paranoia. Dementia and anti-Parkinson pharmacotherapy appear to be frequent, if not universal, risk factors for psychosis.

The treatment of psychosis with Parkinson's may be quite difficult. Neuroleptics and other dopamine antagonists that ameliorate psychosis will exacerbate motor symptoms. Moreover, such patients are generally in an advanced stage of their illness and thus are exquisitely sensitive to medications, with side effects of delirium, orthostatic hypotension, and urinary retention. A forthcoming improvement in the treatment of psychosis in Parkinson's may be clozapine, when it becomes available in the United States. Clozapine is reported to affect dopamine turnover in the limbic system more than in the striatum. Unfortunately, it is associated with a high incidence of side effects such as agranulocytosis (Senn, Jung, Kinz, et al., 1977).

The pharmacotherapy of Parkinson's may itself be the cause of considerable psychiatric morbidity. Anticholinergics, helpful for parkinsonian tremor and rigidity, may produce a toxic confusional state with agitation and impairment of memory. In demented parkinsonian patients, this occurs very frequently, perhaps because the patients already have loss of cholinergic neurons in the nucleus basalis of Meynert (Nakano & Hirano, 1984). Beta blockers such as propranolol, which are prescribed to control action tremors of Parkinson's disease, can also be associated with confusion, depression, and other mental status changes (Avorn, Everitt, & Weiss, 1986).

Dopaminergic agents, such as amantadine, bromocriptine, and L-dopa, may also produce hallucinations, psychosis, and paranoia, and, again, demented patients

appear more sensitive to these effects (Goodwin, 1971). Some patients seem differentially sensitive to psychiatric side effects of different dopaminergic agents, and a switch from bromocriptine to L-dopa, or the converse, could be considered when psychosis develops. Sometimes, a combination of low doses of bromocriptine and L-dopa is better tolerated than a higher dose of either one alone.

Psychiatric side effects are to a certain extent dose related, and it is prudent to use as low a dose of medication as possible to achieve acceptable function. In end-stage Parkinson's the clinician may be faced with the unfortunate choice of producing a patient who can move but is psychotic or a patient with normal affect who is frozen in immobility. Not infrequently the difference in medication to produce either of these two alternatives is very small. At these times a drug holiday may be rational (Weiner, Koller, & Perlik, et al., 1980), although the long-term value of such holidays is debatable. Drug holidays should be conducted in a hospital because the patient may experience pronounced bradykinesia while drug-free and be at risk for pulmonary embolus, aspiration, atelectasis, decubiti, and ileus. The purpose of a drug holiday is to increase sensitivity of striatal dopaminergic receptors that may have altered their receptivity after chronic stimulation by medications.

The treatment of psychiatric illness in parkinsonian patients should have as its goal the improvement of mood and function while avoiding exacerbation of motor symptoms and delirium. Tricyclics have been most frequently reported as helpful for the treatment of depression in Parkinson's disease. Tricyclics, which have monoamine agonist and cholinergic antagonist properties, may also have a direct beneficial effect on motor functions. Imipramine, desipramine, and nortriptyline all have been reported as effective antidepressants (Strang, 1965; Laitinen, 1969; Andersen, Aabro, Gulmann, et al., 1980).

Tricyclics should be started at low dosages and increased gradually. Parkinson's disease is frequently complicated by orthostatic hypotension, so standing blood pressures should be determined frequently.

Electroconvulsive therapy (ECT) has also been reported useful in treating depression in patients with Parkinson's disease. Interestingly, motor symptoms may also improve with ECT, the improvement occasionally antedating the improvement in mood (Lebensohn & Jenkins, 1975; Asnis, 1977). An increase in dopamine turnover, due to ECT, has been postulated as the mechanism of action. Patients may be more sensitive to the development of post-ECT confusion, as are other patients with CNS disorders.

The monoamine oxidase B inhibitor deprenyl has been used to treat Parkinson's disease. By slowing dopamine degradation, deprenyl may prolong the action of L-dopa and sinemet (Birkmayer, Riederer, Youdim, et al., 1975). Deprenyl has also been reported to produce euphoria in Parkinson's patients, perhaps by degradation to amphetamine (Karoum, Chuang, Eisler, et al., 1982).

Other, less selective MAOIs, when combined with Sinemet (Merck, Sharp, & Dohme) or L-dopa, may produce a hypertensive response. Other patients treated with this combination may show a severe exacerbation of orthostatic hypotension. Therefore, standard "psychiatric" MAOIs should be avoided in patients on Sinemet or L-dopa. Parkinson's patients with dementia may have both poor memory and impulsivity and may be at risk for hazardous dietary indiscretions as well. Bromocriptine, a postsynaptic agent, has been used safely with MAOIs. (See also Chapter 4, by Stoudemire and Fogel.)

Monoamine oxidase inhibitors used alone currently show considerable speculative promise to assist also in the prevention and treatment of Parkinson's disease itself. For example, it has been found that monoamine oxidase enzyme B is necessary for MPTP to exert its deleterious effects. MPTP is converted by MAO-B in serotonergic terminals and glial cells to become "MPP+" (1-methyl-4-phenylpyridine), which then enters the dopamine neurons and destroys them (SH Snyder & D'Amato, 1986). If indeed an endogenous or environmental toxin analogous to MPTP is responsible for Parkinson's disease, treatment with MAOIs might avert the progression of the disease.

EPILEPSY

The population of epileptics in the United States, by conservative estimates, numbers over 2 million, yielding a lifetime prevalence of approximately 1 percent, which is roughly equal to the prevalence of schizophrenia and bipolar disorder. Even this estimate may be too low. A European epidemiologic study suggests that two-thirds of the total population of patients with seizures are not under treatment at any given time, one-third because of noncompliance and a remarkable one-third because the epilepsy has never been diagnosed at all (Mesulam, 1985).

Complex partial seizures (CPS), previously referred to by the less accurate term *temporal lobe epilepsy*, are the most common form of epilepsy in adults. Although most complex partial seizures arise from the structures of the temporal lobe, seizures may also arise from the frontal, occipital, or parietal areas or may secondarily involve those areas. The manifestations of complex partial seizures can hence be protean. Moreover, the complex partial epilepsies can be the most difficult to control. While the primary generalized epilepsies usually respond well to anticonvulsants, seizures with a focal onset may be difficult to suppress completely.

The temporal lobe is not uniform, but is composed of several evolutionary and functionally distinct regions. Some of the temporal cortex is involved in auditory and vestibular processing, and to a certain extent in speech (Wernicke's area) and memory; much of the rest of the temporal cortex is densely interconnected by association fibers to other lobes of the brain. Deep within the temporal lobe are major structures of the limbic system, constituting the anatomic substrate of emotion (Papez, 1937). High fevers in infancy appear to cause mesial temporal sclerosis, which underlies an estimated 50 percent of cases of CPS. Closed head trauma, often minor, may be another common cause of CPS. With trauma, the inferomedial and polar surfaces of the brain are injured by the rough surfaces of the skull. Some viruses, chiefly herpes simplex, have a predilection for the temporal lobe. The middle cerebral artery, which supplies most of the temporal lobe, is the usual route for emboli from cardiac and carotid disease. The vasculature of the temporal lobe is vulnerable to compression, and neuronal structures in this region are prone to hypoxia (Glaser, 1964; Ounstead, Glaser, Lindsay, et al., 1985).

The temporal lobe, both cortical and limbic areas, is heavily involved in higher cortical functions such as speech, memory, and affect; damage or seizures in these areas give rise to a number of neuropsychiatric conditions. A seizure is a rapid and synchronous discharge of neurons, and the manifestation of a seizure will correlate with the function of the portion of the brain that is discharging. A discharge in the part of the motor cortex that represents the arm will result in movements of the arm; a discharge in the visual cortex will result in changes in vision. Since the temporal lobe subserves affective, associative, and mnestic functions, a seizure in this region will result in changes in mood, cognition, memory, and behavior (Gloor, Olivier,

Quesney, et al., 1982). The amygdala is particularly epileptogenic, often rapidly involved in a seizure discharge that spreads from other regions of the brain. Experiments on animals indicate that the amygdala is involved in coordination of rage and fear responses, which may underlie certain manifestations of CPS. According to Stevens, Mark, Erwin, et al. (1969) the normal temporal cortex appears to "suppress and modulate primitive automatic emotionally charged patterns of fight, flight, feeling good and sexuality." Most seizures are short-lived. The average complex seizure lasts less than 2 minutes. It would appear, then, that seizure activity could not account for more long-lasting behavioral changes. There are, however, both clinical and theoretical exceptions to this point.

Status epilepticus may occur not only for major motor (grand mal) seizures, but for complex partial seizures as well. Once believed rare, complex partial status is now thought to be of higher prevalence than recognized previously (Van Rossum, Ockhuysen, & Arts, 1985). Partial status may last for a week, or even for 2 months by one report.

Psychomotor status onset is usually acute and presents with an alteration of consciousness, confusion, and an absence of focal neurologic findings. The patient is often initially thought to be suffering from psychosis or some other psychiatric disturbance. Behavior can be bizarre and can be accompanied by subjective feelings of anxiety, paranoia, or euphoria. Prolonged periods of bizarre behavior followed by amnesia for the event can suggest the diagnosis of hysteria (Drury, Klass, Westmoreland, et al., 1985; Lee, 1985; Mayeux, Alexander, Benson, et al., 1979). The EEG documents the epileptic origin of the behavior, and episodes may be terminated with anticonvulsants. *New-onset psychotic symptoms in patients with known epilepsy always constitute an indication for an EEG.*

A seizure discharge may also produce prolonged alterations of the brain and behavior after the actual discharge has ceased. The effects of electroconvulsive treatment bear witness to this point. That this is also true of partial seizures was demonstrated by Stevens and colleagues in 1969. Depth electrodes were placed in the amygdalas; brief stimulation produced changes in mood and behavior that persisted for several weeks. Attendant EEG changes were not seen, confirming that the persisting behavioral changes, although the result of seizure, were not themselves seizures. Among the several changes were severe depression and manic excitability with pressure of speech (Stevens et al., 1969).

Along another line of evidence of persistent behavioral effects of seizures is the concept of *cyclic psychosis*, first noted 50 years ago (Glaus, 1931), when it was observed that some patients experienced periods of psychosis and no seizures, alternating with periods of sanity accompanied by convulsions, which led Glaus and others to conclude that epilepsy and psychosis were "antagonistic." This observation has been reconfirmed many times (Flor-Henry, 1969; Flor-Henry, 1969a; Kirstensen & Sindrup, 1978).

Multiple mechanisms may explain this phenomenon. It is possible that in the periods of psychosis without overt seizures, epileptic activity may persist in deep structures of the temporal lobe, altering function, while the surface EEG remains unchanged or demonstrates only slow waves (Laitinen & Toivakka, 1980). Weiser (1983), using depth recordings, demonstrated ictal rage, hallucinations, and laughter that were not reflected by the surface EEG. Without the use of depth electrodes, such behavior would probably have been regarded as an interictal phenomenon. Persistent epileptic activity cannot, however, explain all interictal behavioral changes.

There is evidence that the brain has homeostatic mechanisms to prevent further seizures. Otherwise, an epileptic focus would seize continuously, but in reality this appears to happen only occasionally. Although some of these inhibitory mechanisms may be local, some appear to be mediated by the corpus callosum, as if one side of the brain were attempting to suppress seizures in the other hemisphere. Perhaps these local and contralateral mechanisms contribute to psychiatric disturbance as well (SS Spencer, Spencer, Glaser, et al., 1984; Stevens, 1983).

That epilepsy is associated with psychiatric disturbance is an ancient notion. Herodotus, writing about an epileptic king, said, "It would not be unlikely that if the body suffered from a great disease the mind was not sound either." Aretaeia of Cappadocia wrote that "they become languid, spiritless, stupid, inhuman, asociable, not disposed to hold intercourse, not to be sociable at any period of life, sleepless, subject to many horrid dreams, without appetite and with bad digestion, pale, of leaden color, slow to learn from torpidity of the understanding and of the senses."

Since then, the association of psychiatric problems with seizures has been the subject of persistent and sometimes vociferous debate. Epilepsy has carried a severe social stigma, which no one wishes to perpetuate, and researchers who have described psychiatric problems as a result of epilepsy have been criticized in this regard. If psychosis, depression, and other psychiatric syndromes, however, are in fact as much a manifestation of an epileptic focus as tonic-clonic movements and staring spells, it would be a disservice to patients to fail to diagnose and treat them.

Trimble (1983) has reviewed the literature on psychiatric disturbance in epilepsy and noted the difficulties in determining the incidence and prevalence of possible associations. One difficulty is the precise delineation and diagnosis of psychiatric syndromes. Such difficulty is of course not unique to the epileptic population. Other problems include separating ictal and interictal symptoms from effects of medication. Despite such difficulties in definition, and in patient selection, a large number of articles attest to various ways in which epilepsy can be complicated by psychiatric disturbance.

Psychosis

It has been estimated that psychosis occurs in approximately 7 percent of patients with epilepsy (McKenna, Kane, & Parrish, 1985). Most of these patients appear to have the origin of their ictus in the temporal lobe (Flor-Henry, 1969b; Stoudemire, Nelson, & Houpt, 1983). There has been argument whether this is true, but given the limitations of localization by scalp EEG (SS Spencer, Williamson, & Bridgers, 1985), and given that the amygdala is easily involved by a seizure disorder regardless of the ictal focus, and that it is known that other, nonconvulsive disorders of the temporal lobe may also result in psychosis (Lishman, 1966), it appears likely that the temporal lobe is etiologic in the production of psychotic disorders. Psychosis appears to develop more frequently, but not exclusively, when seizures originate in the left temporal lobe (Flor-Henry, 1969a,b; Levine & Finklestein, 1982). An excess of left-handedness in psychotic epileptics has also been reported and may suggest a shift in cerebral dominance (Sherwin, Magnan, & Bancaud, 1982).

Chronic interictal psychosis (as opposed to the brief psychotic and confusional states seen with seizures and in the postictal period) has been reported to develop usually some years after the onset of seizures (Slater, Beard, & Glitheroe, 1963) but has also been reported to develop

within much shorter intervals—a month or less (Levine & Finklestein, 1982).

The psychotic disorder associated with epilepsy appears schizophreniform, but with qualifying differences that can assist in differential diagnosis. Many patients have paranoia, occurring in a clear or clouded sensorium, *without* hallucinations, loose associations, and the other accompaniments of true schizophrenia. Other patients may have the positive symptoms of schizophrenia, such as auditory hallucinations and delusions, but usually do not have the negative symptoms, such as withdrawal and affective blunting. The psychosis may be associated with normal affect and the ability to form and maintain social relationships, or may be accompanied by such disturbances of mood such as depression, rage, anxiety, or euphoria (Pond, 1957; Glaser, 1964). Premorbid personality is more likely to have been normal than in "functional" schizophrenia (Toone, Garralda, & Ronma, 1982).

The chronic interictal psychosis of epilepsy does not, as a rule, respond to anticonvulsants (Levine & Finkelstein, 1982; Mendez, Cummings, & Benson, 1984; Stevens, 1983) but may respond to neuroleptics. Highly cholinergic drugs such as chlorpromazine may promote seizures by lowering the seizure threshold and should be avoided (Mendez et al., 1984; Remick & Fine, 1979). Neuroleptics are highly protein bound, and their possible displacement of anticonvulsants from binding sites and consequent effect on free drug levels is largely unknown (GM Simpson & Yadalam, 1985). Moreover, neuroleptics and anticonvulsants may compete for metabolism by the liver, resulting in either increases or decreases in blood levels. Phenothiazines, for example, will elevate phenytoin levels by this mechanism (Vincent, 1980). The opposite effect of anticonvulsants on neuroleptic levels has also been reported. Carbamazepine will cause a decrease in plasma haloperidol levels by an average of 60 percent, which may result in a reemergence of psychosis (Arana, Goff, Friedman, et al., 1986). Phenytoin and phenobarbital have also been reported to reduce haloperidol levels by 50 percent or more and to reduce levels of the thioridazine metabolite mesoridazine (Linnoila, Vivkari, Vaisanen, et al., 1980).As discussed in Chapter 4, relatively nonanticholinergic agents, such as fluphenazine and molindone, are preferred for the treatment of epileptic psychosis. Anticonvulsant levels should be rechecked following dosage changes, in view of possibilities of drug–drug interaction.

Clonazepam has been reported to be helpful in the psychotic disorders of epilepsy (Frykholm, 1985). A long-acting benzodiazepine, clonazepam has a wide spectrum of effects, it has been reported to be effective for seizures, myoclonus, mania (Chouinard, 1985; Dreifuss, 1985), chronic pain, and panic (Beaudry, Fontaine, Chouinard, et al., 1986), as well as psychosis. It may act by elevating serotonin levels or by facilitation of GABA transmission (Browne, 1978). Clonazepam has the advantages of once-a-day dosage and meaningful therapeutic blood levels and does not subject the patient to the risk of tardive dyskinesia.

Resection of the epileptic temporal lobe has not uniformly ameliorated an associated psychosis (Falconer, 1973). More recently, the presence of psychosis has excluded patients otherwise considered for temporal lobectomy (Delgado-Escueta & Walsh, 1985), because the long-term functional outcome of lobectomy appears worse in psychotic patients.

Finally, when the epileptic patient presents with psychosis or any other new psychiatric disturbance, the physician should consider alternative diagnoses. Seizure patients are prone to developing brain tumors, often years after the initial presentation of epilepsy (DD Spencer, Spencer, Mattson, et al., 1984). Psychoses have also

been linked to anticonvulsant toxicity, even with "therapeutic" blood levels (Franks & Richter, 1979). *A comprehensive neurologic reevaluation is therefore indicated whenever an epileptic patient presents with a new major psychiatric syndrome.*

Depression

Several studies, reviewed by Robertson and Trimble (1983), indicate that depression is the most common psychiatric disturbance in epilepsy. Although estimates of prevalence vary between approximately 20 percent and 70 percent most investigators agree that depression occurs in epileptics far more commonly than in the general population (Kogeorgos, Fonagy, & Scott, 1982).

Despite this concurrence of investigators, the phenomenology of depression in seizure patients remains poorly defined. Most studies have rated depression with standardized scales such as the Minnesota Multiphasic Personality Inventory (MMPI) or the Beck Depression Inventory (Perini & Mendius, 1984), or by retrospective tally of assigned diagnoses in hospital records (Schiffer & Babigian, 1984). It remains unclear whether the depression of epilepsy is a mood state alone or is usually accompanied by the changes in sleep, appetite, cognition, libido, and other variables that characterize major mood disorders. Himmelhoch (1984) has done some of the clearest and most detailed descriptions of affective changes that may be seen with epilepsy, and reports that "most patients" have enough atypical or organiform symptoms to vitiate a simple diagnosis of major depressive disorder. In a review of 748 patients referred to a mood disorders clinic, 10 percent were found to have epilepsy. Of these patients, 60 percent had been previously diagnosed as bipolar, 30 percent as dysthymic, and 10 percent as unipolar affective disorder. Lability of affect, paradoxical response to antidepressants, confusional states, and other associated symptoms helped to distinguish these patients from nonepileptics.

Mendez, Cummings, and Benson (1986) reported that patients with epilepsy also have a risk of suicide that is five times higher than the general population and that 30 percent of depressed epileptic patients have attempted suicide.

The etiology of the association of mood disorders with seizures is unknown, but several lines of evidence suggest possible links. It is known from analysis of cerebral cortex resected at temporal lobectomy for intractable seizures that there is a reduction of adrenergic receptors not only in epileptogenic neocortex but also in surrounding, otherwise normal brain (Briere, Sherwin, Robitaille, et al., 1986). Such a reduction in adrenoceptors results in a focal diminution of responsiveness of cortical neurons to norepinephrine. Repeated experimental seizures in rats also lead to reduction in adrenoceptors (Bergstrom & Kellar, 1979). It is tempting to speculate that such a focal change is behaviorally manifested as depression.

Depression may exacerbate seizures by disruption of the sleep architecture. Unipolar depression is associated with a decrease in total sleep time and with sleep continuity disturbance, and both unipolar and bipolar depression have changes in the distribution of sleep stages, which resemble those of sleep deprivation, with shortened rapid eye movement (REM) latency and altered REM distribution. Since sleep deprivation and fatigue are well-known precipitants of convulsions in epileptic patients, it is interesting to speculate whether such changes in sleep underlie an increase in seizure frequency that is often observed when epileptics become depressed.

Phenytoin, phenobarbital, and carbamazepine have all been reported to cause depression, as well as difficulties with memory, concentration, and alertness (Committee on Drugs, 1985). Depression is most common with phenobarbital, less common with phenytoin, and infrequent with carbamazepine, which may actually *improve* mood in epileptic patients. As a general rule, the depressed epileptic on phenobarbital should be switched to a less psychotoxic anticonvulsant.

In children and adolescents and in retarded or brain-injured adults, barbiturates may aggravate hyperactivity, impulsiveness, or aggression. When these behaviors are problematic, an alternate anticonvulsant should thus be substituted.

Phenytoin less consistently causes depression, but some individuals may experience rather severe depression or cognitive impairment. In some cases, these symptoms are due to phenytoin-induced folate deficiency. Phenytoin may also interfere with thiamine effects, so supplementation of both B vitamins and folate is rational for patients on phenytoin. Folate levels should be obtained when psychiatric status changes in a patient on phenytoin without vitamin supplementation.

Phenytoin may produce a number of disfiguring changes in patients' physical appearance, including coarseness of facial features, hirsutism, and gingival hyperplasia. These may produce reactive depression, particularly in adolescents. In general, carbamazepine is preferable to phenytoin in children and adolescents for this reason.

Of all the common anticonvulsants, valproic acid (Depakene or Depakote, Abbott) is least likely to cause cognitive and affective symptoms. Unfortunately, valproic acid is usually not effective for CPS, and its use is chiefly for primary generalized epilepsies.

One disconcerting report suggests that the neuropsychiatric side effects of anticonvulsants may not always be reversible. Bourgeois, Prensky, Palkes, et al. (1983) prospectively studied 72 newly diagnosed epileptic children over 4 years with psychologic interviews and neuropsychiatric tests. Eight of these children suffered a decline in intelligence quotient (IQ) of 10 points or more over the time of the study. Intellectual deterioration did not correlate with seizure frequency per se, as confirmed by others (Ellenberg, Hirtz, & Nelson, 1986), but rather loss of IQ correlated with repeated episodes of drug toxicity.

Such reports would indicate that the physician should attempt to use the minimal number and dosage of anticonvulsants required for seizure control. Recent reports have shown that single-drug therapy is often as effective as the use of two or more anticonvulsants and that it is less toxic (Albright & Bruni, 1985). The interested reader is referred to the recent multicenter cooperative study chaired by Mattson for a comprehensive, detailed, and elegant comparative review of anticonvulsant efficacy and toxicity (Mattson, Cramer, Collins, et al., 1985).

The social stigma of epilepsy remains real and injurious. Although the culture has for the most part disregarded the notion that epilepsy is itself a form of demonic possession, associations with insanity, thoughts of hereditary degeneration, and the vague uneasy feeling that epilepsy is a form of pollution can be voiced by patients and families, who wish the diagnosis concealed. Moreover, the invisibility of the illness interictally, coupled with the often terrifying appearance of the ictus, can deprive the patient of those social benefits and comforts usually afforded the ill person.

At a purely psychologic level, epilepsy can also create difficulties. The knowledge that one has an incurable and perhaps only partially treatable illness, requiring daily medication and frequent physician visits, without prospect of an end, can be demoralizing for some patients. The random, episodic occurrence of some seizures can cause some patients to spend their lives "just waiting for the next seizure," as one patient said, afraid to appear in public, thus complicating employment and education,

as well as creating anxiety in friendships and romantic relationships. Families must also adapt to the diagnosis of epilepsy, and although most of the literature on this subject concerns children, many of the same problems, such as infantilization, enmeshment, and denial, occur with adult patients.

Antidepressants, when employed for the treatment of depression in epilepsy, must be chosen with care. As with neuroleptics, anticholinergic antidepressants such as imipramine and amitriptyline tend to lower the seizure threshold and may result in convulsions (Edwards, 1979). Conflicting reports exist about the safety of desipramine. Although in vitro desipramine appears relatively safe, in overdosage desipramine is reported to cause five times more seizures than other tricyclics (Wedin, Oderda, Schwartz, et al., 1986). Maprotiline also appears to be significantly epileptogenic, although the mechanism of action is unclear (Dessain, Schatzberg, Woods, et al., 1986; Hoffman & Wachsmuth, 1982; Trimble, 1980). If tricyclics are to be used, nortriptylene would be an attractive choice, as it is less anticholinergic than the tertiary tricyclics and has meaningful blood levels. The latter is particularly helpful when pharmacokinetic interactions with anticonvulsants are suspected.

The safest antidepressants for epileptics are probably trazodone and the monoamine oxidase inhibitors. Trazodone, which is highly serotonergic, has no incidence of convulsions in overdosage (Wedin et al., 1986). Trazodone appears well tolerated in the neurologically impaired populations (DM Simpson & Foster, 1986), but its efficacy in depressions of epilepsy has not been specifically reported (Mendez et al., 1984). Initial dosages should be small, 50 mg, and dosages should be increased slowly, as epileptic patients on multiple medications can be exquisitely sensitive to sedation. Even with very cautious increments, patients may be unable to tolerate sufficient medication to produce an antidepressant effect, and in such cases the drug must be discontinued. This also can occur with tricyclics. When trazodone is tolerated and effective, however, it may be the preferable medication for depression in epilepsy because of its safety. Some authors, however, debate the antidepressant potency of trazodone (see Chapter 4).

Monoamine oxidase inhibitors are also well tolerated and effective in depressed epileptics. Monoamine oxidase inhibitors are reported to have anticonvulsant properties by some authors (Prockop, 1959), and proconvulsant properties by others (Tagashira, 1982). In clinical experience, some patients with CPS have a short-lived flurry of sensory auras and increased somnolence, which may clear over days and be replaced by an antidepressant effect. In some, exacerbation of epileptic symptoms persists, and the drug must be discontinued. Patients who can tolerate MAOIs often prefer these drugs because of the relative lack of sedation and anticholinergic side effects. Hypothetical concerns of a possible interaction between MAOIs and carbamazepine, based on the latter's chem-

ical similarity to tricyclics, have not been documented.

Electroconvulsive therapy (ECT) has also been used to treat depression in epileptics. Acutely, the induced convulsion of ECT may both suppress further seizures and reverse depression (Sackeim, 1983), perhaps by evoking of brain inhibitory mechanisms to protect against further seizures. In this line, epileptic patients appear to have a particularly high seizure threshold during the administration of ECT when compared with nonepileptic patients. ECT should probably be reserved for severely ill patients who are refractory to medical treatment and who are at imminent risk for suicide, cachexia, or other major problems (Robertson & Trimble, 1985). Concerns have been raised that ECT, like other seizures, may kindle an epileptic focus leading to the development of a new seizure disorder in nonepileptic patients and, by extension, that it may ultimately exacerbate preexisting seizures (Devinsky, 1983). ECT should not be withheld because of these theoretical concerns, however, if it is strongly indicated psychiatrically.

REFERENCES

Abramowitz JN & Kasdon DL (1982). Recurrent central cord injury. *Neurosurgery, 11*, 543–545.

Adams HP, Butler MJ, Biller J, et al. (1986). Nonhemorrhagic cerebral infarction in young adults. *Archives of Neurology, 43*. 793–796.

Albright P & Bruni J (1985). Reduction of polypharmacy in epileptic patients. *Archives of Neurology, 42*, 797–799.

Andersen J, Aabro E, Gulmann N, et al. (1980). Antidepressive treatment of Parkinson's disease. *Acta Neurologica Scandinavia 62*, 210–219.

Arana G, Goff DC, Friedman H, et al. (1986). Does carbamazepine-induced reduction of plasma haloperidol levels worsen psychotic symptoms? *American Journal of Psychiatry, 143*, 650–651.

Arnold ES, Rudd SM, & Kirshner H (1980). Manic psychosis following rapid withdrawal from

baclofen. *American Journal of Psychiatry, 137*, 1466–1467.

Asnis G (1977). Parkinson's disease, depression and ECT: A review and case study. *American Journal of Psychiatry, 134*, 191–195.

Avorn J, Everitt DE, & Weiss S (1986). Increased antidepressant use in patients prescribed beta-blockers. *Journal of the American Medical Association, 255*, 357–360.

Ball MJ (1984). The morphological basis of dementia in Parkinson's Disease. *Canadian Journal of Neurological Science, 11*, 180–184.

Ballard PA, Tetrud JW, & Langston JW (1985). Permanent human Parkinsonism due to 1-methyl-4-phenyl-1,2,3,6-tetrahydropyridine (MPTP): Seven cases. *Neurology, 35*, 949–956.

Barnett HJM (1980). Progress towards stroke prevention: Robert Wartenberg Lecture. *Neurology, 30*, 1212–1225. 1980.

Barrett L, Drayer B, & Shin C (1985). High-resolution computed tomography in multiple sclerosis. *Annals of Neurology*, *17*, 33–38.

Beal MF, Williams RS, Richardson EP, et al. (1981). Cholesterol embolism as a cause of transient ischemic attacks and cerebral infarction. *Neurology*, *31*, 860–865.

Beaudry P, Fontaine R, Chouinard G, et al. (1986). Clonazepam in the treatment of patients with recurrent panic attacks. *Journal of Clinical Psychiatry*, *47*, 83–85.

Benson DF (1973). Psychiatric aspects of aphasia. *British Journal of Psychiatry*, *123*, 555–6.

Bergstrom DA & Kellar KJ (1979). Effect of electroconvulsive shock on monaminergic receptor binding sites in rat brain. *Nature*, *278*, 464–466.

Birkmayer W, Riederer P, Youdim MBH, et al. (1975). Potentiation of the anti-akinetic effects after L-dopa treatment by an inhibitor of MAO-B, deprenyl. *Journal of Neural Transmission*, *36*, 303–326.

Bogousslavsky J, Fox AJ, Carey LS, et al. (1986). Correlates of brain-stem oculomotor disorders in multiple sclerosis. *Archives of Neurology*, *43*, 460–463.

Bogousslavsky J & Regli F (1986). Borderzone infarctions distal to internal carotid artery occlusion: Prognostic implications. *Annals of Neurology*, *20*, 346–350.

Boller F, Mizutani T, Roessmann V, et al. (1980). Parkinson disease, dementia and Alzheimer disease: Clinicopathological correlations. *Annals of Neurology*, *7*, 329–335.

Bourgeois BFD, Prensky AL, Palkes HS, et al. (1983). Intelligence in epilepsy: A prospective study in children. *Annals of Neurology*, *14*, 438–444.

Briere R, Sherwin AL, Robitaille Y, et al. (1986). Alpha-1 adrenoceptors are decreased in human epileptic foci. *Annals of Neurology*, *19*, 26–30.

Britt RH, Connor WS, & Enzmann DR (1981). Occult arteriovenous malformation of the brainstem simulating multiple sclerosis. *Neurology*, *31*, 901–903.

Browne TR (1978). Drug therapy: Clonazepam. *New England Journal of Medicine*, *299*, 812–816.

Busto R, Harik SI, Yoshida S, et al. (1985). Cerebral norepinephrine depletion enhances recovery after brain ischemia. *Annals of Neurology*, *18*, 329–336.

Caplan LR (1980). "Top of the basilar" syndrome. *Neurology*, *30*, 72–79.

Cascino GD & Adams RD (1986). Brainstem auditory hallucinosis. *Neurology*, *36*, 1042–1047.

Cerebral Embolism Task Force (1986). Cardiogenic brain embolism. *Archives of Neurology*, *43*, 71–84.

Chiappa KH (1980). Pattern shift visual, brainstem auditory and short-latency somatosensory evoked potentials in multiple sclerosis. *Neurology*, *30*, 110–123.

Chouinard G (1985). Antimanic effects of clonazepam. *Psychosomatics*, *26*(Suppl), 7–12.

Committee on Drugs (1985). Behavioral and cognitive effects of anticonvulsant therapy. *Pediatrics*, *76*, 644–646.

Chu AB, Sever JL, & Madden DL (1983). Oligoclonal IgG bands in cerebrospinal fluid in various neurological diseases. *Annals of Neurology*, *13*, 434–439.

Chui HC, Mortimer JA, Slager V, et al. (1986). Pathologic correlates of dementia in Parkinson's disease. *Archives of Neurology*, *43*, 991–995.

Cocito L, Favale E, & Reni L (1982). Epileptic seizures in cerebral arterial occlusive disease. *Stroke*, *13*, 189–195.

Cohen SR, Brooks BR, Herndon RM, et al. (1980). A diagnostic index of active demyelination: Myelin basic protein in cerebrospinal fluid. *Annals of Neurology*, *8*, 25–31.

Cosgrove GR, LeBlanc R, Meagher-Villemure K, et al. (1985). Cerebral amyloid angiopathy. *Neurology*, *35*, 625–631.

Cottrell SS & Wilson SAK (1926). The affective symptomatology of disseminated sclerosis. *Journal of Neurology and Psychopathology*, *7*, 1–30.

Cummings JL & Mendez MF (1984). Secondary mania with focal cerebrovascular lesions. *American Journal of Psychiatry*, *141*, 1084–1087.

Dalos NP, Rabins PV, Brooks BR, et al. (1983). Disease activity and emotional state in multiple sclerosis. *Annals of Neurology*, *13*, 573–577.

Delgado-Escueta AV & Walsh GO (1985). Type I complex partial seizures of hippocampal origin: Excellent results of anterior temporal lobectomy. *Neurology*, *35*, 143–154.

DeMuth GW & Ackerman SH (1983). Alphamethyldopa and depression. *American Journal of Psychiatry*, *140*, 534–538.

Dessain EC, Schatzberg AF, Woods BT, et al. (1986). Maprotiline treatment of depression. *Archives of General Psychiatry*, *43*, 86–90.

Devinsky O, Duchowny MS (1983). Seizures after convulsive therapy, a retrospective case survey. *Neurology*, *33*, 921–925.

DeWitt LD, Buonanno FS, Kistler JP, et al. (1984). Nuclear magnetic resonance imaging in evaluation of clinical stroke syndromes. *Annals of Neurology*, *16*, 535–545.

Dorfman LJ, Marshall WH, & Enzmann DR (1979). Cerebral infarction and migraine: Clinical and radiologic correlations. *Neurology*, *29*, 317–322.

Dreifuss FE (1985). Treatment of seizure disorders and myoclonus. *Psychosomatics*, *26*(Suppl), 30–35.

Drury I, Klass DW, Westmoreland BF, et al. (1985). An acute syndrome with psychiatric symptoms and EEG abnormalities. *Neurology, 35,* 911–914.

Duvoisin RC (1986). Etiology of Parkinsons's disease: Current concepts. *Clinical Neuropharmacology, 9*(Suppl 1), S3–S11.

Ebers GC, Vinuela FU, Feasby T, et al. (1984). Multifocal CT enhancement in MS. *Neurology, 34,* 341–346.

Edwards JG (1979). Antidepressants and convulsions. *Lancet, 22,* 1368–1369.

Elkin CM, Leon E, Grenell SL, et al. (1985). Intracranial lesions in the acquired immunodeficiency syndrome. *Journal of the American Medical Association, 253,* 393–396.

Ellenberg JH, Hirtz DG, & Nelson KB (1986). Do seizures in children cause intellectual deterioration? *New England Journal of Medicine, 314,* 1085–1088.

Erman MK & Guggenheim FG (1981). Psychiatric side effects of commonly used drugs. *Drug Therapy,* Nov., pp 55–64.

Falconer MA (1973). Reversibility by temporal-lobe resection of the behavioral abnormalities of temporal lobe epilepsy. *New England Journal of Medicine, 289,* 451–455.

Farrell MA, Kaufmann JCE, Gilbert JJ, et al. (1985). Oligoclonal bands in multiple sclerosis: Clinical-pathological correlation. *Neurology, 35,* 212–218.

Feeney DM, Gonzalez A, & Law WA (1982). Amphetamine, haloperidol and experience interact to affect rate of recovery after motor cortex injury. *Science, 217,* 855–857.

Finklestein S, Benowitz L, Baldessarini RJ, et al. (1982). Mood, vegetative disturbance, and dexamethasone suppression test after stroke. *Annals of Neurology, 12,* 463–468.

Fisher CM (1982). Lacunar strokes and infarcts: A review. *Neurology, 32,* 871–876.

Flor-Henry P (1969a). Psychosis and temporal lobe epilepsy. *Epilepsia, 10,* 363–395.

Flor-Henry P (1969b). Schizophrenic-like reactions and affective psychoses associated with temporal lobe epilepsy: Etiological factors. *American Journal of Psychiatry, 126,* 148–152.

Flor-Henry P (1983). Determinants of psychosis in epilepsy: Laterality and forced normalization. *Biological Psychiatry, 18,* 1045–1057.

Folstein MF, Maiberger R, & McHugh PR (1977). Mood disorder as a specific complication of stroke. *Journal of Neurology, Neurosurgery and Psychiatry, 40,* 1018–1020.

Franks RD & Richter AJ (1979). Schizophrenia-like psychosis associated with anticonvulsant toxicity. *American Journal of Psychiatry, 136,* 973–974.

Frykholm B (1985). Clonazepam-antipsychotic effect in a case of schizophrenia-like psychosis with epilepsy and in three cases of atypical psychosis. *Acta Psychiatrica Scandinavica, 71,* 539–542.

Gebarski SS, Gabrielsen TO, Gilman S, et al. (1985). The initial diagnosis of multiple sclerosis: Clinical impact of magnetic resonance imaging. *Annals of Neurology, 17,* 469–474.

Geschwind N (1971). Aphasia. *New England Journal of Medicine, 284,* 654–656.

Gilbert JJ & Sadler M (1983). Unsuspected multiple sclerosis. *Archives of Neurology, 40,* 533–536.

Glaser GH (1953). Psychotic reactions induced by corticotropin (ACTH) and cortisone. *Psychosomatic Medicine, 15,* 280–291.

Glaser GH (1964). The problem of psychosis in psychomotor temporal lobe epileptics. *Epilepsia, 5,* 271–278.

Glaus A (1931). Uber Kombinationen von Schizophrenie und Epilepsie. *Z Ges Neurol Psychiatr, 135,* 450–500.

Gloor P, Olivier A, Quesney LF, et al. (1982). The role of the limbic system in experiential phenomena of temporal lobe epilepsy. *Annals of Neurology 12,* 129–144.

Goodwin FK (1971). Psychiatric side effects of levodopa in man. *Journal of the American Medical Association, 218,* 1915–1919.

Grimaldi LME, Roos RP, Nalefski EA, et al. (1985). Oligoclonal IgA bands in multiple sclerosis and subacute sclerosing panencephalitis. *Neurology, 35,* 813–817.

Guberman A & Stuss D (1983). The syndrome of bilateral paramedian thalamic infarction. *Neurology, 33,* 540–546.

Hakim AM & Mathieson G (1979). Dementia in Parkinson disease: A neuropathologic study. *Neurology, 29,* 1209–1214.

Harvey NS (1986). Psychiatric disorders in parkinsonism: 1. Functional illnesses and personality. *Psychosomatics, 27,* 91–103.

Hauser SL, Dawson DM, & Lehrich JR (1983). Intensive immunosuppression in progressive multiple sclerosis. *New England Journal of Medicine, 308,* 173–180.

Heyman A, Wilkinson WE, Hurwitz BJ, et al. (1984). Risk of ischemic heart disease in patients with TIA. *Neurology, 34,* 626–630.

Hier DB, Mondlock J, & Caplan LR (1983). Behavioral abnormalities after right hemisphere stroke. *Neurology, 33,* 337–344.

Hillbom M & Kaste M (1981). Ethanol intoxication: a risk factor for ischemic brain infarction in adolescents and young adults. *Stroke, 12*(4), 422–425.

Himmelhoch JM (1984). Major mood disorders related to epileptic changes. In D Blumer (Ed.): Psychiatric Aspects of Epilepsy. Washington, DC: American Psychiatric Press, pp 271–294.

Hoffman BF & Wachsmuth R (1982). Maprotiline and

seizures. *Journal of Clinical Psychiatry*, *43*, 117–118.

Hornykiewicz O & Kish S (1984). Neurochemical basis of dementia in Parkinson's disease. *Canadian Journal of Neurological Science*, *11*, 185–190.

Huber SJ, Shuttleworth E, & Paulson GW (1986). Dementia in Parkinson's disease. *Archives of Neurology*, *43*, 987–990.

In pursuit of quarry, MS researchers draw on immunology, virology advances (1986). *Journal of the American Medical Association*, *256*, 809–815.

Ishii N, Nishihara Y, & Imamuia T (1986). Why do frontal lobe symptoms predominate in vascular dementia with lacunes? *Neurology*, *36*, 340–345.

Jackson AC, Boughner DR, & Barnett HJM (1984). Mitral valve prolapse and cerebral ischemic events in young patients. *Neurology*, *34*, 784–787.

Jackson JA, Jankovic J, & Ford J (1983). Progressive supranuclear palsy: Clinical features and response to treatment in 16 patients. *Annals of Neurology*, *13*, 273–278.

Jacque C, DeLassalle A, Rancurel G, et al. (1982). Myelin basic protein in CSF and blood. *Archives of Neurology*, *39*, 557–560.

Jambor KL (1969). Cognitive functioning in multiple sclerosis. *British Journal of Psychiatry*, *115*, 765–775.

Jampala VC & Abrams R (1983). Mania secondary to left and right hemisphere damage. *American Journal of Psychiatry*, *140*, 1197–1199.

Javoy-Agid F & Agid Y (1980). Is the mesocortical dopaminergic system involved in Parkinson disease? *Neurology*, *30*, 1326–1330.

Junck L & Marshall WH (1983). Neurotoxicity in radiological contrast agents. *Annals of Neurology*, *13*, 469–484.

Kahana E, Leibowitz V, & Alter M (1971). Cerebral multiple sclerosis. *Neurology*, *21*, 1179–1185.

Karoum F, Chuang LW, Eisler T, et al. (1982). Metabolism of (−) deprenyl to amphetamine and methamphetamine may be responsible for deprenyl's therapeutic benefit: A biochemical assessment. *Neurology*, *32*, 503–509.

Kinkel WR, Jacobs L, Polachini I, et al. (1985). Subcortical arteriosclerotic encephalopathy (Binswanger's disease). *Archives of Neurology*, *42*, 951–959.

Kirshner HS, Tsai SI, Runge VM, et al. (1985). Magnetic resonance imaging and other techniques in the diagnosis of multiple sclerosis. *Archives of Neurology*, *42*, 859–863.

Kirubakaran V, Mayfield D, & Rengachary S (1984). Dyskinesia and psychosis in a patient following baclofen withdrawal. *American Journal of Psychiatry*, *141*, 692–693.

Klawans HL, Stein RW, Tanner C, et al. (1982). A pure parkinsonian syndrome following acute carbon monoxide intoxication. *Archives of Neurology*, *39*, 302–304.

Kogeorgos J, Fonagy P, & Scott DF (1982). Psychiatric symptom patterns of chronic epileptics attending a neurological clinic: A controlled investigation. *British Journal of Psychiatry*, *140*, 236–243.

Komrad MS, Coffey CE, Coffey KS, et al. (1984). Myocardial infarction and stroke. *Neurology*, *34*, 1403–1409.

Kopin IJ (1979). CNS actions of antihypertensive drugs. *Drug Therapy*, Dec, pp 30–40.

Krauthammer C & Klerman GL (1978). Secondary mania. *Archives of General Psychiatry*, *35*, 1333–1339.

Kristensen O & Sindrup EH (1978). Psychomotor epilepsy and psychosis. I. Physical aspects. *Acta Neurologica Scandinavica*, *57*, 361–369.

Kurtzke JF & Hyllested K (1986). Multiple sclerosis in the Faroe islands. *Neurology*, *36*, 307–328.

Kvale JN (1982). Amitriptyline in management of progressive supranuclear palsy. *Archives of Neurology*, *39*, 387–388.

Laitinen L (1969). Desipramine in treatment of Parkinson's disease. *Acta Neurologica Scandinavia*, *45*, 109–113.

Laitinen L & Toivakka E (1980). Slowing of scalp EEG after electrical stimulation of amygdala in man. *Acta Neurochirurgica* (Suppl 30), *80*, 177–181.

Langston JW, Ballard P, Tetrud JW, et al. (1983). Chronic parkinsonism in humans due to a product of meperidine-analog synthesis. *Science*, *25*, 979–980.

Lebensohn Z & Jenkins RB (1975). Improvement of Parkinsonism in depressed patients treated with ECT. *American Journal of Psychiatry*, *132*, 283–285.

Lee SI (1985). Non convulsive status epilepticus. Ictal confusion in later life. *Archives of Neurology*, *42*, 778–781.

Leenders KL, Findley LJ, & Cleeves L (1986). PET before and after surgery for tumor-induced parkinsonism. *Neurology*, *36*, 1074–1078.

Levine DN & Finklestein S (1982). Delayed psychosis after right temporoparietal stroke or trauma: Relation to epilepsy. *Neurology*, *32*, 267–273.

Levine DN & Grek A (1984). The anatomic basis of delusions after right cerebral infarction. *Neurology*, *34*, 577–582.

Link H & Laurenzi MA (1979). Immunoglobin class and light chain type of oligoclonal bands in CSF in multiple sclerosis determined by agarose gel electrophoresis and immuno fixation. *Annals of Neurology*, *6*, 107–110.

Linnoila M, Vivkari M, Vaisanen K, et al. (1980). Effect of anticonvulsants on plasma haloperidol and thioridazine levels. *American Journal of Psychiatry, 137*, 819–821.

Lipsey JR & Robinson RG (1986). Sex dependent behavioral response to frontal cortical suction lesions in the rat. *Life Sciences, 38*, 2185–2192.

Lipsey JR, Robinson RG, Pearlson GD, et al. (1984). Nortriptyline treatment of post-stroke depression: A double blind study. *Lancet, 1*, 297–300.

Lipsey JR, Spencer WC, Rabins PV, et al. (1986). Phenomenological comparison of poststroke depression and functional depression. *American Journal of Psychiatry, 143*, 527–529.

Lishman WA (1978). Organic psychiatry, First Edition. *Blackwell Scientific Publications*, pp 176–187.

Mann D & Yates PO (1983). Pathological basis for neurotransmitter changes in Parkinson's disease. *Neuropathology and Applied Neurobiology, 9*, 3–19.

Mattson RH, Cramer JA, Collins JF, et al. (1985). Comparison of carbamazepine, phenobarbital, phenytoin and primidone in partial and secondarily generalized tonic-clonic seizures. *New England Journal of Medicine, 313*, 145–151.

Mayeux R, Alexander MP, Benson DF, et al. (1979). Poromania. *Neurology, 29*, 1616–1619.

Mayeux R, Stern Y, Cote L, et al. (1984). Altered serotonin metabolism in depressed patients with Parkinson's disease. *Neurology, 34*, 642–646.

Mayeux R, Stern Y, Rosen J, et al. (1981). Depression, intellectual impairment and Parkinson disease. *Neurology, 31*, 645–650.

Mayeux R, Stern Y, Sano M, et al. (1986). The relationship of serotonin to depression in Parkinson's disease. *Annals of Neurology, 20*, 149.

Mayeux R, Stern Y, Williams JB, et al. (1986). Clinical and biochemical features of depression in Parkinson's disease. *American Journal of Psychiatry, 143*, 758–759.

McKenna PJ, Kane JM, & Parrish K (1985). Psychotic syndromes in epilepsy. *American Journal of Psychiatry, 142*, 895–904.

Mendez MF, Cummings JL, & Benson DF (1984). Epilepsy: Psychiatric aspects and use of psychotropics. *Psychosomatics, 25*, 883–894.

Mendez MF, Cummings JL, & Benson DF (1986). Depression in epilepsy, significance and phenomenology. *Archives of Neurology, 43*, 766–770.

Mesulam MM (1985). Principles of behavioral neurology. FA Davis Co, p 291.

Miller BL, Benson DF, Cummings JL, et al. (1986). Late-life paraphrenia: an organic delusional syndrome. *Journal of Clinical Psychiatry, 47*, 204–207.

Miller JR, Burke AM, & Bever CT (1983). Occurrence of oligoclonal bands in multiple sclerosis and other CNS diseases. *Annals of Neurology, 13*, 53–58.

Moore PM & Cupps TR (1983). Neurological complications of vasculitis. *Annals of Neurology, 14*, 155–167.

Mortimer JA, Pirozzolo FJ, Hansch E, et al. (1982). Relationship of motor symptoms to intellectual deficits in Parkinson disease. *Neurology, 32*, 133–137.

Murray GB, Shea V, & Conn DK (1986). Electroconvulsive therapy for poststroke depression. *Journal of Clinical Psychiatry, 47*, 258–260.

Nakano I & Hirona A (1984). Parkinson's disease: Neuron loss in the nucleus basalis without concomitant Alzheimer's disease. *Annals of Neurology, 15*, 415–418.

Noseworthy J, Paty D, Wonnacott T, et al. (1983). Multiple sclerosis after age 50. *Neurology, 33*, 1537–1544.

Ounsted C, Glaser GH, Lindsay J, et al. (1985). Focal epilepsy with mesial temporal sclerosis after acute meningitis. *Archives of Neurology, 42*, 1058–1060.

Papez JW (1937). A proposed mechanism of emotion. *Archives of Neurology and Psychiatry, 38*, 725–743.

Parkinson J (1817). An essay on the shaking palsy. Sherwood, London.

Patel BR, Seth KD, & Meador KJ (1986). Metoclopramide-induced parkinsonism. *Neurology, 36*(Suppl 1), 75.

Perini G & Mendius R (1984). Depression and anxiety in complex partial seizures. *Journal of Nervous and Mental Disorders, 172*, 287–290.

Perry RH, Tomlinson BE, Candy JM, et al. (1983). Cortical cholinergic deficit in mentally impaired parkinsonism patients. *Lancet, 2*, 789–790.

Pond DA (1957). Psychiatric aspects of epilepsy. *Journal of Indian Medical Profession, 3*, 1441.

Poser CM (1985). The course of multiple sclerosis [Letter]. *Archives of Neurology, 42*, 1035.

Prockop DJ, Shore DA, & Brodie BB (1959). Anticonvulsant properties of monoamine oxidase inhibitors. *Annals of the New York Academy of Science, 80*, 643–651.

Pryse-Phillips WEM (1986). The incidence and prevalence of multiple sclerosis in Newfoundland and Labrador, 1960–1984. *Annals of Neurology, 20*, 323–328.

Pullicino P, Nelson RF, Kendall BE, et al. (1980). Small deep infarcts diagnosed on computed tomography. *Neurology, 30*, 1090–1096.

Rafal RD & Grimm RJ (1981). Progressive supranuclear palsy: Functional analysis of the response to methysergide and antiparkinsonian agents. *Neurology, 31*, 1507–1518.

Raichle ME (1983). The pathophysiology of brain ischemia. *Annals of Neurology, 13*, 2–10.

Raisman R, Cash R, & Agid Y (1986). Parkinson's disease, decreased density of 3H-imipramine and 3H-paroxetine binding sites in putamen. *Neurology*, *36*, 556–560.

Rajput AH (1984). Epidemiology of Parkinson's disease. *Canadian Journal of Neurological Science*, *11*, 156–159.

Raymond CA (1986). Diverse approaches to new therapies may hold promise in multiple sclerosis. *Journal of the American Medical Association*, *256*, 685–687.

Reding M, Orto L, Willensky P, et al. (1985). The dexamethasone suppression test, an indicator of depression in stroke but not a predictor of rehabilitation outcome. *Archives of Neurology*, *42*, 209–212.

Reding MJ, Orto LA, Winter SW, et al. (1986). Antidepressant therapy after stroke. *Archives of Neurology*, *43*, 763–765.

Reik L, Smith L, Khan A, et al. (1985). Demyelinating encephalopathy in Lyme disease. *Neurology*, *35*, 267–269.

Remick RA & Fine SH (1979). Antipsychotic drugs and seizures. *Journal of Clinical Psychiatry*, *40*, 78–80.

Riederer P, Birkmayer W, Seemann D, et al. (1977). Brain noradrenaline and 3-methoxy-hydrophenylglycol in Parkinson's syndrome. *Journal of Neural Transmission*, *41*, 241–251.

Riesenberg D (1986). Radiolabeled ligands expand PET exploration of numerous normal, abnormal brain functions. *Journal of the American Medical Association*, *256*, 969–970.

Robertson MM & Trimble MR (1983). Depressive illness in patients with epilepsy: A review. *Epilepsia*, *24*(Suppl), S109–S116.

Robins AH (1976). Depression in patients with parkinsonism. *British Journal of Psychiatry*, *128*, 141–145.

Robinson RG (1979). Differential behavioral and biochemical effects of right and left hemispheric cerebral infarction in the rat. *Science*, *205*, 707–710.

Robinson RG & Bloom FE (1977). Pharmacological treatment following experimental cerebral infarction. *Biological Psychiatry*, *12*, 669–680.

Robinson RG, Kubos KL, Starr LB, et al. (1984). Mood disorders in stroke patients: Importance of location of lesion. *Brain*, *107*, 81–93.

Robinson RG, Lipsey JR, & Price TR (1985). Diagnosis and clinical management of post-stroke depression. *Psychosomatics*, *26*(10), 769–778.

Robinson RG, Lipsey JR, Rao K, et al. (1986). A two-year longitudinal study of post-stroke mood disorders: comparison of acute onset with delayed onset depression. *American Journal of Psychiatry*, *143*, 1238–1244.

Robinson RG & Price TR (1982). Post-stroke depressive disorders: A follow-up study of 103 patients. *Stroke*, *13*(5), 635–641.

Robinson RG, Star LB, Kubos KL, et al. (1983). A two-year longitudinal study of post-stroke mood disorders findings during the initial evaluation. *Stroke*, *14*, 736–741.

Robinson RG, Starr LB, & Price TR (1984). A two-year longitudinal study of mood disorders following stroke, prevalence and duration at six month follow-up. *British Journal of Psychiatry*, *144*, 256–262.

Rodgers J & Stoudemire A (in press). Neuroleptic malignant syndrome and multiple sclerosis. *Psychosomatics*.

Rokey R, Rolak LA, Harati Y, et al. (1984). Coronary artery disease in patients with cerebrovascular disease: a prospective study. *Annals of Neurology*, *16*, 50–53.

Ropper AH & Shafran B (1984). Brain edema after stroke. *Archives of Neurology*, *41*, 26–29.

Rose AS, Ellison GW, Myers LW, et al. (1976). Criteria for the clinical diagnosis of multiple sclerosis. *Neurology*, *2*, 20–22.

Ross ED (1981). The aprosodias. *Archives of Neurology*, *38*, 561–569.

Ross ED & Rush JA (1981). Diagnosis and neuroanatomical correlates of depression in brain-damaged patients. *Archives of General Psychiatry*, *38*, 1344–1354.

Rubin AJ, Kurlan R, Schiffer R, et al. (1986). Atypical depression and Parkinson's disease. Abstract No. P106. *Annals of Neurology*, *20*, 150.

Rundell JR & Wise MG (1985). Neurosyphilis, a psychiatric perspective. *Psychosomatics*, *26*, 287–295.

Sackeim HA, Decina P, Prohovnik I, et al. (1983). Anticonvulsant and antidepressant properties of electroconvulsive therapy: A proposed mechanism of action. *Biological Psychiatry*, *18*, 1301–1310.

Sacks O (1973). *Awakenings* (p. 250). New York: EP Dutton.

Santamaria J, Tolosa E, & Valles A (1986). Parkinson's disease with depression, a possible subgroup of idiopathic parkinsonism. *Neurology*, *36*, 1130–1133.

Schaut J & Schnoll S (1983). Four cases of clonidine abuse. *American Journal of Psychiatry*, *140*, 1625–1627.

Schiffer RB & Babigian HM (1984). Behavioral disorders in multiple sclerosis, temporal lobe epilepsy and amyotrophic lateral sclerosis: An epidemiologic study. *Archives of Neurology*, *41*, 1067–1069.

Schiffer RB, Caine ED, Bamford KA, et al. (1983). Depressive episodes in patients with multiple sclerosis. *American Journal of Psychiatry, 140*, 1498–1500.

Schiffer RB, Hernedon RM, & Rudick RA (1985). Treatment of pathologic laughing and weeping with amitriptyline. *New England Journal of Medicine, 312*, 1480–1482.

Schiffer RB, Wineman M, & Weitkamp LR (1986). Association between bipolar affectve disorder and multiple sclerosis. *American Journal of Psychiatry, 143*, 94–95.

Schoenberg BS, Whisnant JD, Taylor WF, et al. (1970). Strokes in women of childbearing age. *Neurology, 20*, 181–189.

Sears ES, McCammon A, Bigelow R et al. (1982). Maximizing the harvest of contrast enhancing lesions in multiple sclerosis. *Neurology, 32*, 815–820.

Senn HJ, Jung WF, Kinz H, et al. (1977). Clozapine and agranulocytosis. *Lancet, 1*, 547.

Sherwin I, Magnan PP, & Bancaud J (1982). Prevalence of psychosis in epilepsy as a function of the laterality of the epileptogenic lesion. *Archives of Neurology, 39*, 621–625.

Simpson DM & Foster D (1986). Improvement in organically disturbed behavior with trazodone treatment. *Journal of Clinical Psychiatry, 47*, 191–193.

Simpson GM & Yadalam K (1985). Blood levels of neuroleptics: State of the art. *Journal of Clinical Psychiatry, 46*(5, Sec 2), 22–28.

Slater E, Beard AW, & Glitheroe E (1963). The schizophrenia-like psychoses of epilepsy. *British Journal of Psychiatry, 109*, 95–150.

Snider WD, Simpson DM, Nielsen S, et al. (1983). Neurological complications of acquired immune deficiency syndrome: Analysis of 50 patients. *Annals of Neurology, 14*, 403–418.

Snyder AM, Stricker EM, & Zigmond MJ (1985). Stress-induced neurological impairments in an animal model of parkinsonism. *Annals of Neurology, 18*, 544–551.

Snyder SH & D'Amato RJ (1986). MPTP, a neurotoxin relevant to the pathophysiology of Parkinson's disease. *Neurology, 36*, 250–258.

Snyder SH & Reynolds IJ (1985). Calcium antagonist drugs. *New England Journal of Medicine, 313*, 995–1002.

Spencer DD, Spencer SS, Mattson RH, et al. (1984). Intracerebral masses in patients with intractable partial epilepsy. *Neurology, 34*, 432–436.

Spencer SS, Spencer DD, Glaser GH, et al. (1984). More intense focal seizure type after callosal section: The role of inhibition. *Annals of Neurology, 16*, 686–693.

Spencer SS, Williamson PD, & Bridgers SL (1985). Reliability and accuracy of localization by scalp ictal EEG. *Neurology, 35*, 1567–1575.

Stevens J (1973). The anatomy of schizophrenia. *Archives of General Psychiatry, 29*, 177–189.

Stevens JR (1983). Psychosis and epilepsy. *Annals of Neurology, 14*, 347–348.

Stevens JR (1966). Psychiatric implications of psychomotor epilepsy. *Archives of General Psychiatry, 14*, 461–471.

Stevens JR, Mark VH, Erwin F, et al. (1969). Deep temporal stimulation in man. *Archives of Neurology, 21*, 157–169.

Stoudemire A, Nelson A, & Houpt JL (1983). Interictal schizophrenia-like psychoses in temporal lobe epilepsy. *Psychosomatics, 24*, 331–339.

Strang RR (1965). Imipramine in treatment of Parkinsonism: A double-blind placebo study. *British Medical Journal 2*, 33–34.

Surridge D (1969). An investigation into some psychiatric aspects of multiple sclerosis. *British Journal of Psychiatry, 115*, 749–764.

Sweet RD, McDowell FH, Feigenson JS, et al. (1976). Mental symptoms in Parkinson's disease during chronic treatment with levodopa. *Neurology, 26*, 305–310.

Tagashira E, Hiramori T, Urano T, et al. (1982). Specific action of tranylcypromine to precipitate barbital withdrawal convulsions. *Psychopharmacology* (Berlin) *77*, 101–104.

Tolosa ES & Santa-Maria J (1984). Parkinsonism and basal ganglia infarcts. *Neurology, 34*, 1516–1518.

Toone BK, Garralda ME, & Ron MA (1982). The psychoses of epilepsy and the functional psychoses: A clinical and phenomenological comparison. *British Journal of Psychiatry, 141*, 256–261.

Trimble MR (1980). New antidepressant drugs and the seizure threshold. *Neuropharmacology, 19*, 1227–1228.

Trimble MR (1983). Personality disturbances in epilepsy. *Neurology, 33*, 1332–1334.

Van Rossum J, Ockhuysen AA, & Arts RJ (1985). Psychomotor status. *Archives of Neurology, 42*, 989–993.

Vincent FM (1980). Phenothiazine-induced phenytoin intoxication. *Annals of Internal Medicine, 93*, 56–57.

Vincent FM (1985). Tocainide encephalopathy. *Neurology, 35*, 1804–1805.

Walton J (1985). *Brain's Diseases of the nervous system* (pp 307–319). Oxford: Oxford University Press.

Wedin GP, Oderda GM, Schwartz WK, et al. (1986). Relative toxicity of cyclic antidepressants. *Annals of Emergency Medicine, 15*, 797–804.

Weiner WJ, Koller WC, Perlik S, et al. (1980). Drug holiday and management of Parkinson's disease. *Neurology, 30*, 1257–1261.

Weiser HG (1983). Depth recorded limbic seizures and

psychopathology. *Neuroscience and Biobehavioral Review*, *7*, 427–440.

Whitehouse PJ, Hedreen JC, White CL, et al. (1983). Basal forebrain neurons in the dementia of Parkinson disease. *Annals of Neurology*, *13*, 243–248.

Whitlock FA & Siskind MM (1980). Depression as a major symptom of multiple sclerosis. *Journal of Neurology, Neurosurgery and Psychiatry*, *43*, 861–865.

Wood AJ & Feely J (1983). Pharmacokinetic drug interaction with propranolol. *Clinical Pharmacokinetics*, *8*, 253–262.

Young AC, Saunders J, & Ponsford JR (1976). Mental change as an early feature of multiple sclerosis. *Journal of Neurology, Neurosurgery and Psychiatry*, *39*, 1008–1013.

Zubenko GS & Nixon RA (1984). Mood-elevating effect of captopril in depressed patients. *American Journal of Psychiatry*, *141*, 110–111.

Wendy L. Thompson
Troy L. Thompson II

25
Pulmonary Disease

Difficulty breathing has many psychiatric implications. Patients react emotionally to the discomfort of dyspnea, the loss of functional capacity, and the threat of death, while hypoxia, hypercarbia, hyperventilation, respiratory failure, and medications all have direct effects on the brain. Depression is frequently associated with pulmonary disease (Klerman, 1981; Lindegard, 1982). The depression can range from a major depressive episode to a mild dysthymic disorder or an adjustment disorder with depressed mood (WL Thompson & Thompson, 1984). Another psychiatric symptom that frequently accompanies pulmonary disease is anxiety. Most patients with respiratory disease have episodes accompanied by anxiety, when they feel unable to breath adequately. If severe, dyspnea is felt as a sensation of suffocating, strangling, or drowning, and is overwhelmingly frightening, often leading to panic reactions (WL Thompson & Thompson, 1985a). Another frequently associated problem in those with respiratory disease is sexual dysfunction, including inhibited sexual excitement or orgasm, or premature ejaculation. Organic mental disorders often accompany respiratory disease, especially in debilitated patients or geriatric patients who also have many other physical problems.

PSYCHOLOGIC ASPECTS OF PULMONARY DISEASE

The psychologic ramifications of pulmonary disease depend on the specific disease, the age of onset, the etiology of the illness, and the severity of the illness. The psychiatrist must do a thorough assessment of both the individual and the family to determine whether there are specific psychodynamic conflicts, behavioral triggers, or environmental issues that contribute to exacerbations of the respiratory illness or its symptoms (Stoudemire, 1985). It is important to be aware of common familial conflicts or characterologic pathology that may play a role in preventing optimal medical management of the patient (WL Thompson and Thompson, 1985a).

Some pulmonary disease, such as reversible obstructive airways disease (ROAD, or asthma), may have a significant psychosomatic component (Alexander, French, & Pollock, 1968). Early studies in this area hypothesized one specific conflict central to later development of asthma

(French & Alexander, 1939–1941). This conflict was thought to be strong, unconscious dependency wishes toward the mother, coupled with a fear of separation. Although this "specificity hypothesis," associated with asthma and other illnesses with psychosomatic components, is generally considered to be obsolete, the psychodynamic issues set forth by French and Alexander (1939–1941) may still be relevant to some individual patients. For example, a 36-year-old woman was admitted to the hospital for an exacerbation of childhood-onset asthma. She was currently living in another state with her mother, with whom she had a strong symbiotic relationship. It became clear that the wish for and fear of separation from the mother were playing a crucial role in her smoking and taking her medications improperly, "forcing" her to remain at home and not make decisions about emancipating herself. With individual psychotherapy and temporary substitution of the hospital as a transitional object in place of the mother, her asthma became better controlled.

Another important consideration in psychiatric assessment of patients with pulmonary disease is the developmental or life stage during which the patient develops asthma. For example, an infant or child with severe respiratory disease, whether asthma or cystic fibrosis, is likely to be perceived and treated differently by family, friends, and relatives. This may lead to significant impairments in the relationship between the mother and the child and adversely affect advancement through the early stages of development, leading to later susceptibility to the trauma of separation or other psychologic impairment. The patient previously mentioned illustrates this point. It was clear from exploring her childhood history that her severe asthma had fostered the symbiotic relationship and hampered her ability to establish peer relationships, setting the stage for later fears of separation.

Research is currently being done to

assess exactly how these psychodynamic factors could possibly contribute to both the onset and later exacerbations of asthma. The asthmatic reaction is thought to result from a complex interplay between the autonomic nervous system and such substances as epinephrine, norepinephrine, histamine, and prostaglandins (Knapp, 1985; Stein, 1982). The central nervous system is directly involved in stimulating production or regulating metabolism of these substances. Brain stimulation, particularly in the limbic system formation, affects the balance of neurotransmitters, in turn influencing the autonomic nervous system (Martin, Reichlin, & Brown, 1977). This may be the pathway whereby conflicts and emotions affect the development and course of the asthma. Emotional states may be associated with hypothalamic or limbic system alterations that subsequently alter neurotransmitter balance, causing changes in prostaglandin and histamine production and thereby affecting immunologic reactivity.

The experience or fear of suffering respiratory distress with a concomitant sensation of strangling or drowning, along with frequent urgent trips to the emergency room and multiple hospitalizations, understandably can lead to pervasive anxiety in the child and the child's parents. The sedating side effects of some medications, as well as sleep disturbances due to respiratory distress, can impair learning, even when a child is able to attend school. The asthmatic child is often prone to becoming a scapegoat, either among his friends, because of restrictions on activities at school, or at home. Problems may also arise within the family because of the alterations in life-style required by family members dealing with the asthmatic child (Fritz, 1983). For this reason, the family of an asthmatic child deserves a formal psychiatric assessment. Respiratory symptoms in a child may relate to the child's conflicts or fantasies (perhaps around the death of an earlier child by sudden infant death syndrome) or may reflect parental conflicts as well as inherent biologic susceptibility (Wilson, 1981).

Recently, a syndrome of vocal cord dysfunction has been reported, which has usually been misdiagnosed over a period of many years as intractable asthma. Psychiatric disorders are present in most of the patients, and the patients tend to respond best to psychotherapy and to speech therapy (Appelblatt & Baker, 1981; Christopher, Wood, Eckert, et al., 1983).

Most psychologic explanations and analyses of behavioral styles in pulmonary patients have tended to focus on asthmatic patients. Little has been done to explore psychodynamic contributions to chronic obstructive pulmonary disease (COPD) or other chronic pulmonary illnesses. With COPD, instead of directly linking emotions to the disease process, explanations tend to focus on psychologic traits that would lead individuals to engage in behaviors or lifestyles predisposing them to the particular illness. No one has demonstrated, however, unique personality profiles for smokers or coal miners.

Personality traits *have* been found to influence the perception by patients of added resistive loads in breathing. Those who are more dependent and anxious, whether or not they have asthma, tend to have greater thresholds both for inspiration and for expiration than do those who have more adaptive personality styles, or who are rigidly independent (Hudgel, Cooperson, & Kinsman, 1982). These results are not always consistent over time and do not always distinguish between those who have asthma and those who do not. Nonetheless, personality traits can influence effort on pulmonary function tests, which produce less valid results if a full effort is not made.

Regardless of the physiologic severity of the disease, there tends to be a correlation between the *patient's* rating of the severity of the illness and the degree of emotional disturbance found (Plutchik, Williams, Jerrett, et al., 1978). In addition

to this, there appears to be an increasing incidence and severity of neurotic and psychosomatic symptoms associated with an increased amount of asthma medication required to control the disease (Teiramaa, 1978). This finding makes one wonder whether the psychiatric symptoms cause the severity of the asthma to increase and, therefore, increase the amount of medication required, whether the psychiatric symptoms interfere with medical evaluation and patient compliance, or whether the asthma medication is aggravating the psychiatric symptoms. The psychiatric assessment must address these issues. Some of these questions relate to the panic–fear studies of Kinsman and associates (Dirks, Jones, & Kinsman, 1977; Kinsman, Dirks, Dahlem, et al., 1980; Kinsman, Luparello, O'Banion, et al., 1973). These studies have divided panic–fear symptomatology into that which is characterologic and that which is specifically illness-related. Characterologic panic and fear appear to be associated with a basic lack of ego resources and with dependency conflicts, emotional lability, and a tendency toward pervasive anxiety. Patients with characterologic panic relate to a variety of situations in their lives with anxiety, panic, and a sense of helplessness or dependency. By contrast, illness-specific anxiety seems to function as "signal anxiety" and is specific to the situation of breathing difficulties.

Those patients who have both high illness-specific anxiety and high characterologic anxiety tend to have more hospitalizations and lengthier hospital stays and to take higher doses of medications, regardless of the severity of their illness; these factors may lead to increased morbidity and mortality. In contrast, those patients with excessively low panic–fear symptomatology tend to ignore their symptoms and not respond appropriately, or at an appropriate time, to the warning symptoms of their illness. They have a tendency, therefore, to underuse medications, not only those prescribed as needed, but also those prescribed on a regular schedule. They have a tendency to get discharged from hospitals prematurely but also to have a higher rate of rehospitalization; this also leads to higher rates of morbidity and mortality. The patients with the best medical outcome tend to be those with high illness-specific panic–fear, but average levels of characterologic panic–fear. Such patients are able to attend to their respiratory symptoms in a timely and appropriate fashion and to elicit appropriate responses from their medical caregivers as well. Physicians usually do not assess the patient's panic–fear level in determining when to alter medications. Often, when there is an exacerbation, the patient will speak to the physician over the telephone to adjust medications. If the psychiatrist has evaluated the degree of panic–fear present, the psychiatrist can greatly enhance the physician's management of the patient. For example, for high-panic–fear patients, use of a mini-peak flow meter may help establish an objective measure of dyspnea. For the low-panic–fear patient, assistance of a family member may be enlisted. With the high-panic–fear patient, anxiolytics or relaxation techniques may be employed along with psychotherapy to reduce the anxiety. In low-panic–fear patients, therapy around their need for denial and their counterdependent style may be helpful. Primary care by the psychiatrist, with ongoing pulmonary consultation, may be a viable alternative for moderately severe asthmatics with serious characterologic impediments to treatment.

Although these symptoms are described specifically in relation to asthmatic patients, they also seem important in the response of patients to other chronic illnesses, since COPD patients who are coping poorly seem to have a number of factors in common with asthmatic patients. Among these factors are a tendency toward chronic anxiety, which may be related to high panic–fear as well. Such patients seem, in particular, to have a failure to accept their illness and mourn what they have lost, manifested by an inability to shift their expectations and goals. This leads to difficulty in accepting their illness, with related feelings of loss, chronic anxiety, and externalization of responsibility for feelings and behavior; all of which may lead to poor compliance with the medical regimen (Post & Collins, 1981–1982).

Clearly, such variables as psychiatric disturbance, personality structure, reactions to medical caregivers, and expectations about treatment have some prognostic significance for medical outcome (Rutter, 1979), and timely psychiatric intervention can have an important impact. In some COPD patients, anxiety and a fear of shortness of breath (often associated with a fear of death) may result in avoidance of even minimal physical activity. When a patient becomes so fearful about being short of breath, this in and of itself can interfere with the ability to breathe, either by leading to hyperventilation or by increasing the sensation of shortness of breath and decreasing the patient's efficiency in breathing. Any anxiety resulting from the shortness of breath makes the perception of the dyspnea even more acute. Any activity that produces even minimal shortness of breath is therefore avoided as a signal of imminent death (Agle & Baum, 1977).

Reactions to Illness

It has been hypothesized that asthma may be a reaction to some loss or disappointment in the patient's life, and although these observations are a matter of conjecture, many patients with asthma seem to have suffered from some kind of loss or disappointment prior to the onset of their asthma. Disappointments in a close personal relationship have been found to be associated with acute onset of asthma, whereas arrival of a new family member or duration of up to 3 years in marriage has been associated with a more insidious onset of asthma (Teiramaa, 1981). These factors should be considered in the psychiatric evaluation.

The onset of respiratory illness may cause many profound alterations in patients' life-styles and perceptions of themselves and in the reactions of family and friends. As with the amount of panic–fear present, these alterations may also have a significant impact on patients' reactions to their illness, ability or inability to adjust to the illness, and compliance with medical caregivers' recommendations. The type of adaptation patients must make in order to successfully cope with their illness depends on the nature of the illness.

Asthma can be an episodic illness, in which between episodes the patient appears to be a relatively normal individual, and yet the patient must continue to make concessions to his illness in terms of ongoing treatment. COPD and cystic fibrosis, on the other hand, are chronic and often eventually terminal illnesses, wherein the patient can expect little improvement in baseline functioning, but may experience periodic exacerbations. Other chronic respiratory diseases, such as tuberculosis (TB), atypical TB, or other infectious diseases, require coping with a subacute or relatively longstanding illness, but one in which there is both the promise of recovery, with the possibility of return to full function, and the possibility of ongoing impaired function for the rest of the individual's life.

Anxiety

Common to almost all patients with respiratory illness is anxiety related to the sensation of dyspnea, fear of being placed on a respirator, and ultimately a fear of death. One of the most frequent reactions that accompanies onset or recurrence of respiratory illness therefore is anxiety. As mentioned previously, the anxiety may either cause hyperventilation or heighten the individual's perception of dyspnea, which may lead to a vicious cycle. Anxiety can have an impact in a number of ways on the patient's life. Patients may severely restrict their activities, at times becoming agoraphobic. Anxiety may cause an overreporting of symptoms to the physician, leading to increased and often unnecessary use of medications, with their attendant side effects (WL Thompson & Thompson, 1985a). Many COPD patients demonstrate symptoms of anxiety sufficient to interfere with their daily lives (Agle & Baum, 1977). This can have a significant impact on their relations with family members and their ability to continue to work. Anxiety associated with dyspnea may extend to sexual situations as well, making many patients fearful about sexual activities or performance.

Anxiety is not the only cause of sexual dysfunction in patients with chronic respiratory disease. Some COPD patients experiencing sexual inadequacy would have had the same problem regardless of their pulmonary status (Kass, Updegraff, & Muffly, 1972). For other patients, a decrease in pulmonary function is reflected in worsening of sexual function in the absence of identifiable psychiatric factors (Fletcher & Martin, 1982). This phenomenon may be specific to particular patient populations, as it has not been observed in other studies (Agle & Baum, 1977). COPD affects as many as 15 percent of older men, and many of these older patients have other illnesses, such as diabetes, which may affect their sexual performance as well as interfere with the medical management of their respiratory disease. Older patients also tend to take more types of medication than younger patients and thus have an increased risk of side effects and drug interactions, as well as of drug-induced sexual dysfunction (Fritz, 1983).

Other problems with sexual functioning may reflect overall concerns of the patient regarding self-image and self-esteem. As with any chronic illness, there may be a dramatic disruption of the established family roles and interactions, and patients with COPD often feel that their lives are out of their control (Dudley, Sitzman, & Rugg, 1985). In being forced to relinquish many of their usual responsibilities and roles in the family, patients may suffer debilitating loss of self-esteem. Loss of employment may be particularly significant to a head of household, a single parent, or anyone whose sense of self-worth and financial well-being is dependent to a large extent on a job. Some patients may resent being treated as an invalid by family members, and family members as well may have difficulty in adapting to the patient's changed physical status.

An individual who is already anxious about self-esteem may be fearful about initiating sexual contact for fear of withdrawal or rejection by the spouse. Patients may question their sexual prowess and attractiveness to their partners, and many times this may be a justified concern (WL Thompson, 1986). Some patients may respond to their illness by becoming overly dependent on their families and caregivers; this is especially true for those who may have been counterdependent or very dependent in the past. They may also use their illness as an excuse to give up former activities that provoke anxiety or a sense of inadequacy. Those who did not enjoy sexual activity prior to their illness may consciously or unconsciously utilize their sick role as a reason for giving up sex and other unpleasant activities.

Depression

In addition to difficulty with self-esteem, some respiratory patients may also experience significant depression. This may range from an adjustment disorder with depressed mood to a severe and disabling major depression (WL Thompson & Thompson, 1984). Although depression may significantly impair sexual functioning, some depressed individuals may actually desire more close physical contact and feel an increased need to be held and caressed (Hollender & Mercer, 1976). Depression may also predate the illness itself and may thereby complicate the medical management of the illness.

Mood instability is a frequent side effect of many medications that are commonly used to treat chronic respiratory disease, especially corticosteroids. Corticosteroids may decrease the patient's immune response, including the immune response to upper respiratory tract infections, and most patients with chronic respiratory disease will have an exacerbation of their underlying illness whenever they have a superimposed upper respiratory infection. In both monkeys (Reite, Harbeck, & Hoffman, 1981) and humans (Kiecolt-Glaser & Glaser, 1986), depression has also been found to suppress immune response, and thus it may cause more frequent upper respiratory infections (Reite et al., 1981), which will then produce further exacerbation of underlying illness.

The depression of pulmonary patients may be manifested in a variety of ways (Covino, Dirks, Kinsman, et al., 1982), and many physicians have a tendency to view a depression that is related to receiving an emotionally traumatic new diagnosis as understandable and, thus, not to treat it appropriately or vigorously. The symptoms of depression, however—namely, the hopelessness, helplessness, low energy level, guilt, and psychomotor retardation—may interfere with appropriate medical management, regardless of whether the depression is "warranted" or not (See Chapter 2 by Cohen-Cole & Harpe). A chart review study of asthmatic patients found that many had at least fleeting suicidal ideation and that there was a significantly higher incidence of suicide and suicide attempts than in a group of hypertensive patients (Levitan, 1983); this study probably underestimated the actual figures. Suicidal ideation may not be expressed directly, but may be expressed in a more passive fashion by poor adherence to medical treatment.

The diagnosis of major depression may be difficult in patients with symptoms of chronic respiratory disease, since many depressive and pulmonary symptoms overlap, including fatigue, lassitude, weight loss, anorexia, and loss of interest in usual activities. Sleep disturbance may be caused by episodes of sleep apnea or nocturnal coughing, as well as by nocturnal asthma attacks. The depression may be closely associated with the multiple significant losses sustained by an individual with chronic respiratory disease. As mentioned previously, these may include loss of occupation and earning capacity as well as loss of physical strength and changes in physical appearance. Some of these losses are due to the physical wasting caused by chronic illness or to impairment of pulmonary function, and others are attributable to the side effects of medications, especially corticosteroids, taken to treat chronic respiratory disease. The development of moon face, hirsutism, and acne due to steroids may be particularly devastating to some individuals.

Chronic respiratory disease per se does not seem to cause psychotic episodes, although the stress of impending hospitalization, and the resultant breakdown of normal psychologic defenses, may make patients more prone to an episode of mania, depression, or schizophrenia if they are susceptible to these disorders. Again, these psychiatric symptoms may significantly impair medical management. At least one study (Agle & Baum, 1977) found paranoid thinking and paranoid psychoses to be prominent in a sample of patients with COPD. The reason is unknown; perhaps the combination of dyspnea, organic factors, and functional impairment exacerbates paranoid responses.

Alcoholism is also a fairly common problem in patients with COPD. It is difficult to ascertain how much of this is cause and how much of this is effect. Some patients claim that their drinking problem was a response to developing chronic respiratory disease. Chronic alcoholics are susceptible to aspiration pneumonia, which may lead to a chronic respiratory disease, such as bronchiectasis. Most alcoholics are also smokers.

Reactions of Caregivers and Families

In addition to patients' reactions to their illness and the psychiatric disorders that may ensue, the reactions of caretakers or significant others may also have a major impact on the patients. A spouse, like the mother of an asthmatic child (Sperling, 1963), may foster noncompliance because of an inability to accept the patient except when the patient is functioning in a sick role. Family members who have difficulty tolerating the alteration in roles required in the family may become psychiatrically symptomatic themselves or threaten, either consciously or unconsciously, to leave the patient, and this may activate fears of loss and separation. Many adolescent patients with cystic fibrosis appear to have little or no psychiatric symptomatology; however, their mothers tend to be somewhat more depressed than controls (Bywater, 1981).

If the family has a stake in making the patient a scapegoat because of illness or has used the illness to mask other problems in the family, any attempt to make the patient better may be resisted or undermined by the family. In many counterdependent or very dependent patients, the illness may be a means of having dependency needs fulfilled in an acceptable way (WL Thompson & Thompson, 1985a); this may mean dependence both on family and on medical caregivers, which may provoke a countertransference reaction in the medical caregivers. Often, with severely ill asthmatics or patients with terminal COPD, the medical caregiver responds with a sense of hopelessness or even anger at the frequent calls and hospitalizations required by these patients. Anxious patients often provoke the same response, whereas depressed patients may provoke a feeling of depression and hopelessness in the caregiver. This may have serious consequences; for example, it may lead to a "no-code status" for some patients for whom this is inappropriate.

Patients and their families may also have a significant reaction to a need for artificial ventilation. Respirator anxiety is a common problem that can be treated with support, relaxation techniques, or psychotherapy and may require the use of medications. In general, antianxiety drugs or related sedatives are the best initial choice. Neuroleptics are generally reserved for agitated or psychotic patients. Both the patient and the family may respond to an initial episode of respiratory arrest and placement on a respirator with anxiety, but also with the expectation that the patient will improve and will no longer need the respirator (Gale & O'Shanick, 1985). A patient with chronic COPD, however, who has been on a respirator many times, may be more familiar with the treatment but less hopeful about the ultimate outcome. Problems in weaning the patient from a respirator have been found to be associated with interpersonal conflicts as well as depression associated with the illness, fear of death, or anger at having to give up dependence on the respirator (Mendel & Khan, 1980). In addition to these factors, fear of being discharged to a difficult marital or home situation seems to contribute to problems with weaning (Desai, Seriff, Khan, et al., 1976). The technique of weaning is described in Chapter 18, by Goldstein.

BIOLOGIC ASPECTS OF RESPIRATORY DISEASE THAT MAY AFFECT PHYSICAL OR MENTAL FUNCTIONING

Normal alterations in breathing in individuals without respiratory disease do not produce any corresponding subjective sensation of mental change, except during hyperventilation, when an individual may experience dizziness or dissociative feelings. Table 25-1 indicates the psychiatric symptoms associated with various levels of hypoxia and hypercapnia (Gale & O'Shanick, 1985). Many patients with chronic respiratory disease, however, may have had multiple episodes of respiratory arrest or severe hypoxia, which are not manifested by their present arterial blood gas values. These patients frequently present with some cognitive impairment, particularly memory loss and a tendency to "sundown," (getting worse in the evening or at night), especially when hospitalized in an unfamiliar environment. One study (Grant, Heaton, McSweeny, et al., 1982) of patients with hypoxemic COPD found that all of those studied performed significantly worse than controls on virtually all neuropsychologic tests. The higher cognitive functions of abstracting ability and complex perceptual motor integration were most severely affected, and this was found to be correlated with low Pao_2; therefore, it seems that development of organic symptoms is most closely related to hypoxemia.

Patients with chronic respiratory disease and dementia are particularly susceptible to cerebral derangement caused by other superimposed problems. This is especially true of elderly patients, who, as mentioned earlier, tend to have more additional medical problems and to take a larger number of medications than younger patients (TL Thompson, Moran, & Nies, 1983). In addition to the disease itself, the medications usually used to treat the respiratory illness can affect both cognitive and affective functioning. At times it may be difficult to distinguish, however, between a drug effect and the effect of the respiratory illness itself. Sleep apnea with nocturnal oxygen desaturation may cause cognitive impairment whose cause will not be reflected by daytime blood gas values. Sleep apnea should be suspected in a pulmonary patient

Table 25-1
Psychiatric Symptoms Associated with Hypoxia and Hypercapnia

Partial Pressure of O_2	Mental Symptomatology
Hypoxia	
90% of sea level	Altered visual dark adaptation
85% of sea level	Loss of judgment, inappropriate behavior
75% of sea level	Decreased ability to carry out complex tasks
65% of sea level	Impaired short-term memory
50% of sea level	Severe loss of judgment
30–40% of sea level	Unconsciousness

Partial Pressure of Co_2	Mental Symptomatology
Hypercapnia	
Normal	No change
Moderately elevated	Headache, drowsiness, indifference or inattention, Perceptual changes, forgetfulness
Severely elevated	Stupor or coma

Source: Reprinted with permission from Gale J & O'Shanick GJ (1985). Psychiatric aspects of respirator treatment and pulmonary intensive care. *Advances in Psychosomatic Medicine, 14,* 93–108.

with sleep disturbance, a history of snoring and sudden awakening, nocturnal asthma attacks, or worsened pulmonary function tests in the morning. Such patients should be referred for a sleep study in which respiratory movements and oxygen saturation can be continuously monitored. For a more complete discussion of sleep disorders, see Chapter 12, by Regestein.

In the elderly, tuberculosis may present with vegetative signs suggestive of depression. The initial symptoms are often weight loss, lethargy, lack of interest in usual activities, and, at times, confusion. Many of these patients complain of sleep disturbance, which may be a manifestation of night sweats and low grade fever. In elderly patients with systemic symptoms and possible past exposure to TB, a chest X ray is essential, along with sputum cultures for both *Mycobacterium tuberculosis* and atypical forms of tuberculosis, such as *M. avium* and *M. kansasii*. Factors that favor reactivation of dormant disease include immunosuppressive therapy, silicosis, diabetes mellitus, leukemia, lymphomas, gastric

resection, poor nutritional status, severe alcoholism, emotional stress, and acquired immune deficiency syndrome (AIDS) (Moran, 1985).

DIAGNOSTIC AND MANAGEMENT CONSIDERATIONS

Since respiratory dysfunction may significantly affect oxygen saturation, blood pH, and acid–base balance, as well as the oxygen–carbon dioxide ratio, it is imperative to consider an organic etiology for central nervous system (CNS) dysfunction in the face of any psychiatric symptomatology in a respiratory patient. This is especially true if the symptomatology is of recent onset. Especially in older patients, but in most younger patients as well, evaluation should include a thorough screening for other common causes of organic mental disorders, including determination of electrolytes, routine blood chemistries, serum B_{12} and folate, liver and renal function tests, thyroid function tests, venereal disease serology, complete blood count (CBC), urinalysis, and erythrocyte sedimentation rate (ESR) (TL Thompson & Thompson, 1986). The patient should have arterial blood gas determinations done early in the course of an evaluation, along with pulmonary function testing. A detailed medication history must be taken, to completely evaluate drug interactions and the effects that drugs or additives to the drugs may have on respiratory and mental function. It is important to remember that the symptoms associated with chronic respiratory disease, such as fatigue, lethargy, and loss of interest in usual activities, are also frequently signs or symptoms of depression, and that sleep apnea or nocturnal asthma episodes may mimic a sleep disorder due to depression, or vice versa. A history of steroid use and a history of reactions either to high-dose steroids or to steroid withdrawal are also important information to obtain in evaluating chronic respiratory disease patients.

Specific issues to examine during psychatric evaluation of the pulmonary patient include the following:

1. Early family history, including illness in any family member and how the illness affected the family. If the patient was ill, how did this affect family relationships and the patient's role in the family? How did the patient and the family deal with emancipation and separation issues?
2. Current family functioning, including how roles and relationships have shifted since the illness. Direct evaluation of the family provides the best information in this area.
3. Interaction with medical caregivers, including doctor shopping, overdependence, and treatment adherence.
4. Defensive style and object relations, as well as historical evidence for personality disorder.
5. Symptoms of axis I problems, such as

major depression, panic disorder, psychosis, dementia, or delirium.
6. Medications currently in use.
7. Sexual history.

As mentioned earlier, sexual dysfunction frequently accompanies chronic respiratory disease but is not a necessary concomitant of the illness. Especially in asthmatics, some of the sexual dysfunction may be caused by exercise-induced bronchospasm. Prophylactic beta-adrenergic agents can often prevent this bronchospasm.

It is also important to consider the possibility of vocal cord dysfunction, which should be suspected in patients who complain that their throat closes and who on auscultation have upper airway wheezing, which is secondarily reflected to the lungs. They often have a history of asthma refractory to usual medical management. This syndrome is diagnosed through direct visualization of the vocal cords during inspiration and expiration, which shows inappropriate opposition of the cords during breathing. This can have important implications for both psychiatric and medical management of the patient.

During the history taking, the patient's panic–fear level should also be assessed. This may be ascertained by discussing the individual's reactions to asthma attacks and by assessing the patient's overall personality style. At times, however, it may be helpful to give the patient the Asthma Symptom Checklist (Kinsman, et al., 1973) to more fully evaluate the patient's reaction to an asthma attack. The Asthma Symptom Checklist can sometimes help clarify whether or not a patient reacts to an asthma attack with withdrawal and anger, thereby distancing those who may attempt to aid him. This is most useful as an adjunct to the clinical interview.

In general, the dexamethasone suppression test (DST) is not particularly useful in patients with chronic respiratory disease. In those with severe illness whose symptoms most closely mimic those of depression, the patient is generally either on corticosteroids or severely cachectic, and both conditions tend to invalidate DST results. Urinary MHPG levels also have not been standardized for diagnostic purposes and are not routinely recommended (WL Thompson & Thompson, 1985a).

Special Considerations in Psychotherapeutic and Psychopharmacologic Treatment

Often, patients with severe COPD have a very narrow range within which they can maintain their optimal pulmonary status, and they may have difficulty tolerating the emotional stress caused by psychotherapy (Dudley et al., 1985). The chronic respiratory disease patient's fear that a dyspneic episode may be precipitated by stress may interfere with the ability and willingness to participate in psychotherapy; these concerns may become an important focus of the therapy itself if the patient can be engaged. In treating such patients psychotherapeutically, it is important to attempt to disengage the dyspnea–anxiety cycle and to encourage optimal self-care and avoidance of pessimism (Agle & Baum, 1977). It is important to have the patient understand that dyspnea does not necessarily mean imminent danger or death, but can be merely a signal to slow down and pace activities. Physical therapy may need to be combined with psychotherapy in order for this message to reach the patient, and may function as a form of systematic desensitization. Many COPD patients avoid interpersonal contact in order to decrease the amount of stress they experience and, as a result, may become very socially isolated. They may be perceived by others as rude or socially inappropriate, which may elicit negative or frankly hostile responses, further reinforcing the patient's withdrawal. De-

sensitization to social experiences may be useful in treating some patients.

It has been found in asthmatics that the leading factors in precipitating attacks are infection (40 percent), allergy (30 percent), and emotion (30 percent) (Weiner, 1977), so there is clearly a role for psychotherapy in many patients with chonic respiratory disease, to address the emotional component. In general, psychotherapy of these patients may follow the regular patterns and styles of individual, group, family, or behavioral therapy, with a few exceptions.

In COPD patients, the goals of psychotherapy may be somewhat different than in patients with other medical disorders. For patients who associate expressions of affect with dyspnea, an important goal of treatment is for the patient to learn that expressing emotions does not necessarily cause shortness of breath (Dudley et al., 1985). Those who have become more socially isolated may benefit from group therapy, in which they learn that they are not the only persons with their disorder and that others have developed effective means of coping with situations that stress them. Some recommend group or family therapy as the treatment of choice for the COPD patient population (Post & Collins, 1981–1982). Group therapy is most helpful in those who feel most isolated, have little or no social support structure, and cannot tolerate the intensity of individual psychotherapy. Family therapy is recommended when dysfunctional family relationships interfere with medical management or exacerbate the patient's psychopathology.

Oftentimes, an educational approach is very important and useful in helping respiratory patients regain a sense of control over their lives and in lessening the sense of anxiety or panic. Breathing retraining can be helpful in improving ventilation and in combating fears of dyspnea. Education about the proper use of medications, the breathing apparatus, and basic pulmonary physiology requires multiple sessions rather than a one-time intervention. Education and an emphasis on self-care have been demonstrated to result in a decrease in the number of emergency room visits and hospital admissions (Agle, Baum, Chester, et al., 1973).

In asthmatic patients, anxiety caused by dealing with conflicts in psychotherapy may sometimes lead to hyperventilation and may even provoke an asthma attack. This is not a contraindication to psychotherapy, but the patient should come to a psychotherapy session prepared for this eventuality and should bring as-needed (PRN) medications, such as bronchodilator inhalers, to abort an episode. At times, the therapist may have to be more cautious and go more slowly in uncovering significant conflicts to avoid precipitating an attack. Often with these patients, who are very sensitive to emotional stimuli, it is imperative to take a much more active approach than might occur with more standard psychoanalytically oriented psychotherapy.

Though psychoanalysis has been used successfully with some patients with asthma, psychotherapy of all kinds is more effective when combined with pharmacologic therapy and other approaches. In asthmatics, individual psychotherapy is recommended when psychodynamic conflicts play a significant role in preventing the patient from coping most appropriately with the illness. Family therapy may be essential in some cases, especially in children (Liebman, Minuchin, & Baker, 1974) or when a pathologically enmeshed family is involved.

With the advent of the panic–fear studies, it would seem that behavioral therapy might be very helpful in many patients. Even something as seemingly simple as anxiety reduction via relaxation training may be potentially dangerous, however, because decreasing signal anxiety around the illness, thereby decreasing vigilance toward early symptoms, may actually make the patient experience more and worse episodes (Kinsman, Dirks, Jones, et al., 1980).

The choice of therapy is illustrated by the following examples: A patient who is suffering from depression with lowered self-esteem due to an inability to work, who uses a significant amount of denial and a counterdependent stance and who tends to underutilize medication would probably be an appropriate candidate for individual psychotherapy and possibly pharmacotherapy. Chronically anxious patients with little or no insight into the origins of their anxiety would probably do best with behavioral techniques (or antianxiety medication) as an adjunct to supportive group or individual therapy. Efficacy is measured in terms of improvement in medical status, fewer hospitalizations or emergency room visits, improved relationship with the primary physician, satisfaction of the patient and the family, and decrease in psychiatric symptomatology.

In some chronic respiratory disease patients, treatment to aid smoking cessation may be particularly important. No particular treatment method has been proved to be consistently more effective than others. Any form of smoking cessation treatment, however, is usually more effective than no treatment at all (Raw, 1978), and most successful smoking cessation programs have several principles in common. These include an opportunity at the beginning of treatment for the smokers to examine their motives for smoking and for stopping, an explanation of the plan and expectations of the patient, and a brief period of preparation for the day of stopping smoking. Nicotine-containing gum has been used successfully as an adjunct to group and individual approaches, as have hypnosis and behavioral techniques for some patients (Levine & Johnson, 1985). Smoking cessation is discussed in detail in Chapter 15, on habit modification, by Abrams, Raciti, Ruggiero, et al.

Psychiatric Side Effects of Pulmonary Medications

Psychiatric side effects caused by respiratory drugs may range from minimal to severe and incapacitating. Generally, the psychiatric symptoms tend to stop within a few days after the drug is stopped or the dosage is adjusted. The drugs that most frequently produce psychiatric side effects are the corticosteroids. Steroids are used to treat many pulmonary illnesses, ranging from asthma to idiopathic pulmonary fibrosis or sarcoidosis. In patients receiving 40 mg or less of prednisone a day, the incidence of psychosis has been found to be less than 1 percent. The incidence rises steadily, however, to about 18 percent in patients receiving 80 mg or more of prednisone daily (Boston Collaborative Drug Surveillance Program, 1972). The incidence of psychosis may be less if an alternate-day regimen is used. The type of psychiatric symptoms presented by the patient taking steroids tend to be quite varied and may vary within the same patient at different times.

More recent work tends to disagree somewhat with the classic study by Rome and Braceland (1952), which defined four discrete grades of steroid response. Recent research confirms the clinical impression that there are not discrete grades or stages of steroid psychosis. The symptoms of anxiety, agitation, emotional lability, auditory and visual hallucinations, delusions, hypomania, apathy, memory loss, and depression and suicidal ideation tend to fluctuate widely over relatively short periods of time. The onset of steroid psychosis tends to be approximately 5.9 days after the institution of steroid therapy, with twice as many cases occurring in 5 days or less as in 6 days or more (Hall, Popkin, Stickney, et al., 1979). These steroid psychoses can generally be treated with small doses of neuroleptics. Cyclic antidepressants may

worsen the symptoms. The psychiatric symptoms tend to remit rapidly when the steroids are stopped, and such a toxic reaction is not predictive of any future psychiatric disorder.

Steroid psychosis can also occur with withdrawal or reduction of steroids, and patients with such reactions may also exhibit a wide variety of mental symptoms (Sharfstein, Sack, & Fauci, 1982). Steroid withdrawal symptoms can be treated either by increasing the steroids or by reducing the rate of dosage reduction, using psychotropic drugs in small doses if necessary to alleviate psychiatric symptoms.

Theophylline preparations and sympathomimetic bronchodilators may cause jitteriness and a sensation of anxiety, restlessness, and irritability and may interfere with sleep. It is important to distinguish drug-induced "anxiety" from somatic anxiety. Drug-induced symptoms tend to be dose related and temporally related to taking medication. In general, most individuals can tolerate the jitteriness and tremor associated with theophylline and inhaled bronchodilators, especially if the side effects are explained to them. Management consists of lowering the dosage to the minimum required to manage the respiratory illness and, if necessary, altering dosage timing. The specific type of theophylline preparation given may also make a difference, and some patients feel less jittery with one inhaled bronchodilator than another.

Theophylline toxicity, which generally occurs with blood levels greater than 20 μg/ml, is characterized by increased anxiety and severe nausea. It is managed by stopping theophylline until the symptoms abate and the blood level returns to the therapeutic range. A number of other pulmonary drugs may cause psychiatric symptoms, which are listed in Table 25-2 (WL Thompson & Thompson, 1985b).

Some patients who became exceedingly tremulous on theophylline prepara-

Table 25-2
Some Psychiatric Symptoms Casued by Selected Pulmonary Drugs

Drug	Symptoms
Albuterol	Paranoia, hallucinations
Antihistamines	Anxiety, hallucinations, delirium
Atropine	Confusion, memory loss, delirium, tactile, visual and auditory hallucinations, paranoia
Beta$_2$ agonists	Anxiety, insomnia
Cephalosporins	Paranoia, confusion, disorientation
Chloramphenicol	Memory impairment, confusion, depersonalization, hallucinations
Corticosteroids	Depression, mania, emotional lability, hallucinations, paranoia, catatonia
Cycloserine	Depression, anxiety, confusion, hallucinations, paranoia, agoraphobia
Ephedrine	Hallucinations, paranoia
Ethionamide	Depression, psychosis
Gentamicin	Confusion, hallucinations
Isoniazid	Depression, anxiety, paranoia, hallucinations, confusion
Penicillin G procaine	Hallucinations, disorientation, agitation, confusion, bizarre behavior
Phenylephrine	Depression, hallucinations, paranoia
Pseudoephedrine	Hallucinations, paranoia (more in children)
Theophylline	Anxiety, withdrawal, hyperactivity

Source: Reprinted with permission from Thompson WL & Thompson TL, II (1985). Use of medications in patients with chronic pulmonary disease. *Advances in Psychosomatic Medicine, 14*, 136–148.

tions have essential tremor, which is aggravated by theophylline. Benzodiazepine or barbiturate treatment of the tremor may improve the patient's tolerance of theophylline. Beta blockers, the other major treatment for essential tremor, are of course contraindicated in this population.

Adverse Drug Interactions

A number of adverse drug interactions may occur between psychotropic drugs and drugs prescribed for chronic respiratory disease. The most frequent agents involved in these adverse interactions are the monoamine oxidase inhibitors (MAOIs). In patients taking an MAOI, the pressor effects of indirectly acting sympathomimetic amines, such as tyramine, are well known. What is less clear is whether MAOIs enhance the action of epinephrine, since epinephrine is metabolized by both catechol-O-methyltransferase (COMT) as well as monoamine oxidase (MAO) (Baldessarini, 1985). Some of the active metabolites of epinephrine are destroyed by MAO, however, so MAOIs may prolong the action of these active metabolites (Sharman, 1973). MAOIs can also intensify and prolong the central effects of antihistamines and anticholinergic agents (Baldessarini, 1985).

Tricyclic antidepressants can potentiate the anticholinergic effects of atropine (Baldessarini, 1985), which is often used as an inhaled bronchodilator. Tricyclics may also potentiate the pressor effects of epinephrine to a slight degree (Boakes, Laurence, Teoh, et al., 1973). Although epinephrine is no longer the drug of first choice in treating an acute asthmatic exacerbation, care should still be exercised if a tricyclic antidepressant is given to a patient with severe cardiac disease who is receiving concomitant epinephrine injections (Rossing, Fanta, & Goldstein, 1980). Progestational agents are sometimes given to patients with sleep apnea, and may potentiate the action of tricyclic antidepressants by interfering with tricyclics' metabolism by the liver (Baldessarini, 1985). It is safe to use antidepressants, particularly tricyclics, with more selective beta-2 agonists (e.g., terbutaline, metaproterenol, albuterol, and isoetharine).

MAOIs should be avoided if possible when sympathomimetic preparations, such as phenylephedrine, pseudoephedrine, or ephedrine, are used, and should be utilized cautiously with metaproterenol. Neuroleptic drugs (especially those with more pronounced anticholinergic effects, such as thioridazine and chlorpromazine) can have additive anticholinergic effects with atropine or other anticholinergic compounds and may also potentiate the effects of antihistamines (WL Thompson & Thompson, 1985b). Also, although not documented in the literature, there have been several cases in which therapy for atypical tuberculosis, utilizing a six-drug regimen, caused the blood level of imipramine to increase to a toxic level, possibly because of inhibition of the microsomal enzyme system of the liver. Psychotropic drug treatment is discussed extensively in Chapter 4, by Stoudemire and Fogel.

Effects of Psychotropic Drugs on Chronic Pulmonary Disease

Most of the neuroleptics in common usage can be employed with a few cautionary notes in patients with chronic respiratory disease. The use of anxiolytics is quite common in respiratory patients, but it is difficult to assess in advance whether anxiolytic drugs, which have a tendency to depress respiration, will be beneficial or harmful to the patient. There have been variable results reported with the use of anxiolytic drugs in these patients. Promethazine may reduce breathlessness and improve exercise tolerance without altering lung function in certain patients with nonreversible airways obstruction, whereas diazepam may have no effect on breathlessness and may reduce exercise tolerance (Woodcock, Gross, & Geddes, 1981).

The anxiety associated with pulmonary disease must be carefully evaluated in order to try to distinguish psychologically based anxiety from biomedically based anxiety symptoms caused by such factors as hypoxia or medications (Greenblatt, Shader, & Abernethy, 1983). Anxiety may not always be detrimental to the management of chronic respiratory disease; however, in patients who are on a respirator and in many patients with COPD, judicious use of small amounts of benzodiazepines may greatly increase their comfort and decrease their sensation of dyspnea. Many of these patients are elderly or severely debilitated and therefore may require lower than usual doses of benzodiazepines, since sensitivity to benzodiazepine effects increases with aging.

In general, in respiratory patients it is better to use a benzodiazepine with a shorter half-life, such as oxazepam, lorazepam, temazepam, or alprazolam. Respiratory depression may be less likely to result with these agents, and if it does, the adverse effects can be reversed in a shorter interval. Propranolol should be avoided in patients with ROAD, as it causes bronchoconstriction. The use of the new nonsedating, nonaddictive antianxiety agent buspirone should be considered as well as a first line drug, but there is no documented experience with this drug in medically compromised pulmonary patients. Buspirone should not be used with MAO inhibitors.

Antidepressants are also frequently used to treat patients with chronic respiratory disease. The particular antidepressant to be used should be chosen on the basis of its side-effect profile. Patients with compromised pulmonary status, especially COPD or sleep apnea, should generally receive the less sedating drugs. Close attention should be paid in such patients to possible synergistic effects with other sedating drugs, such as antianxiety medications or sedative-hypnotics, which may interact to reduce the respiratory drive. Most antidepressants, however, have little or no effect on respiratory status, and some, such as doxepin, may act as mild bronchodilators. Protriptyline, a tricyclic antidepressant, is often used in patients with sleep-related breathing disorders (WL Thompson & Thompson, 1984, 1985b). However, there are no double-blind, controlled studies demonstrating that protriptyline is superior to any other tricyclic for sleep apnea. Also, since inhaled atropine has been shown to be a potent bronchodilator, either in combination with beta-adrenergic agents or by itself, there is some theoretical benefit in the use of a potent anticholinergic antidepressant in some patients with a degree of reversibility to their symptoms, especially in patients who have nocturnal symptoms. As with the benzodiazepines, the dose of an antidepressant may need to be smaller than in the medically healthy individual. Blood levels should be monitored if severe side effects persist at a relatively low dosage, if there is no response to a supposedly therapeutic dosage, if an increase to a dosage above recommended usual dosage levels is contemplated, or if the patient is on TB medications. (See also Chapter 4 by Stoudemire and Fogel.)

The main concern with neuroleptic use is the provocation of tardive dyskinesia. Antipsychotic medications can cause a tardive dyskinesia that affects the respiratory musculature (Jann & Bitar, 1982). Although this is rare and generally occurs with long-term neuroleptic use, it can be devastating in the patient with reduced respiratory capacity. Also, some of the high-potency neuroleptics, such as haloperidol, may cause bronchoconstriction (Steen, 1976), but otherwise do not tend to have any significant respiratory depressive effect.

Laryngeal dystonia is an extremely rare form of acute dystonic reaction that presents as acute dyspnea. It generally occurs, like other dystonic reactions, within 24–48 hours after therapy is initiated or, in a smaller number of cases, when dosage is increased. High doses are more likely to produce such effects. This can be a life-threatening situation, but the condition responds dramatically to intramuscular injection of antihistaminic or anti-Parkinson agents.

Tartrazine

Tartrazine (FD & C Yellow #5) is a dye used to color many foods, beverages, and drugs, including many psychotropic drugs. In individuals with susceptible airways, tartrazine can provoke severe bronchospasm for up to several hours after it is ingested. While it is not possible to know in advance which individuals will be susceptible to tartrazine, a history of sensitivity to aspirin and of bronchospasm following ingestion of foods that are colored yellow or orange, such as soft drinks, colored candy, or desserts, is suggestive of tartrazine sensitivity (Settipane, 1983). Doses as low as 0.1–0.15 mg of tartrazine have been reported to cause reactions in sensitive individuals. This amount of tartrazine is contained in the usual daily dose of many psychotropic medications (Bedford & Wade-West, 1983). In general, it is best to avoid tartrazine-containing medications in patients with asthma or COPD, unless tartrazine sensitivity has been specifically excluded. Most drugs are available from some pharmaceutical company in a tartrazine-free formulation. Many pharmaceutical companies are in the process of removing tartrazine from all of their formulations. At the present time, drugs are required to be labeled as containing tartrazine; however, if there is doubt, this information can be obtained from the pharmacist or directly from the pharmaceutical company. See Chapter 4, by Stoudemire and Fogel, for a list of antidepressants currently containing tartrazine.

REFERENCES

Agle DP & Baum GL (1977). Psychological aspects of chronic obstructive pulmonary disease. *Medical Clinics of North America, 61,* 749–758.

Agle DP, Baum GL, Chester EH, et al. (1973). Multidiscipline treatment of chronic pulmonary insufficiency 1. Psychologic aspects of rehabilitation. *Psychosomatic Medicine, 35,* 41–49.

Alexander F, French TM, & Pollock G (1968). *Psychosomatic specificity: Experimental study and results* (Vol. 1). Chicago: University of Chicago Press.

Appelblatt NH & Baker SR (1981). Functional upper airway obstruction: A new syndrome. *Archives of Otolaryngology, 107,* 305–306.

Baldessarini R (1985). Drugs and the treatment of psychiatric disorders. In AG Gilman, LS Goodman, TW Rall, & F Murad (Eds), *The pharmacological basis of therapeutics* (7th ed). New York: MacMillan.

Bedford B & Wade-West S (1983). Sensitivity to tartrazine. *British Medical Journal, 286,* 148.

Boakes AJ, Laurence DR, Teoh PC, et al. (1973). Interactions between sympathomimetic amines and antidepressant agents in man. *British Medical Journal, 1,* 311–315.

Boston Collaborative Drug Surveillance Program (1972). Acute adverse reaction to prednisone in relation to dosage. *Clinical Pharmacology and Therapeutics, 13,* 694–697.

Bywater EM (1981). Adolescents with cystic fibrosis: Psychosocial adjustment. *Archives of Disease in Childhood, 56,* 538–543.

Christopher KL, Wood RP, II, Eckert RC, et al. (1983). Vocal cord dysfunction presenting as asthma. *New England Journal of Medicine, 308,* 1566–1570.

Covino NA, Dirks JF, Kinsman RA, et al. (1982). Patterns of depression in chronic illness. *Psychotherapy and Psychosomatics, 37,* 144–153.

Desai G, Seriff N, Khan F, et al. (1976). A multidisciplinary approach to weaning of respirator dependent patients. *Chest, 70,* 424–425.

Dirks JF, Jones NF, & Kinsman RA (1977). Panic-fear: A personality dimension related to intractability in asthma. *Psychosomatic Medicine, 39,* 120–126.

Dudley DL, Sitzman J, & Rugg M (1985). Psychiatric aspects of patients with chronic obstructive pulmonary disease. *Advances in Psychosomatic Medicine, 14,* 64–77.

Fletcher EC & Martin RJ (1982). Sexual dysfunction and erectile impotence in chronic obstructive pulmonary disease. *Chest, 81,* 413–421.

French TM & Alexander F (1939–1941). Psychogenic factors in bronchial asthma. *Psychosomatic Medicine Monograph, 4,* 1–96.

Fritz GK (1983). Childhood asthma. *Psychosomatics, 24,* 959–967.

Gale J & O'Shanick GJ (1985). Psychiatric aspects of respirator treatment and pulmonary intensive care. *Advances in Psychosomatic Medicine, 14,* 93–108.

Grant I, Heaton RK, McSweeny AJ, et al. (1982). Neuropsychologic findings in hypoxemic chronic obstructive pulmonary disease. *Archives of Internal Medicine, 142,* 1470–1476.

Greenblatt DJ, Shader RI, & Abernethy DR (1983). Current status of benzodiazepines. *New England Journal of Medicine, 309,* 354–358, 410–416.

Hall RCW, Popkin MK, Stickney SK, et al. (1979). Presentation of the steroid psychoses. *Journal of Nervous and Mental Disorders, 167,* 229–236.

Hollender MH & Mercer AJ (1976). The wish to be held and the wish to hold in men and women. *Archives of General Psychiatry, 33,* 49–51.

Hudgel DW, Cooperson DM, & Kinsman RA (1982). Recognition of added resistive loads in asthma: The importance of behavioral styles. *American Review of Respiratory Diseases, 126,* 121–125.

Jann MW & Bitar AH (1982). Respiratory dyskinesia. *Psychosomatics, 23,* 764–765.

Kass I, Updegraff K, & Muffly RB (1972). Sex in chronic obstructive pulmonary disease. *Medical Aspects of Human Sexuality, 7,* 33–38.

Kiecolt-Glaser JK & Glaser R (1986). Psychological influences on immunity. *Psychosomatics, 27,* 621–624.

Kinsman RA, Dirks JF, Dahlem NW, et al. (1980). Anxiety in asthma: Panic–fear symptomatology and personality in relation to manifest anxiety. *Psychological Reports, 46,* 196–198.

Kinsman RA, Dirks JF, Jones NF, et al. (1980). Anxiety reduction in asthma: Four catches to general application. *Psychosomatic Medicine, 42,* 397–405.

Kinsman RA, Luparello T, O'Banion K, et al. (1973). Multidimensional analysis of the subjective symptomatology of asthma. *Psychosomatic Medicine, 35*, 250–267.

Klerman GL (1981). Depression in the medically ill. *Psychiatric Clinics of North America, 4*, 301–317.

Knapp PH (1985). Psychosomatic aspects of bronchial asthma: A review. In EB Weiss, MS Segal, M Stein (eds). *Bronchial asthma: Mechanisms and therapeutics* (2nd ed). Boston: Little, Brown.

Levine DJ & Johnson RW (1985). Psychiatric aspects of cigarette smoking. *Advances in Psychosomatic Medicine, 14*, 48–63.

Levitan H (1983). Suicidal trends in patients with asthma and hypertension: A chart study. *Psychotherapy and Psychosomatics, 39*, 165–170.

Liebman R, Minuchin S, & Baker L (1974). The use of structural family therapy in the treatment of intractable asthma. *American Journal of Psychiatry, 131*, 535–540.

Lindegard B (1982). Physical illness in severe depressives and psychiatric alcoholics in Gothenburg, Sweden. *Journal of Affective Disorders, 4*, 383–393.

Martin JB, Reichlin S, & Brown GM (1977). Hypothalamic control of anterior pituitary secretion. *Clinical Neuroendocrinology*, 13–44. Philadelphia: Davis.

Mendel J & Khan F (1980). Psychological aspects of weaning from mechanical ventilation. *Psychosomatics, 21*, 465– 471.

Moran MG (1985). Psychiatric aspects of tuberculosis. *Advances in Psychosomatic Medicine, 14*, 109–118.

Plutchik R, Williams MH, Jr, Jerrett I, et al. (1978). Emotions, personality and life stresses in asthma. *Journal of Psychosomatic Research, 22*, 425–431.

Post L & Collins C (1981–1982). The poorly coping COPD patient: A psychotherapeutic perspective. *International Journal of Psychiatry in Medicine, 11*, 173–182.

Raw M (1978). The treatment of cigarette dependence. In Y Israel, FB Glaser, H Kalant, RE Popham, W Schmidt, & RG Smart (Eds), *Research Advances in Alcohol and Drug Problems*. New York: Plenum Press.

Reite M, Harbeck R, & Hoffman A (1981). Altered cellular immune response following peer separation. *Life Sciences, 29*, 1133–1136.

Rome HP & Braceland FJ (1952). The psychological response to ACTH, cortisone, hydrocortisone and related steroid substances. *American Journal of Psychiatry, 108*, 641–651.

Rossing TH, Fanta CH, & Goldstein DH (1980). Emergency therapy of asthma: Comparison of the acute effects of parenteral and inhaled sympathomimetics and infused aminophylline. *American Review of Respiratory Diseases, 122*, 365–371.

Rutter BM (1979). The prognostic significance of psychological factors in the management of chronic bronchitis. *Psychological Medicine, 9*, 69–70.

Settipane GA (1983). Aspirin and allergic diseases: A review. *American Journal of Medicine, 74*, 102–109.

Sharfstein SS, Sack DS, & Fauci AS (1982). Relationship between alternate-day corticosteroid therapy and behavioral abnormalities. *Journal of the American Medical Association, 248*, 2987–2989.

Sharman DF (1973). The catabolism of catecholamines: Recent studies. *British Medical Bulletin, 29*, 110–115.

Sperling M (1963). A psychoanalytic study of bronchial asthma in children. In HI Schneer, (ed), *The asthmatic child: Psychosomatic approach to problems and treatment*. New York: Harper & Row.

Steen SN (1976). The effects of psychotropic drugs on respiration. *Pharmacology and Therapeutics, 2*, 717–741.

Stein M (1982). Biopsychosocial factors in asthma. In LJ West & M Stein (Eds), *Critical issues in behavioral medicine*. Philadelphia: Lippincott.

Stoudemire A (1985). Psychosomatic theory and pulmonary disease: Asthma as a paradigm for the biopsychosocial approach. *Advances in Psychosomatic Medicine, 14*, 1–15.

Teiramaa E (1978). Psychic disturbances and severity of asthma. *Journal of Psychosomatic Research, 22*, 401–408.

Teiramaa E (1981). Psychosocial factors, personality and acute-insidious asthma. *Journal of Psychosomatic Research, 25*, 43–49.

Thompson TL II, Moran MG, & Nies AS (1983). Psychotropic drug use in the elderly. *New England Journal of Medicine, 308*, 134–138, 194–199.

Thompson TL II, & Thompson WL (1986). Treating dementia in the elderly. *Female Patient, 11*, 62–77.

Thompson WL (1986). Sexual problems in chronic respiratory disease: Achieving and maintaining intimacy. *Postgraduate Medicine, 79*, 41–52.

Thompson WL & Thompson TL II (1984). Treating depression in asthmatic patients. *Psychosomatics, 25*, 809–812.

Thompson WL & Thompson TL II (1985a). Psychiatric aspects of asthma in adults. *Advances in Psychosomatic Medicine, 14*, 33–47.

Thompson WL & Thompson TL II (1985b). Use of medications in patients with chronic respiratory disease. *Advances in Psychosomatic Medicine, 14*, 136–148.

Weiner H (1977). *Psychobiology and human disease*. New York: Elsevier.

Wilson CP (1980–1981). Parental overstimulation in asthma. *International Journal of Psychoanalytic Psychotherapy, 8*, 602–621.

Woodcock AA, Gross ER, & Geddes DM (1981). Drug treatment of breathlessness: Contrasting effects of diazepam and promethazine in pink puffers. *British Medical Journal, 283*, 343–346.

Thomas N. Wise

26
Gastroenterology

Humans have always been fascinated by what they eat, what they excrete, and what disorders upset their gastrointestinal systems. The interplay between psychologic factors and the gastrointestinal system has been accepted for centuries. Among the ancients, potions and purgatives for the alimentary tract were common. The Ebers Papyrus, a medical treatise that dates to 1570 B.C., is devoted primarily to gastrointestinal difficulties (Ghalioungui, 1961). Hippocratic doctrine supported a humoral theory of disease, in which bile was one of the essential humors.

Current culture emphasizes the relationship between emotions and gastrointestinal disease. Media regularly portray stress as a precipitant of abdominal pain; people are warned not to worry or they will "get an ulcer." Behavioral problems such as alcohol ingestion clearly foster gastric, liver, and pancreatic disorders. It has been estimated that 60 percent of the gastroenterologist's clinical activities are devoted primarily to complaints that are of psychologic origin (Switz, 1976).

This chapter will review psychiatric complications associated with diseases of the gastrointestinal tract and will discuss their management.

ESOPHAGEAL DISORDERS

Although esophageal carcinoma, like all cancer, may lead to psychiatric complications, the esophageal disorders of greatest psychiatric interest are the disorders of esophageal motility. Chest pain, difficulty swallowing solids, difficulty ingesting liquids, heartburn, and regurgitation are regularly found in individuals with esophageal motility abnormalities (Reidel & Clouse, 1985). Increased emotional arousal increases respiration as well as swallowing rates, which may augment esophageal distress. Anxiety that increases swallowing rates may thus exacerbate esophageal disorders (Fonagy & Calloway, 1986).

Psychiatric disorders such as mood disorders and generalized anxiety disorder are commonly seen in individuals with esophageal motility disorders (Clouse & Lustman, 1983). This concurs with the finding that individuals with symptomatic hiatal hernias also often have generalized anxiety disorders and depressive disorders (Nielzen, Pettersson, Regnell, et al., 1986). Patients with symptomatic esophageal motility disorders require psychiatric assessment.

Psychopharmacologic and psychotherapeutic treatment of associated anxiety or depression will often substantially alleviate esophageal symptoms. The anticholinergic effects of some psychotropics, however, may aggravate gastroesophageal reflux; if this occurs, a less anticholinergic agent should be substituted, while the symptoms are treated with antacids or H_2 blockers or both. Smoking and heavy coffee drinking, both of which are frequent in psychiatric patients, may exacerbate reflux symptoms.

PEPTIC ULCER DISEASE

The contemporary association between emotional stress and onset of abdominal pain has its roots in the observations of William Beaumont, a Canadian surgeon, who carefully observed the gastric fistula of an injured Canadian lumberjack, Alexis St. Martin. Beaumont documented the correlation between anger and increased gastric fluid output (Beaumont, 1833).

Gastric and duodenal ulcers have different etiologies. Duodenal ulcers may be associated with excess secretion of hydrochloric acid by the stomach; delayed gastric emptying promotes gastric ulcers (Isenberg, 1981). Duodenal ulcers are more frequent in males, but there is no sex bias in gastric ulcers; duodenal ulcers also occur more commonly in people with type O blood.

In addition to peptic ulcer syndromes, there are other types of gastrointestinal ulcers, such as stress ulcers, Cushing's ulcers, and Curling's ulcers, which may result from central nervous system injury, burns, or ingestion of corticosteroids or aspirin. Peptic ulcer disease, however, has been the primary focus of psychosomatic investigation.

Early psychosomatic studies were hampered by imprecise definitions and lacked documentation of ulcer type and location. Franz Alexander (1950) is best known for his psychosomatic hypotheses. He hypothesized that the patient with a duodenal ulcer has frustrated wishes to be loved and cared for, resulting in persistent oral dependent needs. The onset of the ulcer disease occurred when such unsatisfied cravings were augmented by an increase in responsibility or frustrated dependency needs.

Reichsman, Engel, and Segal (1956) quantitatively documented the relationship between gastric acid secretion and affective states of an infant with an esophageal-tracheal fistula; they linked object relations to gastric physiology. To empirically test such single case designs, Weiner, Thaler, Reiser, et al. (1957) investigated 2073 Army inductees, utilizing psychologic testing and serum pepsinogen levels, which correlated with basal rates of gastric acid secretion. Their results supported Alexander's theory in that the Army inductees who later developed duodenal ulceration were those who demonstrated the most intense dependency needs and conflicts with authority. These investigators thus integrated a somatic vulnerability, that is, high baseline pepsinogen levels, with a vulnerable personality characteristic and a stressful life event, such as induction into the Army.

The role of life events in the generation of ulcer disease has also been investigated. A series of studies have suggested that patients with peptic ulcer disease have an increased incidence of stressful life events prior to disease onset (Sapira & Cross, 1982). There is, however, no increased incidence of overt psychopathology (Sandberg & Bliding, 1976). As both alcohol and tobacco consumption have been associated with peptic ulcer disease, the emotional substrates of these addictive behaviors may indirectly link increased peptic ulceration to psychopathology.

Psychologically and behaviorally oriented treatments for peptic ulcer disease are difficult to assess because of significant placebo effects. Since the majority of duodenal and gastric ulcers heal with no medication within 6 weeks, the effects of *any* treatment are relatively difficult to evaluate. Psychologic treatments may nevertheless offer some help in the management of peptic ulcer disease. Chapell, Stefano, Rogers, et al. (1936) utilized dietary management and group therapy with an educational component similar to Buchanan's (1978) two-step methodology for the group treatment of patients with organic illnesses. This method allowed group members to learn about the physiologic aspects of the disease in a formal didactic fashion. The approach promoted discussions of life stresses and difficulties in a group setting. The treated group improved more than untreated controls. More recently, others have documented that stress management training utilizing relaxation therapy and assertiveness training is effective in diminishing ulcer pain and antacid ingestion (Brooks & Richardson, 1980).

Although psychoanalytic psychotherapy offered a research methodology to look at unconscious conflicts presumably associated with peptic ulcer disease, the actual effects of psychoanalytic treatment on the course of the disease are still not clear. One study contended that patients who completed psychoanalysis appeared to have fewer relapses of their disease (Orgel, 1958). The nonrandom design of such studies makes any conclusions impossible. More recently, Sjodin, Svendlund, Ottosson, et al. (1986) investigated the use of combined psychotherapy and pharmacotherapy, utilizing a short-term, dynamically oriented therapeutic approach. The investigators utilized both dynamic and cognitive strategies for patients with peptic ulcer dis-

ease and found that *both* the treatment group and the control group improved. Individuals who underwent psychotherapy, however, had less abdominal pain and, after one year of treatment, appeared to have higher global ratings of both physical health and freedom from emotional complaints than controls. In this model, to allow a therapeutic alliance to develop, treatment was initiated by means of a formal didactic tutorial about the disease. Various life stresses that might have exacerbated the ulcer were reviewed, and exercises in focused problem solving were carried out.

Direct behavioral interventions for peptic ulcer disease are in an experimental stage. Investigators have shown that biofeedback techniques may reduce gastric acid secretion as well as gastric acid motility. Relaxation training may also diminish gastric acid secretion and thus provide a therapeutic rationale for these behavioral interventions. The technical difficulties and cost of such strategies, however, prevent their widespread practical application (Stracher, Berner, Naske, et al., 1975).

Medical management of ulcer disease is the presently accepted approach. The H_2 blockers cimetidine and ranitidine are primary treatments for unperforated ulcer disease. These drugs control gastric acid secretion and can help heal the acute lesion as well as prevent ulcer relapse. There is some evidence, albeit controversial, that ranitidine is more effective in preventing duodenal ulcer relapse (Gough, Bardhan, Crowe, et al., 1984). Side effects of the drugs include confusional states and possibly depression, though depression is poorly substantiated. Initially, it was thought that only cimetidine produced delirium, since it passed the blood–brain barrier. Recently, however, ranitidine has also been documented to cause confusion (Silverstone, 1984). The risk of delirium is greater in elderly patients and in individuals with liver disease. Both drugs also can cause erectile dysfunction, which may limit compliance with the prescribed drug regimen (Assael, Bass, Fischel, et al., 1974). Symptoms remit when the drug is stopped.

Since cimetidine and ranitidine may both cause delirium and depression, the antiulcer drug sucralfate is a safe and effective alternative in susceptible patients. The agent acts locally to coat and protect ulcer sites from gastric acid and has little systemic absorption. The drug is given in a dose of one gram before meals and at bedtime.

Cimetidine has also been associated with elevating blood levels of the tricyclic antidepressant imipramine when the two drugs are used concurrently (see below). Tricyclic antidepressants such as doxepin also possess H_2 receptor blocking capabilities and have been used experimentally as antiulcer agents (Shrivastava, Shah, & Siegal, 1985). The efficacy of these drugs as potent H_2 blockers is controversial, and they should not be considered *primary* treatment, although they may augment and work synergistically with formal medical regimens, particularly in anxious or depressed patients with high psychophysiologic gastrointestinal (GI) reactivity.

Other complications from standard medical interventions for peptic ulcer disease include the milk–alkali syndrome, wherein persistent antacid ingestion and milk drinking create a hypercalcemic state that may cause renal damage as well as the mental symptoms of hypercalcemia. Anticholinergic agents are also utilized in the treatment of peptic ulcer disease; they can precipitate the well-known syndrome of toxicity. Patients with a gastrectomy are vulnerable to B_{12} deficiency, which can present with an organic mood syndrome.

The use of psychotropic agents may be compromised by cimetidine. The levels of benzodiazepines, metabolized primarily by oxidation, and of imipramine may increase because of cimetidine-induced inhibition of the hepatic metabolism of these drugs (Greenblatt, Abernathy, Morse, et al.,

1984; Henaver & Hollister, 1984). The general clinical significance of such slight elevations is doubtful, but the interaction deserves consideration when side effects develop or when patients are otherwise at high risk for toxicity. Lorazepam utilizes an alternative metabolic pathway (glucuronide conjugation), as do oxazepam and temazepam; they are possibly preferred if a benzodiazepine is needed in conjunction with this H_2 blocker (Klotz & Reimann, 1980). Neuroleptic medication may be malabsorbed if taken with cimetidine, and lowered blood levels will thus result (Howes, Pollar, Sourindhriu, et al., 1983). Ranitidine, however, does not impair diazepam clearance (Abernethy, Greenblatt, Eshelman, et al., 1985). It may be given on a twice-daily schedule, in contrast to cimetidine, which is given four times a day. The twice-a-day schedule enhances compliance, so ranitidine is preferable in patients having difficulty with treatment adherence.

ABDOMINAL PAIN OF UNKNOWN ETIOLOGY

Chronic abdominal pain is often seen in medical practice. Patients for whom no clear etiology can be found present a perplexing management problem. Drossman (1982) has reviewed his experience with 24 individuals considered to have psychogenic chronic abdominal pain. His patients were often noted to have evidence of incompletely resolved grief due to prior losses. Most of these patients did not consider their complaints to be of psychologic origin and avoided psychiatric care.

Eisendrath, Way, Ostroff, et al. (1986) noted that patients with psychogenic abdominal pain more often had a past history of somatization of psychologic distress as well as a family history of alcoholism. Patients with medically unexplained abdominal pain deserve psychiatric consultation. Certainly, exploratory surgery should not be performed on such patients without prior psychiatric evaluation. Somatoform and idiopathic abdominal pain syndromes have been recently reviewed elsewhere (Stoudemire & Sandhu, 1987).

The couvade syndrome also presents with acute gastrointestinal symptoms and may be mistaken for organic disease. The syndrome is found in men whose wives are pregnant and is characterized by nausea, vomiting, abdominal bloating, and fatigue (Enoch, Trethowan, & Barker, 1967). Lipkin and Lamb (1982) demonstrated that physicians often miss the relationship of the symptoms to the patient's expected fatherhood. Couvade is best managed by very conservative measures and reassurance that the gastrointestinal difficulties will remit following the birth of the child (Lipkin & Lamb, 1982). Patients refractory to explanation and reassurance require psychiatric assessment and medical psychotherapy.

Before attributing abdominal pain to psychological origins, however, great care should be taken to rule out organic or anatomic etiologies that may have been overlooked in the medical evaluation. Acute intermittent porphyria, for example, presents with a history of chronic abdominal pain (often with a record of multiple negative exploratory laparotomies), peripheral neuropathy, and delirium. Occult intestinal adhesions should also be considered, as well as occult endometriosis in women where the boundaries between abdominal and pelvic pain syndromes are blurred.

HEPATIC DISEASE

Although there are a variety of hepatic diseases due to circulatory abnormalities, biliary obstruction, and hepatotoxic agents, parenchymal liver disease is the most common. The various causes of parenchymal liver disorders include viral hepatitis, neoplastic disease, pyogenic abscesses, genetic errors in metabolism, toxic hepatitis,

and alcoholic cirrhosis. In recent immigrants to the United States from less developed countries, parasitic diseases must always be ruled out.

Alcoholic liver disease, including fatty liver, alcoholic hepatitis, and alcoholic cirrhosis is the most common form of liver disease and ranks among the five leading causes of death in the United States (Galambos, 1979). The major psychologic syndrome seen with alcoholic cirrhosis is portal-systemic encephalopathy (Tarter, Hegedos, Van Thiel, et al., 1985–1986). The psychologic symptoms of hepatic encephalopathy are varied and may be mistaken for nonorganic psychiatric disorders. The early stages of portal-systemic encephalopathy are characterized by cognitive impairment, with difficulties in attention, irritability, and affective lability; later stages are stupor and coma. Sleep disturbances, tremor, asterixis, and motor incoordination are also usual in the early stages. Verbal coherence is often preserved in early encephalopathic states, so a *complete* cognitive verbal status is essential for diagnosis. Read, Sherlock, Laidlaw, et al. (1967) noted that individuals with hepatic encephalopathy were often misdiagnosed as either schizophrenic or bipolar. The electroencephalogram (EEG) may be helpful in doubtful cases if it shows characteristic diffuse slowing of metabolic delirium.

Treatment interventions involve both direct and supportive measures. Pharmacologic approaches, such as oral neomycin and lactulose, are helpful in modifying the encephalopathy. When agitation is severe, low-dose haloperidol can be considered. Benzodiazepines are relatively contraindicated, as they may worsen the encephalopathy. The risk would be greater with those benzodiazepines metabolized by oxidation.

Supportive measures include environmental interventions appropriate to delirium (see Chapter 6) and efforts to educate the family. When the etiology of the liver disease is alcoholic, significant others should be educated regarding the crucial role of abstinence. Because of the encephalopathic patient's cognitive defects, direct confrontation of the patient regarding the alcohol problem is usually unproductive.

Viral infections, most commonly hepatitis B virus, cause serious hepatic disease. In the acute syndrome, transient neuropsychologic changes may occur, which may be manifested behaviorally by irritability, poor concentration, and lethargy (Apstein, Koffe, & Koffe, 1979). Chronic viral hepatitis may produce fatigue and symptoms suggestive of depression. Cyclic antidepressants may help the mood symptoms but may aggravate the hepatitis itself because of their potential hepatotoxicity. For this reason, patients with chronic hepatitis receiving cyclic antidepressants should have weekly liver function tests during the first month of treatment, and then as needed thereafter if hepatic symptoms relapse. Tricyclic blood levels should also be considered, as the hepatitis may impair drug metabolism.

Hepatitis B virus, which can be transmitted by parenteral sources, such as intravenous drug abuse, transfusions, or sexual activity, may affect an individual's social status, leading to social isolation. Psychologic difficulties, such as fatigue, depression, and demoralization, combine with difficulties in sexual functioning because of the fear of transmitting infection. All patients with hepatitis B deserve testing for acquired immune deficiency syndrome (AIDS), as the two diseases are transmitted by the same routes and are prevalent in the same population

Infectious mononucleosis is frequently associated with hepatomegaly. The disorder is due to a primary infection with the Epstein-Barr virus. Psychologic symptoms in infectious mononucleosis include depression, which may mimic a major mood disorder, as well as acute psychotic reactions, which include organic features such as con-

fusion and marked memory loss (Allen & Tilkian, 1986). Pharmacologic treatment of these psychiatric syndromes may be needed; if it is, blood counts and liver enzymes should be monitored during the early weeks of treatment.

A syndrome that has recently been the object of much controversy is the so-called "chronic active Epstein-Barr virus infection," which is characterized by severe cyclic fatigue, sore throat, myalgias, headaches, paresthesias, arthralgias, depression, insomnia, confusion, and gastrointestinal complaints (Buchwald, Sullivan, & Komaroff, 1987). Despite the presence of antibody titers specific to EBV-specific antigens in many of these patients, there is no conclusive evidence that EBV is causally related to the syndrome. Authorities have therefore recommended interpreting antibody titers to EBV with caution until more definitive data are available. Nevertheless, systemic viral syndromes of this nature should be considered in the differential diagnosis of cyclical mood disturbances associated with physical complaints of chronic fatigue and lassitude.

INFLAMMATORY BOWEL DISEASE

Inflammatory bowel disease refers to two processes, ulcerative colitis and regional enteritis, or Crohn's disease (Farmer, 1981). Ulcerative colitis is generally limited to the mucosal lining of the large intestine. Its dominant symptoms are diarrhea and hematochezia. In severe disease states, the individual will present multiple watery stools, which can lead to dehydration and anemia.

Crohn's disease is a transmural process that may affect any point along the alimentary canal but most often involves the distal ileum and proximal colon. Intestinal obstruction, fistulas, and abscesses may occur, causing such symptoms as abdominal pain, fever, and severe weight loss.

Ulcerative colitis increases the risk of colonic cancer to a greater extent than Crohn's disease. Crohn's disease can recur relentlessly despite long periods of apparent remission, whereas ulcerative colitis may actually be cured by colectomy.

Early psychologic investigators attempted to document a specific unconscious conflict for sufferers of both inflammatory bowel diseases. Alexander (1950) proposed a characteristic unconscious conflict in ulcerative colitis patients that represented frustrated aggressive needs. Engel (1955) viewed such patients as extremely sensitive to separation from important individuals in their lives. In such settings of separation, helplessness, and hopelessness, the colitis was exacerbated. Others emphasized stress as a provoking agent in such a disease. Grace, Wolf, and Wolff (1951) noted that ulcerative colitis patients were superficially friendly and needed to please others but were very vulnerable to environmental stress because of their inability to express anger.

Contemporary investigators have tried to partition psychologic factors in Crohn's disease from those in ulcerative colitis. Whybrow, Kane, & Lipton (1968) found that a variety of noxious life changes exacerbated Crohn's disease episodes. Those patients with more depressive symptomatology had a greater length of illness. The essential problem with most of these studies, however, is that it is difficult to separate reactive phenomena from etiologic factors. McKegney, Gordon, and Levine (1970) compared ulcerative colitic patients with those with Crohn's disease and found no significant differences from psychosocial, psychiatric, or behavioral perspectives. They documented that those with more severe physical disabilities had greater depressive symptomatology. As with most other diseases, therefore, psychologic fac-

tors in the *etiology* of the conditions remain speculative.

Two recent, well controlled studies examined psychiatric diagnoses in consecutive cases of ulcerative colitis and Crohn's disease, and compared rates with those obtained in control patients with other chronic medical illnesses. They used structured interviews and operational diagnostic criteria. While ulcerative colitis patients were no more likely than medically ill controls to have psychiatric diagnoses, Crohn's disease patients had significantly higher prevalence of depression than controls. The severity of GI symptoms and psychiatric symptoms were independent, and there was no consistent temporal sequence of involvement. The findings suggest that depression and Crohn's disease are *associated*, but that attribution of causality are not justified (Helzer, et al. 1982, 1984).

The essential differences between regional enteritis—Crohn's disease—and ulcerative colitis must be understood in providing psychologic support for these patients. Specifically, the individual with regional enteritis will have to cope with an uncertain and relentless disease that has exacerbations and remissions. The relatively favorable prognosis of the ulcerative colitis patient after colectomy stands in contrast to that of the Crohn's disease sufferer, whose illness may persist. Thus, psychologic treatment must be directed toward coping with specific life stresses, problems with the actual treatment itself, and the existential nature of the chronic disease (Zisook & DeVaul, 1977). Individuals who become depressed in the setting of chronic bowel pain may benefit from antidepressant medication. Careful behavioral focus on the activities of daily living may help in restoring proper dietary habits and may minimize the exhaustion and the fatigue that occur in a setting of anemia and dehydration. In both ulcerative colitis and Crohn's disease, steroids are often used, leading to their well-known psychologic side effects (Lewis & Smith, 1983).

Utilization of intravenous hyperalimentation is sometimes necessary in fulminant cases of regional enteritis or for individuals with a short bowel syndrome. The psychologic effects of this treatment have been catalogued by Perl, Hall, Dudrick, et al. (1980). Depression, fear, loss of appetite, and marital stress are common in individuals who undergo total parenteral nutrition for periods of a few months or longer. Patients on chronic hyperalimentation have also been found to have mild cognitive impairment. Both mood changes and cognitive dysfunction can thus arise during chronic hyperalimentation. Mood changes should be treated with antidepressants and medical psychotherapy. The detection of cognitive dysfunction should lead to a comprehensive assessment of fluid, electrolyte, and vitamin status, as well as screening for infection related to the central line.

In both ulcerative colitis and Crohn's disease, institution of an ostomy demands significant adaptation by the patient. Patients may react with shame, depression, and anger at the alteration of their excretory system. Prior to surgery, it is most helpful to have ostomy therapists talk to both patient and spouse. Utilization of patient organizations, such as the United Ostomy Association or the National Ileitis and Colitis Foundation, can be an invaluable adjunct to medical treatment. Such groups provide patient advocates who have had personal experience with their own ostomies and can aid the patient with fears about leakage, skin breakdown, odors, and so on. Inclusion of the spouse is important in managing the patient with an ostomy. Dlin and others have noted that men are more comfortable having their wives view their ostomy and appliance whereas women seem to experience more shame and do not like their spouses to see their ostomy (Dlin, Perlman, & Ringold, 1969; Druss, O'Con-

nor, Prudden, et al., 1968). Psychologic complications of ostomy surgery are discussed at length in Chapter 19, by Riether and Stoudemire.

THE IRRITABLE BOWEL SYNDROME

The irritable bowel syndrome is a heterogenous condition of uncertain etiology that accounts for 50 percent of ambulatory cases seen by gastroenterologists (Thompson, 1979). The syndrome is composed of a cluster of bowel symptoms that reflect alternating diarrhea, constipation, and abdominal pain (Thompson, 1979). It may be partitioned into diarrhea-predominant, constipation-predominant, and mixed varieties. Classification of this disorder is difficult because a variety of investigations have shown that normative populations frequently report bowel habits similar to those of patients with operationally defined irritable bowel syndrome (Thompson & Heaton, 1980). It thus may be that patients with irritable bowel syndrome overestimate their excretory problems and seek medical care because of abnormal illness behavior rather than the disease itself. Other data, however, suggest that individuals with irritable bowel syndrome may have abnormal myoelectric activity of the colon, abnormalities of gastric hormones, or food allergies (Wise, 1986). Most investigators, however, would agree that irritable bowel syndrome involves a combination of psychologic and physiologic factors.

Patients with irritable bowel syndrome (IBS) have an increased incidence of psychologic disturbances when compared with those with inflammatory bowel disease (Young, Alpers, & Norland, 1976). This suggests that psychologic illness is associated with the disorder rather than merely a reaction to the discomfort of symptoms. Patients with IBS are more anxious and depressed than normal controls. Latimer,

Sarna, Campbell, et al. (1981) have even postulated that patients with irritable bowel syndrome are as neurotic as psychiatric outpatients and tend to express their symptomatology in somatic terms rather than in psychologic complaints. There is a marked tendency toward hypochondriacal concerns in patients with irritable bowel syndrome, since they view minor illnesses more seriously than other individuals and consult physicians more often for a variety of illnesses.

Various treatments have been utilized for irritable bowel syndrome (Wise, 1986). These include dietary management, with high fiber diets that avoid gas-producing legumes; anticholinergic medication; bulking agents; and utilization of minor tranquilizers or tricyclic antidepressants. Psychotherapy has also been applied. Focal problem-solving therapy techniques, similar to those prescribed for patients with peptic ulcer disease, have been shown to be an effective strategy in modifying such symptoms (Hislop, 1980). Relaxation therapy has also been advocated for reduction of abdominal cramping and bowel symptoms. A combined approach utilizing group therapy, relaxation therapy, and focal problem solving may serve to diminish somatic concerns and anxiety in persons with irritable bowel despite the persistence of symptoms (Wise, Cooper & Ahmed, 1982). In patients with marked hypochondriacal concerns, prevention of doctor shopping and small, but frequent, doses of physician interaction may be useful.

Anxiety and depression must be treated directly, while direct pharmacologic treatment and dietary direction are offered for the somatic aspects of the complaints. As noted earlier, the psychopharmacologic management of irritable bowel often involves use of tricyclics. The use of medications with anticholinergic and sedating side effects, such as doxepin, is preferred for diarrhea-predominant irritable bowel. In subjects with constipation-predominant distress, agents with low anticholinergic effects, such as desipramine, are preferred. Many patients who do not have concurrent major depression will respond symptomatically to relatively low doses (25–75 mg) of a cyclic antidepressant. For antidepressants to be prescribed for irritable bowel patients, it is not necessary that the patient accept a diagnosis of depression. Patients may be told that there is substantial evidence that irritable bowel complaints respond to antidepressants whether or not the patient is clinically depressed. Low-dose antidepressants are also excellent antianxiety agents for this population, often obviating the need for benzodiazepines.

The medical interventions used to treat irritable bowel syndrome are simple and relatively safe, but often considerable trial and error is needed to find the optimal regimen. Primary care provided by the psychiatrist may thus be an option for patients with irritable bowel disease and associated psychopathology. In this model, the gastroenterologist functions as a consultant, and the psychiatrist prescribes *all* medications, including GI remedies.

CARCINOMA OF THE PANCREAS

Carcinoma of the pancreas has long been associated with emotional disorders—in particular, depression (Joffee, Rubinow, Denicoff, et al., 1986). The incidence of depression that predates the discovery of this malignancy varies from 10 to 50 percent. Symptomatology is similar to that of a major mood disorder and may not have somatic or vegetative symptoms. In addition, there may be a positive dexamethasone suppression test as well as a response to cyclic antidepressant medication or ECT in depressions that concur with this neoplasm. Such a cluster of symptoms predates the physical evidence of disease, thus making the malignancy extremely difficult to diagnose. As this malignancy is relatively common in males over 50, the clinician should keep a high index of suspicion for middle-aged males who develop a major mood disorder with no obvious precipitant or premorbid vulnerability characteristics (Fras, Litin and Bartholomew, 1968). The emergence of otherwise unexplained back pain, nausea, or indigestion in a depressed older man should be thoroughly investigated with studies including abdominal ultrasound or abdominal computer tomography (CT) scanning.

COLONIC CARCINOMA

Issues of colonic cancer and of its surgical treatment are discussed in Chapters 23 and 19, respectively.

GENERAL GUIDELINES FOR TREATMENT

Various gastrointestinal disorders will have physiologic phenomena, such as abdominal pain, dyspepsia, or diarrhea, which will occur concurrently with subjective emotional symptoms. To delineate such phenomena it is best that the patient keep a behavioral diary, which is simply a self-report inventory that can be tailored to each patient's specific needs (Kanfer & Saslow, 1965). Elements that need to be included in such a diary are the specific behavior to be monitored (such as abdomi-

nal pain, anxiety, depression, flatulence, or diarrhea), the antecedents of the behavior, and the consequences of the behavior. Such an inventory will allow specific information to be elicited and will allow the patient to make linkages between emotional phenomena and physiologic data. Such a diary can be developed from a small note pad, which can be written in once or twice each day. In addition, dietary patterns and other information that is initially overlooked by the patient can be entered.

The medical psychotherapy of patients with gastrointestinal disorders will combine didactic, insight-oriented, supportive, and behavioral strategies. The therapist must be flexible and understand the physiology of each disease in order to fully comprehend the patient's own experience. Strategies for medical psychotherapy are discussed in Chapter 1, and selection of patients for behavior therapy is discussed in Chapter 14. In addition to these individual interventions, referral of patients with similar illnesses to group therapy may be appropriate, and is especially suitable for socially isolated patients. As noted earlier, gastrointestinal symptoms in many of these patients will "mask" primary Axis I anxiety and depressive disorders of syndromal and subsyndromal proportions. Sorting out this particular group of patients is essential, since many will respond to formal psychiatric interventions despite the presence of multiple psychophysiologic complaints and a relative lack of psychological insight.

REFERENCES

Abernethy DR, Greenblatt DJ, Eshelman FN, et al. (1984). Ranitidine does not impair oxidative or conjugative metabolism: Noninteraction with antipyrine, diazepam, and lorazepam. *Clinical Pharmacology and Therapeutics, 35*, 188–192.

Alexander F (1950). *Psychosomatic medicine.* New York: Norton.

Allen AD & Tilkian SM (1986). Depression correlated with cellular immunity in systemic immunodeficient Epstein-Barr virus syndrome. *Journal of Clinical Psychiatry, 47*, 133–135.

Apstein MD, Koffe E, & Koffe RS (1979). Neuropsychological dysfunction in acute viral hepatitis. *Digestion, 19*, 349–358.

Assael M, Bass D, Fischel RE, et al. (1974). Impotence and peptic ulcer. *International Journal of Psychiatry in Medicine*, 5, 377–387.

Beaumont W (1833). *Experiments and observations on the gastric juice and physiology of digestion.* Plattsburgh, NY: FP Allen.

Brooks GR & Richardson FC (1980). Emotional skills training: A treatment program for duodenal ulcer. *Behavior Therapy*, 11, 198–207.

Buchanan DC (1978). Group therapy for chronically physically ill patients. *Psychosomatics*, 19, 425–431.

Buchwald D, Sullivan JL, & Komaroff AL (1987). Frequency of 'chronic active Epstein-Barr virus infection' in a general medical practice. *Journal of the American Medical Association*, 257, 2303–2307.

Dlin BM, Perlman A & Ringold E (1969). Psychosexual response to ileostomy and colostomy. *American Journal of Psychiatry*, 126, 3–9.

Drossman DA (1982). Patients with psychogenic abdominal pain: Six years observation in the medical setting. *American Journal of Psychiatry*, 139, 1549–1557.

Druss RG, O'Connor J, Prudden JF, et al. (1968). Psychologic response to colectomy. *Archives of General Psychiatry*, 18, 53–59.

Eisendrath SJ, Way LW, Ostroff JW, et al. (1986). Identification of psychogenic abdominal pain. *Psychosomatics*, 27, 705–712.

Engel GL (1955). Studies of ulcerative colitis: 3. The nature of the psychologic process. *American Journal of Medicine*, 19, 231–240.

Enoch MD, Trethowan WH, & Barker JC (1967). *Some uncommon psychiatric syndromes* (pp 56–71). Bristol, England: John Wright.

Farmer RG (1981). Factors in long term prognosis of patients with inflammatory bowel disease. *American Journal of Gastroenterology*, 75, 97–109.

Fonagy P & Calloway SP (1986). The effect of emotional arousal on spontaneous swallowing rates. *Journal of Psychosomatic Research*, 30, 183–188.

Galambos J (1979). Cirrhosis: Epidemiology. In L Smith (Ed), *Major problems in internal medicine* (pp 91–127). Philadelphia: WB Saunders.

Ghalioungui P (1961). *Magic and medical science in ancient egypt.* London: Hodder and Stoughton.

Gough KR, Bardhan KD, Crowe JP, et al. (1984). Ranitidine and cimetidine in prevention of duodenal ulcer relapse. *Lancet*, 2, 659–662.

Grace WV, Wolf S, & Wolff HG (1951). *The human colon* (pp 159–202). New York: Hoeber.

Greenblatt DJ, Abernathy DR, Morse DS, et al. (1984). Clinical importance of the interaction of diazepam and cimetidine. *New England Journal of Medicine*, 310, 1039–1643.

Helzer JE, Stillings WA, Chammas S, et al. (1982). A controlled study of the association between ulcerative colitis and psychiatric diagnoses. *Digestive Diseases and Sciences*, 27(6), 513–518.

Helzer JE, Chammas S, Norland CC, et al. (1984). A study of the association between Crohn's disease and psychiatric illness. *Gastroenterology*, 86, 324–440.

Henaver SA & Hollister LE (1984). Cimetidine interaction with imipramine and nortriptyline. *Clinical Pharmacology and Therapeutics*, 35, 183–186.

Hislop IG (1980). Effect of very brief psychotherapy on the irritable bowel syndrome. *Medical Journal of Australia*, 2, 620–623.

Howes CA, Pollar T, Sourindhriu I, et al. (1983). Reduced steady state plasma concentrations of chloropromazine and indomethacine in patients receiving cimetidine. *European Journal of Clinical Pharmacology*, 24, 99–102.

Isenberg JI (1981). Peptic ulcer. *Disease—A Month*, 28, 1–58.

Joffee RT, Rubinow DR, Denicoff KD, et al. (1986). Depression and carcinoma of the pancreas. *General Hospital Psychiatry*, 8, 241–245.

Kanfer FH & Saslow G (1965). Behavioral analysis. *Archives of General Psychiatry*, 12, 529–538.

Klotz U & Reimann I (1980). Delayed clearance of diazepam due to cimetidine. *New England Journal of Medicine*, 302, 1012–1014.

Latimer PR, Sarna SK, Campbell D, et al. (1981). Colonic motor and myoelectric activity: A comparative study of normal subjects, psychoneurotic patients and patients with irritable bowel syndrome. *Gastroenterology*, 80, 893–910.

Lewis DA & Smith RE (1983). Steroid induced psychiatric syndromes. *Journal of Affective Disorders*, 5, 319–332.

Lipkin M & Lamb GS (1982). The couvade syndrome: An epidemiologic study. *Annals of Internal Medicine*, 96, 509–511.

McKegney FP, Gordon RO, & Levine SM (1970). A psychosomatic comparison of patients with ulcerative colitis and Crohn's disease. *Psychosomatic Medicine*, 32, 153–166.

Nielzen S, Pettersson KI, Regnell G, et al. (1986). The role of psychiatric factors in symptoms of hiatus hernia or gastric reflux. *Acta Psychiatrica Scandinavica*, 73, 214–220.

Orgel SZ (1958). Effect of psychoanalysis on the course of peptic ulcer. *Psychosomatic Medicine*, 20, 117–125.

Perl M, Hall RCW, Dudrick SJ, et al. (1980). Psychological aspects of long-term home hyperalimentation. *Journal of Parental Enteral Nutrition*, 4, 554–560.

Read A, Sherlock S, Laidlaw J, et al. (1967). The neuro-psychiatric syndromes associated with chronic liver disease and an extensive portal-systemic collateral circulation. *Quarterly Journal of Medicine, 36*, 135–150.

Reichsman F, Engel GL, & Segal HL (1956). A study of an infant with a gastric fistula. *Psychosomatic Medicine, 18*, 374–398.

Reidel WL & Clouse RE (1985). Variations in clinical presentation of patients with esophogeal contraction abnormalities. *Digestive Diseases and Science, 30*, 1065–1071.

Sandberg B & Bliding A (1976). Duodenal ulcer in army trainees during basic military training. *Journal of Psychosomatic Research, 20*, 61–74.

Sapira JD & Cross MR (1982). Prehospitalization life change in gastric ulcer versus duodenal ulcer [Abstract]. *Psychosomatic Medicine, 44*, 121.

Shrivastava RK, Shah BK, Siegal H (1985). Doxepin and cimetidine in the treatment of duodenal ulcer: A double-blind comparative study. *Clinical Therapeutics, 7*, 181–189.

Silverstone PH (1984). Ranitidine and confusion. *Lancet, 1*, 1071.

Sjodin L, Svendlund J, Ottosson JO, et al. (1986). Controlled study of psychotherapy in chronic peptic ulcer disease. *Psychosomatics, 27*, 187–200.

Stoudemire A & Sandhu J (1987). Psychogenic/idiopathic pain syndromes. *General Hospital Psychiatry, 9*, 79–86.

Stracher G, Berner P, Naske R, et al. (1975). Effect of hypnotic suggestion of relaxation on basal and betazole-stimulated gastric acid secretion. *Gastroenterology, 68*, 656–661.

Switz DM (1976). What the gastroenterologist does all day. *Gastroenterology, 70*, 1048–1050.

Tarter RE, Hegedos PM, Van Thiel DH, et al. (1985–1986). Portal-systemic encephalopathy neuropsychiatric manifestations. *International Journal of Psychiatry in Medicine, 15*, 265–275.

Thompson WG (1979). *The irritable gut.* Baltimore: University Park.

Thompson WG & Heaton KW (1980). Functional bowel disorders in apparently healthy people. *Gatroenterology, 79*, 283–288.

Weiner H, Thaler M, Reiser MF, et al. (1957). Etiology of duodenal ulcer I. Relation of specific psychological characteristics to rate of gastric secretion (serum pepsinogen). *Psychosomatic Medicine, 19*, 1.

Whybrow PC, Kane TJ, & Lipton MA (1968). Regional ileitis and psychiatric disorders. *Psychosomatic Medicine, 30*, 209.

Wise TN (1986). Psychological management of IBS. *Practical Gastroenterology, 10*, 40–50.

Wise TN, Cooper JN, & Ahmed S (1982). The efficacy of group therapy for patients with irritable bowel syndrome. *Psychosomatics, 23*, 465–469.

Young SJ, Alpers DH, & Norland CC (1976). Psychiatric illness and the irritable bowel syndrome. *Gastroenterology, 70*, 162–166.

Zisook S & DeVaul RA (1977). Emotional factors in inflammatory bowel disease. *Southern Medical Journal, 70*, 716–719.

Norman B. Levy

27
Chronic Renal Disease, Dialysis, and Transplantation

Since the inception of dialysis and renal transplantation, psychiatrists have been involved in rendering care to patients treated by these procedures. Systematic observations have been made that have led to a reasonable body of data upon which to base clinical interventions. The attraction of psychologically trained professionals to this field has been largely due to the need for help of these patients, who are highly stressed by their illness and by technological therapies.

KIDNEY FAILURE AND ITS METHODS OF TREATMENT

The incidence of renal failure is 200 cases for every million people each year, or about 45,000 Americans or 220,000 Chinese each year. This figure includes renal failure caused by systemic illnesses, such as generalized arteriosclerosis and metastatic cancer, in which the treatment of kidney failure would only prolong the agony of life.

The most common causes of kidney failure are chronic glomerulonephritis, chronic pyelonephritis, the congenital kidney diseases such as polycystic kidney disease and Alport's syndrome, lupus nephritis, and diabetic nephrosclerosis. Most of the illnesses that cause kidney failure are not those of older people, but usually occur in young adults. The two basic treatments for chronic renal failure are kidney transplantation and dialysis.

Renal Transplantation

There are two types of transplantation: from a living donor, who is almost always closely related, and from a cadaver. Kidney survival is greater with living, related donors, but availability makes cadavers the more common source of transplantation. Most cadaveric kidneys are "harvested" from the highways; for this purpose, nephrectomies are performed on recently brain-dead individuals. There is some debate in the transplant community concern-

PRINCIPLES OF MEDICAL PSYCHIATRY
ISBN 0-8089-1883-4

583

ing live *un*related donors, such as the spouse of the patient. Some people believe that such donors need not subject themselves to surgery, since cadaveric kidneys survive almost as well. The issue of commercially available organs from individuals who wanted to sell their kidneys brought an outcry in the United States, and such sales have been banned by federal statute.

Immunosuppressants are used postoperatively to inhibit a foreign-body reaction by the recipient, which would otherwise reject the organ. A major medication used for this is prednisone. Recently cyclosporine has been introduced and has been shown to offer substantial additional suppression of rejection. An essential consideration in its use is its cost, about $5000 per year, which is not covered by Medicare at the time of this writing.

Dialysis

The two forms of dialysis are peritoneal and hemodialysis. In peritoneal dialysis, dialysate fluid is introduced into the peritoneal space via an indwelling catheter and removed by the same pathway. Here, the peritoneum serves as a semipermeable membrane. Peritoneal dialysis may be performed intermittently, by a machine in a hospital, or continuously. Continuous ambulatory peritoneal dialysis (CAPD) is done at home and at work. The patient introduces 2 liters of dialysate fluid 3 to 4 times a day and retrieves the fluid by gravity. Hemodialysis may be performed at centers or at satellite units in which there may be varying degrees of self-care. Home dialysis is carried out in the home of the patient. This procedure requires the participation of a spouse, a parent, another relative, or a friend and requires 4–5 hours 3 days each week.

HEMODIALYSIS AND PERITONEAL DIALYSIS: STRESSES

Peritoneal dialysis and hemodialysis are most unusual procedures. In peritoneal dialysis the patient's belly is filled with fluid, which is then permitted to drain off. In hemodialysis a "lifeline" connects the patient's blood supply to a piece of machinery, and blood flows freely between the living and the mechanical. Both procedures place patients in an unusually dependent position, upon the procedure and the people connected with that procedure (Reichsman & Levy, 1972). Changes in the form of treatment may be made, such as switching from a center to the home or from peritoneal dialysis to hemodialysis or vice versa or from either procedure to transplantation. Most patients, however, continue their treatment by the same procedure that they were initially exposed to at the time of onset of renal failure. When a very independent patient is placed on a form of treatment that does not involve a good deal of self-care, psychologic difficulties may ensue (De-Nour, Shaltiel, & Czaczkes, 1968; Levy, 1976). By contrast, the very dependent patient may have emotional problems if pushed into self-care. Only renal transplantation gives patients an opportunity to approach the kind of life they had prior to renal failure, and it is therefore preferable for individuals who have a great need for independence. Astute and compassionate nephrologists assess the character structure of their patients to determine the best form of treatment for each individual (Czaczkes & De-Nour, 1978). This aspect of care will be discussed in the section of this chapter on treatment.

Patients on dialysis are placed on low-sodium, low-potassium, low-protein, and low-fluid diets. For those on hemodialysis the diets mean the virtual elimination of all fruits and vegetables, the eating of only small amounts of meats and fish, and the cessation of drinking directly from a glass in favor of sucking on cracked ice. Patients on peritoneal dialysis usually are given a more lenient diet, since that procedure is more successful than hemodialysis in removing the wastes resulting from eating and drinking. In either form of treatment, most patients find that their diets place them in situations of deprivation. Some people attempt to handle this deprivation by the use of denial, pushing out of mind the necessity of diet and eating freely. Such noncompliant behavior is evident to dialysis unit staff, who can readily monitor and measure dietary indiscretion by serum potassium levels and weight changes between dialysis runs.

Another stress of dialysis results from the lack of respite from treatment or illness (Levy, 1976). Patients are constantly reminded of their illness by receiving treatment either continually or three times a week, being on a restrictive diet, and having to take medications. Most other chronic illnesses afford their victims some "vacation." Patients with metastatic cancer may have periods of being without symptoms, in which they do not require any radiotherapy or chemotherapy. Patients with cardiac conditions often have long periods of being asymptomatic, even if they are disabled.

Patients on dialysis experience a diminution in ability or interest in sexuality, which will be discussed later in this chapter. These changes can be devastating for some patients and are undesirable for most.

About two-thirds of hemodialysis patients who were employed prior to illness no longer work full time (Gutman, Stead, & Robinson, 1981). Most choose to have themselves determined to be disabled, even though they may engage in some part-time activity, which may be on or "off the books." Since disability payments always are less than earnings from employment, the determination of chronic disability has negative economic effects. In the face of less income, patients also have expenses

for which they may not be compensated by various forms of insurance. These include medications, the use of taxis, telephone toll calls, and special diets. Some of these expenses may be paid by Medicaid for those at or near the poverty line. Patients who do not have the benefit of such payment may be placed under economic stress.

Peritoneal dialysis has some special stresses of its own. This treatment distorts the patient's body by infusing fluid into the abdominal space. Although preliminary data seem to show that, in general, patients well tolerate such changes in their bodies, it may be difficult for more narcissistic patients, invested in their bodies, to experience a change in abdominal girth. Patients on peritoneal dialysis face the pain and inconvenience of recurrent episodes of peritonitis, which require hospitalization at a mean frequency of once every 11 months.

PSYCHOLOGIC COMPLICATIONS OF DIALYSIS

Dialysis patients, like virtually all other chronically ill people, experience anxiety and depression, those most common psychologic symptoms of physical illness (Lefebvre, Nobert, & Crombez, 1972). Anxiety may be present during dialysis runs, particularly in hemodialysis. This is so because hemodialysis involves the circulation of blood continuously through a machine in a procedure that may produce major medical complications. Although medical problems also can occur in peritoneal dialysis, such as infections that produce peritonitis, more dramatic complications can occur during hemodialysis, such as stroke and cardiac emergencies.

Early in the history of hemodialysis, patients were dialyzed over periods of 10 hours for each run, and they tended to sleep or attempt to sleep in dialysis units, which were open during the night in order to enable patients to pass their time by sleeping. Insomnia due to anxiety was an exceedingly common symptom in those days. Anxiety may also be expressed by masturbatory behavior, more commonly occurring in men but not restricted to them. Such activity is a method of handling anxiety by a sexual outlet, much like the masturbation seen in men about to face combat situations during war (Reichsman & Levy, 1972). Anxiety may also be seen in connection with the uncertainty patients have about the future, fear about their sexual performance, and fear about their ability to cope with the stress of dialysis and the expectations of dialysis staff and family (Levy, 1983).

Depressed mood and the depressive syndromes occur frequently in these patients. Since depression is a response to loss, it is understandable that it would occur in these patients, who have had loss of strength, energy, sexual ability, work ability, physical freedom, and life expectancy. The evaluation of dialysis patients for depression is complicated by the fact that the signs and symptoms of renal failure and its treatment may be identical to the vegetative signs and symptoms of depression, such as diminished appetite, dryness of the mouth, constipation, and diminished sexual interest and ability. The presence of depressive affects and changes in sleep pattern are most helpful in selecting candidates for antidepressant drug treatment.

Suicide is much more common among dialysis patients than in the general population and probably is more common than in other chronic diseases (Abram, Moore, & Westervelt, 1971; Haenel, Brunner, & Battegay, 1980). Aside from the special stresses of the procedure, another explanation for its prevalence is that these patients have the means for their demise at hand. They may sever their fistulas and exsanguinate or go on potassium binges and not show up for the next two dialysis runs.

Observations have been made that most men on dialysis experience impotence. The frequency of impotence is in the range of 70 percent of adult male patients (Abram, Hester, Epstein, et al., 1975; Levy, 1973). There are problems in both sexes concerning sexual desire, and in women there is a marked diminution in orgasm during sexual intercourse. Men and women both have a marked decrease in frequency of sexual intercourse after being dialyzed, in comparison with their frequency before becoming uremic.

The cause of these sexual problems is not well understood, but they are probably due to physical illness as well as its psychologic complications. Tests of nocturnal penile tumescence suggests a high prevalence of organic, as opposed to purely psychologic, impotence in these patients (Procci, Goldstein, Kletzky, et al., 1983). The cause of the organic sexual impairment is not fully understood. There is a decrease in testosterone and an increase in other hormones, but not enough to explain the extent of patients' sexual difficulties (Antoniou & Shalhoub, 1978; Lim, Auletta, & Kathpolia, 1978; Massry, Goldstein, Procci, et al., 1977). An iatrogenic cause of sexual dysfunction is connected with the use of antihypertensives that may diminish libido in both men and women and cause impotence. Psychologic factors that cause impotence include depression, reversal of family roles, and feelings related to the cessation of urination in male patients (Levy, 1983).

The frequent work disability of male patients often forces the spouse either to return to work or to increase her outside work activity. This places the male patient in a situation of having to participate to a greater extent in household activities such as shopping, cleaning house, and caring for the children. For many patients this is quite acceptable. For many others, however, especially those who are insecure about their masculinity, such a reversal of family roles may lead to feelings of inadequacy and emasculation.

Most patients on dialysis have total cessation of urination. Since the organ of urination in the male is the same as that of sexuality, there may be major psychologic ramifications to having the most often used function of this organ completely stopped (De-Nour, 1969). Here, too, in the more tenuously masculine individual, such a change may be seen as a major blow to his male identity and may affect sexual function. (See also Chapter 13, by Fagan and Schmidt, on sexual dysfunction in the medically ill.)

Uncooperativeness is an important psychologic component and complication for these patients (Levy, 1980). Unfortunately, it is a complication that occurs not infrequently and is a source of stress for the dialysis staff. Questionable "uncooperativeness" may be seen in connection with the desire of patients to challenge the wisdom of procedures and to request other opinions. At times behavior may be unquestionably uncooperative, as in the neglect of diet, the failure to take medication, missed dialysis runs, and the making of openly hostile expressions, such as threats and physical attacks on dialysis staff. Much of this uncooperativeness may reflect displaced anger, with professional caretakers a convenient and relatively safe target.

Organic mental disorders occur in a variety of situations. Patients involved in intellectual activity, especially in a work setting, will tend to note progressive impairment as their day for dialysis approaches. After dialysis they often experience a short period of delirium termed *disequilibrium syndrome*, caused by the rapid change of fluid and electrolytes that has taken place during the dialysis run. This syndrome may last from minutes to hours.

Among the most serious organic mental disorders seen in dialysis patients is *dialysis encephalopathy*. This is an often fatal neurologic syndrome that may occur in patients who have been on hemodialysis for at least 2 years. The early signs are dysarthria, stuttering speech, memory impairment, depression, and psychosis. Patients often develop bizarre limb movements, asterixis, and generalized tremulousness. The disease is progressive and leads to a neurologic death if not successfully treated. Its cause is not fully understood. Aluminum, from trace amounts in dialysate water and from phosphate binding gels, is the most likely culprit (Alfrey, 1986). There are conflicting data, however, concerning aluminum toxicity, since aluminum tends to be present in higher-than-normal quantities in the brain in other, nonrenal dementias, including Alzheimer's disease. Trace amounts of tin and zinc have also been blamed as a cause of this syndrome. The electroencephalogram (EEG) is the most useful diagnostic test for this syndrome, showing typical slow-wave bursts in the early stages (Alfrey, 1986). Treatment of dialysis encephalopathy may include chelation therapy with deferoxamine, reduction in dose of aluminum-containing phosphate binding gels, and use of deionized water (free of aluminum traces) to prepare dialysis solutions. Early cases may be reversible with this treatment (Alfrey, 1986; O'Hare, Callaghan, & Murnaghan, 1983). The psychiatric treatment should address the symptomatic manifestations. Antidepressant and antipsychotic medications should therefore be used when depressive or psychotic syndromes appear.

RENAL TRANSPLANTATION

Renal transplantation is a preferred treatment for exceedingly independent patients. In addition, many nephrologists believe that diabetics are better treated with transplantation than with dialysis, although the transplant procedure itself is associated with a greater morbidity and mortality in diabetic patients. Children, who compose less than 1 percent of the total number of people with renal failure, tend to be better off developmentally with transplantation. Patients who have an identical twin who is in good health are most assured of success in receiving the donated kidney from their twin sibling, without the use either of steroids or of cyclosporine. If one asks nephrologists what method of treatment they would want if stricken with renal failure, they respond, "A live, related donor, if well matched with me." This response can be readily understood because a successful transplantation is the only treatment that can give the patient a life much like that experienced prior to the onset of renal failure. The factors that interfere with the delivery of this form of treatment for a majority of patients with renal failure are the short supplies of available kidneys, both live and cadaveric, and the small number of transplant surgeons (Fox & Swazey, 1974).

The Donor

The selection of the donor is a very difficult matter for the patient with renal failure to handle. The patient expects that people will come forth by themselves, certainly without any personal coaxing. Fortunately, this is usually the case, and it is uncommon for patients with renal failure to confront relatives with their need for the other's kidney. Such a request is usually made by an intermediary person, such as a family member or a physician. Some interesting and unusual things take place in the selection of donors (Fellner & Marshall, 1968). Mothers often want to donate their kidneys to their children, to enable the child to have an opportunity for a new life. At times the "black sheep," usually a sibling of the patient, is selected by the family to undo past badness by making the sacrifice of undergoing surgery and kidney donation.

The decision to donate a kidney is often a very spontaneous one, seemingly without much thought or deliberation as to its consequences, inconvenience, pain, or complications. There has been some debate in renal circles about the long-term complications of a kidney donation (Simmons, 1981; Simmons, Klein, & Simmons, 1977). There is no evidence, however, that having only one kidney places the donor in greater danger of either hypertension or kidney failure.

Preoperatively, the donor is in a situation of being near center stage, as a person whose generosity may make it possible for the patient to lead a new life. Postoperatively, the donor leaves center stage and is replaced by the recipient. Some donors experience a period of "blues" as they perceive what they think is ingratitude in the recipients' preoccupation with their own lives and with the survival of the new kidney. In a follow-up of 130 related donors, it was reported that, in addition to rapidly making the decision to donate, the great majority had no difficulty in coming to that decision and expressed gratification in being donors (Simmons, 1981). Twenty percent of recipients, however, experience unhappiness at never being able to repay the donor in an equivalent manner. If the donor is a male, especially if married, there tends to be some dissatisfaction in having made a donation. If the kidney is viable after a year, there tends to be less dissatisfaction with donation. Remarkably, only 18 percent of donors of rejected kidneys expressed dissatisfaction at having given their kidney for transplantation (Simmons, 1981).

In the case of a cadaveric kidney, matters are a good deal different. As previously mentioned, these kidneys are harvested on the highways from young, brain-dead adults. Like an adopted child in respect to his biologic parents, the recipient is not told much about the donor, usually only the age and sex. Also, like an adopted child, some recipients become very curious about the identity of the donor and may pursue the matter by reading old newspaper articles about automobile accidents and interviewing nurses and other medical people involved in their receiving the kidney. At times recipients experience survivor guilt at having reaped a reward out of the misfortune of another. Psychologic reactions to transplantation are also discussed in Chapter 19 by Riether and Stoudemire.

Organ Rejection or Acceptance

A number of investigators have examined the idea that psychologic factors may play a role in either acceptance or rejection of donated organs (Basch, 1973; Muslin, 1971). It has been reported (Viederman, 1974) that a patient had an organ rejection probably resulting from having given up psychologically. In another study (Eisendrath, 1967), 8 of 11 patients who died following transplant surgery had experienced a sense of pessimism and panic about their transplant to a degree not observed in the surviving recipients. Steinberg, Levy, and Radvila (1981) attempted to test the notion that there is a connection between psychologic acceptance or rejection and physiologic acceptance or rejection by interviewing 26 consecutive recipients and their donors. In a prospective study, an attempt was made to rate the recipients' psychologic acceptance or rejection of the organ. The absence of ambivalence toward the impending surgery and about the donor, realistic expectations concerning the future, reasonable optimism concerning the upcoming operative procedure, and the relative lack of serious psychologic symptoms were considered to favor acceptance of the donated organ. Based on this system, statistical significance was not shown between the predicted outcome, organ rejection or acceptance, and the actual outcome in a one-year follow-up of these individuals.

Postoperative Psychologic Problems

Recipients of kidney transplants have a Sword of Damocles hanging over them in that they live in the shadow of possible organ rejection. The natural forces of the body work to reject foreign substances. The body responds with great vigor to "protect" itself against the transplanted kidney. As time goes on and rejection is not experienced, the recipient feels relieved. The recipient is never, however, completely safe from the possibility of rejection. Also, many diseases causing renal failure can recur in the transplanted kidney, causing another risk to the success of the transplant. Finally, cyclosporine and some antibiotics used to treat opportunistic infections are themselves nephrotoxic. In addition to this stress, the medications needed may cause difficulty. This is particularly true of prednisone, which has to be taken for the rest of the patient's life, initially in large doses and later in relatively small ones. The numerous medical and psychiatric complications of prednisone therapy are well known. Patients with a past personal history of depression or with dysthymic symptoms are more vulnerable to developing a major depressive disorder while receiving prednisone (Levy, 1986). Patients with a history of psychosis or with borderline personalities are more vulnerable to psychosis. These psychiatric complications of steroids should be treated symptomatically. Antidepressant, antipsychotic, and antimanic medications should be given if symptoms warrant them (Levy, 1985). Cyclosporine has not yet been associated with psychiatric side effects, although it has been associated with seizures and tremors, suggesting an effect on the brain. (Canadian Multicenter Transplant Study Group, 1986).

Patients who develop severe psychiatric side effects from steroids might be candidates for immunosuppression with cyclosporine, as cyclosporine-treated patients require less prednisone and azathioprine (Canadian Multicenter Transplant Study Group, 1986). In general, cyclosporine deserves consideration in transplant recipients with severe steroid side effects of any level (Amend, Suthanthiram, & Gambertoglio, 1986).

Patients on prednisone and other immunosuppresants after transplantation are vulnerable to opportunistic infections or may have bacterial infections with fewer systemic signs than usual. New psychiatric symptoms in transplant recipients, particularly if accompanied by cognitive deficit, indicate careful screening for infectious diseases. The psychiatrist's role in initiating the workup is to identify the patient's mental symptoms as being of probable organic origin. When the mental status examination leaves the issue of organic etiology unclear, an EEG may help. (See Chapter 3, by Fogel and Faust, on neurologic assessment.)

The sexual function of patients undergoing renal transplantation is impaired in comparison with function prior to kidney failure, but is usually much better than it was while the patients were on dialysis (Levy, 1973; Salvatierra, Fortmann, & Belzer, 1975). Since posttransplant kidney function may vary, especially in cases of rejection, sexual function may be dependent upon the degree of renal function of the individual. In one study, 46 percent of 56 male transplant patients were either partially or totally impotent (Levy, 1973). The cause of sexual dysfunction in these individuals is not clearly understood, but organic factors seem to be greatly implicated because of hormonal and other changes in renal failure (Procci et al., 1983).

PSYCHOLOGIC TREATMENT CONSIDERATIONS

The psychiatrist's evaluation of the personality and family structure of patients assists in tailoring medical treatment to their psychologic needs. The independent patient should be treated in a self-care hemodialysis unit, with CAPD, or with home hemodialysis, or should receive a transplantation. The narcissistic patient who is very concerned about body shape and appearance should not receive peritoneal dialysis. The patient who is phobic of blood should not be treated by hemodialysis. Since the family plays an essential role in home hemodialysis, in order for such treatment to take place, there needs to be not only sufficient physical space for the machine at the patient's home, but also a consistent supportive "significant other" who is relatively unambivalent about helping with the treatment.

Patients with renal failure should be told that they may develop such problems as depression or sexual dysfunction. If so prepared, the patient, in the face of the presentation of these problems, will tend to see them as complications of treatment and will more readily call them to professional attention (Levy, 1984).

In the case of renal transplantation, patients should be prepared to confront themselves with the complications of prednisone therapy and the continuing threat of possible organ rejection. At times, psychiatric assessment of patients will contribute to a decision not to transplant the patient, because the patient is excessively prone to psychosis or severe depression with prednisone therapy. At other times patients who are at high risk for psychotic reactions postoperatively are transplanted and are carefully monitored by the psychiatrist, with early institution of antipsychotic medication when the early signs of psychosis appear.

The most common specific therapy for the psychologic complications of dialysis and transplantation is medical psychotherapy with or without the use of psychotropic medications. It is important to keep in mind that these patients as a group tend to be deniers of psychologic difficulty and that when a call for help is heard from them there is great need for a rapid response to it. Group therapy has had mixed results in these patients. When successful, this therapy tends to be directed more toward education than uncovering, and is time-limited. A factor of importance in any therapy of these patients is that they feel very much "overdoctored," spending many hours a week with the dialysis procedure. Any form of psychotherapy will have greater success if it takes place in conjunction with clinic visits or dialysis runs (Freyberger, 1983). Psychotherapists may therefore find themselves conducting sessions in a unit in which there is no sound barrier between the patient and others. This situation should not dissuade therapists from continuing, since often the combination of respect for privacy and the involvement of others in their own worlds essentially gives confidentiality of communication, even when the sound of conversation is there to be heard.

Hypnotherapy may help patients deal with problems of pain, appetite, and fluid intake control if they have adequate hypnotic capacity. Patients with active major depression or organic disorders, however, tend to be poor hypnotic subjects.

In the case of sexual dysfunction, careful consideration should be given to the use of behavioral sexual techniques, as described in Chapter 13, by Fagan and Schmidt. Such techniques are based on the fact that people who have sexual dysfunctions tend to withdraw altogether from sexual situations and even avoid non-sexual intimacy with their partners (McKevitt, 1976). This therapy encourages a closeness of partners and attempts to restore sexuality (Berkman, 1978). This restoration is accomplished by assuring the partners that the goal of sexuality is not necessarily intercourse. By sensate focusing and other techniques, patients who have lost confidence in themselves may be able to function better sexually.

The use of psychotropics can and should be an important part of the psychologic treatment of these patients (Levy, 1985). With the exception of barbiturates, almost all psychotropic medicines can be used (Bennett, Muther, Parker, et al., 1980). The problem with barbiturates is that dialysis may produce a withdrawal syndrome due to a sudden drop in barbiturate levels with dialysis. Even lithium, which is both dialyzable and removed by the kidneys, can be used by carefully monitoring blood levels and by giving a single dose, usually 600 mg, after each dialysis run (Lippmann, Manshadi, & Gultekin, 1984; Port, Kroll, & Rosenzweig, 1979; Procci, 1977). Since it is removed by the kidney, in patients who have no kidney function, serum levels should remain constant until lithium is again removed by dialysis. See also Chapter 4 by Stoudemire and Fogel for further discussion of the use of lithium in the medically ill.

A general guideline is that two-thirds of a dosage of a medication given to those with normal kidney function should be given to kidney failure patients. Blood levels of psychotropics should then be obtained if the response is poor or severe side effects develop. With drugs, such as nortriptyline, with a well-established therapeutic range, routine blood levels are justifiable and can be obtained weekly at the time of dialysis until the patient is stabilized clinically. In the choice of medications for these patients, it is best to use those with which there has been great experience in patients with renal failure. Most renal pharmacologists recommend that the monoamine oxidase inhibitors be used with great caution because of their possibility of producing hypertensive episodes. In the case of the use of benzodiazepines, preference should be given to those that have inactive metabolites, such as lorazepam and oxazepam (Brater, 1983).

REFERENCES

Abram HS, Hester LR, Epstein GM, et al. (1975). Sexual functioning in patients with chronic renal failure. *Journal of Nervous and Mental Disease*, *166*, 220–226.

Abram HS, Moore GL, & Westervelt FB, Jr (1971). Suicidal behavior in chronic dialysis patients. *American Journal of Psychiatry*, *127*, 1199–1204.

Alfrey A (1986). Dialysis encephalopathy. *Kidney International*, *29*(Suppl), S-53–S-57.

Amend WJC, Suthanthiram M, & Gambertoglio JG (1986). Immunosuppression following renal transplantation. In MR Gorovy & RD Guttman RD (Eds.). *Renal transplantation*. New York: Churchill Livingstone, pp 73–92.

Antoniou LD & Shalhoub RJ (1978). Zinc in the treatment of impotence in chronic renal failure. *Dialysis and Transplantation*, *7*, 912–915.

Basch SH (1973). The intrapsychic integration of a new organ: A clinical study of kidney transplantation. *Psychoanalytic Quarterly*, *42*, 364–384.

Bennett WM, Muther RS, Parker RA, et al. (1980). Drug therapy in renal failure: Dosing guidelines for adults: 2. Sedatives, hypnotics and tranquilizers; cardiovascular, antihypertensive, and diuretic agents; miscellaneous agents. *Annals of Internal Medicine*, *93*, 286–325.

Berkman A (1978). Sex counseling with hemodialysis patients. *Dialysis and Transplantation*, *7*, 924.

Brater DC (1983). *Drug use in renal disease*. Sydney, Australia: Aidis Health Science Press.

Canadian Multicenter Transplant Study Group (1986). A randomized clinical trial of cyclosporine in cadaveric renal transplantation. *New England Journal of Medicine*, *314*, 1219–1225.

Czaczkes JW & DeNour AK (1978). *Chronic hemodialysis as a way of life*. New York: Brunner/Mazel.

De-Nour AK, Shaltiel J, & Czaczkes JW (1968). Emotional reactions of patients on chronic hemodialysis. *Psychosomatic Medicine*, *30*, 521–533.

DeNour AK (1969). Some notes on the psychological significance of urination. *Journal of Nervous and Mental Disease*, *148*, 615–623.

Eisendrath RM (1967). The role of grief and fear in the death of transplant patients. *American Journal of Psychiatry*, *126*, 381–387.

Fellner CH & Marshall JR (1968). Twelve kidney donors. *Journal of the American Medical Association*, *206*, 2703–2707.

Fox RC & Swazey JP (1974). *The courage to fail: A social view of organ transplants and dialysis*. Chicago: University of Chicago Press.

Freyberger H (1983). The renal transplant patients: Three-stage model and psychotherapeutic strategies. In NB Levy (Ed), *Psychonephrology 2: Psychological problems in kidney failure and their treatment* (pp 259–265). New York: Plenum.

Gutman RA, Stead W, & Robinson RR (1981). Physical activity and employment status of patients on maintenance dialysis. *New England Journal of Medicine*, *304*, 309–313.

Haenel T, Brunner F, & Battegay R (1980). Renal dialysis and suicide: Occurrence in Switzerland and Europe. *Comprehensive Psychiatry*, *21*, 140–145.

Lefebvre P, Nobert A, & Crombez JC (1972). Psychological and psychopathological reactions in relation to chronic hemodialysis. *Canadian Psychiatric Association Journal*, *17*, 9–13.

Levy NB (1973). Sexual adjustment to maintenance hemodialysis and transplantation: National survey of questionnaire. *Transactions; American Society for Artificial Internal Organs*, *19*, 138–142.

Levy NB (1976). Coping with maintenance hemodialysis—psychological considerations in the care of patients. In SG Massry & AL Sellers (Eds), *Clinical aspects of uremia and dialysis* (pp 53–68). Springfield, IL: Charles C Thomas.

Levy NB (1980). The "uncooperative" patient with ESRD, causes and treatment. *Proceedings of the European Dialysis and Transplantation Association*, *17*, 523–530.

Levy NB (1983). Sexual dysfunctions of hemodialysis. *Clinical and Experimental Dialysis and Apheresis*, *7*, 275–288.

Levy NB (1984). Psychological complications of dialysis: Psychonephrology to the rescue. *Bulletin of the Menninger Clinic*, *48*, 237–250.

Levy NB (1985). Use of psychotropics in patients with kidney failure. *Psychosomatics*, *26*, 669–709.

Levy NB (1986). Renal transplantation and the new medical era. *Advances in Psychosomatic Medicine*, *15*, 167–179.

Lim VS, Auletta F, & Kathpolia S (1978). Gonadal dysfunction in chronic renal failure: An endocrinological review. *Dialysis and Transplantation*, *7*, 896.

Lippmann SB, Manshadi MS, & Gultekin A (1984). Lithium in a patient with renal failure on hemodialysis [Letter]. *Journal of Clinical Psychiatry*, *45*, 444.

Massry SG, Goldstein DA, Procci WR, et al. (1977). Impotence in patients with uremia: A possible role for parathyroid hormone. *Nephron*, *19*, 305–310.

McKevitt PM (1976). Treating sexual dysfunction in dialysis and transplant patients. *Health and Social Work*, *1*, 133.

Muslin HL (1976). On acquiring a kidney. *American Journal of Psychiatry, 127,* 1185–1188.

O'Hare JA, Callaghan NM, & Murnaghan DJ (1983). Dialysis encephalopathy. *Medicine, 62,* 129–141.

Port FK, Kroll PD, & Rosenzweig J (1979). Lithium therapy during maintenance hemodialysis. *Psychosomatics, 20,* 130–132.

Procci WR (1977). Mania during maintenance hemodialysis successfully treated with oral lithium carbonate. *Journal of Nervous and Mental Disease, 164,* 355–358.

Procci WR, Goldstein DA, Kletzky OA, et al. (1983). Impotence in uremia: Preliminary results of a combined medical and psychiatric investigation. In NB Levy (Ed), *Psychonephrology 2: Psychological problems in kidney failure and their treatment* (pp 235–246). New York: Plenum.

Reichsman F & Levy NB (1972). Problems in adaptation to maintenance hemodialysis: A four-year study of 25 patients. *Archives of Internal Medicine, 130,* 850–865.

Salvatierra O, Fortmann JL, & Belzer FO (1975). Sexual function in males before and after transplantation. *Urology 5,* 64–66.

Simmons RG (1981). Psychological reactions to giving a kidney. In NB Levy (Ed), *Psychonephrology 1: Psychological factors in hemodialysis and transplantation* (pp 227–245). New York: Plenum.

Simmons RG, Klein SD & Simmons RL (1977). *Gift of life: The social and psychological impact of organ transplantation.* New York: Wiley Interscience.

Steinberg J, Levy NB, & Radvila A (1981). Psychological factors affecting acceptance or rejection of kidney transplants. In NB Levy (Ed), *Psychonephrology 1: Psychological factors in hemodialysis and transplantation* (pp 185–217). New York: Plenum.

Viederman M (1974). The search for meaning in renal transplantation. *Psychiatry, 37,* 283–290.

Michael G. Moran

28
Connective Tissue Diseases

Formerly referred to as the collagen vascular diseases, the connective tissue diseases comprise rheumatoid arthritis, systemic lupus erythematosus, scleroderma, Sjogren's syndrome, various other forms of arthritis, polymyositis, polymyalgia rheumatica, and various vasculitides. Their common clinical features include involvement of connective tissue manifested by inflammation, small vessel damage, serosal surface inflammation, and frequent involvement of the heart, lung, and kidneys. The etiology of many of these illnesses is unknown, but in almost all, autoimmune processes have been implicated, and the laboratory features and diagnosis usually entail the demonstration of immunologic abnormalities. Although the inciting immunologic events are largely unknown, subsequent steps in immunologic pathogenic mechanisms include the formation of antigen–antibody complexes that fix complement, followed by the influx of cellular components of the inflammatory response. Vascular damage and tissue destruction result. The symptoms of the various diseases coincide with the involvement of specific organs or organ systems

and can be quite varied; diagnostic accuracy can be elusive until findings characteristic of the particular disease appear (Rodnan, 1973).

Neuropsychiatric manifestations of these diseases are complex. There are three categorical presentations: direct involvement of, for example, the central nervous system, with affective disturbances, delirium, or other organic mental disorders; psychologic sequelae of the patient's awareness of the illness or its impact; and psychiatric side effects of the drugs used to treat the illness.

LABORATORY DIAGNOSIS IN THE CONNECTIVE TISSUE DISEASES

Although the laboratory findings specific to each disease will be discussed in the sections on the individual illnesses, some general introduction to these tests may be helpful. For the psychiatrist presented with a patient who has psychiatric symptoms, and in whom a connective tissue disease is

PRINCIPLES OF MEDICAL PSYCHIATRY
ISBN 0-8089-1883-4

595

suspected, history and physical findings, as in any other clinical setting, should guide the selection of laboratory tests ordered.

Changes in serum proteins termed *acute phase reactants* are associated with elevation of the *erythrocyte sedimentation rate* (ESR). Elevated ESR is a nonspecific finding that may serve as a rough guide to the activity of several connective tissue diseases: rheumatoid arthritis, systemic lupus erythematosus (SLE), giant cell arteritis, polymyalgia rheumatica, and the vasculitides.

As mentioned before, many of these diseases are felt to be mediated by immunologic changes characterized by the development of antibodies to various self components, such as intranuclear structures. When the antibodies react with appropriate antigen, immune complexes can be formed, with activation of the *complement* sequence. Levels determined reflect an equilibrium between rates of synthesis and catabolism. Serum levels of complement can serve as a rough guide to disease activity most reliably in SLE. All three commonly obtainable assays (CH_{50}, C_4, and C_3) are low in SLE. In drug-induced lupus, complement levels are normal (Volanakis, 1986).

When the clinical picture puts systemic lupus erythematosus in the differential, one thinks of tests to determine the presence of *antinuclear antibody*, of which the LE assay, or "LE prep," was the first. Because of its lack of sensitivity and specificity, it is no longer recommended as a screening test. Fluorescent antinuclear antibody assays (FANA) yield a visual picture of the autoantibody specificity: the nuclei of the patient's test cells fluoresce with patterns categorized as diffuse, speckled, rim, and nucleolar. The rim pattern is associated with antibodies to double-stranded DNA and is most specific for SLE. The nucleolar pattern has been correlated with antibodies to RNA and is seen in scleroderma. Speckled or homogeneous patterns appear in pa-

tients with drug-induced lupus syndromes. Diffuse or homogeneous patterns reflect antibodies to single-stranded DNA. One can also order specific determinations of serum antibodies to double- or single-stranded DNA or, when drug-induced lupus is suspected, to histones (another intranuclear component) (Pincus, 1986).

When evaluating patients whose clinical picture is predominantly arthritic, the physician may want to reconsider rheumatoid arthritis. *Rheumatoid factor* is a term that designates autoantibodies of several classes that react with the Fc portion of autologous IgG. It is a common finding in classical rheumatoid arthritis; its presence is associated with several distinctive clinical features (discussed later). One simply orders "rheumatoid factor"; results are given as titers.

Muscle destruction and inflammation play an important role in some connective tissue diseases, such as polymyositis. Evidence of such inflammation can be found in the serum: intracellular muscle enzymes are liberated by cellular destruction. Aldolase and creatine phosphokinase (CPK) are the tests most commonly ordered. One should ask for "fractionated" CPK. MM patterns reflect CPK of skeletal muscle origin.

SYSTEMIC LUPUS ERYTHEMATOSUS

When the American Rheumatism Association offered criteria for the classification of systemic lupus erythematosus (SLE), it tried to bring order to the understanding of a protean illness. The clinical presentations of the disease are varied and include skin rash (especially the classic malar erythematous rash), polyarthralgias and arthritis, serositis (pericarditis and pleurisy), renal, cardiac, and neurologic abnormalities, and anemia and thrombocytopenia (Tan, 1985) (see Table 28-1).

Table 28-1
Revised Criteria for Classification of SLE

Criterion	Prevalence (%)
Malar rash	57
Discoid rash	18
Photosensitivity	43
Oral ulcers	27
Arthritis	86
Serositis	56
Renal disorder	51
Neurologic disorder	20
Hematologic disorders	59
Immunologic disorder	85
Antinuclear antibody	95

Source: Ball GV (1986). Systemic lupus erythematosus (SLE). In GV Ball & WJ Koopman (Eds), *Clinical rheumatology*. Philadelphia: WB Saunders.
The presence of any four criteria makes the diagnosis.

Women are at much greater risk for contracting SLE then are men, with the prevalence ratio about 8:1. Female sex hormones may modulate the immune response in such a way as to increase the risk of SLE. Increased products of estrone hydroxylation have been found in both male and female SLE patients (Ball, 1986).

In general, non-Caucasian races have a higher prevalence of SLE than Caucasians. Orientals are at three times the risk of Caucasians for getting the disease. Of all groups, black women are at highest risk, being about three to four times more likely to contract SLE than age-matched female controls.

Familial susceptibility seen in SLE seems genetic in etiology. Environmental factors do not appear to be of prime importance in accounting for the frequent patterns of SLE occurrence among close relatives. In one survey of 225 SLE patients, 24 percent had relatives with the disease or another autoimmune illness. Relatives without overt symptoms often have abnormal laboratory immunologic profiles (Ball & Koopman, 1986). Some HLA tissue types (HLA-DR2, HLA-DR3, and HLA-DQ1) have a frequent association with SLE and with certain specific complement component deficiencies (Ahearn, Provost, Dorsch, et al., 1982).

Pathogenesis

Although incompletely understood, the pathogenesis of SLE has been attributed for some time to deposition of circulating immune complexes in the walls of the vessels of affected organs, such as the glomerular vessels of the kidney. Deposition is followed by activation of the complement system, which produces a specific type of cellular inflammatory response that disrupts the vascular structure and lumen. Tissues supplied by the vessels and subject to perivascular inflammation suffer nutrient and oxygen deficits and infarction, causing organ malfunction. Organs involved in this manner in SLE include skin, joints, serous membranes, kidneys, and the nervous system. As will be discussed later, there may be specific instances in which the vascular impairments themselves are not solely responsible for organ malfunction.

Another possible mechanism is the deposition of circulating antigen in the vessel wall, followed by binding of specific antibody, then activation of the complement system and appearance of the inflammatory response. Such a sequence would explain the lack of association between levels of *circulating* immune complexes and the degree of disease activity during exacerbations of SLE (Ball & Koopman, 1986). Laboratory detection of the antibodies specific to components of the cell nucleus, or antinuclear antibodies (ANA), is considered a hallmark of SLE and forms the basis of several important screening tests for the disease.

Laboratory Diagnosis

Autoantibodies have been demonstrated to most of the major known components of the cell nucleus. The LE cell phenomenon is the result of the interaction between antibodies to deoxyribonucleoprotein and the exposed contents of cell nuclei; this reactive mixture is then phagocytized by a polymorphonuclear leukocyte. The distended leukocyte is the LE cell (Hargraves, Richmond, & Morton, 1948). Although it is a relatively easy test to perform, it is neither sensitive nor specific in the diagnosis of SLE. Between 50 to 75 percent of SLE patients will demonstrate the LE cell phenomenon. This test is no longer recommended as a screening test for SLE (Tan, 1985).

The fluorescent antinuclear antibody test (FANA) is much more sensitive as a screening test, being positive in almost all patients with systemic lupus. Titers above 1:160, when associated with clinical signs of disease, are clinically significant and suggest the need for obtaining anti-DNA antibodies for confirmation of the diagnosis of SLE. The homogeneous pattern is common, but has no diagnostic specificity. When FANA is positive in rheumatoid arthritis patients, the pattern is usually speckled, and the titer is low (1:160 to 1:320). Rim patterns, at any titer, are suggestive of the diagnosis of SLE and should also prompt the ordering of anti-DNA antibodies. Among asymptomatic and clinically normal persons, the FANA test is positive at a rate of 2–5 percent; false positives are more common in the elderly. In clinically normal individuals with positive ANA, titers are usually low (less than 1:80) (Pincus, 1986).

A test more specific for systemic lupus detects the presence of antibodies to double-stranded DNA (Ceppelini, Polli, & Celada, 1957). Although only 50–80 percent of SLE patients have the antibodies to double-stranded DNA, the occurrence of these antibodies is seen so seldom in other conditions as to make their presence diagnostic of SLE.

Antibodies to histones (intranuclear polypeptides) are present in about half of all patients with lupus, and in about 75 percent of patients with drug-induced lupus (Pincus, 1986).

Rheumatoid factor is present in a small number of lupus patients (Stage & Mannik, 1973). Almost all patients will demonstrate an elevated erythrocyte sedimentation rate (ESR), which varies somewhat with the activity of the illness. Severe anemia and serum protein abnormalities can also alter the ESR. About 20 percent of SLE patients have a chronic biologic false-positive test for syphilis; it may be positive years before other manifestations of the disease.

The clinician faced with the possible diagnosis of SLE should start with the FANA, since it is the best screening tool. Antibodies to double-stranded DNA confirm the diagnosis, although they are not always present.

Psychiatric Aspects of SLE

Systemic lupus erythematosus is of unknown etiology and is complex, poorly predictable, and often inexorable in its progression. It results in debility, economic suffering, pain, and death. Although it affects up to one million Americans, most people have never heard of it and have no experience with it. One would be hard put to construct a disease that would more severely test the psychologic defenses of its victims. As an understandable consequence, neuropsychiatric complications significantly prolong the medical hospitalizations of these patients (Hall, Stickney, & Gardner, 1981).

The literature on the psychiatric aspects of SLE is confusing; nomenclature varies regarding psychosis, organic brain syndrome, delirium, and "toxic reactions" (Hall et al, 1981; O'Connor, 1959; Stern & Robbins, 1960). Few studies are prospective examinations of the patients. Many are simple chart reviews. In addition, figures for the prevalence of neuropsychiatric disease often omit affective disturbances, such as depressive responses (adjustment disorder with depressed mood, organic mood syndrome, major depressive disorder). Studies are often small, consisting of 20 or fewer patients. Most surveys report the incidence of neuropsychiatric symptoms in SLE as being between 33 and 60 percent (Ball, 1986; Hall et al., 1981; O'Connor, 1959), higher when affective disorders are included. The psychiatrist who wants a firm grasp on the neuropsychiatric aspects of SLE must often make extrapolations from studies of other rheumatic diseases, especially rheumatoid arthritis, about which much has been written. SLE makes cameo appearances in tables and charts outlining medical problems that present with psychiatric symptoms, but rarely gets full attention (Lipkin, 1985).

In some centers, the most common causes of death in lupus patients are neurologic; examples are status epilepticus and intracranial bleeding (Leonhardt, 1966; Rodnan, 1973). Many of the neurologic complications of lupus have psychiatric implications.

From a descriptive standpoint, the clinical presentations of the neuropsychiatric aspects of lupus fall into four categories: delirium, depressive syndromes, seizures, and peripheral nervous system disorders. Each will be discussed in turn, along with aspects of etiology and treatment.

Delirium

The severity of delirium seen in SLE patients can vary widely, from a mildly disturbed level of consciousness and concentration to profound disorganization with agitation and hallucinations. In the literature prior to the advent of DSM-III, some functional psychotic conditions were grouped, along with the severe deliria, under the rubric "psychoses" (O'Connor, 1959; Stern & Robbins, 1960). Lupus itself affects the central nervous system directly, although the mechanisms of symptom production are not always clear. Arteriolar and venular lesions can themselves cause tissue damage, infarcts, and bleeding, as described earlier. An altered blood–brain barrier may permit the entry of antibodies into the brain, with resultant pathogenic interactions with neurons (Zvaifler, 1986). Lupus cerebritis may occur in this fashion.

The most common differential diagnostic problem with delirium in the SLE patient is delineating whether the delirium is secondary to an exacerbation of the primary disease ("lupus cerebritis") or to central nervous system (CNS) infection, metabolic derangement, or corticosteroid side effects. A thorough history, physical examination, and mental status examination early in the course provides a baseline with which subsequent examinations can be compared. Workup of the delirium should include vital signs, a metabolic profile such as SMA-20, and a lumbar puncture with cerebrospinal fluid cell count, glucose, protein, and IgG, and cultures for bacterial and nonbacterial infections.

Diagnosis of CNS lupus as the cause of the delirium must generally follow a thorough search for other causes. There are no specific markers for CNS lupus. Clinically, presentations include meningitis with sterile CSF, and cerebral dysfunction secondary to vasculitis, hemorrhage, or infarct. In contradistinction to some authors' opinions (Lipkin, 1985), serum markers of vasculitic or general disease activity, such as sedimentation rate, ANA titer, or complement level, are not helpful in positively incriminating SLE in the etiology of the CNS symptoms. There may be a diagnostically helpful association, however, between CNS lupus and thrombocytopenia, appearance of new systemic symptoms of lupus coincident with the appearance of the delirium, new dermal vasculitic lesions, and elevation of IgG in the cerebrospinal fluid (Zvaifler, 1986). The EEG is rarely specific; delirium of almost any cause produces diffuse slowing. The cerebrospinal fluid in CNS lupus is generally normal. There are no pathognomonic findings. There may be a mild pleocytosis (usually fewer than 50 mononuclear cells) and a slight elevation of protein (usually less than 80 mg percent per 100 ml).

The treatment of delirium caused by CNS lupus is to give corticosteroids, or to increase the dosage if the patient is already taking them. If steroids have already been increased at the time of the consultation, but the symptoms of delirium preceded the dosage increase, the patient should be observed for a few days at the increased dose, in the hope that the delirium will remit. Acute management of the agitation and psychotic symptoms can be achieved with low doses of neuroleptics. Failure to respond should prompt further historical, physical, and laboratory examination. (See Chapter 6 for a comprehensive discussion of the general topic of delirium and its management. The focus here will be on those features of the differential diagnosis of delirium that have special relevance for the SLE patient.)

Delirium that is due to corticosteroid side effects usually follows a change in dosage, generally a dosage increase. Confusion, alterations in the personality, and occasionally mood changes are seen. The history of recent initiation or increase in dosage of steroids is crucial to the diagnosis. (This principle is applicable to cases of other medications capable of producing delirium, as well.) *Psychotic* delirium from steroids is more frequent at high doses. Treatment includes lowering the dosage of steroids, and adding a small dose of a neuroleptic, for example, 2–4 mg per day of haloperidol (Hall et al., 1981). The occurrence of psychotic delirium in these cases is not reliably predictive of its recurrence should the steroids again be increased (Guze, 1967; Hall, Popkin, Stickney, et al., 1979). A mild delirium accompanied by paranoid ideation and derealization can be seen occasionally in patients rapidly tapered down from a lengthy high-dose course (for example, a drop to 20 mg of prednisone a day from 80 mg a day, in fewer than 4 days) (W. Thompson, May, 1987, personal communication).

Vascular and hemorrhagic sequelae of SLE involvement of the brain include subarachnoid hemorrhage, lupus meningitis (a noninfectious condition of meningeal inflammation, which can present with a typical meningitic picture or that of increased intracranial pressure), or infarcts with stroke symptomatology. All can be associated with delirium; focal lesions from infarction produce the behavioral or motoric symptoms expected from the location of the lesion. Subarachnoid hemorrhage and lupus meningitis are diagnosed by lumbar puncture. Subarachnoid hemorrhage in patients with SLE is usually associated with hypoglycorrachia (Ball, 1986).

Computerized tomography (CT) scans and magnetic resonance imaging (MRI) scans will probably play an increasing role in the differential diagnosis of delirium in these complex clinical situations (Reinitz, Hubbard, & Zimmerman, 1984). In one study using the CT scan, lupus cerebritis was associated with marked atrophy in more than 75 percent of patients. None of the cerebritis patients had normal scans. The control group, SLE patients without CNS symptoms, had normal scans in almost 75 percent of patients (Gaylis, Altman, Ostrov, et al., 1982). Another CT study, however, suggested that there was a stronger association between steroid use and atrophy than between cerebritis and atrophy (Carette, Urowitz, Grosman, et al., 1982). Another group demonstrated atrophy only in cerebritis patients who had symptoms of gradual onset (Weisberg, 1986).

One MRI study suggested three patterns of cerebritis lesions: increased density, suggestive of infarcts; multiple small areas of increased density, suggestive of microinfarcts; and focal gray-matter areas of increased density, which appeared to resolve on subsequent scans. No autopsy findings were reported in this study. Comparison with CT scan in the same group showed greater sensitivity of MRI in the detection of lesions. Of the 7 patients who had lesions on MRI, only 2 had positive CT scan (Aisen, Gabrielsen, & McCune, 1985). Another comparative study showed that the MRI procedure was more sensitive in detecting lesions in SLE patients than was the CT scan. Of the 9 patients studied, MRI found lesions in 8 patients, and CT found lesions in 6. Both techniques showed the 1 patient to be free of lesions, and lesions were of similar degree in 3 additional patients. Three patients showed more areas of involvement on MRI than on CT. In addi-

tion, MRI showed all lesions with greater clarity than did CT (Vermess, Berstein, Bydder, et al., 1983).

Metabolic abnormalities are a potential cause of delirium, especially in those lupus patients with severe renal involvement. Renal failure, with its consequent electrolyte imbalances and often massive fluid and sodium regulatory problems, can produce delirium in the SLE patient. Laboratory examinations reveal elevated blood urea nitrogen (BUN) and creatinine; vital signs show hypertension or postural changes in blood pressure. Physical examination can demonstrate edema in cases of fluid overload, or decreased skin turgor with volume depletion. Dialysis can be an effective treatment for many of the neuropsychiatric symptoms resulting from renal failure. If the dialysis is accomplished too rapidly, with marked shifts in extracellular volume and electrolyte composition, transient affective and cognitive disturbances may result; these are managed with careful observation and small doses of neuroleptics. Liver failure, due to hepatic involvement in lupus, can also produce a refractory delirium that is especially difficult to treat. Close monitoring of diet, judicious use of steroids, and control of intestinal flora with oral antibiotics can be helpful in managing delirium and coma from hepatic failure.

Other sources of delirium in the lupus patient are systemic and CNS infections. Because of their immunocompromised state, lupus patients are susceptible to infection by a variety of pathogens—bacterial, parasitic, and fungal. The use of corticosteroids and immunosuppressive agents such as cyclophosphamide to treat the disease further inhibits the immune system. In many studies, infection is the most common cause of death (Ball, 1986). Sites of entry include the gut, lung, skin, and urinary tract. Hypoxemia in cases of pulmonary infection or fibrosis can worsen the delirium; frequent blood gas determinations are necessary in such instances.

Depressive Syndromes

Observed or self-reported depressive affect is a common finding among SLE patients.The prevalence of affective disturbance is difficult to determine, however, since most studies of prevalence have not been based on standardized diagnostic criteria. Reports suggest 50–80 percent of SLE patients complain of depressed mood at some point during their illness. One large study of ambulatory outpatients revealed self-reported "lowered spirits" in 70 percent of patients. In that same group, Minnesota Multiphasic Personality Inventory (MMPI) results showed abnormal depression scores in 41 percent (Liang, Rogers, Larson, et al., 1984). In order of decreasing frequency, the patients' most frequently reported fears were of worsening disease, of death, and of disability. Limitations imposed by the disease, such as easy fatigability and the necessity of avoiding the sun, were also prominent. Loss of physical functioning, the lack of freedom to plan a family (especially when pregnancy resulted in a relapse), and reductions in social functioning were highly correlated with elevated depression scores. Sexual activity decreased significantly after the onset of the illness.

Some patients felt that the illness had had a positive effect on their lives, having made them aware of their mortality in a new and useful way. This revelatory experience has been described in other settings (Liang et al., 1984; White & Liddow, 1972).

Organic mood syndromes can also occur, either as a result of primary lupus involvement of the brain or secondary to metabolic disturbances or steroid effects (Hall et al. 1981). There is little case material in the literature demonstrating these syndromes in SLE (Gurland, Ganz, Fleiss, et al., 1972).

Dysthymic disorder and adjustment disorders with depressed mood are best treated initially with medical psychotherapy alone; antidepressants should be resumed for patients with vegetative symptoms that persist despite psychotherapy. Organic mood syndromes and major depressive disorders usually require use of antidepressants in addition to measures that address the primary causes: addition of steroids, for cases of CNS involvement, and correction of metabolic problems or drug toxicity when one of the two is felt to be responsible.

Seizures

Convulsions are a common complication with lupus patients, occurring in about 15 percent of cases. Presentations can be focal, akinetic, or grand mal in type. Apart from the morbidity inherent in all seizure disorders, the presence of seizures in SLE correlates with associated peripheral neurologic abnormalities. Convulsions are unlikely to be manifest before SLE is diagnosed but seem to occur early in the course of the illness (Ball, 1986).

Intracerebral hemorrhage (made more likely because of thrombocytopenia), meningoencephalitis, and cerebral infarctions can all produce seizures as complications. Seizures should thus be seen as ominous signs of possible intracranial pathology and should be evaluated with extensive physical and laboratory examinations, including CT or MRI scans. Perhaps the most common cause of seizures in these patients is metabolic and results from uremia (Johnson & Richardson, 1968; Rodnan, 1973). Treatment consists chiefly of hemodialysis. End-stage hepatic failure can also result in convulsions. Use of anticonvulsant medication should not substitute for a thorough evaluation for origins of the seizures. If anticonvulsants are given, they may accelerate the metabolism of steroids and psychotropic drugs. When a patient with SLE who is taking anticonvulsants fails to respond to treatment, drug levels should be checked, and a clinical pharmacologist should be consulted if one is available.

Peripheral Nervous System Disorders

Neurologic disturbances outside the central nervous system are fairly common, especially in those patients with severe disease (Rodnan, 1973). Thrombocytopenia may be a marker for those at greatest risk for these complications, and perhaps for CNS disease as well (Sergent, Lockshin, Klempner, et al., 1975). Peripheral neuropathies, myopathy, and myasthenia gravis are among the clinical presentations. Transverse myelitis is an especially ominous occurrence and can be a cause of death. Arteritis and thrombosis of spinal vessels, spinal subarachnoid hemorrhages, and myelomalacia can also occur, producing varying syndromes of hemiplegia and sensory disturbances. Brachial plexus neuropathy presents with decreased strength and sensation in the arms and hands; CT scan may have a place in its diagnosis (Pillemer, Ashby, Gordon, et al., 1984). Management for most of these complications is supportive, with special attention to the development of infection in those patients who are immobilized or who require surgical measures as part of the treatment. Some of these disorders, such as the uncomplicated peripheral neuropathies, may respond to corticosteroid treatment.

Other neurologic disturbances that can occur with SLE are brain stem strokes, coma, aseptic meningitis, chorea, and encephalomyelitis (Ball, 1986).

Drug-Induced Lupuslike Syndromes

The list of drugs that can produce a syndrome mimicking SLE grows yearly, but procainamide remains the most frequent offender and the best-studied (Blomgren, Condemi, & Vaughan, 1972). The syndrome usually consists of polyarthralgias and arthritis, with occasional pulmonary symptoms. Neuropsychiatric and renal disease are uncommon, but death from severe glomerulonephritis and renal failure have occurred. Positive LE cell reactions and antibodies to double-stranded DNA can be present. Some will develop biologic false-positive tests for syphilis. Antibodies to histones are the most specific test for the drug-induced syndrome, being positive in about 75 percent of patients. Of all patients taking procainamide, about 80 percent will develop antinuclear antibodies; less than 30 percent will develop clinical manifestations of the disease (Ball, 1986). There is probably some association between dosage and likelihood of developing symptoms. Beta blockers, hydralazine, isoniazid, phenytoin, methyldopa, and chlorpromazine are among the other drugs capable of producing drug-induced lupus (Hahn, Sharp, Irving, et al., 1972; Rodnan, 1973).

RHEUMATOID ARTHRITIS

A disease of unknown etiology, rheumatoid arthritis (RA) causes chronic, symmetrical nonsuppurative inflammation of the synovium of the diarthrodial joints, as well as many extra-articular manifestations. Inflammation of the synovium is the primary pathologic event, resulting in pain and swelling, with accumulation of fluid in the joint space. The chronically inflamed synovium is called a *pannus*. Recurrences cause proliferation of the pannus, with invasion and erosion of periarticular bone, gradual destruction of joint cartilage, and weakening of tendons and ligaments. This process results in poorly functioning or nonfunctional joints, immobility, and crippling. In some patients, the disease pursues a malignant course, with rapidly destructive arthritis and diffuse vasculitis. Other variants of the disease are more mild, with frequent remissions and only mild relapses, easily controlled by anti-inflammatory agents.

Rheumatoid arthritis is common; it affects almost 3 percent of the population. Two to three times as many women as men are affected. The disease can present insidiously or rapidly, and large joints are affected initially. With strict application of diagnostic criteria (Ropes, Bennet, Caleb, et al., 1958), one selects a group for whom remissions are infrequent. Gradual progression is the rule, with slight variation in daily and weekly activity of symptoms (Hardin, 1986b).

The prognosis in patients who have persistent RA seems poor, although studies vary as to observed outcomes. Some see RA as producing occupational disability in over half of the patients by 10 years, with most therapeutic endeavors having little effect (Hardin, 1986b). Others demonstrate 50–70 percent employment capability after 10–15 years, with only 10 percent incapacitated (Ragan & Farrington, 1962; Short, Bauer & Reynolds, 1957).

Adult patients often have their first arthritic symptoms in the hands, with pain, swelling, stiffness, and warmth as prominent features. Symptoms are usually worst in the morning. Knees, ankles, wrists, and elbows are involved in the disease process. Bilateral symmetry is the rule in distribution. Subcutaneous nodules may be found along the olecranon processes and the ulna in about one-fourth of patients. Joint deformity is common and is visible in the classic ulnar deviation of the fingers (Rodnan, 1973).

RA is a systemic disease; extra-articular complications develop in over three-fourths of patients and are probably more common in those with high titers of rheumatoid factor (see the subsection on laboratory diagnosis) and with subcutaneous nodules. The exception is neuropsychiatric complications, which seem to be more common in those without rheumatoid factor. Organ involvement can include the heart, lung, eye, and nervous system, as well as certain "systemic" complications. Heart involvement includes percarditis, cardiomyopathy, and valvular lesions (especially aortic). Pulmonary disease can be manifested as pleurisy, rheumatoid nodules in the parenchyma, progressive fibrosis, and pneumoconiosis with nodules (Caplan's syndrome) (Caplan, Payne, & Withy, 1962). In the eye, scleritis and iridocyclitis occur.

Neurologic involvement occurs when neurologic structures or their vascular supply are affected by vasculitis or rheumatoid nodule formation. In addition, joint, ligament, and tendon failure in the area of major nerves can cause compressive neuropathy and myelopathy, seen most commonly in the cases of the median nerve (with thenar wasting), ulnar nerve, and peroneal nerve. Central nervous system involvement is rare, although meningitis and encephalopathy have been reported (Hardin, 1986b). A mild chronic sensory polyneuropathy may be seen, as well as an acute severe sensorimotor neuropathy (Chamberlain & Bruckner, 1970).

Pathogenesis

Although the exact etiology of RA remains unknown, many factors point to its being an immunologically based disease. A microvascular event or injury is probably the first event in the pathogenetic pathway. Synovial membrane proliferation occurs because of repeated inflammation. Local antibody production follows, with immune complex formation between rheumatoid factors and IgGs. The complement sequence is activated, and vascular fluid and cellular components invade the joint space. Proteolytic enzymes are released, with protein destruction and further inflammation. In extra-articular sites, circulating immune complexes may contribute to the pathologic features (Hardin, 1986b; Panush, Bianco, & Schur, 1971).

The strong association of RA with human lymphocyte antigen HLA-DR4 suggests a hereditary immunologic predisposition to the disease. This association is especially notable among Caucasians, blacks, Japanese, and Chicanos but not among Jews (Miller & Glass, 1981).

Systemic complications include the anemia of chronic disease, keratoconjunctivitis sicca, amyloidosis, and Felty's syndrome (leukopenia with splenomegaly). RA patients may have fatigue and myalgias as part of the symptom complex. As the illness progresses, muscle wasting, weight loss, and decreased appetite can occur.

Functional capacity in patients with RA was classified by Steinbrocker, Traeger, and Batterman (1949):

Class I—no impairment, all activities are performed.

Class II—normal duties are performed, but slight limitation or discomfort in one or more joints; no assistive devices are needed.

Class III—only a few duties of job or self-care are possible; assistive devices may be needed.

Class IV—incapacitated, bedridden or wheelchair-bound, no self-care.

Laboratory Diagnosis

The most characteristic laboratory finding in RA is the presence of the rheumatoid factor (RF). Depending on which of the various available tests are used, between 70 and 90 percent of cases that are strictly selected on clinical data will be seropositive. Rheumatoid factor is composed of autoantibodies (chiefly IgM) that react with IgG. Although it is not certain that the ability of RF to form immune complexes is of specific etiologic importance in the disease, evidence is mounting that supports this assertion. Results are reported in titer, and higher titer is correlated with greater likelihood of correct diagnosis of RA, tissue type HLA-DR4, ag-

gressive joint disease, nonneuropsychiatric extra-articular disease, subcutaneous nodules, neuropathy, and Felty's syndrome (Spalding & Koopman, 1986). In the section on psychiatric aspects of the disease, other features of the illness will be discussed relative to seropositivity.

RF is not specific for RA, being found in other chronic inflammatory diseases: infective endocarditis, leprosy, syphilis, sarcoidosis, and tuberculosis. Other rheumatic diseases may have RF as well, including SLE, scleroderma, and polymyositis (Cohen, 1975). Among the general population without rheumatic disease, seropositivity occurs at a rate of about 3 percent. With aging, the prevalence of RF increases, to about 14 percent in men and 9 percent in women over 70 years of age. Titers among the seropositive elderly are low (1:40 to 1:80).

The erythrocyte sedimentation rate is a nonspecific index that may vary proportionally with the activity of the disease. ANA is present in about 30 percent of RA patients, usually in those positive for RF. Speckled patterns are most typical, at titers from 1:160 to 1:320.

Psychiatric Aspects of RA

Psychiatrists may be asked to deal with the psychiatric aspects of RA from at least three different perspectives: emotional predisposition to the illness and any precipitants of exacerbations, the emotional consequences of the disease and its complications, and psychiatric complications of the treatment, especially side effects of medications (Anderson, Bradley, Young, et al., 1985). Physicians may feel that certain psychologic events or stressors bring on exacerbations of the disease. It is not uncommon to have patients report severe emotional distress just before the first clinical evidence of the illness. Also, much early psychiatric work on RA made an attempt to describe a particular personality profile as a risk factor. In addition, the psychiatrist may be consulted regarding the way in which the patient's emotional life affects rehabilitation and treatment efforts. Knowledge of the patient's defensive and adaptive styles is crucial in the long-term management of the case.

Decades of interest in RA as one of the classic "psychosomatic" illnesses have resulted in numerous studies of RA patient's psychologic characteristics (Halliday, 1942; Thomas, 1936). Enthusiasm reigned in the search for a "rheumatic personality" and generated much data. RA patients were characterized as self-sacrificing, masochistic, inhibited, perfectionistic, retiring, and interested in outdoor sports (Moos, 1964; Moos & Solomon, 1964). They were felt to be people whose emotions were "unavailable" to them (Silverman, 1985). Women with RA actively suppressed anger and sexuality; men were depressive. Gardiner (1980) found RA patients to be "more neurotic, more likely to give socially desirable responses, and more prone to psychiatric disturbances" than the general population. Other work seems to contradict these findings, showing that RA patients' personalities hardly differ from a nonpatient population (Cassileth, Lusk, Strouse, et al., 1984; Crown, Crown, & Fleming, 1975). The concept that specific personality types or traits are associated with this disease, as well as other so-called psychosomatic illnesses, is now considered anachronistic.

It is tempting, nevertheless, when speaking of a disease that seems to be immunologically mediated, to look for ways in which the immune system may be affected by stressors in RA patients. Indeed, many have looked for such a causal relationship (Ader, 1981; Solomon, 1969), and effects on the immune system have been found in studies not restricted to RA patients (Rogers, Dubey, & Reich, 1979). Lymphocyte proliferation in response to mitogen stimulation, immunoglobulin con-

centrations, and the course of adjuvant arthritis in rats have been shown to respond to environmental stressors (Amkraut, Soloman, Kraemer, 1971; Silverman, 1985). Natural experiments in man have implied autonomic or other neurologic determinants in the course of RA. Arthritic limbs may improve after denervation; even in disease of long duration, hemiparetic limbs are unaffected (Rodnan, 1973; Silverman, 1985).

A variety of psychologic reactions to the stresses of RA have been described (Kahana & Bibring, 1964; Lipowski, 1975; Meenan, 1981). Forty to 50 percent of RA patients report significant depressive affect on psychologic testing, making depression the most common emotional complaint (Silverman, 1985). Psychotic disturbances are only rarely seen. Some groups found elevated hypochondriasis, depression, and hysteria scales on MMPI in RA patients. The specificity of these findings is low; most chronic disease patients have similar profiles (Polley, Swenson, & Steinhilber, 1970). Although longer duration seems to be associated with greater likelihood of having a profile typical of a patient with chronic disease (Baum, 1982), it appears to be very difficult to select, from psychologic testing, those who will be prone to relapse and the fortunate ones who will have prolonged remissions (Crown, et al., 1975). From psychologic testing alone, it is also impossible to distinguish those patients who are currently severely handicapped from those whose disease is mild (Baum, 1982).

Almost all patients feel that their mobility is undermined, and many rate impaired mobility as their "biggest problem" (Liang et al., 1984). This loss or potential loss of mobility obviously directly affects patients' sense of independence. Such a loss may be especially difficult for the elderly (Weiner, 1975). "Total disability" was rated as the biggest fear by one group of patients (Liang et al., 1984). The psychologic implications of this dreaded consequence are many: untimely dependence on others, fear of burdening others, fear of precipitating a divorce, and loss of control with resulting helplessness are but a few (Cobb, Miller, & Wieland, 1959; Medsger & Robinson, 1972). The repeated losses (of function, ability, mobility, relationships, and sense of body integrity) can produce a state virtually identical to the grief seen in object loss, and it should be treated as such. Medical psychotherapy focused on working through the loss is helpful (see Chapter 1).

Assessment and Treatment Strategies

If symptoms of a major depressive disorder appear, antidepressant medication should be considered (Rimon & Laakso, 1984; Robinson, 1977). Sleep is often disturbed by joint pain and stiffness. Treatment should begin with anti-inflammatory agents, but occasionally patients need sedative-hypnotics (Rogers, 1985).

The importance of taking a sexual history in these patients may be missed by those physicians who do not see the person with RA as still having a sexual life. Even those who are wheelchair-bound may remain sexually active (Yoshino, Uchida, 1981). Fear of imposing on or repulsing a spouse, of becoming too fatigued during sex, or of failing in sexual performance may make sex a conflicted arena for these patients, but many retain their interest (Baum, 1982; Wolpaw, 1960). Sexual partners of RA patients, too, may develop fears about sex: of being too demanding with a sick person or hurting or humiliating the partner. The internist or rheumatologist can play a facilitative role in getting the patient and partner to discuss their fears, or in referring the couple to a psychiatrist for psychotherapy.

Analgesics, used for other than anti-inflammatory effect, may have a place in the treatment of RA. The general experience is that persons with RA rarely become addicted "chronic pain" patients, although we may wonder why (Rogers, 1985; Rogers, Liang, & Partridge, 1982). The alterations in physical appearance in RA are sometimes quite apparent, even to the lay observer. Prominent rheumatoid nodules, or the use of a cane or wheelchair are difficult for many patients to tolerate. Patients may react with shame and attempt to conceal their bodies or restrict their social contacts. Some degree of denial is obviously helpful in any adaptive effort, and some studies of RA patients suggest that those who see themselves as persons other than "arthritic patients" and do not adopt permanent images of themselves as sick (or deformed) may actually have better outcomes (Rogers, Liang, & Partridge, 1982).

Some specific psychological interventions and approaches may be helpful. When the diagnosis is first made, the physician should be aware of the impact of so significant an event; the patient is being told he or she has a chronic, potentially debilitating disease. "Dosing" of the news and allowing the patient to react are essential. Many patients feel guilty and wonder what they might have done to bring this calamity on themselves. An understanding attitude and a clear explanation of the disease are needed. The physician should describe the course of treatment and make it clear that the patient's effort and participation are necessary to achieve a good response. Goals of disease control, not cure, are usually discussed at this point. The aim is the prevention of disability. Most internists (one should also read here *rheumatologists*) can deal with the expectable emotional distress, but they refer to a psychiatrist when anxiety, depression, or denial severely interfere with functioning or participation in the treatment program (Rogers et al., 1982).

The ongoing and chronic financial costs of the illness impose severe burdens on many patients. Loss of insurance and the ability to pursue their regular occupations may aggravate this problem (Baum, 1982; Meenan, 1981). Effects of financial strain may be insidious. Finances are frequently offered as a reason for not buying needed medications, for not making office visits, and for missing physical therapy and other rehabilitation appointments. Patients with advanced RA incur medical expenses that are three times the national average, but they are rarely referred to social service organizations (Meenan, Yelin, Henke, et al., 1978).

Early awareness of how financial difficulties and social problems are interfering with continuing care can enable the physician to intervene and make timely referrals (for example, to social services) that can help restore the patient's full participation in the treatment program (Moran, 1987).

Rehabilitation outcome has been studied extensively in RA patients (Moldofsky & Chester, 1970; Rosillo & Vogel, 1971; Vogel & Rosillo, 1969, 1971). Not surprisingly, patients who are highly motivated tend to have better outcomes. Those who are rated as "intelligent" also fare better in their rehabilitation. Patients who have dysphoric moods that do not correlate with increases in pain have significantly worse outcomes than those with dysphoric moods only at times of pain.

Good rehabilitation outcome is associated with high ego strength on psychologic testing. Poor impulse control is associated with a poor prognosis (Silverman, 1985). Those patients who can be helped to see their treatment goals as adjustable and flexible, rather than rigid, achieve more in rehabilitation programs. A positive attitude toward the rehabilitation personnel is also conducive to good outcome (Rosillo & Vogel, 1971; Vogel & Rosillo, 1969, 1971).

Some centers incorporate as part of their medical treatment teams a psychiatrist, a social worker, and a psychiatric nurse. The social worker can help assess the patient's personal, family, and financial resources, and the psychiatric nurse can help the patient identify stress-inducing situations and design coping strategies. Occupational and physical therapists also have a

crucial role in the overall plan. Staff meetings, with the psychiatrist in attendance, allow early detection of affective disturbances and psychiatric side effects of medications, as well as subtle manifestations of emotional distress that, if not recognized, may mark the beginnings of "noncompliance." This comprehensive approach to the RA patient is especially useful in complex cases (Silverman, 1985).

Psychiatric Side Effects of Medications

In a recent review, Rogers (1985) discusses in detail the psychiatric side effects of drugs used to treat RA, as well as the use of psychotropics in RA patients. Other excellent reviews have appeared (Cuthbert, 1974; Drew, 1962; Lewis & Smith, 1983). The salient points will be discussed here. Three categories of drugs are typically employed to treat RA: simple analgesics, anti-inflammatory drugs, and so-called remittive drugs.

Analgesics are often necessary adjuncts to the commonly used anti-inflammatory medications, most of which are also analgesic in function. Acetaminophen and codeine are typical examples of analgesics. The anti-inflammatory drugs form the foundation of drug treatment, and serve to interdict the pathologic process, although they are generally held to be incapable of inducing a remission. Salicylates were once the standard of this category; they are used in doses higher than those for common analgesia. Nonsteroidal anti-inflammatory drugs (NSAIDs) are now the most commonly used agents of this type; ibuprofen and indomethacin are examples. Corticosteroids also have a place in the treatment of RA, both systemically and locally administered. Those patients with severe disease may be considered candidates for the "remittive drugs." Usually not employed in mild disease because of side effects and expense, these medications work by mechanisms still poorly understood and often require months to demonstrate an effect. Sometimes true induced remission is difficult to differentiate from spontaneous remission. Examples of these drugs include gold sodium thiomalate, D-penicillamine, and the antimalarials (Hardin, 1986b).

Nonpsychiatric side effects of the salicylates are commonly known: gastric irritation, with mucosal erosion and bleeding, as well as disturbed platelet functioning. The local irritation can be somewhat reduced by taking the enteric coated preparations. Blood levels close to 15–30 mg per 100 ml are considered therapeutic; levels are drawn 2–3 hours after the last dose. NSAIDs can cause bone marrow suppression and gastrointestinal distress. Gold toxicity is manifest in renal, skin, and hematologic side effects. D-Penicillamine can cause autoimmune diseases such as SLE. The antimalarials may produce retinal damage.

As for psychiatric side effects, salicylates can cause delirium that can reach psychotic proportions (Greer, Ward & Corbin, 1965). The timing of the occurrence of toxic symptoms correlates poorly with the blood salicylate level, but such levels are helpful in determining the overall severity of the intoxication. Virtually all patients will experience some symptoms of toxicity at blood salicylate levels greater than 50 mg for every 100 ml. The NSAIDs can cause dizziness, vertigo, and headache in up to 50 percent of patients. Sedation and delirium, with associated sleep disruption, have also been reported. Longer-acting agents, such as piroxicam, have half-lives of up to 86 hours and may take 12 days to reach steady state. As a result, side effects may not appear for many days after beginning the medication. The gastrointestinal distress seen with these agents may sometimes be due to anxiety or depression, which would require separate treatment. In other cases, changing to a different NSAID can be helpful. Indomethacin has been reported to pro-duce depressive mood, and both it and ibuprofen can cause a paranoid psychosis (Cuthbert, 1974; Griffith, Smith, & Smith, 1982). NSAIDs can increase steady-state plasma lithium levels. Patients on lithium and NSAIDs should be monitored especially closely during any change of NSAID dose. NSAIDs can also decrease the diuretic and antihypertensive effects of diuretics and beta blockers.

Gold has no known adverse psychiatric effects. Among the antimalarials, psychiatric disturbances seem to be more common with chloroquine than with its hydroxylated form, hydroxychloroquine (Good & Shader, 1977). Affective disturbances, delirium, and suicide have been reported. Steroid side effects have been covered in the section on SLE and in Chapter 6, on delirium.

OTHER CONNECTIVE TISSUE DISEASES

Neuropsychiatric manifestations of other connective tissue diseases generally derive from the patient's psychologic response to the nonneurologic manifestations of the disease. Drug side effects can also present psychiatric concerns; these are similar to those already discussed. In most cases, the central nervous system is not directly involved. Early in the course of most of these diseases, systemic, nonspecific symptoms may dominate the clinical picture. Specific diagnostic evidence may be absent. In this setting, the general internist or rheumatologist may feel that the picture is best explained as a psychiatric illness and may refer the patient. It is then incumbent on the psychiatrist to be aware of the differential diagnositc problem at hand and to be alert to the appropriate measures that are indicated. Several diseases wil be discussed. If specific aspects of an illness are notable, representative features will be discussed.

Progressive systemic sclerosis, or *scleroderma*, affects connective tissue in a widespread manner, causing esophageal dysfunction, pursed and retracted facies, sclerodactyly, and renal and heart disease. Trigeminal neuropathy and peripheral monoeuropathies have been reported. Central nervous system involvement is rare and most commonly appears in end-stage disease, with delirium as a consequence of renal or hepatic failure (Ochtill & Amberson, 1978). ANA are present in over 50 percent, with a nucleolar pattern; one-third are positive for RF.

Polymyositis is a systemic disease of unknown etiology that progressively affects the proximal musculature in an inflammatory process. Symptoms, weakness and pain in various muscle groups, typically present as difficulty climbing stairs or rising from a chair. Serum aldolase and CPK are elevated. The electromyogram (EMG) is abnormal, and muscle biopsy is usually diagnostic. Muscle of the heart and gastrointestinal tract can be involved. Nervous system disease is absent. Early presentations of polymyositis, with malaise, weakness, and weight loss, may be misdiagnosed as a major depressive disorder.

Dermatomyositis is closely related to polymyositis in its pathologic findings and clinical presentation. The dusky red, raised rash seen over the elbows and hand and knee joints separates this entity clinically from polymyositis proper. In addition, those dermatomyositis patients over 40 years of age are at a 50 percent risk of having a carcinoma. The myositis may present as much as 2 years before the malignancy can be detected. Lung cancer and breast cancer are the most commonly associated malignancies.

Primary Sjogren's syndrome results from the inflammatory cell infiltration of the lacrimal and salivary glands, causing xerophthalmia and xerostomia. Secondary Sjogren's syndrome may also appear in association with another connective tissue disease, especially RA. Diagnosis is made by demonstration of abnormally low tear and saliva production and by lacrimal salivary gland biopsy. Neuropsychiatric symptoms can be associated with this disease; they include affective disturbances and alterations in cognitive functioning. A causal connection is not yet clear (Malinow, Molina, Gordon, et al., 1985).

The *vasculitides* are illnesses of widespread systemic distribution, characterized by vascular inflammation, tissue necrosis, and organ dysfunction. Temporal arteritis (TA) is an important example; symptoms include recurrent headaches, tenderness along the temporal artery, and elevated erythrocyte sedimentation rate: readings over 100 are common. Associated symptoms are transient blindness, cerebral ischemic attacks, delirium, and stroke (Cochran, Fox, & Kelly, 1978). Temporal arteritis can be very effectively treated with corticosteroids; high doses (1 mg/kg/day of prednisone equivalent) are considered necessary to prevent blindness and stroke. The patient may need to take the steroids for life. Temporal artery biopsy should be performed on any patient in whom the diagnosis is considered. If the patient has visual symptoms or evidence of transient ischemic attacks, steroids should be begun even before biopsy is performed. Lengthy specimens of the artery (4 to 6 cm) may be necessary, as may be a biopsy of the occipital artery should both temporal arteries be negative.

There is considerable clinical overlap between temporal arteritis and *polymyalgia rheumatica (PMR)* (Allen & Studenski, 1986). Some authors refer to the two as one disease entity (polymyalgia rheumatica/ temporal arteritis). PMR is characterized by aching stiffness of the neck muscles and limb girdles. Apart from the highly elevated ESR, other laboratory tests are normal, including muscle enzymes, muscle histology, and EMG. Physical examination reveals normal muscle strength. These procedures distinguish PMR from polymyositis. Fifty to 60 percent of temporal arteritis patients have PMR, and about 25–75 percent of PMR patients have evidence of arteritis on temporal artery biopsy. Even among those PMR patients without symptoms of arteritis, biopsy is positive in 10–20 percent (Guyton & Ball, 1986).

The sedimentation rates are quite high (100 mm/hour or greater) in 80–90 percent of all PMR/TA patients. The 10–20 percent who have normal ESRs and no clinical symptoms of arteritis are an especially difficult group to diagnose. Other illnesses that may present with limb girdle and neck stiffness and aching include fibrositis (see the following paragraph) and depression. Trigger points may help the physician diagnose fibrositis, and vegetative symptoms and signs may point toward depression. To make matters more complex, PMR patients may respond to doses of steroids as low as 20 mg of prednisone a day, or less. Even NSAIDs may cause symptom improvement. Only high-dose steroids, however, can prevent blindness and stroke in patients with TA. It is clear that the undiagnosed elderly patient with primarily somatic symptoms should be followed closely for progression of symptoms, possibly with serial ESRs, because of the risk of stroke and blindness secondary to TA. In the absence of an elevated ESR (roughly 40 mm/hour for elderly patients), there are no laboratory data that allow one to detect those patients who should have temporal artery biopsies; thus, in the elderly patient with aching muscular complaints and with an ESR above 40 mm/hr, one should be suspicious of PMR/TA and follow the patient closely for the occurrence of new symptoms if low-dose prednisone is used for presumptive PMR without TA (Guyton, Ball, 1986).

Fibrositis, or *fibromyalgia*, is a commonly diagnosed but poorly delineated entity of some disrepute. Symptoms are felt to include widespread myalgias, disturbed sleep, and pain trigger points. (Goldenberg, 1987). There are no reliable diagnostic procedures, although the detection of the trigger point on physical examination may approximate one such test. Emotional distress is felt to be almost universal among these patients, but one wonders whether this is not at least in part the result of repeated attempts to find a satisfactory diagnosis and treatment for their symptoms. Myofascial pain constitutes the main physical finding, typically demonstrable with trigger points, such as at the upper border of the trapezius and at the second costochondral junction. Between 10 and 56 percent of patients have a non-REM sleep disturbance manifested as daytime fatigue and a sense of nonrestorative sleep (Hardin, 1986a). Patient selection variations make sweeping generalizations difficult, but fibrositis patients seem to demonstrate an elevated level of depression on psychologic testing (Hudson, Hudson and Pliner et al., 1985). There has been the suggestion that fibrositis is a depression variant that may be responsive to antidepressant medication (see below).

There are no laboratory tests specific for fibrositis. In the patient with generalized myalgias and arthralgias, the first laboratory test to be performed should be the ESR. If this is elevated, one is not dealing with fibrositis. If the ESR is normal, one needs to consider fibrositis, depression, and PMR/TA with normal ESR. Specific vegetative symptoms or signs would be suggestive of depression. If the presentation is dominated by sleep disorder and trigger points, one must consider fibrositis as the most likely possibility. The group left by these exclusions should be followed closely, as mentioned before, for development of visual or CNS symptoms, which should then be taken as evidence of TA and vigorously treated as such.

For the fibrositis patient, there are few avenues of treatment. Nonpharmacologic measures, such as mild exercise, massage, and biofeedback, are sometimes helpful. Mild analgesics and NSAIDs should be tried but closely managed because of long-term side effects. Analgesics other than NSAIDs may cause severe renal damage when used for long periods. The NSAIDs, however, are usually of little practical help. Since the fibrositis patient may be in pain for years, the physician must closely monitor the analgesic use to help avoid renal toxicity.

Most fibrositis patients seem to derive considerable benefit from treatment of the sleep disorder. This is usually accomplished with tricyclic antidepressants (Hardin, 1986a). One randomized controlled study comparing amitriptyline (25 mg gHS), naproxene (500 mg BID), both medications in combination, and placebo reported significant symptomatic improvement only in the treatment arms containing amitriptyline, hence the tricyclic was felt to be the effective therapeutic agent (Goldenberg, Fleson, & Dinerman, et al., 1986). Other studies have confirmed the effectiveness of low-dose amitriptyline in this disorder (Carette, McCain, & Bell, 1986), although given the increased prevalence of depression in the population, one may assume that patients suffering from major depression were undertreated. Because of the need for sedation, serotoninergically active antidepressants with less anticholinergic effects such as doxepin are the best choice. If "masked" or "somatized" depression is suspected, higher doses of doxepin should be used (150–300 mg/day as tolerated).

First-degree relatives of fibrositis patients appear to have more depressive characteristics than controls (Goldenberg, 1986). "Disturbed" and "chronic pain" patient profiles are other common findings on psychological testing (Ahles, Yunus, Riley, et al., 1984). Physician support, appropriately timed referral to a psychiatrist, the judicious use of psychotherapy and antidepressant medications may provide relief for these patients.

Essential mixed cryoglobulinemia (EMC) is a syndrome comprising the triad of palpable purpura, arthritis or arthralgia, and Raynaud's phenomenon. Cryoglobulins are present and are inferred to be the pathogenetic entities. They are serum proteins, often immunoglobulins, that reversibly precipitate with exposure to cold environmental temperatures. Appearance of the purpura and joint symptoms is precipitated clinically by physical exertion or cold. Renal involvement with vasculitis can cause significant renal disease. The psychiatrist may see the patient because of referral for symptoms without obvious organic basis. Laboratory features include elevated ESR, increased immunoglobulins on serum protein electrophoresis, and mild anemia. If there is renal involvement, renal function tests may be abnormal. Rheumatoid factor is often present in higher titer. The mere detection of cryoglobulins is not diagnostic of EMC; their presence is more often secondary to another disease, such as multiple myeloma, lymphoma, or chronic infection.

Many patients with EMC require no treatment or only NSAIDs. Those with renal or the less common peripheral neurologic involvement (peripheral neuropathy) may require trials of corticosteroids or cytotoxic drugs. Occasionally, plasmapheresis can be helpful.

REFERENCES

Ader R (Ed) (1981). *Psychoneuroimmunology*. New York: Academic Press.

Ahearn JM, Provost JT, Dorsch SA et al. (1982). Interrelationships of HLA-DR, MB, and MT phenotypes, autoantibody expression, and clinical features in systemic lupus erythematosus. *Arthritis and Rheumatism, 25,* 1031

Ahles TA, Yunus MB, Riley SD, et al. (1984). Psychological factors associated with primary fibromyalgia syndrome. *Arthritis and Rheumatism, 27,* 1101–1106.

Aisen AM, Gabrielsen TO, & McCune WJ (1985). MR imaging of systemic lupus erythematosus involving the brain. American Journal of Roentgenology, *144,* 1027–1031.

Allen NB & Studenski SA (1986). Polymyalgia rheumatica and temporal arteritis. *Medical Clinics of North America, 70,* 369–384.

Amkraut AA, Solomon GF, & Kraemer HC (1971). Stress, early experience and adjuvant-induced arthritis in the rat. *Psychosomatic Medicine, 33,* 203–214.

Anderson KO, Bradley LA, Young LD, et al. (1985). Rheumatoid arthritis: review of psychological factors related to etiology, effects, and treatment. *Psychological Bulletin, 98,* 358–387.

Ball, GV (1986). Systemic lupus erythematosus (SLE). In GV Ball & WJ Koopman (Eds), *Clinical rhematology.* Philadelphia: WB Saunders.

Ball GV & Koopman WJ (Eds) (1986). *Clinical rheumatology.* Philadelphia: WB Saunders.

Baum J (1982). A review of the psychological aspects of rheumatic diseases. *Seminars in Arthritis and Rheumatism, 11,* 352–361.

Blomgren SE, Condemi JJ, & Vaughn, JH (1972). Procainamide-induced lupus erythematosus. *American Journal of Medicine, 52,* 338–348.

Caplan A, Payne RB, & Withey JL (1962). A broader concept of Caplan's syndrome relate to rheumatoid factors. *Thorax, 17,* 205–212.

Carette S, McCain GA, Bell DA, et al. (1986). Evaluation of amitriptyline in primary fibrositis. *Arthritis and Rheumatism, 29,* 655–659.

Carette S, Urowitz MB, Grosman H, et al. (1982). Cranial computerized tomography in systemic lupus erythematosus. *Journal of Rheumatology, 9,* 855–859.

Cassileth BR, Lusk EJ, Strouse TB, et al. (1984). Psychological status in chronic illness: A comparative analysis of six diagnostic groups. *New England Journal of Medicine, 311,* 506–511.

Ceppelini R, Polli E, & Celada F (1957). A DNA reacting factor in serum of a patient with lupus erythematosus diffusus. *Proceedings of the Society for Experimental and Biological Medicine, 96,* 572.

Chamberlain MA & Bruckner FE (1970). Rheumatoid neuropathy: Clinical and electrophysiological features. *Annals of the Rheumatic Diseases, 29,* 609–616.

Cobb S, Miller M, & Wieland M (1959). On the relationship between divorce and rheumatoid arthritis. *Arthritis and Rheumatism, 2,* 214–218.

Cochran JW, Fox JH, & Kelly MP (1978). Reversible mental symptoms in temporal arteritis. *Journal of Nervous and Mental Disease, 166,* 446–447.

Cohen AS (1975). *Laboratory diagnostic procedures in the rheumatic diseases.* Boston: Little, Brown.

Crown S, Crown JM, & Fleming A (1975). Aspects of the psychology and epidemiology of rheumatoid disease. *Psychological Medicine, 5,* 291–299.

Cuthbert MF (1974). Adverse reactions to nonsteroidal anti-rheumatic drugs. *Current Medical Research and Opinion, 2,* 600–610.

Drew JF (1962). Concerning the side effects of antimalarial drugs in the extended treatment of rheumatic disease. *Medical Journal of Australia, 2,* 618–620.

Gardiner BM (1980). Psychological aspects of rheumatoid arthritis. *Psychological Medicine, 10,* 159–163.

Gaylis NB, Altman RD, Ostrov S, et al. (1982). The selective value of tomography of the brain in cerebritis due to systemic lupus erythematosus. *Journal of Rheumatology, 9,* 850–854.

Goldenberg DL (1986). Psychologic studies in fibrositis. *American Journal of Medicine, 81,* 67–70.

Goldenberg DL (1987). Fibromyalgia syndrome. *Journal of the American Medical Association, 257,* 2782–2787.

Good MI & Shader RI (1977). Behavioral toxicity and equivocal suicide associated with chloroquine and its related derivatives. *American Journal of Psychiatry, 134,* 798–801.

Greer, HD, Ward HP, & Corbin KB (1965). Chronic salicylate intoxication in adults. *Journal of the American Medical Association, 193,* 555–558.

Griffith JD, Smith CH, & Smith RC (1982). Paranoid psychosis in a patient receiving ibuprofen, a prostaglandin synthesis inhbitor: Case report. *Journal of Clinical Psychiatry, 43,* 499–500.

Gurland BJ, Ganz VH, Fleiss JL, et al. (1972). The study of the psychiatric symptoms of systemic lupus erythematosus: A critical review. *Psychosomatic Medicine, 34,* 199–206.

Guyton JM & Ball GV (1986). Vasculitis. In GV Ball & WJ Koopman (Eds), *Clinical Rheumatology.* Philadelphia: WB Saunders.

Guze SB (1967). The occurrence of psychiatric illness in systemic lupus erythematosus. *American Journal of Psychiatry, 123,* 1562–1570.

Hahn BH, Sharp GC, Irvin WS, et al. (1972). Immune responses to hydralazine and nuclear antigens in hydralazine-induced lupus erythematosus. *Annals of Internal Medicine, 76,* 365–374.

Hall RCW, Popkin MK, Stickney SK, et al. (1979).

Presentation of the steroid psychoses. *Journal of Nervous and Mental Disease*, *167*, 229–236.

Hall, RCW, Stickney SK, & Gardner ER (1981). Psychiatric symptoms in patients with systemic lupus erythematosus. *Psychosomatics*, *22*, 15–24.

Halliday JL (1942). Psychological aspects of rheumatoid arthritis. *Proceedings of the Royal Society of Medicine*, *35*, 455–457.

Hardin JG (1986a). Fibrositis. In GV Ball & WJ Koopman (Eds), *Clinical rheumatology*. Philadelphia: WB Saunders.

Hardin JG (1986b). Rheumatoid arthritis. In GV Ball & WJ Koopman (Eds), *Clinical rheumatology*. Philadelphia: WB Saunders.

Hargraves MM, Richmond H, & Morton R (1948). Presentation of two bone marrow elements: The "tart" cell and the "LE" cell. *Proceedings of the Staff Meetings of the Mayo Clinic*, *23*, 23–28.

Hudson JI, Hudson MS, Pliner LF, et al. (1985). Fibromyalgia and major affective disorder: A controlled phenomenology and family history study. *American Journal of Psychiatry*, *142*, 441–446.

Johnson RT & Richardson EP (1968). The neurological manifestations of systemic lupus erythematosus. *Medicine*, *47*, 337–369.

Kahana RJ & Bibring GL (1964). Personality types in medical management. In RGN Zinbi (Ed), *Psychiatry and medical practice in a general hospital*, (pp 108–123). New York: International Universities Press.

Leonhardt T (1966). Long-term prognosis of systemic lupus erythematosus. *Acta Medica Scandinavica*, *445*, 440–443.

Lewis DA & Smith RE (1983). Steroid-induced psychiatric syndromes—a report of 14 cases and a review of the literature. *Journal of Affective Disorders*, *5*, 319–332.

Liang MH, Rogers M, Larson M, et al. (1984). The psychosocial impact of systemic lupus erythematosus and rheumatoid arthritis. *Arthritis and Rheumatism*, *27*, 13–19.

Lipkin M (1985). Psychiatry in medicine. In HI Kaplan & BJ Sadock (Eds), *Comprehensive textbook of psychiatry* (4th ed, pp 1263–1277). Baltimore: Williams & Wilkins.

Lipowski ZJ (1975). Physical illness, the patient and his environment: Psychosocial foundations of medicine. In S Arieti (Ed), *American handbook of psychiatry* (2nd ed, Vol 4, pp 3–42). New York: Basic Books.

Malinow KL, Molina R, Gordon B, et al. (1985). Neuropsychiatric dysfunction in primary Sjogren's syndrome. *Annals of Internal Medicine*, *103*, 344–350.

Medsger AR & Robinson H (1972). A comparative study of divorce in rheumatoid arthritis and other rheumatic diseases. *Journal of Chronic Diseases*, *25*, 269–275.

Meenan RF (1981). The impact of chronic disease: A sociomedical profile of rheumatoid arthritis. *Arthritis and Rheumatism*, *24*, 544–549.

Meenan RF, Yelin EH, Henke CJ, et al. (1978). The costs of rheumatoid arthritis: A patient-oriented study of chronic disease costs. *Arthritis and Rheumatism*, *21*, 827–833.

Miller ML & Glass DN (1981). The major histocompatibility complex antigens in rheumatoid arthritis and juvenile arthritis. *Bulletin of the Rheumatic Diseases*, *31*, 21–25.

Moldofsky H & Chester WJ (1970). Pain and mood patterns in patients with rheumatoid arhtritis. *Psychosomatic Medicine*, *32*, 309–317.

Moos RH (1964). Personality factors associated with rheumatoid arthritis: A review. *Journal of Chronic Diseases*, *17*, 41–55.

Moos RH & Solomon GF (1964). Personality correlates of the rapidity of progression of rheumatoid arthritis. *Annals of the Rheumatic Diseases*, *23*, 145–151.

Moran MG (1987). Treatment noncompliance in asthmatic patients: An examination of the concept and a review of the literature. *Seminars in Respiratory Medicine*, *8*, 271–277.

Ochtill HN & Amberson J (1978). Acute cerebral symptomatology, a rare presentation of scleromyxedema. *Journal of Clinical Psychiatry*, *39*, 471–475.

O'Connor JF (1959). Psychoses associated with systemic lupus erythematosus. *Annals of Internal Medicine*, *51*, 526–536.

Panush RS, Bianco NE & Schur PH (1971). Serum and synovial fluid IgG, IgA, and IgM antigammaglobulins in rheumatoid arthritis. *Arthritis and Rheumatism*, *14*, 737–747.

Pillemer SR, Ashby P, Gordon DA, et al. (1984). Brachial plexus radiculopathy and computed tomography [Letter]. *Annals of Internal Medicine*, *100*, 619.

Pincus T (1986). Antinuclear antibodies. In GV Ball & WJ Koopman (Eds), *Clinical rheumatology*. Philadelphia: WB Saunders.

Polley HF, Swenson WN, & Steinhilber R (1970). Personality characteristics of patients with rheumatoid arthritis. *Psychosomatics*, *11*, 45–49.

Ragan C & Farrington E (1962). The clinical features of rheumatoid arthritis. *Journal of the American Medical Association*, *181*, 663–667.

Reinitz E, Hubbard D, & Zimmerman RD (1984). Central nervous system diseases in systemic lupus erythematosus: Axial tomographic scan as an aid to differential diagnosis [Letter]. *Journal of Rheumatology*, *11*, 252–253.

Rimon R & Laakso RL (1984). Overt psychopathology

in rheumatoid arthritis: A fifteen-year follow-up study. *Scandinavian Journal of Rheumatology*, *13*, 324–328.

Robinson ET (1977). Depression in rheumatoid arthritis. *Journal of the Royal College of General Practitioners*, *27*, 423–427.

Rodnan GP (Ed) (1973). Primer on rheumatic diseases [Special issue]. *Journal of the American Medical Association*, *224*, 662–812.

Rogers MP (1985). Rheumatoid arthritis: Psychiatric aspects and use of psychotropics. *Psychosomatics*, *26*, 915–925.

Rogers MP, Dubey D, & Reich P (1979). The influence of the psyche and the brain on immunity and disease susceptibility: A critical review. *Psychosomatic Medicine*, *41*, 147–164.

Rogers MP, Liang MH, & Partridge AJ (1982). Psychological care of adults with rheumatoid arthritis. *Annals of Internal Medicine*, *96*, 344–348.

Ropes MW, Bennett GA, Caleb S, et al. (1958). Revision of diagnostic criteria for rheumatoid arthritis. *Bulletin of Rheumatic Diseases*, *9*, 175–176.

Rosillo RH & Vogel ML (1971). Correlation of psychological variables and progress in physical rehabilitation: 4. The relation of body image to success of physical rehabilitation. *Archives of Physical Medicine and Rehabilitation*, *52*, 182–186.

Sergent JS, Lockshin MD, Klempner MW, et al. (1975). Central nervous system disease in systemic lupus erythematosus. *American Journal of Medicine*, *58*, 644–645.

Short CL, Bauer W, & Reynolds WE (1957). *Rheumatoid arthritis*. Cambridge: Harvard University Press.

Silverman AJ (1985). Rheumatoid arthritis. In HI Kaplan & BJ Sadock (Eds), *Comprehensive textbook of psychiatry*, (4th ed). Baltimore: Williams and Wilkins.

Solomon GF (1969). Stress and antibody response in rats. *International Archives of Allergy and Applied Immunology*, *35*, 97–104.

Spalding DM & Koopman WJ (1986). Rheumatoid factor, cryoglobulinemia, and erythrocyte sedimentation rate. In GV Ball & WJ Koopman (Eds), *Clinical rheumatology*. Philadelphia: WB Saunders.

Stage DE & Mannik M (1973). Rheumatoid factors in rheumatoid arthritis. *Bulletin of the Rheumatic Diseases*, *23*, 720–725.

Steinbrocker O, Traeger CH, & Batterman RC (1949). Therapeutic criteria in rheumatoid arthritis. *Journal of the American Medication Association*, *140*, 659–662.

Stern M & Robbins ES (1960). Psychoses in systemic lupus erythematosus. *Archives of General Psychiatry*, *3*, 205–212.

Tan EM (1985). Systemic lupus erythematosus: Immunologic aspects. In DJ McCarty (Ed), *Arthritis and allied conditions* (10th ed). Philadelphia: Lea and Febiger.

Thomas GW (1936). Psychic factors in rheumatoid arthritis. *American Journal of Psychiatry*, *93*, 693–710.

Vermess M, Bernstein RM, Bydder GM, et al. (1983). Nuclear magnetic resonance (NMR) imaging of the brain in systemic lupus erythematosus. *Journal of Computer Assisted Tomography*, *7*, 461–467.

Vogel ML & Rosillo RH (1969). Correlation of psychological variables and progress in physical rehabilitation: 2. Motivation, attitude and flexibility of goals. *Diseases of the Nervous System*, *30*, 593–601.

Vogel ML & Rosillo RH (1971). Correlation of psychological variables and progress in physical rehabilitation: 3. Ego functions and defensive and adaptive mechanism. *Archives of Physical Medicine and Rehabilitation*, *52*, 15–21.

Volanakis JE (1986). The complement system. In GV Ball & WJ Koopman (Eds), *Clinical rheumatology*. Philadelphia: WB Saunders.

Vollhardt BR, Ackerman SH, Grayzel AI, et al. (1982). Psychologically distinguishable groups of rheumatoid arthritis patients: A controlled, single blind study. *Psychosomatic Medicine*, *44*, 358–362.

Weiner CL (1975). The burden of rheumatoid arthritis: Tolerating the uncertainty. *Social Science and Medicine*, *9*, 97–104.

Weisberg LA (1986). The cranial computed tomographic findings in patients with neurologic manifestations of systemic lupus erythematosus. *Computers in Radiology*, *10*, 63–68.

White R & Liddow S (1972). The survivors of cardiac arrest. *Psychiatry in Medicine*, *3*, 219–225.

Wolpaw RL (1960). The arthritic personality. *Psychosomatics*, *1*, 195–197.

Zvaifler NJ (1986). Neuropsychiatric manifestations of SLE, common, hard to identify. *Clinical Psychiatry News*, May, p 26.

Janice L. Petersen

29
Obstetrics and Gynecology

Women turn to their physicians for care of a variety of obstetric and gynecologic problems. The reproductive system, so intimately related to a woman's sense of identity, is highly invested emotionally. The concerned physician, aware of the psychologic implications of obstetric and gynecologic conditions, seeks to treat these as well as the physical symptoms of the patient. With more distressed or problematic patients, the physician or patient may pursue psychiatric consultation for diagnostic and treatment recommendations. This chapter will address the psychiatric aspects of disorders commonly encountered in obstetrics and gynecology.

INFERTILITY

Infertility can be a devastating condition for the 15 percent of American couples that it affects. It is defined as lack of conception after 1 year of unprotected intercourse. Eighty percent of couples achieve pregnancy after 1 year, and an additional 5–10 percent after 2 years (Behrman &

Kistner, 1975). Of those who seek treatment, only 40 percent will be helped by current treatment methods (Collins, Wrixon, James, et al., 1983).

The ability to bear children is an unquestioned expectation of most couples. When this highly valued experience is disrupted by infertility, a major narcissistic injury and sense of loss occurs. Reactions are complex and diverse; they include shock, denial, grief, guilt, anger, anxiety, and depression. The lack of control over such a basic life function is highly distressing.

As the couple realize that they are having difficulty becoming pregnant, they may feel increasingly pressured to perform sexually at the time of ovulation. What formerly was an enjoyable activity becomes a necessary chore; sexual dysfunction may eventually develop and compound the narcissistic injury. If the couple seeks treatment, they must tolerate the physician's inquiry and intervention in ordinarily private experiences. Treatment for the woman may involve daily basal body temperatures, blood or urine samples for

PRINCIPLES OF MEDICAL PSYCHIATRY
ISBN 0-8089-1883-4

617

luteinizing hormone (LH) determinations, oral or intramuscular medications, frequent pelvic examinations, ultrasound examinations (with an uncomfortably full bladder), and laparoscopy or laparotomy; the man's role in treatment may involve urologic evaluation and masturbation on demand for a sperm sample for artificial insemination or in vitro fertilization. Such treatment is expensive, physically taxing, time-consuming, and often depersonalizing. When the woman's period comes at the end of the month despite these efforts, the couple experience a sense of loss and failure.

Women are commonly more distressed by infertility than their spouses, and this difference contributes to difficulties for each partner in understanding the other's reaction. If one member of the pair has been diagnosed as having the problem, that partner may feel particularly injured and guilty, and the other may feel deprived and angry. Their family and friends may have little understanding of what they are experiencing and may make well-meaning but unempathic suggestions. The couple may have great difficulty associating with others who are pregnant or who have children. The infertile couple often feel isolated in their distress. It is not surprising that many such couples experience significant discord, and some will divorce as a result of infertility.

Some contributions to the literature have addressed the issue whether personality factors contribute to infertility. These studies are flawed by lack of adequate control groups and failure to determine whether personality findings were present previously or arose after the infertility emerged. Psychologic causes of infertility, such as psychogenic amenorrhea, nonconsummation, vaginismus, psychogenic impotence, and avoidance of intercourse, account for but a small minority of infertility cases. In gynecologic practice, the most common psychologic management problem is the couple's grief reaction as they face the potential loss of a life goal and try to cope with a stressful treatment plan.

Evaluation of infertility requires a detailed history and examination of both members of the couple. In psychologic evaluation, the psychiatrist should determine why the couple have presented for treatment now, who is most concerned, what life changes have occurred in anticipation of pregnancy, how the problem has affected the marital relationship, how they have coped with it, and what they will do if they do not get pregnant (Downing, in press). Major psychiatric disturbance must be identified and appropriately treated—in particular, major depression that clinical experience suggests is not uncommon in this population.

In dealing with infertility, the psychiatrist should encourage both members of the couple to be involved in the consultation, since infertility is a problem for both of them. The gynecologic and urologic evaluation processes, diagnoses, treatments, and options should be reviewed. If the couple is willing to continue treatment, but is having difficulties coping with it, they may need assistance in negotiating with the gynecologist for a treatment plan that gives them more control, or they may simply need permission to take a break. If the couple's main difficulty is conflict between the spouses, couples therapy may be needed to clarify the issues, each member's contributions to them, and their options in responding to them. If the couple's main difficulty is disagreement over treatment options, for example, whether to pursue artificial insemination by donor, these issues can be explored and worked through, and a plan can be negotiated. For the couple who is considering termination of treatment for infertility, basic grief work may be needed to assist them to come to terms with their loss and to cathect their other options: adoption or child-free living.

PREMENSTRUAL SYNDROME

Premenstrual syndrome (PMS) is a controversial condition that has received much media attention. Patients attribute a wide range psychologic and physical complaints to this disorder. Physicians, however, are much more reluctant to make and treat this diagnosis. Controversy remains because definitive research in this area is lacking. Yet physicians must deal with the many requests for treatment and may request psychiatric consultation for severe premenstrual mood and behavioral problems.

PMS is defined as affective, behavioral, and physical symptoms that occur prior to menses and resolve with the onset of menses or shortly thereafter. The constellation of symptoms varies from patient to patient but generally occurs with consistent timing from cycle to cycle. Twenty to 90 percent of women experience some symptoms premenstrually, and 20 percent of these have symptoms that interfere with functioning. PMS is more common in women in their third and fourth decades, and is more common with increasing parity (Vargyas, in press).

The symptoms attributed to PMS can be classified into three groups (Hamilton, Parry, Alagna, et al., 1984):

1. Psychologic—dysphoria, anxiety, tension, lethargy, irritability, food cravings

2. Somatic—abdominal pain, breast tenderness, bloating, edema, headache, allergic symptoms, skin disorders, decreased coordination

3. Behavioral—avoidance of social contact, altered daily schedules or routines, crying spells, and altered sexual activity.

For some patients, these symptoms are quite disruptive, leading to significant conflict in their roles as wives, mothers, and employees. This can result in guilt and decreased self-esteem, which for some patients leads to a clinical depression and in severe cases to suicidal ideation.

In the evaluation of PMS complaints, it is striking that 50–80 percent are unconfirmed by daily recordings of symptoms for several months (Hamilton et al., 1984). Clinical experience suggests that many women who complain of PMS are experiencing situational adjustment reactions or chronic psychiatric problems. Their distress may be compounded by cultural norms that expect women to care for others while minimizing their own needs. They may be unaware of the true source of their symptoms and may seek the label of premenstrual syndrome to legitimize their difficulties as a physical disorder, which they hope can be treated by their primary physician.

Another surprising aspect of PMS complaints is the high rate of response to nonspecific interventions. Many women are helped by simply recording their symptoms daily and discussing the results with the physician. Furthermore, there is a dramatic placebo response noted in 30–90 percent of subjects in controlled treatment studies (Rubinow & Roy-Byrne, 1984). Despite these observations, there does appear to be a small subgroup of patients with bona fide cyclical symptoms that are unresponsive to supportive interventions and placebo effects and require more specific treatment.

The biological basis of PMS has been the subject of intense scrutiny. Research has centered on identifying possible hormone abnormalities and testing the effects of various treatments. Proposed etiologies have included alterations in levels of estrogen, progesterone, prolactin, aldosterone, prostaglandins, endorphins, thyroid hormones, and catecholamine. Much of this work has been flawed by inadequate diagnostic criteria and control groups (Rubinow & Roy-Byrne, 1984). With efforts to standardize diagnostic criteria and improve experimental design, however, better studies are currently being performed.

Premenstrual syndrome has been linked to mood disorders. There is a significantly higher rate of lifetime incidence of depression, as well as a positive family history of mood disorders in women who seek treatment for PMS (Vargyas, in press). Whether these disorders predispose one to PMS, however, are a result of having it, or are merely associated with it remains to be clarified.

In evaluating the patient with PMS complaints, a detailed history, including the present illness, past medical history, previous psychiatric history and treatment, psychosocial history, and family history, should be obtained. The reason that the patient is now seeking care should be elicited. Since many of these patients are experiencing situational reactions, it is important to understand the patient's current marital, family, and job situations and their influence upon the symptoms. Factors that alleviate or aggravate the symptoms should be explored, particularly the effect of oral contraceptives, pregnancy, and previous treatments. Suicidal ideation and impulse control should be evaluated. Special attention should be given to identifying major psychiatric disorders such as depression, cyclothymic disorder, bipolar disorder (especially the rapid cycling subgroup), anxiety disorders, and severe personality disorders, since these can be exacerbated premenstrually and may present with a chief complaint of premenstrual syndrome. Similarly, one must also rule out other physical conditions, such as dysmenorrhea, endometriosis, thyroid dysfunction, or mastodynia (breast tenderness), that also may be exacerbated premenstrually. A physical examination should be performed. Endocrine tests for various hormones have been recommended in the past, but they are of little value unless there are specific symptoms or signs suggestive of endocrine

disorder, such as hirsutism, markedly irregular periods, galactorrhea, or ovarian cysts.

Once a treatment alliance has been established, the patient can be engaged in clarifying the pattern of the symptoms and instructed on the use of the daily rating forms, which should be recorded for 2–3 months (see Hamilton et al., 1984, for an example of a rating sheet). During this period of observation, the physician can explain that it is important to understand stress in the patient's life and explore ways of coping with it. Although many patients are initially resistant to psychiatric treatment of their problem, they may be able to accept this explanation and participate in medical psychotherapy. Strategies for coping with the symptoms, such as decreasing expectations of oneself and avoiding the scheduling of stressful events in the premenstrual period, should be discussed.

Other basic interventions include improving diet and activity level. Alcohol, caffeine, and recreational drugs must be avoided because they may contribute to lability, fatigue, depression, and somatic symptoms. Careful history with some patients will reveal that episodes of irritability, lability, or hostility occur in the late afternoon, or at times when the patient has a low caloric intake. In such instances, reactive hypoglycemia may be a contributing factor. All patients should be instructed on the practice of regular, balanced meals, including breakfast, lunch, a snack in the late afternoon, and dinner. If weight control is a concern, the patient can eat multiple small meals, rather than saving all her caloric intake for one large meal. Concentrated carbohydrates should be avoided. Salt intake should be reduced for those women with significant edema, weight gain, or bloating. Regular exercise has also been reported to be helpful in improving mood and reducing PMS symptoms. The basis for this is unknown but may be related to stress reduction as the patient changes her priorities or to endorphin release associated with strenuous exercise.

Another conservative measure is to supplement the diet in the last half of the menstrual cycle with pyridoxine, 100 mg twice a day, which can be increased to 300–500 mg a day (Hamilton, et al., 1984; Vargyas, in press). Pyridoxine, a cofactor in the synthesis of serotonin and dopamine, is thought to be relatively deficient when high levels of estrogen are present (Winston, 1973). Although clinical studies have varied in their findings, one controlled, double-blind study found significant improvement in PMS symptoms with the higher doses mentioned above (Day, 1979). The patient must be instructed to avoid using very high doses because neurotoxicity may occur at dosages over 1000 mg a day.

After several months of becoming more aware of themselves and improving diet and exercise, over 30 percent of patients will feel more in control of their symptoms and will not require further treatment (Vargyas, in press). For those who have not responded and who have symptom charts consistent with the rigorous definition of premenstrual syndrome, a number of pharmacologic treatments can be considered. Research on most of these interventions is inconclusive to date (Rubinow & Roy-Byrne, 1984). Yet, clinical experience suggests that, for some, medications are dramatically effective. The physician should adopt an individualized, empirical approach for each patient.

Diuretics. If there is significant edema, weight gain, or bloating, hydrochlorothiazide or spironolactone can be given in standard dosages during the symptomatic part of the cycle.

Ovulation suppressants. Oral contraceptives are the most commonly used preparations for this purpose and are useful for younger patients with few risk factors who can tolerate them and who desire contraception.

Prostaglandin inhibitors (aspirin, NSAIDs). If there is a back-pain or pelvic-pain component to the premenstrual complaints, any drug in this class can be given in standard dosages during the symptomatic part of the cycle.

Progesterone. Although vaginal progesterone suppositories, 100–200 mg twice a day during the symptomatic part of the cycle, have become quite popular for the treatment of PMS, no double-blind, placebo-controlled study demonstrates their efficacy. Use of this agent is therefore questionable. Although some patients are quite emphatic that it is the only treatment that helps them, an empirical trial of progesterone should be reserved for cases that are unresponsive to other modalities. Progesterone suppositories are not commercially available; they must be compounded by a local pharmacist. If they are used, progesterone levels four hours after the morning dose can be used to determine adequacy of treatment trials. The dose of progesterone is increased to produce a level in the upper half of the normal mid-luteal range. If the patient does not respond to this dose, success with progesterone is unlikely.

Anxiolytic agents. Recent unpublished studies suggest that these medications, particularly alprazolam, are useful in treating the anxiety and irritability components of PMS. Low doses, 0.25 mg of alprazolam two or three times a day, can be titrated to the patients' needs during the symptomatic part of the cycle (Vargyas, in press).

Lithium carbonate. If mood liability and depression are prominent, lithium can be adjusted to a therapeutic blood level throughout the month or during the symptomatic part of the cycle.

Antidepressants. For those patients with prominent depressive symptoms, cyclic antidepressants or monoamine oxidase inhibitors in standard dosages can be given continuously throughout the month.

PELVIC PAIN

Pelvic pain is a common complaint in the gynecology clinic. Renaer (1981) has estimated that approximately 25 percent of noncontraceptive gynecologic visits involve some kind of pain complaint and that 50 percent of laparoscopies are done to evaluate pain. Some complaints, such as dysmenorrhea or acute pelvic pain due to ectopic pregnancy, respond to current pharmacologic and surgical treatments. Many types of pelvic pain are chronic, however, and poorly responsive to available treatments. This section will address chronic pelvic pain, defined as pain of greater than 6 months duration, which has been described as "one of the most perplexing problems facing the gynecologist." (Lundberg, Wall, & Mathers, 1973).

The role of personality in pelvic pain has long intrigued clinicians. Many anecdotal reports in the literature lack matched controls or comparisons. Several studies utilizing control groups (Castelnuovo-Tedesco & Krout, 1970; Renaer, Vertommen, Nijs, et al., 1979) show higher levels of psychopathology (hypochondriasis, hysteria, paranoia, psychesthenia, and schizoid features) in patients with pelvic pain than in those without. These characteristics, however, do not discriminate pain patients with clear pelvic pathology from those with none. Furthermore, elevated Minnesota Multiphasic Personality Inventory (MMPI) profiles of both of these groups resembles those of patients with chronic pain in other organ systems (Pasnau, Soldinger, & Andersen, 1985). Whether the psychopathology preceded the pain or is a result of the pain has not been addressed.

Patients with no discernible pelvic pathology compose 17–28 percent of all pelvic pain patients (Kresch, Seifer, Sach, et al., 1984; Renaer, 1980; Rosenthal, Ling, Rosenthal, et al., 1984). Although many theories have been proposed regarding the biologic, psychologic, or psychosomatic etiology of this syndrome, current research remains inconclusive. Clinical experience suggests that this is a diverse group representing a spectrum of biologic and psychologic contributions (Stoudemire & Sandhu, 1987). Beware the assumption that all of these patients have "psychogenic pain." Although a small number of these patients exhibit a conversionlike syndrome, the majority do not. The label "psychogenic" has a pejorative connotation, unfair to the patient and inaccurately suggesting a known etiology. A more appropriate term is *idiopathic pain syndrome* (Williams & Spitzer, 1982). Finally, it should be noted that a history of childhood incest is common in patients with chronic idiopathic pelvic pain and should be thoroughly investigated.

Evaluation of the pelvic pain patient requires a detailed history of the pain complaint, including the location, quality, and course of the pain and any aggravating or alleviating factors. Physical examination and laboratory evaluation are necessary to rule out urologic, gastrointestinal, and musculoskeletal conditions. For all patients with chronic pain, a diagnostic laparoscopy is essential, especially to rule out endometriosis. Psychologic evaluation should address the reasons for the patient's presentation at this time, as well as social history, sexual history, and assessment of secondary gain. Depression and suicidal ideation must be evaluated, as well as the possibility of other major psychiatric pathology. The possibility of somatoform disorders such as somatization disorder should be considered.

Treatment of the patient with a clear etiology for her pelvic pain should focus on acknowledgment of her difficulties, education about her treatment options, and encouragement to maintain maximum activity level. For some, treatment may involve hysterectomy or exogenous hormones that impair fertility, and may present a difficult choice. Others with impaired sexual functioning may need medical psychotherapy or couples therapy to adjust to their situation. Treatment of chronic pain is discussed by Houpt in Chapter 17.

ABORTION

Over 1.5 million abortions are performed in the United States each year. This procedure accounts for 30 percent of the pregnancy outcomes for all females and 45 percent of the outcomes for females aged 11–19 years (U.S. Bureau of the Census, 1985). It is more commonly utilized by unmarried adolescents and young adults and by multiparous women in their late 30s and 40s.

Why do such unwanted pregnancies occur? Adolescent sexuality has become increasingly common in the last 20 years, and most adolescents are not mature enough to take responsibility for contraception. If current trends continue, it is estimated that 40 percent of adolescent girls will become pregnant by age 19 (Guttmacher Institute, 1981). Young adult women may also fail to use contraception in an appropriate way or may ambivalently wish for a pregnancy that they later regret. Often these women are unmarried, with no prospect of marriage to the father of the fetus, and unable to support a child.

Older women who become pregnant may have completed their families and be unwilling to start again. For them and others, contraceptive failures have occurred. Termination of pregnancy may also be sought for reasons of danger to maternal health or knowledge of an abnormal fetus.

Although much has been written about the psychologic sequelae of abortion, the procedure is associated with surprisingly low psychiatric morbidity as measured by incidence of major depression or psychosis (Brewer, 1977; McCance, Olley, & Edward, 1973). Although the woman seeking abortion is often highly distressed before the procedure, this distress subsides rapidly afterward for most. It is not, however, a psychologically painless procedure; many experience guilt and grief in the aftermath. The most frequent complaint 1 year later is a sense of regret, but the majority of women say they would do it again if faced with similar circumstances. Some may experience an anniversary grief reaction, which may occur at the time of the year that the abortion occurred or at the time that the child would have been born. The idea that abortion causes major psychiatric disorders has not held up under critical evaluation; severe postabortion reactions are associated with previous psychiatric difficulties (Ekblad, 1955; Kravitz, Notman, Anderson, et al., 1976). For patients with known major psychiatric disorders, there is no evidence to suggest that therapeutic abortion, if it is desired and accompanied by appropriate psychiatric treatment, leads to an increased rate of subsequent psychiatric hospitalization.

Psychiatric evaluation of abortion patients should include the history of the circumstances of the pregnancy and should explore the patient's relationships with her family and the father of the child. Other issues to be addressed are what the patient thinks about the pregnancy and her options and what kind of support she has. An evaluation for major psychiatric disorders, and for suicidal ideation, must be performed, and appropriate treatment initiated if the evaluation reveals significant psychopathology.

In the United States, counseling for the patient seeking abortion should be routinely provided by the agency or physician providing the procedure. Psychiatric consultation is thus reserved for patients with unusual circumstances, including the following:

1. Major psychiatric disorders such as schizophrenia, bipolar disorder, severe personality disorders, and mental retardation
2. Marked adjustment reactions prior to the procedure
3. Unresolvable conflict between the patient and her family or the father of the fetus
4. Unresolvable ambivalence about whether to have the procedure
5. Persistent contraceptive noncompliance and repeated abortions
6. Marked postabortion reactions
7. Pregnancies that may have resulted from rape or incest

In patients with major psychiatric disorders the concerns involve the following questions: Is this patient competent to make this decision? Will she be able to tolerate the procedure? Is there adequate psychiatric follow-up care? (Competency evaluation is discussed in Chapter 21.) With appropriate counseling and psychiatric treatment, patients with psychiatric disorders are at no additional risk following abortion. Consultation in this instance serves the function of reassuring the gynecologic staff that they are not alone in treating patients with psychiatric disorders, and that appropriate care is being provided.

Patients with severe adjustment reactions, including disorganized behavior, suicidal ideation, or homicidal ideation toward the father of the fetus, require evaluation, crisis intervention, and mobilization of support systems. Hospitalization may be necessary.

Severe conflict between the patient and the family or the father of the fetus may be accompanied by angry, threatening, disorganized, or suicidal behavior. An individual evaluation of each party is then necessary. Clarification of legal rights regarding the abortion decision is useful. The woman has the right to decide about her own body unless she is an unemancipated minor, in which case the parents have the right to make the decision. The dissenting party must then accept the decision. Limits and consequences of inappropriate behavior should be made clear.

Clinical experience suggests that the patient with unresolvable ambivalence strongly wishes to bear the child but is uncertain how she will be able to care for it. Since the time needed to make such a decision may interfere with the feasibility of the abortion, it is useful to empathize with the patient's mixed feelings and suggest that she consider bearing the child to give herself the time to think about it. If she decides that she is unable to care for the child, she can relinquish it after delivery. Psychotherapy then centers on understanding the meaning of the child to the patient and assisting her to determine whether it is realistic for her to keep it. If the patient decides to keep the child under questionable circumstances, the physician should arrange a social service evaluation to monitor the placement and to pursue court-ordered foster care if needed. It is important to recall that ambivalently regarded infants, especially those for whom abortion was considered, are at greater risk for child abuse and neglect.

Clinical experience suggests that patients with contraceptive noncompliance and repeated therapeutic abortions fall into two categories: a chronically disorganized, low-functioning group and a higher-functioning group with neurotic conflicts. For women in the former group, contraceptive noncompliance is just one of many characterologic problems. Although focused counseling about the consequences of repeated abortions and the appropriate use of contraceptives may be helpful, these women should also be confronted about their generalized self-destructive behavior and encouraged to seek psychotherapy.

Women in the latter group need to understand the meaning of the neurotic symptom so that they can find another way of dealing with the conflict. Although the identification and interpretation of the conflict may occur during an initial evaluation session, formal individual psychotherapy is advisable.

Rarely, a patient will demonstrate major psychiatric symptoms after an abortion, such as depression or psychosis. Treatment of these conditions should follow standard approaches for the specific diagnosis, with particular emphasis on the meaning of the loss, mourning it, and dealing with guilt constructively.

PSYCHOLOGIC SIDE EFFECTS OF ORAL CONTRACEPTIVES

Although numerous studies of the psychologic side effects of oral contraceptives (OCPs) have been performed, they are marred by many methodologic flaws (see reviews by Glick & Bennett, 1982; Slap, 1981; Warnes & Fitzpatrick, 1979; Weissman & Slaby, 1973). It is thus difficult to draw conclusions.

Most of the studies reviewed nevertheless suggest that the majority of women taking OCPs do not experience major psychologic side effects. Many, but not all, of the studies, however, report an increased incidence of depression in women taking OCPs. One study reports that OCPs with stronger progestins are associated with an increased incidence of depression and decreased libido (Grant and Pryse-Davies, 1968). Another study suggests that women with premenstrual irritability before starting OCPs have a greater incidence of depression on more strongly estrogenic OCPs and do better on more progestational agents. On the other hand, women without premenstrual irritability did better on more estrogenic pills (Cullberg, 1972). Pyridoxine, a cofactor in catecholamine synthesis, has been reported to be deficient in OCP users (Parry & Rush, 1979; Rose, Strong, Adams, et al., 1972). One double-blind, placebo-controlled study showed that pyridoxine supplementation alleviated depression associated with OCP use (Adams, Rose, Folkard, et al., 1973).

Clinical experience suggests that a small minority of patients on OCPs do complain of marked psychologic side effects. Although the etiology of these complaints cannot be discriminated with certainty, neither can the possibility be ruled out that at least some cases of psychologic symptoms are related to pharmacologic effects of these agents. Evaluation of such complaints should include a complete psychosocial history, to determine if situational reactions are contributory or if major psychiatric illness such as a mood disorder is present.

In the absence of definitive research, the physician can adopt an empirical management approach. If another birth control method is appropriate and acceptable, the patient can discontinue OCPs and shift to it. If she continues to desire the use of OCPs, she can be given a trial of other OCP preparations with a lower estrogen or progestin component (or both). Occasionally a higher estrogen component may be needed (Hatcher, et al., 1986). Another option would be to supplement the OCP with pyridoxine, 20 mg twice a day (Adams et al., 1973). Perhaps most important is developing an alliance with the patient to try to find what works best for her.

POSTHYSTERECTOMY REACTIONS

Hysterectomy is the most common surgical procedure of women and accounts for over 650,000 operations a year (National Center for Health Statistics, 1985). Although some are performed for emergencies and malignancies, most are performed as elective procedures for such indications as endometriosis, menorrhagia, fibroids, dysfunctional uterine bleeding, and chronic pelvic pain. Postoperative psychiatric reactions, particularly depression, have long been associated with hysterectomy. Psychiatric morbidity after hysterectomy has been reported to be 2.5 times more common than after nongynecologic surgery (Richards, 1974).

Alterations in ovarian hormones have been considered a possible etiology for this finding. The incidence of psychiatric disorders following simple hysterectomy, however, is similar to that following combined hysterectomy and bilateral salpingo-oophorectomy, whether or not replacement hormones are provided (Barker, 1968; Gath, Cooper, Bond, et al., 1981; Martin, Roberts, & Clayton, 1980; Richards, 1974). Biologic effects of ovariectomy thus, do not appear to contribute significantly to the development of posthysterectomy psychiatric disorders. Nonetheless, individuals with specific physical symptoms of estrogen deficiency following ovariectomy deserve hormone replacement.

Recent research has compared the preoperative psychiatric functioning of women receiving elective hysterectomies to their postoperative functioning. Multiple studies show a surprising level of psychopathology in the preoperative state (25–57 percent), which drops significantly 6 months to 1 year later (10–35 percent) (Gath, Cooper, & Day, 1982; Lalinec-Michaud & Engelsmann, 1984; Martin et al., 1980; Moore & Tolley, 1976). In these studies hysterectomy appears to improve rather than impair emotional functioning for the majority of women. This improvement may be related to relief of pelvic symptomatology. Nevertheless, a small subgroup does experience a postoperative psychiatric reaction. Age, marital status, number of children, social class, and type of gynecologic pathology do not predict these reactions; the strongest predictor is previous psychiatric history

and preoperative mental state (Gath & Rose, 1985). The hysterectomy may play a precipitating role in bringing these difficulties to the physician's attention.

For the vulnerable woman, hysterectomy may be decompensating for a number of reasons. A grief reaction may be triggered by the loss of the genital organ and the ability to bear children. For the woman whose major source of self-esteem is childbearing, the loss of the uterus means the loss of her feminine identity. For others, damage to the genital means impaired sexuality and loss of sexual value to the spouse. Particularly if her spouse or family has a negative attitude about the procedure and views her as "damaged goods," she will feel injured and devalued.

Psychiatric evaluation may be requested before or after hysterectomy. In addition to a standard history, the evaluator should explore why the procedure is being considered now, what the indications are, and what the patient expects from the procedure, both benefits and detriments. What is the meaning of the hysterectomy for the patient? Did she want more children? Is she afraid of altered relations with her husband? Is she concerned about an altered sense of femininity? What do her husband and family think about the procedure? What previous reactions to stress has she had, and what was helpful in coping? What support systems are available to her? Are there other situational stresses affecting the patient that indicate that surgery should be postponed? The differential diagnosis should include somatization disorder. A disproportionate number of women with this disorder receive hysterectomies, and they are thought to be at risk for unnecessary procedures (Martin, Roberts, & Clayton, 1980).

Psychiatric treatment prior to surgery should include standard pharmacologic and psychotherapeutic approaches to the specific psychiatric diagnosis. If the surgery is elective and the patient would benefit from psychotherapy or psychotropic drugs, the hysterectomy should be postponed. Ventilation, problem solving, and grief work may be needed for life crises occurring coincidentally with the gynecologic problems, such as marital discord, conflicts with adolescent children, concerns about aging parents, or deaths of significant others. Regarding the procedure itself, education and reality testing about its effects can be very helpful. In particular, the patient should know that although many patients are concerned about femininity and sexuality, there is no physical reason why these should be affected. If the patient continues to be distressed about these issues, psychotherapeutic exploration of her concerns is indicated.

For postoperative reactions a similar approach can be taken. Postoperative organic mental disorders must be ruled out. Then medical psychotherapy, which often includes grief work, is offered, supplemented with pharmacologic treatment if a major psychiatric disorder is diagnosed.

MENOPAUSE

A variety of psychologic symptoms, such as irritability, fatigue, depression, and sexual dysfunction, have been attributed to the endocrinologic changes of menopause. The majority of women adjust to menopause without difficulty, yet some become highly symptomatic and seek medical assistance. Although some psychologic complaints temporally associated with menopause are related to situational difficulties, such as the "empty nest syndrome" or marital conflict, other complaints may in fact be precipitated or exacerbated by the fall in estrogen and progesterone levels.

Hormone replacement is an accepted therapy for menopausal women. Not only does estrogen replacement eliminate hot flashes, it also helps prevent osteoporosis (DeFazio & Speroff, 1985) and may reduce

the risk of coronary disease. The epidemiologic association of unopposed estrogen use and endometrial cancer has led to the addition of a progestin to most hormonal replacement regimens for women who have not had hysterectomies.

Although the effect of hormone replacement on psychologic symptoms has been debated, recent data suggest that it can improve psychologic functioning. Several double-blind studies show that sleep disturbance, measured by both subjective complaints and objective episodes of awakening, is improved by estrogen replacement, compared with placebo (Campbell, 1976; Thomson & Oswald, 1977). One review of six double-blind, placebo-controlled studies (Dennerstein & Burrows, 1978) showed that all but one reported a decrease in irritability, fatigue, insomnia, anxiety, and depression when either an estrogen or an estrogen–progestin combination was administered. One large study (Dennerstein, Burrows, & Hyman, 1979) showed ethinyl estradiol (an estrogen) significantly more effective than levonorgesteral (a progestin), a combination of these compounds, or a placebo in improving sexual functioning, depression, fatigue, anxiety, irritability, and insomnia. A recent review concludes that estrogen replacement in menopausal woman improves psychologic functioning but that progestins should be minimized because of possible adverse effects (Dinnerstein, 1987). Estrogen serves as a weak monoamine oxidase inhibitor (MAOI), although the implications of the physiologic effect are not clear for affective stability (Kopera, 1983).

Evaluation of the menopausal woman should include a complete evaluation of all physical and psychologic complaints. A thorough psychosocial history will help evaluate contributions from situational issues. Differential diagnosis should include major mood disorders, personality disorders, anxiety disorders, and substance abuse. Organic mental disorders must also be ruled out, especially thyroid dysfunction. The menopausal woman with marked paroxysmal symptoms, such as dizzy spells and memory lapses, deserves an electroencephalogram (EEG) as a screen for temporal lobe epilepsy, a disorder that can be exacerbated at the menopause.

Pharmacologic treatment involves a number of choices, not only of estrogen and progestin preparations, but also of patterns of administration (see review by Shoupe & Mishell, 1987). The most common regimen now in use is conjugated estrogens, 0.625 mg daily, for days 1–25 of the month, with the addition of medroxyprogesterone acetate, 5 or 10 mg, on the last 10 to 14 days of the estrogen treatment. Another approach, which is becoming more common, is continuous estrogen and progestin treatment. An example of one such regimen would be conjugated estrogens at 0.625 mg daily and 2.5 mg medroxyprogesterone daily or on weekdays only. If psychologic complaints continue that appear related to the hormone therapy rather than some other disorder, an empirical trial of changing the estrogen or progestin dosages (particularly decreasing the progestin), changing to another pattern of administration, or shifting to other preparations can be considered.

If a significant situational component of the complaints is discerned, a referral for appropriate individual, couple, or family therapy should be made.

PSYCHOTROPIC MEDICATIONS IN PREGNANCY

The pregnant woman who requires psychotropic medication for the treatment of a serious mental illness raises a dilemma for the physician. On one hand, management of her mental condition may be very difficult without the benefit of such medication. On the other hand, the potential risks for the fetus include teratogenicity, behavioral teratogenicity, and side effects in the

newborn. Data on these topics are difficult to obtain in a systematic fashion and consist of case series or case reports. Although information is available on malformations and neonatal toxicity, little is known about the long-term behavioral effects of fetal exposure to these agents. Some estimate of risk to the fetus can be made, however. The balance of risks and benefits for each patient must be assessed on an individual basis.

For neuroleptics, there are contradictory reports regarding teratogenicity (Calabrese & Gulledge, 1985; Hauser, 1985). For example, with haloperidol, there are two case reports of limb malformations associated with first-trimester use; yet a study of 100 patients using haloperidol for hyperemesis gravidarum showed no effect on infant mortality or malformation rate. For chlorpromazine, one study of 142 first-trimester exposures showed no increase in malformations, but another study of 304 exposures showed a twofold increase in the rate of malformation. Nevertheless, several reviewers conclude that neuroleptic medication is relatively safe during pregnancy (Briggs, Freedman, & Yaffe, 1986; Calabrese & Gulledge, 1985). Neonatal side effects that have been noted include transient jaundice, sedation, motor excitement, agitation, hypotonia, and extrapyramidal symptoms (Calabrese & Gulledge, 1985).

Similarly, although there are case reports of anomalies associated with tricyclic antidepressants, these agents have not been documented to increase the rate of congenital malformations (Calabrese & Gulledge, 1985). Side effects in the newborn may include cardiac failure, tachycardia, myoclonus, respiratory distress, and urinary retention (Briggs et al., 1986; Calabrese & Gulledge, 1985). A fetal withdrawal syndrome consisting of colic, cyanosis, rapid breathing, and irritability has also been described (Briggs et al., 1986).

Lithium carbonate is the psychotropic medication that shows the best-documented increase in malformations, primarily of heart defects, including Ebstein's anomaly (which affects the tricuspid valve and the right ventricle). Of 217 babies in the Register of Lithium Babies, 7 were stillborn, 2 had Down's syndrome, and 18 had cardiovascular malformations, 6 of those Ebstein's anomaly (Calabrese & Gulledge, 1985). Because of the teratogenic risk of using lithium, alternative approaches to the management of mania should be considered, including neuroleptics and carbamazepine, an anticonvulsant that is low in teratogenicity (Briggs et al., 1986). Side effects of lithium in the newborn include transient cyanosis, lethargy, hypotonia, jaundice, hypothermia, low Apgar scores, and altered thyroid and cardiac function (Briggs et al., 1986). Women of childbearing age who are being considered for lithium treatment should be advised of these risks.

Use of benzodiazepines in the first trimester has been associated with conflicting reports about increased incidence of malformations. Diazepam has been associated with an increased rate of cleft palate (Briggs et al., 1986; Calabrese & Gulledge, 1985). In addition, a syndrome that resembles the fetal alcohol syndrome and results from in utero exposure to benzodiazepines has been described consisting of growth retardation, dysmorphism, malformations of facial regions, and central nervous system dysfunction (Laegreid, Olegard, Wahlstrom, et al., 1987). Because of the possible association with such malformations, and because their use is rarely urgent, benzodiazepines in the first trimester should be avoided (Calabrese & Gulledge, 1985). Side effects in the newborn include central nervous system and respiratory depression (Briggs et al., 1986; Calabrese and Gulledge, 1985). A withdrawal syndrome from diazepam has been described; it consists of irritability, jitteriness, tremor, diarrhea, and vomiting (Rementeria & Bhatt, 1977).

Phenobarbital has been commonly used as a sedating agent during pregnancy. Although its use has been associated with an increased rate of malformation in epileptic patients, it is not thought to pose increased risk in nonepileptic patients (Briggs et al., 1986). It is associated, however, with severe or even fatal hemorrhagic disease in the newborn, as well as withdrawal symptoms (Briggs et al., 1986).

Very little experience with monoamine oxidase inhibitors has been described. One small study reports an increased risk of malformation associated with these agents (Heinonen, Sone, & Shapiro, 1977). MAOIs have been considered contraindicated in pregnancy because of the risk of hypertensive episodes in fetus and mother and the availability of other treatment modalities (Hauser, 1985).

Pharmacologic management of psychiatric illness during pregnancy involves several basic principles. Although the overall risk of psychotropic medication use may be low, it nevertheless entails some uncertainty. The known risk of individual agents should be reviewed with the patient and her spouse. Such information is well summarized in Briggs et al. (1986). The prudent physician and patient will consider whether the psychiatric illness can be managed without medication. Whatever the treatment plan agreed upon, informed consent should be obtained. For some patients with depression or bipolar disorder, electroconvulsive therapy may be an appropriate alternative. Neuroleptics and carbamazepine should be considered as an alternative to lithium for bipolar patients, since teratogenic effects have not been conclusively documented. If medication is deemed necessary, postponement until the end of the first trimester is advisable if at all possible. After the first trimester, fetal organ differentiation is completed and is much less vulnerable to teratogenic effects. Use the medication with the lowest toxicity, and find the lowest effective dosage.

For those patients who do take medications throughout the pregnancy, consider tapering the dosage near the expected time of delivery to decrease the chance of severe side effects in the newborn. The pediatrician should be alerted to the maternal medication use so that appropriate neonatal care can be rendered.

ELECTROCONVULSIVE THERAPY IN PREGNANCY

In general, electroconvulsive therapy (ECT) is considered safe during pregnancy (Fink, 1981; National Institute of Mental Health Consensus Conference, 1985; Repke & Berger, 1984; Varan, Gillieson, Skene, et al., 1985; Wise, Ward, Townsend-Parchman, et al., 1984). This conclusion is drawn from a series of case reports in the literature rather than from controlled studies. There is nevertheless a striking absence of reported untoward effects. Because of the teratogenic risk of pharmacotherapy, ECT may actually be safer for the fetus in the first trimester, but again controlled studies are lacking (Remick & Maurice 1978). Developmental follow-up on children who were in utero during ECT has shown no abnormalities (Forssman, 1955; Impastato, Gabriel, & Landaro, 1964; Sobel, 1960).

Recommendations for safe ECT in the pregnant patient include a complete physical and pelvic examination, an obstetrician on the treatment team, and fetal monitoring for third-trimester patients (Remick & Maurice, 1978). ECT is relatively contraindicated in patients at high risk of premature labor. Depending on maternal and fetal risk factors, some patients may require endotracheal intubation; electrocardiograph (EKG) monitoring; arterial blood-gas measurements; Doppler ultrasonography of fetal heart rate; tocodynamometer recording of uterine tone; and tests of fetal lung maturity. Glycopyrrolate may be safer than

atropine, if an anticholinergic premedication is needed (Wise et al., 1984). (See also Chapter 5, by Weiner and Coffey, on ECT.)

PSYCHOTROPIC DRUGS IN LACTATION

Numerous case reports have shown little accumulation of psychotropic drugs in breast milk. This information has led the American Academy of Pediatrics (1982) to conclude that ingestion of psychotropic drugs by a lactating mother represents little risk to the infant. Single cases have been reported, however, of infant lethargy and weight loss due to accumulation of diazepam and of infant lethargy due to chlorpromazine (American Academy of Pediatrics, 1982). Long-term effects of infant exposure to psychotropic agents has not been studied.

Psychotropic drugs should be administered during lactation only if necessary for maternal health. If one of these agents is indicated, the patient should be informed of the uncertainty regarding long-term effects on the infant and given the option of discontinuing breast feeding. If breast feeding is continued, the lowest possible dosage of medication should be utilized, and the infant monitored for untoward effects.

A recent report studied desipramine and its metabolite 2-hydroxydesipramine in human breast milk and in the nursing infant's serum during administration of 300 mg/day to the mother (Stancer & Reed, 1986). Even though it was estimated that the infant in this study was ingesting 1/100 of the dose of the mother each day (6 mg/kg), derived from the milk, no detectable levels of either metabolite could be detected in the infant's serum. Other studies focusing on tertiary tricyclic antidepressants have failed to find detectable serum levels in nursing infants of mothers taking these medications, indicating levels less than 10 ng/ml (Bader & Newman, 1980).

One clinical report, however, described an 8-week-old nursing infant with respiratory depression that appeared to correlate with accumulation of the desmethyl metabolite of doxepin after the dose in the mother had been increased from 10 mg/day to 75 mg/day; doxepin itself was undetectable in the child's serum (Matheson, Pande, & Alertsen, 1985). The consensus of opinion, however, is that imipramine, desipramine, amitriptyline and the monoamine oxidase inhibitor tranylcypromine can be, in general, safely given to nursing mothers (Ananth, 1978). More detailed reviews of the literature may be found in articles by Ananth (1978) and Stancer and Reed (1986).

PREVENTION OF CHILD ABUSE AND NEGLECT

There has been a revolution in our awareness of child abuse and neglect in the last twenty years. Although efforts to detect child abuse and neglect are usually centered in the pediatric clinic, high-risk families can often be identified during pregnancy in the prenatal clinic as well. The obstetrician may turn to the psychiatric consultant for assistance in evaluating and coordinating the treatment of such patients. Early identification allows more effective intervention. One large, controlled study (Gray, Cutler, Dean, et al., 1979) showed that for high-risk families such interventions as regular pediatric appointments every 2 weeks, encouragement to call when problems arose, referrals for appropriate medical and mental health treatment, and lay health visitors significantly reduced the incidence of serious injuries, from 10 percent in the control group to 0 percent in the experimental group.

Known risk factors for child abuse and neglect include (1) abuse and neglect in the patient's background, (2) abuse, failure to thrive, relinquishment, or foster care for previous children, (3) previously expressed desire to abort or relinquish the current pregnancy, (4) history of mental illness, (5) mental retardation, (6) history of institutionalization, (7) history of spouse abuse, (8) alcohol or drug abuse, (9) chaotic living situation, (10) criminal record, (11) social isolation, (12) lack of financial resources, (13) age less than 17 years, (14) lack of anticipative behavior, (15) abnormal expectations of the child, and (16) single parenthood (Aycub & Pfeifer, 1977; Gray et al., 1979; Soumenkoff, Marnefe, Gerard, et al., 1982). Such psychosocial risk factors should be explored during the prenatal history. Another important souce of information about potential abuse is the observation of parental reactions to the infant at the time of delivery and during the immediate postpartum period. A hostile, negative, or disappointed reaction is significantly correlated with later abuse (Gray et al., 1979).

Evaluation of the high-risk patient should involve a thorough history to assess strengths and vulnerabilities, especially impulse control. Particular attention to current stresses and living situation will clarify the social interventions that may be needed. Determine the supports available to the patient, including the father of the child, the patient's family, her friends, and social agencies, such as a community mental health center. The patient's wishes and fantasies about the baby should be explored, as well as her plans for providing appropriate food, clothing, and shelter for the infant. Major mental illnesses, such as schizophrenia, mood disorders, substance abuse, and severe personality disorders, should be identified and treated. The possibility of mental retardation should also be considered.

Management of these patients requires a comprehensive psychosocial approach. Major categories of interventions include (1) developing an alliance, (2) solving social problems, (3) improving parenting behavior, (4) treating mental disorders, (5) coordinating postpartum follow-up, and (6) obtaining court-ordered measures. Since a number of health professionals may become involved in such a case, coordination of the various efforts by the psychiatrist is invaluable.

Developing an alliance is the single most important factor in working with women or couples at risk for child abuse and neglect. Many of them have been abused and neglected themselves and may react with suspicion and hostility at the physician's concern. Many are pleased, however, that someone is taking an interest in them. An essential aspect of the therapeutic alliance is continual positive reinforcement of the patient's self-esteem and acknowledgment of her efforts to be a good parent. It is also important to encourage the patient's connection to the clinic staff by calling the patient to reschedule missed appointments and by encouraging her to call if problems arise. In many ways the patient needs the clinic staff members to serve as models for her own parenting behavior.

Assisting the patient to solve problems in a structured manner is another important intervention. Clarify any existing problems with finances, the living situation, or support systems. Many women need information about the services that are available and the steps they must take to get them. They may need encouragement in making an appointment with social services to pursue Medicaid, food stamps, and Aid to Families with Dependent Children (AFDC). They may need suggestions about budgeting and places to stay. Sometimes an arrangement can be made with family, the father of the child, or friends to provide resources, financial and otherwise. Other potential supports can be explored and engaged.

A third area for therapeutic attention is the development of the parenting identity and behavioral repertoire. The health professional's mirroring of the patient's wish to be a good mother and promoting the patient's interest in anticipative behaviors, such as getting a crib and baby clothes, helps build that aspect of the self. The patient's fantasies about what the child will be like should be explored, and reality testing or problem solving provided when needed. If the patient is amenable, parenting classes at community agencies can be considered as an additional way of educating her and providing support.

For those prenatal patients with a diagnosed mental disorder, specific psychiatric treatment should be arranged. If the consulting psychiatrist chooses to provide such care, appointments can be scheduled to coincide with the prenatal clinic visits. The issues of termination of therapy after delivery and arrangements for subsequent treatment must also be addressed.

Coordination of postpartum follow-up is needed in many other areas as well. The inpatient obstetrical nursing staff needs to be informed about high-risk patients so that they can observe interactions and provide maximum education and support. The pediatric clinic staff also needs to be advised of the patient's situation so that an appropriate alliance can be formed. Many patients will benefit from postpartum outreach to their homes by a visiting nurse. In some areas volunteer workers may be available to provide a supportive, nonthreatening relationship during the postpartum period.

For those patients who are seriously disturbed and either unable to take care of themselves or in imminent danger of harming their infants, a court-ordered intervention must be obtained. A certification for involuntary inpatient psychiatric treatment should be considered if the patient is gravely disabled or dangerous to self or others, including the fetus. If the patient does not require hospitalization, yet there is grave concern about her ability to care for the child, a protective custody order can be sought that requires foster home placement or child protection services monitoring. Clinical experience suggests that the courts are quite interested in the information and opinions provided by the psychiatrist. Since the court generally wishes to preserve the mother–infant relationship, it may use compliance with a proposed treatment plan as a condition of regaining custody. Such conditions of custody can have a powerful structuring and motivating effect on the mother.

Although helping families at high risk for child abuse and neglect is often complicated and time-consuming, there is significant potential for reducing serious injury and even death. Perhaps our present efforts will decrease the incidence of child abuse and neglect for the next generation.

SUBSTANCE ABUSE AND PREGNANCY

Substance abuse is of special concern in pregnant women because of the increased incidence of fetal loss, malformation, and growth retardation and because of neonatal abstinence syndromes (Zuspan & Rayburn, 1986). Substance abuse is also associated with poor general health and nutrition for the mother, and an increased frequency of complications of labor and delivery (Zuspan & Rayburn, 1986). Women substance abusers may demonstrate low self-esteem, impulsiveness, and provocative behavior that impedes adherence to medical treatment. The obstetrician may request psychiatric consultation for assistance in managing these patients and arranging appropriate treatment plans.

Perhaps the most common error in dealing with substance abuse is failure to identify it. A substance abuse history should be routinely obtained in the prenatal history as well as in every psychiatric consultation. Other tip-offs to substance abuse include requests for drugs, evidence of intoxication, and suggestive physical findings, such as "tracks," a perforated nasal septum, or stigmata of liver disease. The substance abuse history should explore the history of drug use, the current pattern of use, the presence of tolerance and withdrawal symptoms, the perceived beneficial effect of substance use, and social factors that reinforce substance use. A thorough psychosocial evaluation should inquire about the patient's current financial status and living situation, as well as the attitudes of significant others and the availability of potential supports. Since substance abuse may serve the function of self-medicating an underlying psychiatric disorder, differential diagnosis should include mood disorders, personality disorders, anxiety disorders, and psychoses. See Chapter 10 for further discussion of the evaluation and treatment of alcohol and drug abuse.

Establishing an alliance is the most important step in treating substance abuse. Whatever clinicians' personal reactions, they should avoid being judgmental. The patient should be informed about confidentiality of medical evaluation and treatment. Responsiveness to the patient's concerns can be conveyed by open-ended interview techniques for at least part of the interview. If she indicates that she is concerned about the risk to the baby, this concern can be reinforced and used to help her maintain motivation to seek treatment. Once an empathic interaction has been established, the diagnosis of substance abuse can be clarified. For some patients, recognition of this problem will be a genuine surprise. Others will be relieved that someone is taking an interest. Some, however, will deny the problem and require a more confrontational approach: "I realize that you aren't concerned about drinking every day, but it is definitely harmful to you and the baby, and you need help with it. Let's try to understand why this is so hard to think about." (See excellent discussion by Senay, 1983.)

The patient will benefit from education about the nature of substance abuse and the type of treatment and life changes that will be needed. The fact that dealing with a substance abuse problem is a long-term process should be explained. Inpatient detoxification may be indicated. Residential treatment programs should be recommended if they are available. Education about the referrals to long-term support programs such as Alcoholics Anonymous or Narcotics Anomymous should be included. The patient may need considerable support to deal with her reactions to such treatment programs and to pursue treatment in these settings.

Treatment for some substance abuse disorders must be modified during pregnancy. For those patients with narcotic abuse, rapid withdrawal should be avoided, since it is associated with an increased incidence of fetal loss. Methadone maintenance titrated to a low dosage, 20–30 mg, has been recommended in this group to block craving for street drugs as well as the withdrawal syndrome (Zuspan & Rayburn, 1986). For alcohol-dependent patients, a gradual detoxification on long-acting benzodiazepines or phenobarbital is indicated despite some reports of increased rate of malformations associated with these agents. The use of disulfiram, however, is contraindicated in pregnancy because of its toxic effects on the fetus (Briggs et al., 1986).

Another important intervention is understanding the patient's social situation so that changes that support drug-free living can be made. Some patients may need assistance in obtaining Medicaid, food stamps, or AFDC. Others may need assistance in finding a place to stay apart from substance abusing acquaintances. Potential non-substance-using supports, such as family and friends, should be explored. The patient's significant other should be included in the evaluation process. If the expectant father is also a substance abuser, an attempt to engage him in treatment should be made as well.

Some substance-abusing women are disorganized, self-destructive, and noncompliant. Such behavior raises the question of potential child abuse and neglect after delivery. In this instance the local social service agency should be advised of the high-risk situation, and a court-ordered evaluation and protective custody order considered (see previous section, on prevention of child abuse).

Although dealing with substance-abusing patients can be emotionally taxing and time-consuming, the physician can render a very important service by being willing to be concerned. Not only may the child be spared the untoward effects of maternal substance abuse, but the alliance achieved during prenatal care may create a crucial turning point in the mother's life.

Tobacco Use in Pregnancy

As cigarette smoking has become increasingly prevalent among women of childbearing age, birth defects similar to the fetal alcohol syndrome have emerged as a potential complication of smoking during pregnancy. Smoking during pregnancy is also associated with prematurity and low birth weight (Nieburg, Marks, McLaren, et al., 1985). Smokers who become pregnant should thus not only be counseled to stop smoking, but should be referred for smoking cessation interventions if they are unable to stop on physician's advice alone. The use of nicotine-containing gum is contraindicated during pregnancy because of toxic effects on the fetus. Smoking cessation interventions are discussed further in Chapter 15.

PREGNANCY LOSS

Over one million women a year experience an unsuccessful pregnancy. A surprisingly high percentage of pregnancies result in loss: 15–20 percent in miscarriage,

1 percent in stillbirth, and 1 percent in perinatal death (Borg & Lasker, 1982; Friedman & Gradstein 1982). Furthermore, with modern, highly sensitive pregnancy tests, women are increasingly aware of early pregnancy loss.

Even an early pregnancy is a child for a woman who desires one. Thus, loss of the pregnancy can be like the loss of a beloved person. The normal grieving reaction may include a sense of shock and disbelief, intense sadness and crying, anger toward the physician and others, somatic symptoms of weight loss, sleep disturbance, and decreased sexual interest, and guilt and a sense of inadequacy at having been unable to sustain the fetus ("what did I do wrong?"). The woman will usually have a much more pronounced reaction to miscarriage than her spouse. Her bodily changes make the pregnancy a more tangible reality for her. The husband's subdued reaction may cause the woman to feel isolated and abnormal in her grief. Friends and family members, unless they have suffered miscarriage themselves, may have little sympathy for the patient and may minimize the patient's distress with the comment "Well, you can get pregnant again." The grief reaction will be most intense in the first few weeks after the loss and will continue for several months, gradually subsiding. After 6 months, severe symptoms that continue to disrupt the patient's previous level of functioning should be considered a pathologic grief reaction and deserve a full psychiatric evaluation.

Pregnancy loss in the second or third trimester, after fetal movement has been felt and an ultrasound image seen, is associated with even more intense grieving because of the increased attachment to the physically perceived fetus. Stillbirth and perinatal death are even more intense losses. Carrying the child for 9 months and preparing her life for the new arrival, the woman invests a great deal emotionally in the child. Instead of the expected happy event, the woman must face loss, the reactions of family and friends, the making of funeral arrangements, and the return home to an empty crib. She may be unable to tolerate being on an obstetric unit, where she can see other women and their newborns. Such a loss can exacerbate preexisting marital conflict, especially when grief-handling styles are not complementary, and may lead to marital discord, sexual dysfunction, and, in some cases, divorce.

Late fetal loss, stillbirth, and perinatal death are also difficult for physicians and nurses, who may be overwhelmed by the patient's feelings and their own personal reactions. They also may feel a sense of guilt, wondering if there was something they could have done to prevent the loss. The lack of control that occurs with fetal demise is especially disturbing for medical professionals, who are accustomed to being in control. They may react by blaming the patient or minimizing the patient's loss. It is crucial that the staff members handle their own reactions in a constructive way, because the patient and her spouse are vulnerable to their comments and depend on them for emotional support.

Although psychologic factors are not thought to be contributory to fetal loss in general, there is evidence that women with multiple spontaneous abortions significantly improve their chances of carrying a pregnancy to term with medical psychotherapy, particularly psychotherapy that facilitates grieving of the previous losses (Tupper & Weil, 1962).

Psychiatric treatment of pregnancy loss involves a number of interventions. The events of the pregnancy, the fetal loss, and subsequent circumstances should be reviewed. The explanation for the loss should be discussed, and any uncertainties about the events clarified, especially regarding the patient's being at fault. The single most important factor in facilitating a grief reaction is allowing and empathizing with the patient's feelings. At times this may feel overwhelming, but it is very useful and deeply appreciated by the patient. She should be educated that she is not mentally ill but that she is experiencing a normal grief reaction, and that it will be very intense at first and then gradually subside over several months. If the spouse and the family can be involved in the evaluation and similarly informed, they will be better able to work through their own grief and support the patient as well.

If there has been a stillbirth or perinatal death, the couple should be helped to decide whether they should see and hold the body, take a picture of it, and name the child. Although the couple may wish to "forget" the unfortunate event, they should be educated that many couples have later found it helpful to have tangible memories of their child (Harmon & Macey & Harman, in press). They may need support in making funeral arrangements. The psychiatrist can also help them anticipate the potential reactions of friends and family, so that the couple are less vulnerable to unempathic comments. It is also useful to anticipate with the couple how they may feel when they return home and what they will do with any preparations they have made for the child.

The psychiatrist can also talk with obstetric staff members to assess their reactions and allow ventilation so that they will be better able to deal with the patient. Some hospitals routinely arrange case conferences to review these cases and provide support for the staff.

After discharge, the couple, especially the woman, should be encouraged to call if they become overwhelmed. Follow-up appointments 1 week and 1 month after discharge should be arranged; more frequent appointments should be arranged if the couple or the woman desires them.

The question when to seek a new pregnancy may be raised. Although the wish to replace the lost child and urgency related to other conditions, such as infertility, may push the couple to seek a new pregnancy immediately, these concerns must be balanced against the importance of grief reaction resolution in facilitating attachment to a new child. Particularly for third-trimester losses, stillbirths, and perinatal losses, the couple should be advised of this and encouraged to give themselves some time, perhaps 6 months, before seeking a new pregnancy (Macey & Harmon, in press).

POSTPARTUM PSYCHIATRIC DISORDERS

Postpartum psychiatric disorders span a spectrum of conditions that occur from a few days to several months after delivery. The three main categories are

1. "Maternity blues," a transient condition affecting 50–80 percent of new mothers within the first week after delivery and usually resolving within 2–3 weeks. It is characterized by emotional lability (particularly tearfulness and irritability), sleep disturbance, fatigue, and mild confusion.
2. Postpartum depression, a condition that is more common than generally realized, affecting 10–15 percent of new mothers. Its initial presentation may resemble "the blues," but it is distinguished by its persistence beyond the first postpartum month and by the greater severity of symptoms. This condition is consistent with DSM-III-R criteria for major depression or bipolar disorder, depressed.
3. Postpartum psychosis, a much less common condition, affecting only 0.1 percent of new mothers. It is defined as a psychosis occurring within 6 months of delivery and is consistent with DSM-III-R diagnoses of brief psychotic reaction, schizophreniform disorder, schiz-

ophrenia, and bipolar disorder with manic episode (Inwood, 1985).

The role of biologic contributions to these disorders has long intrigued clinicians. The biologic changes associated with childbirth, particularly the rapid drop of estrogen and progesterone levels, have been hypothesized to affect central nervous system neurotransmitter levels and to play a "predisposing, if not causal role" in the etiology of these disorders (Campbell and Winokur, 1985). Efforts to prevent and treat these disorders with hormone replacement have, however, yielded equivocal results. Genetic vulnerability does seem to play a role, since there is an increased lifetime incidence of depression and a higher rate of positive family histories of mental disorders in those who develop postpartum disorders (Campbell and Winokur, 1985). Psychosocial factors also affect the development of these disorders. Risk factors include an unwanted pregnancy, an unstable or absent marital relationship, and a lack of social supports. Women who have had a complicated delivery or a premature, abnormal, sick, or "difficult" child are more at risk for postpartum disorders, as are those who have lost the child through stillbirth or perinatal death (Pitt, 1985). Women who have a poor relationship and identification with their mothers are also thought to be more at risk for psychologic difficulties (Melges, 1968).

Psychiatric evaluation of postpartum disorders should include a detailed history of the pregnancy, the delivery, and postpartum adjustment, as well as information about past psychiatric illness, family history, and social history, especially the availability of such supports as the father of the child, family members, and friends. A complete mental status examination should be performed. Although organic mental syndromes are now uncommon sequelae of childbirth, they must be ruled out. Postpartum endocrine disorders, such as hypo-thyroidism due to thyroiditis and pituitary insufficiency, should be considered. A thyrotropin (TSH) level is advisable; endocrine consultation is relevant if abnormal vital signs or laboratory values suggest pituitary disease. The presence of psychotic symptoms, such as delusions and hallucinations, should be addressed. The woman's ability to care for the child must also be evaluated. Reports of difficulty feeding and of infant weight loss may be early indicators of failure to thrive. Special attention must be given to evaluating suicidal or infanticidal ideation, as these constitute psychiatric emergencies.

The mainstays of treatment for the "maternity blues" are education and reassurance that it will subside in a matter of weeks. If, however, symptoms last longer than 3–4 weeks, vigorous evaluation should be pursued.

Management of a postpartum depression involves the standard approaches to major depression, including psychotherapy and medication. If the patient can be treated as an outpatient, support systems must be mobilized to help provide appropriate care for the child. If psychiatric hospitalization is needed, consider admitting the child concurrently in order to facilitate maternal–infant attachment and reinforce mothering behavior in the patient. Involve the father as much as possible in the treatment plan. If the child is not admitted, arrangements of the child's care must be made with the father, family, friends, or social services.

The treatment of postpartum psychosis also requires standard treatment approaches for the specific diagnosis. Because of the unpredictable nature of psychosis, most of these patients will require hospitalization. As already mentioned, care for the child must be arranged. If the mother's mental condition appears to be chronic, questions about her ability to care for the child are likely to be raised during

discharge planning. For some patients, social services will need to be involved at this
time, to evaluate the need for foster care or
a supervised placement of the child with the

mother. For others, regular pediatric follow-up will be needed to monitor the situation. If visiting nurse service is available, it
can also provide support and monitoring.

REFERENCES

Adams P, Rose D, Folkard J, et al. (1973). Effect of
pyridoxine on depression associated with oral
contraceptives. *Lancet*, 7809.

American Academy of Pediatrics, Committee on
Drugs (1982). Psychotropic drugs in pregnancy
and lactation. *Pediatrics*, *69*, 241–244.

Ananth J (1978). Side effects in the neonate from
psychotropic agents excreted through breast feeding. *American Journal of Psychiatry*, *135*, 801–
805.

Aycub C & Pfeifer D (1977). The prophylaxis of child
abuse and neglect. *Child Abuse and Neglect*, *1*,
71–75.

Bader TF & Newman K (1980). Amitriptyline in
human breast milk and the nursing infant's serum.
American Journal of Psychiatry, *137*, 855–856.

Barker MG (1968). Psychiatric illness after hysterectomy. *British Medical Journal*, *2*, 91–95.

Behrman S & Kistner R (1975). *Progress in infertility*.
Boston: Little, Brown.

Borg S & Lasker J (1982). *When pregnancy fails*.
Boston: Beacon Press.

Brewer C (1977). Incidence of post-abortion psychosis: A prospective study. *British Medical Journal*,
1, 476–477.

Briggs G, Freedman R, & Yaffe S (Eds) (1986). *Drugs
in pregnancy and lactation* (2nd ed). Baltimore:
Williams and Wilkins.

Calabrese J & Gulledge A (1985). Psychotropics during pregnancy and lactation: A review. *Psychosomatics*, *26*, 413–426.

Campbell S (1976). Double blind psychometric studies
on the effects of natural estrogens on post-menopausal women. In S Campbell (Ed), *Management of menopause and post-menopausal years*.
Lancester, England: MTP Press.

Castlenuovo-Tedesco P & Krout B (1970). Psychosomatic aspects of chronic pelvic pain. *Psychiatry in
Medicine*, *1*, 109–126.

Collins J, Wrixon W, James L, et al. (1983). Treatment
independent pregnancy among infertile couples.
New England Journal of Medicine, *309*,
1201–12005.

Cullberg J (1972). Mood changes and menstrual symptoms with different gestagen/estrogen combina-

tions. A double blind comparison with placebo.
Acta Psychiatrica Scandinavia, *236*, 1–86.

Day JB (1979). Clinical trials in the premenstrual
syndrome. *Current Medical Research and Opinion*, *6*(Suppl 5), 40–45 (1979).

DeFazio J & Speroff L (1985). Estrogen replacement
therapy: Current thinking and practice. *Geriatrics*, *40*, 32.

Dennerstein L (1987). Psychologic and sexual effects.
In D Mishell (Ed), *Menopause: Psychology and
pharmacology*, Chicago: Year Book Publishers.

Dennerstein L Dennerstein & Burrows G (1978). A
review of studies of psychological symptoms
found at the menopause. *Maturitas*, *1*, 55–64.

Dennerstein L, Burrows G, & Hyman G (1979). Hormone therapy and affect. *Maturitas*, *1*, 247.

Downing J (in press). Impaired fertility. In JL Petersen, E DalPozzo, MP Weissberg, et al. (Eds),
*Pregnancy: Psychological issues and their man-
agement*. Philadelphia: WB Saunders.

Ekblad M (1955). Induced abortion on psychiatric
grounds; follow-up study of 479 women. *Acta
Psychiatrica Scandinavica*, (Suppl 99), 1–238.

Fink M (1981). Convulsive and drug therapies of
depression. *Annual Review of Medicine*, *32*, 405–
412.

Forssman H (1955). Follow-up of sixteen children
whose mothers were given electric convulsive
therapy during gestation. *Acta Psychiatrica
Neurologica Scandinavica*, *30*, 437–441.

Friedman R & Gradstein B (1982). *Surviving pregnancy loss*. Boston: Little, Brown.

Gath D, Cooper P, Bond A, et al. (1982). Hysterectomy and psychiatric disorder: II. Demographic,
psychiatric and physical factors in relation to
psychiatric outcome. *British Journal of Psychiatry*, *140*, 343–350.

Gath D, Cooper P, & Day A (1982). Hysterectomy and
psychiatric disorder: I. Levels of psychiatric morbidity before and after hysterectomy. *British
Journal of Psychiatry*, *140*, 335–342.

Gath D & Rose N (1985). Psychological problems and
gynecological surgery. In R Priest (Ed), *Psychological disorders in obstetrics and gynecology*.
London: Butterworth.

Glick ID & Bennett S (1982). Psychiatric complications of progesterone and oral contraceptives. *Journal of Clinical Psychopharmacology, 1,* 350–367.

Grant E & Pryse-Davies J (1968). Effects of oral contraceptive on endometrial monoamine oxidase and phosphates. *British Medical Journal, 3,* 777–780.

Gray JD, Cutler C, Dean J, et al. (1979). Prediction and prevention of child abuse and neglect. *Journal of Social Issues, 35*:127–139.

Allan Guttmacher Institute (1981). *Teenage pregnancy: The problem that hasn't gone away.* New York: Alan Gluttmacher Institute.

Hamilton J, Parry B, Alagna S, et al. (1984). Premenstrual mood changes: A guide to evaluation and treatment. *Psychosomatics, 14,* 426–435.

Hatcher R, Guest F, Stewart F. et al. (1986). *Contraceptive technology 1986-87. 13 ed.* New York: Irvington Publishers.

Hauser L (1985). Pregnancy and psychotropic drugs. *Hospital and Community Psychiatry, 36*(8), 817–818.

Heinonen O, Sone D, & Shapiro S (1977). *Birth defects and drugs in pregnancy* (pp 336–337). Littletoon, MA: Publishing Sciences Group.

Impastato D, Gabriel A, & Landaro H (1964). Electric and insulin shock therapy during pregnancy. *Journal of Nervous and Mental Disorders, 25,* 542–546.

Inwood D (1985). The spectrum of postpartum psychiatric disorders. In D Inwood (Ed), *Postpartum psychiatric disorders.* Washington, DC: American Psychiatric Press.

Kopera H (1983). Sex hormones and the brain. In D Wheatley (Ed.) *Psychopharmacology and sexual disorders.* Oxford: Oxford University Press, pp 50–67.

Kravitz A, Notman M, Anderson J, et al. (1976). Outcome following therapeutic abortion. *Archives of General Psychiatry, 33,* 725–733.

Kresch A, Steifer D, Sach L, et al. (1984). Laparoscopy in 100 women with chronic pelvic pain. *Obstetrics and Gynecology, 64,* 672–674.

Laegreid L, Olegard R, Wahlstrom J, et al. (1987). Abnormalities in children exposed to benzodiazepines in utero. *Lancet, 1,* 108–109.

Lalinec-Michaud M & Engelsmann F (1984). *Psychosomatics, 25,* 550–558.

Lundberg W, Wall J, & Mathers J (1973). Laparoscopy in evaluation of pelvic pain. *American Journal of Obstetrics and Gynecology, 42,* 872–876.

Macey T & Harmon B (in press). Perinatal loss. In J Petersen, E DalPozzo, M Weissberg, et al. (Eds), *Pregnancy: Psychological issues and their management.* Philadelphia: WB Saunders.

Martin R, Roberts W, & Clayton PJ (1980). Psychiatric status after hysterectomy: One year prospective follow-up. *Journal of the American Medical Association, 244,* 350–353.

Matheson I, Pande H, & Alertsen AR (1985). Respiratory depression caused by N-desmethyldoxepin in breast milk [Letter]. *Lancet, 2,* 1124.

McCance C, Olley P, & Edward V (1973). Long-term psychiatric follow-up. In Y Horobin (Ed), *Experience with abortion.* London: Cambridge University Press.

Melges F (1968). Postpartum psychiatric syndromes. *Psychosomatic Medicine, 30,* 95–108.

Moore J & Tolley D (1976). Depression following hysterectomy. *Psychosomatics, 17,* 86–89.

National Center For Health Statistics (1985). *Detailed diagnosis and surgical procedures for patients discharged from short stay hospitals, United States, 1983* (Vital and Health Statistics Series 13, No. 82). Washington, DC: U.S. Government Printing Office.

National Institute of Mental Health Consensus Conference Electroconvulsive Therapy (1985). *JAMA,* Vol. 254:15, *Journal of the American Medical Association, 254,* 2103–2108.

Nieburg P, Marks JS, McLaren NM, et al. (1985). The fetal tobacco syndrome. *Journal of the American Medical Association, 253,* 2998–2999.

Parry B & Rush A (1979). Oral contraceptives and depressive symptomatology: Biologic mechanisms. *Comprehensive Psychiatry, 20,* 347.

Pasnau R, Soldinger S, & Andersen B (1985). Pelvic pain. In R Priest (Ed), *Psychological disorders in obstetrics and gynecology.* London: Butterworth.

Pitt B (1985). The puerperium. In R Priest (Ed), *Psychological disorders in obstetrics and gynecology.* London: Butterworth.

Rementeria J & Bhatt K (1977). Withdrawal symptoms in neonates from intrauterine exposure to diazepam. *Journal of Pediatrics, 90,* 123–126.

Remick R & Maurice W (1978). ECT in pregnancy. *American Journal of Psychiatry, 125,* 761–762.

Renaer M (1980). Chronic pelvic pain without obvious pathology in women. *European Journal of Obstetrics, Gynecology, and Reproductive Biology, 10,* 415–463.

Renaer M (1981). *Chronic pelvic pain in women.* Berlin: Springer-Verlag.

Renaer M, Vertommen H, Nijs P, et al. (1979). Psychological aspects of chronic pelvic pain in women. *American European Journal of Obstetrics and Gynecology, 134,* 75–80.

Repke J & Berger N (1984). Electroconvulsive therapy in pregnancy. *Obstetrics and Gynecology, 63*(Suppl 3), 39S–41S.

Richards DH (1974). A post-hysterectomy syndrome. *Lancet, 2,* 983–985.

Rose D, Strong R, Adams P, et al. (1972). Experimental vitamin B_6 deficiency and the effect of estrogen containing oral contraceptives on tryptophean metabolism and vitamin B$_6$ requirements. *Clinical Services*, *42*, 4655.

Rosenthal R, Ling F, Rosenthal T, et al. (1984). Chronic pelvic pain: Psychological features and laparoscopic findings. *Psychosomatics*, *25*, 833–841.

Rubinow D & Roy-Byrne P (1984). Premenstrual syndrome: Overview from a methodologic perspective. *American Journal of Psychiatry*, *141*, 163–172.

Senay E (1983). *Substance abuse disorders in clinical practice*. Inc., Littleton, MA: John Wright, PSG.

Shoupe D & Mishell D (1987). Therapeutic regimens. In D Mishell (Ed), *Menopause: Physiology and pharmacology*. Chicago: Year Book Publishers.

Slap G (1981). Oral contraceptives and depression. *Journal of Adolescent Health Care*, *2*, 53–64.

Sobel D (1960). Fetal damage due to ECT, insulin coma, chloromazine, and reserpine. *Archives of General Psychiatry*, *2*, 606–610.

Soumenkoff G, Marnefe C, Gerard M, et al. (1982). A coordinated attempt for prevention of child abuse at the antenatal care level. *Child Abuse and Neglect*, *6*, 87–94.

Stancer HC & Reed KL (1986). Desipramine and 2-hydroxydesipramine in human breast milk and the nursing infant's serum. *American Journal of Psychiatry*, *143*, 1597–1600.

Stoudemire A & Sandhu J (1987). Psychogenic/idiopathic pain syndromes. *General Hospital Psychiatry*, *9*, 79–86.

Thomson J & Oswald I (1977). Effect of estrogen on the sleep mood and anxiety of menopausal women. *British Medical Journal*, *2*, 1317–1319.

Tupper C & Weil RJ (1962). The treatment of habitual aborters by psychotherapy. *American Journal of Obstetrics and Gynecology*, *83*, 421–424.

U.S. Bureau of the Census (1985). *Statistical abstract of the United States, 1986*. Washington, DC: U.S. Government Printing Office, 1985.

Varan L, Gillieson M, Skene D, et al. (1985). ECT in an acutely psychotic pregnant woman with actively aggressive (homicidal) impulses. *Canadian Journal of Psychiatry*, *30*, 363–367.

Vargyas J (in press). The premenstrual syndrome. In C Beckman (Ed), *Clinical manual of obstetrics and gynecology*. Norwalk, CT: Appleton-Century-Crofts.

Warnes H & Fitzpatrick C (1979). Oral contraceptives and depression. *Psychosomatics*, *20*, 187–194.

Weissman M & Slaby A (1973). Oral contraceptive and psychiatric disturbance: Evidence from research. *British Journal of Psychiatry*, *123*, 513–518.

Williams J & Spitzer R: Idiopathic pain disorder: A critique of pain-prone disorder and a proposal for a revision of the DSM-III category psychogenic pain disorder. *Journal of Nervous and Mental Disease*, *170*, 415–419.

Winston F (1973). Oral contraceptives, pyridoxine and depression. *American Journal of Psychiatry*, *130*, 1217–1224.

Wise M, Ward S, Townsend-Parchman W, et al. (1984). Case report of ECT during high risk pregnancy. *American Journal of Psychiatry*, *141*, 99–101.

Zuspan F & Rayburn W (1986). Drug abuse during pregnancy. In W Rayburn & F Zuspan (Eds), *Drug therapy in obstetrics and gynecology*. Norwalk, CT: Appleton-Century-Crofts.

Gregory J. O'Shanick
David F. Gardner
Susan G. Kornstein

30
Endocrine Disorders

Psychiatric symptomatology in endocrine disorders has long been recognized. Cognitive, affective, and behavioral changes were noted in the earliest accounts of Addison (1868), Cushing (1932), Sheehan (1939), and others. These symptoms often precede or present simultaneously with the more definitive signs and symptoms of endocrine disease and may confuse even the most astute diagnostician. Symptoms may be mislabeled in early stages as "neurotic" in nature, and in more advanced stages as dementia or psychotic disorders. Particularly in the elderly, in whom the physical manifestations of an endocrinopathy may not be evident and the mental changes mistaken for senility, the diagnosis of an endocrine disorder may easily be missed.

In this chapter, we will focus on the endocrine disorders in which psychiatric syndromes are most often encountered, specifically, those involving the thyroid, adrenal glands, and disorders of calcium homeostasis. We will also examine complications of abnormal pituitary function, diabetes mellitus, hypoglycemia, and pheochromocytoma. The emphasis of the

chapter will be on the differential diagnosis of the psychiatric syndromes and on screening diagnostic studies. Our contention that, whenever possible, treatment should first be directed at the underlying endocrine disorder, as resolution of the psychiatric disturbance usually follows, is not universally shared. Some clinicians hold that when disabling mental symptoms exist, psychotropics should be used until endocrine homeostasis is achieved. Where solid scientific evidence exists for either efficacy or significant complications of such use, these studies will be highlighted.

HYPERTHYROIDISM

Hyperthyroidism (or thyrotoxicosis) is the clinical syndrome resulting from the chronic exposure of body tissues to excessive quantities of thyroid hormones. Surveys estimate the incidence to be 1–2 cases for every 1000 persons each year, with women affected approximately seven times more frequently than men. The peak incidence in women is between 20 and 40 years of age.

The most common cause of hyperthyroidism is Graves' disease, an autoimmune disorder characterized by diffuse thyroid enlargement and extrathyroidal manifestations involving primarily the eyes (ophthalmopathy) and the skin (dermopathy). Graves' disease, toxic nodular goiter, and thyroiditis account for more than 95 percent of all cases of hyperthyroidism. Other causes include thyrotropin-secreting pituitary tumors, struma ovarii, and trophoblastic tumors. The differential diagnosis should also include consideration of excessive doses of exogenous thyroid hormone, on either an iatrogenic or factitious basis.

Although the symptoms of hyperthyroidism will vary from patient to patient, the following are most often reported: nervousness, increased sweating, heat intolerance, fatigue, dyspnea, palpitations, weight loss with increased appetite, eye symptoms, muscle weakness, hair loss, and hyperdefecation. Irregular menses may be observed, with either cycle duration or interval abnormalities. The term "apathetic" hyperthyroidism describes the atypical hyperthyroid patient, who lacks many of the classic symptoms of this disorder. These patients are usually elderly and present with unexplained weight loss, weakness, and cardiovascular manifestations (Kathol, Turner, & Delahunt, 1986). The diagnosis is often overlooked because these patients lack the more typical symptoms of nervousness and heat intolerance.

The patient's general appearance may be the first clue that thyroid hyperfunction is present. The typical patient is hyperactive and appears to have lost weight; speech is often rapid and rambling. Other important physical findings include tachycardia (occasionally atrial fibrillation), warm, smooth, moist skin, fine hair, thyroid enlargement, fine tremor of the hands, and hyperactive deep tendon reflexes. Lid retraction and lid lag may be seen in all hyperthyroid patients, but infiltrative eye changes (i.e., exophthalmos) are specific for Graves' disease. The nature of the thyroid enlargement will depend on the etiology of the hyperthyroidism.

Mental changes in hyperthyroidism are common and may be the initial complaint (Hall, 1983). The most frequent psychiatric presentation is anxiety with irritability, emotional lability, a feeling of apprehension, and inability to concentrate. Cognitive changes include short attention span, distractibility, and decreased recent memory, but the impairment is generally less severe than in hypothyroidism. Psychosis is also less common and less severe, with a prevalence of up to 20 percent in severe hyperthyroidism. There may be rapid speech and psychomotor agitation or frank psychosis with paranoid and grandiose delusions. In thyroid storm, visual hallucinations and delirium are not uncommon.

Symptoms of hyperthyroidism are most frequently misdiagnosed as anxiety disorders (Greer, Ramsay, & Bagley, 1973). Features that help to distinguish hyperthyroidism from an anxiety disorder include the findings of cognitive impairment, tachycardia, fatigue accompanied by a desire to be active, constant rather than intermittent anxiety, and palms that are warm and dry, as opposed to cool and clammy. Apathetic hyperthyroidism may be mistaken for a primary depressive disorder or dementia (Kathol, et al., 1986). Other common misdiagnoses of hyperthyroidism include anorexia nervosa, bipolar disorder, schizophrenia, psychotic depression, and organic mental disorders of other etiology. In the case of a maniclike presentation of hyperthyroidism, treatment with lithium produces dramatic short-term improvement; however, rapid relapse into the hyperthyroid state occurs (Cowdry, Wehr, Zis, et al., 1983; O'Shanick & Ellinwood, 1982).

The diagnosis is hyperthyroidism rests

on the demonstration of elevated concentrations of circulating thyroid hormones. An elevated *free* thyroxine (T4) concentration in a patient with appropriate signs and symptoms is sufficient for diagnosis. Elevation of the *total* T4 concentration is not diagnostic, as alterations in serum thyroxine binding globulin (TBG) may increase the total T4 concentration without affecting the free hormone concentration. In most clinical laboratories, the free-T4 concentration is estimated by using the free thyroxine index (FTI), although there are now several techniques for direct free-T4 determinations. A normal serum free-T4 concentration does not exclude the diagnosis of hyperthyroidism, and if there remains a strong clinical suspicion, a serum triiodothyronine (T3) level should be determined. The syndrome of hyperthyroidism with a normal free-T4 concentration and an elevated T3 concentration has been called T3-thyrotoxicosis and probably accounts for about 5 percent of all hyperthyroid patients. Finally, recently developed highly sensitive thyrotropin (TSH) assays can now discriminate between the low TSH levels sometimes seen in normals and the markedly depressed levels observed in hyperthyroid patients.

A rare patient will present with suspicious signs and symptoms and borderline results on all of the above studies. The thyrotropin releasing hormone (TRH) test (see Appendix A) may be valuable in such a patient, as a normal TSH response to TRH virtually excludes the diagnosis of hyperthyroidism. A blunted or absent response, however, does not conclusively prove the diagnosis. Blunted responses to TRH have been documented in euthyroid patients with nodular goiters, depressed patients, alcoholics during and after withdrawal, patients with anorexia nervosa, patients experiencing massive weight loss, and normal men over the age of 60. It should be noted as well that transient hyperthyroxinemia has been demonstrated in some patients with acute psychiatric disorders (Spratt, Pont, Miller, et al., 1982). The fact that these abnormalities resolve without any specific therapy suggests that these patients are not truly hyperthyroid, and the significance of this finding is currently unclear.

A detailed account of therapy for hyperthyroidism is beyond the scope of this review. Although the ultimate goal in all patients is restoration of the euthyroid state, initial therapy is often symptomatic in nature. Beta-adrenergic blocking agents have no direct effect on thyroid hormone secretion, but they do effectively reverse many of the signs and symptoms of hyperthyroidism. Patients report improvement in nervousness, palpitations, sweating, and tremor, as well as improvement in their overall sense of well-being. Definitive therapy in most patients will be either antithyroid drugs (propylthiouracil or methimazole) or radioactive iodine. The role of surgery is quite limited, reserved primarily for children and adolescents and pregnant women not responding to or having an allergic reaction to antithyroid drugs. As thyroid function returns to normal, anxiety, affective symptoms, and cognitive deficits improve. Organic impairment may persist in patients with severe or prolonged illness (Kathol et al., 1986).

Use of psychotropic medications in hyperthyroid patients should be tempered by the risk of potentially lethal complications. Tricyclic antidepressants may evoke cardiac arrhythmias (Blackwell & Schmidt, 1984). Although no definitive studies currently exist, potential sensitization of tissues to catecholamines by coincident exposure to high concentration of thyroid hormone may be the cause of this phenomenon (Whybrow & Prange, 1981). Phenothiazines may intensify tachycardia (Foldes, Nagy, Kertai, et al., 1959). When indicated for management of severe psychiatric symptoms, conservative regimens should be employed, with frequent monitoring of blood levels and electrocardiograms. Adrenergic blockers may also be useful for symptomatic relief, although the risk of further psychiatric complications must be considered (Utiger, 1984).

Persistence of depressive symptoms for greater than 4–6 weeks after normalization of thyroid serum values may indicate the evolution of a major depressive episode requiring more aggressive biologic intervention with either antidepressants or electroconvulsive therapy. Assuming that restoration of thyroid hormone homeostasis will in all situations correct the accompanying mood disturbance is naive at best and may prolong unnecessarily the psychiatric morbidity of these patients. As noted below in the discussion of hypothyroidism, premature use of antidepressants may induce rapid cycling (Cowdry, Wehr, Zis, et al., 1983).

HYPOTHYROIDISM

Hypothyroidism is a clinical syndrome of diverse etiologies, which have in common a decrease in circulating thyroid hormone concentrations. It is a common disorder, occurring most frequently in women between the ages of 40 and 60. Overall prevalence is about 1 percent in women and 0.1 percent in men. The prevalence of the disorder appears to increase significantly after age 60, and may be as high as 6 percent in elderly women. The most common cause of hypothyroidism in adults in the United States is autoimmune thyroiditis (Hashimoto's thyroiditis). Hypothyroidism is also common following both radioactive iodine treatment or surgery for hyperthyroidism. Although iodine deficiency is an important cause of hypothyroidism in many parts of the world, it is extremely rare in industrialized societies. Less common causes of hypothyroidism include external irradiation, medications (e.g., lithium, antithyroid drugs, excess iodine), and in-

volvement of the thyroid in malignancies. Finally, hypothyroidism may be secondary to disorders of the pituitary or of the hypothalamus and is then called secondary or tertiary hypothyroidism, respectively.

Classic symptoms of hypothyroidism include weakness, fatigue, cold intolerance, weight gain, constipation, hair loss, menstrual disturbances (oligomenorrhea and menorrhagia), hoarseness, and muscle aches, stiffness, and pain. Cerumen in the external auditory canals is also decreased. Typical physical findings include bradycardia, dry, cool skin, facial puffiness, thickened tongue, slow speech, peripheral edema, pallor, and delayed relaxation of the deep tendon reflexes. Onset of signs and symptoms is subtle and insidious and often goes unnoticed by the patient and relatives. This is particularly true in the elderly, in whom a clinical diagnosis of hypothyroidism may be extremely difficult. Because of the high prevalence of the disorder in the elderly and its subtle manifestations in this age group, some have advocated routine screening for hypothyroidism in all patients over age 60.

Mental disturbance is a prominent feature of hypothyroidism and may be the presenting complaint. Multiple psychiatric symptoms have been described (Goggans, Allen, & Gold, 1986). Progressive cognitive dysfunction characterized by slowness in comprehension and impairment of attention, recent memory, and abstract thinking is often found. Affective disturbance is perhaps the most common clinical presentation, with dysphoric mood, psychomotor retardation or agitation, sleep disturbance, crying spells, anhedonia, decreased libido, and suicidal thoughts common. A maniclike state, with agitation, paranoid ideation, and hypersexuality, has been reported. Insidious personality changes may be noted, such as irritability, suspiciousness, anxiety, and social withdrawal. Severe and longstanding or rapidly progressive disease may present with generalized agitation, paranoid delusions, auditory or visual hallucinations, and clouded sensorium.

Given the wide range of psychiatric presentations and the usual subtlety of physical findings, the diagnosis of hypothyroidism can be easily missed. Personality changes may be mistaken for neurosis, cognitive changes for dementia, affective disturbance for major mood disorder (depression or mania), and psychotic features for schizophrenia or an acute paranoid state. Studies have shown that a significant number of patients referred to psychiatrists for treatment of a "primary" depression have overt, mild, or subclinical hypothyroidism (Gold, Pottash, & Extein, 1981).

Definitive diagnosis of hypothyroidism in the patient with suggestive signs and symptoms requires laboratory confirmation. Typically, depression of both the serum total-T4 and the free-T4 concentrations is found. Diagnosis of primary hypothyroidism (i.e., hypothyroidism due to intrinsic thyroid disease) is confirmed by the presence of an elevated serum TSH concentration. Patients with milder degrees of hypothyroidism may have T4 and free-T4 concentrations within the normal range, and the diagnosis can be made with certainty only by finding an elevated serum TSH. This may also be true in patients who are on supplemental exogenous thyroid replacement regimens at an insufficient dose to produce a totally euthyroid state. The patient with low serum thyroid hormone levels and a normal TSH concentration should be suspected of having underlying hypothalamic-pituitary disease and requires referral for further evaluation of this possibility. As the basal serum TSH concentration is almost always elevated in patients with primary thyroid failure, TRH testing is usually unnecessary. An occasional patient with a borderline TSH elevation, however, may show an exaggerated TSH response to TRH, confirming the diagnosis of hypothyroidism.

The diagnosis of Hashimoto's disease can be confirmed by the presence of circulating antithyroid antibodies. The most sensitive test for the diagnosis of this autoimmune disorder is the antithyroid microsomal antibody determination. High titers of antithyroid antibodies in a patient with primary hypothroidism or goiter are strongly suggestive of Hashimoto's disease. Patients with Hashimoto's disease are at increased risk for other autoimmune endocrine disorders, including Addison's disease, hypoparathyroidism, type I diabetes mellitus, and premature ovarian failure. As these conditions are quite rare, however, screening should be limited to patients with suspicious signs and symptoms.

Certain psychotropics can confound thyroid function tests. High doses of benzodiazepines can give false normal thyroid function tests (Baron, 1967; Harvey, 1967; Marzollo, 1963). Chronic lithium therapy can cause elevated TSH and exaggeration of the TRH response (Smigan, Wahlin, Jacobson, et al., 1984). Should symptoms of hypothyroidism occur, the patient, if possible, should have lithium discontinued. If this is not clinically feasible or if the condition is not corrected by lithium withdrawal, replacement with T4 is advised.

Replacement therapy in hypothyroid patients should be in the form of 1-thyroxine, with the usual adult daily dose in the 0.1–0.2 mg range. The usual starting dose is 0.05 mg a day, with 0.025–0.05-mg increases at 2–3 week intervals. Higher initial doses and more rapid dose increases may precipitate serious cardiovascular side effects, particularly in the elderly (Hoffenberg, 1986). The goal of therapy should be to restore the serum TSH to the normal range, regardless of the etiology of the deficiency.

With thyroid hormone replacement, both physical and mental symptoms improve, although emotional and cognitive disturbances may persist for weeks to months. When disease has been long standing, residual cognitive deficits may exist (Whybrow & Hurwitz, 1976). Psychotic symptoms usually clear within 2–3 weeks, especially if an antipsychotic medication is added. Exacerbation of the psychosis may occur early in the course of replacement therapy. If thyroid replacement is given in too high a dose or too rapidly, an acute organic psychosis may be precipitated (Mason, 1968).

If affective symptoms persist after a euthyroid state has been achieved, psychiatric intervention may be indicated (Wilson & Jefferson, 1985). Use of tricyclic antidepressants or lithium while the patient is still hypothyroid will not augment resolution of symptoms and may induce rapid cycling (Cowdry, Wehr, Zis, et al., 1983; O'Shanick & Ellinwood, 1982). An additional concern is the sensitivity of hypothyroid patients to the hypotensive and anticholinergic side effects of tricyclic antidepressant medications. Phenothiazines must also be used with great caution, as they may precipitate myxedema coma (Jones & Meade, 1964). Use of benzodiazepines is not typically associated with untoward effects in this group, although at least one report exists of concurrent obstructive sleep apnea and hypothyroidism (McNamara, Southwick, & Fogel, 1987). In these situations, use of benzodiazepines may worsen the sleep apnea and, hence, the organic mood symptoms.

CUSHING'S SYNDROME

Cushing's syndrome is best defined as the signs and symptoms associated with prolonged exposure to inappropriately elevated plasma glucocorticoid levels. It may occur spontaneously (endogenous hypercortisolism) or secondary to the chronic administration of glucocorticoids for suppression of a variety of inflammatory disorders. Spontaneous Cushing's syndrome may be caused by excessive pituitary adreno-

corticotropin (ACTH) secretion (Cushing's disease), benign or malignant adrenal neoplasms, or ectopic ACTH production by nonendocrine malignancies. In adults, Cushing's disease accounts for 60–70 percent of all cases, adrenal tumors for approximately 20 percent, and the ectopic ACTH syndrome for the remaining 10–20 percent.

Clinical manifestations of endogenous hypercortisolism include truncal obesity, moon facies, hypertension, muscle wasting and weakness, easy bruising, purple striae, facial plethora, hirsutism, acne, menstrual irregularities (usually amenorrhea), peripheral edema, and impotence. Hyperpigmentation is most prominent in the ectopic ACTH syndrome but may also be present in Cushing's disease. Metabolic consequences include glucose intolerance, osteoporosis, and hypokalemic alkalosis. Psychiatric disturbances occur in over 50 percent of patients (Starkman & Schteingart, 1981).

Although in the past psychiatric findings have been attributed to the disruption of physical and social function caused by disfigurement, mental symptoms in fact, often precede any physical signs or symptoms. A wide range of psychiatric symptoms have been reported, and marked variation of symptomatology may occur in the course of a single patient's illness (Starkman, Schteingart, & Schork, 1981). Depression is the most frequent presentation, accompanied by insomnia, irritability, crying spells, low energy, poor concentration and memory, anhedonia, decreased libido, and suicidal ideation. Psychomotor retardation may alternate with periods of agitation. Rapid mood fluctuations, with episodes of acute anxiety, may be seen. Euphoria and manic excitement are rare, occuring typically prior to the onset of depression, sometimes with an intervening period of remission. Psychoses are usually depressive, but paranoid states and schizophreniform syndromes also occur. Organic mental states with confusion and disorientation are seen

(Whelan, Schteingart, Starkman, et al., 1980). Medical complications of the illness, such as electrolyte disorders, diabetic ketosis, and hypertensive encephalopathy, may cause additional mental impairment.

Cushing's syndrome can present a difficult diagnostic challenge to even the most astute clinician, because of the marked diversity of its clinical manifestations. With the frequency of psychiatric symptoms as initial complaints, patients are often misdiagnosed as having major depression, mania, bipolar depression, schizophrenia, and a variety of other organic, toxic, or metabolic conditions. Definitive diagnosis requires the demonstration of cortisol overproduction and an abnormality in the suppression of cortisol secretion.

Two convenient tests are available for outpatient screening of patients with suspected Cushing's syndrome. The overnight dexamethasone suppression test (see Appendix B) involves the administration of 1 mg of dexamethasone at 11:00 P.M. and the measurement of plasma cortisol at 8:00 A.M. the following morning. Normals will show suppression of the plasma cortisol concentration below 5 μg/dl, and a normal result virtually excludes the diagnosis of Cushing's syndrome. False positive results (i.e., plasma cortisol levels greater than 5 μg/dl in the absence of Cushing's syndrome) may occur in obesity, depression, acute stress, alcohol withdrawal, and pregnancy and in patients taking estrogens or phenytoin. Determination of the 24-hour urinary free-cortisol excretion is another excellent screening test, although it requires adequate patient compliance for a meaningful result. Patients demonstrating abnormalities on either of the screening tests just described need referral for more definitive diagnostic studies.

Some depressed patients show significant abnormalities of the hypothalamic-pituitary-adrenal axis, resulting in sustained hypercortisolism. Use of the dexamethasone suppression test (DST) has been advocated for diagnosis of melancholia (Carroll, Feinberg, Greden, et al., 1981). Although many false positives and false negatives exist, the *psychiatric* DST differs from the *endocrine* DST in that 4:00 P.M. and 11:00 P.M. postdexamethasone cortisol values are the central concern. Late escape (i.e., failure to suppress plasma cortisol concentration below 5 μg/dl) from normal suppression at either time is strongly correlated with melancholia. (The sensitivity of this test is approximately 50 percent in carefully selected populations). Current evidence finds the DST to be less useful in clinical settings than in research endeavors (Hirschfeld, Koslow, & Kupfer, 1983). Occasionally depressed patients may be impossible to distinguish from patients with true Cushing's disease, even with formal dexamethasone suppression testing. Recent studies suggest that there are differences in ACTH responsiveness to corticotropin-releasing hormone between depressed patients and those with Cushing's disease, differences that allow diagnostic separation (Chrousos, Schuermeyer, Doppman, et al., 1985; Gold, Loriaux, Roy, et al., 1986).

Successful therapy of Cushing's syndrome depends on an accurate determination of the cause of the hypercortisolism. In patients with primary adrenal tumors or the ectopic ACTH syndrome, treatment is generally directed at removing the underlying neoplasm. Although therapy for pituitary-dependent Cushing's syndrome or Cushing's disease remains controversial, in most centers transsphenoidal pituitary surgery has become the treatment of choice. In patients without an obvious pituitary tumor, total hypophysectomy or bilateral adrenalectomy may be necessary. As cortisol levels are reduced to normal, psychiatric symptoms usually remit. Low doses of neuroleptics or electroconvulsive therapy may be helpful for symptomatic relief. Use of tricyclic antidepressants may precipitate a manic episode and should be

Table 30-1
Equivalent Steroid Doses

Steroid	Dose (mg)
Cortisone	5
Hydrocortisone	4
Prednisone	1
Methylprednisolone	0.8
Triamcinolone	0.8
Dexamethasone	0.15

employed only if depression is severe or persists after cortisol levels are normalized.

Exogenous, or iatrogenic, Cushing's syndrome results from the prolonged administration of either ACTH or supraphysiologic doses or glucocorticoids. As many as 5 percent of patients receiving high doses of glucocorticoids develop significant psychiatric symptoms at some time during their treatment (Boston Collaborative Drug Surveillance Program, 1972). Occurrence of these symptoms is clearly related to the dose of drug administered. Patients receiving more than 50 mg per day of prednisone or its equivalent (see Table 30-1) are at greater risk. Premorbid personality, history of previous steroid psychosis, or history of previous psychiatric disorder did not affect risk in one series (Hall, Popkin, Stickney, et al., 1979).

Physical manifestations of exogenous Cushing's syndrome are similar to those of endogenous Cushing's, except that myopathy, glucose intolerance, and osteoporosis tend to be more prominent. Cataracts and aseptic necrosis of the femoral head may also be seen, which are rare in endogenous Cushing's syndrome. Hypertension is less common, and signs of masculinization and hyperpigmentation do not occur.

Mental changes can be seen at any point during the course of glucocorticoid therapy but are most common in the first 4–6 hours after ACTH administration or within 4–6 days after oral administration of steroids. Alterations in mood are the most

common problem, with euphoria occuring in 75 percent of cases, often accompanied by irritability, increased appetite, increased libido, and insomnia. A prodromal state of "cerebral excitability" has been reported by many patients (Goolker & Schein, 1953). Depression is infrequent but may be severe, with significant suicidality, and may follow a period of euphoria. One-third of patients show cognitive disturbance (Whybrow & Hurwitz, 1976). Some patients present with a "spectrum psychosis," marked by rapid shifts of symptoms ranging from affective to schizophreniform to organic. These symptoms may include agitation, emotional lability, distractibility, memory impairment, pressured speech, mutism, auditory and visual hallucinations, delusions, and body image distortions.

Diagnosis of exogenous Cushing's syndrome is based on the history of ingestion of supraphysiologic doses of glucocorticoids. Measurement of 8:00 A.M. plasma ACTH concentrations will reveal subnormal values, although similar low values will be seen in patients with primary adrenal neoplasms causing Cushing's syndrome.

Following cessation of glucocorticoid therapy, spontaneous recovery of psychiatric and behavioral symptoms occurs in 2 weeks to 7 months (Hall et al., 1979). Reduction of dosage alone may cause symptoms to remit. Treatment with low to moderate doses of neuroleptics results in significant improvement with or without discontinuation of steroids and dramatically shortens the duration of the psychotic state (Hall et al., 1979). Electroconvulsive therapy may also be useful, whereas tricyclic antidepressants have been reported to cause exacerbation of symptoms (Hall, Popkin, & Kirkpatrick, 1978). Prophylactic treatment with lithium at psychiatric doses reduced the psychiatric complications in one study of patients receiving ACTH for multiple sclerosis (Falk, Mahnke, & Poskanzer, 1979). No conclusive selection criteria exist. Although the study of Hall et al. (1979) suggests no correlation of previous psychosis on steroids to subsequent events, prophylaxis of patients with previous steroid psychosis would appear intuitively prudent.

ADDISON'S DISEASE (ADRENOCORTICAL INSUFFICIENCY)

Inadequate secretion of adrenal corticosteroid hormones may either result from primary adrenal disorders (Addison's disease) or be secondary to inadequate ACTH secretion (secondary adrenal insufficiency). Although in the past tuberculosis was the major cause of Addison's disease, 75 percent of all new cases fall into the idiopathic category. Most of these cases are believed to represent autoimmune adrenal destruction. Other causes include fungal diseases (especially histoplasmosis), metastatic tumor, adrenal hemorrhage associated with anticoagulant therapy, sepsis (meningococcemia), infiltrative disorders (amyloidosis, sarcoidosis, hemochromatosis), and previous adrenal surgery.

Typical clinical manifestations of Addison's disease include generalized weakness and fatigability, weight loss, anorexia, vomiting, hyperpigmentation, abdominal pain, hypotension with orthostatic dizziness, nonspecific muscle and joint aching, and perceptual abnormalities. Common laboratory features include hyperkalemia and hyponatremia, and an occasional patient will manifest hypercalcemia. In patients with secondary adrenal insufficiency associated with hypothalamic-pituitary dysfunction, hyperkalemia and hyperpigmentation will be absent.

Mental changes are observed in 60–90 percent of patients with Addison's disease (Cleghorn, 1951; Engel & Margolin, 1941). Development of symptoms is insidious and often precedes the more classic somatic features. Early manifestations include apa-

thy, social withdrawal, fatigue, irritability, negativism, and poverty of thought. Moderate to severe depression is present in 30–50 percent of patients. Often there is cognitive impairment, particularly of memory. Mental changes tend to be episodic and fluctuating in severity. In Addisonian crisis, delirium may occur, with confusion, disorientation, and frank psychosis (Ettigi & Brown, 1978). Because of the slow onset of illness and the frequent initial appearance of psychiatric symptoms, the diagnosis of Addison's disease may be overlooked. Common misdiagnoses include depression, hypochondriasis, and conversion disorders. Autoimmune thyroiditis may coexist with autoimmune Addison's disease. As potentially lethal complications (i.e., Addisonian crisis) can occur with thyroid replacement alone in this situation, a high index of suspicion should be maintained for their coexistence.

The diagnosis of adrenal insufficiency can be suspected on the basis of a low 8:00 A.M. plasma cortisol concentration or decreased 24-hour urinary free-cortisol or 17-hydroxycorticosteroid excretion. Definitive diagnosis is made by ACTH stimulation studies. The rapid ACTH test with synthetic ACTH (Cortrosyn) is an excellent outpatient screening study, with a normal result virtually excluding the diagnosis of primary or secondary adrenal insufficiency. An abnormal result, however, needs confirmation, and the patient should be referred for definitive studies with prolonged ACTH infusions.

Treatment of Addison's disease with both glucocorticoid and mineralocorticoid replacement produces rapid resolution of mood and cognitive disturbances. Organic psychoses may persist for several weeks. Only rarely do irreversible mental changes occur. Psychotropic medications should not be employed except with great caution, as they are likely to exacerbate hypotension (Thompson, 1973).

HYPERPARATHYROIDISM

Primary hyperparathyroidism is a clinical syndrome characterized by hypercalcemia due to excessive secretion of parathyroid hormone (PTH). The prevalence of the disorder may be as high as 1:1000, with females more commonly affected than males. It is the most common cause of hypercalcemia in the ambulatory care population. Approximately 85 percent of cases are due to a single parathyroid adenoma and 15 percent to parathyroid hyperplasia. Rarely, hypercalcemia is associated with multiple adenomas or a parathyroid carcinoma. In hospitalized patients, an underlying malignancy is the most common cause of hypercalcemia. The neoplasms most commonly implicated are lung, breast, prostate, kidney, and multiple myeloma. Other causes of hypercalcemia include hyperthyroidism, sarcoidosis, drugs (thiazides, lithium, vitamin D), Addison's disease, and immobilization.

Clinical manifestations of hyperparathyroidism are extremely variable. Many patients are entirely asymptomatic, and the diagnosis is suspected only at the time of a "routine" serum calcium determination. In other patients, the symptoms are subtle and their onset is insidious. Patients may complain of nonspecific muscle weakness, fatigue, anorexia, nausea, constipation, headaches, thirst, and vague abdominal and musculoskeletal pains. Finally, patients may present with more acute symptoms associated with a kidney stone, peptic ulcer disease, pancreatitis, or a pathologic fracture.

Reports of the occurrence of psychiatric symptoms in hyperparathyroidism vary from 5 percent to 65 percent. Generally, changes in mental status parallel the degree of elevation of serum calcium (Borer & Bhanot, 1985). In mild hypercalcemia, personality changes, loss of spontaneity, and lack of initiative are typical complaints. In moderate hypercalcemia (12–16 mg/dl),

symptoms are principally depressive, with dysphoria, anhedonia, apathy, anxiety, irritability, impaired concentration and recent memory, and sometimes suicidal ideation. In severe hypercalcemia (16–19 mg/dl) or following a precipitous rise in serum calcium, psychotic and organic symptoms predominate, including confusion, disorientation, catatonia, agitation, paranoid ideation, delusions, and auditory and visual hallucinations. Above 19 mg/dl, stupor and coma are common. In some patients, significant elevations in serum calcium have been reported without observable mental changes.

In view of the insidious onset and frequent lack of specific symptomatology, the diagnosis of hyperparathyroidism is often overlooked ("Calcium Metabolism," 1977). Common misdiagnoses include neuroses, hypochondriasis, mood disorders, schizophrenia, and various organic mental disorders. Correction of hypercalcemia results in rapid reversal of many of the psychiatric manifestations (P Peterson, 1968). A trial of oral phosphate therapy that induces a detectable reduction in serum calcium with concurrent reversal of psychiatric symptoms may be useful in defining whether parathyroid surgery will be helpful. No published data appear to exist on this issue.

A serum calcium determination remains the single best screening test for hyperparathyroidism. Serial determinations may be necessary in patients with borderline calcium elevations, to determine whether the diagnosis of hyperparathyroidism should be pursued. An "ionized" calcium determination may be helpful in patients with abnormalities in serum albumin concentrations. Definitive diagnosis of hyperparathyroidism requires the exclusion of other causes of hypercalcemia and the demonstration of an elevated serum PTH concentration. Patients on chronic lithium therapy may present a clinical picture indistinguishable from primary hyperparathyroidism. Discontinuation of lithium in these patients should result in a return of serum calcium levels to the normal range.

HYPOPARATHYROIDISM

Hypoparathyroidism is characterized by a decrease in the serum calcium concentration in association with hyperphosphatemia. The most common cause of hypoparathyroidism is accidental damage to or removal of parathyroid glands during thyroid surgery or radical neck dissection for cancer. Other etiologies include severe magnesium deficiency (often associated with alcoholism), parathyroid aplasia (Di George's syndrome), trauma, and after neck irradiation; it may also be idiopathic (probably autoimmune). Pseudohypoparathyroidism is a rare hereditary disorder in which there is decreased end-organ responsiveness to PTH. Other conditions that may cause hypocalcemia include alcoholism, malabsorption syndromes, vitamin D deficiency, pancreatitis, and renal failure.

As in hyperparathyroidism, symptoms of hypoparathyroidism tend to be nonspecific and insidious in onset (Fonseca & Calverley, 1967). Early complaints of lethargy, muscular weakness, and paresthesias may be followed by attacks of tetany, carpopedal spasms, and athetoid movements. In later stages, laryngeal stridor and generalized seizures may occur.

Psychiatric findings in hypoparathyroidism occur in 30–50 percent of patients. The rapidity of change in serum calcium and other electrolytes seems to be the most important factor in determining the severity of symptoms. Common complaints include anxiety, depression, irritability, emotional lability, social withdrawal, phobias, and obsessions. In severe cases, delirium with confusion, disorientation, agitation, paranoia, and auditory and visual hallucinations may be present. Intellectual deterioration is found in one-third of patients with primary

hypoparathyroidism, the result of a long duration of illness prior to diagnosis and treatment. In surgically induced hypoparathyroidism, cognitive changes are rare, as the condition is usually treated promptly.

Symptoms of hypoparathyroidism may be mistaken for neuroses, hypochondriasis, conversion disorders, anxiety disorders, depression, schizophrenia, dementia, and other organic mental states. The diagnosis of primary hypoparathyroidism is confirmed by the findings of a low serum calcium concentration in association with a low serum PTH level.

Treatment of hypoparathyroidism consists of vitamin D and oral calcium supplements. Normalization of serum calcium results in symptomatic improvement. When intellectual impairment is present, residual cognitive deficits often persist. With regard to the use of psychotropic medications, patients with hypoparathyroidism have shown an increased sensitivity to acute dystonias secondary to phenothiazines (Schaaf & Payne, 1966).

DISORDERS OF GLUCOSE METABOLISM

Both hyperglycemia and hypoglycemia can produce significant behavioral disturbances. A variety of psychosocial factors have impact on metabolic control in the diabetic patient (Boehnert & Popkin, 1986). Recent evidence indicates that the type of stress (acute vs. chronic) may govern abnormal glucose metabolism in type I diabetics (Kemmer, Bisping, Steingruber, et al., 1986). Acute stress, in this study, did not disturb metabolic control in these patients. Changes anecdotally reported in the literature (Bernstein, 1986) may relate to more subtle compliance lapses in individuals experiencing stressful and distracting external events.

Hyperglycemia results in symptoms often misdiagnosed in early states as hypochondriasis (Pennebaker, Cox, Gonder-Frederick, et al., 1981). Polyuria, polyphagia, and polydipsia often coexist with anorexia, fatigue, and visual changes (primarily blurring). Ketoacidosis rarely (in fewer than 5 percent of cases) presents with delirium, whereas hyperosmolar nonketotic states more often present with altered mental status. Schizophreniform and depressive syndromes have been observed. A significant diagnostic dilemma exists in the patient whose sole presenting symptom is impotence (Martin, 1981). Diabetic autonomic neuropathy and vascular disease may coexist with psychogenic etiologies, particularly depressive. Presence of morning erections, situation-specific impotence, and abrupt onset may indicate significant psychogenic components. Clinical polysomnography with assessment of nocturnal penile tumescence (NPT), as well as penile arterial Doppler studies will often define organic importance in the diabetic patient (Karacan, Salis, Ware, et al., 1978).

Longstanding diabetes is associated with a variety of microvascular (retinopathy, nephropathy), macrovascular (coronary artery, cerebrovascular, and peripheral vascular disease), and neuropathic complications. These complications, in turn, influence the use of psychotropic agents. For example, anticholinergic activity of the antipsychotics and antidepressants may have adverse effects in patients with diabetic gastroparesis or neurogenic bladders, exacerbating vomiting and urinary retention, respectively. Use of metoclopramide may also result in extrapyramidal side effects. Alpha-adrenergic blocking activity of some psychotropic agents may worsen orthostatic hypotension. Selection of agents with low anticholinergic and alpha-adrenergic blocking profiles in selected patients may be critical to successful overall management. Tricyclic antidepressants should be used with caution in the diabetic patient with organic heart disease and a predisposition to cardiac arrhythmias. Cau-

tion should govern the use of beta blockers in these patients, as they may mask autonomic symptoms due to hypoglycemia.

Diabetes may be associated with a variety of painful neuropathic syndromes. The most common diabetic neuropathy is a bilateral, symmetric, predominantly sensory syndrome characterized by paresthesias (e.g., tingling and numbness) and loss of sensation. Superimposed on this relatively asymptomatic condition, however, may be numerous painful neuropathies, typically associated with burning and shooting pains in the lower extremities. Anticonvulsants (phenytoin, carbamazepine) have shown some success in the treatment of these pain states. The role of antidepressant and antipsychotic therapy for these pain syndromes remains controversial (Maciewicz, Bouckoms, & Martin, 1985). Recent studies favor the use of tricyclic antidepressant agents whose net effect is to increase the availability of serotonin at the synapse (e.g., amitriptyline, doxepin, trazodone, imipramine). Inconsistencies abound, however, with regard to the need for "antidepressant" dosages in these situations (Kvinesdal, Molin, Frland, et al., 1984). Careful monitoring of nondepressed patients indicates that therapeutic benefit may be derived from "subtherapeutic" doses of these agents. The issue of anticholinergic activity is essential to optimizing clinical care. Use of neuroleptics such as fluphenazine and haloperidol for chronic neuropathic pain has been less encouraging. Concern related to the development of tardive dyskinesia in these patients has relegated this therapy to only the most severe cases in which other therapeutic modalities have failed. Refractory situations have been reversed in some patients with lidocaine infusion.

Hypoglycemia

Hypoglycemia is best defined by the following clinical triad: (1) plasma glucose less than 50 mg/dl, (2) appropriate symptoms, and (3) relief of symptoms by glucose administration. *Reactive* (postabsorptive) *hypoglycemia* refers to hypoglycemia occuring within 5 hours of food ingestion. *Fasting*, or *spontaneous*, *hypoglycemia* occurs more than 6 hours after food ingestion (Berger, 1975). Fasting hypoglycemia may be associated with a variety of disorders, including insulin-secreting tumors of the pancreatic islets, nonislet cell neoplasms, severe liver or renal disease, endocrine deficiency states such as hypoadrenalism and hypopituitarism, and drug or toxin ingestion (e.g., alcohol, salicylates). Perhaps the most commonly encountered form of hypoglycemia is iatrogenic, associated with either excessive insulin or sulfonylurea administration. Finally, the differential diagnosis must include surreptitious self-administration of insulin. Such factitious disorders (Munchausen syndromes) are well documented in the literature and should be considered in all patients prior to pancreatic exploration for an islet cell tumor. The presence of anti-insulin antibodies and low C-peptide levels strongly suggest factitious hypoglycemia.

Hypoglycemic symptoms are generally divided into two categories—beta-adrenergic and neuroglycopenic (Pennebaker et al., 1981). Beta-adrenergic or catecholamine-mediated symptoms may include tachycardia, anxiety, diaphoresis, tremor, weakness, hunger, and palpitations. Symptoms may be suggestive of a panic disorder. An inadequate glucose supply to the central nervous system—neuroglycopenia—may result in faintness, headaches, blurred vision, lethargy, confusion, bizarre behavior, seizures, and coma. Considerable controversy exists as to whether irritability, fugue, amnesia, and automatisms are directly related to hypoglycemia (Anderson & Lev-Ran, 1985).

Perhaps the major clinical issue regarding hypoglycemia is its overdiagnosis. Reactive hypoglycemia has become a fashionable diagnosis to account for numerous poorly defined physical and psychologic ills, including depression, anxiety, fatigue, sexual dysfunction, and loss of vitality. The diagnosis of hypoglycemia should *not* be made on the basis of results of an oral glucose tolerance test. Ideally, patients should be evaluated with a plasma glucose determination at the time of symptoms after a normal mixed meal. The oral glucose challenge is a very "unphysiologic" stimulus rarely encountered by most patients in their daily lives. In addition, symptoms during an oral glucose tolerance test rarely coincide with the nadir of the plasma glucose concentration.

An important issue in the psychopharmacologic management of patients with hypoglycemia is the risk of beta-blocker therapy. Early misdiagnosis of panic disorder or anxiety disorders and treatment with agents whose action blocks the normal response to hypoglycemia may prevent subjective experience of potentially lethal hypoglycemia.

DISTURBANCES OF PITUITARY FUNCTION

Pituitary disorders may be divided into those associated with pituitary hormone hypersecretion (hyperpituitarism) and those associated with inadequate pituitary hormone secretion (hypopituitarism). Hyperpituitarism is most often associated with pituitary adenomas, although dopaminergic blockade due to neuroleptic therapy is an important cause of hyperprolactinemia (Cohen, Greenberg, & Murray, 1984). The disfigurement caused by excessive growth hormone secretion (acromegaly) may inflict some degree of social inhibition, although there are few data in the literature regarding psychopathology in these patients. Hyperprolactinemia states associated with amenorrhea, galactorrhea, decreased libido, and apathy may suggest multiple psychologic illnesses, varying from depression to anorexia nervosa to pseudocyesis (Peterson & O'Shanick, 1985).

Hypopituitarism may result from a variety of destructive processes. In the past, postpartum hemorrhage with hypotension, resulting in pituitary infarction (Sheehan's syndrome), was a common cause of hypopituitarism. More common etiologies today include large pituitary adenomas, pituitary surgery, irradiation, and post-head-injury pituitary dysfunction (Horn & Sandel, 1986). Primary hypothalamic disorders may result in secondary pituitary dysfunction. Clinical manifestations of hypopituitarism reflect target gland deficiencies (i.e., hypothyroidism, hypoadrenalism, and hypogonadism). Diagnosis of hypopituitarism is frequently delayed because of the nonspecific nature of the symptoms and their often insidious onset. Psychologic symptoms may include amotivation, dysphoria, and cognitive impairment. Schizophreniform or periodic psychoses have rarely been reported in the absence of acute organic confusional states.

The diagnostic studies utilized in the evaluation of patients with suspected pituitary dysfunction include a variety of provocative and suppression tests, which are beyond the scope of this chapter. Screening studies should include assessment of target gland function: thyroid function, 8:00 A.M. cortisol, and testosterone (in males). Use of psychotropic agents is suggested only after correction of the abnormal secretion.

PHEOCHROMOCYTOMAS

Pheochromocytomas are rare, catecholamine-secreting tumors that arise most often from adrenomedullary chromaffin cells. The estimated incidence in the hypertensive population is less than 0.1 percent. There is a slight female preponderance, with most patients presenting prior to age 50. Clinical manifestations include hypertension (sustained or paroxysmal), palpita-

tions, headaches, diaphoresis, nausea, vomiting, tremor, and anxiety. Cardiac arrhythmias and hypertensive crises account for the significant incidence of sudden death in untreated patients. The paroxysms characteristic of this disorder may be confused with seizures, anxiety attacks, and hyperventilation. There is also occasional confusion with another hypermetabolic state, hyperthyroidism.

Psychologic symptoms occur, although a recent study finds minimal true overlap with anxiety disorders as defined by DSM-III (Starkman, Zelnik, Nesse, et al., 1985). Affective lability is most commonly described in association with signs of sympathetic arousal. Diagnosis depends on the demonstration of increased levels of catecholamines or their metabolites or both in urine and blood. Perhaps the best screening test for this disorder is a 24-hour urine collection for metanephrine, although a normal result in a patient with suspicious symptoms will require additional investigation. It should also be remembered that pheochromocytomas may present as part of the multiple endocrine neoplasia, type II, syndrome, which also includes hyperparathyroidism and medullary carcinoma of the thyroid.

CONSULTATION BETWEEN ENDOCRINOLOGY AND MEDICAL PSYCHIATRY

As noted above, evaluation of endocrinopathies has traditionally occured following demonstration of *systemic* signs and symptoms. Skin changes, electrolytic and metabolic disturbances, and other pathophysiologic evidence of hormonal abnormalities have become the "activation threshold" for diagnostic workup. Expanding awareness of cognitive and behavioral changes associated with endocrinopathies and the evidence of neuroendocrine mechanisms in psychiatric disorders may obscure the most appropriate point for endocrine evaluation. Personal experiences of the psychiatrist will determine the levels of comfort and confidence in administering and interpreting endocrine tests. If psychiatrists, for whatever reasons, choose not to pursue a limited endocrine evaluation when clinically indicated, they should seek endocrine consultation *and* provide a detailed justification of the need for consultation. With collaboration, both the psychiatrist and the endocrinologist should define limits of confidence with regard to organic mental disorders due to endocrine dysfunction.

SUMMARY

Endocrine disturbances frequently mimic psychiatric disturbances. "High-risk" groups, which require careful endocrine evaluation, include

1. Patients with affective symptoms and coexistent cognitive dysfunction, especially geriatric patients
2. Patients with inconsistent or atypical presentation of psychiatric disorders
3. Patients with symptoms of dementia
4. Patients with known preexisting endocrine abnormalities
5. Patients with affective symptoms after closed head injury

ACKNOWLEDGMENTS

The authors wish to acknowledge the tireless efforts and understanding of Ivy Joyner, without whose help this chapter would have been impossible.

APPENDIX A

TRH Stimulation Test

1. Administer an IV bolus of 500 μg of TRH.
2. Draw blood (10 ml) for TSH at 0 (baseline), 15, 30, 45, and 60 min.

In normal individuals, TSH increases by 7–15 μU/ml. Some variability may occur based on age and sex.

APPENDIX B

Dexamethasone Suppression Test (for major affective disorders)

1. Administer 1.0 mg dexamethasone orally between 10:00 P.M. and midnight.
2. Draw blood (10 ml) for plasma cortisol at 8:00 A.M., 4:00 P.M., and 11:00 P.M. on the following day.

In normal individuals, plasma cortisol remains below 5 μg/dl for all 3 samples (if radioimmunoassay method is used).

REFERENCES

Addison T (1868). On the constitutional and local effects of disease of the suprarenal capsules. In S Wilkes & E Daldey (Eds.), *A collection of the published writings of Thomas Addison* (Vol. 36). London: New Sydenham Society.

Anderson RW & Lev-Ran A (1985). Hypoglycemia: The standard and the fiction. *Psychosomatics*, 26, 38–47.

Baron JM (1967). Chlordiazepoxide (Librium) and thyroid function tests. *British Medical Journal*, 1, 699–700.

Berger H (1975). Hypoglycemia: A perspective. *Postgraduate Medicine*, 57, 81–85.

Bernstein RK (1986). Psychological stress and metabolic control in Type I diabetes mellitus [Letter]. *New England Journal of Medicine*, 315, 1293–1294.

Blackwell B & Schmidt GL (1984). Drug interactions in psychopharmacology. *Psychiatric Clinics of North America*, 7, 625–636.

Boehnert CE & Popkin MK (1986). Psychological issues in treatment of severely non-compliant diabetics. *Psychosomatics*, 27, 11–20.

Borer MS & Bhanot VK (1985). Hyperparathyroidism: Neuropsychiatric manifestations. *Psychosomatics*, 26, 597–601.

Boston Collaborative Drug Surveillance Program (1972). Acute adverse reaction to prednisone in relation to dosage. *Clinical Pharmacology*, 13, 694–697.

Calcium metabolism and mental disorder [Editorial] (1977). *Psychological Medicine*, 8, 557–560.

Carroll BJ, Feinberg M, Greden JF, et al. (1981). A specific test for the diagnosis of melancholia: Standardization, validation, and clinical utility. *Archives of General Psychiatry*, 38, 15–22.

Chrousos GP, Schuermeyer TH, Doppman J, et al. (1985). Clinical applications of corticotropin-releasing factor. *Annals of Internal Medicine*, 102, 344–358.

Cleghorn RA (1951). Adrenal cortical insufficiency: Psychological and neurological observations. *Canadian Medical Association Journal*, 65, 449–454.

Cohen LM, Greenberg DB, & Murray GB (1984). Neuropsychiatric presentation of men with pituitary tumors (the "four A's"). *Psychosomatics*, 25, 925–928.

Cowdry RW, Wehr JA, Zis AP, et al. (1983). Thyroid abnormalities associated with rapid-cycling bipolar illness. *Archives of General Psychiatry*, 40, 414–420.

Cushing H (1932). The basophil adenomas of the pituitary body and their clinical manifestations. *Johns Hopkins Medical Journal*, 50, 137–195.

Engel GL & Margolin SG (1941). Neuropsychiatric disturbances in Addison's disease and the role of impaired carbohydrate metabolism in production of abnormal cerebral function. *Archives of Neurology and Psychiatry*, 45, 881–884.

Ettigi PG & Brown GM (1978). Brain disorders associated with endocrine dysfunction. *Psychiatric Clinics of North America*, 1, 117–136.

Falk WE, Mahnke MW, & Poskanzer DC (1979). Lithium prophylaxis of corticotropin-induced psychosis. *Journal of the American Medical Association*, 241, 1011–1012.

Foldes J, Nagy J, Kertai P, et al. (1959). Effect of chlorpromazine in thyroid activity. *Acta Medica Academiae Scientiarum Hungaricae*, 14:371–378.

Fonseca O & Calverly J (1967). Neurological manifestations in hypoparathyroidism. *Archives of Internal Medicine*, 120, 202–206.

Goggans FC, Allen MR, & Gold MS (1986). Primary hypothyroidism and its relationship to affective disorders. In I Extein & MS Gold (Eds), *Medical mimics of psychiatric disorders*. Washington, DC: American Psychiatric Press.

Gold MS, Pottash ALC, & Extein I (1981). Hypothyroidism and depression: Evidence from complete thyroid function evaluation. *Journal of the American Medical Association*, 245, 1919–1922.

Gold PW, Loriaux DL, Roy A, et al. (1986). Responses to corticotropin-releasing hormone in the hypercortisolism of depression and Cushing's disease: Pathophysiologic and diagnostic implications. *New England Journal of Medicine*, 314, 1329–1335.

Goolker P & Schein J (1953). Psychic effects of ACTH and cortisone. *Psychosomatic Medicine*, 15, 589–613.

Greer S, Ramsay I, & Bagley C (1973). Neurotic and thyrotoxic anxiety: Clinical, psychological, and physiological measurements. *British Journal of Psychiatry*, 122, 549–554.

Hall RCW (1983). Psychiatric effects of thyroid hormone disturbance. *Psychosomatics*, 24, 7–18.

Hall RCW, Popkin MK, & Kirkpatrick B (1978). Tricyclic exacerbation of steroid psychosis. *Journal of Nervous and Mental Disorders*, 166, 738–742.

Hall RCW, Popkin MK, Stickney SK, et al. (1979). Presentation of the "steroid psychoses." *Journal of Nervous and Mental Disorders*, 167, 229–236.

Harvey RF (1967). Drugs and thyroid function tests. *British Medical Journal*, 1, 52.

Hirschfeld RMA, Koslow SH, & Kupfer DJ (1983). The clinical utility of the dexamethasone suppression test in psychiatry: Summary of a NIMH workshop. *Journal of the American Medical Association*, 250, 2172–2174.

Hoffenberg R (1986). Hypothyroidism. In SM Ingbar & LE Braverman (Eds), *Werner's The thyroid* (5th ed, pp 1255–1265). Philadelphia: JB Lippincott.

Horn LJ & Sandel ME (1986). Anterior pituitary dysfunction after traumatic brain injury: A preliminary report of 30 patients [Abstract]. *Postgraduate Course of Rehabilitation of the Brain-Injured Adult and Child, 10th Annual Conference/International Head Injury Association Inaugural Meeting* (pp 199–200). Williamsburg, VA: Medical College of Virginia.

Ingbar SH & Woeber KA (1983). Diseases of the thyroid. In RA Petersdorf, RD Adams, E Braunwald, et al. (Eds), *Harrison's principles of internal medicine* (10th ed). New York: McGraw-Hill.

Jones JH & Meade TW (1964). Hypothermia following

chlorpromazine therapy in myxedematous patients. *Gerontologia Clinica*, 6, 252–256.

Karacan I, Salis PJ, Ware JW, et al. (1978). Nocturnal penile tumescence and diagnosis in diabetic impotence. *American Journal of Psychiatry*, 135, 191–197.

Kathol RG, Turner R, & Delahunt J (1986). Depression and anxiety associated with hyperthyroidism: Response to antithyroid therapy. *Psychosomatics*, 27, 501–505.

Kemmer FW, Bisping R, Steingruber HJ, et al. (1986). Psychological stress and metabolic control in patients with Type I diabetes mellitus. *New England Journal of Medicine*, 314, 1078–1084.

Kvinesdal B, Molin J, Frland A, et al. (1984). Imipramine treatment of painful diabetic neuropathy. *Journal of the American Medical Association*, 251, 1727–1730.

Maciewicz R, Bouckoms A, Martin JB (1985). Review: Drug therapy of neuropathic pain. *Clinical Journal of Pain*, 1, 39–49.

Martin LM (1981). Impotence in diabetes: An overview. *Psychosomatics*, 22, 318–329.

Marzollo M (1963). Librium in the treatment of some states of hyperthyroidism. *Minerva Medicine*, 54, 1609–1614.

Mason JW (1968). A review of psychoendocrine research on the pituitary-thyroid system. *Psychosomatic Medicine*, 30, 666–681.

McNamara E, Southwick SM, & Fogel BS (1987). Sleep apnea and hypothyroidism presenting as depression in two patients. *Journal of Clinical Psychiatry*, 48, 165–165.

O'Shanick GJ & Ellinwood EH (1982). Persistent elevation of thyroid stimulating hormone in women with bipolar affective disorder. *American Journal of Psychiatry*, 139, 513–514.

Pennebaker JW, Cox DJ, Gonder-Frederick L, et al. (1981). Physical symptoms related to blood glucose in insulin-dependent diabetics. *Psychosomatic Medicine*, 43, 489–500.

son LG & O'Shanick GJ (1985). Psychiatric symptoms in endocrine diseases. *Postgraduate Medicine*, 77, 233–239.

son P (1968). Psychiatric disorders in primary hyperparathyroidism. *Journal of Clinical Endocrinology and Metabolism*, 28, 1491–1495.

Schaaf M & Payne C (1966). Dystonic reactions to prochlorperazine in hypoparathyroidism. *New England Journal of Medicine*, 275, 991–994.

Sheehan HL (1939). Simmonds disease due to post partum necrosis of the anterior pituitary. *Quarterly Journal of Medicine*, 8, 277–307.

Smigan L, Wahlin A, Jacobson L, et al. (1984). Lithium therapy and thyroid function tests, a prospective study. *Neuropsychobiology*, 11, 39–43.

Spratt DI, Pont A, Miller MB, et al. (1982). Hyperthyroxinemia in patients with acute psychiatric disorders. *American Journal of Medicine*, 73, 41–48.

Starkman MN & Schteingart DE (1981). Neuropsychiatric manifestations of patients with Cushing's syndrome. *Archives of Internal Medicine*, 141, 215–219.

Starkman MN, Schteingart DE, & Schork MA (1981). Depressed mood and other psychiatric manifestations of Cushing's syndrome: Relationship to hormone levels. *Psychosomatic Medicine*, 43, 3–18.

Starkman MN, Zelnik TC, Nesse RM, et al. (1985). Anxiety in patients with pheochromocytomas. *Archives of Internal Medicine*, 145, 248–252.

Thompson WF (1973). Psychiatric aspects of Addison's disease: Report of a case. *Medical Annals of the District of Columbia*, 43, 62–64.

Utiger RD (1984). Editorial retrospective: Beta-adrenergic antagonist therapy for hyperthyroid Graves' disease. *New England Journal of Medicine*, 310, 1597–1598.

Whelan TB, Schteingart DE, Starkman MN, et al. (1980). Neuropsychological deficits in Cushing's syndrome. *Journal of Nervous and Mental Disorders*, 168, 753–757.

Whybrow PC & Hurwitz T (1976). Psychological disturbance associated with endocrine disease and hormone therapy. In EJ Sachar (Ed), *Hormones, behavior, and psychopathology* (pp 124–143). Washington, DC: Raven.

Whybrow PC & Prange AJ (1981). A hypothesis of thyroid-catecholamine receptor interaction. *Archives of General Psychiatry*, 38, 106–113.

Wilson WH & Jefferson JW (1985). Thyroid disease, behavior and psychopharmacology. *Psychosomatics*, 26, 481–492.

Michael G. Moran

31

Psychologic and Neuropsychiatric Aspects of Acquired Immune Deficiency Syndrome

EPIDEMIOLOGY

Infection with the virus named human immunodeficiency virus (HIV), formerly called HTLV-III, is a necessary event in the pathophysiologic sequence leading to the clinical entity AIDS, or acquired immune deficiency syndrome. At a recent international congress of AIDS researchers, evidence was presented that indicates that the infection will ultimately lead, in every case, to AIDS. HIV is easily inactivated by heat and commonly used disinfectant techniques. It resembles a lentivirus of sheep, visna virus, which causes a chronic and degenerative neurologic disease (Shaw, Harper, Hahn, et al., 1985). Infection occurs by the potential victim's intimate contact with virus-laden body fluids of an infected person. Sexual intercourse, especially anal intercourse, intravenous (IV) use of infected needles, and administration of

virus-containing blood and blood products are understood to be the most frequent modes of virus transmission. The virus can also be transmitted in utero (Ammann 1985; Rubinstein, Sicklick, Gupta, et al., 1983; Scott, Buck, Leterman, et al., 1984).

The acronym denotes AIDS to be a *syndrome*, not a disease. First described in 1981 (Gottlieb, Schroff, Schanker, et al., 1981; Masur, Michelis, Greene, et al., 1981), it is defined as a deficiency in cellular immunity that is usually followed by the occurrence of opportunistic infections, such as *Pneumocystis carinii* pneumonia (PCP), Kaposi's sarcoma, or both. Laboratory examination of T-cell populations reveals a fall in the T4/T8 ratio (Gottlieb, 1984; Schroff, Gottlieb, Prince, et al., 1983). Absolute T-helper cell count is low, with the diagnostic criterion set at fewer than 400 cells/mm^3 (Centers for Disease Control, 1984; Landesman, Ginzburg, &

Weiss, 1985). AIDS-related complex (ARC) is a syndrome that comprises patients who are infected with HIV and demonstrate chronic lymphadenopathy, with depletion of T-helper cells. This group, not having opportunistic infections or neoplasms, does not meet the criteria for AIDS (CDC, 1985).

Laboratory techniques now allow the detection of antibody to HIV and the virus can be cultured in specialized research laboratories. An immune response to past contact with the virus can thus be documented, but verification of infectivity is not easily accessible. A person recently infected with the virus may be viremic, and infectious, but not yet demonstrate circulating antibody (Wong-Staal & Gallo, 1985). The most sensitive procedure to detect presence of antibody is the enzyme-linked immunosorbent assay (ELISA). It is almost 99 percent specific and is 97 percent sensitive. The Western Blot procedure is even more specific for antibody to HIV (Weiss, Goedert, Sarngadharan, et al., 1985). The antibody is present in a very small number of apparently healthy persons in the general population (Brun-Vezinet, Rouzioux, Montagnier, et al., 1984; Cheingsong-Popov, Weiss, Dalgleish, et al., 1984).

New cases of AIDS currently occur at a rate of approximately 1000 a month. Within 2–8 weeks after infection with HIV, the ELISA test becomes positive (Cooper, Gold, MacLean, et al., 1985). The average incubation period, the time from point of infection to diagnosis of AIDS, varies with the mode of infection. For adult patients infected via blood transfusion, it is 29.6 months. For homosexual males whose route of infection is thought to be primarily oral and anal sexual intercourse, the average incubation period is 38 months. The upper limit in the sample was 65 months, however, and the design of the study could not exclude even longer incubation periods in individual cases (Francis, Jaffe, Fultz, et al., 1985).

Several groups have been identified as at greatest risk for acquiring AIDS and ARC. Bisexual and homosexual men make up 72 percent of all AIDS patients. Of this group, 74 percent are white, and 8 percent are IV drug users. Of the heterosexual IV drug users (17 percent of all AIDS cases), 80 percent are nonwhite. Women represent about 7 percent of AIDS patients, fewer than 1000 cases, 53 percent of them being IV drug users (CDC, 1985). Other women at risk include prostitutes and sexual partners of men at risk (Ginzburg & MacDonald, 1986; Harris, Small, Klein, et al., 1983; Redfield, Markham, Salahuddin, et al., 1985a; Redfield, Markham, Salahuddin, et al., 1985b). Recipients of blood and blood product transfusions represent 2.3 percent of AIDS patients. Recreational drug use, especially use of inhaled nitrates, is seen with a high frequency among AIDS patients. Whether it represents a factor adding to the risk of acquiring the disease or is merely a marker for a life-style that is risk-promoting is not yet clear (Goedert, 1984).

In terms of geographic distribution, four cities dominate the demographic picture: New York (the metropolitan area has 40 percent of all cases), San Francisco, Los Angeles, and Miami.

PSYCHOLOGIC ASPECTS OF AIDS

With any psychic insult, the timing of its occurrence and the affected person's defensive structure, past psychic development, and support from friends and caregivers modify the psychologic response to the injury. Public awareness and characterization of AIDS are such that even among the general population, not currently thought to be at risk, the illness exerts a psychologic effect, which includes panic, phobic avoidance of persons in or thought to be in high-risk groups, and at times even calls for quarantine measures. Within groups at high risk, those not infected with the virus but faced with the prospect of possible infection may agonize about their future. In the case of male homosexuals, conflict about their choice of life-style may result in guilt, the acting out of denial about their risk of exposure, depression, or condemnation of other homosexuals (Forstein, 1984; Malyon & Pinka, 1983; McKusick, Hortsman, & Coates, 1985; SF Morin & Batchelor, 1984; Wolcott, Fawzy, & Pasnau, 1986). If there is preexisting severe distress or character pathology, contracting AIDS may be a choice taken as a route to act on unconscious self-destructive impulses to commit suicide (Frances, Wikstrom, & Alcena, 1985). Other AIDS patients with severe character pathology will seek opportunities to possibly infect other people through unsafe sex practices or sharing of needles.

After the diagnosis of AIDS, reactions of individual patients vary, but often include denial, abject sadness and despondency, sense of a loss of hope for any remnants of health, and panic. When one adds to this clinical picture the presence of delirium (from many possible sources), drug use, and attendant alterations in impulse control, the potential emotional and behavioral panorama seen in the AIDS patient becomes quite complex. The psychiatrist must adopt an approach that allows the conceptualization of symptoms and bodily and behavioral signs in an extensive differential diagnostic schema. Previous experience with cancer patients may be of empiric use to the clinician (Wolcott et al., 1986).

After diagnosis, the progression of psychologic symptoms can indeed be "malignant" (Wolcott et al., 1986). Dealing with a life-threatening illness, uncertainty about the implications of the diagnosis, social isolation, and guilt about previous life-style face almost every AIDS patient. If discharge from the hospital does occur, fear of death and dying, of exposure of life-style, of contagion, and of loss of self-esteem and physical attractiveness cause tumult in the

effort to maintain identity as a gay man (SJ Morin, Charles, & Malyon, 1984). Depression is the most commonly stated reason for a request for inpatient psychiatric consultation, and among hospitalized AIDS patients, disorders with depressive affect are common: major depression, dysthymic disorder, and adjustment disorder with depressed mood (Dilley, Ochtill, Perl, et al., 1985).

Before diagnosis, many of these patients were young and active men; they now face what is often a prolonged and agonizing illness, requiring medication and repeated hospitalizations. It is common for relationships with lovers, family, and friends to suffer under the strain imposed by the massive changes that occur (Ferrara, 1984). In some cases, employers and landlords have reacted in a frightened and angry way to an employee's or tenant's AIDS diagnosis and have fired or evicted the patient. The loss of employment usually means the loss of health insurance, and it adds a substantial financial burden to the patient's medical and emotional burdens.

In response to the diagnosis of other fatal diseases, a patient often reestablishes contact with parents and siblings, becoming quite dependent on their support, if not their presence, for the ordeal ahead. In contrast, AIDS patients seem to seek out their families, or succeed in making contact, in only a minority of cases. Least often successfully recovered is the male homosexual patient's relationship with his father (Christ, Wiener, & Moynihan, 1986). The patient's (or family's) wish to keep secret the sexual life-style of the patient adds to the growing estrangement and isolation of the newly diagnosed person with AIDS. Sustaining this secret requires considerable psychic energy and, over time, exacts its toll. The lovers of homosexual men with AIDS, anxious about their own health, can become so frightened or angry that the relationship with the patient is seriously threatened (SF Morin & Batchelor, 1984).

Alienated, unwanted, fired, and evicted, the AIDS patient feels expendable (Cohen & Weisman, 1986).

One perspective involves broadly grouping the psychiatric presentations of AIDS patients into two categories: (1) mild chronic depression, with features seen in the DSM-III-R disorders major depressive disorder, adjustment disorder with depressed mood, and dysthymic disorder; and (2) acute psychosis, with features seen in the DSM-III-R disorders schizophreniform disorder, acute paranoid disorder, brief reactive psychosis, mania, and major depression with psychotic features. In both presentations, close attention to the possible organic and neurologic contributions to the psychiatric symptoms is emphasized. Perry and Jacobsen (1986) demonstrate with case examples the pitfalls of ascribing all the patient's emotional and behavioral symptoms and signs to psychologic causes, resulting in the neglect of the presence of organic and neuropsychiatric complications. This differential may be most difficult early in the course of the deliria and dementias to be discussed later, in which symptoms of lethargy, depressive affect, lack of motivation, disturbed mentation, and personality changes can deflect clinical interest from the neuropsychiatric syndromes (Hoffman, 1984; Perry & Jacobsen, 1986).

BIOLOGIC ASPECTS OF THE ILLNESS THAT AFFECT PSYCHOLOGIC FUNCTIONING

The biological effects of AIDS manifest themselves in two major neuropsychiatric syndromes: delirium and dementia. Most AIDS patients will develop dementia before death. Up to one-third of AIDS patients will have other neurologic complications before they die (Bredesen & Messing, 1983; Navia & Price, 1986). Almost 10 percent may present with neurologic symptoms up to 12 months before any clinical evidence of the immunologic deficits (RM Levy, Pons, & Rosenblum, 1984). Two-thirds demonstrate brain abnormalities at autopsy (Welch, Finkbeiner, Alpers, et al., 1984). Of hospitalized AIDS patients, almost 30 percent meet DSM-III-R criteria for delirium, and about 12 percent meet the criteria for dementia (Perry & Tross, 1984). Delirium and dementia will be discussed in detail.

Delirium

Causes of delirium in AIDS patients include intracranial infections, a diffuse encephalopathy, systemic infections (with viremia, bacteremia, or fungemia, or combinations), hypoxemia, volume depletion, electrolyte imbalance, and medication side effects (Gottlieb, Groopman, Weinstein, et al., 1983; Jordan, Navia, Petito, et al., 1985).

Intracranial infections occur in a high proportion of patients. In one study, 31 of 50 patients with neurologic symptoms had central nervous system (CNS) infections (Snider, Simpson, Nielsen, et al., 1983). The lesion in cellular immunity leaves the AIDS patient vulnerable to opportunistic infections, capable of causing delirium, that are seen in cancer patients and patients on immunosuppressive therapy; agents of intracranial infection include fungi, especially *Cryptococcus neoformans*, and protozoa, especially *Toxoplasma gondii*. With *Cryptococcus*, one often sees meningitic syndromes: altered mental status, irritability, seizures, diplopia, and vomiting. Intracerebral mass lesions are unusual, and computer-assisted tomography (CAT) scans demonstrate no structural changes (Whelan, Kricheff, Handler, et al., 1983). Diagnosis is made by examination of the cerebrospinal fluid, which reveals the pleocytosis of aseptic meningitis, the organism, and possibly the presence of cryptococcal antigen. As noted in Chapter 3, cryptococcal antigen tests may yield false negative results, and multiple large-volume cultures may be needed to isolate the organism (Davis, 1985). *Toxoplasma* can cause diffuse (meningitic) and localized (mass lesion) syndromes. The patient may be irritable and have a disturbance of sensorium. Less commonly, motor or sensory deficits will be evident, from a mass (toxoplasmoma) and its associated edema (Alonso, Heiman-Patterson, & Mancall, 1984; Horowitz, Bentson, Benson, et al., 1983). Incontinence, coma, and a picture of dementia can also occur. Diagnosis can be made by finding the organism in cerebrospinal fluid sediment. Indirect hemagglutination and indirect fluorescent antibody tests are probably the most reliable serologic tests for detection of toxoplasmosis. Tests which detect the presence of *Toxoplasma* antigen are being devised; these may allow identification of disseminated infection (Remington & McCleod, 1985). If a mass lesion is present, it may be visible on CT scan, but must be differentiated from other causes of mass lesions in the AIDS patient.

In addition to HIV itself and CMV, other viruses play a significant role in AIDS morbidity and mortality. Transient aseptic meningitis caused by these viruses can present initially as a delirium, and lumbar puncture may reveal the meningitic process. Serologic detection of antibodies to cytomegalo-virus (CMV) occurs in many AIDS patients and is usually not helpful in assigning etiology of an acute meningitic or encephalopathic picture (Pagano & Lemon, 1985). Other agents that cause aseptic meningitis include those of the herpesvirus group: Epstein-Barr, varicella zoster, and herpes simplex. Herpes simplex may produce a mass lesion with accompanying clinical signs and symptoms.

The majority of those with infections have the picture of diffuse encephalopathy, the course of which becomes subacute or chronic (descriptively, a dementia). The same two viruses have been implicated in the etiology of this syndrome: the AIDS virus itself (HIV), the CNS manifestations of which will be discussed in greater detail in the section on dementia, and, less commonly, cytomegalovirus. Early features for both acute viral encephalopathies include mental status changes with altered memory, variations in alertness, apathy, depressive affect, irritability, and loss of mental and verbal acuity and spontaneity. Inappropriate, impulsive, paranoid, and psychotic behavior can occur and can be associated with hallucinations (Navia & Price, 1986). Certainty as to viral etiology is not established until autopsy. Cerebrospinal fluid analysis is typically nonspecific, revealing only mononuclear pleocytosis with or without elevations in protein (Britton & Miller, 1984; Hawley, Schaefer, Schulz, et al., 1983).

Systemic infections can result in the seeding of the bloodstream with viruses, bacteria, fungi, or combinations. Fever may occur, when the patient is able to mount this response, and delirium can result. Repeated diarrhea, of nonspecific etiology or from microbial gastrointestinal infection (including candidiasis), causes esophageal and intestinal wall lesions which readily permit microbial access to the bloodstream. Other portals of entry are the upper and lower respiratory tract, skin lesions, and seeding from sites of intracranial infection.

Hypoxemia is most commonly due to severe pulmonary infection with *Pneumocystis carinii*. The patient is severely dyspneic and may be febrile, with a cough that is often nonproductive. The chest roentgenogram typically shows minimal involvement, especially when compared with clinical appearance of the patient and the arterial O_2, which is invariably low. Mentation can be severely affected unless adequate oxygen supplementation is supplied. Obviously, other fulminant pulmonary infections can produce severe hypoxemia and, hence, delirium.

Volume depletion and electrolyte imbalance often results from the severe episodic diarrhea that these patients experience. The possible causes have been discussed. Alone, or in combination with other factors mentioned, they can result in delirium, probably accompanied by orthostatic faintness or syncope.

In the differential diagnosis of delirium in the AIDS patient, acute exacerbations or the initial presentations of the following, more chronic conditions are also to be considered: progressive multifocal leukoencephalopathy (Miller, Barrett, Britton, et al., 1982; Reichert, O'Leary, Levens, et al., 1983), seizure disorder, stroke, and mass lesions.

Dementia

When one excludes from demented AIDS patients those whose dementia is caused only by the chronic sequelae of such factors as mass lesions, hypoxemia, and meningitis, those left demonstrate findings at autopsy that suggest HIV itself as the causative agent. Patients in one study, ranging in age from 4 months to 49 years, with debilitating dementia and encephalopathy, were examined at autopsy. One-third had evidence of active HIV brain infection (Shaw et al., 1985). Morphologic and genetic relatedness has been demonstrated between HIV and visna virus, a lentivirus that causes a chronic degenerative neurologic disease in sheep. Homosexual men, both with (JA Levy, Shimabukuro, Hollander, et al., 1985) and without AIDS (Goldwater, Synek, Koelmeyer, et al., 1985), who had severe neurologic symptoms have been shown to have cerebrospinal fluid containing HIV in one case and seropositivity for HIV antibody and autopsy evidence of subacute encephalopathy in another.

Neuropathologic studies of the brains of AIDS patients with dementia demonstrate chiefly subcortical and white-matter changes, with sparing of cortical gray matter—hence, the term *subcortical dementia* (Cummings & Benson, 1984). Perivascular collections of macrophages, lymphocytes, and multinucleated giant cells are particularly striking. Glial nodules and inclusion bodies are present but are not the hallmark of the dementia as once thought. Inclusions do occur in cytomegalovirus infections, which can result in dementia in AIDS patients. This infection seems to be a secondary event, however, and not a common cause of the dementia in AIDS (Navia & Price, 1986).

Among those patients with dementia, one-fourth present with the dementia before other signs and symptoms of AIDS. At the time of their presentation, they tend to have clinically detectable disturbances in immune function, as demonstrated by abnormal T-cell ratios.

In the initial stages, the dementia can be difficult to diagnose and is easily mistaken for depression, reactive despondency, or an adjustment disorder. Loss of mental acuity, mild confusion, and concentration deficits can be accompanied by impairment in rapid movements, leg weakness, gait ataxia, and dysarthria. Hyperreflexia and tremor can be present. The bedside mental status exam may reveal only mild psychomotoric slowing, or the patient may be agitated and delirious (Navia & Price, 1986). Laboratory tests, electroencephalogram, and CAT scan may be normal in the early stages.

Most patients rapidly deteriorate. Within a few months, the steady advance of the dementia brings the patient to a severely debilitated state. Staring vacantly, the patient may be unaware of the illness or its severity. Patients are significantly slowed and may become mute. There may be periods of psychotic agitation. They are susceptible to delirium from many causes. Confusion and cognitive deficits become severe. Motor abnormalities progress to include truncal ataxia, seizures, spastic weakness, and, in some, paraplegia or quadriparesis (Navia & Price, 1986).

Early confirmation of the diagnosis is almost impossible using laboratory tests: none are specific. The electroencephalogram shows diffuse slowing, as in most organic states. Cerebrospinal fluid analysis may be normal or show only mild elevations in protein with a mononuclear pleocytosis. CT scan may be normal, but ventricular enlargement and cortical atrophy are common, even early (Navia & Price, 1986; Perry & Jacobsen, 1986). High-resolution CT scans with contrast material enhancement are superior to nonenhanced CT scans in differentiating lesions from surrounding edema, in discriminating between lesions in close proximity, in locating lesions for biopsy, and in judging lesion activity. Magnetic resonance imaging (MRI) is superior to CT scanning in evaluation of white-matter lesions and detection of small lesions surrounded by edema (Post, Sheldon, Hensley, et al., 1986).

Morbidity from the dementia is high. If a treatment for the immune deficiency caused by HIV is developed before a treatment for the infection itself (especially brain infection), there may continue to accumulate a population of young patients who face the possibility of a life spent in need of near total care.

Other Neurologic Problems Associated with AIDS

A vacuolar myelopathy similar to that seen in severe vitamin B_{12} deficiency has been described in AIDS patients and may cause leg weakness, gait disturbances, and incontinence (Petito, Navia, Cho, et al., 1985). Other spinal cord syndromes may produce similar clinical pictures (Goldstick, Mandybur, & Bode, 1985).

Neoplastic changes also occur in AIDS, some similar to those seen in other illnesses

marked by depressed immunity. Kaposi's sarcoma and lymphomas of the diffuse undifferentiated, immunoblastic, and B-cell types, are examples (CDC, 1982; Levine, Meyer, Begandy, et al., 1984; Penn, 1981; Scully, 1983). All have been reported to occur in the central nervous system of AIDS patients.

Cranial nervous syndromes have been reported, which involve facial and optic nerves and are caused by infectious agents and by neoplasms. Cryptococcus and other fungi can involve the meninges and cranial nerves (Snider et al., 1983). Peripheral nerve involvement can include distal neuropathies and Landry-Gullain-Barre syndrome (Gapen, 1982; Snider et al., 1983). Opthalmologic involvement points to a poor prognosis in AIDS patients (Khadem, Kalish, Goldsmith, et al., 1984).

Neurologic complications of AIDS are summarized in Table 31-1.

PRACTICAL DIAGNOSIS AND MANAGEMENT

Medical and psychiatric problems often first bring the AIDS patient to a physician's attention. Neurology and infectious diseases consultations are usually necessary at some point in the course of the illness. Nurses have daily and intense contact with the patients as they administer prescribed treatment. Social workers may assist in family treatment regarding issues of adjustment to illness and death and provide services associated with finding housing and care outside the hospital. Hospital staff, from respiratory therapists to dietary consultant, all have necessary contacts with the patient. Countertransference responses at any point in this vast system (and this is not an all-inclusive list) can interrupt or preclude delivery of appropriate care. Hospital- and system-wide programs have been developed, the aim of

Table 31-1
Neurological Complications of AIDS

Infections	Symptoms	Signs	CT Scan	CSF	Treatment
HIV Encephalopathy	Depression, personality change, gait difficulty	Encephalopathy, apathy, cerebellar findings	Normal or diffuse atrophy	Little or no inflammation	Experimental
HIV Aseptic meningitis	Headache, fever	Meningismus	Normal	Lymphocytic pleocytosis	Experimental
HIV Polyneuropathy	Paresthesias, distal weakness	Stocking-glove hypesthesia, hyporeflexia	Normal	Little or no inflammation	Experimental
HIV Myelopathy	Leg weakness, incontinence	Spastic paraparesis	Normal	Little or no inflammation	Experimental
Herpes simplex encephalitis	Confusion, fever, nausea	Encephalopathy, seizures	Variable	Generally inflammatory	Acyclovir
Cryptococcal meningitis	Headache, fever, nausea	Variable meningeal findings	Normal	Variable inflammation but positive crypto antigen culture	Amphotericin-B +/− Flucytosine
Toxoplasmosis	Headache, confusion, weakness	Encephalopathy, seizures, variable focal findings	Multiple ring-enhancing lesions	Little or no inflammation	Pyrimethamine plus sulfadiazine
Tumors: Non-Hodgkin's lymphoma	Variable	Variable depending upon location	Intensely enhancing lesions	Variable, occasionally cytology positive	Radiation, Chemotherapy

Source: Reproduced with permission from Hollander H (1986). Neurologic complications of AIDS. *The San Francisco General Hospital AIDSfile, 1*(3), 2.

which is the coordination of multidisciplinary treatment (Cohen & Weisman, 1986).

From the foregoing discussion of medical aspects of AIDS, one can appreciate the need for a high index of suspicion for organic and neurologic complications of the illness. In outpatient clinics and on inpatient units, medical and nursing staff must be well informed about dementia and delirium. Early in the course of the illness, evidence of such complications may be fleeting. Language and cognitive disturbances secondary to delirium and dementia will impede the very reporting of symptoms. Affective disruptions and personality changes may alienate the patient from family and friends, as well as from caregivers. (Holland & Tross, 1985). Such problems should always be viewed in the context of the illness, as potential signs of further progression—for example, of brain involvement (Wolcott et al., 1986). The effectiveness of any therapeutic or management effort will have to take into specific account the patient's current and likely future neurologic status.

Flow sheets that allow rapid scanning of the progress of the patient's mental and affective status are useful in both inpatient and outpatient settings. The psychiatrist can be helpful in familiarizing nonpsychiatric staff with such evaluative techniques as the mental status examination and its proper recording. Subtle behavioral and sensorial changes may precede florid delirious states; the electroencephalogram and even formal cognitive testing may not yet register the changes at such times (Hoffman, 1984). When delirium occurs, one should proceed with a careful differential diagnosis that includes a meticulous search of the patient's medication list, an examination of the vital signs, and a review of the most recent laboratory findings, looking for evidence of correctable metabolic insults. Every AIDS patient with unexplained delirium should have a lumbar puncture (LP) and, if the diagnosis remains obscure, a CT

scan. After such a review has taken place, and appropriate adjustments made in, for example, the patient's fluid, electrolyte, or oxygenation status, standard use of low-dose neuroleptic medication may help manage behavioral disturbances and psychotic symptoms (Lipowski, 1980; McEvoy, 1981). As with any demented or delirious patient, one should use caution in the prescribing of psychotropic, especially neuroleptic, medication. Although no studies to date document the incidence of adverse effects in the use of neuroleptics in AIDS-dementia patients, clinical experience suggests a greater likelihood of parkinsonian, sedating, and alpha-blockade side effects in this group. In addition, there is speculation that these patients may be at increased risk for neuroleptic malignant syndrome and other severe extrapyramidal reactions when prescribed neuroleptics. A more detailed discussion of the diagnosis and management of delirium will be found in Chapter 6.

The psychosocial management of the demented AIDS patient is especially problematic (Loewenstein & Sharfstein, 1983–1984). As the dementia progresses, the patient becomes more withdrawn and less interactive and becomes more susceptible to delirium. With communication halted, the staff's fantasies and fears about the patient may flourish to fill the void, further complicating adequate care delivery. Advance planning, which takes into timely account the patient's impending death, often gets overlooked in the rush to manage the many crises that occur. The psychiatrist can play a crucial role in bringing to discussion issues that, if left unattended, could become another crisis; these include putting affairs in order regarding insurance and wills, the intermittent process of life review and mourning the loss of health and life, and making informed decisions about life-sustaining and heroic medical measures (Dilley, Shelp, & Batiki, 1986).

AIDS strikes young people in almost

all cases. The occurrence of the illness at a life stage at which neither death or dying is part of the typical experience builds in a psychologic unpreparedness that ripples throughout the management of the case: caretakers, perhaps young themselves, may overidentify with patients and avoid them; part of the intense rage felt by patients and close friends and relatives is related to the sense of gross unfairness about the striking down of a young person by a horrible illness (some of the critical and abusive attacks on homosexual AIDS patients, that they "deserve" the illness, comes from a need to deal with the issue). This is not to say that contracting AIDS as an elderly person is a psychologically easy task. Unexpected revelations about the patient's homosexuality, sudden disruption in relationship with lovers, avoidance by important persons in the patient's life, and the sense of expendability are all evident in the psychic pain of such patients (Cohen & Weisman, 1986; Polan, Hellerstein, & Amchin, 1985).

The illness so dominates the patient's life that the patient may feel he or she is *becoming* the illness: a lethal, gruesome, contagious plague. Preoccupation with other gays' behavior, a reformist and reforming resolve, and an aloof critical posture, alternating with devastating self-criticism and severe depressive affect, may be seen. Such draining self-attacks, especially if unconscious and not dealt with in psychotherapy, add to a pervasive physical and psychologic exhaustion. Much of the psychologic work to be done is approachable in the outpatient setting, either in groups or in individual treatment. In the early phases of the illness, the patients often request information, access to support groups consisting of gays in similar medical stages, and, sometimes, psychotherapy. After the impact of severe dementia or recurrent delirium, the patient's apparent wishes and needs change.

The presence of family and friends seems noticed and appreciated by many patients, but the patients rarely ask for psychotherapeutic treatment and probably benefit little from it (Wolcott et al., 1986).

As the focus on the patient intensifies, the family, friends, and lovers are often ignored. They watch as someone close to them deteriorates, often suddenly and swiftly, losing health, personality, and, finally, life (Dilley, 1984). Up to one-third of hospitalized AIDS patients will spend half of their remaining lives in hospitals (Rivin, Monroe, Hubschuman, et al., 1984). Lovers, guilty about possibly having transmitted the illness or terrified that they might catch or already have caught the illness, may withdraw or seek to make the patient feel guilty. Depending on the family's and friends' awareness of the patient's sexual orientation, their reactions can range from indignant surprise and horror to shock and feelings of helplessness. Again, the ultimate response may be withdrawal from the patient. Specific supportive measures and interventions are needed from the psychiatrist. Ultimately, family, friends, and lovers may then be better able to contribute what they can to the support of the patients, especially in the form of their presence. When this is not possible without undue conflict, rage toward the patient, or anxiety, recommendations may be made for psychotherapy of significant others. Referrals to other centers, to support groups, or to social workers for family treatment must be done carefully, with attention to the significant others' reactions and degree of acceptance of the referral, to avoid *their* feeling rejected.

Another group severely affected by repeated and frustrating contact with persons with AIDS is hospital staff. Frustrated by inexorable progression of the disease and repeated deaths of patients whom they come to know, their sense of professional identity and effectiveness can be undermined. If the life-styles of the homosexual and drug-using AIDS patients shock, offend, or disgust the staff member, countertransference acting out can be particularly aggressive: inappropriate use of intramuscular injections, restraints, restrictions on visitation, slowness to respond to calls, forgetting to take vital signs. The fear of contracting AIDS leaves many staff frightened of having *any* association with the patient. Admissions and business office representatives may refuse to interview the patient. Union support for these refusals has been observed (Cohen & Weisman, 1986; Perry, 1985). In-service training and information sessions can be helpful in alleviating some of the phobia surrounding these patients (Batten, 1983). During the consultation process, empathic attention by the psychiatrist to countertransference issues can help reduce the staff's acting out.

SPECIAL CONSIDERATIONS IN PSYCHOTHERAPEUTIC AND PSYCHOPHARMACOLOGIC TREATMENT

Similarities between AIDS, with its medical and psychosocially "malignant" characteristics, and cancer have been discussed at length elsewhere (Wolcott et al., 1986). The literature on the psychiatric aspects of cancer, as pointed out by those authors, is likely to be of great use to psychiatrists dealing with persons with AIDS. There are, however, psychologic issues of particular importance that concern AIDS patients, stemming from special qualities of the illness.

Fantasies about AIDS, shared by many persons, powerfully influence our feelings and behavior with patients afflicted with the illness. The fears of contagion are one example peculiar to AIDS; these fears, heightened by lack of an effective cure,

have been legitimized by the federal government in the form of regulations permitting firing of persons with AIDS. Fear of contagion itself is offered as reason enough to fire or relocate such persons.

In most societies, the sick are allowed certain privileges, such as accommodation for days missed at work because of illness. Such privileges appear to be denied the AIDS patient (Christ et al., 1986).

Intimacy with friends, relatives, and lovers is virtually eliminated by the diagnosis of AIDS (or, for that matter, ARC). All of the psychologic needs that are normally met by physical contact suffer severe disruption, if not severance, at the announcement of the diagnosis. Measures taken for infection precaution, especially when they include gowns, gloves, and masks, in spite of lack of indication, can only promote a sense of loneliness. Few other illnesses impose such psychologic isolation on their victims. Certain sexual practices do not transmit AIDS and may be employed safely by AIDS patients and their partners. A guide to the safety of sexual practices is set out on Table 31-2.

Because of the complexity of the illness and the variety of its complications, multiple caregivers and consultants, including psychiatrists, are often involved. The *model of primary care*, with one physician assuming chief responsibility and importance with the patient, is difficult to maintain. One can speculate that the effects on the patient of such necessarily fragmented care probably only add to feelings of alienation, isolation, and expendability.

Those persons with AIDS who are not homosexual men are most likely to be intravenous drug users. This group of patients is typically viewed by caretakers as difficult because of their demands and apparent sense of entitlement and may constitute another group felt to be "deserving" of AIDS (Cohen & Weisman, 1986).

Chronic inpatient care and hospice fa-

Table 31-2
Guidelines on Sexual Practices and AIDS*

Safe	Possibly Safe	Unsafe
Body massage	Anogenital contact with condom	Anogenital receptive contact without condom
Hugging	Orogenital contact without ejaculation	Anogenital insertive contact without condom
Body rubbing	French kissing	Anomanual contact
Mutual masturbation	External urine contact	Anodigital contact
Social dry kissing	Penile-vaginal contact with condom	Orogenital receptive contact with ejaculation
Using one's own sex toys, dildoes	Orovaginal contact	Oroanal contact
		Anal or oral contact with urine
		Penile-vaginal contact without condom
		Sharing sex toys, dildoes
		Unsafe sexual contact with multiple partners

Source: Adapted with permission of the publisher from Campbell JM (1985). Safe sex guidelines for risk reduction. In JM Campbell & WL Warner (Eds), *Medical evaluation of persons at risk for AIDS*. San Francisco: San Francisco AIDS Foundation.

Note: These guidelines are intended for sexually active men or women who have had multiple sex partners since 1978.

* Note: "safe-sex" guidelines are dependent on seropositive status of each partner; specific guidelines for "safe-sex" may be modified as transmission data with AIDS increases. More analytic research is needed to confirm what actually determines "safe-sex" and the level of safety that condoms provide. (Goedert, 1987)

cilities can be of great use to the dying AIDS patient, but such arrangements may be extremely hard to find. Many long-term care facilities refuse these patients admission and even evaluation because of fears of contagion and stigma.

AZT (3'-azido-3'-deoxythymidine), an analogue of thymidine, has been demonstrated to have virustatic activity in AIDS and ARC patients (Yarchoan, Klecker, Weinhold, et al., 1986). No behavioral or affective side effects have yet assumed prominence, but headache and confusion have been reported. This drug has just recently been implemented on a wide-scale basis as a palliative treatment for AIDS.

In some states, AIDS is a reportable illness, and many gay active organizations have expressed concern that the names of the patients might be used in a discriminatory way. There has even been expressed the concern that the necessary breaches of confidentiality that occur during surveillance research on the syndrome are potentially harmful to the patient's welfare. Proposals regarding measures for the maintenance of confidentiality have been set forth (Novick, 1984).

REFERENCES

Alonso R, Heiman-Patterson T, & Mancall EL (1984). Cerebral toxoplasmosis in acquired immune deficiency syndrome. *Archives of Neurology, 41,* 321–323.

Ammann AJ (1985). The acquired immune deficiency syndrome in infants and children. *Annals of Internal Medicine, 103,* 734–737.

Batten CP (1983). Nursing the patient with AIDS. *Canadian Nurse, 79,* 19–22.

Bredesen DE & Messing RO (1983). Neurological syndromes heralding the acquired immune deficiency syndrome. *Annals of Neurology, 14,* 141.

Britton CB & Miller JR (1984). Neurologic complications in acquired immune deficiency syndrome (AIDS). *Neurologic Clinics, 2,* 315–339.

Brun-Vezinet F, Rouzioux C, Montagnier L, et al. (1984). Prevalence of antibodies to lymphadenopathy-associated retrovirus in African patients with AIDS. *Science, 226,* 453–456.

Centers for Disease Control (1982). Diffuse, undifferentiated non-Hodgkins lymphoma among homosexual males—United States. *Morbid Mortal Week Report, 31,* 277–279.

Centers for Disease Control (1984, December 31). *Weekly surveillance report, acquired immune deficiency syndrome (AIDS).*

Centers for Disease Control (1985, November 25). *Weekly surveillance report, acquired immune deficiency syndrome (AIDS).*

Cheingsong-Popov R, Weiss RA, Dalgleish A, et al. (1984). Prevalence of antibody to human T-lymphotropic virus type III in AIDS and AIDS-risk patients in Britain. *Lancet, 2,* 477–480.

Christ GH, Wiener LS, & Moynihan MT (1986). Psychosocial issues in AIDS. *Psychiatric Annals, 16,* 173–179.

Cohen MA & Weisman HW (1986). AIDS: Biopsychosocial approach. *Psychosomatics, 27,* 245–249.

Cooper DA, Gold J, MacLean P, et al. (1985). Acute AIDS retrovirus infection. Definition of a clinical illness associated with seroconversion. *Lancet, 1,* 537–540.

Cummings JL & Benson F (1984). Subcortical dementia—review of an emerging concept. *Archives of Neurology, 41,* 874–879.

Davis CE (1985). Cryptococcus. In AI Braude, CE Davis, & J Fierer (Eds), *Infectious diseases and medical microbiology* (pp 564–571). Philadelphia: WB Saunders.

Dilley JW (1984). Treatment interventions and approaches to care of patients with acquired immune deficiency syndrome. In SE Nichols & DG Ostrow (Eds), *Psychiatric implications of acquired immune deficiency syndrome.* Washington, DC: American Psychiatric Press.

Dilley JW, Ochtill HN, Perl M, et al. (1985). Findings in psychiatric consultations with patients with acquired immune deficiency syndrome. *American Journal of Psychiatry, 142,* 82–86.

Dilley JW, Shelp EE, & Batiki SL (1986). Psychiatric, ethical issues in care of AIDS patients. *Psychosomatics, 27,* 562–566.

Ferrara AJ (1984). My personal experience with AIDS. *American Psychologist, 39,* 1285–1287.

Forstein M (1984). The psychosocial impact of the acquired immunodeficiency syndrome. *Seminars in Oncology, 11,* 77–82.

Frances RJ, Wikstrom T, & Alcena V (1985). Contracting AIDS as a means of committing suicide. *American Journal of Psychiatry, 142,* 656.

Francis DP, Jaffe HW, Fultz PN, et al. (1985). The natural history of infection with the lymphadenopathy-associated virus human T-lymphotropic virus type III. *Annals of Internal Medicine, 103,* 719–722.

Gapen P (1982). Neurological complications now characterizing many AIDS victims. *Journal of the American Medical Association, 248,* 2941–2942.

Ginzburg HM & MacDonald MG (1986). The epidemiology of human T-cell lymphotropic virus, type-III. *Psychiatric Annals, 16,* 153–166.

Goedert JJ (1984). Recreational drugs: Relationship to AIDS. *Annals of the New York Academy of Sciences, 437,* 192–199.

Goedert JJ (1987). What is safe sex? Suggested standards linked to testing for human immunodeficiency virus. *New England Journal of Medicine, 316,* 1339–1341.

Goldstick L, Mandybur TI, & Bode R (1985). Spinal cord degeneration in AIDS. *Neurology, 35,* 103–105.

Goldwater PN, Synek BJ, Koelmeyer TD, et al. (1985). Structures resembling scrapie-associated fibrils in AIDS encephalopathy. *Lancet, 2,* 447–448.

Gottlieb MS (1984). Nonneoplastic AIDS syndromes. *Seminars in Oncology, 11,* 40–46.

Gottlieb MS, Groopman JE, Weinstein WM, et al. (1983). The acquired immunodeficiency syndrome. *Annals of Internal Medicine, 99,* 208–220.

Gottlieb MS, Schroff R, Schanker HM, et al. (1981). *Pneumocystis carinii* pneumonia and mucosal candidiasis in previously healthy homosexual men: Evidence of a new acquired cellular immunodeficiency. *New England Journal of Medicine, 305,* 1425–1431.

Harris C, Small CB, Klein RS, et al. (1983). Immunodeficiency in female sexual partners of men with the acquired immunodeficiency syndrome. *New England Journal of Medicine*, *308*, 1181–1184.

Hawley DA, Schaefer JF, Schulz DM, et al. (1983). Cytomegalovirus encephalitis in acquired immunodeficiency syndrome. *American Journal of Clinical Pathology*, *80*, 874–877.

Hoffman RS (1984). Neuropsychiatric complications of AIDS. *Psychosomatics*, *25*, 373–400.

Holland JC & Tross S (1985). The psychosocial and neuropsychiatric sequelae of the acquired immune deficiency syndrome and related disorders. *Annals of Internal Medicine*, *103*, 760–764.

Horowitz SL, Bentson JR, Benson F, et al. (1983). CNS toxoplasmosis in acquired immunodeficiency syndrome. *Archives of Neurology*, *40*, 649–652.

Jordan BD, Navia BA, Petito C, et al. (1985). Neurological syndromes complicating AIDS. *Frontiers of Radiation Therapy and Oncology*, *19*, 82–87.

Khadem M, Kalish SB, Goldsmith J, et al. (1984). Ophthalmologic findings in acquired immune deficiency symdrome (AIDS). *Archives of Ophthalmology*, *102*, 201–206.

Landesman SH, Ginzburg HM, & Weiss SH (1985). Special report: The AIDS epidemic. *New England Journal of Medicine*, *312*, 521–525.

Levine AM, Meyer PR, Begandy MK, et al. (1984). Development of B-cell lymphoma in homosexual men: Clinical and immunologic findings. *Annals of Internal Medicine*, *100*, 7–13.

Levy JA, Shimabukuro J, Hollander H, et al. (1985). Isolation of AIDS-associated retroviruses from cerebrospinal fluid and brain of patients with neurological symptoms. *Lancet*, *2*, 586–588.

Levy RM, Pons VG, & Rosenblum ML (1984). Central nervous system mass lesions in the acquired immunodeficiency syndrome (AIDS). *Journal of Neurosurgery*, *61*, 9–16.

Lipowski ZJ (1980). *Delirium: Acute brain failure in man*. Springfield, IL: Charles C Thomas.

Loewenstein RJ & Sharfstein SS (1983–1984). Neuropsychiatric aspects of acquired immune deficiency syndrome. *International Journal of Psychiatry in Medicine*, *13*, 255–260.

Malyon AK & Pinka AT (1983). Acquired immune deficiency syndrome: A challenge to psychology. *Professional Psychology*, *7*, 1–11.

Masur H, Michelis MA, Greene JB, et al. (1981). An outbreak of community acquired *Pneumocystis carinii* pneumonia: Initial manifestation of cellular immune dysfunction. *New England Journal of Medicine*, *305*, 1431–1438.

McEvoy JP (1981). Organic brain syndrome. *Annals of Internal Medicine*, *95*, 212–216.

McKusick L, Horstman W, & Coates TJ (1985). AIDS and sexual behavior reported by gay men in San Francisco. *American Journal of Public Health*, *75*, 493–496.

Miller JR, Barrett RE, Britton CB, et al. (1982). Progressive multifocal leukoencephalopathy in a male homosexual with T-cell immune deficiency. *New England Journal of Medicine*, *307*, 1436–1438.

Morin SF & Batchelor WF (1984). Responding to the psychological crisis of AIDS. *Public Health Reports*, *99*, 4–9.

Morin SJ, Charles KA, & Malyon AK (1984). The psychological impact of AIDS on gay men. *American Psychologist*, *39*, 1288–1293.

Navia BA & Price RW (1986). Dementia complicating AIDS. *Psychiatric Annals*, *16*, 158–166.

Novik A (1984). At risk for AIDS: Confidentiality in research and surveillance. *IRB A Review of Human Subjects Research*, *6*, 10–11.

Pagano JS & Lemon SM (1985). The herpesviruses. In AI Braude, CE Davis & J Fierer (Eds), *Infectious diseases and medical microbiology* (pp 470–477). Philadelphia: WB Saunders.

Penn I (1981). Depressed immunity and development of cancer. *Journal of Experimental Immunology*, *46*, 459–474.

Perry S (1985). Irrational attitudes toward addicts and narcotics. *Bulletin of the New York Academy of Medicine*, *61*, 706–729.

Perry S & Jacobsen P (1986). Neuropsychiatric manifestations of AIDS-spectrum disorders. *Hospital and Community Psychiatry*, *37*, 135–142.

Perry SW & Tross S (1984). Psychiatric problems of AIDS inpatients at the New York hospital: Preliminary report. *Public Health Reports*, *99*, 200–205.

Petito CK, Navia BA, Cho ES, et al. (1985). Vacuolar myelopathy pathologically resembling subacute combined degeneration in patients with the acquired immunodeficiency syndrome. *New England Journal of Medicine*, *312*, 874–879.

Polan HJ, Hellerstein D, & Amchin J (1985). Impact of AIDS-related cases on an inpatient therapeutic milieu. *Hospital and Community Psychiatry*, *36*, 173–176.

Post MJD, Sheldon JJ, Hensley GT, et al. (1986). Central nervous system disease in acquired immune deficiency syndrome: Prospective correlation using CT, MR imaging, and pathologic studies. *Radiology*, *158*, 141–148.

Redfield RR, Markham PD, Salahuddin SZ, et al. (1985a). Frequent transmission of HTLV-III among spouses of patients with AIDS-related complex and AIDS. *Journal of the American Medical Association*, *253*, 1571–1573.

Redfield RR, Markham PD, Salahuddin SZ, et al. (1985b). Heterosexually acquired HTLV-III/LAV disease (AIDS-related complex and AIDS): Epidemiologic evidence for female-to-male transmission. *Journal of the American Medical Association, 254*, 2094–2096.

Reichert CM, O'Leary TJ, Levens DL, et al. (1983). Autopsy pathology in the acquired immune deficiency syndrome. *American Journal of Pathology, 112*, 357–382.

Remington JS & McCleod R (1985). Toxoplasmosis. In AI Braude, CE Davis & J Fierer (Eds), *Infectious diseases and medical microbiology* (pp 1521–1535). Philadelphia: WB Saunders.

Rivin BE, Monroe JM, Hubschuman BP, et al. (1984). AIDS outcome: A first follow-up [Letter]. *New England Journal of Medicine, 311*, 857.

Rubinstein A, Sicklick M, Gupta A, et al. (1983). Acquired immunodeficiency syndrome with reversed T4/T8 ratios in infants born to promiscuous and drug-addicted mothers. *Journal of the American Medical Association, 249*, 2350–2356.

Schroff RW, Gottlieb MS, Prince HE, et al. (1983). Immunological studies of homosexual men with immunodeficiency and Kaposi's sarcoma. *Clinical Immunology and Immunopathology, 27*, 300–314.

Scott GB, Buck BE, Leterman JG, et al. (1984). Acquired immunodeficiency syndrome in infants. *New England Journal of Medicine, 310*, 76–81.

Scully RE (1983). Weekly clinicopathological exercises: Case 32-1983. Case records of the Massachusetts General Hospital. *New England Journal of Medicine, 309*, 359–369.

Shaw GM, Harper ME, Hahn BH, et al. (1985). HTLV-III infection in brains of children and adults with AIDS encephalopathy. *Science, 227*, 177–182.

Snider WD, Simpson DM, Nielsen S, et al. (1983). Neurological complications of acquired immune deficiency syndrome: Analysis of 50 patients. *Annals of Neurology, 14*, 403–418.

Weiss SH, Goedert JJ, Sarngadharan MG, et al. (1985). Screening test for HTLV-III (AIDS agent) antibodies: Specificity, sensitivity, and applications. *Journal of the American Medical Association, 253*, 221–225.

Welch K, Finkbeiner W, Alpers CE, et al. (1984). Autopsy findings in the acquired immune deficiency syndrome. *Journal of the American Medical Association, 252*, 1152–1159.

Whelan MA, Kricheff II, Handler M, et al. (1983). Acquired immunodeficiency syndrome: Cerebral computed tomographic manifestations. *Radiology, 149*, 477–484.

Wolcott DL, Fawzy FI, & Pasnau RO (1986). Acquired immune deficiency syndrome (AIDS) and consultation-liaison psychiatry. *General Hospital Psychiatry, 7*, 280–292.

Wong-Staal F & Gallo RC (1985). Human T-lymphotropic retroviruses. *Nature, 317*, 395–403.

Yarchoan R, Klecker RW, Weinhold KJ, et al. (1986). Administration of 3'-azido-3'-deoxythymidine, an inhibitor of HTLV-III/LAV replication, to patients with AIDS or AIDS-related complex. *Lancet, 1*, 575–580.

Part III

Medical-Psychiatric Units

Alan Stoudemire
Barry S. Fogel

32

Organization and Development of Combined Medical-Psychiatric Units: Part 1

In the past five years, interest has increased in the development of specialized inpatient settings for combined psychiatric and medical treatment. While several program descriptions (Fogel, 1985; Fogel, Stoudemire, & Houpt, 1985; Goodman, 1985; Hoffman, 1984; Koran & Barnes, 1982; Molnar, Fava, & Zielezhy, 1985; Stoudemire, Brown, McLeod, et al., 1983; Stoudemire, Kahn, Brown, et al., 1985; Withersty, Shemo, Waldman, et al., 1980) and one comparative study (Fogel et al., 1985) have been published, comprehensive guidelines for the development of medical-psychiatric units (MPUs) have not yet appeared in the literature. This chapter, along with Chapter 33, provides a systematic approach to organizing and operating these units, based on the authors' experience in developing and managing them in different settings, and in consulting to hospitals considering forming combined inpatient programs.

Issues addressed in this chapter include selection and admission of patients, architectural and physical environment,

medical and diagnostic therapeutic resources required, psychiatric therapy and the therapeutic milieu, and roles of other mental health disciplines on the unit.

The term *medical-psychiatric unit* has been applied to a number of different entities. In this chapter, we will discuss units that are oriented toward the admission and treatment of patients with combined medical and psychiatric illness, that attempt to integrate medical and psychiatric care, and that emphasize a disease model of psychopathology. Units so defined may take a variety of forms, depending on their administrative environment, the nature of the local medical and psychiatric communities, and the orientation of their leadership. Because of this heterogeneity, and because descriptions and empirical studies of MPUs are few, our guidelines can be regarded only as an informed view, rather than as final conclusions based on adequate data. Nonetheless, we believe that the guidelines may offer a valuable starting point for those considering an MPU, and constitute a framework for debate and further study.

PRINCIPLES OF MEDICAL PSYCHIATRY
ISBN 0-8089-1883-4

SELECTION AND ADMISSION
OF PATIENTS

By definition, MPUs maintain their distinctive patient population by promoting the admission of patients with combined medical and psychiatric illness. In most cases, the units will exclude some classes of psychiatric patients who do not have concurrent medical illness. Recruitment of suitable patients is facilitated by close links between the unit and the general hospital psychiatric consultation-liaison service. A second source of patients is affiliation with a free-standing psychiatric hospital or Community Mental Health Center (CMHC), which may transfer to the MPU patients too medically ill to be cared for in traditional psychiatric inpatient settings. A third source may be other psychiatric units in the same hospital, if these exist. Finally, direct referrals from community physicians may be promoted by disseminating information about the unit's distinctive therapeutic capabilities.

Depending on the administrative environment and other resources available in the community, some MPUs will not fill completely with patients with combined disease. These units will admit some physically healthy psychiatric patients to fill their remaining beds. Ideally, these would be patients who could benefit from a predominantly medical model of treatment, and who are not so behaviorally threatening that they would disrupt the medical treatment being administered to other patients (Molnar et al., 1985). Patients to be excluded include those who are too physically ill to be managed with the available level of medical coverage (Fogel, 1985; Koran & Barnes, 1982; Molnar et al., 1985), and those whose behavioral problems cannot be managed with the available staffing and physical environment. In systems where alternatives exist, it is also wise to consider excluding patients with severe dispositional problems unlikely to be resolved even with effective psychiatric treatment (Goodman, 1985).

Different MPUs may target different populations. One group common to all MPUs consists of patients with depression and concurrent medical disease (Fogel et al., 1985; Koran, 1985). Because medical illness may complicate somatic antidepressant treatment and because severe depression may interfere with patients' cooperation with medical treatment, these patients often require hospital admission, and usually will benefit from conjoint medical-psychiatric treatment. Further, depressive symptoms and symptoms of medical disease may overlap, creating difficult diagnostic problems best resolved by careful inpatient observation and antidepressant trials. (Anderson & Sivesind, 1985).

In the public sector, a common medical-psychiatric population consists of patients with chronic schizophrenia and concurrent physical disease (Molnar et al., 1985). Chronically mentally ill populations, particularly if indigent, may have a very high prevalence of inadequately treated medical disease (Hall, Gardner, Stickney, et al., 1980). Special medical-psychiatric settings may be particularly useful in identifying and addressing their problems.

The typical MPU will supplement its core patient population with other patients according to the unit's administrative auspices, the capacity of the unit to effectively treat particular problems, and the therapeutic capacities of other clinical services in the area. Other problems treated on MPUs include psychiatric complications of neurologic disease (stroke, epilepsy, parkinsonism, head trauma), delirium, eating disorders with significant medical complications, behaviorally complicated dementia, chronic pain, paroxysmal behavioral disorders of unknown etiology, factitious illness, somatoform disorders, and physical illness combined with complex family or psychosocial problems that interfere with the patient's ability to cooperate with necessary medical treatment.

In selecting clinical populations to be served, the unit leadership may wish to consider the following questions. Which categories of potential medical-psychiatric patients are poorly served by the existing system? Service to these patients would be unlikely to compete with existing institutions, and therefore might be welcomed by the community. For which classes of patients would reimbursement be adequate? Would contracts with local CMHCs or psychiatric hospitals be possible or desirable? What are the special competences and interests of the attending staff contemplated for the unit? Would residents or other trainees serve on the unit? If so, what would their training needs be? What coverage for urgent medical problems would be available?

Once the target populations are determined, a system of priorities for admission can be set up. The priority system may take into account urgency of the clinical problem, diagnosis, length of time on the waiting list, and the current location of the patient. It may be advantageous to grant a high priority to patients awaiting transfer to the MPU from medical and surgical services within the general hospital. Doing so creates goodwill among the medical staff, facilitating further referrals to the unit. Also, by solving difficult management problems, it develops support for the unit among hospital administrators and physicians of other specialties.

As noted above, patients may need to be excluded if they are too physically ill for the unit's medical coverage or are too behaviorally disturbed to be managed in the MPU environment. In addition to these exclusions, most adult MPUs will decline to admit children and adolescents, except in extraordinary situations. Sixteen may be taken as a rough lower bound for admission.

Medical-psychiatric units with a relatively small number of beds need to screen their patients prior to admission for potential disposition problems. Evaluating long-term disposition needs prior to admission will help avoid tying up the unit's beds with numerous long-stay patients who would benefit only marginally from the unit's unique, intensive resources. However, exclusion of patients with dispositional problems may be unnecessary if the unit has its own strong links with a variety of community resources (Hoffman, 1984).

Whatever admission criteria and priority system are chosen, some admission decisions are likely to be difficult. While many gatekeeping decisions can be made by the nurse in charge, problem cases will require intervention by the medical director. Systems problems are minimized if the hospital administration and the head of the psychiatry department unequivocally support the medical director's authority to decline admission to patients thought inappropriate for the unit.

ARCHITECTURAL AND PHYSICAL ENVIRONMENT

The ideal physical environment of an MPU provides safety for delirious and behaviorally disturbed patients, facilitates the rendering of medical services, and provides a pleasant environment suitable for the relatively long hospital stays often required by complex multiproblem patients.

Safety features are essential not only for suicidal patients, but also because delirious persons may impulsively harm themselves (Wolff & Curran, 1935). Safety features include shatterproof windows, breakaway curtain rods, and electrical outlets that disconnect if tampered with. For units with semiprivate bathrooms, lockable water taps may be useful.

Medically relevant features of patient rooms will vary with the patient populations served. If the MPU is to handle acute medical illness, desirable features would include adequate lighting for bedside examination, outlets for oxygen and for suction, and adjustable hospital beds.

In addition to adequate common areas for group dining, activities, educational programs, family meetings, group therapy, and occupational therapy, additional space will be needed for staff meetings and conferences. Sufficient storage space for medical equipment and supplies is essential. The care of complex medical-psychiatric patients often requires frequent small conferences among professionals of different disciplines and specialties to coordinate care. One or two small conference rooms in addition to on-site professional offices for the medical director, social worker, head nurse, and trainees afford privacy and quiet for conferences and interviews. Finally, an adequate staff lounge not only improves morale, but also facilitates communication between the different caretakers of complex patients. The overall space requirements do not differ much from those of the *ideal* psychiatric ward described by Barton and Barton (1983), but they do exceed the space available on less-than-ideal general hospital psychiatric units.

DIAGNOSTIC AND MEDICAL THERAPEUTIC RESOURCES

The diagnostic and medical therapeutic capabilities of MPUs will vary with their intended populations. For units with a relatively high level of medical problems, or with a substantial proportion of neuropsychiatric patients, essential diagnostic capabilities would include neuropsychological testing, EEG, CT scanning, and plasma level monitoring for medical and psychiatric drugs.

In these units, two essential treatment

capabilities are intravenous drug therapy and ECT. The ability to give I.V. therapy is a virtual sine qua non of an MPU. Electrotherapy is frequently the treatment of choice for patients with severe depressive disorders and concurrent cardiac disorders, and for patients with psychotic depression so severe that nutrition and hydration have become impaired, thus requiring a medical-psychiatric admission (Fink, 1979). Oxygen should be available if patients with heart failure or lung disease are to be admitted. Nutritional support services such as tube feedings and total parenteral nutrition may be needed if severely malnourished patients are to be accepted.

Depending on the level of medical specialization desired, monitoring devices might be considered. With adequate medical coverage, cardiac monitoring may improve the safety of psychotropic drug treatment of patients with moderately unstable heart rhythm. On units accepting neuropsychiatric patients, EEG telemetry or 24-hour ambulatory EEG monitoring may be an extremely valuable tool for diagnosing patients with paroxysmal behavioral disorders or a mixture of epileptic and psychiatric symptoms (Feldman, Paul, & Cummins-Ducharme, 1982).

PSYCHIATRIC THERAPY AND THE THERAPEUTIC MILIEU

In keeping with contemporary general hospital psychiatric practice, medical-psychiatric inpatients usually receive pharmacologic or somatic therapy for their psychiatric disorders (Sederer, 1983). However, psychosocial therapies are no less important for medically ill patients, and may comprise the full range of treatments, including short-term individual psychotherapy, behavioral therapy, family therapy, hypnosis, relaxation instruction, and biofeedback. In psychotherapy, issues of adaption to physical illness and disability arise frequently. These include conflicts over dependency, grief reactions to loss of function, and angry or guilty feelings toward principal caretakers. Some form of family intervention is needed in almost every case. Because the patients' physical illnesses often place family members in caretaking roles, lack of knowledge, poor communication, or hostility among family members may have major effects on the patients' physical health and activity level.

The varying physical capacities and functional limitations of medical-psychiatric patients preclude a conventional therapeutic milieu with standardized expectations for all patients. Instead, expectations must be individualized (Anderson & Sivesind, 1985). Existing MPUs have adopted a variety of milieu features for specific subsets of their populations, and have found them helpful. These include the following.

Group Psychotherapy

Short-term psychotherapy groups, usually led by nonphysicians, may concentrate on issues of adaptation to illness, activity versus passivity, and communication skills. Groups for the elderly may include a reminiscence or life-review component (Kaminsky, 1984). These groups usually exclude patients with impaired impulse control, intolerance of extreme stimulation, muteness, or major cognitive impairment (Rutchick, 1983).

Group Education Programs and Discussion Groups

These can focus on topics such as depression and its physical symptoms, stress management, coping with chronic disability, alcohol issues, or the use of psychotropics. Some units have augmented these programs with videotapes or films.

Occupational, Physical, and Recreational Activity Groups

Physical mobilization and exercise is crucial for depressed patients with chronic medical illness. These patients usually are less active than would be ideal for their physical and mental health but may be too demoralized to exercise regularly. Traditional psychiatric unit activities such as games or crafts can provide welcome recreation for patients undergoing a course of ECT or a prolonged drug trial in the hospital (Goodman, 1985).

Ward Meetings

While patient participation in unit government would be inappropriate for a medically acute unit, ward meetings two or three times per week to orient new patients, to facilitate patients' leave-taking, and to share information about events on the ward can be valuable. These ward meetings are similar to the "community meetings" of traditional general hospital psychiatric units (Leeman, 1983) but are less process-oriented (Fogel, 1985; Goodman, 1985).

Process Groups for Staff

Staff groups are popular on many psychiatric units and MPUs. These groups may help resolve intrastaff conflicts that might otherwise interfere with patient care (Abrams, 1969). In our opinion, having a designated leader or facilitator enhances the productivity of such groups.

ROLES OF OTHER MENTAL HEALTH DISCIPLINES

A multidisciplinary treatment team best addresses the many complex needs of patients with combined disease. While team members of different disciplines may all practice psychotherapy, and all may have a role in the administration of the unit, each discipline has a unique contribution to make. In contrast to some traditional psychiatric units, overall direction of the unit must be the responsibility of the physician, because the patients are physically ill, and a medical model of diagnosis and treatment is being practiced.

The active participation of nursing staff in treatment planning facilitates the integration of physical care and psychotherapy. A nurse clinical specialist with both medical and psychiatric background can be invaluable not only as a milieu coordinator, but also as a supervisor for nurses on difficult cases and as an organizer of special in-service training when unfamiliar medical issues are dealt with on the unit.

Patients with combined psychiatric and medical problems frequently require complex social work interventions. Patients with physical disabilities may require services such as vocational rehabilitation or home health care. Those patients who do need placement may be particularly hard to place (Gruenberg & Willemain, 1982), and the placement task may include first matching the patient's needs with the facility's program and then persuading the facility to accept the patient. One MPU (Hoffman, 1984), reported success from ongoing liaison with specific community agencies.

For those patients who have intact families, brief family therapy is often needed for the best outcome. Early and thorough family assessment can identify potential barriers to the patient's returning home, as well as family resistances to alternative methods of managing the patient's illness. Brief family intervention can reduce the rate of institutional placements of MPU patients. The social worker requires not only skills in family assessment and therapy

but also considerable medical sophistication, so that realistic problems of the patient's physical illness can be distinguished from fears, misinformation, or distortions connected with a family's resistance to change (Wallace, Goldberg, & Slaby, 1984).

Consulting psychologists with expertise in neuropsychology, personality assessment, and principles of behavior therapy are valuable resources. Psychologists' skills in behavior therapy frequently are needed to tailor programs for patients with learned maladaptive behavior such as conditioned psychophysiologic vomiting, and to design contingency management contracts for eating disorder patients and patients with drug abuse problems. Neuropsychological assessment is particularly valuable in quantifying and characterizing patients' cognitive impairment, permitting the development of therapeutic programs that take those impairments into account. However, formal neuropsychological testing usually is not necessary for distinguishing "functional" from "organic" etiologies for disease. Both factors are operative in most medical-psychiatric patients, and medical tests and consultations are more valuable than psychological tests in uncovering specific treatable causes of organic impairment. Formal personality assessment can be particularly helpful in defining the psychopathology behind a screen of somatic symptoms (Stoudemire et al., 1985), and in identifying personality traits and disorders that would require special management to avoid destructive acting-out on the unit.

ACKNOWLEDGMENTS

This chapter was previously published in *Psychosomatics*, 27 (5), May 1986, and is reprinted with permission.

REFERENCES

Abrams GM (1969). Defining milieu therapy. *Archives of General Psychiatry*, *21*, 553–560

Anderson S & Sivesind D (1985). Depressed elderly in the inpatient psychiatric milieu. In CA Rogers & J Ulsafer-Van Lanen (eds), *Nursing interventions in depression* (pp 195–220). Orlando: Grune & Stratton.

Barton WE & Barton GM (1983). Ward administration. In WE Barton & GM Barton (Eds), *Mental health administration, priciples and practice* (Vol 2, pp 537–557). New York: Human Sciences Press.

Feldman RG, Paul NL, & Cummins-Ducharme J (1982). Videotape recording in epilepsy and pseudoseizures. In TL Riley & A Roy (Eds), *Pseudoseizures* (pp 122–134). Baltimore: Williams & Wilkins.

Fink M (1979). Risk-benefit analysis. In *Convulsive therapy: Theory and practice* (pp 51–58). New York: Raven Press.

Fogel BS (1985). A psychiatric unit becomes a psychiatric-medical unit: Administrative and clinical implications. *General Hospital Psychiatry*, *7*, 26–35.

Fogel BS, Stoudemire A, & Houpt JL (1985). Contrasting models for conjoint medical and psychiatric inpatient treatment: Psych/med vs med/psych. *American Journal of Psychiatry*, *142*, 1085–1089.

Goodman B (1985). Combined psychiatric-medical inpatient units: The Mount Sinai model. *Psychosomatics*, *26*, 179–189.

Gruenberg LW & Willemain TR (1982). Hospital discharge queues in Massachusetts. *Medical Care*, *20*, 188–200.

Hall RCW, Gardner ER, Stickney SK, et al. (1980). Physical illness manifesting as psychiatric disease. Analysis of a state hospital inpatient population. *Archives of General Psychiatry*, *37*, 989–995.

Hoffman RS (1984). Operation of a medical-psychiatric unit in a general hospital setting. *General Hospital Psychiatry*, *6*, 93–99.

Kaminsky M (1984). *The uses of reminiscence. New ways of working with older adults.* New York: Haworth Press.

Koran LM (1985). Medical-psychiatric units and the future of psychiatric practice. *Psychosomatics*, *26*, 171-175.

Koran LM & Barnes LEA (1982). The Stanford comprehensive medical unit: Integrating psychiatric and medical care. In JM Kuldau (Ed), *New directions for medical health services: No. 15. Treatment for psychosomatic problems (pp 61–73).* San Francisco: Jossey-Bass.

Leeman CP (1983). The therapeutic milieu. In LI Sederer (Ed), *Inpatient psychiatry diagnosis and treatment* (pp 222–233). Baltimore: Williams & Wilkins.

Molnar G, Fava GA, & Zielezny MA (1985). Medical-psychiatric unit patients compared with patients in two other services. *Psychosomatics*, *26*, 193–209.

Rutchick IE (1983). Group psychotherapy. In LI Sederer (Ed), *Inpatient psychiatry diagnosis and treatment* (pp 250–263). Baltimore: Williams & Wilkins.

Sederer LI (1983). *Inpatient psychiatry diagnosis and treatment.* Baltimore: Williams & Wilkins.

Stoudemire A, Brown JT, McLeod M, et al. (1983). The combined medical specialties unit: An innovative approach to patient care. *North Carolina Medical Journal*, *44*, 365–367.

Stoudemire A, Kahn M, Brown JT, et al. (1985). Masked depression in a combined medical–psychiatric unit. *Psychosomatics*, *26*, 221–228.

Wallace SR, Goldberg RJ, & Slaby AE (1984). *Clinical social work in health care. New biopsychosocial approaches.* New York: Praeger.

Withersty DJ, Shemo JPD, Waldman RH, et al. (1980). Evaluating a conjoint psychiatric-medical inpatient unit: A one-year follow-up study of depressed patients. *Journal of Clinical Psychiatry*, *41*, 156–158.

Wolff HG & Curran D (1935). Nature of delirium and allied states. The dysergastic reaction. *Archives of Neurology and Psychiatry*, *13*, 1175–1215.

Barry S. Fogel
Alan Stoudemire

33
Organization and Development of Combined Medical-Psychiatric Units: Part 2

NURSE STAFFING AND TRAINING

To provide holistic nursing care and to promote the greatest flexibility in assignment of staff to patients, the nursing staff of a medical-psychiatric unit (MPU) should consist entirely of registered nurses who combine superb psychiatric nursing abilities with the broadest possible range of medical/surgical nursing skills. However, practical limitations on budget and recruitment may necessitate some compromise. A staff consisting mostly of RNs with some nursing assistants and practical nurses can deliver adequate care (Fogel, 1985; Goodman, 1985). Instead of all nurses being generalists, some may have particularly strong medical/surgical nursing skills while others are most experienced in behavioral and psychotherapeutic interventions. While formal psychiatric nursing training and experience is not absolutely necessary for the majority of nurses (Fogel, 1985; Goodman, 1985), the presence of a few senior nurses with extensive psychiatric experience can contribute greatly to the management of behaviorally difficult patients, particularly if those nurses enjoy giving physical care and enthusiastically support the model of combined medical and psychiatric treatment.

Many unit directors have told us that the personal qualities of nurses matter as much as their formal training. One personal quality particularly valued by the directors is flexibility. Rigid personality traits, of almost any type, or rigid adherence to a particular model of treatment, are virtually incompatible with the constantly shifting demands placed on the medical-psychiatric nurse. A common experience of MPU directors is that nurses lacking in flexibility often choose to leave conjoint care settings in favor of more traditional medical or psychiatric environments.

The ideal staff:patient ratio will depend on the target population and acuity level of the unit, but some suggestions can be made for units intending to have a high

685

proportion of patients with nontrivial medical illness. First, no fewer than six total nursing hours should be available per patient day. This amount, which is roughly comparable to one full-time equivalent nurse per bed, has been described by Barton and Barton (1983) as the minimum necessary for first-rate psychiatric care, totally apart from considerations of concurrent medical illness. Second, the evening and night shifts need strong coverage because medical-psychiatric patients often have sleep disturbances, and because medical symptoms often are especially troublesome at night. A one-to-five staff-to-patient ratio on the night shift has proved adequate on the Brown University (Rhode Island Hospital) and Emory University units.

To best integrate physical and psychotherapeutic treatment, and to best facilitate teamwork, one or two nurses on each shift should carry most of the nursing care responsibility for each patient, and those nurses should be regularly involved in treatment planning and in meetings with caretakers from other disciplines. However, since many physical care tasks need to be undertaken on an MPU, assignment of these tasks has to be somewhat flexible. Dividing the nursing staff into practice groups sharing the care of a specified group of patients is one way to provide flexibility while maintaining consistency in the psychological approach to the patient (Burn & Tonges, 1983).

PSYCHIATRIC STAFF AND QUALITY ASSURANCE FOR PSYCHIATRIC CARE

Either an open or a closed psychiatric staff is compatible with successful operation of the MPU. The principal advantage of an open staff is a broad range of community referrals to the unit when community-based practitioners can admit patients. Closed staffs offer the advantages of greater

cohesion and potentially better quality assurance, as well as a quicker response to crises when the psychiatric staff is based on or near the unit.

If an open staff model is selected, the unit needs quality assurance mechanisms to compensate for community-based psychiatrists' varied training and more limited physical availability. Mechanisms include special continuing medical education programs on medical-psychiatric topics, consultation by the medical director, and frequent systematic critical reviews of all cases. The medical director, head nurse, and psychiatric resident can make periodic rounds on all patients, addressing issues of psychiatric-medical liaison, changes in medical status, and emergence of drug side effects. Regular medication chart rounds are helpful for critical review of the polypharmacy that so often is unavoidable in patients with multiple illnesses. Finally, on-site availability (with decision-making authority) of at least one psychiatrist, whether a resident, the medical director, or a hospital-based staff psychiatrist, helps minimize the escalation of crises.

PSYCHIATRIST-INTERNIST RELATIONS AND PROVISION OF MEDICAL COVERAGE

When MPUs operate under psychiatric auspices, the psychiatrist is the attending physician and head of a multidisciplinary, multispecialty team. Psychiatrists, with formal training in the management of teams, usually are best qualified to serve as team captains. Also, it may be easier for a medically-oriented psychiatrist to communicate with consultants about issues of physical illness than for a nonpsychiatrist to discuss complex behavioral and psychodynamic issues (Fogel & Goldberg, 1983–1984; Fogel, Stoudemire, & Houpt, 1985). However, having an internist on salary either as a co-director or as a liaison internist can enhance the quality of medical care and promote more frequent collaboration in decision-making and treatment planning (Goodman, 1985; Stoudemire, Brown, McLeod, et al., 1983).

To estimate medical coverage needs, one may divide patients into three broad categories. The first category comprises patients with severe medical illness in addition to psychiatric illness, who definitely require the daily attendance of an internist (or other medical or surgical specialist). The second group comprises patients who require frequent but not daily attention from the internist or surgeon, such as persons with diabetes or congestive heart failure needing periodic readjustments of a medical regimen, or persons recovering from trauma who need periodic changes in orthopedic management. The third group consists of patients who require initial diagnostic consultations or medication adjustment, and then do not need to be seen on a regular basis by a nonpsychiatric physician.

While patients may shift from one category to another during a course of treatment, units with specified target populations and stable referral patterns do develop somewhat consistent distributions of medical acuity that permit planning of medical coverage. Units with a high proportion of patients in the first two categories of acuity may need a salaried liaison internist and/or medical house staff specifically assigned to the MPU and regularly involved in patient care. Exceptional units may deal with high medical acuity by having a medical director and/or attending staff members with dual training both in psychiatry and in medicine or neurology. Regardless of acuity, all MPUs must be prepared to provide emergency medical treatment for major problems such as cardiac arrhythmia, status epilepticus, and respiratory failure. This need can be met either by medical house staff coverage, or by an arrangement with a medical or surgical group that provides coverage elsewhere in the hospital.

Units not equipped to handle a high proportion of medically acute patients still may occasionally accept medically acute patients if there is adequate emergency coverage. However, such patients put additional stress on consultants, the emergency coverage system, and the nursing staff. Thus, their admission would seem desirable only when the expected benefit to the patient is proportional to the stress imposed.

Financial arrangements between psychiatrists and internists jointly involved in caring for patients should be clarified in advance. In all but the most medically complicated cases, the psychiatrist usually spends more time with the patient than the internist (Fogel et al., 1985). For this reason, it usually is more efficient for the psychiatrist to directly bill third parties for the daily attending fee, while the internist or subspecialist bills the patient for follow-up over and above the initial consultation. In our experience, medical follow-up fees usually are paid, and major medical plans often cover a substantial part of them.

ROLE OF THE UNIT MEDICAL DIRECTOR

The medical director of an MPU is the linchpin of the service, and his or her importance cannot be overestimated. Because of the complex administrative interfaces of an MPU and the complex illnesses of the patients, numerous situations arise that require the director's presence and judgement. For this reason, the medical director requires a salary with no less than one half of his or her income noncontingent on direct patient care. Setting up an MPU is a nearly full-time job, and the ongoing operation of the unit of ten to 20 beds may easily consume 20 hours per week, exclusive of direct service to individual patients.

There are three alternate models for the medical direction of an MPU. In one model, the medical director is a psychiatrist who is also extensively trained either in internal medicine or in neurology, and who is responsible for both psychiatric and medical quality assurance. In the second model, a psychiatrist and an internist share responsibility for medical direction of the unit. In the third model, the psychiatrist is the medical director, and a part-time liaison internist has delegated functions that include medical quality assurance and the rendering of medical care to some or all of the patients. A potential fourth model, comprising an internist director with a part-time liaison psychiatrist, has not been followed by any of the units that have reported program descriptions.

Regardless of the model chosen, the psychiatrist medical director requires substantial medical experience, continuing interest in the psychiatric-medical interface, and belief in a disease model of psychopathology. Many director of existing units came to their jobs from consultation-liaison psychiatry. The advantages of a dually-trained medical director are the potential for the creative synthesis of treatment approaches made possible by dual training, and the economy of requiring only one base salary. The other two approaches, while somewhat more costly, have salient benefits. First, an internist can more easily remain current in the broad field of internal medicine than can a dually-trained chief who must also keep up with developments in psychiatry. Second, replacements for psychiatrists and internists may be easier to find than replacements for dually-trained directors. Thus, co-directorship or the liaison internist approach may enhance administrative stability.

The medical director's duties include gatekeeping, quality assurance, staff supervision, training, continuing medical education, troubleshooting and the provision of consultations in difficult cases. The medical director also is responsible for liaison with referring sources in the community, public relations for the unit, and assistance with the resolution of legal and ethical problems in patient care.

In addition to requiring salary support and space on the unit, the medical director requires secretarial support. Conservatively, a half-time secretary would be needed if the medical director were involved neither in research nor in private practice; if the medical director did engage in these activities, a full-time secretary would be needed.

ADMINISTRATIVE INTERFACES

With the Department of Psychiatry

The MPU requires sufficient autonomy to adopt policies and procedures appropriate for its special population. It must preserve the ability to keep its own "gate."

With the Hospital Administration

Because MPUs often require different staffing and supplies from ordinary psychiatric units, and often involve different lengths of stay and criteria for utilization review, a personal relationship between the unit chief and a specific hospital administrator is helpful in anticipating, preventing, and solving administrative problems.

With the Community and Community Mental Health Centers

General hospital psychiatric units often are expected to serve as a place of disposition for indigent patients and clients of community mental health centers (CMHCs) (Richman & Harris, 1985). Our experience suggests that CMHCs and other referring sources are most interested in having an MPU available as a resource for their most complex and refractory patients with combined disease. If reasonable numbers of these patients are accepted by an MPU, there may be greater understanding by the referring source when the unit turns down other patients for whom alternate dispositions are feasible.

With Third-Party Payors

Insurance companies and utilization reviewers are not always familiar with the medical-psychiatric model and with the need for many time-intensive professional services to optimally treat patients with combined illness. To ensure adequate reimbursement for services, and to minimize difficulties with utilization review departments, detailed documentation of the patients' multiple impairments is crucial. Also, it may be useful for the medical director to meet with insurance company officials, professional review organizations, and the hospital utilization review department prior to the establishment of a unit, and periodically thereafter, to minimize the emergence of major problems. Regular monitoring of medical records by the medical director and/or senior nursing staff may help ensure that documentation is adequate for utilization review and for justification of the expense of conjoint medical-psychiatric treatment.

With the Legal System

An important consideration in organizing an MPU is whether the unit will be subject to legal requirements to accept involuntary patients for treatment. In some states, new general hospital psychiatric units may be subject to such requirements. If local mental health regulations require the indiscriminate acceptance of involuntary patients by the MPU, the unit must provide adequate staffing and facilities for

seclusion and restraint to permit the safe conduct of medical procedures on other, less acutely disturbed patients. Alternatively, in a region where a more specialized MPU seemed desirable, the unit director might negotiate for a total or partial exemption from a legal requirement to accept involuntary patients. A third option would be for the MPU to accept only those medically ill patients whose medical treatment could not be easily disrupted by the violent actions of other patients. In this case, the use of intravenous medication and fluids might be limited.

Once an MPU is in operation, legal issues must be faced concerning the involuntary treatment of delirious patients. Delirious patients often receive involuntary treatment in traditional medical settings (Applebaum & Roth, 1984). Medical-psychiatric units often treat delirious patients who may refuse needed medical diagnostic or therapeutic interventions because of an organically-based inability to adequately comprehend and judge their situation. In medical settings, delirious patients usually are treated without recourse to mental health laws and formal guardianship procedures, but in traditional psychiatric settings statutes regarding involuntary treatments must be applied. Therefore, the medical director of an MPU needs to clarify with legal counsel and state mental health authorities whether or not the consent requirements of state mental health laws would apply to the medical as well as the psychiatric treatments administered to patients on the unit. If they did, the ability of the unit to respond to the urgent medical problems of delirious patients might be impaired.

Even with no statutory impediment to addressing the medical problems of delirious patients without formal guardianship, there still are ethical and common law problems to be faced. Truly emergent medical problems in grossly delirious patients can be treated without formal consent, by extension of the legal doctrine of implied consent. When the situation is not emergent, the proposed intervention is risky, and the patient objects to the intervention, it is necessary to obtain guardianship. In intermediate cases, medical second opinions and discussions with family members may be reasonable, although these have no formal sanction. The medical director must be well informed about local standards and legal precedents in this area, so as to be able to advise the psychiatric, medical, and nursing staff when crises arise. A commonsense approach based on common law principles is described in a recent article (Fogel, Mills, & Landen, 1986). However, because states and localities differ considerably, medical directors should obtain legal consultation, as well as review relevant articles and texts on competency and informed consent.

FINANCIAL ISSUES

Financial questions regarding MPUs may pertain to direct costs, indirect costs, recovery of costs, costs avoided, and cost-effectiveness.

The direct cost of treatment on an MPU may be greater than the direct cost of treatment on a traditional psychiatric unit with the same psychiatric level of acuity and the same intensity of therapeutic milieu. The cost may be relatively higher because more medical equipment and supplies are required, because the staff will probably consist mainly of registered nurses, and because a relatively high staffing level is needed on nights, evenings, and weekends if medically unstable patients are to be accepted. The requirement for a salaried medical director must also be considered in assessing direct costs. Indirect costs of MPUs may reflect the greater utilization of general hospital services, such as the laboratories, operating room, radiology department, and patient transport, by patients with active medical illness.

In the private sector, costs potentially can be better recovered for MPUs than for traditional psychiatric units. First, many of the ancillary services utilized by medical-psychiatric patients are well reimbursed and may yield a profit to the hospital. Second, a high-quality MPU in a private setting may be able to attract a large proportion of well-insured patients. However, recovery of costs is sensitive to local rate-setting arrangements and prospective payment contracts, so no generalization is appropriate.

Having an MPU may be money-saving to the host hospital, particularly if its target population is distinct from the population served by other medical or psychiatric beds in the same hospital. If the target population is noncompetitive and currently underserved in the community, establishment of an MPU may lead to a higher total occupancy rate for the hospital, thereby permitting better recovery of fixed costs. Further, if the MPU is Diagnosis-Related Groups-(DRG) exempt, it may provide an internal disposition for some Medicare patients who would otherwise be DRG outliers. These patients' costs could be recovered in full for their stays on the MPU as long as the unit's total costs fell within the Medicare cap. Finally, availability of the unit as an internal disposition may minimize the need for costly special observation of medically ill patients who are acutely suicidal or behaviorally disturbed.

In large public sector hospitals, the development of an MPU may permit clustering of the medically ill patients, possibly reducing staffing and medical coverage requirements for other units, as well as minimizing the time-consuming administrative difficulties that may arise when treating combined medical-psychiatric patients on medical wards or on traditional psychiatric units.

The issue of cost-efficiency of conjoint

medical-psychiatric care is open. While many MPU directors believe that conjoint treatment may resolve problems that would otherwise become chronic and costly, hard evidence to support this belief does not exist. Cost-effectiveness studies for MPUs are needed, but will pose significant methodologic problems because of the heterogeneity of their patient populations.

The possible extension of prospective payment systems for the inpatient treatment of psychiatric disorders raises the natural question of whether an MPU can be operated under a DRG system. The authors have argued elsewhere (Fogel et al., 1985) that a therapeutically oriented MPU is not consistent with the current Medicare DRG system, because normative lengths of stay for psychiatric patients are too short, and because the medical-psychiatric population has an even greater variance in length of stay and resource utilization than does an uncomplicated psychiatric population. DRGs have not been shown to be predictive of resource utilization and length of stay for general psychiatric patients, and are likely to be even less helpful for patients with combined medical and psychiatric illness. As opposed to a rigid prospective payment system, concurrent review or prior authorization systems for cost control would not necessarily threaten MPUs. The severity and complexity of the patients problems might even facilitate justification of hospital treatment, under a fairly administered system of prior or concurrent review. An MPU operated under the current DRG system would have to limit its goals to diagnosis and stabilization, with treatment to be continued in another setting.

CONCLUSION

A number of scientific, societal, and economic forces have converged to shift psychiatric practice back to its medical roots. These factors include advances in biological psychiatry, competition from nonmedical psychotherapists, increasingly narrower criteria for hospitalizing patients, and increased demands for documentation by third-party payors. Medical-psychiatric units may provide ideal settings for psychiatrists to rediscover and use their special medical skills and to provide integrated care for a complex patient population. The guidelines offered in the two parts of this article are intended for assessing the feasibility of these units and to assist in their creation.

ACKNOWLEDGMENTS

This chapter was previously published in *Psychosomatics*, *27*(6), June 1986, and is reprinted with permission.

REFERENCES

Appelbaum PS & Roth LH (1984). Involuntary treatment in medicine and psychiatry. *American Journal of Psychiatry*, *141*, 202–205.

Barton WE & Barton GM (1983). Ward administration. In WE Barton & GM Barton (Eds), *Mental health administration: Principles and practice* (Vol 2, pp 537–557). New York: Human Sciences Press.

Burn ED & Tonges MC (1983). Professional nursing practice in acute care settings. *Nursing Administration Quarterly*, *8*, 65–75.

Fogel BS (1985). A psychiatric unit becomes a psychiatric—medical unit: Administrative and clinical implications. *General Hospital Psychiatry*, *7*, 26–35.

Fogel BS & Goldberg RJ (1983–1984). Beyond liaison: A future role for psychiatry in medicine. *International Journal of Psychiatry in Medicine*, *13*, 185–192.

Fogel BS, Mills MJ, & Landen JE (1986). Clinicolegal aspects of treating delirious patients. *Hospital and Community Psychiatry*, *37*, 154–158.

Fogel BS, Stoudemire A, & Houpt JL (1985). Contrasting models for conjoint medical and psychiatric inpatient treatment. *American Journal of Psychiatry*, *142*, 1085–1089.

Goodman B (1985). Combined psychiatric-medical inpatient units: The Mount Sinai model. *Psychosomatics*, *26*, 179–189.

Richman A & Harris P (1985). General hospital psychiatry: Are its roles and functions adjunctive or pivotal? *General Hospital Psychiatry*, *7*, 258–266.

Stoudemire A, Brown JT, McLeod M, et al. (1983). The combined medical specialties unit: An innovative approach to patient care. *North Carolina Medical Journal*, *44*, 365–367.

Index

693

neuroleptic malignant
 syndrome from, 456
 tardive dyskinesia from, 455–
  456
 pregnant, treatment of, 456–457
 psychopharmacology of, 454–
  456
 surgery and, 457
Schizophreniform disorder in
 epilepsy, 540
Scleroderma, 610
Sclerosis, progressive systemic,
 609–610
Sedating neuroleptics, for agitation
 in dementia patients, 153
Sedation of delirious patients,
 neuroleptics for, 90–91
Sedative-hypnotic abuse, 244
 in chronic pain patients, 393
Sedatives, withdrawal from,
 anxiety in, 179–180
Seizure(s). See also Epilepsy
 complex partial, 537–538
 in systemic lupus
  erythematosus, 602–603
Seizure disorders
 anticholinergic effects of cyclic
  antidepressants in, 85–86
 sleep disorders and, 280–281
Self-esteem, bolstering, in anxiety-
 suppressing
 psychotherapy, 14–15
Self-help programs for cancer
 patient, 512–513
Self-management techniques in
 chronic pain
 management, 398–399
Self-monitoring for compliance
 problems, 359–360
Self-regulation in neurological
 assessment, 66
Self-regulation methods for
 anxiety, 195–197
Self-scrutiny, willingness for, in
 psychotherapy diagnosis,
 13
Senile dementia, sleep disorders
 and, 281
Sensitivity in depression diagnosis,
 27
Sensitization, covert, in behavioral
 therapy, 340–341
Sensorimotor functions,
 neuropsychological
 assessment of, 65
Sensory augmentation in dementia
 management, 150
Serotoninergic alteration in

Parkinson's disease, 533
Sexual counseling for cancer
 patient, 513–514
Sexual desire, disorders of, 309
 treatment of, 321
Sexual dysfunction in medically
 ill, 307–325
 drugs causing, 317–318t
 elaboration of, 308–320
  endocrine studies in, 313–314
  intracavernosal injection in,
   319
  medical history in, 313, 314t,
   315t, 316t, 317–318t
  neurologic assessment in,
   315–316
  nocturnal penile tumescence
   studies in, 316, 319
  psychiatric interview in, 311,
   312
  psychologic assessment in,
   320
  vascular studies in, 314–315
 medical conditions causing,
  314t, 315t, 316t
 physical examination of,
  components of, 313t
 sexual response pattern and,
  208–211
 treatment issues on, 320–325
  for disorders
   of desire, 321
   of excitement, 321–323
   of orgasm, 323
   of resolution, 323
  medical-surgical, 321–323
  psychologic, 323–325
Sexual excitement disorders, 309–
 310
 treatment of, 321–323
Sexual functioning
 after ostomy surgery, 439–440
 dialysis and, 585, 586–587
 in pelvic exenteration patient,
  437–438
 in pulmonary patients, 557–558,
  562
 renal transplantation and, 590
 in rheumatoid arthritis, 607
 in spinal cord injury patient,
  431–434
 urologic surgery and, 436–437t
Sexual history, 312t
Sexual practices, AIDS and, 660–
 661, 668, 670t
Sexual response pattern, sexual
 disorder and, 308–311
Shaping procedure

in behavioral therapy, 336–338
 for compliance problems, 360
Shunting for hydrocephalus in
 dementia, 143
Signal anxiety, 6
Single photon emission computed
 tomography (SPECT) in
 neurologic assessment, 56
Sjögren's syndrome, primary, 610
Sleep
 bodily clocks and, 271–272
 disorders of
  in dementia, 151–152
  in medically ill, 271–293
  dyssomnias as, 273–283.
   See also Dyssomnias
 epidemiology of, 271
 physiology of, 271–273
 non–rapid-eye-movement, 272
 quality of
  for aged, 288–290
  improving, 288–292
   drug adjustments in, 288
   hospitalization routines for,
    291
   hyperarousal avoidance in,
    290
   psychopathology
    management in, 290–291
   scheduling adjustments in,
    290
 rapid-eye-movement, 272
 regulation of, 272–273
Sleep apnea, 277–278
 brain disease and, 281
 cognitive impairment from, 560–
  561
 diabetes mellitus and, 279
 hypertension and, 279
 obstructive, androgens and, 280
 whiplash and, 281
Sleep chart in dyssomnia
 evaluation, 286, 287
Sleep history in dyssomnia
 evaluation, 283, 285
Sleep hygiene, 292–293
Smoking
 biobehavioral basis for, 354
 as cardiovascular risk factor,
  348, 354–357
 in pregnancy, 634
 treatment of, 354–357
  compliance with, 357–360
  intermediate interventions for,
   356
  maintenance strategies in, 357
  maximal interventions for,
   356–357